Postgraduate Orthopedics
An Exam Preparatory Manual

Postgraduate Orthopedics
An Exam Preparatory Manual

FOURTH EDITION

Manish Kumar Varshney
MS(Orthopedics) DNB(Orthopedic Surgery) MNAMS MRCS(Glasgow)
Assistant Professor and Incharge Head
Department of Orthopedics
SMVD Institute of Medical Excellence
Senior Consultant
SMVD Narayana Superspeciality Hospital
Reasi, Jammu and Kashmir, India

Co-Author
Mohinder Singh Chib
MS(Orthopedics)
Consultant Orthopedics
Gupta Hospital
Kathua, Jammu and Kashmir, India

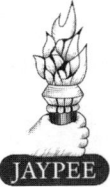

JAYPEE BROTHERS MEDICAL PUBLISHERS
The Health Sciences Publisher
New Delhi | London

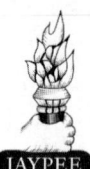

Jaypee Brothers Medical Publishers (P) Ltd

Headquarters
EMCA House, 23/23-B
Ansari Road, Daryaganj
New Delhi 110 002, India
Landline: +91-11-23272143, +91-11-23272703
+91-11-23282021, +91-11-23245672
e-mail: jaypee@jaypeebrothers.com

Corporate Office
4838/24, Ansari Road, Daryaganj
New Delhi 110 002, India
Phone: +91-11-43574357
Fax: +91-11-43574314
e-mail: jaypee@jaypeebrothers.com

Overseas Office
JP Medical Ltd.
83, Victoria Street, London
SW1H 0HW (UK)
Phone: +44-20 3170 8910
e-mail: info@jpmedpub.com

EU GPSR Authorised Representative
Logos Europe, 9 rue Nicolas Poussin
17000, La Rochelle, France
Phone: +33 (0) 6 67 93 73 78
e-mail: contact@logoseurope.eu

Website: www.jaypeebrothers.com
Website: www.jaypeedigital.com

© 2026, Jaypee Brothers Medical Publishers

The views and opinions expressed in this book are solely those of the original contributor(s)/author(s) and do not necessarily represent those of editor(s) or publisher of the book.

All rights reserved. No part of this publication may be reproduced, stored or transmitted in any form or by any means, electronic, mechanical, photocopying, recording or otherwise, without the prior permission in writing of the publishers.

All brand names and product names used in this book are trade names, service marks, trademarks or registered trademarks of their respective owners. The publisher is not associated with any product or vendor mentioned in this book.

Medical knowledge and practice change constantly. This book is designed to provide accurate, authoritative information about the subject matter in question. However, readers are advised to check the most current information available on procedures included and check information from the manufacturer of each product to be administered, to verify the recommended dose, formula, method and duration of administration, adverse effects and contraindications. It is the responsibility of the practitioner to take all appropriate safety precautions. Neither the publisher nor the author(s)/editor(s) assume any liability for any injury and/or damage to persons or property arising from or related to use of material in this book.

This book is sold on the understanding that the publisher is not engaged in providing professional medical services. If such advice or services are required, the services of a competent medical professional should be sought.

Every effort has been made where necessary to contact holders of copyright to obtain permission to reproduce copyright material. If any have been inadvertently overlooked, the publisher will be pleased to make the necessary arrangements at the first opportunity.

Inquiries for bulk sales may be solicited at: jaypee@jaypeebrothers.com

Postgraduate Orthopedics: An Exam Preparatory Manual / Manish Kumar Varshney

First Edition: 2020

Fourth Edition: **2026**

ISBN: 978-93-7202-770-9

Printed in India at K. K. Printers, Kundli, Haryana-131 028.

Dedicated to

*All my students, my teachers from whom I learned Orthopedics,
both my sons—Siddhant and Mrigank who taught me how to teach,
and my loving wife—Neeta,
who spared me from my homely duties while being engaged in preparing this book.*

Preface to the Fourth Edition

It is with great satisfaction and academic humility that I present the fourth edition of *"Postgraduate Orthopedics: An Exam Preparatory Manual"*. This edition continues the mission set forth in the first—to serve as a focused, concept-driven guide for postgraduate students preparing for theory examinations in orthopedics, particularly the DNB and MS formats.

Over the past 15 years, the landscape of orthopedic education has evolved, and so has the nature of questions posed in theory exams. This compilation reflects that progression, offering structured, thematic answers to a wide array of previously asked questions. Rather than merely providing rote responses, the book emphasizes **"conceptual clarity"**, encouraging students to understand the underlying principles and develop a strategic approach to answering theory questions effectively.

The answers herein are designed to act as **"cues"**—not definitive endpoints. They aim to guide students in framing relevant, coherent, and clinically contextual responses. While many answers are based on established texts such as Essential Orthopedics: Principles and Practice, a significant portion has been freshly written or adapted to reflect the nuances of question framing and the integration of multiple subtopics. Readers are strongly encouraged to cross-reference with **current textbooks, peer-reviewed journals, and authoritative guidelines**, as orthopedic knowledge is dynamic and continually refined.

This edition retains the organizational structure that groups similar questions together, allowing for streamlined revision and thematic learning. It is my earnest request that students use this manual as a **springboard for deeper study**, not as a substitute for comprehensive textbooks or mentorship. The goal is to foster exam readiness through understanding, not memorization.

As we move forward, I remain committed to updating and expanding this resource in response to new questions and emerging concepts. I hope this edition continues to ease the burden of exam preparation and inspires a more thoughtful, confident approach to orthopedic theory.

Wishing all aspirants clarity of thought, precision in writing, and success in their academic journey.

Manish Kumar Varshney

Preface to the First Edition

It gives me immense pleasure to introduce the first edition of book *Postgraduate Orthopedics: An Exam Preparatory Manual* for aspirants of a postgraduate degree in the faculty of orthopedics. This book is intended to help the students in framing and answering questions in orthopedics asked in theory examinations. The book is basically compiled on the theoretical questions asked in DNB examinations over past 10 years. This is also similar to pattern asked in the MS Orthopedic examination. The book is divided into six chapters covering core orthopedics (including trauma) and general surgical and allied medical conditions. The organization would help students understand the variedness of questions asked on a topic or similar topics. Also the students will not have to shuffle through pages across the book had we arranged the questions year-wise. So readers will find all similar questions at one place, making the learning easy. The answers are primarily based on the book *Essential Orthopedics: Principles and Practice* however, nearly 30% of the answers have been written afresh due to demands of question organization or multiple topics/questions framed in the main question.

It is my erstwhile request to the readers to LEARN from the book about the technique of answering questions and make it a revision source for examinations; while core orthopedic learning should always be based on standard theoretical books, recent advances from dedicated journals and most respectful teachers in the field. No attempt should be made to cram the answers as it is as uniqueness is lost and it defies the basic purpose of facultative learning. These and similar resources are only a guide to understanding the topics, easing the examination fear and focusing on the skills of answering the questions. Kindly develop good learning from conventional and standard orthopedic sources. No work can encompass the futuristic questions and knowledge; kindly remain updated with current knowledge which is fast changing and the pace of changes ousts any written compilation. We will be working on incorporating newer questions as they are asked in examinations soon to expand the text further regularly.

All the best for postgraduate examination preparation and learning feast.

Manish Kumar Varshney

Acknowledgments

I would like to thank Shri Jitendar P Vij (Group Chairman), Mr Ankit Vij (Managing Director), Mr MS Mani (Group President), Mr Sabyasachi Hazra (Director—PG and PNR Publishing), Ms Pooja Bhandari [Director—Production (Books and Journals)], Ms Nikita Chauhan (Publishing Manager) and the staff of M/s Jaypee Brothers Medical Publishers (P) Ltd, New Delhi, India.

Contents

1. **General Topics** — 1
2. **General Orthopedics** — 79
3. **Orthopedic Trauma** — 335
4. **Regional Orthopedics** — 464
5. **Neoplasia** — 812
6. **Miscellaneous Topics and Recent Advances** — 867

   Index — *893*

CHAPTER 1

General Topics

(This chapter covers questions asked with respect to the medical and surgical associations of orthopedics including complications of orthopedic injuries/procedures. Also, some research-based questions and ancillary diagnostic modalities used are covered.)

1.1 MEDICAL/SURGICAL/EMERGENCY MEDICINE TOPICS/COMPLICATIONS IN ORTHOPEDICS (Q1–32)

1. Explain the role of Virchow's triad in the pathogenesis of deep vein thrombosis (DVT).

Ans: Virchow's triad **(Fig. 1.1.1)** defines the three critically important factors amalgamating into development of DVT, these are:
1. *Venous blood stasis*: This seems to be the most important component as stasis initiates venous thrombi even without evidence of endothelial injury and stasis may by itself result in increased viscosity.
2. *Abnormalities of vessel wall*: Vessel damage may result from intrinsic or extrinsic trauma to endothelium exposing the underlying media and collagen basement membranes that activate the coagulation cascade.
3. *Abnormal activation of coagulation pathway or a hypercoagulable state*: This results from altered blood component structure where increase in circulating tissue activation factor, combined with a decrease in circulating plasma antithrombin and fibrinolysins, may result in certain metabolic conditions.

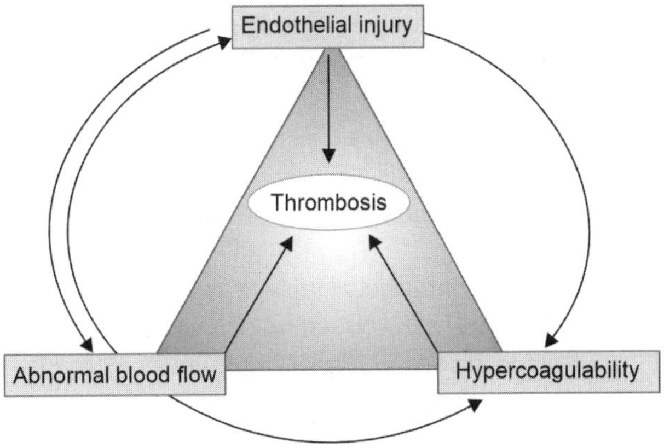

Fig. 1.1.1: Virchow's triad and interplay between the three components in pathogenesis of deep vein thrombosis.

Role of stasis: In a normal blood flow, the blood does not move in a cylindrical column. The central stream moves fastest and consists of leukocytes and red cells. The platelets are present in slow-moving laminar stream adjacent to central stream, while peripheral most stream consists of slow moving cell-free plasma close to endothelial layer. In stasis, the platelets fall out of the intermediate column and come in contact with endothelium called pavementation and margination. Due to reduced movement, adenosine diphosphate (ADP) gets released leading to further platelet aggregation. This results in formation of a temporary plug and then the whole clotting system gets activated propagating the thrombus. Stasis may occur in hypercoagulable states (blood dyscrasias or carcinoma), low cardiac output, obesity, advanced age, prolonged bed rest, postpartum period, dehydration, polycythemia, long surgical procedures, especially under general anesthesia (GA), fractures or injuries of lower limbs, left and right ventricular failure, and use of estrogens.

Abnormalities of vessel wall: Endothelial injury exposes subendothelial connective tissues (collagen, elastin, fibronectin, laminin, and glycosaminoglycans), which are thrombogenic and play an important role in initiating thrombosis by extrinsic pathway.

Abnormal activation of coagulation pathway or a hypercoagulable state: Occurrence of thrombosis in some conditions such as in nephritic syndrome, advanced cancers, extensive trauma, burns, and during puerperium is explained on basis of hypercoagulability that occurs due to increase in coagulation factors, increase in platelet count and their adhesiveness, and decreased levels of coagulation inhibitors.

2. Enumerate the risk factors for developing deep venous thrombosis.

Ans: The risk factors for development of DVT can be summarized and grouped as follows:
- Acquired includes:
    - *Previous DVT*: The single most powerful risk marker (25% patients)
    - Age [the annual incidence of venous thromboembolism (VTE) rises with each decade over the age of 40 years]
    - Obesity
    - Immobilization longer than 3 days
    - Major surgery (especially orthopedic) lasting > 2 hours in previous 4 weeks
    - Long plane or car trips (> 4 hours) in previous 4 weeks
    - Mass effect on iliac veins:
        - Cancer
        - Pregnancy
        - Congenital anomaly
    - Stroke
    - Postpartum period
    - Acute myocardial infarction (AMI)
    - Congestive heart failure (CHF)
    - Sepsis
    - Nephrotic syndrome
    - Ulcerative colitis
    - Multiple trauma
    - Burns
    - *Trauma*: Endothelial injury can convert the normally antithrombogenic endothelium to become prothrombotic:
        - *Central nervous system (CNS)/spinal cord injury*: Abbreviated Injury Scale (AIS) ≥ head/neck
        - *Mechanical injury to veins*: Lower extremity fractures—multiple long bone fractures (≥ 3)
        - Severe pelvic fracture (posterior elements) + long bone fracture
        - Glasgow Coma Scale (GCS) ≤ 8
        - Injury Severity Score (ISS) ≥ 15
        - Hip and knee arthroplasty (manipulation of nearby major veins)
        - Inflammation-induced alteration in endothelial function [as in patients with coexisting urinary tract infection (UTI) or respiratory tract infection (RTI)]
    - Oral contraceptives
    - Estrogens
    - Heparin-induced thrombocytopenia (HIT)
    - Intravenous (IV) drug abuse
- *Congenital includes*:
    - Systemic lupus erythematosus (SLE) and the lupus anticoagulant
    - Behçet syndrome
    - Homocystinuria
    - Polycythemia rubra vera
    - Genetic mutations in blood coagulation cascade
    - Genetic thrombocytosis and thrombophilia
    - Inherited disorders of coagulation/fibrinolysis—altered factor VIII, factor IX, factor XI, and prothrombin, antiphospholipid syndrome
    - Antithrombin III deficiency

- Protein C deficiency
- Protein S deficiency
- Prothrombin 20210A mutation
- Factor V Leiden
- Dysfibrinogenemias and disorders of plasminogen activation

3. Describe clinical features of deep vein thrombosis (DVT) in a bedridden patient.

Ans: The *most common symptoms* and *signs* of DVT, but none of them specific include the following:
- *Edema*: It is the most specific sign. Thrombus that extends above the bifurcation of iliac veins produces bilateral leg edema.
- *Leg and calf pain*: Occurs in 50% of patients but is nonspecific. Calf pain may be reproduced or provoked on dorsiflexion of the foot (*Homan's sign*).
- Reddish purple hue of lower limb from venous engorgement and obstruction includes:
  - Phlegmasia alba dolens (painful white inflammation), which is characterized by pale affected extremity, often having poor or even absent distal pulses—it may be confused with acute arterial occlusion, but the presence of edema, petechiae, and superficial vein distention suggest DVT.
  - Phlegmasia cerulea dolens (painful blue inflammation)—the leg is usually markedly edematous, painful, and cyanotic.
- *Calf tenderness*: Occurs in 75% of patients, it is usually confined to the calf muscles. The tenderness may extend in the medial thigh along with the course of deep veins. The size, location and extent of the thrombus have no correlation with the pain and tenderness felt.
- Increased temperature or erythema in the area of DVT (may be confused with cellulitis).
- Clinical symptoms of pulmonary embolism (PE) as the primary manifestation occur in 10% of patients with confirmed DVT.
- *Superficial thrombophlebitis*: Palpable, indurated, cord-like, and tender subcutaneous venous segment.

4. Discuss the management of deep vein thrombosis (DVT).

Ans: (Partly from Joint consensus document from the European Society of Cardiology.)

Any question asking for "management" must include both diagnosis and proper treatment.

Diagnosis: DVT stands for "deep vein thrombosis." Clinical signs and symptoms of DVT are highly variable and nonspecific. The "suspicious symptoms" include—pain, swelling, increased skin vein visibility, erythema, and cyanosis accompanied by unexplained fever. Wells criteria should be used to stratify patients with DVT. Enzyme-linked immunosorbent assay (ELISA) for D-dimer is a good test to exclude patients with low suspicion of DVT or those with DVT having unlikely pretest probability. D-dimer is elevated (> 500 ng/mL) in most patients, but it is not specific. In DVT, it remains elevated for 7 days. D-dimer results should be used as follows:
- A negative D-dimer rules out DVT in patients with low-to-moderate risk and a Wells score ≤ 2.
- All patients with positive test and moderate-to-high risk of DVT require a diagnostic study [Doppler ultrasonography (USG)].

Doppler USG is recommended as the first-line imaging method for DVT diagnosis in all patients with positive D-dimer or with likely DVT pretest probability (Wells score); but it is highly operator dependent. The major criterion for detecting venous thrombosis is failure to compress the vascular lumen. Venous ultrasound (US) should be proposed also in case of confirmed PE for initial reference venous imaging, useful in case of DVT recurrence suspicion, or for further stratification in selected patients.

Ascending contrast venography (phlebography) had been the gold standard, but Doppler USG is more user-friendly and noninvasive. Venous computed tomography (CT), impedance plethysmography, and radiofibrinogen method are very accurate but reserved for specific circumstances only (high suspicion but Doppler negative, iliac vein thrombosis, etc.) and not routinely used.

Treatment: In general, the leg is kept elevated to 15° and anticoagulation treatment is usually begun with heparin [or low-molecular-weight heparin (LMWH)] and continued with warfarin (direct oral anticoagulation can also be begun).

- Patients with proximal DVT should be anticoagulated for at least 3 months. Also, patients with isolated distal DVT who are at high risk of recurrence are also anticoagulated as for patients with proximal DVT. Decision to discontinue or extend anticoagulation is always individualized, balancing risk of recurrence against bleeding and also considering the patients' preferences and compliance.
- Patients with isolated distal DVT who are at low risk of recurrence are given shorter treatment for 4–6 weeks with lower doses. Doses in these patients may be adjusted on USG surveillance.
- In the absence of contraindications, direct oral anticoagulants should be preferred as first-line anticoagulant therapy in noncancer patients with proximal DVT. LMWH is recommended for initial and long-term treatment in cancer patients. LMWH is overall superior to unfractionated heparin (UFH). For acute DVT, initial anticoagulation should be one of the following regimens: (1) apixaban 10 mg twice a day for 7 days, then 5 mg twice a day; (2) dabigatran 150 mg twice a day after a 5- to 10-day lead-in course of LMWH; (3) edoxaban 60 mg daily (30 mg, if creatinine clearance is 30–50 mL/min or potent proton-pump inhibitor abuse after a 5- to 10-day lead-in course; (4) rivaroxaban 15 mg twice a day for 21 days, then 20 mg daily; or (5) warfarin with a goal international normalized ratio (INR) 2–3 days and LMWH for 5–10 days (until INR > 2).
- Adjuvant catheter-directed thrombolysis may be considered at specialized centers in selected patients with iliac vessel or femoral DVT, symptoms < 14 days, and life expectancy > 1 year. Primary acute DVT stenting or mechanical thrombus removal alone is not recommended. Vena cava filters may be considered, if anticoagulation is contraindicated; their use in addition to anticoagulation is not recommended.
- Compression therapy associated with early mobilization and walking exercise should be considered to relieve acute venous symptoms.
- In pregnancy, USG is recommended as first-line DVT imaging test. LMWH is recommended for initial and long-term treatment during pregnancy. Anticoagulant treatment should be continued for at least 6 weeks after delivery with a total of 3 months of treatment.
- *Venous thromboembolism recurrence*: Vienna model, the DASH score, and HERDOO-2 can be used to assess VTE recurrence. Secondary prophylaxis for recurrent DVT is given with low-dose aspirin, apixaban 2.5 mg twice a day, or rivaroxaban 10 mg daily. In general, anticoagulation is preferred over aspirin therapy.
- For upper extremity DVT, US is the diagnostic modality of choice and treatment is similar to lower extremity DVT.

5. **Describe chemical prophylaxis of deep vein thrombosis (DVT) with pros and cons of each modality.**

Ans: (*Note*: "Prophylaxis" is completely different from "treatment" of DVT, understand this difference.)

Antiplatelet drugs (like Clopidogrel):

Pros:
- Simple administration
- Tested drug
- No need for monitoring INR
- Low side effects.

Cons:
- Low efficacy
- Dosage still unclear
- Need to be combined with other modalities.

Vitamin K antagonists (like Coumarin):

Pros:
- Known dosage that can be titrated with effect in individual patients
- Known and studied drugs
- Oral drugs.

Cons:
- Long onset of action and also long residual activity after discontinuation
- The necessity to monitor INR values frequently
- The long half-life that may require vitamin K reversal in incidents of hemorrhage
- Narrow therapeutic window
- Prominent drug and dietary interactions
- Most unexpected but sure variable patient response
- Hemorrhagic complications are reported in up to 3–5% of patients on warfarin prophylaxis. "Warfarinization" for orthopedic surgeries.

Low-molecular-weight heparins (like enoxaparin):

Pros:
- Most studied drugs
- Established efficacy for prevention and treatment
- Low complication profile.

Cons:
- Injection form may not be preferred by patients
- Hemorrhage
- Hematuria
- Hypersensitivity reactions
- Urticaria
- Rash
- Hematoma
- Anaphylaxis
- Prolonged clotting time
- Thrombocytopenia
- Irritation
- Ulceration
- Hyperkalemia
- Necrosis
- Pain
- Osteoporosis
- Reversible alopecia.

Contraindications for the use of LMWH:
- Hypersensitivity to drug
- Hemophilia
- Severely compromised renal function
- Severely compromised liver function
- Bacterial endocarditis
- Gastric ulcer (active disease)
- Uncontrolled high blood pressure.

Factor Xa direct inhibitors (like fondaparinux):

Pros:
- Rapid onset of action, so no need for bridging therapy
- Short half-life, so easy control of anticoagulant effect
- Little or no food interaction, so no dietary restrictions like warfarin
- Predictability of anticoagulation effect without a need for routine coagulation monitoring.

Cons:
- *Prohibitively* high cost resulting in poor compliance (apixaban is exception, as it is relatively much cheaper)
- *No* monitoring is possible
- *No* specific antidote
- *Serious* bleeding in renal-impaired patients and elderly > 80 years. If glomerular filtration rate (GFR) is 15–30 mL/min, prefer warfarin as anticoagulant.

Direct thrombin inhibitor and dabigatran etexilate:

Pros: *As for factor Xa inhibitors.*

Cons:
- Patients with mechanical prosthetic valves
- Presence of pathological bleeding
- Known hypersensitivity reaction
- Dabigatran should be used with caution in elderly patients aged over 75 years and in patients with active peptic ulcer, bleeding, and renal diseases due to risk of bleeding. For same reason, use of alcoholic beverages is prohibited.
- Drug interactions may occur with warfarin, clopidogrel, ticlopidine, streptokinase, urokinase, quinidine, rifampicin, antiarrhythmic drugs, calcium-channel blockers, nonsteroidal anti-inflammatory drugs (NSAIDs), and antifungal drugs.

6. Mechanism of action of various anticoagulants and precautions required during their use.

Ans: Flowchart 1.1.1: Provides the mechanisms of action of various anticoagulants according to their site of action.

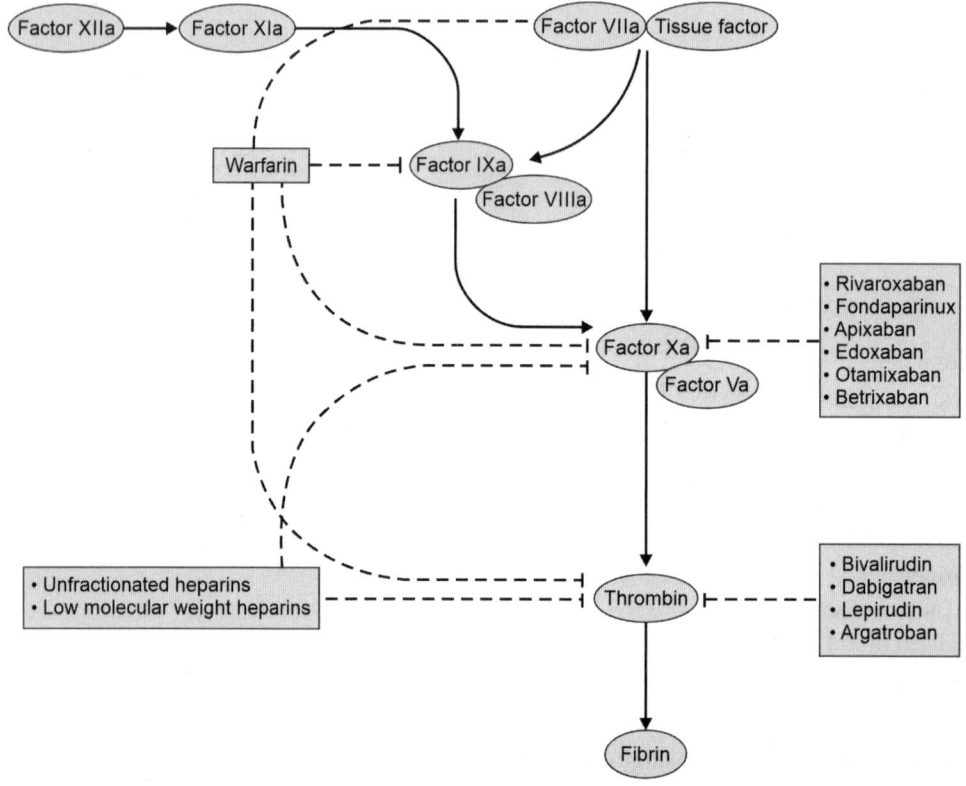

Flowchart 1.1.1: Site of action for various anticoagulants indicating their mechanism of action.

Precautions:

Warfarin: Due to delayed effect (1–3 days), it is used for maintenance.
- Regular monitoring of prothrombin time (PT), INR needed.
- Given during pregnancy can cause fetal warfarin syndrome.

Appropriate dosing precaution is needed during the following as they increase effect of oral anticoagulants:
- *Debility, malnutrition, malabsorption, and prolonged antibiotic therapy*: The supply of vitamin K to liver is reduced in these conditions.
- *Liver disease, chronic alcoholism*: Synthesis of clotting factors may be deficient.
- *Hyperthyroidism*: The clotting factors are degraded faster.
- Newborns have low levels of vitamin K and clotting factors (there should be no need of these drugs in neonates anyway).

Following factors decrease effect of oral anticoagulants:
- *Pregnancy*: Plasma level of clotting factors is higher.
- *Nephrotic syndrome*: Drug bound to plasma protein is lost in urine.
- Genetic warfarin resistance.

Drug interactions: Many drugs interact with oral anticoagulants so their simultaneous prescription should be carefully monitored.

- *Increased effect of warfarin*:
  - Broad-spectrum antibiotics reduce vitamin K production.
  - Newer cephalosporins (cefamandole, moxalactam, and cefoperazone) warfarin-additive action.
  - Aspirin—synergistic hypoprothrombinemic action and also displace warfarin from protein-binding site.
  - Sulfonamides, indomethacin, phenytoin, and probenecid—displace warfarin from plasma-protein binding.
  - Chloramphenicol, erythromycin, celecoxib, cimetidine, allopurinol, amiodarone, metronidazole, tolbutamide, and phenytoin—inhibit warfarin metabolism.
  - Liquid paraffin (habitual use)—reduces vitamin K absorption.
- *Reduced anticoagulant action*:
  - Barbiturates (but not benzodiazepines), rifampin and griseofulvin induce the metabolism of oral anticoagulants.
  - *Oral contraceptives*: Increase blood levels of clotting factors.

Indirect thrombin inhibitors:
- Needs monitoring by activated partial thromboplastin time (aPTT).
- LMWH and fondaparinux does not need monitoring.
- Heparin should not be mixed with penicillin, tetracyclines, hydrocortisone, or noradrenaline in the same syringe or infusion bottle.
- Hematomas are more common with intramuscular injection—this route should not be used for heparin administration.

7. Describe thromboprophylaxis in orthopedics.
Ans: Kindly see the answers above.

8. Discuss various methods of preventing DVT following total knee replacement (TKR). Discuss their merits and demerits.
Ans: *(One should understand that management of DVT and prevention of DVT are altogether different aspects, so must not be confused.)*

Giving prophylaxis after TKR is highly controversial at least for the regimen preferred by surgeons. At one extreme, some do not give any prophylaxis; while at other extreme, routine multidrug prophylaxis is given to all patients for a substantial duration. Most, however, adjust their dose, drug, and regimen duration in between these extremes. A general guide is to first stratify the patients based on Wells score.
- Patients with a score of 1 or less (low-risk) require early and aggressive mobilization. No specific prophylaxis is required for these patients.
- A patient having a score of 2 or less has 1–2% risk of developing clinical PE. Successful prevention strategies in this group consist of LMWH (low-dose), graduated compression stockings (GCS) or IPC (intermittent pneumatic compression), antiplatelet drugs (alone), or oral agents (direct Xa inhibitors).
- High-risk patients have a score of 3 or 4. The risk of PE occurring is 2–4%. Successful prevention strategies in this group consist of LMWH (higher doses), GCS or IPC with antiplatelet drugs, oral agents (+GCS or IPC or antiplatelet drugs).

- The highest-risk patients have a score of 5 or greater. The estimated risk of clinical PE is 4–10% and fatal PE is 0.2–5%. Successful prevention strategies include LMWH (higher doses), fondaparinux, and coumarins (to maintain INR 2.5–3). It may be prudent to combine GCS or IPC with LMWHs.

The usual guidelines for a patient post-TKR are as follows:

Prophylaxis is "usually" recommended for all patients. Administer LWMH 12–24 hours postoperatively, and continue for 14 days. The biggest advantage of LMWHs is that they do not require monitoring of either aPTT or INR, the half-life is longer (compared to UFH) and effect is more consistent, so that lesser dose adjustments are needed (in fact standard doses are administered). The hemorrhagic complications are less. LMWHs have gradually replaced heparin for prophylaxis and treatment of DVT (this might change with the increasing use of oral Xa inhibitors).

Complications with LMWH therapy are:
- Hemorrhage
- Hematuria
- Hypersensitivity reactions
- Urticaria
- Rash
- Hematoma
- Anaphylaxis
- Prolonged clotting time
- Thrombocytopenia
- Irritation
- Ulceration
- Hyperkalemia
- Necrosis
- Pain
- Osteoporosis
- Reversible alopecia.

Contraindications for the use of LMWH are:
- Hypersensitivity to drug
- Hemophilia
- Severely compromised renal function
- Severely compromised liver function
- Bacterial endocarditis
- Gastric ulcer (active disease)
- Uncontrolled high blood pressure.

Relative contraindications (need special monitoring) are:
- Renal impairment
- Metabolic acidosis
- Patient on potassium-sparing medications
- Hypoaldosteronism
- Diabetes mellitus
- Spinal or epidural anesthesia.

Alternative medications for DVT prophylaxis after total knee arthroplasty (TKA) are:
- *Fondaparinux*: Fondaparinux (direct selective inhibitor of factor Xa), which requires only a single-daily subcutaneous dose, is required. Fondaparinux is not associated with HIT. It is contraindicated in chronic renal failure patients having creatinine clearance < 30 mL/min. No specific antidote to fondaparinux is available.

- *Rivaroxaban/apixaban*: Rivaroxaban can be used in high-risk groups (e.g., fragile patients, cancer patients, and patients with a large clot).
- Dabigatran
- GCS/IPC/foot pumps + Aspirin (AAOS)
- Foot pumps or GCS or IPC alone can be used for contraindications to pharmacotherapy.

Aspirin alone is not recommended as is warfarin, unless it has been given otherwise for therapeutic measure (as in previous cardiac surgery).

(Detailed discussion on each modality can be referred to Chapter 18: Deep Vein Thrombosis of the book Essential Orthopedics: Principles and Practice, 2nd edition.)

9. Discuss low-molecular-weight heparin with its indications and monitoring during treatment.

Ans: Low-molecular-weight heparins are lower molecular-weight moieties that contain the active ATIII-binding site. They exhibit their action mainly by anti-IIa and anti-Xa activity. The biggest advantage of LMWHs over regular heparin is that they do not require regular monitoring of either aPTT or INR (except in special circumstances), the half-life is longer (compared to UFH) and their effect is more consistent, so that lesser dose adjustments are needed. General indications (orthopedic and nonorthopedic) for use of LMWH are:

- *Treatment and prophylaxis of DVT and PE*: These drugs are mainly used for deep venous thrombosis prophylaxis, management, and aversion of complications and are highly effective. They are routinely prescribed in major lower limb or pelvic trauma/postsurgery and now also indicated for prevention of upper limb venous thrombosis. Patients with high risk for developing DVT are also prescribed LMWH prophylaxis.
- Along with aspirin, it is used in combination for unstable angina.
- It is also used in disseminated intravascular coagulation (DIC) (defibrination syndrome).
- They are of little value in cerebral thrombosis once neurological deficit has occurred, but these can be used to decrease the occurrence of stroke.
- They do not cross the placenta and are the anticoagulant of choice during pregnancy.
- To maintain patency of cannulae and shunts in dialysis patients, and in extracorporeal circulation.

Monitoring: Normally in therapeutic doses, regular monitoring of LMWH therapy is not recommended and not routinely performed. Only in certain special circumstances like in patients with renal impairment (altering metabolism of LMWH) which incurs the risk of accumulation, or at extremes of weight or age where the patient may get under- or overdosed, respectively, do we need to monitor the LMWH therapy? Monitoring may also be needed, if desired effect is not seen as in recurrent thrombosis or in cases needing intense anticoagulation. The following are the common methods recommended for monitoring LMWH therapy:

- Activated clotting time (ACT) point-of-care test is the preferred test in patients needing intense anticoagulation such as cardiopulmonary bypass. This is to ensure sufficient level of anticoagulation before beginning invasive procedure and also determine complete reversal following the procedure. At this level of anticoagulation, aPTT is rendered useless because the blood is virtually nonclottable for this test. ACT is equivalent to whole-blood PTT adapted to reflect an intense degree of anticoagulation.
- *Anti-factor Xa (anti-FXa)*: This is considered the gold standard test to monitor LMWH effect in prophylaxis/treatment of VTE. Because LMWH has predominantly anti-FXa activity, the anti-FXa assay reflects the activity responsible for their therapeutic effects in the body and indirectly tells about the expected effect of therapy. Longer LMWHs have higher direct FIIa inhibition than smaller molecules that are more specific to FXa inhibition, thus measuring anti-FXa would somewhat underestimate the anticoagulation effect of larger molecules in clinical use.
- Activated partial thromboplastin time values vary a lot between laboratories complicating the dose-effect titration.
- *Thrombin generation*: There is emergent interest in the use of this test for monitoring LMWH therapy, as it may be superior to the aPTT. Measurement of the area under the thrombin generation curve reflecting the endogenous thrombin potential (ETP) determines physiologically relevant amount of thrombin formed upon in vitro activation of coagulation that can be linearly inhibited by dose-dependent drug administration.

10. Describe the metabolic acidosis.

Ans: Metabolic acidosis is characterized by a reduction in plasma bicarbonate and a consequent rise in hydrogen ion concentration producing a low serum pH (< 7.35). The partial pressure of carbon dioxide in blood is reduced secondarily by hyperventilation.

There are three major pathogenic mechanisms:
1. Excess of endogenous acid—diabetic ketoacidosis, lactic acidosis, shock, methanol poisoning, and salicylate poisoning
2. Loss of bicarbonate—renal tubular acidosis, diarrhea, fistulae, and ureterosigmoidostomy
3. Inadequate acid excretion—chronic renal failure, distal renal tubular acidosis, and acute renal failure.

Clinical features and causes: In severe cases, there is deep sighing respiration (Kussmaul breathing). There is a shift to right of the oxyhemoglobin dissociation due to acidosis reducing the oxygen carrying and delivery capacity of blood. After 6 hours, however, the red cell levels of 2,3-DPG (2,3-Diphosphoglycerate) reduce shifting the oxygen dissociation curve back to normal. Peripheral vasodilatation of arterioles due to sympathetic overactivity and fall in cardiac output may result in a fall in blood pressure (BP), and this is accentuated by depression of myocardial contractility (due to hyperkalemia) and vasoconstriction of pulmonary arteries (increased PAP). There is, in addition, resistance to effects of catecholamines. Hyperkalemia is due to shift out of K^+ out of cells, and in chronic acidosis, bone resorption ensues. Severe acidosis may be associated with drowsiness, confusion, and coma.

One should be vigilant as to the cause of anion gap acidosis that can be elicited by observing signs. Specific toxins produce "toxidromes," viz., "cherry-red" flushing of cyanide poisoning, tachypnea in salicylate toxicity; jaundice, spider angiomas, palmar erythema, caput medusae of liver disease in ethanol, methanol, or polyethylene glycol ingestions; afferent pupillary defect indicates severe methanol poisoning. Methanol poisoning also produces mydriasis, a retinal sheen and hyperemia of the optic disk. Ethylene glycol metabolism can lead to cranial nerve palsies and tetany from oxalate-induced hypocalcemia. Septic shock-like findings indicate lactic acidosis. Patients with diabetic ketoacidosis present with altered mental status, abdominal pain, and signs of volume depletion. Patients with renal failure have findings of uremia (altered mental status, asterixis, pleural effusions, and pericardial friction rubs).

Diagnosis: In diabetics with diarrhea and renal disease, one should be suspicious of metabolic acidosis. Immediately, the blood samples for electrolytes, albumin, and an arterial blood gas, and a metabolic panel including blood urea nitrogen (BUN), creatinine, calcium, magnesium, and glucose should be obtained. In the setting of a low pH with low bicarbonate and high-anion gap, the diagnosis is usually made. Additionally, one finds low partial pressure of carbon dioxide and high serum potassium levels. To identify underlying cause, order can be placed for serum lactic acid, β-hydroxybutyrate (for ketoacidosis), and a comprehensive toxicology screen (acetaminophen, salicylate, ethylene glycol and isopropyl alcohol, and ethanol levels). Standard infectious workup including blood and urine cultures should be obtained. Electrocardiogram (ECG) may show signs of hyperkalemia (tall T-waves) or QTc prolongation caused by hypocalcemia from ethylene glycol toxicity. Urine anion gap and osmolar gap may be ordered in special circumstances like methanol, ethylene glycol, or isopropyl alcohol ingestion (they increase osmolar gap).

The anion gap must be measured from the formula:

$$\text{Serum AG} = Na - (Cl^- + HCO_3^-)$$

This subtracts the major measured anions (chloride and bicarbonate) from the major measured cation (sodium). Value > 12 mEq/L indicates positive anion gap acidosis (correct for hypoalbuminemia by increasing anion gap by 2.5 mEq/L for 1 g/dL reduction of albumin). Anion gap would result either from a fall in unmeasured cations (as seen in hypomagnesemia or hypocalcemia) or a rise in unmeasured anions. This can be caused by salicylate or alcohol consumption or in uremia, lactic acidosis (infection/septic), or ketoacidosis (diabetic, alcoholic, and starvation) as mentioned in the earlier text. Other uncommon causes include rhabdomyolysis or cyanide poisoning.

Treatment: The main aim of treatment is to correct the underlying disorder. Initiate supportive treatment (e.g., fluids, oxygen, and treatment for hyperkalemia) immediately. Sodium bicarbonate may be given in severe acidosis and is often considered to be a method to speed up return of bicarbonate levels to normal. It may be useful in mineral acidosis (hyperchloremic metabolic acidosis) where there are no endogenous acid anions, which can be metabolized by the liver; in other etiologies, it is useless or may even be harmful. In renal failure with metabolic acidosis, dialysis may be necessary.

In alcohol poisoning, correction of acidosis to prevent the effects of toxic metabolites (bicarbonate is administered in a bolus dose followed by an infusion), alcohol dehydrogenase inhibition by fomepizole or ethanol, treatment with enzymatic co-factors, and consideration of hemodialysis in patients with severe acidosis or end-organ damage. Alkalization of the serum and urine is the mainstay of therapy for salicylate poisoning. Reduced organ perfusion is the most common cause of lactic acidosis in shock, infection, etc., so it must be managed. Removal of culprit toxin in type B lactic acidosis is imperative. For type D-lactic acidosis, treatment of gut bacterial overgrowth is primary. Administration of bicarbonate in lactic acidosis is controversial. For cyanide poisoning, antidotes like hydroxocobalamin, sodium thiosulfate, and induction of methemoglobinemia are usually initiated in combination.

11. Describe gate control theory of pain. What is transcutaneous nerve stimulation and what are its indications?

Ans: The psychologist Ronald Melzack and the anatomist Patrick Wall proposed the "gate control theory of pain" in 1965. Due to variable perception of pain among individuals and its different nature depending on type of injury, site of origin, and abstract conditions like time of day/night, emotional variance, etc., it became slowly understood that pain is NOT a PURE sensation rather it is modulated by interaction of various neurons into the pain receptor neuron. According to the pain gate theory, a "gate system" in CNS opens and closes to allow the pain signals pass to the brain for processing or to block them at the start (usually Rexed laminae I and II of spinal cord). This theory also explains occurrence of phantom pain, chronic pain, and pseudo pain sensation when actually there is no painful stimulus. Gate control theory of pain was the first systematic attempt to discuss pain transmission.

Gate at spinal cord level: Nociceptors are free nerve endings embedded in tissue that get stimulated by tissue damaging stimuli [mechanical (prick, cut, and deep pressure), thermal, electrical, inflammation, etc.]. Nerve fibers with smaller diameter (Aδ and C) carry pain stimuli to the spinal cord "gate mechanism." The gate mechanism according to the theory is located in the spinal cord. The marginal zone and substantia gelatinosa nuclei (corresponding to Rexed laminae I and II, respectively) are responsible for pain modulation/control mechanism before being transmitted/relayed by lateral spinothalamic tract. The "gate" is apparently controlled by nerve fibers with larger diameter, which carry other stimuli such as touch that pass through the same gate. The larger nerves inhibit the transmission of pain signals by smaller nerves through the gate. When pain sensation is produced in any part of the body, its intensity and type perception will hence be dependent on the other afferents particularly the touch fibers reaching the posterior column of spinal cord that also get activated. Here, the touch impulses generally inhibit the release of substance-P by the pain fibers ending on substantia gelatinosa. So, the pain sensation is suppressed. Thus, the gating of pain in posterior gray horn level is similar to presynaptic inhibition. This is the mechanism of pain relief by rubefacients and counterirritants. Dorsal column fibers also send collaterals to the cells of substantia gelatinosa in the posterior gray horn. Thus, some of the impulses ascending via dorsal column fibers pass through the collaterals and reach substantia gelatinosa further controlling (positive/negative modulation) the gate.

Gate control at higher center: The nociceptive stimuli that pass through spinal gate are transmitted by spinothalamic tract to ventrobasal nuclei of the thalamus (some also pass through spinoreticular tract). In the thalamus and brainstem, the periaqueductal gray matter and the raphe nucleus (midbrain) modulate pain transmission (principally involving endogenous opioids—the enkephalins, endorphins, and dynorphins) that is further modulated in the cerebral cortex and thalamus by emotions. The midbrain nuclei form part of the descending pain suppression system (also involving opioids) that positively modulate substantia gelatinosa inhibiting pain transmission.

These complex relationships indicate that relative excitation and inhibition at different levels affect whether a nociceptive stimulus would be perceived and still ultimately its nature would be altered by human thoughts, beliefs, and emotions.

Transcutaneous electric nerve stimulation (TENS): TENS uses pulsed electric current through the skin to stimulate sensory nerves and underlying muscle that provide pain relief by inhibiting the "pain gate," reducing muscle spasm and counterirritant action. TENS may also act through the release of endogenous opioids via collateral pathway. For gate pathway modulation, three strategies are used—one is activation of Aβ pathway, another is activation of alternative opioid pathway by low frequency stimulation, and last is combining both the mechanisms. For Aβ fiber stimulation, generally,

10–30 mA of current is used at 90–130 Hz. Stimulation of large Aβ fibers activate the dorsal horn and action potentials from small diameter afferent nociceptors (Aδ and C fibers) are selectively suppressed. Direct stimulation of Aδ fibers by using a low-frequency current (2–5 Hz) activates the opioid mechanisms by releasing encephalin that blocks the noxious sensory pathway in a negative inhibitory loop. Combination approach is used by delivering high-frequency (100 Hz) "bursts" at rate of 2–3 bursts per second. The latter frequency additionally also activates Aδ fibers to cause release of endogenous opioids, while the high-frequency bursts stimulate the Aβ fibers. The chief problem with the combination approach is the uneasy sensation that is not very much acceptable to patients.

Precautions and contraindications:
- Patients allergic to the metal and/or gel used
- Patients with pacemakers and implanted electronic devices
- Patients with dermatitis or skin lesion at site of application of electrode
- Patients with epilepsy
- Do not apply electrodes over eyes or anterior aspect of neck or abdomen (especially in pregnant females).

12. **What is disseminated intravascular coagulation? Write a note on etiopathogenesis, clinical features, prevention, and management.**

Ans: Disseminated intravascular coagulation, also known as consumption coagulopathy and defibrination syndrome, is an acute or chronic bleeding disorder caused by abnormal consumption of prothrombin, fibrinogen, and clotting factors (mainly coagulation factors V, VIII, and platelets) occurring in a variety of conditions. The chronic form usually presents with venous thrombotic and embolic manifestations, while the acute form manifests as bleeding.

Etiopathogenesis: Usually, the exposure of tissue factor to blood activates coagulation pathway that if unregulated disseminates causing widespread consumption of prothrombin and fibrinogen. Formation of diffuse thrombus or microthrombi traps platelets and also utilizes the coagulation factors. As is normal for this physiological process to counteractivate fibrinolytic pathway system [facilitated also by release of tissue plasminogen activator (tPA) from endothelial cells due to obstructed microvascular flow] rendering the used coagulation substrates a waste. There, hence, occurs acute deficiency of coagulation system and normal homeostasis is deranged tilting the balance toward hypocoagulation predisposing to bleeding diathesis. The pathogenesis is illustrated in the adjacent **Flowchart 1.1.2**.

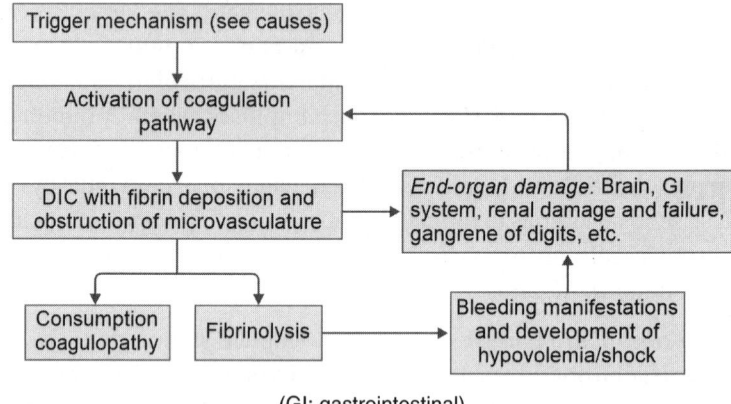

Flowchart 1.1.2: Pathogenesis of disseminated intravascular coagulation (DIC).

(GI: gastrointestinal)

Causes: Lot of clinical circumstances may cause development of DIC, the following are common causes:

Acute form (over hours or days) is seen in:
- Infections—septicemia, especially due to gram-negative infections (gram-negative endotoxin causes activation of tissue factor pathway), meningococcal infections, malaria, and fungal infections.
- Obstetric causes—saline-induced abortions, septicemia, preeclampsia, retained dead fetus, abruption placentae, and amniotic fluid embolism. The placental tissue has prominent tissue factor activity that may cause activation of coagulation cascade.
- Malignancies—adenocarcinoma of pancreas or prostate and acute myeloid leukemia are known to precipitate DIC.
- Miscellaneous—snake bite, major surgery or trauma, heat stroke, shock-causing ischemic tissue injury, burns, massive intravascular hemolysis, frostbite, etc.

Chronic form (over weeks or months) is seen in:
- Malignancies
- Aortic aneurysms
- Large cavernous hemangiomas (Kasabach–Merritt syndrome).

Clinical manifestations of rapidly evolving DIC are usually gastrointestinal (GI) bleeding, genitourinary bleeding, bleeding from operative site, skin, and mucous membrane bleeding (purpura, petechiae), persistent bleeding from skin puncture sites (IV cannulation, etc.), and ecchymosis from sites of parenteral injections. The patient may report chest pain and shortness of breath. There may be development of headaches, speech changes, paralysis (an inability to move), dizziness, and trouble speaking, and understanding in cerebral embolism. Chronic form usually presents as thromboembolism (pain, redness, warmth, and swelling in the lower leg).

Investigations: Suspect DIC in any case of unexplained bleeding or VTE. Obtain complete hemogram with peripheral smear, coagulation panel, D-dimer assay, and cultures as needed. There is low erythrocyte sedimentation rate (ESR), thrombocytopenia, prolonged PT and aPTT, reduced plasma fibrinogen level (two consecutive measurements), elevated levels of fibrin degradation product and D-dimers and schistocytes [due to mechanical disruption of red blood cells (RBCs)] on peripheral smear. Factor VIII assay may be done in cases of suspected massive hepatic necrosis. In chronic form, obtain Doppler study of lower limbs and echocardiography (may show leaflet vegetations).

Management: It should be handled with urgency and the priority of management lines are as follows:
- Eliminate underlying cause by rigorous treatment (broad-spectrum antibiotic treatment of suspected gram-negative sepsis, evacuation of the uterus in abruptio placentae), and correction of precipitating factors.
- As a second line of management, replacement of coagulation factors and platelets by fresh whole blood, fresh frozen plasma (FFP), cryoprecipitate, or platelet concentrates may be considered in severe bleeding and ensuing hypovolemia. It has also to be considered in cases requiring emergent surgical intervention.
- *Inhibition of coagulation process*: Heparin is indicated in thrombotic manifestations (especially the chronic form or slowly evolving DIC to stop consumption coagulopathy). It should be given after correction of bleeding risk.

Prevention: Primary prevention is by early treatment of conditions or disorders known to precipitate DIC. Both early identification and prompt treatment of these conditions or disorders are required to reduce the chance of developing DIC. Secondary prevention is by actively and aggressively treating the underlying disease and restoration of normality in deranged coagulation systems.

13. Describe Sudeck's osteodystrophy.

Ans: "Sudeck's atrophy/osteodystrophy" term applies to the radiological appearance of osteoporosis in a patient of complex regional pain syndrome (CRPS). A number of clinical syndromes appear under this heading, including *Sudeck's atrophy, reflex sympathetic dystrophy (RSD), algodystrophy, shoulder–hand syndrome,* and, particularly after a nerve injury, *causalgia*. CRPS is a syndrome of regional pain where pain is usually disproportionate to the injury, and the affected area will also have sensory, motor, autonomic, and trophic (skin and bone) changes. CRPS may occur with or without injury, and severity of trauma has no relationship with occurrence of CRPS.

Incidence of CRPS possibly increases with age. Females are affected more than males with ratio of 3:1. The arm is affected in about 60% of cases and the leg in about 40%. The disease resolves spontaneously in 74% cases in the 1st year and 23–36% within 6 years of treatment.

Basically, it was divided into two types based on the presence of nerve lesion; now, a third group has been included where CRPS criteria are partially fulfilled.
1. *Type I*: When there is no evidence of nerve injury. RSD, Sudeck's atrophy, reflex neurovascular dystrophy (RND), or algoneurodystrophy all come under this category.
2. *Type II (causalgia)*: When there is obvious nerve damage (partial or complete).
3. *CRPS-NOS (not otherwise specified)*: When the criteria for CRPS are partially met and the condition (signs and symptoms) cannot be explained by any other disease.

Pathogenesis: *Pathophysiology*—Some individuals are more susceptible than others to develop CRPS. The definitive factors responsible for the occurrence and final course of CRPS are not known; however, history of asthma, migraine and angiotensin-converting enzyme (ACE)-inhibitors group of antihypertensive drugs, which increase the availability of substance P and bradykinin, have been identified as risk factors for CRPS.

There is evidence that supraspinal mechanisms are involved in the pathophysiology of CRPS. After injury, activated cutaneous nociceptors induce retrograde depolarization of small-diameter primary afferents through axon reflex. This causes the release of neuropeptides such as substance P and calcitonin-gene-related peptide (CGRP) from sensory terminals in the skin. These neuropeptides are primarily responsible for CRPS. The exact origin and development of the disorder are unclear, though a few hypotheses have been proposed to elaborate the understanding. The hypotheses regarding pathogenesis of CRPS are:
- Induced neurogenic inflammation
- Autonomic dysfunction
- Neuroplasticity within CNS.

Clinical features: Reflex sympathetic dystrophy can have predominantly inflammatory features, sympathetic features or could be a mix of the two. Apart from the varied features, there is a temporal evolution of the disease. The symptoms usually initially manifest near the site of injury and are often minor. Patient complains of spontaneous pain described as simple aching or burning to throbbing shooting or stabbing. Moving or touching the limb is often painful. Patients may also present with muscle spasms, local swelling, and sensitivity to air, water, touch, and vibrations with abnormally increased sweating. On examination, there may be change in skin temperature (usually hot but sometimes cold) and color (reddish violet) along with joint tenderness or stiffness and/or restricted/painful movements. The motor changes include weakness, distal tremors, dystonia, and myoclonus.

Radiologically, softening and thinning of bones (osteoporosis) especially periarticular but usually "cat bite" lesions are seen. Over a period of time, loss of function, muscle, and limb atrophy become evident with trophic changes like reduced and abnormal nail growth, thin and glossy skin associated with reduced elasticity, and ulceration. Over prolonged period of immobility, contractures and fibrosis develop in the nearby joints. Due to long-standing and progressive nature of disease, patients often have associated psychological and psychiatric disturbances.

Though infrequent but falls, presyncope and syncope may be seen.

Diagnosis: The features that suggest diagnosis of CRPS according to International Association for the Study of Pain are as follows:
- The presence of an initiating noxious event or a cause of immobilization may or may not be present.
- Pain is disproportionate to any known inciting event.
- Presence of edema, changes in the skin blood flow or abnormal sudomotor activity in the region of pain (can be sign or symptom)
- The diagnosis of CRPS is by exclusion (no other conditions that would otherwise account for the degree of pain and dysfunction).

Some diagnostic tests in cases that fall as borderline for CRPS include:
- Sympathetic blockade
- Thermography
- Sweat testing
- Quantitative sensory testing and autonomic testing
- Radiological changes
- Three-phase bone scanning.

Treatment: Treatment should be started as early as possible; if the condition is allowed to persist for more than a few weeks, it may become irreversible. In the acute stage, physical therapy is the most important factor in reversing the syndrome. In subacute and chronic stages, it works to improve pain and function and helps to prevent joint stiffness and contractures. Mild cases often respond to a simple regimen of reassurance, anti-inflammatory drugs, and physiotherapy.

Other conservative measures include the administration of corticosteroids, calcium channel blockers, and tricyclic antidepressants. Mirror box therapy may benefit in early CRPS.

If there is no improvement after a few weeks, and as a first measure in severe cases, sympathetic blockade often helps. This can be done by one or more local anesthetic injections to the stellate or the appropriate lumbar sympathetic ganglia, or by regional block with guanethidine given intravenously to the affected limb. However, the effectiveness of these measures is unpredictable and somewhat doubtful.

A small percentage of patients go on complaining of pain and impaired function almost indefinitely. More aggressive methods like spinal cord stimulation, neuraxial techniques, sympathetic denervation, Botox injections, psychotherapy, relaxation techniques, and hypnosis may all be exhausted before labeling patient unresponsive and resistant.

14. Discuss stages of complex regional pain syndrome and also mention its criteria for staging of complex regional pain syndrome (CRPS).

Ans:

Stages: The symptoms of CRPS and its evolution can be divided into three stages (Bonica's) that has limited therapeutic and prognostic relevance:

1. *Stage 1: Acute (it begins immediately after injury for up to 3 months)*: This stage has a good prognosis and it is reversible. Severe burning pain at the site of injury, associated muscle spasm, joint stiffness, and restricted mobility are characteristics of this stage. Increased hair and nail growth and changes in skin (red, warm, swollen, dry, and inflamed) may be seen due to vasodilatation. At later stage, color may change to mottled with marked hyperhidrosis. In patients with low severity, this stage lasts only for few weeks. At this stage, it can subside spontaneously or respond rapidly to treatment such as physical therapy or intervention by pain specialist.
2. *Stage 2: Subacute or dystrophic (6 weeks–1 year)*: The pain intensity increases. Swelling spreads; hair growth diminishes; nails become cracked, brittle, grooved, and spotty (mainly due to vasospasm); osteoporosis becomes severe and diffuse; joints thicken and muscles get atrophied.
3. *Stage 3: Atrophic (6 months to may be forever)*: With the progression of disease, irreversible changes in the skin and bones occur and unresolved pain may involve the entire limb. Marked muscle atrophy may occur with severely limited mobility of the affected area and flexion contractures. Skin is atrophied, waxy, very thin, and ulcerated. The limb has "woody" feel on examination. The nails become brittle. Occasionally, the limb is displaced from its normal position. Severe osteoporosis with washed-out appearance of bone is seen in radiographs.

Criteria:

International Association for Study of Pain Diagnostic Criteria:
- The presence of an initiating noxious event or a cause of immobilization may or may not be present.
- Pain is disproportionate to any known inciting event.
- Presence of edema, changes in the skin blood flow, or abnormal sudomotor activity in the region of pain (can be sign or symptom).
- The diagnosis of CRPS is by exclusion (no other conditions that would otherwise account for the degree of pain and dysfunction).

Budapest diagnostic criteria:
- Presence of continuous pain which is disproportionate to any inciting event.
- Complaints of at least one symptom in three (clinical diagnostic criteria) or four (research diagnostic criteria) of the following categories:
  - *Sensory*: Hyperesthesia or allodynia
  - *Vasomotor*: Temperature asymmetry and/or skin color changes and/or skin color asymmetry
  - *Sudomotor or edema*: Edema and/or sweating changes, or sweating asymmetry
  - *Motor or trophic*: Decreased range of motion and/or motor dysfunction (weakness, tremor, or dystonia), and/or trophic changes (hair, nails, or skin)

- Presence of at least one sign at time of diagnosis in two or more of the following categories:
  - *Sensory*: Hyperalgesia to pinprick and/or allodynia to light touch, deep somatic pressure, or joint movement (usually nonpainful)
  - *Vasomotor*: Asymmetry of temperature and/or skin color changes
  - *Sudomotor or edema*: Edema and/or sweating changes and/or asymmetrical sweating
  - *Motor or trophic*: Decreased range of motion and/or motor dysfunction, i.e., muscle weakness, tremors, or dystonia and/or trophic changes (hair, nails, or skin)
- No other condition or diagnosis that could better explain the signs and symptoms.

[The diagnosis of CRPS is by exclusion and it should be differentiated with diseases of similar clinical signs and symptoms. As a diagnostic rule, there should be at least one symptom in all four symptom categories and at least one sign (observed at evaluation) in two or more sign categories.]

15. Enumerate the clinical criteria to diagnose CRPS. Enumerate the principles of managing such cases.

Ans: *Clinical criteria to diagnose*:

International Association for Study of Pain Diagnostic Criteria
- The presence of an initiating noxious event or a cause of immobilization may or may not be present.
- Pain is disproportionate to any known inciting event.
- Presence of edema, changes in the skin blood flow, or abnormal sudomotor activity in the region of pain (can be sign or symptom).
- The diagnosis of CRPS is by exclusion (no other conditions that would otherwise account for the degree of pain and dysfunction).

Budapest diagnostic criteria: There should be at least one symptom in at least three symptom categories and at least one sign (observed at evaluation) in two or more sign categories:
- Presence of continuous pain which is disproportionate to any inciting event.
- Complaints of at least one *symptom* in three (clinical diagnostic criteria) or four (research diagnostic criteria) of the following categories:
  - *Sensory*: Hyperesthesia or allodynia
  - *Vasomotor*: Temperature asymmetry and/or skin color changes and/or skin color asymmetry
  - *Sudomotor or edema*: Edema and/or sweating changes, or sweating asymmetry
  - *Motor or trophic*: Decreased range of motion and/or motor dysfunction (weakness, tremor, or dystonia), and/or trophic changes (hair, nails, or skin)
- Presence of at least one *sign* at time of diagnosis in two or more of the following categories:
  - *Sensory*: Hyperalgesia to pinprick and/or allodynia to light touch, deep somatic pressure, or joint movement (usually nonpainful)
  - *Vasomotor*: Asymmetry of temperature and/or skin color changes
  - *Sudomotor or edema*: Edema and/or sweating changes and/or asymmetrical sweating
  - *Motor or trophic*: Decreased range of motion and/or motor dysfunction, i.e., muscle weakness, tremors, or dystonia and/or trophic changes (hair, nails, or skin)
- No other condition or diagnosis that could better explain the signs and symptoms.

Principles of management: The diagnosis is based on clinical criteria and no further investigation is actually needed. The radiographs may be obtained to ascertain bone union before initiating therapy. Sometimes differentiation from other conditions may need documentation and bone scan may be obtained if infection is to be ruled out. Electrodiagnostic studies may be obtained to rule out neural injury. The treatment aims primarily at:
- Pain control
- Desensitization
- Regaining function

The common flow of interventions and modalities to achieve the therapeutic aim is presented in **Flowchart 1.1.3**.

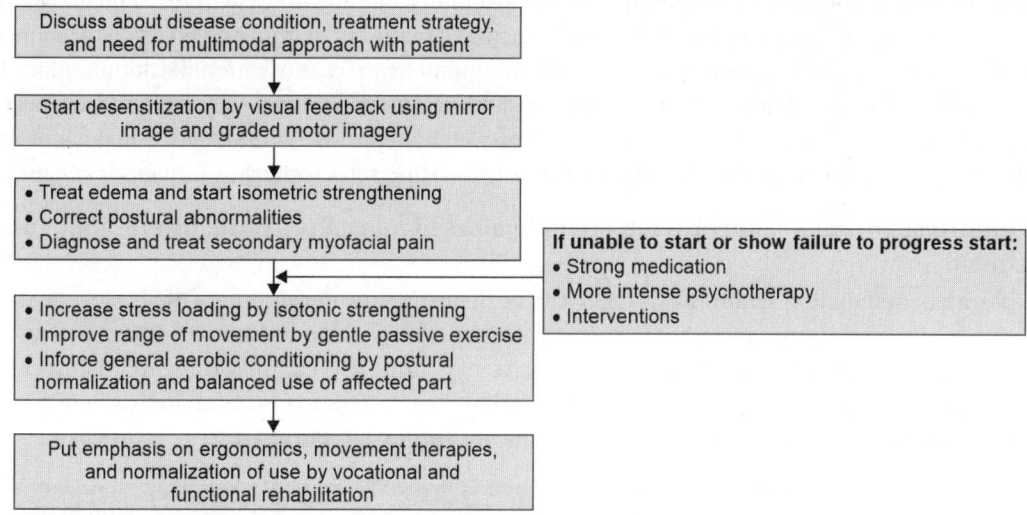

Flowchart 1.1.3: Stepwise interventions and modalities used to control complex regional pain syndrome.

16. Describe gram-negative septicemia.

Ans: Septicemia is an alarming condition with often disastrous consequences, if not treated expeditiously. Gram-negative septicemia attracted attention for its poorer outcomes from last decade of 20th century where it produced higher mortality and was difficult to control compared to gram-positive sepsis. It is much more commonly associated with severe sepsis and septic shock and it has been found that adults with septic shock more frequently used to have gram-negative sepsis. Distinctive immunophysiological processes have been identified associated with gram-negative septicemia that leads to such catastrophic progression.

Theories for pathophysiology:

- *The intravascular stimulus hypothesis* suggests invasion through a normal or damaged epithelium into bloodstream by the gram-negative bacteria that produces systemic inflammatory responses. Endotoxins play a major role in activation of multiple inflammatory pathways to cause systemic effects, promptly involving tumor necrosis factor-α (TNF-α), and interleukins (ILs). TNF-α acts synergistically with IL-1 or γ-interferon or both to trigger a systemic inflammatory response and cause damage to the vascular endothelium. This causes increased vascular permeability (bradykinins), leukocyte-endothelial adhesion, and activation of complement and clotting pathways (particularly factor XII—Hageman factor) progressing at a faster rate simultaneously to ultimately result in multiorgan failure (MOF).
- The other theory suggests that the MOF and shock result from neuroendocrine dysregulation and mediators released into the bloodstream from the infected tissues. Circulating bacteria or endotoxin are not needed as direct stimuli for intravascular inflammation.

Markers for septicemia and shock: It has been identified that elevated levels of IL-6 and C-reactive protein (CRP) are associated with septic shock compared to sepsis or severe sepsis. Septic shock patients usually have gram-negative septicemia and higher mortality. These inflammatory responses may be generated in response to exogenous pathogen-associated molecular patterns and to endogenous signals of tissue and cell injury (alarmins). Among the alarmins, high-mobility group box 1 has been described as a mediator of sepsis that can be targeted for therapy. Procalcitonin is a better marker than CRP levels that identify sepsis 24–28 hours earlier on an average.

Treatment: It is imperative to start appropriate antimicrobial therapy that is guided by blood cultures and antibiogram of the hospital. Empirical drug therapy has to be instituted commonly, as the results of culture sensitivity are available only at 49–72 hours while most deaths occur within 2 days of septic shock. Usually, a combination therapy is instituted that comprises aminoglycoside and expanded spectrum cephalosporin or antipseudomonal penicillin. The latter is preferred in patients with neutropenia, burns, or infection related to respiratory therapy. In case of resistance to cephalosporins, imipenem, or meropenem is used depending on hospital practice. Treatment of fluid and electrolyte balance to manage shock is important that may also be supplemented with sympathomimetics in case of shock like dobutamine, dopamine, or noradrenaline. Use of corticosteroids and naloxone is still elusive but latter has been frequently used to counter endotoxic shock. Coagulopathy should be controlled with low-molecular-weight heparins. Granulocyte transfusions have not been extensively supported for benefit in survival. Immunotherapy against lipopolysaccharide antigens is still under evolution.

17. **What is multisystem organ failure? What are indicators of mortality? Write briefly about diagnosis and management.**

Ans: The multiple organ dysfunction syndrome (MODS) can be defined as the development of physiological derangement involving two or more organ systems (such that homeostasis can no longer be maintained without active intervention), *not* involved in the primary disorder that resulted in intensive care unit (ICU) admission, and arising in the wake of a potentially life-threatening physiologic insult. It is a process rather than a single event. As an indicator of mortality, MODS score is calculated based on parameters as shown in the adjacent **Tables 1.1.1 and 1.1.2**.

TABLE 1.1.1: The multiple organ dysfunction syndrome (MODS) score.

Organ system	0	1	2	3	4
Respiratory system:					
pO_2/FiO_2 ratio without reference to the use or mode of mechanical ventilation, and without reference to the use or level of PEEP	>300	226–300	151–225	76–150	≤75
Renal system:					
Serum creatinine (µmol/L)	≤100	101–200	201–350	351–500	>500
Liver and biliary system:					
Serum bilirubin (µmol/L)	≤20	21–60	61–120	121–240	>240
Cardiovascular system:					
Pressure-adjusted heart rate (heart rate × RAP/mean BP)	≤10.0	10.1–15.0	15.1–20.0	20.1–30.0	>30.0
Hematology					
Platelet count (10^3 per mL)	>120	81–120	51–80	21–50	≤20
Central nervous system:					
Glasgow coma score	15	13–14	10–12	7–9	≤6

(FiO_2: fraction of inspired oxygen; PEEP: positive end-expiratory pressure; pO_2: partial pressure of oxygen; RAP: right atrial pressure)

TABLE 1.1.2: Relative prognostication importance of MODS score to mortality.

MODS score	Mortality
0	0
9–12	25
13–16	50
17–20	75
>20	100

(MODS: multiple organ dysfunction syndrome)

Diagnosis: Diagnosis of MODS is mainly clinical, which is supplemented by laboratory tests and imaging modalities:
- *In hepatic dysfunction:* If ischemic hepatitis—jaundice, increased transaminase, and increased serum bilirubin. If acalculous cholecystitis—right hypochondrial pain and tenderness, abdominal distention, unexplained fever, and loss of bowel sounds.

- *In pulmonary dysfunction,* there are symptoms suggestive of acute respiratory distress syndrome (ARDS).
- *In renal dysfunction,* there are azotemia, fluid and electrolyte imbalance, decreased creatinine clearance, and fluid volume overload.
- *In cardiovascular system (CVS)* due to cardiac hypoperfusion, there is decrease in the contractility of the myocardium, with fall in cardiac output and stroke volume and inability to maintain the BP without vasopressors.
- *In DIC,* there are microvascular clotting and hemorrhage in organ systems.
- *CNS dysfunction,* there are impaired mentation, confusion, altered level of consciousness, delirium, and psychosis and abnormal bispectral electroencephalography (EEG) monitoring.
- Muscle wasting, severe weight loss, hyperglycemia, hypertriglyceridemia, increased serum lactate, hypoalbuminemia, decreased prealbumin and serum transferrin, and decreased retinol-binding protein.
- *In immune dysfunction,* there are nosocomial infection, pyrexia, and decreased lymphocyte anergy.

Treatment: At present, there is no specific treatment of MODS. The treatment modality is mainly supportive to correct the underlying disorder and optimize physiology. The principles for the treatment of MODS are:
- Early recognition
- *Control of infection*: Incision and drainage of any abscess, antibiotics—sepsis—identification and treatment of the source of infection, volume resuscitation, vasopressors, and inotropes, if evidence of hypoperfusion.
- *Maintenance of tissue oxygenation*: Mechanical ventilation and increasing tissue perfusion. Control of bleeding, maintenance of hemoglobin 8–10 g/dL.
- Nutritional/metabolic support.

18. What is fat embolism, detail its management following fracture shaft of femur in a young adult in emergency department?

Ans: Fat embolism occurs due to release of lipid from medullary canal of large bones upon injury into free circulation that causes clinical abnormalities by virtue of mechanical or metabolic consequences.

Presentation: Respiratory failure, cerebral dysfunction, and skin petechiae generally develop 24–72 hours after trauma. Initially, larger fat globules cause mechanical occlusion of multiple blood vessels, which is transient and even incomplete as the fat globules are never capable of completely obstructing microcirculation due to their fluidity and deformability. It is the hydrolysis of fat into more irritable fatty acids that cause late systemic manifestations of fat embolism syndrome (FES).

- *Cardiopulmonary*:
  - Persistent tachycardia
  - Tachypnea, dyspnea, and hypoxemia are the earliest to manifest and seen in 75% of patients. They are liable to progress to respiratory failure in 10% of the cases.
  - High-grade fever.
- *Dermatologic*:
  - The characteristic petechial rash develops in about 20–60% of cases.
  - Petechial rashes are seen in mucous membrane (oral), the conjunctiva, and skin folds of the neck and axilla. Usually, they appear within first 36 hours.
- *Neurologic*:
  - The common presentation is an acute confusional state. Focal neurological signs, such as aphasia, apraxia, hemiplegia, visual field disturbances, anisocoria, seizures, and decorticate posturing, are also sometimes seen.
  - Fundoscopic examination reveals retinal hemorrhages with intra-arterial fat globules.
- *Other miscellaneous findings*:
  - Right heart failure pattern is common on an ECG.
  - Myocardial ischemia causing reduced efficacy of myocardium.
  - Macular edema causing scotomata associated with soft fluffy retinal exudates (Purtscher's retinopathy).
  - Features of DIC.
  - Oliguria, lipiduria, proteinuria, or hematuria.

Diagnosis: FES is mainly a clinical diagnosis, whereby other causes are systematically excluded.
- *Schonfeld's criteria* **(Table 1.1.3)**:
  – Cumulative score > 5 requires diagnosis.

TABLE 1.1.3: Schonfeld's criteria.	
Criteria/clinical feature	*Score*
Petechiae	5
Chest X-ray changes (diffuse alveolar infiltrates)	4
Hypoxemia (PaO$_2$ < 9.3 kPa)	3
Fever (> 38°C)	1
Tachycardia (> 120 bpm)	1
Tachypnea (> 30 bpm)	1
(PaO$_2$: partial arterial pressure of oxygen)	

- *Lindeque's criteria*: According to Lindeque et al., FES can be diagnosed on the basis of respiratory system involvement alone.
  – Sustained pO$_2$ < 8 kpa
  – Sustained pCO$_2$ > 7.3 kpa
  – Sustained respiratory rate > 35 breaths/min, in spite of sedation
  – Increased work of breathing, dyspnea, tachycardia, and anxiety.

Laboratory studies: Laboratory tests in FES are mostly nonspecific:
- *Arterial blood gas*: Unexplained increase in pulmonary shunt fraction (P alveolar O$_2$ – P arterial O$_2$) and difference is strongly suggestive of the syndrome, especially if it occurs immediately after 24–48 hours.
  – Arterial blood gas analysis also reveals hypoxia, with a PaO$_2$ of < 60 mm Hg along with hypocapnia—paCO$_2$ < 30 mm Hg.
- *Hematocrit, platelet count, and fibrinogen*: Fall in hematocrit occurs within 24–48 hours and is due to intra-alveolar hemorrhage. Coagulation abnormalities are all nonspecific.
- *Demonstration of fat globules*: Sensitivity and negative predictive value of this test are very low to be of any concrete use in diagnosis and are more of academic interest. Fat globules in the urine are as such common after bone injuries or polytrauma.

Imaging:
- *Plain chest radiographs*: Some demonstrable X-ray findings appear within 24–48 hours of onset of clinical findings and these are as follows:
  – Diffusely distributed bilateral pulmonary infiltrates
  – "Snow storm" appearance of fleck-like pulmonary shadows
  – Prominent pulmonary bronchiolar markings
  – Enlargement of the right side of the heart.
- High-resolution chest CT for PE demonstrates three main patterns, which are described as follows:
  1. Ground-glass opacities with interlobular septal thickening
  2. Ground-glass opacities in geographic distribution
  3. Nodular opacities.

Treatment: No specific treatment is available for FES. Most modalities aim to provide adequate symptomatic relief:
- Maintain adequate tissue oxygenation and pulmonary ventilation.
- Maintain hemodynamic stability.
- Blood products should be only instituted as clinically indicated and not irrationally.
- *Adequate fluid balance*: It is better to restrict fluid intake and increase the use of diuretics to minimize fluid accumulation in the lungs, provided circulation is not compromised. This latter part of maintenance of intravascular volume is really important otherwise shock can further exacerbate lung injury caused by FES, so only "excess fluid" is restricted.

- Institute prophylaxis for DVT according to institutional policy.
- *Fracture stabilization*: Early immobilization of fractures should be done and operative treatment is more beneficial than the conservative one. Raised intraosseous pressure during orthopedic procedures is quite common, so a practice of damage control orthopedics (DCO) would tend to control FES—it is believed. This would reduce the insult from intravasation of intramedullary fat and other debris in a homeostatically unstable patient further compromising his physiology.

Medication: No drug is found completely useful for FES and controversies exist:
- *Steroids*:
  - Decrease inflammatory reaction in lungs caused by free fatty acids.
  - Decrease capillary leakage by stabilizing lysosomal and capillary membrane.
  - Prophylactic dose of methylprednisolone—1.5 mg/kg IV—can be administered every 8 hours for six doses.
- Alcohol, albumin, aprotinin, and hypertonic glucose all are proposed for treatment of FES, but they are found to be of no use.

19. How will you clinically differentiate between cerebral signs as a result of head injury versus fat embolism? Describe in brief about the management of fat embolism syndrome.

Ans: In fat embolism, the signs and symptoms more closely resemble those of stroke.

The common presentation is an acute confusional state. Focal neurological signs, such as aphasia, apraxia, hemiplegia, visual field disturbances, anisocoria, seizures, and decorticate posturing, are also sometimes seen. Fundoscopic examination reveals retinal hemorrhages with intra-arterial fat globules. These signs indicate focal deficits.

In a case of head injury instead there is commonly loss of consciousness for several minutes to hours. There is associated headache that may worsen. Patients report nausea/vomiting and there could be a history of convulsions and seizures. The person may be difficult to awaken from sleep and slowly deteriorate in vocal and motor response to stimuli. These signs indicate more global involvement of cerebrum.

Management of fat embolism is written in answer above.

20. Describe pathophysiology of fat embolism.

Ans: The exact mechanism producing fat embolism is not known; different theories have been proposed. They may act singly or in combination with each other. Mainly two theories about fat embolism exist:

1. *Mechanical theory (Gassling et al.)*: According to this theory, traumatic injury forces liquefied fat droplets from disrupted bone marrow into torn venules. These droplets then enter into the pulmonary capillary beds serving as a primary reservoir and migrate through arteriovenous shunts to the brain. Microvascular deposition of droplets produces local ischemia by occlusion of the vessels and inflammation by virtue of reactive nature of the lipid. This leads to concomitant release of inflammatory mediators as a reaction to both ischemia and ongoing inflammation which proceeds platelet aggregation in the capillaries setting up a vicious loop of ischemia. Ischemia also gets facilitated by simultaneous release of vasoactive amines.
2. *Biochemical theory*: Explains nontraumatic forms. A number of biochemical mechanisms are proposed for this theory that are as follows:
   - *Toxic theory*: Baker suggested that local hydrolysis of fat emboli by lung lipase generates chemically toxic free fatty acids, which causes severe inflammatory changes by producing endothelial damage, inactivation of lung surfactant, and increasing lung permeability. They can also enter into systemic circulation causing multiorgan dysfunction.
   - *Obstructive theory*: This theory states that hormonal changes caused by trauma and/or sepsis in the patient leads to systemic release of free fatty acids as chylomicrons. Subsequently, chylomicrons coalesce because of elevated acute-phase reactant in these patients, such as CRPs, which leads to embolization and causes the physiologic reactions as described earlier.

21. Define nonunion. Discuss management of diaphyseal gap nonunion with 5 cm bone loss in a young adult.

Ans:

Definition: Nonunion of fracture is said to exist when the fracture shows clinically, radiologically, and biologically no signs of progression to repair itself after prolonged duration [US Food and Drug Administration (FDA) considers this as

9 months with failure of progression for 3 consecutive months] for the type, site, and pattern of fracture and will not unite unless radical alteration in management is undertaken.

In 1986, for purposes of testing bone-healing devices, a US FDA panel defined nonunion as "established when a minimum of 9 months has elapsed since injury and the fracture shows no visible progressive signs of healing for 3 months."

The methods that can be deployed for management of gap nonunion are:
- Acute docking + bone lengthening (external bone transport) by Ilizarov method
- Acute docking + bone grafting and fixation—causes shortening and is unacceptable, even in forearm shortening of 4 cm is acceptable but the critical defect in question is 5 cm, so this may not be acceptable except in frailest elderly patient who cannot bear with cumbersome procedures
- Out of label use of Masquelet technique
- Lengthening over nail.

(Details of Ilizarov procedure and other techniques can be read from the book Essential Orthopedics: Principles and Practice, 2nd edition.)

22. Management strategies in nonunion of tibia.

Ans: Treatment of tibial shaft nonunions: Key principles and strategies

Union rates by treatment modality:
- Closed bone grafting (hypertrophic nonunions): 72.1–87.8%
- Internal fixation: ~98%
- Electrical stimulation: 78.8%

Treatment selection factors:
- Vascularity (hypervascular vs. avascular)
- Alignment (acceptable vs. malaligned)
- Presence of infection, defect, or deformity

Specific Treatment Methods
- Partial fibulectomy and weight bearing
    - *Indication*: Fibular healing preventing tibial compression
    - *Advantages*:
        - Simple, preserves vascularity
        - Allows weight-bearing stimulation
        - Permits future grafting/fixation if needed
    - *Technique*:
        - Resect 2.5 cm fibular segment
        - Align tibia, apply long leg walking cast (6 weeks)
    - *Failure risks*: Nonweight-bearing, pseudarthrosis, prior external fixation
- Posterolateral bone grafting
    - *Indication*: Infected nonunions or large defects
    - *Union rate*: 80–90% (5–7 months average)
    - *Advantage*: Single, nondestructive procedure
- Percutaneous bone marrow injection
    - *Role*: Adjunct for biological stimulation (not a stability solution)
    - *Often combined with*: Demineralized bone matrix (DBM)
    - *Requires*: Concurrent stabilization (cast, nail, or fixator)

Internal Fixation Options
- Intramedullary nailing (IMN)
    - *Preferred for*: Diaphyseal nonunions with intact medullary alignment

- *Benefits*:
    - Closed technique preserves vascularity
    - Reaming provides endosteal grafting effect
- *Caution*:
    - Higher infection risk if prior external fixation or open fracture
    - Avoid in infected nonunions
- Plate Fixation
    - *Best for*: Correcting deformity, tension-side application
    - *Technique*:
        - Lag screws + compression plating
        - Limited periosteal stripping to preserve blood supply
    - *Risks*: Infection, implant failure (avoid in prior infection)

External Fixation (Ilizarov/Taylor Spatial Frame)
- *Indications*:
    - Infected nonunions
    - Severe deformity/bone loss (bone transport)
- *Advantages*:
    - Minimally invasive, adjustable correction
    - High union rates in complex cases

Conclusion
- *Hypervascular nonunions*: Fixation alone is often sufficient
- *Avascular nonunions*: Require decortication + grafting
- *Infection*: External fixation or staged protocols preferred

23. Discuss causes of nonunion of fractures. Describe types of nonunion and classify them. Discuss various modalities used to diagnose nonunion.

Ans: Causes:

Systemic factors:
- Age (elderly)
- Malnutrition (albumin < 3.4 g/dL; lymphocyte count < 1,500/mm^3)
- Corticosteroid therapy
- Immunosuppressive treatment
- Systemic disease (hepatic and renal)
- Diabetes mellitus (secondary to neurovascular compromise)
- Metabolic bone disease
- Anticoagulants
- NSAID therapy
- Burns
- Smoking
- Alcohol
- Radiation

Local factors:
- *Fracture related*:
    - Site (fracture neck of femur, scaphoid, capitellum, fracture neck of talus, lateral condyle of humerus fractures, and diaphyseal fractures of distal third tibia)
    - Open
    - Infected

- Comminuted
- Segmental
- Fractures of irradiated bone
- Intra-articular fractures
- *Treatment related*:
  - Inadequate reduction
  - Inadequate immobilization
  - Inadequate fixation
  - Inadequate blood supply
  - Inadequate soft tissue cover
  - Interposition of soft tissue
  - Inadequate apposition "distraction"

Classification: For clinical evaluation and mobility at nonunion site, the nonunions have been classified into:
- *Mobile (or lax) nonunion*: The arc of motion > 7° with radiological defect > 1 cm.
- *Short-stiff (nonmobile) nonunions*: The arc of motion ≤ 7° (classically < 1 cm defect radiologically) at nonunion site that is quite adequately bridged by fibrocartilage to resist movements grossly. Often only micromotion can be elicited; even the patient may bear weight partially in such cases.

For practical purpose, the nonunion can be simply classified into:
- Infected nonunion (with active or quiescent infection)
- Noninfected nonunions.

Noninfected nonunions: The noninfected nonunions have been classified variedly by different authors. The most popular system is the modified Muller and Judet classification given by *Weber and Cech*.

Hypervascular nonunion:
- *Elephant foot*: They have hypertrophic callus formation and result from either inadequate fixation/immobilization or premature weight bearing.
- *Horse hoof*: The ends are mildly bulbous exceeding the thickness of bone and result from moderately unstable fixation.
- *Oligotrophic*: The ends are not hypertrophic but callus is absent and result from inadequate apposition, displaced fracture, and distracted fragments with adequate vascularity.

Avascular nonunion:
- *Torsion wedge nonunion*: The intermediate butterfly (wedge) fragment has compromised blood supply that heals to one main fragment of bone but not to other.
- *Comminuted (necrotic) nonunion*: Has one or more necrotic fragments in between that fails to unite to any fragment and remains isolated disrupting the continuity of the repair process.
- *Defect (gap) nonunion*: In open fractures or sequestration process of long-standing osteomyelitis, the intermediate fragment or a part of bone is lost in full circumference (differentiating from torsion wedge or necrotic nonunion).
- *Atrophic*: The ends of bone are osteoporotic and atrophic due to lack of trophic factors and loss of blood supply.

Paley classification of nonunion specifically deals with legs bones and is based on bone loss, fracture laxity, deformity, and shortening.
- Type A (< 1 cm bone loss)
  - *A1*: Mobile deformity
  - *A2*: Fixed deformity
    - *A2-I*: Stiff nonunion without deformity
    - *A2-II*: Stiff nonunion with fixed deformity
- Type B (> 1 cm bone loss)
  - *B1*: Bony defect no shortening
  - *B2*: Shortening but no defect
  - *B3*: Both (shortening with defect)

Diagnosis:

Radiographs: Radiographs should be obtained always in two perpendicular planes and oblique views are also helpful sometimes. Stress views for demonstration of deformation at fracture site objectively demonstrate nonunion. Typically, the varus-valgus and anteroposterior (AP) stress are employed. Radiographs show some characteristic features:
- Marked sclerosis of ends with rounding-off appearance
- Medullary canal closed
- Diffuse osteoporosis of both fragments
- Fracture gap persists and widened due to unsuccessful bridging.
- Proximal end convex and distal end concave (pseudoarthrosis)

Computed tomography: Any doubt for cortical continuity can be readily evaluated with high-resolution CT and 3D-reconstruction. It is especially useful for oblique and spiral fractures.

Magnetic resonance imaging (MRI): MRI can be used for evaluation of vascularity of the fragments and small bones. Especially, bones susceptible for osteonecrosis due to fracture (scaphoid, talus, and head of femur) should be evaluated using MRI.

Bone scan:
- Used to detect the presence of synovial pseudoarthrosis—a cold cleft is seen between two areas of high uptake.
- Scintigraphy is employed to assess nonunion biological activity and infection.
- Scintigraphy is a particularly a useful technique to distinguish hypervascular active nonunion and nonresponsive avascular nonunions.
- Indium scans are more sensitive and specific for diagnosing infections.

Positron emission tomography scan: Positron emission tomography scan increases the sensitivity and specificity when combined with bone scan and MRI for diagnosing infection and vascularity but the cost is a prohibiting factor.

Laboratory investigations are aimed to find infection at the nonunion site and include ESR, CRP, and total leukocyte count (TLC). Renal and liver functions are other investigations that can be done to find risk factors. For choosing surgical treatment, nutritional status of the patient should also be evaluated.

24. Explain stove-in chest.

Ans: Stove-in chest is a severe and complex type of flail chest due to blunt or crush injury producing depression of the chest. This results in breathing problem and altered chest expansion. The clinical features and management are like flail chest only.

Pathophysiology: There is depression of chest wall with ribs broken at multiple levels. The chest wall becomes discontinuous and is unable to function as a closed chamber. There is inward movement of broken segment during inspiration and reverse happens during expiration—*paradoxical breathing*.

Clinical features: These paradoxical movements prevent usual expansion of lungs (the chest wall fails to pull lungs into inflation) and, hence, reduce ventilatory lung surface area. This produces respiratory dysfunction.

Mediastinal flutter: Paradoxical and nonphysiological movement of mediastinum during different phases of breathing occurs, often causing kinking of great vessels and sudden cardiac arrest.

In case of one-sided stove-in chest, pendular movements of air from one lung to other would occur, thus preventing atmospheric air to get into both injured and normal lungs despite best efforts of the patient and it produces respiratory failure. The "hypoventilation" thus created causes carbon dioxide retention and ultimate respiratory failure.

Investigations: Chest X-ray to identify fracture segment, blood grouping (for substituting blood loss), arterial pO_2, pCO_2 monitoring, and serum electrolytes.

Treatment: The patient is managed on emergent basis following the Advanced Trauma Life Support (ATLS) protocol securing airway, breathing, and circulation (ABC). Specific management includes:
- Intercostal tube drainage
- Applying clips to fracture ribs and fixing above and below to normal ribs

- Antibiotics
- Blood transfusion, IV fluids
- Bronchodilators, steroids for circulatory support
- Ventilator support with intermittent positive pressure ventilation (IPPV) is essential, as lungs need to be inflated from within
- Thoracotomy is not routinely indicated but should be performed when required.

25. What are principles of management including recent advances in treatment of flail chest?

Ans: Principles:

Principles for initial management:
- Minimize further injury to the underlying lung
- Provide adequate analgesia
- Maintain oxygenation
- Controlled fluid resuscitation

Principles for definitive management:
- Analgesia is the mainstay.
- Intubation and ventilation if hypoxic
- *Chest tube insertion*: To treat hemo/pneumothorax
- *Rib fracture fixation*: On a case-to-case basis
- *Proper rehabilitation with physiotherapy*: To build musculature, reposition the chest wall.

Recent advances:
- Early use of noninvasive ventilation (NIV) appears to be well tolerated in select hemodynamically stable blunt trauma patients. For those patients requiring intubation, airway pressure release ventilation is an excellent mode to decrease the risk of posttraumatic acute lung injury.
- Despite its increasing use, there continue to be conflicting results about the role of surgical rib fixation for the treatment of flail chest. No advantage could be demonstrated for operative fixation of rib fractures. Future studies are needed before rib fixation is embedded or abandoned in clinical practice.
- The Indian Society of Critical Care Medicine (ISCCM) guidelines for use of NIV in acute respiratory failure due to chest trauma—the three randomized controlled trials (RCTs) studies have shown that when NIV is used in patients with chest trauma is beneficial (reduced infectious complications and ICU/hospital stay) when compared with use of high-flow oxygen through a mask or endotracheal intubation and invasive mechanical ventilation. Recommendation is that NIV may be used in traumatic flail chest along with adequate pain relief.
- Extracorporeal CO_2 removal targeting hypocapnia is a potential adjunct in management of extensive flail chest undergoing nonsurgical management as it is hypothesized that this therapy will suppress the respiratory drive sufficiently, to permit synchronous mechanical ventilation allowing rib fracture healing in awake patients with extensive bilateral flail chest.

26. Discuss management of multiple rib fractures with hemothorax.

Ans: Hemothorax is collection of blood in pleural space resulting from blunt or penetrating trauma to chest wall and containing structures such as ribs, lung parenchyma, minor veins, and, rarely, arterial injury.

Diagnosis: Small and moderate hemothorax needs radiological or other evaluation and may be missed clinically. Clinically, detectable hemothorax is usually large enough to prompt emergent treatment. Additionally, evaluate for crepitus—indicating rib fracture, segmental collapse—stove-in chest, flail chest and paradoxical breathing, contusion, number, bruising, and depth and extent of penetrating injuries. There is reduced chest expansion, dullness to percussion, and reduced breath sounds and unless massive there is no mediastinal or tracheal shift. In supine position, most of the signs are absent due to dorsal settling of the blood. Chest X-ray demonstrates fluid level with classical meniscus but only in an erect film. Obliteration of costophrenic angle indicates 400–500 mL of blood in cavity. In supine radiographs, there may be diffuse opacification of the hemithorax. (FAST) Focused assessment with sonography for trauma (FAST) US is sensitive enough to detect 200 mL of blood but may be difficult to interpret, if there is additional pneumothorax or subcutaneous emphysema. CT scans are now more readily available in emergencies and indispensable to know the cause of hemothorax and can even detect small collections ≈50 mL. Currently, they are indicated in polytrauma and to differentiate hemothorax from pulmonary contusion, aspiration syndrome, etc.

Treatment: Start with ATLS protocol of airway, breathing, circulation, disability, exposure, and resuscitation. In a clinically identified hemothorax (massive hemothorax), emergent treatment by intercostal chest tube insertion is done with aggressive resuscitation. Usually, dark-colored blood indicates venous bleed, while arterial bleed is suspected with cherry red blood and it is an ominous sign possibly urgently needing a thoracotomy in first instance itself. Emergent thoracotomy is also possibly needed if initial blood drained exceeds 1,000 mL in first go. If bleeding continues (venous bleed: 200–250 mL blood per hour for 4–5 hours) or features of shock develop, urgent thoracotomy has to be considered. The bleeding may be delayed or may recur after several days. Indications for thoracotomy—initial volume of blood loss is not as important as the amount of ongoing bleeding, drainage is > 1,000 mL or 200 mL each hour for 3 hours, suspected clotted hemothorax (opacity persisting on chest X-ray even after intercostal tube).

Multiple rib fractures without flail chest: Strapping is occasionally necessary, that can be done with intermittent use of Velcro rib belt. Epidural analgesia is standard for pain management in these patients.

Multiple rib fractures with flail chest: Ribs fracture at two places and become indrawn during inhalation leading to paradoxical respiration and respiratory failure. One needs to use sea gull prosthesis for anterior type of flail chest. Lateral flail chest is treated by chest stabilization. Rarely, surgical stabilization is indicated. Intermittent positive pressure respiration (IPPR) intubation is newer method for physiological stabilization. It is called as internal pneumatic fixation.

27. Describe tension pneumothorax—causes, manifestation, and management.

Ans: Pneumothorax is presence of air in pleural cavity. Tension pneumothorax is the build-up of air in the pleural cavity in a way that it exerts positive pressure on mediastinal and intrathoracic structures. The mechanism is formation of one-way valve allowing air to enter the pleural space during inspiration, coughing, sneezing, and straining but not allowing it to escape. Large amount of air gets trapped in the pleural space and the intrapleural pressure becomes much higher than the atmospheric pressure. Open penetrating trauma to the chest is the usual cause whereby chest wall tissue or parietal pleura forms the valve flap. Lung lacerations may also produce tension pneumothorax where the communication between pleura and lung persists leaking air into the cavity but not allowing it to return through lungs. Insidious pneumothorax may develop in patients with ventilator support in ICU who are kept on positive pressure ventilation. Lastly, rapidly developing and refractory tension pneumothorax may develop in injury to large airway where bronchopleural fistula develops. In such situation, even chest tube drainage may not relieve the tension pneumothorax, as the air flow is voluminous (thus refractory to usual treatment).

Critical concern: The high intrapleural pressure results in compression of the underlying lung as well as gross shift of mediastinum to the opposite side with consequent compression of the opposite lung also. It also reduces venous return by compressing the vena cava, resulting in circulatory instability that may quickly result in traumatic arrest if not corrected promptly.

Examination findings: Clinically, these patients present with rapidly progressive breathlessness, central cyanosis, rapid and thready pulse, and signs of peripheral circulatory failure. The chest is hyperexpanded that moves little if any with breathing, there is tympanic note on percussion, auscultation reveals total absence of breath sounds, and on palpation, there is prominent tracheal shift. One can see prominent neck veins due to venous congestion and the central venous pressure (CVP) is raised. The patient is hypotensive, and in late cases, one finds pulseless electrical activity (ECG present but no pulses) and death can occur within minutes from asphyxia and circulatory collapse.

Radiology: Chest X-ray demonstrates pneumothorax, tracheal deviation away from pneumothorax, mediastinal shift away from pneumothorax, and depression of hemidiaphragm. In bilateral tension pneumothorax, both sides pleural cavity is absent and trachea is central. Conspicuously, the mediastinum is thinned out and one would be surprised by the "absence" or minimal cardiac shadow.

Treatment: It is an acute medical emergency. Prompt diagnosis is to be done, and based on clinical suspicion, treatment with emergent chest decompression is instituted immediately. One may not wait for chest X-ray. Following are the methods of chest decompression in tension pneumothorax:
- *Needle thoracostomy*: This is done by the introduction of a wide-bore cannula (14 or 16 G, recommended) or needle (not recommended, use only if cannula not available) inserted in the 2nd intercostal space in midclavicular line. The needle is removed leaving the sheath within cavity; the other end of cannula may be attached to long rubber tubing the end of which is placed underwater in a bottle. Usually, there is a gush of air that converts tension pneumothorax into simple pneumothorax. A better alternative is introduction of an intercostal chest tube drainage as soon as emergent decompression with cannula is done.
- *Intercostal chest tube drainage*: This is the definitive management of tension pneumothorax and placement is also quite fast. Although it is preferable to needle thoracostomy, but in a hemodynamically unstable patient, the extra minutes needed for its insertion may threaten the patient's life, so needle thoracostomy as a prior procedure in such patients is recommended.

28. Describe thoracic outlet syndrome (TOS).

Ans: Thoracic outlet syndrome can be defined as a group of various disorders resulting from compression of the neurovascular bundle in the thoracic outlet region, producing various signs and symptoms in the neck, shoulder, and upper limbs.

Etiology: Thoracic outlet syndrome can occur mainly because of four causes; more than one cause may affect the patient simultaneously.
1. *Congenital anomalies*: These may be bone anomalies such as presence of cervical rib, prolonged transverse process of C7 cervical vertebra, elevation of the scapula, fibrous anomalies like presence of transversocostal and costocostal fibrous bands, and muscular anomalies like abnormal insertion of scalenus anterior muscle or sickle-shaped scalenus medius muscle.
2. *Posttraumatic causes*: Like fracture of the clavicle or upper ribs, hyperextension neck injuries and shoulder injuries (whiplash injury), and injuries to the scalene muscle with their subsequent fibrosis.
3. *Functional acquired causes*: They are thought to be the most common causes of TOS. These include adoption of abnormal postural habits, drooping shoulder conditions, heavy breasts, hypertrophy of the scalene muscles, decreased tone of trapezius and rhomboids, rapid weight loss due to vigorous physical activity, etc.
4. *Other acquired causes*: Tumors like Pancoast tumor, osteomyelitis, and exostosis of the first rib are rare causes.

Clinical presentation:

Neurological symptoms:

Most of the patients present with one of the neurological symptoms (95–98%). They may range from mild pain and sensory changes to limb- or life-threatening complications.

Neurological TOS (NTOS) can be divided into two groups—true NTOS, associated with true neurological deficits (mainly muscular atrophy), and symptomatic TOS, associated with symptoms of TOS without any neurological, radiological, or electrophysiological abnormalities. Most of the patients belong to latter group.

The main symptoms are pain, paresthesia, numbness, and/or weakness. The symptoms of the NTOS do not follow dermatomal or myotomal pattern. They can be categorized according to area or roots of the brachial plexus involved. If the upper plexus (C5–C7) is involved, the patient presents with ipsilateral neck or ear pain, pain over the face, mandible and occipital region, headache, and pain over the clavicular and pectoral region moving toward trapezius and deltoid down lateral arm. If the lower plexus (C8–T1) is involved, patient presents with pain over AP aspect of shoulder radiating down to the medial side of arm, forearm, and hand in the fourth and fifth fingers.

The general features of NTOS include headache with pain in the occiput area, exacerbation of pain with overhead activities or carrying heavy objects, numbness, and paresthesia in the upper limbs. The patient may develop progressive weakness and dysfunction of the hands.

The timing of the symptoms is also important. Some patients may awake in the night because of paresthesia in the upper limb, the reason is thought as return of normal sensation after release of compression of the perineural blood supply to the brachial plexus (known as "release phenomenon"). Other patients have pain throughout the daytime because of using prolonged posture resulting in increased tension or compression on the brachial plexus (known as "compressors"). In trauma cases, the brachial plexus injury leading to NTOS results in Erb-Duchenne—like palsy, if the upper plexus is involved, and Klumpke's palsy, if the lower plexus is involved. NTOS must be differentiated from other pathologies of the upper arm such as carpal tunnel syndrome and cervical radiculopathy.

Arterial symptoms:
The symptoms are due to compression of the subclavian artery or its branches, mainly by the cervical rib.

The compression of the subclavian artery results in "poststenotic" arterial aneurysm. Thromboembolization may occur and dislodgment of clot results in distal ischemia and arm fatigue. With overhead activities, pallor, weak, or absent pulses and coolness of the upper extremity result. All these symptoms worsen by exposure to cold. If vertebral artery is compressed, postural vertigo, balance difficulties, falls and drop attacks, diplopia, syncope, etc., may be present. Blood pressure difference between affected and nonaffected arm of greater than 20 mm Hg is sometimes noted, which indicates arterial involvement.

Venous symptoms:
Symptoms are due to compression of subclavian and axillary vein between clavicle and the first rib, and mainly seen in young athletes involved with sports requiring frequent overhead activities. The symptoms include sudden spontaneous swelling of the upper limb, cyanosis of the arm, feeling of heaviness in arm, hand, and fingers, and pain in the upper extremity. Distended veins in the shoulder or chest are noted. Rarely, PE may occur.

Physical examination: In inspection, asymmetry of the shoulders, drooping shoulders, and large breasts should be noted. During palpation, supraclavicular fossa for tenderness and scalene muscles for increased tone should be palpated. The base of the examination is formed by stress tests or provocative tests, though it should be noted that they have low specificity, sensitivity, and predictive value.
- *Adson's test*: The anterior and middle scalene muscles are tensed in this test to see their compressive effects over axillary artery. If the pulse is obliterated, it is due to middle scalene muscle. This test has high false-positive results.
- *Halstead's maneuver*: Disappearance of radial pulse indicates the compression of the neurovascular bundle by the cervical rib and the test is positive.
- *Wright's hyperabduction test*: Disappearance of the radial pulse indicates the compression of the neurovascular bundle between pectoralis minor and the rib cage.
- *Roos test*: Patient of TOS may not be able to keep both the arms in elevated position because of ischemic, vascular type of pain.
- *Retroclavicular Spurling's test*: Tingling or numbness in the tested limb indicates the positive test.

Diagnostic studies:
- *X-rays*: Cervical rib, elongated process of C7 vertebra, Pancoast tumor, healed old fracture, etc.
- *Arteriography*: It demonstrates extrinsic arterial compression.
- *Venography*: Ascending brachial venography is the most definitive examination, if venous thrombosis is suspected.
- *Electromyography*: They are mainly indicated to rule out other pathologies such as cervical radiculopathy, carpal tunnel, and cubital tunnel syndrome.
- *Magnetic resonance imaging*
- *Duplex USG*: It is the most dominant noninvasive test for vascular TOS. In arterial TOS, the waveforms are reduced, but the velocities are either increased like in stenosis or absent like in complete occlusion.

Treatment: *Nonoperative*—conservative treatment including NSAIDs, strengthening and stretching exercises, US, transcutaneous nerve stimulation, occupational therapy, and biofeedback is sufficient for most of the patients and it must be the initial treating approach for the patient of TOS. If the symptoms do not respond to conservative treatment or worsen while the treatment, surgical intervention becomes necessary.

Treatment of neurogenic TOS:
- *Physical therapy*: Physical therapy relieves the pressure on the thoracic outlet by correcting postural abnormalities and improving muscle imbalance.
- *Medications*: NSAIDs such as aspirin, ibuprofen, and naproxen are used to reduce pain and inflammation of TOS.

- *Surgery*: If the symptoms persist despite the conservative therapy and interferes with activities of daily living, surgical decompression of the thoracic outlet becomes necessary.

Treatment of venous TOS:
Thrombolytic and anticoagulation medicines are started to reduce the risk of blood clot formation, to dissolve the already formed clot, and to reduce the risk of PE. In patients with compression of the vein, surgical correction becomes necessary depending on the severity of the compression.
- *Thrombolytic medications*: They are used to promote lysis of the already formed clot and the thrombus in the occluded vessels.
- *Anticoagulant medications*: This group includes drugs such as warfarin, heparin, LMWH, and fondaparinux. They are used to treat acute arterial and venous occlusion.
- *Surgery*: As stated earlier, surgery may be necessary along with medications to correct the symptoms. The venous stenosis is corrected with angioplasty (< 2 cm long lesion) or venous bypass surgery (>2 cm long lesion).

Treatment of arterial TOS:
- *Surgery*: Surgery may be required to decompress the space, like with removal of the first rib or with lysis of the abnormal fibrous bands. If the artery is injured, surgery may be necessary to repair the artery.
- *Thrombolytic medications*: It is given as the same way as described above for venous TOS.

Other medications: Other temporary treatment modalities are intra-articular or intramuscular cortisone injections and "scalene block" with the Botox injections that may provide relief for 3–4 months.

Operative treatment: Only few of the patients with NTOS require surgical treatment, but most of the patients with venous or arterial TOS eventually need surgical decompression. If conservative measures fail and the symptoms persist, surgical treatment may become necessary. It is mainly done to decompress the thoracic outlet. The procedure can be performed by either transaxillary approach, supraclavicular approach, or by infraclavicular approach. With any of the approach, the goal of the surgery may involve:
- Partial or complete removal of the scalene muscles
- Removal of the first thoracic rib
- Removal of any supernumerary abnormal rib
- Removal of the fibrous band causing compression of the neurovascular bundle
- Removal of the subclavian artery aneurysm, if present, and reconstruction of the artery.

(For details of tests and surgery, kindly refer to Chapter 118 of the book Essential Orthopedics: Principles and Practice, 2nd edition.)

29. Discuss etiopathogenesis of thoracic outlet syndrome.

Ans: The TOS may present in different forms, viz., neurological, arterial, and venous forms due to predominant involvement of respective structures. The symptoms of the NTOS do not follow dermatomal or myotomal pattern. They can be categorized according to area or roots of the brachial plexus involved. If the upper plexus (C5–C7) is involved, the patient presents with ipsilateral neck or ear pain, pain over the face, mandible and occipital region, headache, pain over the clavicular and pectoral region moving toward trapezius and deltoid down lateral arm. If the lower plexus (C8–T1) is involved, patient presents with pain over AP aspect of shoulder radiating down to the medial side of arm, forearm, and hand in the fourth and fifth fingers.

Arterial TOS arises due to compression of subclavian artery or its branches. The compression of the subclavian artery results in "poststenotic" arterial aneurysm. Thromboembolization may occur and dislodgment of clot results in distal ischemia and arm fatigue. With overhead activities, pallor, weak or absent pulses and coolness of the upper extremity result.

Venous TOS occurs due to compression of subclavian and axillary vein between clavicle and the first rib, mainly seen in young athletes involved with sports requiring frequent overhead activities like in swimmers, water polo, baseball players, etc. The symptoms include sudden spontaneous swelling of the upper limb, cyanosis of the arm, feeling of heaviness in arm, hand, and fingers, and pain in the upper extremity. Distended veins in the shoulder or chest are noted. Rarely, PE may occur.

30. Describe pathoanatomy of thoracic outlet syndrome.

Ans: Neurological and vascular symptoms and signs in the upper limbs may be produced by compression of the lower trunk of the brachial plexus (C8 and T1) and subclavian vessels between the clavicle and the first rib. The subclavian artery and lower brachial trunk pass through a triangle based on the first rib and bordered by scalenus anterior and medius. These neurovascular structures are made taut when the shoulders are braced back and the arms held tightly to the sides; an extra rib (or its fibrous equivalent extending from a large costal process), or an anomalous scalene muscle, exaggerates this effect by forcing the vessel and nerve upward.

(Further details can be read from the 3rd edition of the book, Essential Orthopedics: Principles and Practice, Chapter on Thoracic Outlet Syndrome.)

31. Define cervical rib. Describe its etiopathogenesis, clinical features, and management.

Ans:

Definition: The cervical rib is a supernumerary rib that arises usually from the 7th and rarely from the 6th or 5th cervical vertebrae. It is frequently bilateral.

Etiopathogenesis: In the embryo, the size of nerves is much larger in proportion to the ribs than they are in the fully developed human being. When the nerves are unusually large, as they are in the cervical region, they interfere with the development of costal processes. The brachial plexus has two distinct types of arrangement:

1. The prefixed plexus has a well-developed 4th cervical root and a small 1st thoracic root. Formation of a costal process encounters little resistance from the small 1st thoracic nerve root. As a result, there develops a rib extending from the transverse process of the 7th cervical vertebra varying in size from a small rudimentary rib to a complete rib extending forward to articulate with the sternum or the costal cartilage of the 1st thoracic rib. Where the rib is underdeveloped, a fibrous band may extend from its outer extremity to the 1st thoracic rib, usually attaching near the scalene tubercle. Intercostal muscles, nerves, and vessels are usually associated with a completely formed cervical rib.
2. A postfixed plexus receives few fibers from the 4th cervical root but has a large, well-developed 1st thoracic nerve root. Formation of a costal process is less likely in such cases.

Clinical features: Symptoms can occur at any age but often are initiated under conditions effecting descent of shoulder girdle. Clinical features are there of ulnar nerve distribution pointing to the lower trunk of the plexus.

- *Symptoms*: Pain and paresthesia occur in the ulnar aspect of the hand and the little and ring fingers. Less commonly symptoms can be felt in the whole hand. Pain may be dull aching or sharp. Sensation of tingling in forearm and hand which patient describes as falling asleep is due to circulatory deficiency and is associated with diminution of radial pulse. Patient complains of weakness of hand, clumsiness in use of fingers, and dropping of objects. Symptoms accentuated by downward displacement of shoulder girdle.
- *Signs*: It may be possible to feel bony prominences of cervical rib at the base of neck. Failure to palpate does not rule out this syndrome, since a fibrous band may be the offender. The irritated plexus is tender to deep pressure lateral to and behind the sternocleidomastoid. Muscles supplied by lower trunk may be atrophied commonly the lumbricals and interossei. Flexion at metacarpophalangeal (MCP) joints, extension at interphalangeal (IP) joints, abduction and adduction of fingers, and adduction of thumb are weak. Less commonly the thenar muscles namely abductor pollicis brevis and opponens pollicis are involved. Sensation is diminished over ulnar aspect of forearm and volar aspect of little finger and ulnar half of ring finger. Diminished circulation is evidenced by coldness, pallor, cyanosis, and reduced volume of radial nerve.
    - Adson sign intensifies the symptoms by increasing tension on scalenus anterior and narrowing the rib-muscle interval. The patient rotates the chin toward the affected side, elevates the chin, and hyperextends the neck and then takes a deep breath. This increases pain and paresthesia and often obliterates the radial pulse.
    - A palpable, pulsatile mass with bruit detected in supraclavicular fossa suggests an aneurysmal dilatation of subclavian artery. Trophic changes include a thin glossy skin, ulcerations, ridging, and brittleness of nails. Localized areas of gangrene indicate that embolism to a distal artery has occurred, usually in the lower region of forearm, palm, or finger.
- *X-rays*: A cervical rib is found extending outward from the 7th cervical transverse process. It may be small or rudimentary or large and fully developed. The condition is often bilateral.

Treatment: Elevation of shoulder girdle releases tension on the brachial plexus and the axillary artery. When symptoms are minimal, conservative treatment may be tried. It consists of exercises designed to increase the tone of trapezius and levator scapulae. The arm is placed at rest in elevated position. Activities requiring lifting are avoided. Often symptoms are severe, and surgical removal of the rib is necessary.

32. Explain battered baby syndrome (BBS).

Ans:

Definition: Battered baby syndrome or battered child syndrome (BCS) refers to nonaccidental injuries sustained by a child as a result of physical abuse, usually inflicted by an adult caregiver.

Demographics: The highest percentage of child abuse occurs between birth and 2 years of age. The total abuse rate of children is 25.2 per 1,000 children, with physical abuse accounting for 5.7 per 1,000. Physical abuse can be in the form of internal injuries, cuts, burns, bruises, and broken or fractured bones or a combination of these. BCS is found at every level of society, although the incidence may be higher in lower-income households.

Causes:
- Lack of education
- Single parenthood
- Alcoholism or other drug addictions
- Psychological and traditional beliefs:
  - Child as a property that can be handled any way
  - Abusers have been themselves abused during childhood.

Identification and diagnosis: In any child younger than 2-year-old with a significant fracture and a questionable history (delayed visit to emergency) or mechanism of injury (imprint abrasion, scald marks, and bite marks), child abuse should be suspected. Multiple areas of large ecchymoses in different stages of resolution (from black and blue to brown and green) are pathognomonic of child abuse. Similarly, multiple fractures in different stages of healing almost always indicate child abuse. To rule out this possibility, a bone scan or a skeletal survey generally is indicated. CT, MRI, and US evaluations also may be beneficial, especially in children with suspected head trauma. Other less common findings include skin burns, ocular changes, hematuria, and abdominal signs. The most common sites of fractures caused by child abuse are the humerus, tibia, and femur. Epiphyseal-metaphyseal (corner) fractures are almost always pathognomonic of child abuse because the pulling and twisting forces necessary to produce these injuries rarely are accidental. Rib fractures are found to have a positive predictive value of nonaccidental injury of 95% in children younger than 3 years of age and are the only skeletal manifestation of abuse in almost 30% of children.

Standard skeletal survey for suspected child abuse:

Minimum required views
- Anteroposterior views of entire skeleton
- Dedicated views of hands and feet
- Lateral views of appendicular skeleton—skull and spine.

Specificity of skeletal trauma for child abuse:

High specificity
- Classic metaphyseal fractures
- Posterior rib fracture
- Scapular fracture
- Spinous process fracture
- Sternal fracture.

Moderate specificity
- Multiple fractures, especially bilateral
- Fractures in various stages of healing
- Epiphyseal separation
- Vertebral body fracture or separation

- Digital fracture
- Complex skull fracture.

Prognosis: Failure to recognize child abuse may result in a 25% risk of repeat abuse and a 5% risk of death.

Management: Immediately report suspected child abuse and arrange quarantine. Definite knowledge or a specific diagnosis is not required. The orthopedic surgeon should protect a child who has a fracture caused by child abuse and should inform the parents of his or her legal responsibility to report any suspicion to authorities. Both physical and psychological therapies are often recommended as treatment for the abused child.

The use of educational programs to teach caregivers good parenting skills and to be aware of abusive behaviors so that they seek help for abusive tendencies is critical to stopping abuse.

1.2 POLYTRAUMA DAMAGE CONTROL ORTHOPEDICS AND TRANSFUSION MEDICINE (Q33–60)

33. Briefly discuss about the principles and priorities in managing polytrauma.

Ans: *Principles* of managing polytrauma in brief are as follows:

Team approach is essential for the management of different and varied organ systems. The care can be divided into four stages:

1. *Immediate care*: Follow ATLS guidelines. Resuscitate patient and stabilize.
2. *Acute care*: It includes mainly lifesaving procedures to control hemorrhage (embolization, pelvic external fixation, etc.), respiratory support, and circulatory support with revaluation. Practice of DCO begins here.
3. *Intermediate care*: Skeletal stabilization as a part of DCO, nutritional support, and pain control.
4. *Definitive care*: Comprehensive management of injuries and rehabilitation.

It should be borne in mind that there is trimodal peak distribution of trauma mortality:

- Most deaths occur during 1st hour after injury, mostly due to CNS injury (approximately 50%), followed by exsanguination (approximately 20%).
- Second peak during 1–4 hours after injury also known as *"golden period"*. The most common cause of death in this period is hypovolemic shock.
- Third peak several weeks later. Patient dies of late complications such as sepsis and multiple organ failure.

Early death is caused by severe trauma to vital organs (severe head injury or cardiac insult) or more importantly due to missed opportunity to treat potentially manageable life-threatening injuries. Late death is a result, often, of MOF when the compensatory mechanism becomes complicated and down-spiral with improperly managed organal damage. Polytrauma management begins at the injury site itself (prehospital) with raising alarm and informing approachable services, rescue, and transportation of resuscitated patient preferably on spine board supervised by paramedics. To prevent life-threatening complications, a mandatory schema is followed under expert guidance. Hospital management of polytrauma victim is prioritized to life salvage, limb salvage, and then functional salvage. As stated earlier, team approach is a must to determine the operative plan for the polytrauma patient on immediate basis and to put it in action. Each of the members of the trauma team should be assigned a specific task, so that the patient would be treated as a whole simultaneously and not by treating one injury after another. To this effect, the team leader has following functions:

- Assess the clinical situation
- Gather information
- Direct the setup of the operating room
- Treatment needs from other faculties
- Determine priorities
- Set limits on time and complexity of procedures.

Setting priorities in management of polytrauma: Triage is the most essential aspect of prioritizing the patient *(details in Chapter on Polytrauma of the book Essential Orthopedics: Principles and Practice, 2nd edition)*. Once done and as soon as the patient is received in emergency bay, cervical stabilization followed by ABCs of trauma management begins. The so-called ABCs of trauma reflect priorities in primary survey for initial trauma management.

- Cx, always assume cervical spine injury in conscious and unconscious patient—always stabilize first (cervical collar—hard) and use backboard. Once evaluation for cervical spine is completed then remove board.
- A—Airway management with protection of the cervical spine
- B—Breathing and ventilation
- C—Circulation with hemorrhage control
- D—Disability—neurologic status, and
- E—Exposure/environment (remove clothes to evaluate external wounds but avoid hypothermia).

Each of these areas is addressed simultaneously by the trauma team. The primary survey usually takes no longer than a few minutes, unless procedures are required. Treatment is simultaneously provided, while evaluation is being done.

34. **A. Describe pathophysiology of polytrauma patient.**
B. Discuss principles of damage control orthopedics (DCO) versus early total care (ETC).

Ans:

A. The pathophysiology is best summarized in the Consensus definition of the American Association for the Surgery of Trauma and the German Trauma Society (2014). This incorporates both anatomical and physiological parameters—two or more injuries having AIS > 2 in different regions + one or more of the following five physiological parameters:
  1. Hypotension [systolic blood pressure (SBP) ≤ 90 mm Hg]
  2. Consciousness (GCS ≤ 8)
  3. Acidosis defined as base excess < –6.0
  4. Coagulopathy (INR) ≥ 1.4
  5. Age > 70 years

  Beyond this, one can understand the pathophysiology in terms of differing ideologies—ETC versus DCO and hence the specific needs.

B. *Damage control orthopedics versus early total care*: It was considered the ideal approach to treat orthopedic injuries by doing "definitive fixation" of all fractures in one trip to the operating room. This approach is called early total care and was widely used in the 80s to efficiently use the operating theater resources and perform surgeries with one set on investigations and anesthetic exposure. The complications were found higher when this approach was used especially in polytrauma patients. The ETC school emanated from the finding that patients previously managed by conservative methods (say cast or traction for fracture shaft femur) fared worse than the early definitely operated patients. The development of newer methods of osteosynthesis also favored the concept of "early definitive management." These patients were found to have less pulmonary complications (pneumonia, ARDS), reduced length of ICU, FES, and hospital stay, compared to patients with delayed surgery. Though popular and practiced for more than a decade opposing views came in since 1990s and concept of ETC was challenged. In unstable patients, ETC was associated with an unexpectedly high rate of pulmonary complications. In light of associated risks and benefits of ETC, some moderation was needed and concept of "damage control" emerged. The concept of "damage control" comes from US Navy, in reference to keeping afloat a badly damaged ship by procedures to limit flooding, stabilize the vessel, isolate fires and explosions, and avoid their spreading.

There are four phases of DCO:
1. Acute phase—lifesaving procedures are performed.
2. Second phase is aimed to control hemorrhage, temporary stabilization of major skeletal fractures, management of soft tissue injuries, while minimizing the degree of surgical insult to the patient.
3. Phase three consists of a monitoring period in ICU/high-dependency unit (HDU).
4. Last phase comprises definitive fixation.

The shift from ETC to DCO comes from better understanding of systemic inflammatory response syndrome (SIRS) followed by a period of recovery mediated by a counter-regulatory anti-inflammatory response (CARS). Initial traumatic injury induces an inflammatory response followed sometimes by an excessive CARS that produces a prolonged and deleterious immunosuppressed state. This initial traumatic injury is called the "first hit" and predisposes the patient to a potential risk of deterioration after surgery (that actually produces a "second hit"). In polytrauma patients, the recognition of high levels of inflammatory markers favors the DCO application in order to prevent the effects of the "second hit" inflammatory reaction. IL6 is considered the most specific prognostic indicator (discussed later) and early high levels of IL6 have been associated with the development of organ failure (measuring IL6 has become a routine in dedicated trauma centers). Thus, the type of initial stabilization and timing of definitive osteosynthesis modulate these adverse events. Initial stabilization came to be highly relied upon external fixation. Simple stabilization with splints and casts, however, is also effective except for lower extremities like shaft femur fractures. For these, skeletal traction has been found to be equal to external fixation in terms of ARDS, MODS, pneumonia, deep VTE PE development, as well as ICU stay and death rate. The timing for definitive osteosynthesis has been set at "window of opportunity" between 5th and 10th days. Now both DCO and ETC are challenged and instead a more logical approach of early appropriate care (EAC) is being practiced.

(Learn more about EAC from chapter 24 of the book Essential Orthopedics Principles and Practice, 3rd edition, 2022)

35. Prehospital care of a polytrauma patient.

Ans: The concept of prehospital care of polytraumatized patient was initiated by Kirschner in 1950s. The following are some of the prehospital measures necessary to stabilize the patient that may be even initiated at the scene of incidence like:

- Treatment of hypoxia
- Achieving normoventilation
- Shock therapy for controlling cardiac rhythm

However, these illnesses and disorders in unmonitored settings like site of accident can be only recognized by a well-trained and experienced emergency physician or specialized doctor who has mastered the diagnosis of critical illnesses or injuries. The management for critical illness often needs endotracheal intubation and management of hemorrhagic shock on-site for which emergency anesthesia may also be needed. Thus expert experienced emergency physicians are able to quickly and safely treat life-threatening polytrauma patients out of the hospital. One needs to limit the underestimation of injury so whenever in doubt greater injury severity should be assumed. The following are common guides that indicate severe injury and may indicate need for shock treatment:

- Pedestrians/cyclists versus cars (> 30 km/h)
- High energy trauma
- Deformation of a vehicle by > 50 cm
- Thrown out of the vehicle
- Death of an inmate
- Fall from > 3 m height
- Explosion
- Entrapment/burial

The following are some general guidelines for emergency on-site management commonly performed.

- Prevent and manage the "lethal triad" of hypoxia, hypotension and hypercapnia with adequate measures for life-saving treatment priority.
- Mannitol or hypertonic saline solutions are needed for suspected raised intracranial pressure and herniation (rapid change in consciousness, mydriasis, and hyperventilation)
- Tension pneumothorax should be rapidly decompressed using needle decompression or mini-thoracotomy.
- For abdominal injuries, penetrating injuries should be left in place for possible tamponade effect.
- Mechanical stabilization of unstable pelvis should be achieved to reduce hemorrhage and hypotension.
- Cervical spine and spinal stabilization are a priority especially in patients with neurological deficit, pain or tight muscles in spine and intoxication.
- Bleeding from extremity should be controlled by tourniquet application.

36. Describe triage and its role in the management of polytrauma patients.

Ans: In trauma management, triage is used when the number of casualties is greater than can be managed simultaneously by the medical personnel available. There are two stages applicable in the prehospital environment: A *triage sieve* and a *triage sort*.

The triage sieve is a quick and uncomplicated system based on simple clinical observation of a casualty's ability to walk, breathe, and maintain peripheral perfusion. It can be performed by trained, but nonclinical, personnel. Usually, the triage sieve is conducted in pairs and basic medical interventions can be instituted during the triage-like application of tourniquets and homeostatic dressings for catastrophic hemorrhage, opening the airway and placing unconscious, but breathing, casualties into the recovery position.

The triage sort is performed by trained clinical staff using physiological measurements to score casualties and place them into priority groups. Both triage systems place casualties into four color-coded priority categories as shown in **Table 1.2.1**.

TABLE 1.2.1: Standard color coding of bands used in triage.		
Priority 1	Immediate	Red
Priority 2	Urgent	Yellow
Priority 3	Delayed	Green
Priority 4	Dead	Black

37. Describe acute respiratory distress syndrome (ARDS).

Ans: The American-European Consensus Conference (AECC) defined ARDS as *"An acute condition characterized by bilateral pulmonary infiltrates and severe hypoxemia in the absence of evidence for cardiogenic pulmonary edema."* ARDS can be simply defined as noncardiogenic pulmonary edema.

Pathophysiology: ARDS is associated with diffuse alveolar damage and lung capillary endothelial injury. The disease is usually described in two phases:
1. The early phase which is described as being exudative.
2. The late phase which is fibroproliferative in character.

Etiology: Major risk factors associated with the development of ARDS includes:
- Sepsis
- Trauma, with or without pulmonary contusion
- Burns
- Massive transfusion
- Bacteremia
- Fractures, particularly multiple fractures and long bone fractures
- Pneumonia
- Drug overdose
- Postperfusion injury after cardiopulmonary bypass
- Fat embolism
- Aspiration
- Near drowning
- Pancreatitis

Presentation: Patients developing ARDS are often critically ill associated with the involvement of multisystem organ failure. It usually presents with acute onset of dyspnea with the sensation of rapid shallow breathing and hypoxemia giving the feeling of not able to get enough air to breathe. It is necessary to enquire about any of the risk factors or any event, which possibly can cause ARDS. The event may be sepsis, massive transfusion, acute pancreatitis, aspiration, trauma, or any other possible cause. The symptoms usually start within hours to days of an inciting event and typically ARDS develops within 12–48 hours of the event.

Physical findings: Physical findings are often nonspecific, and patient has tachypnea and tachycardia owing to the rapid shallow breathing and hypoxemia. The patient may be febrile or hypothermic. Patients on ventilator require high fraction of inspired oxygen and high positive end expiratory pressure. Thorough clinical examination should be done to differentiate ARDS from cardiogenic pulmonary edema by carefully looking for signs of CHF such as raised jugular venous pressure, murmurs, gallops, and edema of the dependent part.

Diagnosis:
- *Severity*: Oxygenation
  - *Mild*: 200 mm Hg < PaO_2/FiO_2 < 300 mm Hg
  - *Moderate*: 100 mm Hg < PaO_2/FiO_2 < 200 mm Hg
  - *Severe*: PaO_2/FiO_2 < 100 mm Hg
- *Onset*: Acute
- *Chest radiograph*: Bilateral alveolar or interstitial infiltrates
- *Absence of left atrial hypertension*: Pulmonary capillary wedge pressure (PCWP) < 18 mm Hg or no evidence of increased left atrial hypertension.

Treatment: First and foremost is identification and treatment of the cause as early as possible. Immediate goals are supportive care and the prevention of complications. The mortality of patients with ARDS is usually not due primarily to respiratory failure. Most patients die from secondary infections, other organ failures, or the complications of prolonged hospitalization.

Mechanical Ventilation:
Although mechanical ventilation has lifesaving potential, it can also aggravate lung injury. Trials show that lung injury occurs because of two processes: (1) Recurrent alveolar collapse, and (2) Repeated alveolar over distention. So, to minimize the lung injury it is recommended to use lung protective ventilator strategy, which includes low tidal volume (6 mL/kg of predicted body weight), limitation of plateau pressure (< 28–30 cmH_2O), and appropriate positive end-expiratory pressure (PEEP). In ARDS, the presence of alveolar and interstitial fluid and the loss of surfactant can lead to a marked reduction of lung compliance, so a high-end expiratory pressure is required to prevent alveolar collapse at end expiration and to maintain oxygenation. PEEP is usually set to minimize FiO_2 (inspired O_2 percentage) and maximize PaO_2 (arterial partial pressure of O_2). Although high PEEP does improve lung function but no mortality benefit has been seen. Oxygenation can also be improved by inverse ratio ventilation in which inspiration is kept for a longer duration than expiration leading to trapping of more air in the lung causing dynamic hyperinflation, which maintains end expiratory pressure similar to PEEP.

Recruitment maneuvers that transiently increase PEEP to "recruit" atelectatic lung can also increase oxygenation but a mortality benefit has not been established.

Fluid Management:
Fluid management is one of the most difficult measures to manage in septic shock patients with ARDS as vascular and epithelial permeability is increased in ARDS. Conservative fluid management is highly recommended after hemodynamic stabilization in ARDS patients. A conservative fluid management strategy maintains a relatively low CVP which is associated with the need for fewer days of mechanical ventilation.

Neuromuscular Blockade:
In ARDS patients, sedation alone is not adequate to maintain synchrony with the mechanical ventilation, so early neuromuscular blockade for at least first 48 hours is recommended with cisatracurium besylate. This not only increased the rate of survival but also increases ventilator free days.

Glucocorticoids—initially used to counteract the pulmonary inflammation but recent evidences do not recommend the use of glucocorticoids in ARDS.

Prevention: Although multiple risk factors for ARDS are known, no successful preventive measures have been identified. Careful fluid management in high-risk patients may be helpful. Because aspiration pneumonitis is a risk factor for ARDS, taking appropriate measures to prevent aspiration (e.g., elevating the head of the bed and evaluating swallowing mechanics before feeding high-risk patients) may also prevent some ARDS cases.

38. Describe damage control surgery in orthopedics.

Ans: It was considered the ideal approach to treat orthopedic injuries by doing "definitive fixation" of all fractures in one trip to the operating room. This approach is called early total care and was widely used in the 80s to efficiently use the operating theater resources and perform surgeries with one set on investigations and anesthetic exposure.

The complications of ETC were found higher especially in polytrauma patients. The ETC School emanated from the finding that patients previously managed by conservative methods (say cast or traction for fracture shaft femur) fared worse than the early definitely operated patients. The development of newer methods of osteosynthesis also favored the concept of "early definitive management". These patients were found to have less pulmonary complications, reduced length of ICU and hospital stay (LOS) compared to patients with delayed surgery, but careful analysis showed that in unstable patients, ETC was associated with an unexpectedly high rate of pulmonary complications and increased mortality.

The concept of "damage control" emanated where immediate and ongoing damage is controlled to improve patient condition to a level where definitive management would carry lesser risk. There are four phases of DCO:
1. Acute phase—lifesaving procedures are performed.
2. Second phase is aimed to control hemorrhage, temporary stabilization of major skeletal fractures, management of soft-tissue injuries, while minimizing the degree of surgical insult to the patient.
3. Phase three consists of a monitoring period in ICU/HDU.
4. Last phase comprises definitive fixation.

The shift from ETC to DCO comes from better understanding of SIRS followed by a period of recovery mediated by a CARS. Initial traumatic injury induces an inflammatory response followed sometimes by an excessive CARS that produces a prolonged, deleterious immunosuppressed state. This initial traumatic injury is called the "first hit" and predisposes the patient to a potential risk of deterioration after surgery (that actually produces a "second hit"). In polytrauma patients, the recognition of high levels of inflammatory markers favors the DCO application, in order to prevent the effects of the "second hit" inflammatory reaction. IL-6 is considered the most specific prognostic indicator and early high levels of IL-6 have been associated with the development of organ failure (measuring IL-6 has become a routine in dedicated trauma centers). Thus, the type of initial stabilization and timing of definitive osteosynthesis modulate these adverse events. The timing for definitive osteosynthesis has been set at "window of opportunity" between 5th and 10th days. During days 2–4, immunological changes keep occurring along with unsuitable fluid shift and local tissue edema making it unsuitable. After 15 days, the contamination rate around the pins has been found to be a significant cause of infection. Thus, DCO avoids provoking a severe inflammatory response while fulfilling the goals of sufficient stabilization of fractures to prevent further tissue damage and the potential compartment syndrome, while allowing the patient to be mobilized for tests and improved pulmonary care.

- Pain control is an important aspect to additionally stabilize the sympathetic hyperactivity and drug combinations are usually required; IV paracetamol and continuous infusion techniques are in fashion.
- Whether a limb should be reconstructed or amputated is decided by severity of injury, expertise of the surgeon, available resources, and socioeconomic status of the patient. Reconstruction has advantages like original limb is saved, but having disadvantages of long rehabilitation, prolonged hospital stay, economic burden, repeated operations, and difficulties to family.

In specific situations, the fracture treatment should be deferred (follow DCO):
- Head injury with GCS < 8
- Massive intracranial bleeding
- Severe thoracic trauma
- Hemodynamically unstable with uncompensated cardiac function
- Blood dyscrasias
- Hypothermia < 32°C.

39. What is a second-hit phenomena?

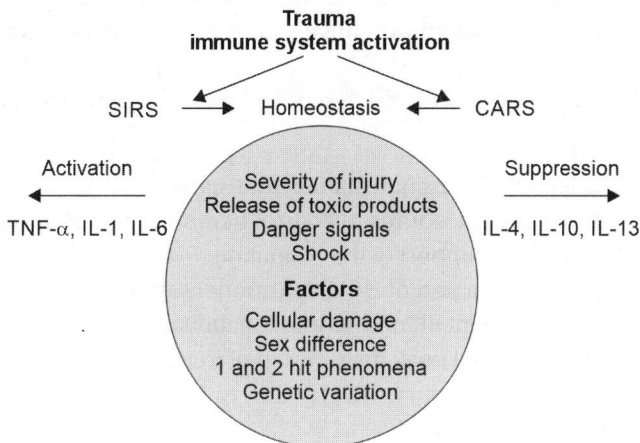

Fig. 1.2.1: Factors associated with the "second hit" phenomena.
(CARS: Counter-regulatory anti-inflammatory response syndrome; SIRS: systemic inflammatory response syndrome; TNF: tumor necrosis factor)

Ans: In a patient with multiple injuries, viz., association of femoral shaft fractures with other injuries, including head, chest, abdominal and pelvic trauma, there is increased potential for developing fat embolism, ARDS, and MOF. The risk of systemic complications can be significantly reduced by early stabilization of the fracture, usually by a locked intramedullary nail. However, surgery to introduce a reamed intramedullary nail may produce untoward effects in those with severe chest injuries, especially when carried out within 24 hours of the fracture. It is thought that the trauma of surgery and blood loss induces inflammatory changes that may increase both morbidity and mortality—this phenomenon is called "*the second hit*," referring to a second episode of trauma, albeit surgical, on the patient **(Fig. 1.2.1)**.

Consequently, in the multiple injured patient, particularly one with severe chest trauma, prompt stabilization with an external fixator may be wise; the fixator can be exchanged for an intramedullary nail when the patient's condition stabilizes. The timing of this second procedure is still problematic and largely undefined, resting on clinician's experience.

Some guidance can be sought from measurement of circulating levels of IL-6, a proinflammatory cytokine when the levels start to decrease, it should be safe to perform "second hit" interventions. Clinically, this occurs around 5–7 days after admission, but this window is by no means applicable to all patients nor is it conclusive at this time.

First-hit phenomena refers to the primary injury response of the body by stimulation of various inflammatory mediators in the immediate aftermath of trauma.

40. (A) Define polytrauma. (B) Explain clinical presentation, complications, and general principles of management of polytrauma.

Ans:

A. *Definition of polytrauma*: Polytrauma is defined specifically as injury to two major systems, along with one bony injury or one major system injury along with two major long bone fractures. Unstable pelvic fractures by themselves are also included in polytrauma as most often they are associated with internal organ injury. Polytrauma is a product of multisystem injury that induces profound pathophysiological changes and their cumulative effects could be life-threatening. In general, 65% of polytrauma patients had cerebral injuries, 58% thoracic trauma, and 81% extremity fractures of which one-third are open injuries. Polytrauma is the most common cause of death between 15 and 45 years of age. Merely having multiple bony injuries in a single patient is not polytrauma.

Objectively, polytrauma is defined as:
- Injury to several (≥ 2) physical regions or organ systems, where at least one injury or the combination of several injuries is life-threatening with the severity of injury being > 15 or 17 (commonly followed) on the scale of the ISS. ISS > 16 = major trauma (mortality 10%). This value of ISS depicting major trauma is however highly variable ranging from 15 to 26 depending on various reports.

- Anatomic injury score > 2 in at least two body regions.

B. The patient of polytrauma usually presents with unstable vitals hemodynamically or they may be borderline normal. These patients are tricky as any delay in resuscitation is hugely detrimental and one may lose precious opportunity to optimize patient.

Team approach is essential for the management of different and varied organ systems.

The care can be divided into four stages:
1. *Immediate care*: Follow ATLS guidelines. Resuscitate patient and stabilize.
2. *Acute care*: It includes mainly lifesaving procedures to control hemorrhage (embolization, pelvic external fixation, etc.), respiratory support, and circulatory support with revaluation. Practice of DCO begins here.
3. *Intermediate care*: Skeletal stabilization as a part of DCO, nutritional support, and pain control.
4. *Definitive care*: Comprehensive management of injuries and rehabilitation.

It should be borne in mind that there is trimodal peak distribution of trauma mortality:
- Most deaths occur during 1st hour after injury, mostly due to CNS injury (approximately 50%), followed by exsanguinations (approximately 20%).
- Second peak during 1–4 hours after injury also known as "golden period". The most common cause of death in this period is hypovolemic shock.
- Third peak several weeks later. Patient dies of late complications such as sepsis and multiple organ failure. Early death is caused by severe trauma to vital organs (severe head injury or cardiac insult) or more importantly due to missed opportunity to treat potentially manageable life-threatening injuries. Late death is a result, often, of MOF when the compensatory mechanism becomes complicated and down-spiral with improperly managed organal damage. Polytrauma management begins at the injury site itself (prehospital) with raising alarm and informing approachable services, rescue, and transportation of resuscitated patient preferably on spine board supervised by paramedics. To prevent life-threatening complications, a mandatory schema is followed under expert guidance.

Hospital management of polytrauma victims is prioritized to life salvage, limb salvage, and then functional salvage. As stated earlier, team approach is a must to determine the operative plan for the polytrauma patient on immediate basis and to put it in action. Each of the members of the trauma team should be assigned a specific task, so that the patient would be treated as a whole simultaneously and not by treating one injury after another. To this effect, the team leader has following functions:
- Assess the clinical situation
- Gather information
- Direct the setup of the operating room
- Treatment needs from other faculties
- Determine priorities
- Set limits on time and complexity of procedures.

For further details, kindly see Answer to Question 33.

41. Discuss trauma associated coagulopathy (TAC).

Ans: TAC is typically defined as a coagulopathy that arises in the context of traumatic injuries, particularly in cases of severe blunt or penetrating trauma. TAC is a complex and often life-threatening condition that occurs in severely injured patients. It is characterized by a paradoxical increased tendency to bleed due to a combination of several factors that disrupt the normal hemostatic mechanisms. It can manifest rapidly after the initial injury and may lead to significant morbidity and mortality.

Pathophysiology

The pathophysiology of TAC is multifactorial and may include the following components:
- *Acute coagulopathy of trauma*: This specific form of TAC occurs shortly after trauma and may result from:
  - *Hypoperfusion and hypoxia*: Reduced blood flow and oxygen delivery can impair the function of platelets and coagulation factors.
  - *Acidosis*: Metabolic acidosis can inhibit the clotting cascade and lead to a dysfunctional coagulation response.

- *Dilutional coagulopathy*: Massive fluid resuscitation can dilute clotting factors and platelets, impairing hemostasis.
- *Microvascular injury*: Tissue damage can lead to the exposure of thrombogenic substances and dysregulation of the coagulation cascade.
- *Trauma-induced inflammation*: Severe trauma triggers a systemic inflammatory response, which can lead to:
  - *Disseminated intravascular coagulation*: Overactivation of coagulation can result in the formation of microthrombi and contribute to bleeding.
  - *Imbalance of coagulation and anticoagulation factors*: Alterations in the delicate balance between procoagulant and anticoagulant forces can lead to impaired hemostasis.
- *Platelet dysfunction*: Severe trauma can cause alterations in platelet function due to:
  - *Endothelial injury*: Damage to endothelial cells may prevent normal platelet adhesion and aggregation.
  - *Coagulopathy due to severe injury*: Trauma can impair platelet activation and responsiveness.
- *Contributing factors*: Several factors may exacerbate TAC, including:
  - *Severity of injury*: More severe injuries often lead to more pronounced coagulopathy.
  - *Preexisting conditions*: Patients with liver disease, anticoagulant use, or clotting disorders may be at greater risk.
  - *Temperature*: Hypothermia can impair coagulation processes and further contribute to coagulopathy.
  - *Transfusion practices*: Large-volume crystalloid resuscitation without appropriate replacement of blood components can worsen dilutional coagulopathy.

Diagnosis
- *Clinical evaluation*: Assessing for signs of hypovolemic shock and coagulopathy (e.g., prolonged bleeding from wounds).
- *Laboratory tests*: Routine tests may include:
  - Prothrombin time and aPTT
  - Platelet count
  - Fibrinogen levels [thromboelastography (TEG) or rotational thromboelastometry (ROTEM) may be used to assess the overall hemostatic function more comprehensively].

Management
- *Early recognition*: Rapid identification of coagulopathy and initiation of appropriate treatment are crucial.
- *Resuscitation*:
  - *Hemorrhagic shock management*: Focus on controlling bleeding through surgery, if necessary.
  - *Fluid resuscitation*: Use balanced resuscitation strategies with a focus on early use of whole blood, packed red blood cells (PRBCs), FFP, and platelets (massive transfusion protocols).
- *Coagulation factor replacement*:
  - Administer FFP and cryoprecipitate to replenish clotting factors, fibrinogen, and other components crucial to hemostasis.
  - *Tranexamic acid (TXA)*: Use of antifibrinolytics like TXA can reduce mortality when administered early.
- *Optimize temperature*: Prevent and manage hypothermia through warming measures.
- *Monitor and adjust therapy*: Regularly monitor coagulation status and adjust transfusion strategies based on results.
- *Multidisciplinary approach*: Collaboration between trauma surgeons, anesthesiologists, hematologists, and critical care teams is vital for optimal management.

42. How do you classify polytraumatized patients?

Ans: *Some questions are so incomplete and nonspecific that it is not possible to understand what is being asked. Does this question ask types of polytrauma or classifications used to assess polytrauma?* Anyways—some investigators crudely suggest that at least two anatomical regions have to be injured for a patient to be identified as having polytrauma. Objectively polytrauma is defined as:
- Injury to several (≥ 2) physical regions or organ systems, where at least one injury or the combination of several injuries is life-threatening (Tscherne et al.) with the severity of injury being > 15 or 17 (commonly followed) on the scale of the ISS **(Box 1.2.1)**. ISS ≥16 = Major trauma (mortality 10%). This value of ISS depicting major trauma is however highly variable ranging from 15 to 26 depending on various reports.

- Because of the variability in ISS, the "polytrauma" definition of Butcher and colleagues using the AIS ≥ 3 for at least two different body regions seems more reasonable and feasible for identifying polytrauma patients.
- *The new Berlin definition*: Cases with an AIS ≥ 3 for two or more different body regions and one or more additional variables from five physiologic parameters:
  1. Hypotension (SBP ≤90 mm Hg)
  2. Unconsciousness [GCS score ≤ 8)
  3. Acidosis (base excess ≤ –6.0)
  4. Coagulopathy (partial thromboplastin time ≥ 40 sec or INR ≥ 1.4)
  5. Age (≥ 70 years)

> **Box 1.2.1:** Injury severity score
>
> Six regions:
> 1. Head and neck
> 2. Face
> 3. Thorax
> 4. Abdomen
> 5. Extremity
> 6. Pelvis
>
> Scoring: 1—Minor, 2—Moderate, 3—Severe, 4—Life-threatening, 5—Critical, 6—Fatal
>
> *Each region*: Abbreviated injury scale (AIS)—Injury severity score (ISS) is the sum of the squares of the highest AIS scores from three of the six body region. AIS six automatically converts the ISS to 75.

43. What are the advanced trauma life support (ATLS) guidelines in polytrauma management? Describe the principles of early total care in polytrauma and its indications.

Ans: *ATLS guidelines*: As soon as the patient has received cervical stabilization followed by ABCs of trauma, management begins. The so-called ABCs of trauma reflect priorities in primary survey for initial trauma management.
- Cx, always assume cervical spine injury in conscious and unconscious patient—always stabilize first (cervical collar—hard) and use backboard. Once evaluation for cervical spine is completed then remove board.
- A—Airway management with protection of the cervical spine
- B—Breathing and ventilation
- C—Circulation with hemorrhage control
- D—*Disability*: Neurologic status
- E—Exposure/environment (remove clothes to evaluate external wounds, but avoid hypothermia).

Each of these areas is addressed simultaneously by the trauma team. The primary survey usually takes no longer than a few minutes, unless procedures are required. Treatment is simultaneously provided, while evaluation is being done.

Airway: Airway and breathing are handled first and no other procedures are initiated until the airway is secured. To check the patency of airway, the simplest way is to ask the patient—how he or she is feeling. If responds verbally—he or she has an intact airway, is breathing, is thinking, and, therefore, has a pulse. If unresponsive, airway patency should be checked. Assess the airway by:
- *Listening air movement (nose/mouth and chest movement)*: Snoring or gurgling suggests partial airway obstruction.
- *Look for intercostal retraction*: Look for chest expansion, listen and feel for air movement.
- Observe for foreign body obstruction in the oropharynx—stridor.
- Check for gag reflex—watch for swallowing.
- Use chin-lift or nasopharyngeal airway (chin-lift maneuver must not be used in confirmed cervical spine injury). Cricothyrotomy may be done in emergent situations, if there is obstruction near vocal cords that cannot be immediately removed or bag-mask ventilation is not possible. This achieves 3Ps:
  1. Airway patency
  2. Aspiration protection
  3. Positive pressure ventilation.

Any foreign bodies that are seen should be removed. Blind mouth sweep must not be performed. Secretions and blood should be suctioned.

Indications for intubation are:
- GCS < 8
- Inability to maintain ventilation
- Apnea
- Severe maxillofacial injury.

Breathing: For breathing, respiratory rate and depth should be assessed; cyanosis is a late feature. Oxygen at 6–10 L/min via a nonrebreathing face mask should be given. Patient should be ventilated, if needed, with rescue breaths, a bag-valve device (bagging the patient), or a ventilator. Look for trachea and deviation to one side.

Circulation: To assess circulation, one should look for the level of consciousness, skin temperature, color, nail bed capillary refill time, and rate and quality of the pulses. External bleeding should be controlled with direct pressure without inadvertent use of tourniquet. Blood should be sent for basic laboratory studies. Resuscitation should be done with two large-bore (14–16 G) IV catheters (antecubital—femoral—subclavian or jugular) using warmed fluids (Ringer's lactate is the fluid of choice—bolus 1–2 units or in children 20 mL/kg) and PRBCs, if necessary. Amount of the fluid to be given is decided by blood pressure monitoring, CVP monitoring, and urine output monitoring. The initial aim is to maintain a palpable radial pulse, which will need a SBP of 70–80 mm Hg. If there is any suspicion of head injury, the SBP should be maintained > 90 mm Hg in order to maintain cerebral perfusion. Crude measure for fluid replacement is 3:1, i.e., 3 mL fluid for 1 mL blood loss. It is imperative to warm the fluids to 39°C to prevent hypothermia:

- Blood pressure, pulse oximetry, blood gas monitoring, and electrocardiogram (ECG) are used as adjuncts. Urinary catheters and nasogastric tubes may be placed.
- Upon completion of primary survey, response to resuscitation is assessed. Shock should be promptly identified.
- Hemorrhagic shock is treated with volume replacement. The extent of blood loss is best assessed by the response to initial fluid bolus (lactated Ringer's solution or normal saline: 1–2 L for adults, 20 mL/kg for children). Maintain urine output: 0.5 mL/kg in adults and 1 mL/kg in infants.

Assess the response to fluid loading as follows:
- *Rapid response*: Hemodynamic returning to normal. Usually, loss is < 20%.
- *Transient response*: 20–40% loss, needs blood transfusion.
- *No response*: Surgical intervention for blood loss (always look for pericardial effusion).
  – If the patient's vital signs are weak or absent, severe blood loss (> 40%) is suspected, and additional transfusion with untyped blood is required. If a transient response is noted, but vital signs begin to deteriorate again, moderate blood loss (20–40%) is suspected, and blood should be secured for potential transfusion requirements (type-specific or cross-matched as available). O-negative blood can be used for life-threatening situations or if type matched blood is unavailable.
  – In patients requiring massive blood transfusion, FFP, and platelets should be arranged urgently and transfused to improve survival and to decrease overall requirement of the packed cells.
  – If the patient is severely hypotensive (SBP < 70 mm Hg) and not responding to resuscitation, they should be taken to the operating theater immediately.

Always assume cervical spine injury in unconscious and also conscious patient needs CT scan for documentation in unconscious patient. Alert patient with normal neurology and no neck pain in conscious patient indicates a stable spine and X-rays are not needed. Flaccid paralysis with incontinence suggests spinal shock.

A quick neurological examination should be performed by assessing the patient's level of consciousness, pupillary size and reaction, and gross motor functioning. The GCS is the most commonly used rating system.

Hypoxia, hypotension, hypothermia or hyperthermia, and hypoglycemia in a polytrauma patient must be suspected and looked for.

The patient should be exposed by removing all clothes. Hypothermia should be controlled with adequate warming or blankets.

Adjuncts to the primary survey are:
- *Radiography*: The "trauma triple" is a portable cervical spine lateral view, AP chest, and AP pelvis radiographs. By these three X-rays, an idea about the potentially dangerous conditions can be obtained in minimal time.
- *Laboratory studies*: Hemogram, complete blood count including differential count, electrolytes level, assessment of renal function, and urine analysis including toxicology screen should be obtained.
- *Blood preparations*: Blood grouping and typing should be done, and according to severity of trauma and shock, 2–4 units of RBCs should be cross-matched.

Disability:
- A—Alert
- V—Vocal response
- P—Responds to pain
- U—Unresponsive to all stimuli—*three causes* are hypoxia, hypovolemia, and head injury.

Secondary survey is said to begin after primary survey; however, practically it is often completed during the process of treating priorities identified in primary survey. There is no specific sequence of trauma patient management and it keeps on changing with the priorities identified by expert from time to time.

Focused patient history should be taken. History should include at least following mnemonic SAMPLE:
- Symptoms—pain, difficulty in breathing, heaviness in chest, dizziness, and other symptoms
- Allergies to any specific drug/drugs
- Medications regularly taken and taken before the event
- Past history of any surgery/medical diseases
- Last meal timing of last meal is necessary in emergency management to determine the risk of aspiration.
- Events responsible for trauma.

The survey is postponed till the patient is hemodynamically stable. The more serious injuries are addressed first so as to gradually help the patient to recover, e.g., a head injury will get priority over assessment of closed tibial fracture, which can be splinted till head injury is managed. For secondary survey of the head, neck, and trunk, CT scanning has become a necessity and it should be done on urgent basis. Now, it is possible to obtain the scan and the reports within even 30 minutes of patient's arrival in centers of excellence.

- Pelvic injury should be suspected whenever there is pain in the pelvic region or leg length discrepancies. AP pelvic radiographs should be taken as soon as the primary survey is completed. Pelvic injuries are serious and marker of high-energy injury.

  Hypovolemic shock in these patients is multifactorial and patients may have blood loss from associated thoracic, intra-abdominal, or extremity injuries.

- Pelvic fractures are frequently associated with urethral injuries, especially the AP compression injuries. Clinical findings suggestive of urethral injuries are presence of blood at the meatus, perianal hematoma, and history of hematuria.
- Gentle one attempt of catheterization should be done in patients of pelvic fractures without above findings.

Principles of ETC (also see Answer to Question 38):
The ETC (early total care) School emanated from the finding that patients previously managed by conservative methods (say cast or traction for fracture shaft femur) fared worse than the early definitely operated patients. The development of newer methods of osteosynthesis also favored the concept of "early definitive management." These patients were found to have less pulmonary complications, reduced length of ICU and hospital stay compared to patients with delayed surgery. It was considered the ideal approach to treat orthopedic injuries by doing "definitive fixation" of all fractures in one trip to the operating room. This approach is called ETC and was widely used in the 80s to efficiently use the operating theater resources and perform surgeries with one set on investigations and anesthetic exposure. Though popular and practiced for more than a decade, opposing views came in 1990s and it was introspected, if ETC is really as successful as thought since in unstable patients, it was associated with an unexpectedly high rate of pulmonary complications.

Indications: It has to be individualized and not recommended unless the institute is versed in managing complications and has specialists available for management. If optimum care can be given for management of all injuries within 36 hours then one may institute ETC to patients with:
- Lactate of < 4.0 mmol/L
- pH ≥ 7.25
- Base excess ≥ −5.5 mmol/L

44. **A. Describe steps and algorithm of pediatric and adult basic cardiac life support.**
   B. Describe steps and algorithm of pediatric and adult advanced cardiac life support.

Ans: Basic Life Support (BLS) for Adults and Pediatrics—Step-by-Step Algorithm

Basic cardiac life support (BCLS) is a critical emergency procedure performed to maintain circulation and oxygenation in cardiac arrest victims until advanced care arrives.

Basic Life Support for Adults:

(Applies to adolescents and older)

Steps:
1. Ensure safety
   - Check for hazards before approaching (e.g., electrical, traffic).
2. Assess responsiveness
   - Tap shoulders and shout, "Are you okay?"
   - If unresponsive, call for help and activate emergency response (e.g., dial local emergency number).
3. Check breathing and pulse (Simultaneously if trained)
   - Look for chest rise, listen for breaths, feel for a pulse (carotid artery, 5–10 sec).
   - If no normal breathing or pulse → Start cardiopulmonary resuscitation (CPR).
4. Begin CPR (C-A-B sequence)
   - *Chest compressions (C)*:
     - *Position*: Heel of one hand on the lower half of the sternum, other hand on top.
     - *Rate*: 100–120 compressions/min.
     - *Depth*: At least 5 cm (2 inches).
     - Allow full chest recoil.
   - Airway (A)
     - *Head-tilt chin-lift (if no trauma) or jaw thrust (if trauma suspected).*
   - Breathing (B)
     - *Give 2 rescue breaths (1 second each, visible chest rise).*
     - *Mouth-to-mouth or bag-mask ventilation if available.*
5. Use an automated external defibrillator (AED)
   - Turn on AED, attach pads, follow voice prompts.
   - Analyze rhythm → Shock if advised [for shockable rhythms: Ventricular fibrillation (VF)/pulseless ventricular tachycardia (pVT)].
   - Resume CPR immediately after shock (or if no shock advised).
6. Continue CPR until
   - Return of spontaneous circulation (ROSC).
   - Advanced medical help takes over.
   - Victim shows signs of life.

Pediatric BLS (Infants and Children):

(Infants: < 1 year/Children: 1–puberty)

Key differences from adult BLS:
1. For unresponsive child/infant
   - If alone, perform 5 cycles (2 min) of CPR before calling emergency services (except in witnessed sudden collapse).
   - If with a helper, send them to call for help immediately.
2. Compression technique
   - *Infants (< 1 year)*:
     - Two-finger technique (for lone rescuer) or two-thumb encircling hands (for two rescuers)
     - Depth: ~4 cm (1.5 inches)
   - *Children (1–puberty)*:
     - Use one or two hands (depending on size)
     - Depth: ~5 cm (2 inches)
3. Compression-to-ventilation ratio
   - *Single rescuer*: 30:2 (same as adult)
   - *Two rescuers*: 15:2 (for better oxygenation)

4. Rescue breaths
   - Cover mouth and nose for infants
   - For children, use mouth-to-mouth (pinch nose)
   - Gentler breaths (avoid overinflation)
5. AED use
   - Use pediatric pads if available (reduce energy dose).
   - If unavailable, use adult AED (better than no shock).

Advanced Cardiac Life Support (ACLS) for Adults and Pediatrics—Step-by-Step Algorithm

Advanced cardiac life support builds upon BLS with additional interventions, including advanced airway management, medications, and rhythm-specific treatments.

Adult ACLS Algorithm:

Key steps:
1. Immediate recognition and BLS initiation:
   - Confirm unresponsiveness, no breathing/pulse.
   - Start high-quality CPR (100–120 compressions/min, depth ≥ 5 cm).
   - Attach AED/defibrillator as soon as possible.
2. Assess rhythm (shockable vs. nonshockable):
   - Shockable rhythms:
     – Ventricular fibrillation
     – Pulseless ventricular tachycardia
   - Nonshockable rhythms:
     – Asystole
     – Pulseless electrical activity (PEA)
3. Shockable rhythm (VF/pVT)—algorithm
   - *1st shock*: Biphasic 120–200 J (monophasic 360 J)
   - Resume CPR immediately for 2 min.
   - Epinephrine 1 mg IV/intraosseous (IO) every 3–5 min
   - 2nd shock after 2 min CPR
   - Amiodarone 300 mg IV/IO (or lidocaine 1–1.5 mg/kg if amiodarone unavailable)
   - Repeat shocks every 2 min while continuing CPR.
4. Nonshockable rhythm (asystole/PEA)—algorithm
   - Continue CPR (no shock delivered)
   - Epinephrine 1 mg IV/IO every 3–5 min
   - Search for reversible causes (Hs and Ts):
     – Hypoxia, hypovolemia, hypo/hyperkalemia, hypothermia
     – Toxins, tamponade (cardiac), tension pneumothorax, thrombosis [pulmonary embolism (PE)/myocardial infarction (MI)], trauma
5. Advanced airway management
   - Endotracheal intubation or supraglottic airway [e.g., laryngeal mask airway (LMA)]
   - Confirm placement with waveform capnography [end-tidal carbon dioxide (ETCO$_2$)]
   - Ventilate at 10 breaths/min (continuous compressions)
6. Return of spontaneous circulation management
   - *Postcardiac arrest care*:
     – Maintain BP [mean arterial pressure (MAP) ≥ 65 mm Hg], oxygenation (SpO$_2$ 92–98%), normothermia.
     – Targeted temperature management (TTM) if comatose (32–36°C for 24 h).
     – Treat underlying cause [e.g., percutaneous coronary intervention (PCI) for ST-elevation myocardial infarction (STEMI)].

Pediatric ACLS Algorithm:
(Infants < 1 year, Children 1–puberty)
Key differences from adult ACLS:
1. Initial BLS focus (before ACLS)
   - If alone, perform 5 cycles (2 min) of CPR before calling for help (unless witnessed collapse).
   - *Compression-to-ventilation ratio*:
     - *Single rescuer*: 30:2
     - *Two rescuers*: 15:2
2. Defibrillation energy doses
   - *First shock*: 2 J/kg
   - *Subsequent shocks*: 4 J/kg
   - Use pediatric pads if available (if not, use adult AED).
3. Medication dosing
   - *Epinephrine IV/IO*: 0.01 mg/kg (1:10,000, 0.1 mL/kg) every 3–5 min
   - *Amiodarone IV/IO*: 5 mg/kg (max 300 mg) for VF/pVT
   - *Lidocaine alternative*: 1 mg/kg
4. Reversible causes (Pediatric Hs and Ts)
   - Hypovolemia, hypoxia, hypoglycemia, hypo/hyperkalemia, hypothermia
   - Toxins, tamponade, tension pneumothorax, thrombosis (rare), trauma
5. Advanced airway management
   - *Endotracheal tube (ET) tube size*: (Age/4) + 4 (uncuffed) or (Age/4) + 3.5 (cuffed)
   - *Ventilation rate*:
     - *With advanced airway*: 1 breath every 2–3 sec (8–10 breaths/min)
6. ROSC management
   - Avoid hyperoxia (SpO_2 94–99%).
   - Glucose check (treat hypoglycemia).
   - Consider extracorporeal membrane oxygenation (ECMO) in refractory cases [e.g., extracorporeal cardiopulmonary resuscitation (ECPR) for in-hospital arrest].

45. Describe the treatment of a borderline patient of polytrauma. What is hypotensive resuscitation?
Ans:
Borderline patient: "Borderline" patient represents the most controversial category in which the choice between ETC and DCO remains uncertain. Pape coined the term "borderline" to describe a patient who is apparently in stable condition before surgery, but who deteriorates unexpectedly and develops organ dysfunction postoperatively. The following are criteria suggested in literature to define and evaluate a borderline patient:
- Polytrauma ISS 20 and additional thoracic trauma (AIS 2)
- Polytrauma with abdominal/pelvic trauma (Moore 3) and hemodynamic shock (initial blood pressure 90 mm Hg)
- ISS 40 or above in the absence of additional thoracic injury
- Radiographic findings of bilateral lung contusion
- Initial mean pulmonary arterial pressure 24 mm Hg
- Pulmonary artery pressure increases during intramuscular nerve (IMN) by 6 mm Hg.

Presence of any one of the above criteria shifts the management to DCO side, else ETC can be undertaken. If expected surgical time is 6 hours or more then DCO should be followed.

Hypotensive resuscitation: This is used in a patient of traumatic shock. This is observed in conscious patients maintaining adequate organ perfusion. It has been shown that aggressive volume replacement can exacerbate bleeding before the hemorrhage is controlled. This has emphasized on permitting low blood pressures (i.e., SBP = 90 mm Hg or mean BP = 50 mm Hg) in trauma patients with hemorrhagic shock until the bleeding is controlled. This strategy has been shown to reduce resuscitation volumes and increase survival rates.

46. Discuss borderline polytrauma. Mention clinical and investigative parameters to decide whether the patient should be managed by early total care (ETC) or damage control orthopedics (DCO).

Ans: Kindly see Answer to Question above.

47. What are the effects of polytrauma on respiratory physiology?

Ans: ARDS and FES may occur due to polytrauma.

ARDS: ARDS is defined as "*an acute condition characterized by bilateral pulmonary infiltrates and severe hypoxemia in the absence of evidence for cardiogenic pulmonary edema.*"

ARDS can be simply defined as noncardiogenic pulmonary edema.

Physical findings are often nonspecific, and patient has tachypnea and tachycardia owing to the rapid shallow breathing and hypoxemia. The patient may be febrile or hypothermic. Patients on ventilator require high fraction of inspired oxygen and high positive-end expiratory pressure. Thorough clinical examination should be done to differentiate ARDS from cardiogenic pulmonary edema by carefully looking for signs of CHF such as raised jugular venous pressure, murmurs, gallops, and edema of the dependent part.

Fat embolism: FES is a constellation of physiological abnormalities of cardiorespiratory and neurocognitive system produced as a result of blockage of vascular system by fat droplets. The clinical presentation is usually delayed by 2–3 days so one must be vigilant in diagnosing the disorder.

Kindly also see Answers to Questions 15 and 16 above for fat embolism.

48. Discuss fluid management and clinical monitoring of a polytrauma patient with hemorrhagic shock.

Ans: Source of bleeding should be identified as soon as possible and treatment should be done as per norms of hypovolemic shock. Antibiotics should be started as soon as possible and crystalloid fluids are given to combat hypoperfusion and hypotension.

- *Fluid resuscitation in trauma patients with uncontrolled bleeding*: Because uncontrolled exsanguinating hemorrhage is the leading cause of death in hemorrhagic shock, the following practices are being adopted to limit the extent of bleeding in cases of massive blood loss (defined as the loss of one blood volume in 24 hours). These practices are part of an overall approach known as damage control resuscitation.

It includes:
- *Hypotensive resuscitation*: This is observed in conscious patients maintaining adequate organ perfusion. It has been shown that aggressive volume replacement can exacerbate bleeding before the hemorrhage is controlled. This has emphasized on permitting low blood pressures (i.e., SBP = 90 mm Hg or mean BP = 50 mm Hg) in trauma patients with hemorrhagic shock until the bleeding is controlled. This strategy has been shown to reduce resuscitation volumes and increase survival rates.
- *Hemostatic resuscitation*: Traditionally, it was practiced to give 1 unit of FFP for every 6 units of RBCs. But after the discovery that severely injured trauma victims often have a coagulopathy on presentation the practice has changed to giving 1 unit of FFP for every 1–2 unit of RBCs. In trauma patients, transfuse 1–2 L of crystalloid bolus. If profound shock is recognized early, blood transfusion should be started with uncross-matched blood. Resuscitation with fluid or blood products must not delay the operative procedure to control the ongoing bleeding.

Fluid replacement: Upon initial presentation, it is necessary to place one or two large-bore (≥ 16 G) peripheral IV catheters with initial rapid infusion of either isotonic saline (although care must be taken to avoid replacement with excess chloride) or a balanced salt solution such as Ringer's lactate (being cognizant of the presence of potassium and potential renal dysfunction). No additional benefit from the use of colloid has been demonstrated, and apart from being expensive thus, increasing the cost of the treatment, in trauma patients, it is associated with a higher mortality, particularly in patients with traumatic brain injury.

- If "mean" arterial pressure is < 60–65 mm Hg, SBP is < 90 mm Hg, or evidence of tissue hypoperfusion is present, an IV fluid challenge (20–40 mL/kg crystalloid or colloid) should be given rapidly. The infusion of 2–3 L of salt solution over 20–30 minutes should restore normal hemodynamic parameters. After achieving hemodynamic stability, a bolus of 500 mL every 30 minutes titrated to MAP or measurement of preload is recommended.

- Persistent hemodynamic instability implies that shock has not been reversed and/or there is significant ongoing blood or other volume losses. Continuing acute blood loss, with hemoglobin concentrations declining to ≤ 100 g/L (10 g/dL), should initiate blood transfusion, preferably as fully cross-matched recently banked (< 14 days old) blood. Resuscitated patients are often coagulopathic due to deficient clotting factors in crystalloids and banked PRBCs.
- Early administration of component therapy during massive transfusion (FFP and platelets) approaching a 1:1 ratio of PRBC/FFP appears to improve survival.
- In cases of extreme emergencies, type-specific or O-negative packed red cells may be transfused. Once the patient has been stabilized and hemorrhage is controlled, blood transfusions should not be continued unless the hemoglobin is < 7 g/dL.

Role of vasopressors: If the patient remains hypotensive even after administration of appropriate amount of fluid, vasopressors such as norepinephrine, dopamine, should be administered to restore adequate systemic arterial pressure while the diagnostic evaluation is ongoing but only after blood volume has been restored. Increases in peripheral vasoconstriction with inadequate resuscitation leads to tissue loss and organ failure.

However, vasopressors may also mask hypovolemia when they increase blood pressure.

- If the volume status cannot be defined or the hemodynamic condition requires repeated fluid challenges or vasopressor treatment, a central venous catheter should be placed to determine ventricular filling pressure, intravascular volume status, and central venous oxygen saturation.
- Based on these data, patients can usually be classified and managed according to their hemodynamic and oxygen transport patterns.
- These catheters had previously been used in critically ill patients to guide response to volume and vasopressor therapy, but data emerged suggesting that pulmonary artery catheters (PACs) increased mortality, prompting further studies. Thus, the routine use of PACs cannot be recommended. However, in some complex situations, PACs may be useful in distinguishing between cardiogenic and septic shock.

The following additional clinical monitoring is mandatory:
- *Chest*: If injury to lung parenchyma, great vessels of lung or cardiac wounds is suspected, bilateral chest tubes should be inserted. If bleeding is > 1,500 mL immediately or > 200 mL/h for > 3 hours, prompt operative intervention is required.
- *Abdomen*: In patients with abdominal trauma, abdominal pain, peritonitis, or abdominal distention suggests intra-abdominal hemorrhage. Focused abdominal US or diagnostic peritoneal lavage should be done. Prompt operative intervention is necessary in ongoing intra-abdominal bleeding.
- *Retroperitoneum/pelvis*: In patients with open book or distracted pelvic fractures, there is loss of significant amounts of blood into the retroperitoneum. If pelvic fracture is suspected or diagnosed, a pelvic binder should be immediately placed. Angiography with embolization can be done to stop bleeding.
- *Long bones*: Damaged control orthopedics should be applied in long bone fractures. Immediate reduction and temporary stabilization should be done with definitive management later on.
- *External*: If there is extensive soft tissue injury with source of blood loss, debridement, and pressure bandage should be applied. In case of clean wounds, primary suturing should be done with running interlocking sutures.

49. Hemorrhagic shock: Discuss pathophysiology in a 23-year-old polytrauma.

Ans: *Pathophysiology*: The metabolic rates of brain and heart are high and they have low storage of energy substrate so these organs are critically dependent on continuous supply of oxygen and nutrients. To maintain this homeostasis, body has complex physiological response which decreases blood supply to intestine and liver and maintains blood and oxygen supply to brain and heart.
- *Afferent signaling*: With decrease in blood volume, CNS sends several afferent signals to maintain homeostasis. Baroreceptors of carotid bodies and aortic arch, volume receptors of atria and chemoreceptors that senses O_2 tension, CO_2 and pO_2, all sense the changes due to hypoperfusion and sent afferent signals to hypothalamic-pituitary-adrenal (HPA) axis-leading to release of vasopressin and autonomic nervous system (ANS) leading to initiate compensatory mechanisms.

- *Cardiovascular*: Cardiovascular system acts through neuroendocrine pathways in response to hypoperfusion. Activation of ANS results in activation of α1 and β1 receptors. Activation of α1 receptors results in vasocompression with selective shunting of blood to brain and heart. Activation of β1 receptors causes increase in heart rate (HR) and cardiac output. But, this effect blunts in neurogenic shock due to loss of sympathetic input and in cardiogenic shock due to deranged heart function. The result of above cardiogenic mechanisms is twofold:
    1. *Hypoperfusion*: It is essential for cellular viability to have adequate delivery and utilization of oxygen and the failure to deliver or utilize oxygen is the most important step in the pathogenesis of shock. The systemic circulation is usually autoregulated; systemic arterial pressure is inversely proportional to the diameter of the vessel so that the flow is maintained. Normally, systemic vascular resistance increases to compensate the decreased cardiac output in order to maintain the normal MAP. Despite the near-normal blood pressure, however, the patient is in "cryptic shock" because of tissue hypoperfusion. The metabolic rates of brain and heart are high and they have low storage of energy substrate so these organs are critically dependent on continuous supply of oxygen and nutrients. Blood flow to these organs is carefully regulated and maintained over a wide range of blood pressures. Whereas in other organs, such as the intestine or liver, autoregulation is not as tightly maintained as heart or brain.
    2. *Vasodilatation*: During shock, in areas of hypoperfusion both the inflammatory and clotting cascades may be triggered. Hypoxic vascular endothelial cells activate white blood cells (WBCs), which bind to the endothelium inflammatory mediators [e.g., cytokines, leukotrienes, and TNF] and release directly damaging substances (e.g., reactive O_2 species). Some of these mediators bind to cell surface receptors and activate nuclear factor kappa B (NFκβ), which leads to production of additional cytokines and nitric oxide (NO), a potent vasodilator. Inflammation is more pronounced in septic shock than other forms because of the actions of bacterial toxins, especially endotoxin. Potent inflammatory mediators cause vasodilatation of capacitance vessels leading to pooling of blood and hypotension because of relative hypovolemia. Localized vasodilation increases vascular permeability and may shunt blood past the capillary exchange beds, causing focal hypoperfusion despite normal cardiac output and BP. Blood flow to microvessels including capillaries is reduced even though large-vessel blood flow is preserved in settings of septic shock in order to maintain blood flow to vital organs.
- *Neuroendocrine*: Several hormones are released in response to hypoperfusion. From adrenal medulla, epinephrine and norepinephrine are released, which increase vasomotor tone. Renin-angiotensin aldosterone system is activated and vasopressin is released from hypothalamus which increases water reabsorption from kidney. Cortisol and glucagon are released which increase catabolic rate at cellular level.
- *Immunologic and inflammatory*: It mainly occurs in septic shock, but to some extent, it occurs in all types of shock. In this proinflammatory state, there is release of important mediators such as cytokines, complement, oxygen radicals, eicosanoids, and NO. Important cytokines are TNF-α, IL-1, IL-2, and IL-6.
- *Cellular effects*: Amount of oxygen required by the tissues to avoid anaerobic metabolism is known as the oxygen demand. Normally, systemic oxygen delivery is sufficient to fulfil oxygen demand so that systemic oxygen consumption is not altered by or dependent on changes in delivery. However, if systemic oxygen delivery drops below a critical value, it is maintained by a compensatory increase in oxygen extraction ratio, which maintains systemic oxygen consumption at an adequate level to meet systemic oxygen demands. When oxygen supply to the cells decreases to critical level, aerobic metabolism is switched to anaerobic one, with decreased production of adenosine triphosphate (ATP) and accumulation of lactate. With depletion of ATP supply, energy dependent mechanisms of the cell such as enzyme synthesis, DNA repair, and signal transduction fails. Na+/K+ ATPase fails and cellular swelling with subsequent lysis occurs due to water accumulation. Acidosis leads to changes in local microcirculation, and with activation of neutrophils, proinflammatory damage aggravates.

An oxygen delivery dependency also exists in patients with sepsis, trauma, and ARDS and after resuscitation from prolonged cardiac arrest. These patients have systemic oxygen delivery in the normal or elevated range but an impairment of oxygen utilization. This condition of tissue hypoxia is a result of ineffective distribution of blood flow or a defect in the utilization of substrate at the microcirculatory or subcellular level. This process is believed to be an important mechanism of cellular damage in various forms of shock.

50. Define shock. Discuss management of shock in a polytrauma patient.

Ans: Shock is a state of decreased perfusion of the body resulting in inadequate supply of oxygen and nutrients to the tissues leading to dysfunction of the normal cellular milieu, and if not treated promptly resulting in cell death.

Quantification of hypoperfusion
- *Oxygen debt*: Cells require oxygen for all aerobic mechanisms. When oxygen supply declines to a critical level, oxygen demands of the cells are not fulfilled by the oxygen supply leading to oxygen debt. It correlates directly with degree and duration of hypoperfusion and survival in hypovolemic patients. Its direct measurement is difficult, so other measures of hypoperfusion are necessary.
- *Lactate and base deficit*: Compared to cardiac output, blood pressure, and volume loss, lactate levels (chemical marker of impaired tissue perfusion) and arterial base deficits are better indicators of oxygen debt and to decide therapy. Elevated serum lactate in setting of acute blood loss is presumptive evidence of hemorrhagic shock. Accumulation lactate in low-flow state is result of decreased clearance. Lactate level of > 4 mM/L is usually life-threatening (normal up to 2 mM/L).

Management proper
The injured patient with shock is assumed to have hypovolemic shock until proven otherwise.
- *Airway, breathing, and circulations*: In initial approach, always look for ABC. Secure the airway and ventilate the patient for adequate oxygen delivery, insert two large-bore IV cannulas, halt external hemorrhage with pressure temporarily, and prevent hypothermia with adequate warming and warm IV fluids. Because the Trendelenburg position may impair gas exchange and promote aspiration, an alternative is to elevate the legs to 45° above the horizontal plane while in the supine position will move 150–750 mL of blood out of the legs and toward the heart, thereby serving as a built in fluid challenge. Cardiac monitoring can detect myocardial ischemia or malignant arrhythmias, which can be treated by standard ACLS protocols. Unresponsive or minimally responsive patients should have their glucose checked immediately and if their glucose level is low, 1 ampoule of 50% dextrose intravenously should be given. An arterial line should be placed for continuous blood pressure measurement, and a Foley catheter should be inserted to monitor urinary output.
- *Hypovolemic and hemorrhagic shock*: In trauma patients, transfuse 1–2 L of crystalloid bolus. If profound shock is recognized early, blood transfusion should be started with uncross-matched blood. Resuscitation with fluid or blood products must not delay the operative procedure to control the ongoing bleeding.
    - *Fluid replacement*: Upon initial presentation, it is necessary to place one or two large-bore (≥ 16 G) peripheral IV catheters with initial rapid infusion of either isotonic saline (although care must be taken to avoid replacement with excess chloride) or a balanced salt solution such as Ringer's lactate (being cognizant of the presence of potassium and potential renal dysfunction). No additional benefit from the use of colloid has been demonstrated, and apart from being expensive thus, increasing the cost of the treatment, in trauma patients, it is associated with a higher mortality, particularly in patients with traumatic brain injury.
        - If "mean" arterial pressure is < 60–65 mm Hg, SBP is < 90 mm Hg, or evidence of tissue hypoperfusion is present, an IV fluid challenge (20–40 mL/kg crystalloid or colloid) should be given rapidly.
        - Persistent hemodynamic instability implies that shock has not been reversed and/or there is significant ongoing blood or other volume losses. Continuing acute blood loss, with hemoglobin concentrations declining to ≤ 100 g/L (10 g/dL), should initiate blood transfusion, preferably as fully cross-matched recently banked (< 14 days old) blood.
        - Resuscitated patients are often coagulopathic due to deficient clotting factors in crystalloids and banked PRBCs. Early administration of component therapy during massive transfusion (FFP and platelets) approaching a 1:1 ratio of PRBC/FFP appears to improve survival.
        - *Role of vasopressors*: If the patient remains hypotensive even after administration of appropriate amount of fluid, vasopressors, such as norepinephrine, dopamine, should be administered to restore adequate systemic arterial pressure while the diagnostic evaluation is ongoing but only after blood volume has been restored.
    - Hemorrhagic shock patients can be classified as responders, transient responders, and nonresponders, with last two types having increased severity of shock due to continued bleeding and deterioration of condition. They require prompt operative or endovascular intervention to stop the bleeding.

- *Chest*: If injury to lung parenchyma, great vessels of lung or cardiac wounds are suspected, bilateral chest tubes should be inserted. If bleeding is > 1,500 mL immediately or > 200 mL for > 3 hours, prompt operative intervention is required.
- *Abdomen*: In patients with abdominal trauma, abdominal pain, peritonitis, or abdominal distention suggests intra-abdominal hemorrhage. Focused abdominal US or diagnostic peritoneal lavage should be done. Prompt operative intervention is necessary in ongoing intra-abdominal bleeding.
- *Retroperitoneum/pelvis*: In patients with open book or distracted pelvic fractures, there is loss of significant amounts of blood into the retroperitoneum. If pelvic fracture is suspected or diagnosed, a pelvic binder should be immediately placed. Angiography with embolization can be done to stop bleeding.
- *Long bones*: Damaged control orthopedics should be applied in long-bone fractures. Immediate reduction and temporary stabilization should be done with definitive management later on.
- *External*: If there is extensive soft tissue injury with source of blood loss, debridement, and pressure bandage should be applied. In case of clean wounds, primary suturing should be done with running interlocking sutures.

- *Traumatic shock*: Source of bleeding should be identified as soon as possible and treatment should be done as per norms of hypovolemic shock. Antibiotics should be started as soon as possible and crystalloid fluids are given to combat hypoperfusion and hypotension.
  - *Fluid resuscitation in trauma patients with uncontrolled bleeding*: Because uncontrolled exsanguinating hemorrhage is the leading cause of death in hemorrhagic shock, the following practices are being adopted to limit the extent of bleeding in cases of massive blood loss (defined as the loss of one blood volume in 24 hours). These practices are part of an overall approach known as damage control resuscitation. It includes:
    - *Hypotensive resuscitation*: This is observed in conscious patients maintaining adequate organ perfusion. It has been shown that aggressive volume replacement can exacerbate bleeding before the hemorrhage is controlled. This has emphasized on permitting low blood pressures (i.e., SBP = 90 mm Hg or mean BP = 50 mm Hg) in trauma patients with hemorrhagic shock until the bleeding is controlled. This strategy has been shown to reduce resuscitation volumes and increase survival rates.
    - *Hemostatic resuscitation*: Traditionally, it was practiced to give 1 unit of FFP for every 6 units of RBCs. But after the discovery that severely injured trauma victims often have a coagulopathy on presentation the practice has changed to giving 1 unit of FFP for every 1–2 unit of RBCs.
- *Vasogenic shock*:
  - *Septic shock*: Septic shock is present in trauma patient in late cases or when infection is prevalent. The first step is to correct hypoperfusion by giving IV fluids typically beginning with 1–2 L of normal saline over 1–2 hours. To avoid pulmonary edema, the CVP should be maintained at 8–12 cmH$_2$O. Vasopressors such as epinephrine and norepinephrine are used when hypotension persists after fluid resuscitation.
    - Underlying infection must be treated on prompt basis. Source of infection should be identified and treated accordingly whether medically or surgically. Thorough debridement is done and broad spectrum antibiotics are started. Pus should be drained and any devitalized tissues should be removed. Pus should be sent for culture and antibiotic sensitivity testing.
    - As soon as culture and sensitivity report become available, antibiotics should be changed to sensitive one. If no organisms are found, empiric antibiotic therapy should be stopped and close follow-up should be started.
    - Mechanical ventilation is required in majority of patients who have septic shock because acute lung injury is the most common complication. Lung-protective ventilation, which is defined as the mechanical ventilation that minimizes lung injury by using a relatively low tidal volume (such as < 6 mL/kg of predicted body weight), decreases mortality from acute lung injury and ARDS.
    - Immunomodulatory therapy and use of protein C are under experiment at present in treatment of septic shock.
    - For a successful outcome, early goal-directed therapy is recommended; these measures should be initiated within 1 hour of the patient's presentation with severe sepsis or septic shock (the physician should be prompt in diagnosing hence!).
- *Neurogenic shock*: As common with other forms of shock, fluid resuscitation is the initial treatment of choice. Excessive volume of fluid may be required to retain normal hemodynamic functions, if given alone. In persistent hypotensive patients, once hemorrhage has been ruled out, vasopressors (to augment vascular resistance) like neither adrenaline

nor phenylephrine are useful. The latter is preferred because of its pure alpha agonistic activity. Generally, patients recover well within 48 hours of the initial treatment.
- *Obstructive shock*: These patients present with rapidly deteriorating condition requiring emergent steps to save the patient. Tension pneumothorax should be treated promptly by needle thoracostomy and chest tube insertion. Cardiac tamponade may require thoracotomy in extreme conditions, but if the patient is stable, cardiac window should be made.

51. Define neurogenic shock following spinal cord injury. Discuss in detail about clinical methods to diagnose level of spinal cord injury.

Ans:

Definition: Neurogenic shock is a combination of hypotension, bradyarrhythmia, and temperature dysregulation due to peripheral vasodilatation seen after cervical and high thoracic spinal cord injury. The manifestations are a result of autonomic instability (sudden loss of sympathetic tone, with preserved parasympathetic function).

Clinical methods:
American Spinal Injury Association (ASIA) form is commonly used for assessment of spinal level and documentation.

Sensory examination is performed with light touch, then pinpricks (using a sterile needle), beginning at the head and neck and progressing distally, to examine specific dermatome distributions. The following dermatomes are important landmarks:
- The nipple line (T4)
- Xiphoid process (T7)
- Umbilicus (T10)
- Inguinal region (T12, L1)
- Perineum and perianal region (S2, S3, and S4).

Evidence of sacral sensory sparing establishes the diagnosis of an incomplete spinal cord injury.

Motor examination should be systematic, beginning with the upper extremities. During motor examination, it is important to differentiate between complete and incomplete spinal cord injuries and pure nerve root lesions. After examination of the extremities and trunk, the presence or absence of sacral motor sparing should be determined by voluntary rectal sphincter or toe flexor contractions. If voluntary contraction of the sacrally innervated muscles is present with sacral sensation, the prognosis for recovery of motor function is good. The presence of an anal reflex without sacral sensation is consistent with a complete injury. Finally, reflexes should be documented. Hyperreflexia, clonus, and pathological reflexes, such as a Babinski reflex in the lower extremities or a Hoffman sign in the upper extremities, indicate chronic spinal cord compression. Penile erection and incontinence of the bowel or bladder suggest a significant spinal injury.

The Key Muscle Groups Used in ASIA Motor Source Evaluation of Spinal Cord Injury are detailed in **Table 1.2.2**:

TABLE 1.2.2: The key muscles tested to determine involvement of specific myotome indicating the injury level in ASIA scoring.

Level	Muscle Group
C5	Elbow flexors (biceps, brachialis)
C6	Wrist extensors (extensor carpi radialis longus and brevis)
C7	Elbow extensors (triceps)
C8	Finger flexors (flexor digitorum profundus to the middle finger)
T1	Small finger abductors (abductor digiti minimi)
L2	Hip flexors (iliopsoas)
L3	Knee extensors (quadriceps)
L4	Ankle dorsiflexors (tibialis anterior)
L5	Long toe extensors (extensor hallucis longus)
S1	Ankle plantarflexors (gastrocnemius, soleus)

52. Classify different types of hemorrhagic shock.

Ans: The clinical features of hemorrhagic shock entirely depend on amount of blood lost which has been classified by the American College of Surgeons (Table 1.2.3):

- *Class I*: ≤15% of the blood volume loss (or ≤ 10 mL/kg). It is usually fully compensated by transcapillary refill. Clinical findings are minimal or absent.
- *Class II*: 15–30% of the blood volume loss (or 10–20 mL/kg). This represents the compensated phase of hypovolemia, where BP is maintained by systemic vasoconstriction. Postural changes in pulse rate and blood pressure may be evident, but these findings are inconsistent, and the hypovolemia can be clinically silent.
- *Class III*: Loss of 30–40% of the blood volume (or 20–30 mL/kg). This marks the onset of decompensated phase of hypovolemia, where the vasoconstrictor response is no longer able to sustain blood pressure and organ perfusion. The clinical consequences can include evidence of impaired organ perfusion (e.g., cool extremities, oliguria, and depressed consciousness), supine hypotension, and evidence of anaerobic metabolism (i.e., lactate accumulation in blood).
- *Class IV*: Loss of > 40% of the blood volume (or > 30 mL/kg). This degree of blood loss results in profound hypovolemic shock, which may be irreversible. Clinical manifestations include MOF and severe metabolic (lactic) acidosis. Perfusion of the CNS is well maintained until shock becomes severe. Hence, mental obtundation is an ominous clinical sign.

TABLE 1.2.3: Comparison of characteristics of classes of hemorrhagic shock.

Characteristic	Class I	Class II	Class III	Class IV
Blood loss (mL)	Up to 750	750–1,500	1,500–2,000	>2,000
% volume loss	Up to 15	15–30	30–40	>40
Pulse rate (per min)	<100	>100	>120	>140
Blood pressure	Normal	Normal	Decreased	Decreased
Pulse pressure	Normal or increased	Decreased	Decreased	Decreased
Respiratory rate (per min)	14–20	20–30	30–40	>35
Urine output (mL/h)	>30	20–30	5–15	Negligible
Mental status	Slightly anxious	Mildly anxious	Anxious, confused	Confused, lethargic
Fluid replacement	Crystalloid	Crystalloid	Crystalloid and blood	Crystalloid and blood

53. Tabulate differences between septic and hypovolemic shock.

Ans: Table 1.2.4 *Compares the hypovolemic from septic shock.*

TABLE 1.2.4: Comparative differences between hypovolemic and septic shock.

Features	Hypovolemic shock	Septic shock
Systemic vascular resistance	Increased	Decreased
Pulse	Weak, thready	Bounding pulse
Skin	Cool, pale, moist skin	Pink, warm, flushed skin
Altered coagulation status	Sometimes present	Often present
Cutaneous vasoconstriction	Often absent	Present
Serology	Reduced blood counts	Raised leukocyte counts, raised ESR, CRP, procalcitonin
Fluid challenge	Responds if promptly introduced	Refractory to fluid challenge
Management	Restore blood volume	Control sepsis, restore peripheral vascular resistance and cardiac pumping

(CRP: C-reactive protein; ESR: erythrocyte sedimentation rate)

54. Define blood component therapy. Enumerate and mention uses of various blood fractions.

Ans: Mostly, patients require transfusion for specific causes like treating anemia, or reduced platelet counts or replacing clotting factors in bleeding disorders, etc. This makes use of whole blood superfluous and actually wastes the fraction of blood that was actually not needed in the patient. The therapeutic use of specific portions/components (better called fraction) of blood, e.g., factor 8 concentrate, packed red cells, or platelets rather than whole blood to treat a specific deficiency, is hence in wide practice and logical.

The various blood components, which are commonly used in clinical practice, are:

- *Packed RBCs*: These are used to raise the oxygen-carrying capacity of blood and are used in normovolemic patients of anemia without cardiac disease. One unit of PRBCs is expected to raise hemoglobin (Hb) by 1.2 g/dL.
- *Platelets*: Transfusion of platelets is done in patients of thrombocytopenia who have hemorrhage. This can be given to a patient with platelet count below 10,000/µL.
- *Fresh frozen plasma*: It contains plasma proteins and coagulation factors such as albumin, protein C and S, and antithrombin. FFP transfusion is indicated in patients of coagulation failure and thrombotic thrombocytopenic purpura (TTP).
- *Cryoprecipitate*: It is a source of insoluble plasma proteins, fibrinogen, factor 8, and vWF. Indications of cryoprecipitate are for patients requiring fibrinogen, factor 8, and vWF.

(Details of each can be obtained from Chapter 24: Transfusion Medicine of the book Essential Orthopedics: Principles and Practice, 2nd edition.)

55. Explain autologous transfusion.

Ans: It is collection of patient's own blood cells for transfusing back the same after processing. In an attempt to reduce the incidence of allogeneic blood transfusion reactions, various ways have been determined to use patient's own blood. Preoperative blood donation can be utilized in elderly patients, although there is higher risk of iatrogenic preoperative anemia and more serious cardiovascular complication. However, it decreases risk of viral infections; the risk of bacterial contamination still remains.

There are four methods of autologous transfusion:

1. *Intraoperative cell salvage*: Blood is collected from suction, surgical drains, or both and retransfused back to the patient after filtration or washing.
2. *Preoperative autologous donation (PAD)*: Blood is collected in advance of an elective procedure, stored in the blood bank, and transfused back to the patient when required. Some have used erythropoietin to increase the hemoglobin preoperatively to improve the yield.
3. *Acute normovolemic hemodilution (ANH)*: Blood is collected immediately prior to surgery and blood volume restored by crystalloid or colloid. The blood is then retransfused toward the end of surgery once hemostasis is achieved. It is mainly used in cardiac bypass surgery.
4. *Postoperative cell salvage (PCS)*: It is a rarely used system and not recommended except in rarest of circumstances. Here, the blood from wound drains of total hip arthroplasty or total knee arthroplasty is filtered or processed in an automated system, then reinfused to patient.

Indications of autologous blood transfusion:

- Major elective orthopedic surgery, cardiovascular surgery, obstetric surgery, and gastrosurgery.
- When anticipated blood loss is > 20% in any surgery.
- Blood collected in abdominal cavity due to organ rupture or during surgery.
- Jehovah's Witness who is not willing to accept allogeneic blood.

56. A. Blood conservation strategies in major orthopedic surgeries.
B. Role, mechanism of action and recommended dose of tranexamic acid.

Ans:
A. Autologous blood transfusion has been written in Answer to Question above. The other method of blood conservation is by increasing hematocrit judiciously preoperatively by using erythropoietin and iron supplements.
B. Tranexamic acid (Kindly also see Answer to Question 78 in the following text):

Role: It has been used for prevention of excessive bleeding in:
- Overdose of fibrinolytics
- After cardiopulmonary bypass surgery
- After tonsillectomy, prostatic surgery, tooth extraction in hemophiliacs.
- Menorrhagia, especially due to intrauterine contraceptive device (IUCD).
- Recurrent epistaxis, ocular trauma, and bleeding peptic ulcer.

Mechanism of action: It is a drug of class antifibrinolytics. It inhibits plasminogen activation and dissolution of clot. Like epsilon amino caproic acid (EACA), it binds to the lysine-binding site on plasminogen and prevents its combination with fibrin and is 7 times more potent.

Recommended dose: 10–15 mg/kg 2–3 times a day or 1–1.5 g TDS oral 0.5–1 g TDS by slow IV infusion.

57. Discuss principle of tranexamic acid in management of polytrauma.
Ans: Written in answers above.

58. Describe methods of reducing risks in blood transfusion.
Ans: Various risks of blood transfusion involve immunological and non-immunological reactions. These can be reduced by following methods:
- Prior to receiving a blood transfusion, patient's red cells are typed for ABO and Rh status using commercially available reagents.
    - During front typing or forward typing, the donor's red cells are reacted with antibodies directed against the A, B, and D antigens.
    - Blood grouping is confirmed during back typing in which donor serum is tested for the presence of anti-A and anti-B antibodies. Following blood grouping, recipient serum or plasma is screened for red cell antibodies. The alloantibody is tested by mixing patients serum that contains the major antigens of the blood group and whose extended phenotype is known as O blood group RBC. If an antibody is present in the serum, it will react with the screening cell and cause red cell agglutination. Naturally occurring ABO antibodies do not interfere with antibody identification because screening cells are type O.
    - Cross-matching is used to make sure that the specific donor blood that will be used during a transfusion does not react with a patient's blood. It is basically a transfusion done in a test tube. The process may take 45 minutes to an hour and should be done ideally at least 3 days prior to the transfusion to be accurate. The tests are also used on pregnant women in order to prevent hemolytic disease of the newborn (HDN).
- Volume overload in massive transfusions or in renal patients can be done by constant monitoring and giving diuretics.
- Allergic reactions can be reduced by using irradiated blood or leukoreduced products in sensitive patients or patients with immunodeficiency. Universal leukoreduction has been found to prevent complications like febrile nonhemolytic transfusion reactions; platelet refractoriness due to human leukocyte antigen alloimmunization; and transmission of *Cytomegalovirus*.
- Thorough screening of blood and products for designated infections (hepatitis B surface antigen, hepatitis B virus core antibody, hepatitis C virus antibody, human T-lymphotropic virus 1 and 2 antibody, human immunodeficiency virus 1 and 2, and syphilis) is mandatory and cannot be skipped at any cost.
- Transfusion-associated acute lung injury can be reduced by using male-only plasma.
- Blood products should only be used for designated indications.

59. Transfusion mismatch.
Ans: *Absurdly asked incomplete question but the students must answer to pass. The following should be a reasonable answer in my opinion.*

Definition
Any unfavorable and harmful transfusion-related event occurring in a patient during or after transfusion of blood or its components is called transfusion reaction. This may arise out of mismatch or immune incompatibility or nonimmune related reaction arising out of various reasons not related to identifiable mismatch. The following are common causes of transfusion mismatch:

- Wrong identification of patient
- Incorrect sample identification
- Wrong blood or component issued
- Administration error
- Technical error
- Storage error

Due to transfusion mismatch, the following types of reactions may be seen:

- *Immune-mediated*:
  - *Hemolytic reactions*: Most severe type of transfusion reactions
    - Immediate (intravascular)—hemolysis occurring within few minutes to 24 hours usually due to ABO incompatibility
    - Delayed (extravascular)—these are rare and occur due to minor blood grouping components such as Kell, Duffy, Rh, and MNS incompatibility causing hemolysis within few hours to 3–7 days in liver and spleen. They are identified by fall in hemoglobin despite transfusion, rise in bilirubin and renal failure.
  - *Nonhemolytic reactions*:
    - Febrile nonhemolytic transfusion reaction
    - Urticarial transfusion reaction
    - Anaphylactic transfusion reaction
    - Noncardiogenic pulmonary edema (transfusion-related acute lung injury, TRALI)
    - Circulatory overload
    - Graft versus home disease (GVHD)
- *Nonimmune-mediated reactions*:
  - Immediate
  - Delayed

Hemolytic immediate transfusion reactions are most serious and are clinically identified by:
- Fever, chills, pain at transfusion site
- Hypotension
- Chest and flank pain
- Nausea/vomiting
- Dyspnea
- Hemoglobinuria
- Renal failure
- Shock and DIC

These are managed by immediately stopping transfusion, preventing renal failure by mannitol and stopping immune reaction by instilling steroid and antihistaminics for symptomatic control. Management of blood pressure is a priority.

60. Describe terrible triad of death.

Ans: The lethal triad of hypothermia, acidosis, and coagulopathy has been recognized as a significant cause of death in patients with traumatic injuries. Ultimately, this triad results in worsening hemorrhage and eventual death. A thorough understanding of triad is needed to manage patients. It serves as a cornerstone for all interventions provided to the bleeding trauma patient. If left untreated, hypothermia, acidosis, and coagulopathy bring about and propagate each other in collateral damaging vicious circle, eventually resulting in a predictable but irreversible progression toward death.

Consequences of hypothermia:
- Decreased cardiac output and myocardial ischemia
- Decreased cardiovascular response to catecholamines
- Impaired tissue oxygen delivery
- Arrhythmias, e.g., atrial and ventricular fibrillation
- Decreased function of coagulation factors and platelets to make clot and thus stop hemorrhage

- Decreased number and function of WBCs
- Increased risk of wound infection, pneumonia, and sepsis.

Consequences of severe acidosis:
- Decreased cardiac output and arterial BP
- Decreased cardiovascular response to catecholamines
- Reduced threshold for developing ventricular fibrillation
- Hyperventilation
- Decreased strength and increased fatigue of respiratory muscles
- Decreasing mental status and coma
- Decreased function of coagulation factors and platelets to make clot and thus stop hemorrhage

Management:
- Triad begins and ends with bleeding, so find bleeding and stop it.
- Make every effort to expose only those body parts that need examination. Cover the rest of the parts to prevent hypothermia.
- Limit crystalloids, as these contribute to patient's acidosis and dilute the remaining clotting factors.
- Maintain tissue perfusion and avoid overly aggressive fluid administration, which can dislodge the clot and worsen hemorrhage.
- If possible, administer warm fluids (40°C).
- Measure prehospital lactate levels when available to more accurately detect cryptic shock in trauma patients with normal vital signs. $ETCO_2$ may also be a useful marker.
- Monitor and maximize oxygenation.
- Treat causes of hypoventilation to prevent respiratory acidosis.
- Administer tranexamic acid to prevent clot breakdown and thus decrease blood loss from vulnerable sites.

1.3 MEDICAL TOPICS IN ORTHOPEDICS (Q61–69)

61. **Discuss diagnosis of gout, newer drugs in gout, and its specific indications.**

Ans: The term gout is used to represent a heterogeneous group of diseases found exclusively in the human species related to elevated uric acid levels.

Diagnosis: The American College of Rheumatology has suggested 11 criteria (clinicoradiological) and the presence of six or more suggests that gout is present.
1. More than one attack of active arthritis
2. Maximum inflammation develops within one day
3. Oligoarthritis attack
4. Redness observed over joint
5. First metatarsophalangeal joint painful or swollen (podagra)
6. Unilateral first metatarsophalangeal joint attack
7. Unilateral tarsal joint attack
8. Tophus (proven or suspected)
9. Hyperuricemia—serum uric acid levels are elevated (> 7 mg/dL in males and > 6 mg/dL in postmenopausal females). However, during an acute attack, serum uric acid may be normal in 50% cases.
10. Asymmetrical swelling within a joint on radiography—sharply punched out round to oval defects situated in the marginal areas of the joint that are surrounded by a sclerotic border. The appearance of clasp-like erosions in a distribution that is typical for gout is nearly pathognomonic. Periarticular osteopenia is absent and joint space is preserved in gout.
11. Complete termination of an attack.

Synovial fluid examination by polarized microscopy can demonstrate urate crystals. They are seen as slender, needle-shaped, and negatively birefringent structures.

Newer medications: Apart from the routine drugs such as allopurinol, oxipurinol, and probenecid, some newer drugs have been introduced in the market for treatment of gout and include:
- *Febuxostat*: It decreases production of uric acid by selectively inhibiting the enzyme xanthine oxidase. It is indicated for chronic gout in the intercritical period and has been found to be superior in reducing serum urate levels in stage 2 or 3 chronic kidney disease. There is a labeled warning concerning cardiovascular safety with the use of febuxostat.
- *Lesinurad*: It is a selective uric acid reabsorption inhibitor (SURI) that is used in combination with febuxostat or allopurinol whose gout is not controlled by current medications. The drug works by inhibiting a protein called urate transporter 1 (URAT1), which is responsible for the majority of uric acid reabsorption by the kidneys. Because of different mechanism of action of lesinurad from xanthine oxidase inhibitors (XOIs), it can be even prescribed as a fixed dose combination drug with XOIs.
- *Rasburicase*: It is recombinant urate oxidase that increases metabolism of uric acid.
- Pegloticase is another similar drug that is pegylated to increase duration of action.
- *BCX4208*: This is under development for reduced uric acid synthesis. The drug acts by inhibiting purine nucleoside phosphorylase (PNP) enzyme of the purine salvage pathway.
- *Interleukin 1 blockers*: These drugs are relevant in controlling the acute flare-ups that are partly mediated by IL-1. Study on rilonacept and canakinumab suggests symptomatic improvement in patients failing to respond to NSAIDs and colchicine in acute gout flares.

62. Describe pathogenesis and management of gout.

Ans: Kindly also see Answer to Question 61.

Pathogenesis: Prolonged hyperuricemia at concentrations yielding supersaturation (generally, serum uric acid > 7.0 mg/dL) leads to precipitation of crystals in soft tissues. This process is facilitated by trauma or microtrauma/surgery, dietary changes, acute illness, dehydration, and administration of serum urate-lowering medications. Monosodium urate (MSU) crystals deposit in synovium and are coated with a variety of serum proteins, notably immunoglobulins. These attract and enhance phagocytosis by polymorphonuclear (PMN) leukocytes which due to inability to disintegrate the crystals produce uncontrolled inflammation enhanced by chemoattractants, including IL-1 and a specific PMN-derived crystal-induced chemotactic factor. PMN lysis occurs due to crystals further releasing lysosomal contents causing indiscriminate tissue damage and symptoms.

Management: Medicines are the mainstay of treatment both in acute stage and chronic one.
- The treatment is aimed primarily at terminating the acute attack as fast and as gently as possible, to reverse or prevent complications of crystal deposition and to prevent recurrences of acute arthritis.
- Nonsteroidal anti-inflammatory drugs are the mainstay for controlling inflammation during acute attack or flare. Few NSAIDs also have uricosuric effect (etodolac, etoricoxib) and can be of clinical value.
- Corticosteroids (through various routes) have been found to be highly effective in controlling the acute flares.
- For acute severe attack (VAS of ≥ 7 on scale of 10), initial combination therapy with full dose of either: (1) colchicine and NSAIDs; (2) oral corticosteroids and colchicine; or (3) intra-articular steroids with all other modalities have been recommended. Colchicine has a low therapeutic index and usually an oral dose of 0.5 or 0.6 mg is taken hourly until one of three things occurs: (1) Joint symptoms ease; (2) Nausea, vomiting, or diarrhea develops; or (3) The patient has taken a maximum of 10 doses. If 10 doses are taken without benefit, the diagnosis should be questioned. Colchicine inhibits E-selectin mediated adhesiveness for neutrophils and diminishes neutrophil L-selectin expression, random motility, chemotaxis, PLA2 activation, and IL-1 expression, and the chemotactic factors CCF and LTB4.
  For chronic gout, the pharmacotherapy is primarily directed to reduce the serum uric acid levels and prophylaxis for acute attack:
- Reduction of the serum urate concentration is achieved pharmacologically by:
  – Increasing the renal excretion of uric acid (uricosuric agents) or
  – By decreasing uric acid synthesis.
- For those patients with gout who excrete < 800 mg of uric acid per day and have normal renal function, reduction of serum urate concentration can be achieved equally well with a xanthine oxidase inhibitor or a uricosuric drug.

Allopurinol is probably the drug of choice because it can be used with fewer restrictions compared to uricosuric agents in most cases.
- Uricosuric agents such as probenecid are indicated in patients < 60 years with hyperuricemia and urinary excretion of < 800 mg/24 hours on a regular diet, satisfactory renal function, no renal calculi and absence of polypharmacy. These agents are ineffective with compromised renal function and GFR of < 30 mL/minute.
- Concomitant colchicine or NSAID cover should be used to prevent acute attacks due to crystal dissolution and reprecipitation.
- Fenofibrate may provide an attractive option for those subjects with both hyperuricemia and hyperlipidemia additionally, given in combination it suppresses the acute flare associated with rapid lowering of uric acid levels seen with allopurinol.
- In certain situations (urate excretion > 1,000 mg/day, urate nephropathy, nephrolithiasis, prophylaxis for tumor lysis syndrome, gout with renal insufficiency (GFR < 60 mL/min) and allergy to or failure of uricosurics), an inhibitor of xanthine oxidase is clearly the drug of choice in the gouty patient. It is effective in virtually all cases of hyperuricemia but is typically indicated for:
    - Patients with either renal insufficiency or a 24-hour urinary uric acid excretion of greater than 1,000 mg/day
    - Noncompliance or failure to respond to with uricosuric agents
    - A history of renal calculi of any type and a urinary uric acid excretion of greater than 600 mg/24 hours
    - Prophylaxis or treatment of tumor lysis syndrome.
- Febuxostat is also not reincorporated into nucleotides and does not regulate pyrimidine metabolism. It has been found superior in reducing serum urate levels in stage 2 or 3 chronic kidney disease patients compared to allopurinol.
- Uricase therapy has been tried and is still evolving. Expression of uricase enzyme ceased in human during evolution. The therapy is based on premises that the enzyme converts uric acid to allantoin (along with one hydrogen peroxide molecule) which is much more soluble and the fact that rodents that express uricase have uric acid levels less than 1 mg/dL. The therapy is associated with oxidative stress (hydrogen peroxide) producing methemoglobinemia and hemolysis that could be substantial in patients with G6-PD deficiency.

63. **What is pseudogout? Discuss its pathology, clinical features, and treatment. Differentiate between gout and pseudogout.**

Ans: Pseudogout is a nonurate crystal arthropathy caused by deposition of calcium pyrophosphate dihydrate ($Ca_2P_2O_7 \cdot 2H_2O$, or CPPD) crystals in the loose, avascular connective tissue matrices of articular hyaline cartilage, fibrocartilage nous menisci, and of certain ligaments and tendons that are particularly susceptible to calcification.

Pathology: Pyrophosphate is probably generated in abnormal cartilage by enzyme activity at chondrocyte surfaces; it combines with calcium ions in the matrix where crystal nucleation occurs on collagen fibers. The crystals grow into microscopic "tophi," which appear as nests of amorphous material in the cartilage matrix. *Chondrocalcinosis* is most pronounced in fibrocartilaginous structures (e.g., the menisci of the knee, triangular ligament of the wrist, pubic symphysis and intervertebral disks) but may also occur in hyaline articular cartilage, tendons, and periarticular soft tissues. From time to time, CPPD crystals are extruded into the joint where they excite *an inflammatory reaction* similar to gout. The long-standing presence of CPPD crystals also appears to influence the development of *osteoarthritis* in joints not usually prone to this condition (e.g., shoulders, elbows, and ankles). Characteristically, there is a hypertrophic reaction with marked osteophyte formation. Synovitis is more obvious than in "ordinary" osteoarthritis.

Clinical features: Clinically, CPPD affects a similar population to that of osteoarthritis. CPPD is very often clinically silent, but is a biomarker of aging, connective tissue degeneration, and low-grade inflammation. In most patients, CPPD appears to represent a systemic articular and soft-tissue pathophysiology disorder in aging as supported by the GOAL study. It becomes more prevalent with age and affects about 5% of the population. The disease may be asymptomatic, acute, subacute, or chronic or may cause acute synovitis superimposed on chronically involved joints. The clinical features in many cases are very similar to osteoarthritis: joint pain, crepitus, and stiffness after prolonged rest. However, radiographic evidence of CPPD at one joint is frequently associated with CPPD at distant joints, whether osteoarthritis is present or not.

CPPD has a predilection for joints different from typical osteoarthritis although knee is still the most frequent joint involved. But it is interesting to note that knee osteoarthritis, but not hip osteoarthritis, is associated with radiographic evidence of CPPD at distant joints. These joints susceptible for CPPD disease include the radioscaphoid joint, the scapho-trapezio-trapezoidal (STT) joint, the MCP joints (particularly, the second and third), the patellofemoral joint, and the talonavicular joint. There is no clear correlation between the extent of calcification and progression of CPPD. CPPD is polyarticular in around 70% patients and radiographic demonstration of punctate and/or linear radiodense deposits in fibrocartilaginous joint menisci or articular hyaline cartilage (called *chondrocalcinosis*), the diagnosis of CPPD disease is supported over osteoarthritis.

Other features that help make the diagnosis of CPPD over osteoarthritis include:
- Axial involvement
- Sacroiliac erosions
- Cortical erosions of femur
- Osteonecrosis of medial femoral condyle.

It should be borne in mind that chondrocalcinosis is also seen in calcium oxalate deposition. CPPD also has a tendency to present with occasional flares where patients develop acute inflammation in the joint, swelling from a joint effusion and erythema.

Other clinical manifestations of CPPD deposition include:
- Worsening of typical forms of osteoarthritis
- Neuropathic arthritis-like induction of severe destructive disease, e.g., the Milwaukee shoulder
- Rheumatoid arthritis (RA)-like production of symmetric synovitis (sometimes seen in familial forms with early onset),
- Ankylosing spondylitis-like intervertebral disk and ligament calcification with restriction of spine mobility that mimics (also seen in hereditary forms)
- Spinal stenosis (most commonly seen in the elderly)
- Rarely periarticular tophus-like nodules

Treatment: Approaches aim to control the acute attacks and lessen chronic and anatomically progressive sequelae of crystal deposition. There is no specific treatment for idiopathic CPPD deposition disease. NSAIDs, steroids through various routes of administration, colchicine, synthetic adrenocorticotropic hormone (ACTH) are mainstays for controlling acute attacks. Chloroquine has been found to be effective in treating polyarticular crystal deposition disease. Patients with pseudorheumatoid disease may potentially respond to methotrexate (MTX). Arthroscopic irrigation and colchicine help in osteoarthritic CPPD deposition disease. Novel targeting therapies include probenecid that suppresses ANK-induced and transforming growth factor beta (TGF)-β-induced increases in extracellular inorganic pyrophosphate in vitro. Phosphocitrate is an inorganic pyrophosphate analog that inhibits nitric oxide (NO)-induced calcification of cartilage and suppresses cell-stimulation and recruitment in hyaluronic acid and CPPD crystal deposition. Phosphocitrate also suppresses the ankylosing features of crystal deposition disease but has low bioavailability and needs to be given parenterally. Bisphosphonates (pyrophosphate analogs) can be beneficial in some cases of idiopathic infantile arterial and periarticular calcification, including disease associated with PC-1/NPP1 deficiency.

The differences between pseudogout and gout are given in **Table 1.3.1**.

TABLE 1.3.1: Differences between pseudogout and gout.	
Pseudogout	**Gout**
The classical features are found in large joints	Smaller joints of hands and feet are predominantly affected
The patients have pain similar to osteoarthritis and degenerative joint disease; inflammation is minimal	Pain characteristically has an intense inflammatory component, felt throughout day but increasing in morning or with change in weather
The margins of joint are irregular (enlarged joints) with osteophytes and bony swelling	The joints are inflamed and tender with classical signs
Radiologically chondrocalcinosis is seen in advanced cases in the form of fine calcified cartilage line	Serologically patients have elevated uric acid levels
Examination of joint fluid reveals calcium pyrophosphate crystals	The patients have characteristic uric acid needle-like crystals

64. Enumerate bleeding disorders. How will you manage a grossly arthritic knee in hemophilia?

Ans: *Bleeding disorders*: The bleeding disorders may arise from one of the following reasons:
- Platelet abnormality—idiopathic thrombocytopenic purpura (ITP), Glanzmann thrombasthenia, Bernard–Soulier syndrome, and antiplatelet drugs.
- Vascular abnormality—hereditary hemorrhagic telangiectasia, Ehlers–Danlos syndrome, Marfan syndrome, and scurvy.
- Coagulation disorders—Von Willebrand disease, hemophilia A and B, and factor 11 deficiency.
- Acquired—liver disease, uremia, hyperglobulinemia, and DIC.

Management of hemophilic arthropathy knee: Intra-articular hemorrhages are the most common manifestations of spontaneous bleeding in patients with hemophilia. Hemophilic arthropathy may also develop in patients with thrombopathy, thrombocytopenia, or von Willebrand disease (vWD). Ankle, knee, and elbow joints are most commonly affected. The "blood" is a strong irritant of synovium and engenders chronic synovitis with acute exacerbations. These changes are persistent due to hemosiderin deposition within synoviocytes and stroma. The friable villous hypertrophic synovium is further susceptible to recurrent hemorrhages and vicious cycle ensues. Iron is a potent stimulator of proinflammatory cytokines that produce synovitis and also has a direct toxic effect on cartilage. This leads to development of degenerative arthropathy that produces often rapidly in absence of treatment and persistent intra-articular milieu. Synovial proliferation produces joint swelling that persists for long and patients have painful joints due to inflammation limiting the ROM making joints stiff in long run. Hemorrhagic joint effusions also cause increased blood flow to the bone around the joint possibly due to inflammation. There is epiphyseal overgrowth (and early fusion) and other bony changes due to persistent inflammation causing limb length discrepancy.

Diagnosis: Clinically, patients have enlarged, swollen, stiff, and painful joints combined with wasting of surrounding muscles. There is subnormal gain in height due to premature epiphyseal fusion. Severe intramuscular hemorrhages may produce "hemophilic pseudotumor" formation in unusual cases. The characteristic radiographic appearance includes:
- Joint effusions (acute hemorrhages)
- Periarticular osteoporosis
- Enlarged epiphysis (distal femoral more prominent)
- Relatively thinned diaphysis
- Degenerative changes viewed as loss of joint space
- Widened intercondylar notch in knee
- Squaring of inferior patellar pole
- Flattened condylar surfaces of femur.

Radiological staging can be done using Arnold–Hilgartner system:
Stage 1—soft tissue swelling
Stage 2—periarticular osteoporosis
Stage 3—subchondral cyst but joint mostly well-formed
Stage 4—narrowing of joint space
Stage 5—severe arthritis of affected joint.

Magnetic resonance imaging is quite sensitive in early diagnosis as it easily picks the hemosiderin signals. There is characteristic demonstration of siderotic synovitis in the form of thickened synovium with low signal due to hemosiderin susceptibility effect. Cartilage erosions are also quite evident. Arthritic changes are evident in most by second to third decade depending on disease severity.

Hematological investigations are needed for quantification of factor deficiency and staging of hemophilia. Also, one needs investigation to screen for factor VIII inhibitors.

Treatment: *Supportive and conservative treatment* primarily comprises of replacement of the deficient factor (VIII, costly) or FFP (factor IX) started as soon as the prodromal symptoms develop to maintain 50% of activity. This is also required when planning a major surgery. Patients receiving cryoprecipitate are at risk of developing HIV and hepatitis B and C infection so factor VIII concentrate is the preferred modality. The patients undergoing joint replacement should be

monitored for deficient factor levels; presence of high titers of factor VIII inhibitor is a contraindication to this surgery. Desmopressin may be used in mild cases of factor VIII deficiency. The usual recommendations for maintenance of factor VIII levels are as follows:
- For rigorous physiotherapy—maintain at least 20% of levels
- For prevention of intramuscular hematoma formation—at least 30% of the levels
- For acute hemarthrosis and soft tissue surgery—at least 40–50% of the levels
- For surgery on bone—maintain 100% preoperative levels and following 1 week of surgery.

Synoviorthesis (Radionucleotide/chemical synovectomy): Intra-articular injection of either yttrium-90 (^{90}Y), gold (^{198}Au), rhenium (^{186}Re) or phosphorous-32 (^{32}P) as a radioactive agent is used for synovial tissue destruction. Because of the concerns of radiation and subsequent development of malignancy chemical synovectomy may be preferred with osmic acid, etc.

Operative management comprises of one of the following modalities as needed:
- *Synovectomy (arthroscopic preferred but open may also be done)*: It is needed for recurrent hemarthrosis and proliferative synovitis not responding to conservative management. It also helps in limiting pain and swelling.
- *Total joint arthroplasty/arthrodesis*: It is indicated in end-stage arthropathy with gross joint destruction.
- *Osteotomy*: It may be needed to restore alignment and correct deformity around knee, hip or ankle.

65. Define hemophilic cyst.

Ans: Hemophilic cyst is also known as hemophilic pseudotumor first described by Starker in 1918. These basically develop from chronically evolving hematoma slowly expanding the bone in severe forms of the disease. The hematoma fails to coagulate while its feeder would continue pumping blood into the cavity. Most develop in muscles or intermuscular planes while some may develop in bone(s) (femur, pelvis, tibia, and bones of the hand) or subperiosteally *de novo*. They are an uncommon feature of the disease occurring in 1–2% cases only and that too with severe deficiency of factor. Patients between 20 years and 70 years of age with severe forms of hemophilia A (factor VIII deficiency) and hemophilia B (factor IX deficiency, or Christmas disease) develop this complication and being X-linked recessive genetic disorders, pseudotumors are found almost exclusively seen in men. Typical appearance is of an encapsulated, chronic, and slowly expanding hematoma that may erode adjacent bone if it develops in muscle with broad tendinous insertion. Internal calcification or ossification may be seen. Osseous pseudotumors are uniformly lytic expansile lesions that grow usually eccentrically but may involve complete bone segments replacing the native tissue. Osseous trabeculae traverse the lesion and reactive sclerosis is seen at the margins. Dystrophic calcification or ossific foci may be also seen. Subperiosteal bone formation is also common confusing the lesion to neoplasia. Pathologically, the mass consists of blood products in various stages of evolution and has a fibrous capsule that contains hemosiderin-laden macrophages. The lesion by itself is painless however pressure on adjacent structures may cause pain and neuropathy may occur due to neural compression. Large tumors may produce joint contractures and/or compartment syndrome and functio lesia.

Complications of pseudotumors:
- Exsanguination due to rupture of pseudotumor and bleeding
- Infection and fistula formation
- Pathological fracture of bone
- Compartment syndrome
- Neuropathy.

Treatment: Recent or evolving pseudotumors from ongoing hemorrhage respond best to conservative management and immobilization along with clotting factor replacement. Surgery is mostly not indicated for them unless some emergent complication is developing like compartment syndrome. Surgical management is indicated for older pseudotumors that fail to respond with conservative measures. Radiation therapy is not recommended unless surgery is contraindicated in patients failing on conservative therapy.

66. What are pseudotumors?

Ans: Kindly see Answer to Question 65 above.

67. Discuss the bleeding disorders in orthopedic practice. Discuss hemophilia pseudotumor and its management.

Ans: Kindly see Answers to Questions 64 and 65 above.

68. What are the clinical, radiological, and lab features of sexually acquired reactive arthritis (SARA)? Discuss briefly its management in a young adult male.

Ans: Clinical features of sexually acquired reactive arthritis:

The SARA presents with a clinical spectrum ranging from isolated, transient monoarthritis to severe multisystem disease. Patients typically exhibit:
- Asymmetric lower limb oligoarthritis
- Conjunctivitis
- Dysuria

Arthritis usually lasts 3–5 months but may extend up to 1 year. Chronic heel pain, low back pain, sacroiliitis, and ankylosing spondylitis are common sequelae. Dysuria may be attributed to *Chlamydia trachomatis* or sterile pyuria related to bowel infections. Approximately 20% of patients with inflammatory bowel disease develop reactive arthritis.

Radiological Features:
- MRI findings may include sacroiliac and vertebral changes similar to ankylosing spondylitis. Peripheral joint involvement may show features of erosive arthritis.

Laboratory Features:
- Tests for HLA-B27 are positive in roughly 75% of patients with sacroiliitis. Elevated ESR may occur during active disease. The causative organism can often be identified in urethral fluids or fecal specimens, and serological tests may reveal antibodies.

Management of SARA:
Diagnosis should be considered in young adults presenting with acute or subacute lower limb arthritis, especially following genitourinary or bowel infections. Initial management focuses on treating the underlying infection, particularly *Chlamydia trachomatis*. While treating the infection may not alleviate reactive arthritis, antibiotics like tetracycline can reduce recurrence risk.

Symptomatic management includes:
- Analgesics and NSAIDs
- Corticosteroid injections for aggressive inflammatory responses
- Disease-modifying antirheumatic drugs (DMARDs) if symptoms persist
- Topical steroids for associated uveitis
- There is some evidence that treatment of *Chlamydia* infection with tetracycline for periods of up to 3 months can reduce the risk of recurrent joint disease.

69. A. What are the causes of inflammatory arthritis?

B. Mention in brief the risk factors, clinical features, investigations, and management of psoriatic arthritis.

Ans:
(A) The various causes of inflammatory arthritis are:
- Monoarthritis—gout, septic arthritis, tuberculous arthritis
- Oligoarthritis—gout, spondyloarthropathy [(1) ankylosing spondylitis (AS), (2) psoriatic arthritis (PsA), (3) reactive arthritis, (4) arthritis associated with inflammatory bowel disorders (enteropathic arthritis), and (5) undifferentiated spondylarthritis (SpA)], psoriasis
- Polyarthritis—SLE, psoriasis, RA

(B) *Risk factors*:
- *Genetic predisposition*: A significant body of research indicates that genetic factors play a pivotal role in the development of PsA. A family history of psoriasis or psoriatic arthritis substantially increases the risk, suggesting a

hereditary component. Specific human leukocyte antigen (HLA) alleles, particularly HLA-B27, have been implicated in the pathogenesis of PsA, although the association is less pronounced than in ankylosing spondylitis. Additional susceptibility loci have been identified in genome-wide association studies, highlighting the multifactorial genetic landscape of PsA.

- *Environmental triggers*: Environmental factors also contribute to the onset of PsA in genetically predisposed individuals. Notably, skin trauma, such as that resulting from cuts, abrasions, or surgical procedures, can precipitate a flare of psoriasis, subsequently leading to the development of PsA, a phenomenon referred to as the Koebner phenomenon. Other environmental triggers may include infections, particularly streptococcal infections, which can initiate or exacerbate psoriatic skin lesions and potentially trigger arthritic changes.
- *Obesity*: An increasing body of evidence underscores the association between obesity and the risk of developing psoriatic arthritis. Adipose tissue is known to produce proinflammatory cytokines and adipokines, which may exacerbate systemic inflammation, thereby contributing to the pathogenesis of PsA. The correlation between obesity and the severity of psoriatic disease further emphasizes the importance of weight management in at-risk populations.
- *Metabolic syndrome*: Comorbidities associated with metabolic syndrome, including hypertension, dyslipidemia, and type 2 diabetes, have been correlated with an increased risk of PsA. This relationship may be mediated through shared inflammatory pathways that underpin both metabolic dysfunction and psoriatic disease.
- *Age and gender*: PsA can manifest at any age; however, it commonly presents in adults aged 30–50 years. The condition appears to affect men and women at roughly equal rates, although certain subtypes, such as arthritis mutilans, may exhibit a higher prevalence in men. Hormonal factors may also influence disease onset, particularly in women, where fluctuations in estrogen levels could modulate inflammatory responses.
- *Smoking and alcohol consumption*: Lifestyle factors, such as smoking and excessive alcohol consumption, have also been implicated in the development of PsA. Smoking is recognized as an independent risk factor, potentially due to its role in enhancing systemic inflammation and altering immune responses. Similarly, alcohol may exacerbate inflammation and interfere with the efficacy of treatments for psoriasis.

Clinical features:
Patients with psoriatic arthritis may exhibit a range of joint involvement patterns. These patterns can include arthritis predominantly affecting the distal IP joints, arthritis mutilans, asymmetrical large joint oligoarthritis, as well as presentations that closely resemble RA or ankylosing spondylitis. Notably, cutaneous or nail psoriasis typically precedes the onset of arthritis; however, subclinical lesions, such as those found in the natal cleft or umbilicus, may often go unnoticed.

The progression of psoriatic arthritis can vary significantly, with some cases advancing slowly while others may exhibit rapid deterioration, potentially entering quiescent phases. In certain instances, particularly among female patients, joint involvement may present symmetrically, leading to clinical presentations that can be indistinguishable from seronegative RA. Asymmetrical swelling of two or three fingers might indicate a combination of IP arthritis and tenosynovitis.

Sacroiliitis and spondylitis are observed in approximately one-third of patients, with these manifestations sometimes being the predominant feature, creating a clinical picture akin to that of ankylosing spondylitis. Furthermore, heel pain due to enthesitis is a common complaint among these patients, reflecting the disease's association with spondyloarthropathies. In advanced cases, both the spine and peripheral joints may be affected, leading to severe deformations of fingers and toes due to erosion and instability of the IP joints, characteristic of arthritis mutilans. Additionally, ocular inflammation is reported in roughly 30% of patients, further underscoring the systemic implications of this condition.

Investigations:
Imaging: *X-ray* examination may show severe destruction of the IP joints of the hands and feet; changes in the large joints are similar to those of rheumatoid disease. Sacroiliac erosion is fairly common; if the spine is involved the appearances are identical to those of ankylosing spondylitis.

Ultrasound scanning and *MRI* may show greater definition of the extent and activity of synovitis.

Special investigations: Tests for rheumatoid factor are almost always negative. HLA-B27 occurs in 50–60%, especially in those with overt sacroiliitis.

Management:

Diagnosis: The Caspar criteria for psoriatic arthritis:
A patient must have inflammatory articular disease (joint, spine, or entheseal) with 3 points from any of the following five categories:
1. Evidence of current psoriasis (assigned 2 points) a personal history of psoriasis, or a family history of psoriasis (assigned 1 point each)
2. Typical psoriatic nail dystrophy
3. Negative rheumatoid factor
4. Either current dactylitis or a history of dactylitis (demonstrated by rheumatologist)
5. Radiographic evidence of juxta-articular new bone formation (excluding osteophytes) in the hand or foot

Treatment: The treatment of PsA is directed at controlling the inflammatory process. Patients are often treated with NSAIDs for PsA, but to date evidence supporting the use of NSAIDs for PsA is scarce. In patients with severe skin inflammation, medications such as MT, retinoic acid derivatives, or psoralen plus ultraviolet light (PUVA) should be considered which are effective for both skin and joint affections. DMARDs such as sulfasalazine, MTX, and cyclosporine are also commonly used for patients with PsA but the effects are modest. Strong evidence has emerged supporting the use of anti-TNF-α agents for the treatment of PsA and biological agents might be considered first-line therapy. Prompt and dramatic resolution of both arthritis and skin lesions has been considered with etanercept, infliximab, adalimumab, and golimumab. Tofacitinib is a very good freely available agent that produces dramatic relief in skin and joint symptoms with sustained benefit. The clinical response is more dramatic than in RA, and delay of radiographic disease progression has been demonstrated. Paradoxically, rare cases have been reported of exacerbation or de novo appearance of psoriasis precipitated by anti-TNF therapy for a variety of conditions, the therapy can be continued despite this. Sustained benefits for patients with skin and joint disease were seen at 1 year in a trial using infliximab. Etanercept was also found to reduce joint symptoms, improve psoriatic lesions, and inhibit radiographic progression of disease at 1 year. Adalimumab showed similar efficacy with significantly improved joint and skin manifestations and a reduction in irreversible structural damage on radiographs. The anti-T-cell biologic agent alefacept, in combination with MTX, has shown benefit in both PsA and psoriasis. Ustekinumab, a monoclonal antibody to the shared IL-23/IL-12p40 subunit, has shown promise in treating both psoriasis and PsA in early clinical trials. The surgical treatment is aimed at restoring painless mobility of joints, though results are inferior to other groups. Patients with PsA may have skin involvement in the proposed surgical incision. Because local bacterial contamination may increase the risk of infection, it is recommended that the skin be treated aggressively with topical agents or ultraviolet light before any surgical procedure.

1.4 RESEARCH IN ORTHOPEDICS (Q70–82)

70. Describe randomized control trial.

Ans: Determined efforts have been made to use scientific technique to evaluate methods of treatment and prevention. An important advancement in this field has been the development of an assessment method, known as randomized control trial (RCT), which is really an epidemiologic experiment. RCTs have questioned the validity of widely used conventional approaches in medicine like use of oral hypoglycemic agents, varicose vein stripping, tonsillectomy, hospitalization of all patients of myocardial infarction, etc. and also many other preventive and therapeutic procedures. RCTs are considered to be the most reliable form of scientific evidence in the clinical literature that may influence practice. It is considered the gold standard for a clinical trial. RCT are typically used to test the effectiveness of different medical interventions, especially those having clinical equipoise ("genuine uncertainty within the expert medical community for following or choosing the preferred treatment"). These can be of three types depending on the organization of study based on "visibility" of treatment to observer and subjects:
- *Unblinded*: The interventionist and study subjects, both are aware of the treatment given, usually done in surgical trials.
- *Single blind*: A study is single blind, if subjects being treated are unaware of which treatment (including any control) they are receiving.
- *Double blind*: A study is considered double blind, if in addition to single blinding, the investigators of outcome variables are also unaware of type of treatment the subjects are actually receiving.

Typically, in an RCT, the randomly designed groups (two or more) of subjects are allocated treatment(s) (or no treatment) and are followed in exactly the same way differing in terms of primary question variable(s) or intervention (parallel design). A crossover design is better than a parallel design in which the study is repeated on the individual with reversed parameters (if treated early then now made control or vice versa for example) **(Flowchart 1.4.1)**. There is usually a washout period between the two periods to allow any residual effect of previous treatment (carryover) to dissipate. These crossover designs are more precise, as the variation within the individual is much less than the variation between individuals, and they require lesser number of individuals to decipher the effect but they are impractical in surgical therapies. The basic steps in conducting an RCT include the following [it is best to follow CONSORT (consolidated standards of reporting trials) guidelines]:

- Setting a relevant study question and formulating a hypothesis
- Drawing up a protocol and determining sample size based on expected type I and type II errors and outlining the outcome criteria that will answer the question or will be needed for hypothesis evaluation
- Selecting reference and experimental populations—sampling after carefully defining the inclusion and exclusion criteria
- Randomization of study population and blinding—randomization is a statistical procedure by which the participants are allocated into groups usually called study and control groups. Randomization is an attempt to eliminate bias and allow for comparability. It gives the greatest confidence that the groups are comparable so that like can be compared with like. It ensures that the investigator has no control over allocations of participants to either study or control group, thus minimizing selection bias

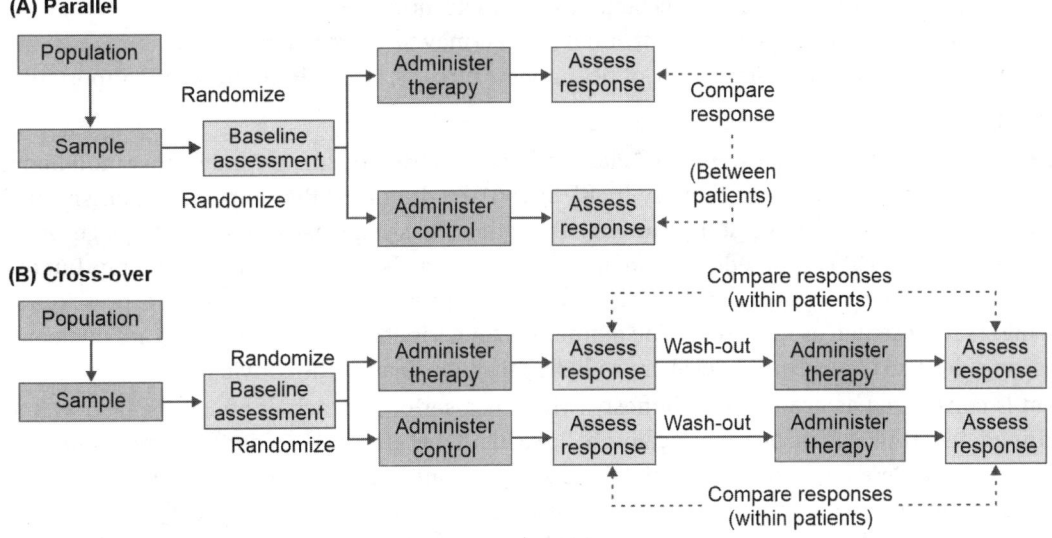

Flowchart 1.4.1: Randomized control study designs.

- Manipulation or intervention + follow-up
- Data collection and analysis of outcome measure.

(Further details on the individual steps further reading can be done from Chapter 12—Biostatistics, Ethics and Research Methods of the book Essential Orthopedics: Principles and Practice, 2nd edition.)

71. Write short notes on:
   A. Impact factor
   B. Plagiarism.

Ans: A. Impact factor (IF): It is basically an average measure reflecting the average number of citations to recent articles published in the journal. The impact factor (IF, or more precisely the 2-year impact factor) was devised by Eugene Garfield in late 1950s. It is being published since the 1960s (previously by Institute for Scientific Information®); now the reporting is done by Clarivate Analytics Journal Citation Reports® on a yearly basis. There are other measures [viz., Citescore, Eigenfactor, Google Scholar Metrics, SCImago Journal and Country Rank (SJR), Source normalized impact per paper

(SNIP), etc.] for ranking the value of journals but IF is considered the most relevant benchmark to compare the relative importance of peer-reviewed journals.

Impact factor is principally calculated as the average number of times articles from a particular journal published in the past 2 years, which have been cited in that particular year (current year of determination). An impact factor of 1 would mean that on an average, the articles published 1 or 2 year ago have been cited one time.

Importance of impact factor: It has gained acceptance as a quantitative measure of journal quality. It is used commonly for managing scientific library collections. The major dilemma is to define "citable articles" as a variety of articles that are published in journals from expert opinions to randomized comparative/control trials. In general, original research articles and review articles are included for determination of IF, but editorials containing lengthy reference list with good new knowledge content are also included.

Controversies and limitation of IF:
- Inherent to the usage, scientific journals rank higher than clinical journals; review journals score higher than original articles, though the content may not really qualify for "truly" higher impact factor.
- It does not measure impact of 1 article but a mean of all articles—may be partly taken care of by SNIP.
- A time lag exists as using the 2-year reference period (may be covered by 5-year impact factor calculation)
- High impact factor is likely in journals covering large areas of basic research than subject-specific journals (may be taken care by using SJR)
- Index is heavily skewed toward English language journals
- There is no distinction between positive and negative (critical) citations
- Calculation of impact factor is not corrected for self-citations
- Journal's internet access increases its impact factor as it attracts more readers
- Impact factor does not describe quality of individual papers (may be corrected by SNIP)
- Impact factor says nothing about stringency of peer review process, which is another very important parameter of journal quality.

B. Plagiarism: (Latin: plagiarius = kidnapper): "Plagiary" (derived from plagiarius and further modified to plagiarism now) was used to describe someone of "literary theft" in 1601 by dramatist Ben Jonson. Plagiarism in simple terms represents copying and/or publishing another author's thoughts, ideas, expression or even language, and representing as one's own original work. Different medical regulatory bodies/councils have their own definitions but in common, all have the common notion that plagiarism involves deliberate appropriation of the works (idea, expression, study, or even language) of others represented as one's own. The definitions for various aspects of this fraud are unclear however, and there are unclear rules and consensus for legal or professional action against the convict.

Plagiarism is considered as academic dishonesty, which is a serious breach of ethics of practice, and constitutes copyright infringement (that can be possibly legally challenged on this ground). Plagiarism appears similar to copyright violation but there is a difference in plagiarism that there is "gain in author's reputation" ("how much gain" is difficult to quantify in terms of "losses" to the original author—so the legal procedure falls weak) by work done by someone else, so it does not directly come under jurisdiction. In copyright violation, the author use work without consent that is protected by copyright holder and is liable to be directly challenged in court of law. In medical literature, there have been several instances (and are also coming up) where students, professors, and various researchers have used partially or completely the work done by someone else for their publication or thesis work. This amounts to academic fraud and dishonesty. Though difficult to challenge in court of law, there are chances of stringent action and even expulsion of the doer if the authority takes cognizance and sincere effort to stop such activities establishing examples for future. The practice of copying gained momentum with the increase in the published literature due to availability of online tools and also partly due to peer pressure for publication and gaining reputation. The following are considered as an act of plagiarism in general:
- Publishing or expressing someone else's work as your own in part or whole
- Not placing a quotation in quotation marks!
- Providing incorrect information about the source of a quotation
- Copying concepts, words, study material, process or ideas from someone else without giving credit
- Copying the sentence structure but modifying words (without giving credit).

Some people even resort to *self-plagiarism* (recycling fraud) where the author publishes one's own work in identical or nearly identical form at various places without acknowledging or citing the original work. These are duplicate or multiple publications, but are difficult to identify because there is a fair acceptance among the fraternity to limited reuse of work. Self-plagiarism embroils dishonesty, but not a theft per se. People argue that the term self-plagiarism in a misnomer as plagiarism involves copying others work so "self" represents oxymoron. Self-plagiarism is thought to represent specific forms of unethical conduct like dual or redundant publication.

72. Discuss the role of medical ethics in orthopedics.

Ans: The code for medical ethics for orthopedic surgeons have been comprehensively developed by the American Academy of Orthopaedic Surgeons (AAOS), the revised version as published in 2011 is as follows (no change has been made in the published text available online also with AAOS):

- **The Physician-Patient Relationship**
  - The orthopedic profession exists for the primary purpose of caring for the patient. The physician-patient relationship is the central focus of all ethical concerns.
  - The physician-patient relationship has a contractual basis, and is based on confidentiality, trust, and honesty. Both the patient and the orthopedic surgeon are free to enter or discontinue the relationship within any existing constraints of a contract with a third party. An orthopedist has an obligation to render care only for those conditions that he or she is competent to treat.
  - The orthopedist shall not decline to accept patients solely on the basis of race, color, gender, sexual orientation, religion, or national origin or on any basis that would constitute illegal discrimination.
  - The orthopedic surgeon may choose whom he or she will serve. An orthopedic surgeon should render services to the best of his or her ability. Having undertaken the care of a patient, the orthopedic surgeon may not neglect that person. Unless discharged by the patient, the orthopedic surgeon may discontinue services only after giving adequate notice to the patient so that the patient can secure alternative care. Both orthopedic surgeons and patients may have contracts with managed care organizations, and these agreements may contain provisions, which alter the method by which patients are discharged. If the enrollment of a physician or patient is discontinued in a managed care plan, the physician will have an ethical responsibility to assist the patient in obtaining follow-up care. In this instance, the orthopedic surgeon will be responsible to provide medically necessary care for the patient until appropriate referrals can be arranged.
  - It is not ethical for an orthopedic surgeon to sever his or her relationship with a patient because of failure of a treatment or because no further operative treatment is indicated. The orthopedic surgeon is ethically obligated to assist the patient in transferring care to a specialist appropriate to treat the problem.
  - When obtaining informed consent for treatment, the orthopedic surgeon is obligated to present to the patient or to the person responsible for the patient, in understandable terms, pertinent medical facts, and recommendations consistent with good medical practice. Such information should include alternative modes of treatment, the objectives, risks, and possible complications of such treatment, and the complications and consequences of no treatment.

- **Personal Conduct**
  - The orthopedic surgeon should maintain a reputation for truth and honesty. In all professional conduct, the orthopedic surgeon is expected to provide competent and compassionate patient care, exercise appropriate respect for other healthcare professionals, and maintain the patient's best interests as paramount.
  - The orthopedic surgeon should conduct himself or herself morally and ethically, so as to merit the confidence of patients entrusted to the orthopedic surgeon's care, rendering to each a full measure of service and devotion.
  - The orthopedic surgeon should obey all laws, uphold the dignity and honor of the profession, and accept the profession's self-imposed discipline. Within legal and other constraints, if the orthopedic surgeon has a reasonable basis for believing that a physician or other healthcare provider has been involved in any unethical or illegal activity, he or she should attempt to prevent the continuation of this activity by communicating with that person and/or identifying that person to a duly-constituted peer review authority or the appropriate regulatory agency. In addition, the orthopedic surgeon should cooperate with peer review and other authorities in their professional and legal efforts to prevent the continuation of unethical or illegal conduct.

- Because of the orthopedic surgeon's responsibility for the patient's life and future welfare, substance abuse is a special threat that must be recognized and stopped. The orthopedic surgeon must avoid substance abuse and, when necessary, seek rehabilitation. It is ethical for an orthopedic surgeon to take actions to encourage colleagues who are chemically dependent to seek rehabilitation.
- Orthopedic surgeons should promote their own physical and mental well-being by maintaining healthy lifestyles. They should be attuned to evolving mental or physical impairment, both in themselves and in their colleagues, and take or encourage necessary measures to ensure patient safety. These measures might include medical intervention, professional counseling, or in situations where reasonable offers of assistance are declined, reporting the impairment to appropriate authorities.

- **Conflicts of Interest**
  - The practice of medicine inherently presents potential conflicts of interest. When a conflict of interest arises, it must be resolved in the best interest of the patient. The orthopedic surgeon should exercise all reasonable alternatives to ensure that the most appropriate care is provided to the patient. If the conflict of interest cannot be resolved, the orthopedic surgeon should notify the patient of his or her intention to withdraw from the relationship.
  - If the orthopedic surgeon has a financial or ownership interest in a durable medical goods provider, imaging center, surgery center or other healthcare facility where the orthopedic surgeon's financial interest is not immediately obvious, the orthopedic surgeon must disclose that financial interest to the patient. The orthopedic surgeon has an obligation to know the applicable laws regarding physician ownership, compensation, and control of these services and facilities.
  - When an orthopedic surgeon receives anything of value, including royalties, from a manufacturer, the orthopedic surgeon must disclose this fact to the patient. It is unethical for an orthopedic surgeon to receive compensation (excluding royalties) from a manufacturer for using a particular product. Fair market reimbursement for reasonable administrative costs in conducting or participating in a scientifically sound research clinical trial is acceptable.
  - An orthopedic surgeon reporting on clinical research or experience with a given procedure or product must disclose any financial interest in that procedure or product if the orthopedic surgeon or any institution with which that orthopedic surgeon is connected has received anything of value from its inventor or manufacturer.
  - Except when inconsistent with applicable law, orthopedic surgeons have a right to dispense medication, products, assistive devices, orthopedic appliances, and similar related patient-care items, and to provide facilities and render services as long as their doing so provides a convenience or an accommodation to the patient without taking financial advantage of the patient. Ultimately, the patient must have the choice of accepting the dispensed medication, products or patient-care items or obtaining them outside the physician's office.

- **Maintenance of Competence**
  - The orthopedic surgeon continually should strive to maintain and improve medical knowledge and skill, and should make available to patients and colleagues the benefits of his or her professional attainments. Each orthopedic surgeon should participate in relevant continuing medical education activities.

- **Professional Relationships**
  - Good relationships among physicians, nurses, and other healthcare professionals are essential for good patient care. The orthopedic surgeon should promote the development and utilization of an expert healthcare team that will work together harmoniously to provide optimal patient care.
  - The professional conduct of the orthopedic surgeon may be scrutinized by local professional associations, hospitals, managed care organizations, peer review committees, and state medical and/or licensing boards. These groups merit the participation and cooperation of orthopedic surgeons.
  - Orthopedic surgeons are frequently called upon to provide expert medical opinions or testimony. In providing opinions, the orthopedic surgeon should ensure that the opinion provided is nonpartisan, scientifically correct, and clinically accurate. The orthopedic surgeon should not offer opinions concerning matters about which the orthopedic surgeon is not knowledgeable. It is unethical for an orthopedic surgeon to accept compensation that is contingent upon the outcome of litigation.

- **Relationship to the Public**
  - The orthopedic surgeon should not publicize himself or herself through any medium or form of public communication in an untruthful, misleading, or deceptive manner. Competition between and among surgeons and other healthcare practitioners is ethical and acceptable.
  - Professional fees should be commensurate with the services provided. It is unethical for orthopedic surgeons to bill individually for services that are properly considered a part of the "global service" package where defined, i.e., services that are a necessary part of the surgical procedure. It is unethical for orthopedic surgeons to submit billing codes that reflect higher levels of service or complexity than those that were actually required. It is unethical for orthopedic surgeons to charge for services not provided.
  - Physicians should be encouraged to devote some time and work to provide care for individuals who have no means of paying.
  - The orthopedic surgeon may enter into a contractual relationship with a group, a prepaid practice plan, or a hospital. The physician has an obligation to serve as the patient's advocate and to ensure that the patient's welfare remains the paramount concern.
- **General Principles of Care**
  - The orthopedic surgeon should practice only within the scope of his or her personal education, training, and experience. If an orthopedic surgeon contracts to provide comprehensive musculoskeletal care, then he or she has the obligation to ensure that appropriate care is provided in areas outside of his or her personal expertise.
  - It is unethical to prescribe, provide, or seek compensation for unnecessary services. It is unethical not to provide services that are medically necessary. It is unethical to prescribe controlled substances when they are not medically indicated. It is also unethical to prescribe substances for the sole purpose of enhancing athletic performance.
  - The orthopedic surgeon should not perform a surgical operation under circumstances in which the responsibility for diagnosis, care, or decision-making is delegated to another who is not qualified to undertake it.
  - When a patient submits a proper request for records, the patient is entitled to a copy of such records as they pertain to that individual. Charges should be commensurate with the services provided to reproduce the medical records. Certain correspondence from insurance carriers or attorneys may call for conclusions on the part of the orthopedic surgeon. As such, a reasonable fee for professional services is permissible.
- **Research and Academic Responsibilities**
  - All research and academic activities must be conducted under conditions of full compliance with ethical, institutional, and governmental guidelines. Patients participating in research programs must have given full informed consent and retain the right to withdraw from the research protocol at any time.
  - Orthopedic surgeons should not claim as their own intellectual property that which is not theirs. Plagiarism or the use of others' work without attribution is unethical.
  - The principal investigator of a scientific research project or clinical research project is responsible for all aspects of the research, including reporting. The principal investigator may delegate portions of the work to other individuals, but this does not relieve the principal investigator of the responsibility for work conducted by the other individuals.
  - The principal investigator or senior author of a scientific report is responsible for ensuring that appropriate credit is given for contributions to the research described.
- **Community Responsibility**
  - The honored ideals of the medical profession imply that the responsibility of the orthopedic surgeon extends not only to the individual but also to society as a whole. Activities that have the purpose of improving the health and well-being of the patient and/or the community in a cost-effective way deserve the interest, support, and participation of the orthopedic surgeon.

73. Describe levels of evidence in research methodology.

Ans: Kindly see the answer above.

74. Define hierarchy of evidence. Define broad principles of each level of evidence.

Ans: For established evidence-based medicine (EBM) understanding, the relative authority of presented "evidence" is important before adapting the same in practice. Before accepting any research or study outcome, one needs to have answer to simple question—"Is this the best available evidence?" Determining the "levels of evidence" helps in making the decision fast and consistently. For best decision, the levels must be easily available and in conformity to universal practice. These are commonly used to produce clinical practice guidelines that are published time and again with evolving evidence. Because a universal truth is highly unlikely in medical practice, one needs to know and believe the least harmful method/treatment at least. These evidences are classified to minimize therapeutic harm to patients by using evidence that is least likely to be wrong. Based on the Oxford Centre for Evidence-based Medicine Levels of Evidence **(Table 1.4.1)**, as given in the instructions to author for publication in Journal of Bone and Joint Surgery the following is a good acceptable guide.

TABLE 1.4.1: The accepted levels of evidence in medical literature based on Oxford Centre for evidence-based medicine.

	Therapeutic studies: Investigating the results of treatment	*Prognostic studies: Investigating the outcome of disease*	*Diagnostic studies: Investigating a diagnostic test*	*Economic and decision analysis: Developing an economic or decision model*
Level I	• Randomized controlled trial (significant difference. No significant difference but narrow) • Confidence interval • Systematic review of level I randomized controlled trials (studies were homogeneous)	• Prospective study • Systematic review of level I studies	• Testing of previously developed diagnostic criteria in series of consecutive patients (with universally applied reference "gold standard") • Systematic review of level I studies	• Clinically sensible costs and alternatives; values obtained from many studies; multiway sensitivity analyses • Systematic review of level I studies
Level II	• Prospective cohort study • Poor quality randomized controlled trial (e.g., < 80% follow-up) • Systematic review of level II studies • Nonhomogeneous level I studies	• Retrospective study • Study of untreated controls from a previous randomized controlled trial • Systematic review of level II studies	• Development of diagnostic criteria based on basis of consecutive patients (with universally applied reference "gold standard") • Systematic review of level II studies	• Clinically sensible costs and alternatives; values obtained from many studies; multiway sensitivity analyses • System review of level II studies
Level III	• Case-control study • Retrospective study • Systematic review of level III studies		• Study of nonconsecutive patients (no consistently applied reference "gold" standard") • Systematic review of level III studies	• Limited alternatives and costs; poor estimates • Systematic review of level III studies
Level IV	Case series (no or historical control group)	Case series	• Case-control study • Poor reference standard	No sensitivity analyses
Level V	Expert opinion	Expert opinion	Expert opinion	Expert opinion

75. Describe evidence-based medicine (EBM).

Ans: *Definition*: Evidence-based medicine implies the explicit, judicious, and reasonable use of latest, substantiated, and best evidence used for deciding optimal care of individual patients that integrates clinical experience/information with the current best available research on a defined question. This is a life-long process based on problem-based learning aimed to provide cost-effective and better care. With the increasing use of newer modalities and web-based interaction, EBM has grown by leaps and bounds but with rapid growth, some polluting literature is also available that has less or sometimes no credibility. This makes it imperative to set guidelines for reporting analysis or evaluation of existing or newer modalities/techniques. Nonstandardization and enormous options for similar conditions hence brings variability of expression and management of individual patients due to lack of appropriate frames, systems, and strategies, which will more efficiently influence the professional conduct. One method of improving the evidence available is to categorize its derivation into ranks according to the strength of their freedom from various biases. Thus, the classification of EBM emerged that has following ranks/levels of evidence:

1. *Level I*: Evidences obtained by meta-analysis of several randomized controlled research (RCR).
2. *Level Ib*: Evidences from only one RCR.
3. *Level IIa*: Evidences from well-designed controlled research RCR.
4. *Level IIb*: Evidences from one quasi-experimental research.
5. *Level III*: Evidences from nonexperimental studies (comparative research and case study), according to some, for example textbooks.
6. *Level IV*: Evidences from experts and clinical practice.

This considers that EBM be derived from scientific evidence for diagnostic or therapeutic procedures and relying on clinical experience or intuition is avoided. Best evidence is by far available in the form of well-organized large population blinded RCT or a systematic review of RCTs **(Fig. 1.4.1)**. Though it is difficult to determine what is true, but still with current evidence, we would come as close to the truth as possible using the available resources at least virtually. Next best is the prospective-matched cohort study where appropriate control is compared to a treatment group (and better if crossed) to study the question in interest. Then comes the case-controlled study where similar evidence is searched on a retrospective basis. Cross-sectional studies and meta-analysis are used only in specific instances. An example of increasing levels of evidence is presented in the adjoining figure that can be used to substantiate the strength of answer to question of interest.

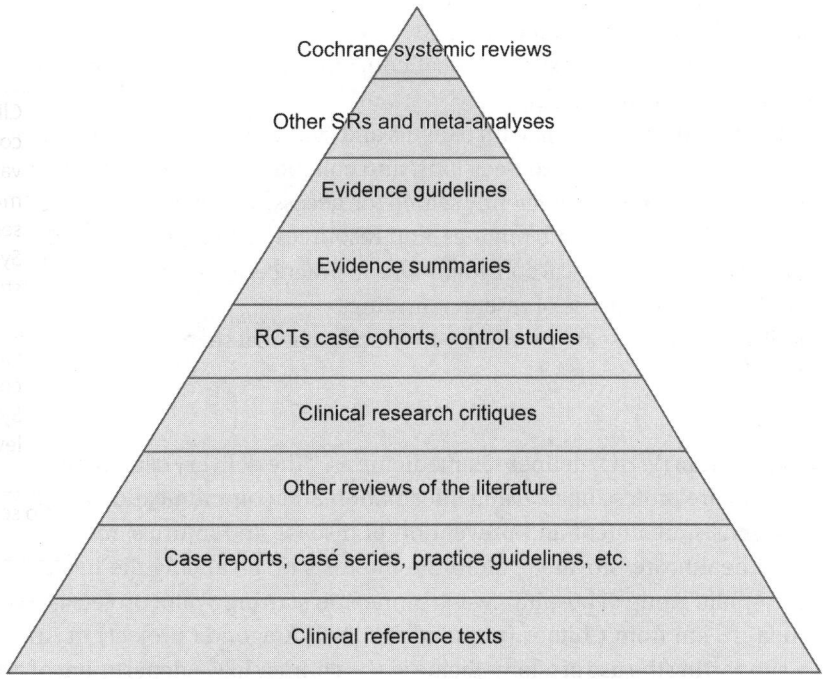

Fig. 1.4.1: Evidence-based medicine pyramid.
(RCTs: randomized controlled trials; SRs: systematic reviews)

Practice of EBM: There is a particular way to enact EBM. Foremost is the will to practice EBM and come out of the false realm of "my experience" and intuition. The following is a general method to practice EBM in any field:
- Identify the problem.
- Synthesize an answerable and fixed end-point question with input and output parameters.
- Search and research literature (articles, reviews, meta-analysis, practice guidelines, systematic reviews, etc.) for available resources and level of evidence available to answer the question. If a high-level research is available that

satisfies the question, then proceed to practice as below else one has to take the path of determining evidence based on own research and study.
- Produce concise answer to the question based on search or study.
- Use evidence by formulating protocol/formulary/guideline, etc., to improve the diagnosis/treatment/care.

76. Describe attributes required to practice evidence-based medicine.

Ans: Evidence-based medicine (EBM) is an approach to medical practice that emphasizes the use of the best available research evidence in making clinical decisions. It requires a combination of skills and attributes for effective practice. Here are some key attributes required to practice evidence-based medicine:
- *"Critical thinking"*: The ability to evaluate the validity and relevance of research findings critically. This includes assessing the quality of studies, understanding biases, and interpreting statistical data.
- *"Research literacy"*: Understanding how to read and interpret medical literature, including clinical trials, systematic reviews, and meta-analyses. This also involves familiarity with different study designs and their strengths and limitations.
- *"Clinical expertise"*: A solid foundation of medical knowledge and clinical skills is necessary to apply research findings to individual patient care effectively. This includes diagnostic skills and familiarity with current clinical guidelines.
- *"Patient-centered care"*: Being able to integrate the best research evidence with clinical expertise and patient values. This means considering patients' preferences, concerns, and unique circumstances when making clinical decisions.
- *"Lifelong learning"*: A commitment to continuous professional development and staying current with new research findings and evolving medical practices. This includes engaging with ongoing education, such as attending conferences and workshops or participating in professional networks.
- *"Statistical proficiency"*: Understanding basic statistical concepts is essential for interpreting research studies and assessing their applicability to clinical practice.
- *"Interpersonal skills"*: Effective communication with patients and colleagues is crucial. This involves explaining research findings, guiding patients in making informed decisions, and collaborating with other healthcare professionals.
- *"Information retrieval skills"*: The ability to efficiently search for, access, and manage medical literature and guidelines. This includes knowledge of databases, search engines, and resources relevant to clinical decision-making.
- *"Ethical understanding"*: Awareness of ethical considerations in practice, including issues related to informed consent, patient autonomy, and the responsible use of research findings.
- *"Adaptability"*: The ability to adapt research evidence to specific clinical scenarios and to adjust to new information as it becomes available.

77. Explain telemedicine.

Ans: The World Health Organization (WHO) defines telemedicine as, "The delivery of healthcare services, where distance is a critical factor, by all healthcare professionals using information and communication technologies for the exchange of valid information for diagnosis, treatment and prevention of disease and injuries, research and evaluation and for the continuing education of healthcare providers, all in the interests of advancing the health of individuals and their communities." In India, the Apollo group of hospitals was a pioneer in starting a pilot project at a secondary level hospital in a village called Aragonda, 16 km from Chitoor (population 5,000, Aragonda project) in Andhra Pradesh. Currently various organizations are supporting the use of telemedicine in the country like—department of information technology, the Indian Space Research Organization (ISRO), the North Eastern Council (NEC) telemedicine program for north-east, Apollo hospitals, and Asia heart foundation with active state and central government involvement.

Advantages of telemedicine:
- Accessibility to faraway areas where live programs are difficult to organize.
- Patients need not travel long distance for regular follow-ups, saving time and costs.
- Multiple centers can be connected simultaneously so communication between health providers can also be established.
- The platform can be used for continuing medical education and training.
- Surveillance and public awareness can be raised using the system.
- Public healthcare programs and schemes can be monitored and issues sorted out fast instead of calling for meetings.
- Surgery can be delivered through robotic systems (futuristic).

Methods of telemedicine delivery:
- *Store and forward method*: Here the images and data stored at a place are pushed to the other user for interpretation/evaluation at a different time and results are then sent back. This is a common example in teleradiology, telepathology, etc.
- *Interactive telemedicine*: Here both the ends have active participants taking part in live discussions/techniques through a videoconference. The participation is real time and can take upon clinical and nonclinical (research, monitoring, and surveillance) aspects.

Infrastructure requirements:
- ISDN: Integrated services digital network
- T-1: This is used to transmit the voice and data digitally
- Plain old telephone services
- Internet and internet-based services

Challenges for implementation on large scale:
- Financial viability and continuing aid
- Fear of unknown among patients and doctors
- Dissatisfaction due to lack of healing touch and personal examination by doctors
- Poor literacy rate
- Technical constraint

78. **Explain the mechanism of action of tranexamic acid. Discuss its pharmacodynamics and kinetics along with its role in prevention of excessive bleeding.**

Ans: Tranexamic acid is an antifibrinolytic hemostatic drug with chemical formula $C_8H_{15}NO_2$.

Mechanism of action: It binds to both the strong and weak binding lysine binding sites (kringle domain) on plasminogen competitively inhibiting its activation to plasmin (fibrinolysin). Thus the formation of fibrin from fibrinogen is inhibited as also conversion of procoagulant factor V and VIII to activated factors V and VIII because they all need fibrinolysin enzyme. At high concentrations, it also acts as a direct inhibitor of plasmin noncompetitively. These actions are similar to aminocaproic acid but with nearly 10 times the potency.

Pharmacodynamics and kinetics: Approximately 30–50% oral drug is absorbed and is unaffected by food intake. The plasma protein binding is 3% (mainly to plasminogen, minimal to albumin if any) of the therapeutic levels with volume of distribution of 9–12 L. Only 5% of drug is metabolized while most is secreted through renal route.

Uses:

It has been used for prevention of excessive bleeding in:
- Overdose of fibrinolytics
- After cardiopulmonary bypass surgery
- After tonsillectomy, prostatic surgery, tooth extraction in hemophiliacs
- Menorrhagia, especially due to intrauterine contraceptive device (IUCD)
- Recurrent epistaxis, ocular trauma, bleeding, peptic ulcer.
- Orthopedic and joint replacement surgery to reduce intraoperative and postoperative bleeding
- Familial angioedema (The drug inhibits activation of complement C1).

In orthopedics, tranexamic acid helps decrease the postoperative soakage, seroma, and serous fluid formation in wound and leads to wound healing with reduced risk of infection as this accumulated fluid is a good culture media for organisms to grow and cause wound infection, wound dehiscence and septicemia. It is given before any major surgical procedure, e.g., Arthroplasties and trauma cases where intraoperatively excessive bleeding is expected.

Dosage is 500 mg IV injection given slowly thrice a day for the first day and switched to oral dose of 500 mg thrice daily for 3 days.

Adverse effects: Main side effects are nausea, diarrhea, fever, and stomach pain/discomfort. Headache, giddiness, and thrombophlebitis of injected vein are other adverse effects.

Contraindications: The drug is avoided in following patients:
- Increased risk of blood clotting
- Fluid accumulation in brain
- Retinal vein clotting
- Myocardial infarction
- Valvular heart disease
- Pulmonary artery disease

79. Discuss liquid culture (MGIT) used to grow mycobacteria.

Ans: MGIT is abbreviation for *M*ycobacteria *G*rowth *I*ndicator *T*ube. It is a rapid liquid culture method as compared to the conventional solid culture methods used to grow mycobacteria. It consists of round bottom tubes containing 4 mL of modified Middlebrooks 7H9 broth which has an oxygen sensitive fluorescent sensor at the bottom.

When mycobacteria grow, they deplete the dissolved oxygen in the broth and allow the indicator to fluoresce brightly in a 365-nm UV light.

Positive signals are obtained in 10–12 days. MGIT can also be used as a rapid method for the detection of drug-resistant strains of *Mycobacterium tuberculosis* directly from acid-fast smear-positive samples as well as from indirect drug susceptibility studies.

A big disadvantage of liquid culture system is that they are more prone to contamination. It means that other bacteria can enter the system more easily and jade results.

Advantages over BACTEC:
- Cheaper
- No problem of radioactive waste disposal

80. What is the role of liquid culture [mycobacteria growth indicator tube (MGIT)] in diagnosis and management of osteoarticular tuberculosis (TB)?

Ans: Mycobacteria growth indicator tube) contains 7 mL of modified Middlebrook 7H9 Broth base + OADC enrichment + PANTA antibiotic mixture. This has been one of the most commonly used liquid media for the cultivation of mycobacteria from pulmonary and extrapulmonary samples. The tubes can be manually monitored for growth of mycobacteria or can be deployed in automated systems like BACTEC (Becton Dickinson) using fluorescent indicators to identify mycobacterial culture. The fluorescent compound used in the MGIT is sensitive to the dissolved oxygen in broth and does not show up until sufficient oxygen remains in liquid culture medium. Once the organism start growing oxygen is used up and fluorescence increases that can be detected by microMGIT fluorescence or Wood's lamp UV source reader. The BACTEC MGIT 960 System incorporates MGIT and incubate them at 37° scanning the tubes every 60 minutes for increased fluorescence. Tubes that do not show fluorescence by 42nd day are discarded as negative.

Thus, MGIT has diagnostic utility for identifying *M. Tuberculosis* infection.

Utility in management of osteoarticular TB: The culture broth can be supplanted with various antitubercular drugs and if the bacterium fails to grow then it indicates drug-susceptibility. Similarly, drug-resistance is indicated thus helping in identifying drug-resistant, multi-drug resistant, extensively drug-resistant (XDR), and total drug resistant variants.

81. Write briefly on the role of interventional radiology in orthopedics. Support with at least two examples in detail.

Ans: Interventional radiology entails use of image-guided, minimally invasive procedures for diagnosis or treatment. The technique is being increasingly used to save lives in emergency orthopedic care while it is also used for elective procedures for improved safety and better surgical procedure. The following are some of the uses:
- *Role in arterial vascular injuries*: Vascular injuries may occur during arthroplasty procedures (total knee, shoulder, and hip arthroplasties) especially in revision surgery or in patients with peripheral vascular injuries, renal failure, metastatic disease, or arteriosclerosis—they present early with signs of acute limb ischemia, including pain, pallor, pulselessness, paresthesia, and paralysis in arterial occlusion or intraoperative hemorrhage or hematoma formation postoperatively in cases of arterial laceration. Management is commonly done with open surgical repair, open thrombectomy, or

bypass grafting, however endovascular approach using embolization or covered stents offers faster approach with lower morbidity. Arterial occlusion may be managed with pharmacomechanical thrombectomy, catheter-directed pharmacological thrombolysis, or angioplasty with or without stenting.

- Late vascular complications are not uncommon especially with complicated surgeries and unconventional reconstructions. Aneurysm formation for example is seen with Ilizarov wires, screw tips, etc., multiple surgeries done for osteomyelitis and related complications risk formation of mycotic aneurysms. Such pseudoaneurysms, arteriovenous fistula or hypertrophic vascular synovium presents insidiously with persistent pain and swelling weeks to months after the initial procedure. Pseudoaneurysm after TKR commonly forms in popliteal region and is palpable as a pulsatile mass, it can be easily managed with coil embolization, thrombin injection or stent graft exclusion.
- Recurrent hemarthrosis following TKR may be due to impinging hypertrophic proliferative synovium causing recurrent bleeding and is managed by angiographic identification and embolization of genicular artery especially if the synovium is hypervascular.
- Pulmonary embolism from DVT in cases of pelvic, hip or knee surgery can be managed by placing inferior vena caval filter.
- Orthopedic oncology has found a special place for endovascular procedures. Preoperative angiography to identify major blood supply to the malignant tumor provides apt avenue for its embolization thus reducing the vascularity of tumor and better surgical field. Also, this may reduce the size of tumor making it easier to approach in difficult sites such as pelvis, spine, and scapular/axillary region. Giant cell tumors arising near epiphyseal regions and those from sacrum are most amenable to this technique. Palliative embolization for unresectable tumors or highly aggressive metastatic disease (renal/thyroid/hepatocellular carcinoma) helps in controlling pain.
- Innovative pain control embolization of neovascularization in inflammatory conditions such as knee osteoarthritis, shoulder adhesive capsulitis, Achilles tendinopathy, and plantar fasciitis has been done using transcatheter arterial embolization of abnormal neovessels (imipenem/cilastatin sodium and 75 μm Embosphere particles).

Patients needing prolonged antibiotic therapy for infected arthroplasty or recalcitrant osteomyelitis may be implanted with peripherally inserted central catheters, tunneled central lines (Hickman lines) and implantable ports.

82. Hospital/biomedical waste disposal management.

Ans: Biomedical waste is defined as any waste, which is generated during the diagnosis, treatment or immunization of human beings or animals, or in research activities pertaining thereto or in the production or testing of biologicals.

Categories of biomedical waste in India (Table 1.4.2).

TABLE 1.4.2: Categorization of biomedical waste in India.

Category	Waste Content	Components	Method of treatment and disposal
Category no. 1	Human anatomical waste	Human tissues, organs, body parts	Incineration/deep burial
Category no. 2	Animal waste	Animal tissues, organs, body parts carcasses, bleeding parts, fluid, blood and experimental animals used in research, waste generated by veterinary hospitals colleges, discharge from hospitals, animal, houses	Incineration/deep burial
Category no. 3	Microbiology and biotechnology waste	Wastes from laboratory cultures, stocks or specimens of microorganisms live or attenuated vaccines, human and animal cell culture used in research and infectious agents and industrial laboratories, wastes from production of biologicals, from research toxins, dishes and devices used for transfer of cultures	Local autoclaving/microwaving/incineration
Category no. 4	Waste sharps	Needles, syringes, scalpels, blades, glass, etc. that may cause puncture and cuts. This includes both used and unused sharps	Disinfections chemical treatment/autoclaving/microwaving and mutilation shredding

Contd...

Contd...

Category	Waste Content	Components	Method of treatment and disposal
Category no. 5	Discarded medicines and cytotoxic drugs	Wastes comprising of outdated, contaminated and discarded medicines	Incineration/destruction and drugs disposal in secured landfills
Category no. 6	Solid waste	Items contaminated with blood, and body fluids including cotton, dressings, soiled plaster casts, lines, beddings, other material contaminated with blood	Incineration, autoclaving/microwaving
Category no. 7	Solid waste	Wastes generated from disposable items other than the waste sharps such as tubing's catheters, intravenous sets, etc.	Disinfections chemical treatment/autoclaving/microwaving and mutilation shredding
Category no. 8	Liquid waste	Waste generated from laboratory and washing, cleaning, housekeeping and disinfecting activities	Disinfections by chemical treatment and discharge into drains
Category no. 9	Incineration ash	Ash from incineration any biomedical waste	Disposal in municipal landfill
Category no. 10	Chemical waste	Chemicals used in production of biologicals, chemicals used in disinfection, as insecticides, etc.	Chemical treatment and discharges into drains

Color coding and type of container for disposal of biomedical wastes (Table 1.4.3)

TABLE 1.4.3: Color coding of containers for various types of biomedical waste.

Color coding	Type of container	Waste category	Treatment options
Yellow	Plastic bag	1, 2, 3, 6	Incineration/deep burial
Red	Disinfected container/ plastic bag	3, 6, 7	Autoclaving/Microwaving/Chemical treatment
Blue/white translucent	Plastic bag (puncture proof container)	4, 7	Autoclaving/Microwaving/Chemical treatment Destruction/Shredding
Black	Plastic bag	5, 9, 10	Disposal in secured landfill

CHAPTER 2

General Orthopedics

2.1 ANATOMY OF BONE CARTILAGE AND JOINT (Q1–14)

1. Describe:
   A. The histology of growth plate.
   B. Factors causing growth disturbance.
   C. Principles of guided growth modulation.

Ans:

A. The fully developed cartilaginous growth plate (physis) in the human long bone is referred as an organ by many researchers. The physis can be divided into three components **(Fig. 2.1.1)**:
   1. The *cartilaginous component* of growth plate contains three predominant regions:
      i. *Reserve zone:* It contains spherical, single or paired chondrocytes involved in matrix production. They are full of glycogen and have predominantly anaerobic environment due to low PO_2.

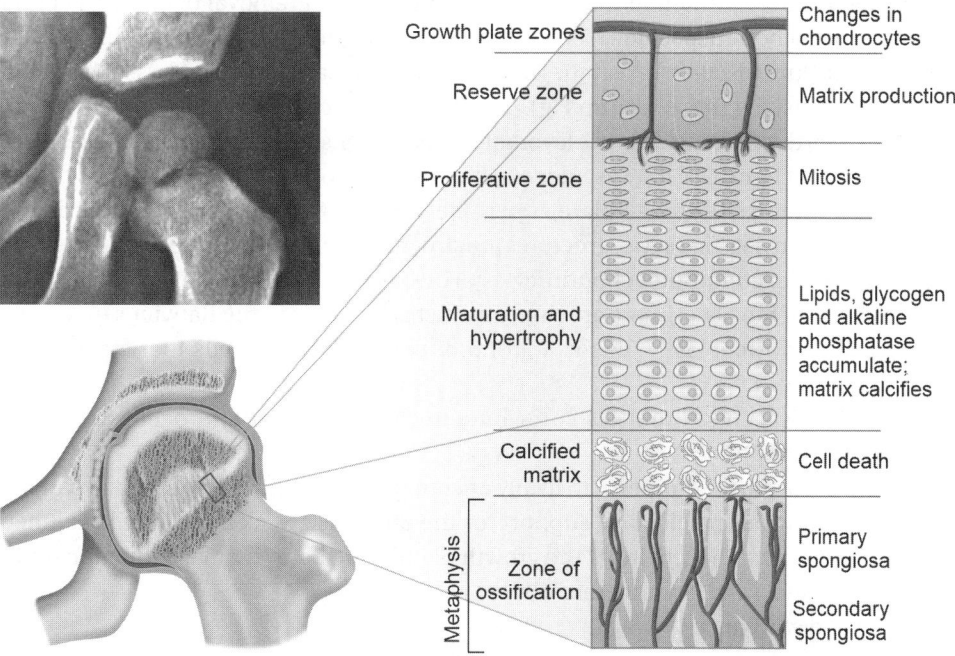

Fig. 2.1.1: Components of physis.

   ii. *Zone of chondrocyte proliferation:* This zone serves three purposes—matrix production, cellular proliferation and longitudinal growth. Latter is equal to the combination of former two. It has flattened chondrocytes arranged in distinct columns. The endoplasmic reticulum occupies progressively increasing percent of the cytoplasmic area that rises from 14.9% at the top of the zone to 40.1% at the bottom of the zone of chondrocyte proliferation. Biochemical analysis reveals that this zone contains the highest content of hexosamine, inorganic pyrophosphate and has the highest lysosomal activity. The chondrocytes in this zone are the only cells of growth plate that divide (proliferate). Due to heavy demand and consumption, oxygen tension is maintained higher in the proliferating zone of physis at mean of 57 mm Hg (± 5.8 mm Hg) compared to any other zones.

    iii. *Zone of chondrocyte hypertrophy:* This zone has three discrete functional and histological regions namely the *maturation zone, degenerative zone,* and *zone of provisional calcification.* The function of this zone is to prepare the matrix for calcification and to calcify the matrix. The chondrocytes show progressive vacuolation and increase in size with disintegration. The mitochondria instead of forming adenosine triphosphate (ATP) start to accumulate calcium. The initial calcification (seeding) occurs at the bottom of the hypertrophic zone (zone of provisional calcification) within physis. This is initiated by matrix vesicles around which then mineralization progresses.

The following sequence of events occurs for final calcification:
- Mitochondrial calcification
- Reduction of nutrients and oxygen supply to the hypertrophic chondrocyte with mitochondrial death
- Anaerobic glycolysis (this occurs due to distance from vascular supply, and hence oxygen tension in this hypertrophic zone is very low to a mean of 24.3 ± 2.4 mm Hg). All the stored glycogen is consumed
- Calcium is released from mitochondria
- Nucleation of mineralization in matrix vesicles
- Matrix calcification

2. The *bony component or metaphysis* serves few important functions. It is involved in vascular invasion of transverse septa at the bottom of cartilaginous portion of growth plate providing blood supply, the other functions are new bone formation and bone remodeling. It has two predominant components: (1) *the primary spongiosa* and (2) *the secondary spongiosa.* There is internal (histologic) remodeling with removal of calcified cartilage bars (primary spongiosa) and lamellar bone deposition (secondary spongiosa). The external or anatomic remodeling gives funnel shape to metaphysic (funnelization). Near the transverse septa separating metaphyseal from cartilage component there is low oxygen tension (19.8 ± 3.2 mm Hg). The low oxygen tension inhibits white blood cell (WBC) activity which is highly oxygen dependent, while it is favorable for pathogens. This may explain the reason for hematogenous osteomyelitis in ends of bone and not vascular stasis per se; the concept is still, however, challenged.

3. A *fibrous sheath* surrounds the growth plate at periphery that comprises perichondrial ring of LaCroix and the ossification groove of Ranvier. These two structures are structurally different and serve different functions. It appears that the groove of Ranvier contributes chondrocytes to the physis for the growth in diameter (appositional growth or latitudinal growth) of the plate. There are three distinct cell groups in the Ranvier's ossification groove:
   i. Progenitor cells for osteoblasts—this is a group of densely packed cells that forms the bony band in the perichondrial ring.
   ii. Undifferentiated cells and fibroblasts contribute to appositional chondrogenesis and are responsible for diametrical growth of physis.
   iii. Fibroblasts cover the groove and serve to firmly anchor the perichondrium of hyaline cartilage to growth plate.

The perichondrial ring provides mechanical support for the otherwise weak bone-cartilage junction of the growth plate. It is a dense fibrous band that encircles the growth plate at the bone-cartilage junction and in which collagen fibers run vertically, obliquely and circumferentially.

B. Factors causing growth disturbance:
- Trauma
- Metabolic
  - Rickets
  - Glycogen storage disorders
- Congenital
  - Epiphyseal dysplasias

- Developmental disorders—tibia vara and coxa vara
- Hormonal disorders
  - Acromegaly
  - Thyroid and parathyroid disorders.

C. Growth modulation involves exploitation of the physeal response to stress (Hueter–Volkmann law). According to this principle, excessive compression leads to tissue atrophy and inhibits the physeal growth, whereas decreased compression and moderate distraction enhances osteogenesis promoting bone growth. The effect is such that a physis subjected to angulatory forces will show retarded growth at the compression side **(Fig. 2.1.2)** and increased growth at the distraction side (tensile forces). Finely analyzed the bone is adapting itself in the direction of applied force and is in congruence with Wolff's law.

This principle is especially useful for guided growth method where the growth on the convex side of deformity is restricted by temporarily halting the growth. When the deformity is corrected then restriction can be removed for normal limb growth. Also this method can be applied for permanent methods when at a calculated time the physis growth is permanently halted on the convex side of deformity until fusion.

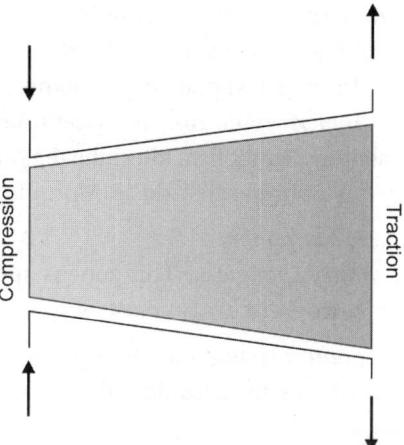

Fig. 2.1.2: Hueter–Volkmann law. Physis (growth plate) grows more on the tensile side compared to compression side.

2. Describe the structure of physis with suitable diagram. Classify physeal injuries.

Ans: Structure of physis (with diagram) has been described in answer above.

Classification of Physeal Injuries

Classification (Salter and Harris classification) of physeal injuries has been described in **Table 2.1.1**.

TABLE 2.1.1: Classification of physeal injuries—Salter and Harris classification.	
Type I	A transverse fracture through the growth plate typically through the hypertrophic zone. This manifests as increased width of physis. As the germinal portion remains intact there is no growth disturbance
Type II	A fracture through the growth plate and the metaphysis, sparing the epiphysis
Type III	A fracture through growth plate and epiphysis, sparing the metaphysis. The line of fracture passes from hypertrophic zone of physis and exits through epiphysis damaging the germinal layer. Being intra-articular prompt reduction and fixation is mandatory. Tillaux fracture is a typical example
Type IV	A fracture through all three elements of the bone, the growth plate, metaphysis and epiphysis. The straight fracture line passes through the whole width of physis and is prone to growth disturbances at healing by virtue of linear bony bar formation
Type V	A compression fracture of the growth plate due to crushing force. This results in a decreased height of the growth plate radiologically. The growth disturbance is very common and has a poor prognosis
Type VI (Rang, 1968)	Injury to the peripheral portion of the physis (zone of Ranvier) and a resultant bony bridge formation which may produce an angular deformity
Type VII (Ogden, 1982)	Isolated injury of the growth plate only—no involvement of epiphysis or metaphysis
Type VIII (Ogden, 1982)	Isolated injury of the metaphysis at the primary and secondary spongiosa region with possible impairment of endochondral ossification
Type IX (Ogden, 1982)	Injury of the periosteum (periosteal avulsion—usually iatrogenic) which may impair intramembranous ossification

3. Discuss clinical significance of physeal zones.

Ans: Cartilage component:

Reserve zone: Diastrophic dwarfism, pseudoachondroplasia, and Kniest syndrome affect this region. Basically, defects of collagen and proteoglycan synthesis or structure involve this zone (also other zones).

Proliferative zone: Susceptible to tensile stresses. Achondroplasia and hypochondroplasia, gigantism, malnutrition, Cushing's, syndrome, and irradiation affect this zone.

The slip in slipped capital femoral epiphysis (SCFE) occurs between proliferative and hypertrophic zones.

Hypertrophic zone is susceptible to shear stress and various lysosomal storage diseases. Metabolic disorders of calcium metabolism affect the region of provisional calcification. The maturation and degenerative regions are involved in mucopolysaccharidosis (Morquio and Hurler syndrome).

Bony component

Primary spongiosa: This zone is susceptible to compressive stresses. Metaphyseal chondrodysplasia (persistence of hypertrophic cells) and osteomyelitis (OM) develop here.

Secondary spongiosa: Osteopetrosis, osteogenesis imperfecta, scurvy, and metaphyseal dysplasia (Pyle disease and disorder of funnelization) develops here.

4. Discuss management of physeal injury in children.

Ans: Any physeal injury may result in growth disturbance, although it is more common after Salter-Harris types III, IV, and V fractures. Mostly types I and II fractures can be treated by closed reduction.

- Types III and IV fractures often require open reduction and internal fixation to reposition the fragments anatomically and to fix them securely so that growth in the physis may continue and the joint may be congruous. In type V fractures, the cartilage cells of the physis are crushed, and regardless of the form of treatment, growth disturbance can occur. A type V fracture usually is diagnosed only in retrospect when a growth disturbance develops.
- If a fracture involves a physis, the parents should be informed fully at the time of fracture concerning the possibility of growth disturbance.
- A type II distal femoral physeal fracture that is significantly displaced often results in growth arrest and angular deformity. A gentle closed anatomical reduction of this fracture is required to avoid crushing or otherwise injuring the germinal cells in the physis in the proximal fragment; even so, the physis may close prematurely. Many authors indicate that nondisplaced types III and IV distal tibial fractures can be treated closed.
- Crossing the physis with any form of fixation should be avoided if possible. In type III and IV fractures, the pins should cross the epiphysis in the fractured areas, and in types II and IV fractures, they should cross the metaphysis rather than the physis if possible.

5. Describe the types of cartilage. Also, describe the physiology and ultrastructural characteristics.

Ans:

Types of cartilage:
- Hyaline—most common, found in ribs, nose, trachea, and articular cartilage
- Fibrous—found in intervertebral disks, and ligaments
- Elastic—pinna, epiglottis, and larynx.

Physiology: It is a known fact that the articular cartilage is avascular so in any case the metabolism is anaerobic and that too scanty due to paucity of cellular components. Despite this, it is important to maintain a constant environment in the tissue given the high level of wear and tear of cartilage that would occur throughout the life. Subchondral bony plate separates articular cartilage from the richly vascular subchondral spaces so there is no direct nutritional supply. Articular cartilage derives its nutrition from diffusion through the synovial fluid. Due to the absence of specialized nutritional supply, the cartilage matrix itself takes over the function of selecting nutrition offered. Cartilage matrix restricts diffusion of molecules by their size, charge, and molecular configuration. Though not consistently seen (due to dynamic nature), it is estimated that the mean pore size within the extracellular matrix (ECM) is about 6.0 nm. The anaerobic metabolism of chondrocytes can be altered by a variety of factors. These affect the immediate microchemical and mechanical environment of chondron. Cytokines and various growth factors mediate the intercellular communications. The factors have autocrine, paracrine and endocrinal influence. Alteration in the cytokine milieu as is seen in diseases such as rheumatoid arthritis (RA), osteoarthritis, and osteoporosis due to altered production causes abnormal responses by cartilage cells. They also affect the underlying bone. Some of identified cytokines affecting articular cartilage are:

- *Insulin-like growth factors (IGFs):* IGF-1 (somatomedin C) and IGF-II are trophic to articular cartilage and stimulate deoxyribonucleic acid (DNA) and cartilage matrix synthesis. They are mostly important in immature cartilage of growth plate, but also play determinant role in adult articular cartilage.
- *Transforming growth factors (TGFs):* TGFβ 1–3 stimulate synthesis of proteoglycans while suppressing the type II collagen synthesis. It stimulates synthesis of plasminogen activator inhibitor-1 and tissue inhibitor of matrix metalloproteinases (MMPs), protecting the cartilage from degradation.
- *Acidic and basic fibroblast growth factors (aFGF and bFGF):* They may be involved in cartilage repair as they stimulate DNA synthesis in chondrocytes.
- *Interleukins (ILs):* IL-1β, IL-6 and IL-8 stimulate chondrocyte as regards the synthesis, secretion and maintenance of proteoglycans into the ECM by them.
- *Tumor necrosis factor (TNF):* TNF-α plays a role in the degradation and synthesis of matrix macromolecules, especially metabolism of proteoglycans.
- *Colony-stimulating factor (CSF):* Macrophage CSF stimulates cartilage repair following injury.
- *Others:* Prostaglandins and parathyroid hormone-related peptide (PTHrP) affect healing of cartilage, especially the degenerative one.

The cartilage macromolecules once formed are rarely recycled. For example, proteoglycan turnover can take up to 25 years and is mostly limited to late adult life. The half-life of collagen ranges from several decades to 400 years. Once damaged, new chains and macromolecules need to be synthesized and integrity restored. MMPs like the collagenases, gelatinases and stromelysins, and the cathepsins primarily the cathepsin B and D are mainly involved in cartilage turnover. These enzymes have specific functions, principles of which are:

- Degradation of aggrecan by cathepsins
- Degradation of helical collagen fibrils by collagenase that acts at a single site
- Stromelysin degrades the protein core of aggrecan causing disintegration of the molecule
- Gelatinase acts as scavenger and digests denatured types II and IV collagen which is seen in elderly. Gelatinase also digests fibronectin, elastin, and collagen types V, VII, X, and XI to make up space for further protein synthesis and incorporation.

Metalloproteinases are secreted as latent proenzymes that remain inactive until activated extracellularly. This process is inhibited by matrix metalloproteinase inhibitor (MMPI). Inactivation of MMP is an emerging trend in prevention of joint degenerative disorders (osteoarthritis) and even RA. Some antibiotics like doxycycline and minocycline have been found to be useful to this effect.

Ultrastructural characteristics (**Fig. 2.1.3**): Hyaline cartilage is the chief component of articular cartilage typically (fibrocartilage is seen in repair of damaged articular cartilage, callus, and at tendon-ligament insertion; fibroelastic cartilage is seen in menisci) and is 1–4 mm thick. It is composed of a dense ECM that comprises the main tissue and only a thin distribution of *chondrocytes*. The cartilage cells or chondrocytes are surrounded immediately by pericellular matrix containing proteoglycan and noncollagenous proteins (no collagen), completely engulfing the chondrocyte. Surrounding this is the territorial matrix containing collagen fibrils possibly providing mechanical protection to chondrocytes during loading. As a functional unit, the chondrocyte along with its pericellular microenvironment form the "chondron". The chondron has been classically considered to represent primary

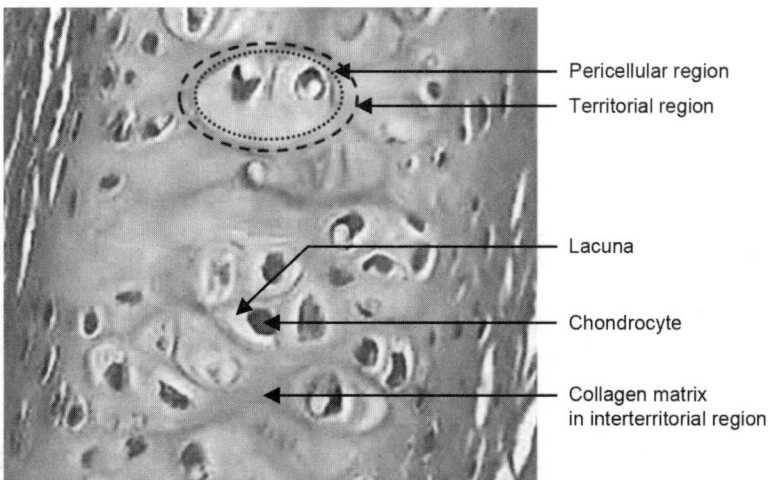

Fig. 2.1.3: Cartilage structure.

structural, functional, and metabolic unit of articular and other hyaline cartilages. The concept of the chondron historically was introduced by Benninghoff (1925) who identified it using polarized light microscopy. Later these structural units were released from tibial cartilage in the mid-1980s by Poole et al., demonstrating the individuality of chondrons. This finding conclusively established that chondron is a microanatomical unit defining the adult articular cartilage. Grossly each chondron is made up of a single chondrocyte that is attached peripherally to transparent pericellular glycocalyx. This is then further enclosed within a fibrillar pericellular capsule serving together as a basic structural unit. Macrostructurally, the chondrocytes are distributed in different zones of articular cartilage together with ultrastructural matrix of collagen fiber and ECM. There are five discrete zones in a hyaline cartilage primarily depending on the collagen fibers alignment, which impart each zone particular function biomechanically.

1. *Superficial zone (gliding zone and tangential collagen fibers)*—resistant to shear; has few, if any, metabolic activity. It has the lowest proteoglycan and highest water content and is covered by fine layer called "lamina splendens".
2. *Transitional zone (middle zone and oblique collagen fibers)*—resistant to compression, active metabolism of chondrons, and ECM proteins.
3. *Radial zone (deep zone and vertical collagen fibers)*—resistant to compression, collagen synthesis, and crosslinking zone. It has the highest proteoglycan content and lowest water.
4. *Tidemark*—resistant to shear.
5. *Calcified zone*—basically acts to anchor articular cartilage and subchondral bone and prevents transport of nutrients from underlying bone.

When examined under low power microscopy (10×), three theoretical regions can be identified within each zone—(1) the pericellular region, (2) the territorial region, and (3) the interterritorial region (largest region comprising collagen fibrils with specific spatial distribution in different zones and proteoglycan) which is responsible to most of material properties of cartilage.

6. Describe morphology of articular cartilage and changes that occur in articular cartilage in osteoarthritis.

Ans: The different zones of articular cartilage are described in Answer to Question 5. **Figure 2.1.4** (Zone 1) illustrates these different zones of cartilage.

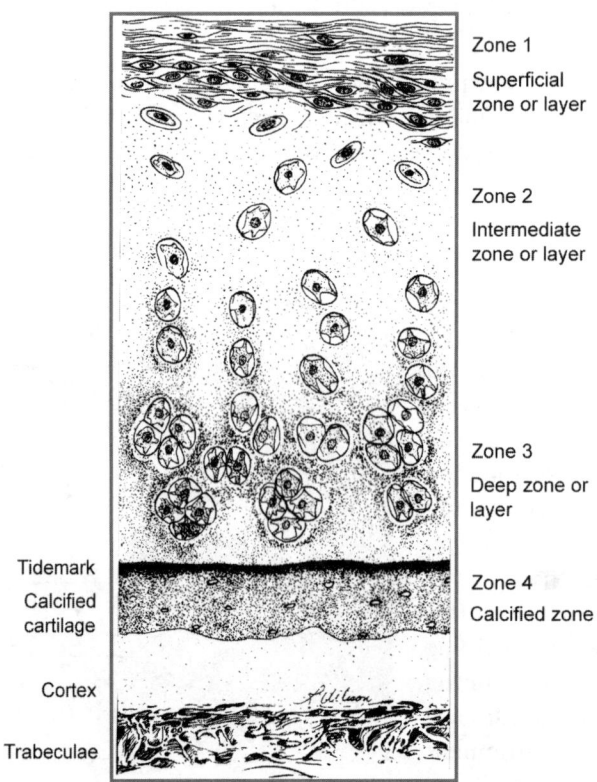

Fig. 2.1.4: The different zones of articular cartilage.

Changes in osteoarthritis: There is an imbalance between the catabolic and anabolic pathways of cartilage metabolism in osteoarthritis. The catabolic pathways are commonly associated with proinflammatory proteins, including IL-1β, TNF-β, IL-17, macrophage inflammatory protein-1β (MIP), etc. Proteinases (such as cysteine proteinases, metalloproteinases, and serine proteinases) are upregulated in response to stress on cartilage. There is impairment of production of new extracellular matrix proteins by chondrocytes under the influence of cytokines while increased degradation of the products already present. Matrix metalloproteinases (MMPs) have been linked to development of osteoarthritis due to their effect on cartilage degradation. *Traumatic insult* and increased IL-1 stimulate chondrocytes to undergo cell division "cloning") and start repair, producing increased quantities of collagen, metalloproteinases and proteoglycans. This leads to thickening of cartilage in the very early stages of osteoarthritis (because of increased proteoglycan accumulation) but the repaired tissue has qualitatively inferior type 1 collagen and has increased fibronectin. Patchy sclerosis and osteophytes however, reduce bone elasticity transferring increasing loads to the cartilage causing further damage. With passage of time, however, because of continuing cell damage and the release of cathepsins and metalloproteinases there is a loss of cartilage. Synovitis occurs in reaction to degraded cartilage and bone and soluble matrix proteins.

The osteoarthritic changes are found to progress in following stages:

Stage 1: Proteolytic breakdown of the cartilage matrix along with altered chondrocyte metabolism. The chondrocytes produce increased number of catabolic enzymes (metalloproteinases such as collagenase and stromelysin) destroying the cartilage matrix. The production of protease inhibitors [tissue inhibitors of metalloproteinases (TIMP) 1 and 2] is reduced.

Stage 2: Fibrillation and erosion of the cartilage, releasing the degenerated and altered proteoglycan and collagen fragments into synovial fluid producing inflammatory reaction.

Stage 3: Chronic inflammatory reaction in the synovium. Production of metalloproteinases, IL-1, and TNF-β by synovial macrophages; further increasing the cartilage breakdown. Other proinflammatory molecules such as free radicals may also be a factor in Stage 3.

Stage 4: With the loss of cartilage, there is alteration in the joint architecture, and compensatory bone overgrowth to distribute pressure over a larger surface area. These changes, however, further irritate the synovium and a vicious cycle gets laid down.

7. Classify cartilage injury according to configuration and severity.

Ans: Classification of articular lesions by configuration (Bauer and Jackson) is given in **Table 2.1.2**.

TABLE 2.1.2: Classification of articular lesions by configuration (Bauer and Jackson).

Type	Configuration
I	Linear
II	Stellate
III	Flap
IV	Crater
V	Fibrillation
VI	Degrading

Classification of articular cartilage lesions by severity is given in **Table 2.1.3.**

TABLE 2.1.3: Classification of articular lesions by severity.

Grade	Outerbridge	Modified outerbridge	International Cartilage Repair Society (ICRS)
0	Normal cartilage	Intact cartilage	Intact cartilage
I	Softening and swelling	Chondral softening or blistering with intact surface	Superficial (soft indentation or superficial fissures and cracks)

Contd...

Contd...

Grade	Outerbridge	Modified outerbridge	International Cartilage Repair Society (ICRS)
II	Fragmentation and fissures in area <0.5 inch in diameter	Superficial ulceration, fibrillation, or fissuring <50% of depth of cartilage	Lesion less than half the thickness of articular cartilage
III	Fragmentation and fissures in area > 0.5 inch in diameter	Deep ulceration, fibrillation, fissuring, or chondral flap >50% of cartilage without exposed bone	Lesion more than half the thickness of articular cartilage
IV	Exposed subchondral bone	Full-thickness wear with exposed subchondral bone	Lesion extending to subchondral bone

8. Explain the structure of bone with illustrative diagram.

Ans: Bone is a composite tissue consisting of organic matrix, inorganic minerals, cells, and water. Biologically, it is a dynamic mesenchymal (specialized connective) hard tissue that undergoes continuous formation, deformation, and remodeling throughout life. The size of bone increases by growth (*skeletal modeling*) during initial life till physeal closure but the shape of bone changes throughout life by virtue of the dynamic process of *remodeling*. Remodeling gives capacity to bone to repair itself and renew the lost internal structures from wear and tear process. It also enables bone to adapt itself to changing environment resulting from altered activity levels and aging. Bone per se consists of predominant inorganic component (60%) and organic component (40%).

- The inorganic portion comprises crystalline calcium phosphate salts, present in the form of hydroxyapatite $[Ca_{10}(PO_4)_6(OH)_2]$ with minor contribution from carbonates, fluorides, and other magnesium salts.
- The organic component is dominated by type I collagen that forms the basic architecture of bone on which inorganic portion is deposited. Support to collagen is provided by derived protein components like proteoglycans, glycoproteins, phospholipids, and phosphoproteins that serve specific functions.

Both the components give bone its unique mechanical, biological, and electrical properties. Loss or inadequacy of mineral component (osteomalacia or rickets) or organic component (like osteogenesis imperfecta) produces structurally weak bones that fail easily. The human and primate bones comprise typical distribution of hard (compact) bone outside, supported internally by biologically more active (cancellous) bone that has nine times the metabolic activity. This distribution of hard (cortical/compact bone) and weaker (cancellous bone) components in tandem gives bone mechanical advantage of discrete rigidity and flexibility together **(Flowchart 2.1.1)**.

Flowchart 2.1.1: Broad constituents of bone.

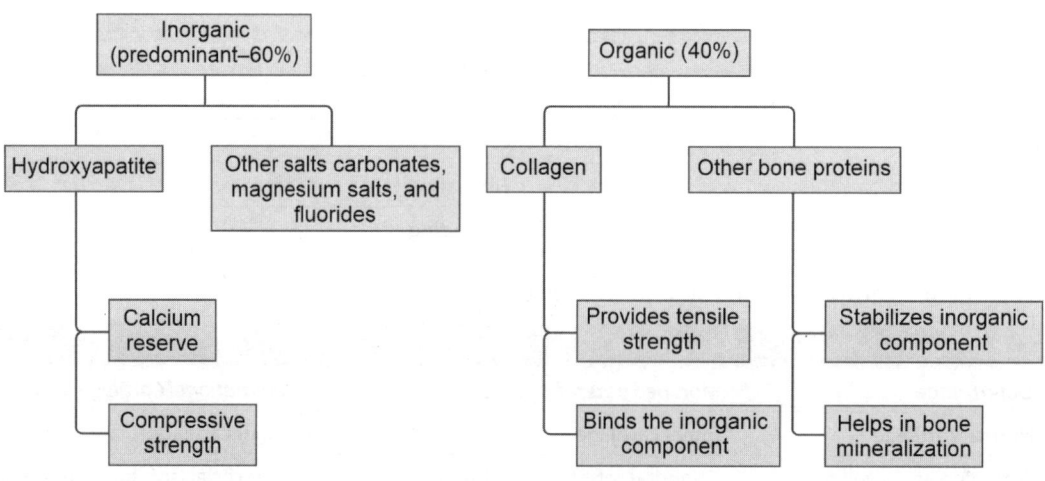

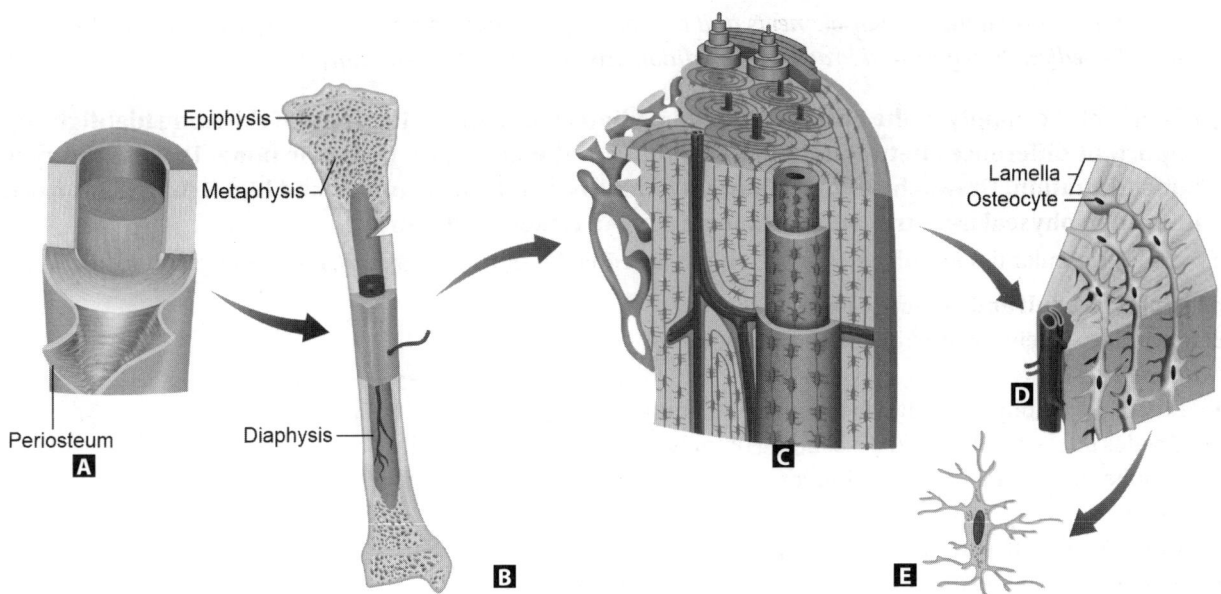

Figs. 2.1.5A to E: Gross appearance to microstructure of bone.

Gross appearance to microstructure of bone: The cortex forms a cylinder encircling the medullary cavity and is in turn covered by the periosteum (*see* **Fig. 2.1.5A**). Illustrated **Figures 2.1.5A to E** show the dispositions of cortical and cancellous components of human bone in a typical long bone (tibia here), the cancellous bone typically occupies the epiphysis and metaphysis of a long bone while cortical bone predominates in the diaphysis. The microstructure of mature cortical (compact) bone comprises concentric rings around Haversian (longitudinal) and Volkmann (transverse) canal system within the osteoid also shown are the osteocytes arranged in the lamellations that form the largest network of cells connecting skeletal system to the outside environment through their processes and also maintains homeostasis within bone.

The bone can be divided into following *anatomical parts* (these are also functionally and physiologically distinct units):
- Epiphysis
- Metaphysis
- Diaphysis
- Bone marrow
- Periosteum
- Endosteum

Based on collagen fiber arrangements, bones have two distinct histological appearances—(1) woven bone and (2) the lamellar bone.
1. *Woven bone:* Woven bone is also called immature bone, coarse bundled bone or sometimes fiber bone. It is made from randomly oriented collagen fibers in interlacing or "burlap" (coarse canvas) fashion, with numerous osteoblasts and osteoprogenitor cells (so-called immature bone cells).
2. *Lamellar bone:* Lamellar (thin plate) bone (mature bone) on polarized light microscopy has characteristic well-organized arrangement of collagen fibers seen as parallel bundles (2–4 μm) of deposited bone. Lamellar bone develops during remodeling of immature bone by replacement of the latter.

Cellular elements of bone: Osteoblasts, osteocytes, and osteoclasts are predominant cells in bone. Osteoblasts serve the purpose of bone formation (osteogenesis), while osteoclasts are mainly accountable for bone resorption; their combined action contributes to progressive mineralization and remodeling.

The osteocytes maintain the milieu of bone and its homeostasis through vast network of canalicular system that communicates with external environment through Haversian system.

(For additional details on the cellular elements and anatomical divisions of bone kindly refer to Chapter 1 of the book Essential Orthopedics: Principles and Practice, 2nd edition. Also one may add vascularity of bone.)

9. **Discuss blood supply to the bone (adult and pediatric) and draw diagrams of the same highlighting the important differences between the blood supply of the adult and pediatric bone. Discuss the types of bone formation. Draw a histologic diagram of physis-epiphysis complex and highlight the zone usually injured in physeal fractures and pathologic zone in rickets and scurvy.**

Ans: Bone is a vascular tissue with a rich blood supply essential for nutrition, growth, remodeling, and repair.

Blood supply to adult and pediatric bone

Adult long bones receive blood from three main sources:

1. *Nutrient artery*:
   - Enters the diaphysis (shaft) via the nutrient foramen.
   - Divides into ascending and descending branches in the medullary cavity.
   - Supplies the medullary cavity, inner two-thirds of cortex, and metaphysis.
2. *Periosteal arteries*:
   - Tiny vessels from surrounding muscles or soft tissue
   - Penetrate the periosteum to supply the outer one-third of cortex.
   - Important in fracture healing
3. *Metaphyseal and epiphyseal arteries* (Separate in pediatric bones while in adults they communicate to form epimetaphyseal system):
- In adults, the epiphysis (end of the bone) and metaphysis (region between the epiphysis and diaphysis) are supplied by separate arteries derived from periarticular vascular networks.
- These vessels penetrate the bone at the epiphysis and metaphysis, forming an anastomosis with medullary vessels.
- In adults, the epiphyseal plate is closed (replaced by an epiphyseal line), so there is no barrier between metaphyseal and epiphyseal blood supplies, allowing some vascular continuity.
- In children, the pattern is similar, but with a key difference due to the presence of the growth plate (physis).

Differences between adult and pediatric bone blood supply (Highlighted in **Table 2.1.4***):*
- The epiphyseal and metaphyseal circulations are separate because the physis acts as a barrier.
- The nutrient artery still supplies the diaphysis and part of the metaphysis.
- The epiphysis is supplied separately via epiphyseal arteries.
- This separation has clinical implications:
  - Infections like osteomyelitis often localize to the metaphysis in children due to sluggish blood flow and lack of phagocytosis in that area.
  - Pediatric fractures near the growth plate (Salter–Harris fractures) can disrupt epiphyseal blood supply → growth disturbances.
  - Adult fractures rely more on periosteal blood supply for healing – minimize periosteal stripping during osteosynthesis

TABLE 2.1.4: Differences in blood supply of adult and pediatric bone.

Feature	Pediatric bone (Fig. 2.1.6)	Adult bone (Fig. 2.1.7)
Growth plate (Physis)	Present—separates blood supply	Fused—allows communication
Metaphysis and epiphysis	Supplied by different vessels	Communicating vessels after fusion
Risk of infection	Higher in metaphysis	Lower in metaphysis
Fracture healing	Fast due to active periosteum	Slower, periosteum less active
Risk of ischemia	Growth arrest if epiphyseal vessels damaged	Lower risk of growth-related issues

General Orthopedics

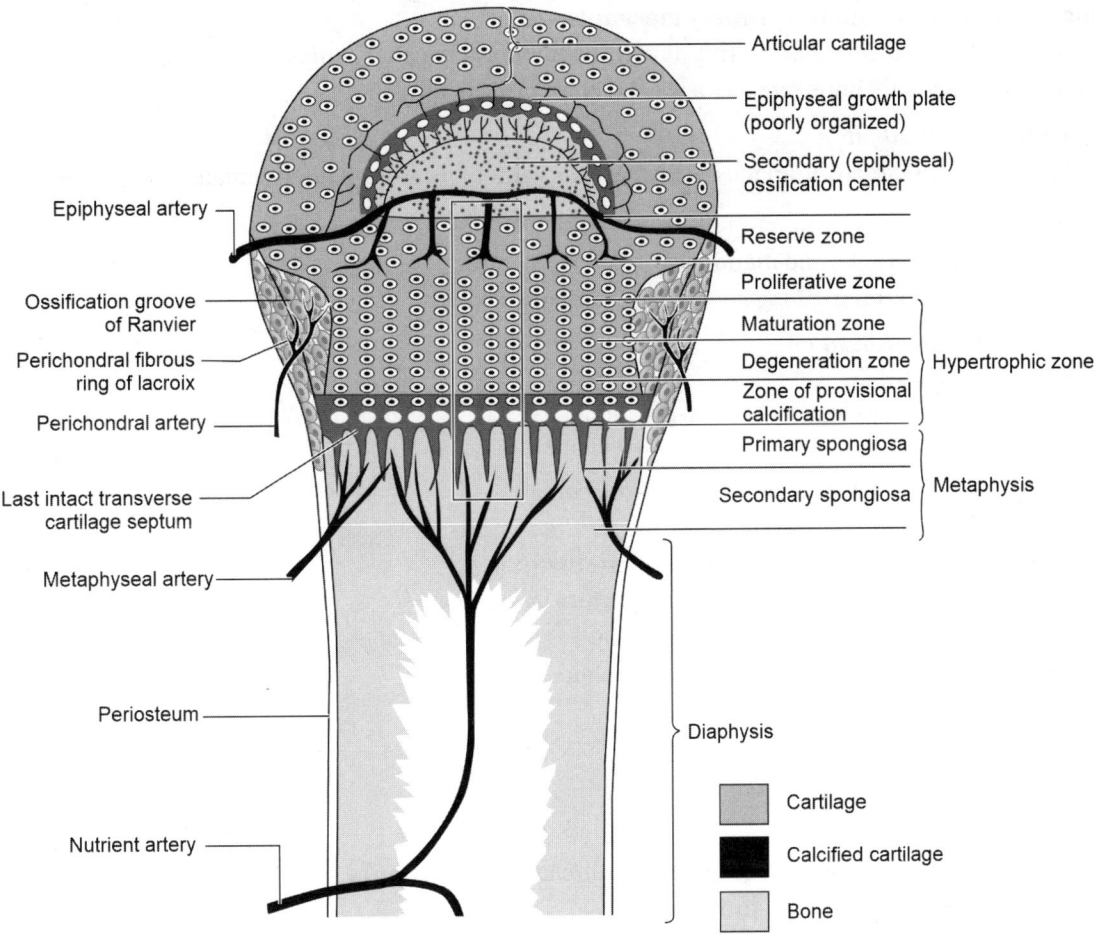

Fig. 2.1.6: Diagram illustrating blood supply of pediatric bone.

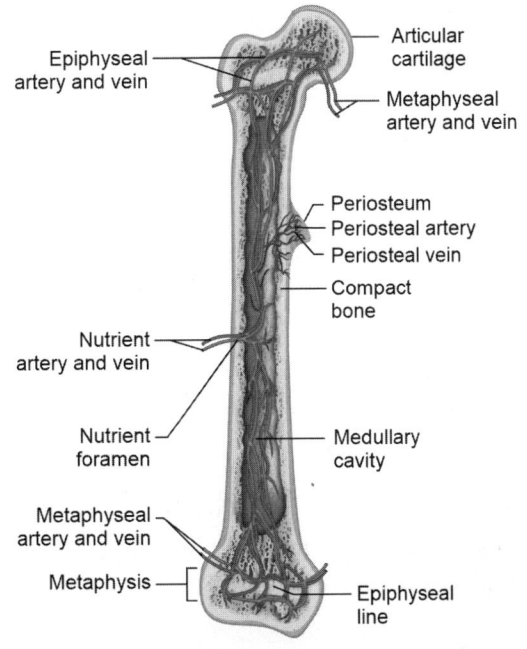

Fig. 2.1.7: Diagram illustrating the blood supply of adult bone.

Bone formation occurs through two primary mechanisms:
1. *Intramembranous ossification:* Bone forms directly within mesenchymal connective tissue.
2. *Endochondral ossification:* Bone replaces a pre-existing cartilage model.

1. Intramembranous ossification

Definition: Bone develops directly from mesenchymal cells without a cartilage intermediate.

Key locations:
- Flat bones (e.g., skull, clavicle, and mandible)
- Also contributes to *thickening of long bones* (appositional growth).

Steps of intramembranous ossification
1. Mesenchymal condensation
    - Mesenchymal stem cells cluster at the ossification site
2. Osteoblast differentiation
    - Mesenchymal cells → osteoprogenitor cells → osteoblasts
3. Osteoid secretion and mineralization
    - Osteoblasts secrete osteoid (unmineralized bone matrix).
    - Calcium phosphate deposits → osteoid hardens into *woven bone.*
4. Trabecular formation and periosteum development
    - Woven bone remodels into trabecular (spongy) bone.
    - Outer mesenchyme condenses into *periosteum.*
5. *Compact bone formation*
    - Trabeculae at the surface fuse into *compact bone.*

Clinical relevance:
- Defects cause cleidocranial dysplasia (impaired skull/clavicle formation).
- Critical for fracture callus formation during healing.

2. Endochondral ossification

Definition: Bone replaces a hyaline cartilage template.

Key Locations:
- Most bones (long bones, vertebrae, and pelvis)

Steps of endochondral ossification:
1. *Cartilage model formation:*
    - Mesenchymal cells → chondroblasts → hyaline cartilage model
2. Primary ossification center (diaphysis):
    - Chondrocytes hypertrophy → secrete alkaline phosphatase → calcify matrix
    - Blood vessels invade, bringing osteoblasts → replace cartilage with *woven bone.*
3. Secondary ossification centers (epiphyses):
    - After birth, centers form in epiphyses
    - Growth plate *(physis)* remains between diaphysis and epiphysis.
4. Growth plate zones (pediatric bone):
    - *Resting zone* (reserve chondrocytes)
    - *Proliferative zone* (chondrocyte mitosis → longitudinal growth)
    - *Hypertrophic zone* (chondrocytes enlarge and matrix calcifies)
    - *Ossification zone* (osteoblasts replace cartilage with bone)
5. Epiphyseal closure (adult bone):
    - Growth plate ossifies → bone lengthening stops

Clinical relevance:
- *Achondroplasia:* FGFR3 mutation → disrupted growth plate function → dwarfism
- *Rickets/vitamin D deficiency:* Poor cartilage mineralization → growth deformities

Histological diagram of physis-epiphysis complex highlighting the zone usually injured in physeal fractures and pathologic zone in rickets and scurvy is illustrated in **Figure 2.1.8**.

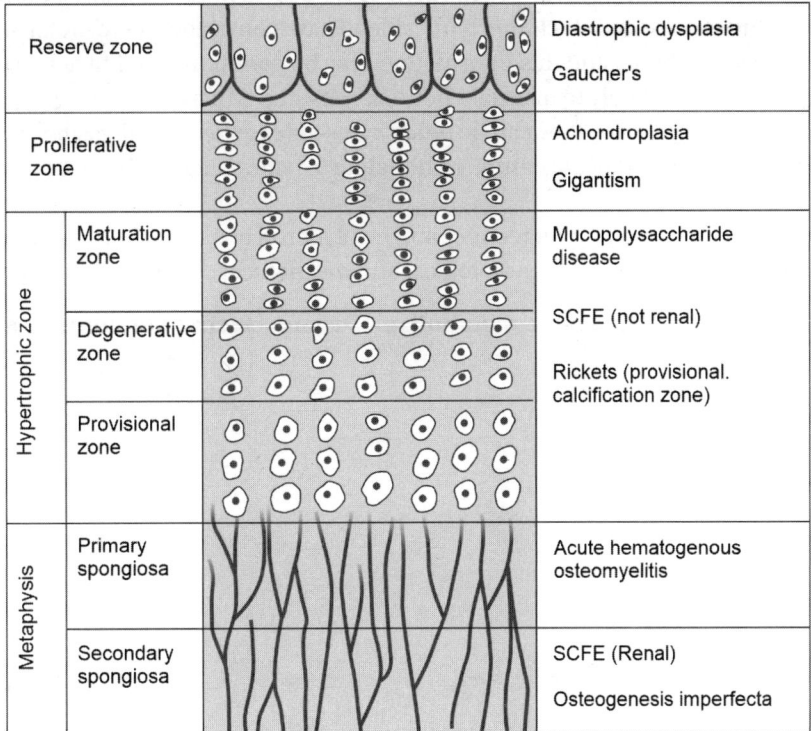

Fig. 2.1.8: Histologic diagram of physis-epiphysis complex highlighting the zone usually injured in physeal fractures and pathologic zone in rickets and scurvy.
Courtesy: Dr ShaJi.

10. What are osteocytes?

Ans: They are the most abundant cells of bone (90–95% of all bone cells). Around 10% of the embryonic osteoblastic population is lost by getting trapped and enclosed in their own synthesized matrix. Nestled within their bony lacunae, they remain anything but passive. Through delicate cytoplasmic processes, they maintain a profound network of communication, both among themselves and with the surface lining cells entwined in the fabric of the bone.

Their precise role, shrouded in mystery, may yet hold significant implications for the dynamics of bone biology. Under the influence of parathyroid hormone (PTH), they could play a pivotal part in bone resorption, engaging in a process known as "osteocytic osteolysis," while simultaneously facilitating the transport of calcium ions. Furthermore, emerging hypotheses suggest that these cells are attuned to mechanical stimuli, acting as sentinels that sense changes in stress and strain. In this capacity, they relay vital information to the active osteoblasts, which can then adjust their osteogenic activities in response to the biomechanical landscape.

1. *Transition from osteoblasts:* Osteocytes can be considered as "spent" osteoblasts that have become embedded within the bone matrix after their role in bone formation is complete. Although they are no longer active in forming new bone, they continue to play important roles in bone health.
2. *Location and communication:* Osteocytes reside in small cavities known as lacunae within the bone. They extend slender cytoplasmic processes through tiny channels called canaliculi, allowing them to communicate with each other and with surface osteoblasts and lining cells. This communication is crucial for coordinating bone remodeling and maintenance.

3. *Functions:*
   a. *Bone resorption:* They may be involved in the process of bone resorption through osteocytic osteolysis, particularly under the influence of PTH, which helps to regulate calcium levels in the body.
   b. *Calcium ion transport:* Osteocytes may also facilitate the transport of calcium ions, contributing to overall calcium homeostasis.
4. *Response to mechanical stimuli:* Osteocytes are thought to be sensitive to mechanical forces and play a role in mechanotransduction, the process by which mechanical loads are converted into cellular signals. They can detect changes in stress and strain on bone, and this information may be communicated to active osteoblasts, prompting them to adjust their activity accordingly to maintain bone density and structure.
5. *Aging and resorption:* As osteocytes age, they can be phagocytosed (engulfed and digested) by osteoclasts during the bone resorption process. This is a part of the natural remodeling of bone, where old or damaged bone is replaced with new bone tissue.

In summary, osteocytes are crucial for the maintenance and regulation of bone metabolism, serving as a communication hub within the bone matrix and responding to physiological and mechanical changes within the skeletal system.

11. **Mention various factors regulating bone metabolism. Discuss electric phenomena and electrical charges in bones.**

Ans:
- *Endocrine factors:*
  - Parathyroid hormone
  - Calcitonin
  - Vitamin D
  - Vitamin A
  - Gonadal hormones
  - Growth hormone
- *Growth factors:*
  - Transforming growth factor-β
  - Bone morphogenic proteins
  - Insulin-like growth factors 1 and 2
  - Other growth factors such as platelet-derived growth factor (PDGF) and fibroblast growth factor (FGF)

Electric phenomena and electrical charges in bones:
The "electrical properties" of bone depend on a number of factors. The bone is "dielectric" (applying voltage produces current across ends determining the "capacitance") and "anisotropic" (charge flowing in all directions in a branching pattern rather than unidirectional flow in a metal wire/rod) with respect to its electrical properties. This means that they are semiconductive (dielectric) themselves but properties differ, "impedance" is lowest in the longitudinal direction and highest in the radial direction.

The electrical properties of fully hydrated bone are significantly different from those of dry and partially wet bone and these properties are highly frequency dependent, they also vary with moisture content, methods of measurement, temperature, and pH of the fluid.

In general, the cancellous bone has lower resistance than cortical bone. The metaphysis of long bones is negatively charged in relation to diaphysis. The fracture site is more electronegative than surrounding bone. "Conductance" is a property of the bone marrow and a normal value indicates establishment of intramedullary (IM) canal. Piezoelectricity is a coupled field effect meaning application of stress/strain are coupled to electrical field generating current and polarization (like thermoelasticity—application of heat produces expansion and vice versa). These gradient effects are now referred to as "flexoelectric;" however, the term piezoelectric effect will be used here for common understanding. Bones exhibit "piezoelectric properties" meaning that when stress is applied to the bone, the bone produces a current within itself—the piezoelectric effect, this is due to deformation of hydroxyapatite (HA) crystals.

Under the effect of a tensile strain, the bone develops electronegativity at the compression site (electrons grouped nearer) while it becomes electropositive at the tension side (electrons deviate farther). Reverse piezoelectric effect (an applied current produces material compression) is a property exhibited by some materials exhibiting piezoelectric effect such as bone. This piezoelectric property implies that a voltage could be applied to the bone and the bone itself would compress (develops strain). Compression across fracture improves healing (mechanical property of bone) but the dielectric property (capacitance) would lead to generation of current with the applied voltage and could damage the cells if it exceeds the impedance. So, it is imperative that standard protocols must be used. Compact bone in addition exhibits a permanent electric polarization as well as "pyroelectricity" (which is a change of polarization with temperature) determined by polar structure of collagen and orientation in bone. Electric properties and variation with fracture occurrence (development of electronegativity) and restoration (of electrical properties) with healing have been exploited to develop impedance imaging that may possibly indicate development of nonunion or delayed union early. Conductance measures indicate fracture healing at 8 weeks but the values depend tremendously on the cross-sectional area and volume of bone. Inductance, though independent of these variables, is still not standardized.

12. Describe mechanism of electrically induced osteogenesis.

Ans: Like most incidental findings in medical science the mechanism of new bone formation through electrical or magnetic field is largely unknown. cAMP and alteration in intracellular calcium levels have been implicated but never consistently confirmed. Stimulation by "direct current" stimulates neo-osteogenesis by direct effect of current, release of hydroxyl ions locally (chemical reaction), reducing vicinity PO_2 and increased pH. Low PO_2 stimulates new bone growth and higher pH favors calcium deposition. The mechanisms of "inductive coupling" and "capacitive coupling (CC)" are even more unclear but possibly related to direct effect of the current.

Direct current: Constant application of 20 µA at 1 V to cathode applied directly to the bone surface (Dwyer/Wickham) induces bone by electric, chemical and mechanical effect. The anode is placed in the adjacent soft tissue or skin surface. Electric current is the primary stimulator but the production of hydroxyl ions (electrochemical) locally increases the pH and lowers pO_2 at cathode. This prevents bone resorption and increases bone formation by stimulating the osteoblastic activity. There is additionally production of H_2O_2 at cathode which enhances osteoclast differentiation. Osteoclast bone resorption additionally stimulates the osteoblasts.

The H_2O_2 may also stimulate the macrophage to secrete VEGF that indices angiogenesis and fracture healing. Direct current stimulation may induce formation of BMP 2, 6 and 7 by osteoblasts to stimulate bone formation. Mechanical effects of cathode insertion and electrode movement can possibly help bone formation. Inflammatory reaction (stage I of fracture repair) is produced in the tissue. The method is invasive and vigilant measures and regular monitoring needs to be done to prevent infection. Direct current leads to warming effect in tissues and blistering at anode while pitting at cathode. This may also be responsible to inflammatory effect at fracture site at low strengths. Brighton used similar DC current but applied to percutaneous electrodes reporting bone union in 84% uncomplicated (no infection or synovial pseudoarthrosis) cases.

Inductive coupling or pulsed electromagnetic field (PEMF) developed by Bassett et al.: Here a time-varying electric field is applied to a pair of coils placed on opposite sides of fractured extremity. This produces time-varying magnetic field between coils and in turn secondary time-varying electric field of 10 µA/cm^2 at 20 mV gets generated in the tissues. PEMF acts by both electrical and mechanical influence on the bone. Electrical current helps as described in the direct current, while pulsed electrical field generates piezoelectric effect compressing and relaxing the fracture site. This generates micromotion and compressive strain at the fracture site. This induces calcification of fibrocartilage and hyaline cartilage (fibrous tissue is not induced at all). PEMF has also been found to upregulate the genes related to bone formation (*HOXA10 and AKT1*), collagenous and noncollagenous matrix proteins (*COL1A and SPARC*), genes for cytoskeletal component (FN1 and VCL), and genes at transductional level (*CALM1 and p2RX7*) in in-vitro cell culture of osteoblasts. They are also found to downregulate the genes related to degradation of extracellular matrix (MMP-11 and DUSP4). PEMF has direct inhibitory influence on parathyroid hormone (PTH) signaling. The PEMF prevents store of cAMP to build up inside cell normally associated with PTH activity. This increases increased calcium uptake by the cell. Also, there is direct increase in intracellular levels by a mechanism different from CC. This is a noninvasive method but requires frequent and prolonged sittings and visits to hospital. Double-blinded studies have shown efficacy of PEMF on osteotomy healing and delayed union.

Capacitive coupling (CC): A time-varying electric field is applied to paired electrodes (not coils), generating time-varying electric field (capacity coupled generators) across tissue in a symmetrical sine wave pattern with peak-to-peak amplitude of 5 V and frequency of 60 kHz. This is due to dielectric property of bone. This produces average electric field of 80 mV/cm (range 20–150) at 5–10 mA in the fracture callus. Here, the role of any magnetic field (as in inductive coupling) is negligible. CC causes an increase in cytosolic calcium through voltage gated calcium channels increasing intracellular calcium. This enhances calmodulin stores and induces cell proliferation and callus formation and maturation. CC also enhances bone formation by activation of bone formation through expression of mRNA for BMP 2, 4, 5, 6 and 7. Collagen synthesis and production of cAMP is induced in the tissues enhancing calcification on reparative stage.

13. Explain the blood supply of long bones and effects of various modalities of fixation on this.

Ans: Bone receives around one-fifth (10–20%) of the cardiac output.
The two predominant vascular systems for blood supply **(Fig. 2.1.9)** include:
1. The periosteal system
2. The endosteal system (misnomer as there is no endosteum, better called *intramedullary system*).

Minor contributions come from:
1. Epimetaphyseal system
2. Articular ligaments (like obturator ligament in hip).

Periosteal system: The periosteal system (also called accessory nutrient arterioles) supplies only the outer third of the cortex. Entire long bone except its cartilage ends is covered by periosteum with deficiencies only in the region of capsular attachments and nutrient vessels. The outer layer of periosteum consists of fibrous tissue that is predominantly supportive and imparts stiffness to it. The periosteum is thick in children due to the presence of active cambium (cellular layer) with blood supply in the form of *longitudinal arterioles* incorporated within. However, with aging the cambium gets hypotrophied and becomes thin, also the vascularity reduces with absence of prominent longitudinal arterioles.

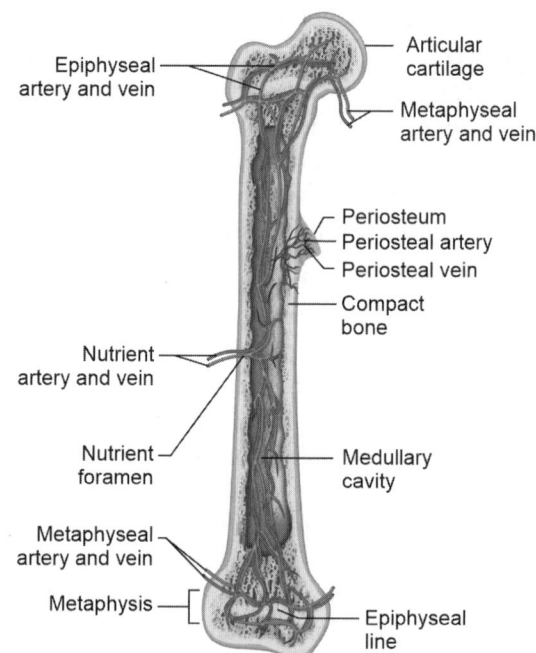

Fig. 2.1.9: Blood supply of long bones.

Effects of surgery:
- This has important surgical implications with respect to higher incidence of nonunion and delayed union in fractures fixed after ripping periosteum, especially in adults. Over most of the surface of long bones in an adult, the periosteum is loosely attached beneath muscle bellies.
- In vascular stress situations like acute embolism of the intramedullary system or reaming of intramedullary canal, the blood flow of the periosteum increases many fold compensating for the loss in blood supply. In such situations, the blood flow becomes *centripetal*.

Intramedullary system: Diaphyseal nutrient arteries (one or two) enter through the cortical bone often in an oblique direction. The common ports of nutrient artery entry are the fascial regions firmly attached to the diaphysis of long bones or along anatomical bony ridges like linea aspera of the femur. The principal nutrient artery to bone is formed of these afferent vessels. The afferent vessels after entering the intramedullary system divide into ascending and descending branches that supply inner two-thirds of the cortex (outer thirds being supplied by periosteal supply) and whole of the medullary cavity. The intramedullary and periosteal systems of blood supply anastomose freely.

Effects of surgery:
- The system gets damaged during reaming as for intramedullary reaming making the blood supply centripetal and increasing periosteal (and metaphyseal artery) and muscular blood flow. This improves chances of formation of periosteal callus formation and maturation.
- Damage to intramedullary blood supply would cause osteonecrosis in critical bones especially in bones that are exclusively supplied by this system only (like scaphoid and talus).

Metaphyseal and epiphyseal arteries: This system supplies blood to the ends of bones, diaphysis being supplied by the above-mentioned systems. They arise as principal branches from adjacent articular supply or periarticular plexus. This system also freely anastomoses with the diaphyseal or intramedullary system terminating in bone marrow, trabecular bone, cortical bone and articular cartilage. In immature skeleton, growth plate (end-plates of cartilage component of physis) separates these arteries from intramedullary system. Near the growth plate (physis) a few vessels make hairpin bend and retreat back upon themselves, while most enter into an open circulation. In the past, this arrangement of hairpin bends was considered to reduce the rate of blood flow to cause localization of blood-borne bacteria and serve as focus of onset of hematogenous osteomyelitis, especially in children.

Throughout life of individual this layer remains dormant and atrophic until activated by specific stimulus like trauma and surgery.

14. Discuss anatomy of joint capsule and its surgical importance.

Ans: *Anatomy:* Synovial joints consist of fluid-filled cavity containing hyaline cartilage-lined bone ends enclosed in a tough fibrous capsule joining and surrounding the adjoining bony surfaces. The joint capsule is lined by a synovial membrane that secretes the synovial fluid.

The synovial joint is covered all around by *joint capsule* forming the outermost layer. There are two connective tissue layers in the joint capsule. The outer fibrous layer is made up of collagen fibers. The fibrous capsule is thickened at places forming intrinsic ligaments that are different from ligaments outside the capsule (extrinsic ligaments).

Both types of ligaments provide vital additional stability to the synovial joint. The fibrous layer surrounds the joint and attaches to the periosteum of the adjacent bones. The joint capsule is supplied by a number of somatic sensory fibers for sensations of proprioception, pressure, pain, and vibration. Sometimes the joint capsule may be deficient to allow for passage of structures in/out of the joint such as the biceps tendon in shoulder joint. The synovial membrane "itself in the" inner layer of joint capsule and is poorly innervated and but highly vascularized.

Surgical importance:
- Stabilization of joint, distribution of biomechanical load, protection of the joint by limiting normal range of motion. The joint helps stabilization by preventing:
  – Movement beyond normal range(s)
  – Excessive laxity
- Proprioceptors of joint capsule help in maintaining joint position awareness.
- The capsule provides a base for synovial membrane. The synovial membrane secretes joint fluid so capsule helps indirectly in maintaining joint biology.
- Joint capsule serves as bearers of intrinsic joint ligaments while the extrinsic ligaments are spanned across the joint capsule. During surgical exposures, the disposition of capsule and ligaments has to be maintained for proper functioning of the joint.
  – The ligaments and joints should be adequately repaired to maintain joint stability.
  – Avulsed joint capsules disrupt the smooth joint motion that is synchronized with muscular contractions so repair of the capsule is imperative.
- Excessive lax joint capsule may occur after repeated joint dislocations in which case they have to be retightened by appropriate measures. Capsules that are lax by virtue of inherent disorders or collagen disorders would not benefit from surgical procedures so must be differentiated and refrained from surgery.

2.2 FRACTURE REPAIR AND ITS ENHANCEMENT, BONE BANKING (Q15–29)

15. Describe various types of fracture healing.

Ans:

A. *Intramembranous repair (direct bone healing, gap healing):* There is no callus formation (primary fracture repair) and the bone heals directly without any intervening tissue or callus mainly due to rigid fixation. Bones when apposed together anatomically under physiological compression loads heal without any intervening tissue. This is the ideal situation for fracture repair and is the natural course when the gap is below critical limit of 400 μm (some take it to

500 μm). The cutting cones cross from one side to another across the fracture (**Fig. 2.2.1**) and following ossification front heals the fracture in turn. The healing passes through the following stages:
- Resorption of bone ends
- *Fibrous tissue formation:* Fibrous tissue forms from the healing hematoma or lying down of inflammatory tissue at the gap
- *Maturation to lamellar bone:* The advancing osteoclastic migration front in the form of cutting cones cross the fracture site and the fibrous tissue followed by the osteoblastic ossification front and thin capillary vessels that seal the gap.

B. Second type is *creeping substitution* (term first used by Phemister) and is primarily seen in cancellous bone. It is typical of intra-articular and periarticular fractures stabilized by rigid fixation anatomically. Creeping substitution is also seen during incorporation of cancellous bone graft. Creeping substitution is the process of resorption of the trabecular network of bone and lying of new bone by appositional ossification on the surface of the scaffold hence left (both processes occurring simultaneously). Gross architecture of the bone is maintained hence the scaffold (dead trabecular bone) is copy-pasted (substituted) by new living bone.

C. *Repair with bone callus formation (endochondral repair, secondary bone healing, indirect bone healing)* is the most common type of bone healing and is typical of diaphyseal

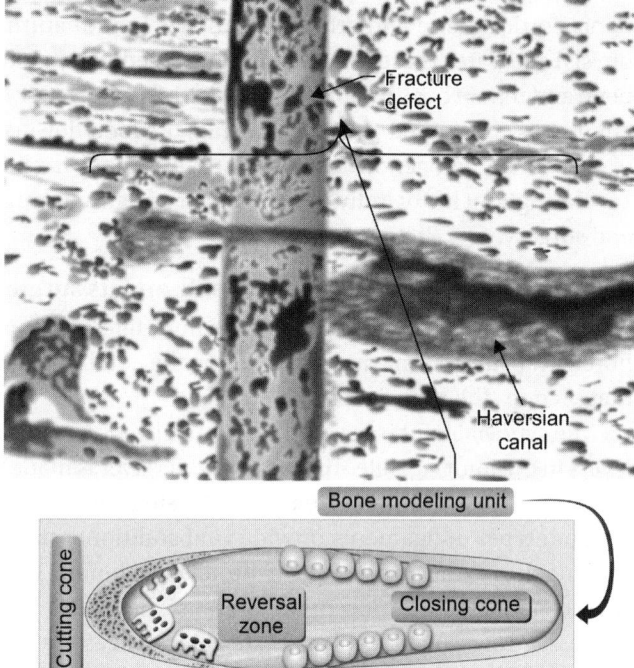

Fig. 2.2.1: "Cutting cone" healing of bone. The bone remodeling unit traverses across the compressed fracture producing primary healing.

fractures that pass through formation of intermediary stage of callus formation. Callus is a preossification cartilage tissue that forms in response to controlled motion rather micromotion at the fracture site. Endochondral fracture repair process is also termed secondary bone repair (because there is need for "intermediate tissue" the callus) and can be broadly classified into three main stages as below:

1. *Reactive stage (inflammatory stage):* This stage is akin to inflammatory response seen in response to tissue injury and comprises of two phases:
    i. *Hematoma formation and induced inflammation:* Hematoma immediately forms due to blood leak into surroundings from disrupted vessels, periosteum and endosteum. This hematoma is vastly responsible for further stages and osteogenesis as demonstrated by Mizuno et al. They demonstrated that as early as 4th day the hematoma has "osteogenic power" that progressively increases. Osteoblast progenitors are recruited by osteogenic induction of undifferentiated cells from bone marrow and mesenchymal cells from "cambium" layer of periosteum. Osteoclasts come from hemopoietic cells of bone marrow. Bone morphogenetic proteins (BMPs) help in differentiation of cells to osteoblasts, osteoclasts and osteocytes. These cells then migrate to fracture focus. Mineralization is controlled by systemic factors regulating calcium and phosphorus metabolism. Inflammation usually reaches its peak at 48 hours and then is modulated according to the treatment a fracture is receiving.
    ii. *Granulation tissue formation:* The hematoma is infiltrated by developing vessels from surrounding healing tissue under effect of vascular endothelial growth factor (VEGF) and FGF. The proliferating fibroblasts (that survive ischemia) along with ingrowing vessels evolve into fibrovascular granular tissue rich in type II collagen. This stage lasts some 2 weeks.
2. *Reparative stage:* This stage essentially comprises of reparative tissue deposition and can be divided into following phases:
    i. *Callus formation:* Callus is the bone regenerative tissue that forms in response to micromotion at the bone injury site aimed to naturally unite the two opposed stabilized bone ends. Formation of callus reduces the

interfragmentary strain by increasing surface area and thus improving local environment toward healing. There are two histologically varied forms of callus that can be recognized:

   a. *Soft callus (primary callus):* After 2 weeks at the fracture site, the cells deposit hyaline cartilage, and as the focus solidity increases the cartilaginous cells hypertrophy and cartilage progressively mineralizes by endochondral ossification. There are three types of callus formation at the site of fracture. (1) "Periosteal bridging callus" typically develops in the above described fashion. In addition to the periosteal callus a slowly developing (2) "intramedullary callus" is laid down from inside the bone supplied by medullary arterial system. This has double concave shape with periphery adhered to endosteum and is the predominant response during "gap repair". (3) Third type is the "intercortical uniting callus" occupying the space between the opposed cortices of fractured ends. Its size is totally dependent on reduction and apposition of bone ends so that it is absent in compressed plating. Apart from above a fourth type of tissue is also seen called "external soft tissue" response (not a true callus) that develops from vascular mesenchymal tissue like muscles and is important in fracture repair as absence of the same has been cited as one of the reasons for nonunion of distal third tibial fractures. The mineralization progresses from immature bone bridge toward focus. The fracture during this stage is "sticky", i.e., it is deformable (can be angulated) but not displaceable (ends cannot be separated) by physiologic loads. Supervised mobilization can begin during this stage.
   b. *Hard callus:* As the immature bone grows strong the woven bone gradually transforms into primary lamellar bone. This bone, however, grows in many directions. The transformation usually commences in 4th week and finishes around 16th week. The amount of callus formation is dependent primarily on oxygen tension but also on strain pattern (treatment) at the fracture site.

   ii. *Consolidation (lamellar bone deposition):* There is resorption of bone ends with bridging callus formation. The fracture line becomes vague. The process of formation of lamellar bone in hyaline cartilage is termed endochondral ossification. Mineralization of fracture callus is an essential step in bone formation that depends on degradation of proteoglycans affected by endopeptidase and deposition of crystals affected by alkaline phosphatase.

3. *Remodeling:* Remodeling is the process of slow restoration of normal bone structure, passing through stages of primary lamellar bone (multidirectional osteons) to secondary lamellar bone (longitudinal osteons). The stage starts during reparative stage and continues even after clinical bone union (up to 7 years). Remodeling is based on the special units called "bone modeling units" described by Frost. This structural modification continues indefinitely according to the functional load and stress pattern on the bone (Wolff's law).

16. Examples of intramembranous ossification and enchondral ossification.

Ans: Depending on the mode of fixation used for osteosynthesis the bone may undergo intramembranous or enchondral repair **(Table 2.2.1)**.

TABLE 2.2.1: Different types of bone repair based on fixation mode.	
Type of stabilization	*Predominant type of repair*
Plaster of Paris cast	Enchondral ossification
DCP plating	• Gap repair without compression • Primary cortical repair (Haversian remodeling) with compression • Enchondral repair can occur on opposite side
Locked plating in rigid mode and compression	Primary cortical repair
Open reduction and locked plate in "elastic mode"	Combination of primary cortical repair and enchondral repair (predominates)
MIPPO	Enchondral repair
Intra-articular fractures fixed with plate	Creeping substitution at cancellous surface and primary cortical repair (no callus)
Intramedullary nail	Early periosteal callus and enchondral repair. Late intramembranous repair
External fixator	• *Elastic*: Enchondral repair through periosteal bridging callus • *Rigid*: Primary cortical repair
Wire loops	Creeping substitution at cancellous bone and endochondral repair at diaphysis

17. Define bone remodeling.

Ans: Kindly see the answer above for definition and details.

18. A. Describe fracture healing.
   B. Describe the various factors influencing fracture healing.
   C. Differentiate between rheumatoid arthritis and osteoarthritis.

Ans:

A. "Fracture repair" or healing [if not augmented (by fixation or BMP) or interfered (gross displacement, loss of vascularity, etc.)] is a systemic and organized cascade of regenerative tissue formation with influences of local and systemic factors. For a successful fracture repair, appropriate cells need to be recruited with simultaneous activation of appropriate genes at a right time in a correct anatomical location. Fracture repair is essentially a "regenerative" process rather than healing as the defect is actually replaced by new bone and not by scar tissue (so fracture "healing" could be a misnomer). The potential of skeleton to regenerate is astounding. Notwithstanding with the healing of other adult tissues that leave a scar tissue, new bone is formed, replaced and continuously remodeled/modeled until the original site of injury is barely recognizable.

Surrounding soft tissue injury is an important determinant to fracture repair by virtue of maintaining good blood supply to the region. Repair may be disrupted at start (slow union), or initially (delayed union) or interrupted (nonunion) anytime during the process depending on healing of surrounding soft tissue and synchronization of bone repair. Colloquially, it is said that fracture is a soft tissue injury where the bone is incidentally broken.

Types of fracture healing have been described in detail in answer above.

B. The various factors that affect fracture healing are as follows:

Local factors:
   – Type of bone (reduced with pathologic fractures)
   – Type of fracture (open and comminuted, bone loss)
   – Intra-articular fracture
   – Surrounding soft tissue injury and devascularization
   – Single or both bone fracture (maintained fibula can produce tibial nonunion)
   – Soft tissue interposition and distraction
   – Local bone pathologies like cysts, fibrous dysplasia, malignancies (neoplastic cells keep eating away the repair response and cells)
   – Infection (misdirection of energy and inflammatory cells to counter infection rather than healing of bone)
   – Venous stasis
   – Type of treatment and fixation (rigid, soft, tissue stripping, etc.)

Systemic factors:
   – Age
   – Activity level (immobilization in the form of bed rest, "space" flight)
   – Nutritional status
   – Hormonal factors
   – Vitamin and mineral deficiencies
   – Diseases like diabetes mellitus, anemia, neuropathies
   – Drugs [nonsteroidal anti-inflammatory drugs (NSAIDs), cytotoxic chemotherapy, fluoroquinolones, phenytoin, calcium channel blockers, steroids and tetracyclines]
   – Smoking
   – Alcohol abuse
   – Head injury

C. Differences between RA and osteoarthritis have been shown in **Table 2.2.2**.

TABLE 2.2.2: Differences between rheumatoid arthritis and osteoarthritis.

Criteria	Rheumatoid arthritis	Osteoarthritis
Pathogenesis	Autoimmune synovial disorder; usually inherited but *de novo* cases increasing in frequency	Usually degenerative loss of cartilage, genetic involvement not strongly documented
Involvement	Usually symmetrical	Asymmetrical
Joints affected	Usually small joints initially but later large joints	Usually large joints and in patients with diathesis smaller joints of hands are also involved
Joint swelling	Common with morning stiffness (>1 hour)	Swelling in acute exacerbations only. Stiffness <1 hour more common, returns at end of day and after activity
Systemic involvement	Common with systemic symptoms (fatigue, fever, loss of appetite, etc.) and disease also is mostly polyarticular	Either none or minimal, disease is also pauci- or monoarticular
Inflammatory signs	Common	Only in acute exacerbations
Deformity	Common with disease progression especially in small joints of hands and feet	Deformity of large joints is typical—like varus for knees
Inflammatory markers in blood	Usually raised	Normal commonly
Age at onset	Any age mostly begins in middle age (35–50 years)	Usually presents later in life (>60 years)
Treatment	Mostly pharmacological treatment. Surgery reserved for deformity correction	Mostly conservative with support to joints and physiotherapy. Surgery for advanced degenerative joints that cripple functionality

19. Describe the primary and secondary fracture healing.

Ans: Kindly see Answer to Question 15 above.

20. Explain the methods used for augmentation of fracture healing.

Ans: Fracture repair may not progress the ideal way always and various methods are utilized to improve or enhance the fracture repair. These are broadly classified into:
- Biophysical stimulation (mechanical and electrical methods)
- Biological methods.

The various "biophysical methods" rely on the interactions between biophysical stimuli and cellular responses to effect bone repair or enhance the callus maturation. The basis of using various methods is the effect of mechanical stimulation on induction of fracture repair or at least alteration of its pathway. Repetitive loading under small strain and high frequency or overloading through excessive exercise causes bone hypertrophy. This was also influenced by the direction and magnitude of mechanical stimulation. It is envisaged that mechanical stimuli possibly alter cytoplasmic processes or paracrine influences on the cells and if it is so then mechanical stimulation can consistently produce desirable effects. The commonly used methods are discussed as follows:
- Ultrasound
- Electrical stimulation
- Extracorporeal shock wave therapy (ESWT)
- Mechanical stimulation
  - Distraction histiogenesis (osteogenesis)
  - Controlled axial micromotion
  - Intermittent pneumatic soft tissue compression
  - Functional cast bracing of Sarmiento
- Biological methods
  - Osteoconductive
    - Bone graft substitutes

- Osteoinductive
    - Bone morphogenetic proteins
    - Platelet-rich plasma
    - Conditioned plasma
- Osteogenic
    - Bone grafts
    - Bone marrow infiltration
- Systemic agents
    - Prostaglandins
    - Fibronectin

(The above is only a list of the various methods—for details on each method kindly refer to Chapter 2 of the book Essential Orthopedics: Principles and Practice, 2nd edition.)

21. **Enumerate the biologic and biophysical technologies for the enhancement of fracture repair. Also discuss the use of BMP in orthopedics.**

Ans: Biologic and biophysical techniques are written above.

Role of BMP: Bone morphogenetic proteins seem to be involved in the regulation of cell proliferation, survival, differentiation and apoptosis, but their hallmark is their ability to induce bone, cartilage, ligament, and tendon formation at both heterotopic and orthotopic sites. This is affected by inducing differentiation of multipotent mesenchymal stem cells into osteoblasts and osteochondrogenic lineages. Recombinant human BMP-2 (rhBMP-2) blocks the differentiation of osteoblast precursor cells into myoblasts or adipocytes. Sampath and collaborators demonstrated that when osteogenic protein-1 (OP-1; BMP-7) is added to cultures of bone cells enriched with osteoblasts at different stages of differentiation, it stimulates cell proliferation, collagen synthesis, induction of alkaline phosphatase, parathyroid hormone (PTH)-mediated production of cyclic adenosine monophosphate (cAMP), and osteocalcin synthesis. The effects of BMP are mediated by canonical and noncanonical signaling mediated by the C-terminal peptide binding to receptor. At the cellular level, the BMPs migrate along concentration gradient inducing differentiation and proliferation along defined spatial arrangement. The cells are stimulated to form chondrocytes within 5–7 days that upon capillary invasion get calcified and replace with bone in 9–12 days. The mineralized bone gains functional bone marrow elements by 14–21 days. Clinically, rhBMP-7 (OP-1) has been approved as alternative to allograft for treatment of nonunion which was extended in 2004 to its use as an alternative to allograft for posterolateral spine fusion. The rhBMP-2 (infuse) has been approved for use in anterior lumbar interbody fusion with a fusion device (LT-Cage—lumbar tapered titanium interbody fusion device). In 2008, this has been extended to its use for posterolateral lumbar pseudoarthrosis, open tibia shaft fractures with intramedullary nail fixation. There is, however, extensive off label use of BMP (cervical discectomy and fusion, etc.) which has recently raised concern particularly as to hypertrophic bone formation at the site and induction of colon cancer and Barrett's esophagus. Various delivery systems have been evaluated notable of which are demineralized bone matrix (DBM), poly lactic and glycolic acid, hyaluronic acid gel, ceramics, calcium phosphate-based cements, depot injectable carriers, viral vectors and gene guns. Carrier for BMP needs to maintain a critical threshold concentration of BMP at implantation site for the required period (temporal distribution), act as scaffold over which bone growth can occur and contain the BMP at the localized site and prevent extraneous bone formation (spatial containment). The current typical dosage of rhBMP-7 is 3.5 mg which is generally administered bound to 1 g of bovine collagen granules acting as scaffold. The complications of BMP like excess bone formation and immunologic response (anticollagen and anti-rhBMP protein formation) are linked to the dose administered. Apart from bone formation, BMP could help in cartilage regeneration in osteochondral defects and reverse diabetic renal disease. For anterior interbody fusion, a total dose of 4.2–12 mg of rhBMP-2 at concentration of 1.5 mg/mL is recommended. The recommended total dose of OP-1 as humanitarian device exemption for recalcitrant posterolateral fusion nonunion is 7 mg for both sides. The recommended dose of OP-1 for recalcitrant long bone nonunions is 7 mg. Recent studies have identified specific BMP antagonists (i.e., noggin and chordin) and members of the DAN family (i.e., gremlin and follistatin). These antagonists may be used therapeutically in pathological conditions characterized by excessive bone formation.

22. Describe the types of bone grafts. What are the principles of bone banking? Describe the bone graft substitutes.

Ans:

Types:
- *Multiple cancellous (or corticocancellous) chips:* Most widely used for stacking, stuffing voids, filling defects, nonunion, delayed union, fusion, etc. in onlay fashion. It has highest osteogenic potential. It can be morcellized and used for impaction bone grafting (amount is the limiting factor). Ilium is the most common site for procurement proximal and distal femur, proximal and distal tibia, distal radius and olecranon can be used as required.
- *Single onlay cortical grafts:* Treatment of nonunions before development of good internal fixation methods. Tibia or split fibula was commonly used. Spinal fusion (rare) is the only modern use, principally because of donor site morbidity and development of fixation.
- *Dual onlay cortical bone graft (of Boyd 1941):* Classically described for congenital pseudoarthrosis tibia.
- *Inlay bone grafting:* Principally described as a sliding and graft reversal inlay technique to treat nonunion tibia by Albee (superseded now by rigid fixation and cancellous bone grafting). Extended indications in current practice are typically utilized for ankle arthrodesis and anterior spinal fusion. Typically, local tibia, fibula, ribs or iliac crest are used.
- *H-grafts:* Typically used for anterior cervical spine in past and uncommonly for scaphoid nonunion.
- *Dowel grafts and peg grafts:* Corticocancellous grafts used in past for treatment of nonunions in regions where onlay grafting is not possible. Carpal scaphoid nonunions have also been treated by cancellous pegs prepared from dense bone. Nowadays, vascularized pedicle or free grafts are commonly used.
- *Medullary grafts:* Intramedullary fibula provides two additional cortices for screw purchase. With locked screw plate constructs the utility has reduced.
- Hemicylindrical grafts
- *Fibular head graft:* This is typically used to recreate distal radius articular surface. In cases where distal radius is sacrificed as in giant cell tumor same side fibula is harvested and fixed in a reversed fashion.
- *Vascularized pedicle grafts:* These grafts carry their own vascular supply so that the incorporation and remodeling is faster. Local rotation pedicle grafts are more popular as they are easy to use like periosteal and muscle pedicle-based grafts for hip, scaphoid (pronator quadratus based), intercompartmental supraretinacular artery-based bone pedicle for scaphoid. Free microvascular fibular grafts can be placed at remote site for femoral neck and other diaphyseal defects following tumor excision, infection or traumatic bone loss are popular but require expertise.
- Intercalary graft.

Principles of bone banking: The general principles of bone banking are written here (for details kindly see Answer to Question 25)
- Thorough informed and written consent
- Securing respect for the donor—intention and good faith of donor party
- Guarantee of free will decision for the donor
- Donation must be on a nonprofit basis
- Protection of personal data
- Fulfillment of donor's good intentions
- Provision of information
- Institutional protocol, procurement, set-up, processing, etc. are detailed in Answer to Question 27.

Bone graft substitutes: "Bone graft substitutes" are material that can be used in place of bone grafts but are purely osteoconductive unless they act as carrier for delivery of some inductive materials like BMP. Typically, they are comprised of silicon, calcium or aluminum.
- *Calcium-based products are widely used:*
  - *Calcium phosphate-based grafts (tricalcium phosphate, TCP):* Calcium phosphate naturally occurs in bone as hydroxyapatite (HA) [$(Ca_5(PO_4)_3OH$ or $Ca_{10}(PO_4)_6OH_2)$]. Synthetic HA is osteoconductive but very slow to absorb taking years to incorporate. Calcium phosphate-based grafts are hence synthesized in different forms to improve

biological characteristics and are available as ceramics, powders and cements. "Ceramics" are highly crystalline structures created by a process known as "sintering" (heating nonmetallic mineral salts at temperatures greater than 1,000°C). They have the advantage of incorporating at a slower rate than calcium sulfate materials but faster than HA. Recommended pore size is 100–150 µm. Higher pore size permits faster ingrowth but reduces strength. This results in a faster degradation of the mineral substitute. Mineral substitutes with a smaller pore size allow the platelets and leukocytes to congregate within the pores and secrete cytokines to induce and implement bone formation. Mineral substitutes are osteoconductive only; however, they may be combined with DBM (osteoinductive) or bone marrow aspirate (BMA) (osteogenic) to form a composite bone graft substitute. TCP is one such bioceramic that is available in alpha and beta forms. A number of materials have been produced by substituting ions like silicate, carbonate, fluoride, magnesium and strontium. Silicate substituted calcium phosphate results from substitution of the phosphate ions by silicate ions.
- Coralline ceramics are formed by thermochemically treating coral with ammonium phosphate, leaving TCP with a structure and porosity that are similar to those of cancellous bone. Pore size and porosity are important characteristics of bone graft substitutes. Calcite (magnesium-containing calcium carbonate) is obtained from sea urchins having characteristics similar to bone HA.
- Calcium sulfate and calcium carbonate are not very popular for bone grafting. Calcium sulfate is commonly known as "plaster of Paris" as it was used in Paris for coating walls to make them fire resistant. Calcium sulfate ($CaSO_4.2H_2O$) partially dehydrates to produce a hemihydrate ($CaSO_4.½H_2O$). Calcium sulfate rapidly absorbs within few weeks following insertion and has been used clinically as autograft extender in short segment posterolateral spinal fusions.
- *Bioactive composites:*
    - *Silicate-based grafts:* Available as bioactive glasses are usually now available for carrier purpose and have good structural strength.
    - Bioactive composite of polyethylene reinforced with HA has been used for orbital floor repair and as middle ear implants.
    - Newer materials being studied include biodegradable polymers like polylactic and glycolic acids that are completely degraded by hydrolysis later into nontoxic metabolites eliminated as CO_2 and water.
- Aluminum-based grafts like aluminum oxide bind to bone in response to stress and strain between implant bone interfaces.

23. What are the advantages and disadvantages of bone graft substitutes?

Ans: (*One should read the bone graft substitutes listed and described in detail in Chapter 2 of the book, Essential Orthopedics: Principles and Practice, and enumerate them here*).

Advantages:
- No additional surgery or anesthesia time
- Reduced morbidity in the form of pain and delayed mobilization due to graft harvesting
- No risk of development of incisional hernia and additional site for infection
- No risk of vascular or neurological injury
- No risk of wound complications
- Unlimited quantity available
- No threat to cosmesis
- No risk of transmitting infection (as is with allograft)
- Available in various sizes and forms—can be tailored for need

Disadvantages:
- Added cost
- Limited osteoinduction capacity
- Take very long to get incorporated
- Sterilization concern—can transmit infection if not sterilized well
- Needs strict quality control

24. Discuss allograft bone and their types, their processing, characteristics and antigenicity. Describe Urist stages of allograft healing.

Ans: An allograft is bone tissue transplanted from one individual to another of the same species, usually a cadaver donor. It is widely used in orthopedic surgery to repair or replace bone defects, especially when autograft (self-bone) is not feasible.

Types of allograft bone: The main types are—

A. *Structural allografts*:
- Provide mechanical strength.
- *Examples:* Femoral head, cortical bone shafts, whole bone segments.
- Used in spinal fusions, tumor resections, and reconstruction.

B. *Nonstructural (particulate) allografts*:
- Used primarily for filling bone defects and aiding fusion.
- *Examples*:
    - Cancellous chips
    - Cortical cancellous mix
    - Demineralized bone matrix (DBM)

Allograft bone is classified based on its preparation, structure, and intended use:

1. *Fresh-frozen allografts:* Bone is harvested from a donor, cleaned, and frozen at −70–80°C without further processing.
   - *Uses:* Commonly used in structural applications like large bone defects, joint reconstruction, or spinal fusion (e.g., femoral heads and long bones).
   - *Advantages*:
     - Retains biomechanical strength and some osteoinductive properties (due to preserved growth factors).
     - Minimal processing preserves bone architecture.
   - *Disadvantages*:
     - Higher risk of disease transmission and immunogenicity compared to other types.
     - Requires strict storage conditions (deep freezing).

2. *Freeze-dried (lyophilized) allografts:* Bone is dehydrated through lyophilization (freeze-drying) to remove water content, then stored at room temperature or refrigerated.
   - *Uses:* Used in nonstructural applications like filling bone voids, dental procedures, or as bone graft extenders (e.g., cancellous chips and cortical powder).
   - *Advantages*:
     - Long shelf life (up to 5 years) and easy storage.
     - Reduced antigenicity due to removal of cellular components.
   - *Disadvantages*:
     - Reduced biomechanical strength compared to fresh-frozen allografts.
     - Limited osteoinductive potential due to processing.

3. *Demineralized bone matrix (DBM):* Bone is processed to remove mineral content (calcium phosphate), leaving a collagen matrix enriched with growth factors (e.g., bone morphogenetic proteins, BMPs).
   - *Uses:* Used in bone void fillers, spinal fusion, and craniofacial reconstruction.
   - *Advantages*:
     - Highly osteoinductive due to preserved growth factors.
     - Available in various forms (e.g., putty, gel, and powder) for versatility.
   - *Disadvantages*:
     - Lacks structural integrity; not suitable for load-bearing applications.
     - Variable osteoinductive potential depending on processing and donor factors.

4. *Cancellous allografts:* Derived from cancellous (spongy) bone, typically processed as fresh-frozen or freeze-dried chips or granules.
   - *Uses:* Bone void filling, non-load-bearing defects, and augmentation in joint replacements.

- *Advantages*:
  - Porous structure promotes osteoconduction (scaffold for new bone growth).
  - Good integration with host bone
- *Disadvantages*:
  - Limited mechanical strength
  - Slow incorporation compared to autografts
5. *Cortical allografts:* Derived from cortical (compact) bone, often processed as struts, wedges, or rings.
   - *Uses:* Structural support in spinal fusion, fracture repair, or joint reconstruction
   - Advantages:
     - High mechanical strength for load-bearing applications
     - Provides structural stability.
   - *Disadvantages*:
     - Slower incorporation due to dense structure
     - Limited osteoinductive potential
6. *Osteochondral allografts:* Include bone and adjacent cartilage, typically fresh-frozen to preserve cartilage viability.
   - *Uses:* Joint surface reconstruction (e.g., knee and ankle) in cases of cartilage defects or osteochondral lesions.
   - *Advantages*:
     - Restores both bone and cartilage, preserving joint function.
     - Suitable for young, active patients.
   - *Disadvantages*:
     - High immunogenicity due to cartilage and cellular components
     - Limited availability and complex storage requirements

Characteristics of allograft bone

Allograft bone is characterized by its biological and mechanical properties, which determine its clinical utility:
1. *Osteoconduction:*
   - Allografts provide a scaffold for host bone cells to grow into, guided by the porous structure of cancellous bone or the matrix of DBM.
   - Cortical allografts offer less osteoconduction due to their dense structure.
2. *Osteoinduction:*
   - DBM is highly osteoinductive due to growth factors (e.g., BMPs) that stimulate mesenchymal stem cells to differentiate into osteoblasts.
   - Fresh-frozen allografts retain some osteoinductive potential, while freeze-dried and cortical allografts have minimal to none.
3. *Osteogenesis:*
   - Allografts lack viable cells, so they do not provide osteogenesis (direct bone formation by living cells).
4. *Biomechanical properties:*
   - Cortical allografts provide high mechanical strength for load-bearing applications.
   - Cancellous allografts and DBM are weaker and used in nonstructural roles.
   - Fresh-frozen allografts retain near-native strength, while freeze-drying reduces strength by ~10–20%.
5. *Integration:*
   - Allografts integrate more slowly than autografts due to the absence of living cells.
   - Incorporation occurs via "creeping substitution," where host cells gradually replace the graft with new bone.

Antigenicity of allograft bone

Antigenicity can lead to graft rejection or failure.
1. *Sources of antigenicity:*
   - *Cellular components:* Bone marrow, blood cells, and soft tissues in fresh allografts contain antigens (e.g., major histocompatibility complex, MHC, and molecules) that can trigger an immune response.
   - *Cartilage:* Osteochondral allografts retain cartilage, which is immunogenic due to chondrocytes and matrix proteins.
   - *Collagen and proteins:* The collagen matrix in DBM has low antigenicity, but residual proteins (e.g., BMPs) may provoke a mild response.

2. *Impact of processing on antigenicity:*
   - *Fresh-frozen allografts:* Highest antigenicity due to preserved cellular components. Immune responses may include inflammation or graft rejection, though rare in bone due to its low immunogenicity compared to organs.
   - *Freeze-dried allografts:* Reduced antigenicity due to removal of cellular elements and dehydration, making them less likely to provoke an immune response.
   - *Demineralized bone matrix:* Minimal antigenicity, as demineralization removes most immunogenic components, leaving primarily collagen and growth factors.
   - *Sterilization:* Irradiation or chemical processing further reduces antigenicity but may not eliminate it entirely.
3. *Immune response:*
   - Immune reactions may manifest as local inflammation, delayed incorporation, or, in rare cases, graft resorption.
   - Osteochondral allografts have a higher risk of immune rejection due to cartilage components, sometimes requiring immunosuppressive therapy in joint reconstruction.
4. *Strategies to minimize antigenicity:*
   - Thorough cleaning to remove marrow and soft tissues.
   - Processing (e.g., freeze-drying and demineralization) to eliminate cellular components.
   - Matching donor and recipient for major blood groups or HLA types in rare cases (e.g., osteochondral grafts).
   - Use of DBM or highly processed allografts in immunologically sensitive patients.

Processing of allografts

The goal is to remove cellular elements while preserving biomechanical properties.

A. *Harvesting*:
   - From screened cadaveric donors under aseptic conditions.
B. *Sterilization*:
   - Gamma irradiation, ethylene oxide, or supercritical CO_2.
   - Must balance between antigen removal and preserving bone strength.
C. *Preservation*:
   - Fresh-frozen
   - Freeze-dried (lyophilized)
   - Cryopreserved
D. *Demineralization (for DBM)*:
   - Removes mineral component, leaving behind collagen + growth factors (e.g., BMPs).
E. *Packaging and Storage*:
   - Fresh-frozen allografts require deep-freeze storage.
   - Freeze-dried and DBM allografts are stored at room temperature or refrigerated.
   - Packaging ensures sterility and traceability (e.g., lot numbers, donor information).
F. *Quality control*:
   - Testing for microbial contamination and biomechanical properties.
   - Compliance with regulatory standards (e.g., FDA) ensures safety and efficacy.

Described by *Marshall R. Urist,* the healing of allografts (particularly cortical) occurs in *four distinct stages:*

Stage 1: Inflammatory stage
- Hematoma and inflammation
- Infiltration by macrophages and fibroblasts
- Resorption of necrotic tissue

Stage 2: Revascularization
- Capillary ingrowth from host bone
- Important for graft incorporation
- Begins at the interface and proceeds inward

Stage 3: Osteoinduction and remodeling
- Recruitment of mesenchymal stem cells

- Differentiation into osteoblasts under influence of growth factors (e.g., BMPs)
- New bone formation begins on graft scaffold

Stage 4: Replacement and remodeling
- Gradual resorption of the graft and replacement with host bone.
- Slow process (months to years).
- *Creeping substitution:* simultaneous resorption and new bone formation

25. What is Phemister bone grafting?

Ans: Phemister described a technique of onlay bone grafting for established nonunions in which the graft is placed subperiosteally across the fragments without mobilizing the fragments. Besides being simple to do, its advantages were that the blood supply of the fragments and the normal impacting forces of the fracture were not disturbed. Forbes described a modification of the Phemister technique. Using this modification, he obtained union after the first operation in 27 of 29 nonunions of the tibia. The modified Phemister grafting involved developing osteoperiosteal flaps and keeping the long pencil-like matchstick grafts (corticocancellous) beneath the flaps. Additionally, to traverse across the nonunion site and facilitate osteogenesis, longitudinal troughs were dug—a process called shingling. The edges of shingles were everted to increase surface area. Petaling was also added as described by Uthoff that involved raising petal-like osteoperiosteal flaps on both sides of the nonunion transverse to shingles. These procedures additionally increased the surface area and helped in increasing the vascularity with enhanced approach to the regenerative cells improving chances of achieving union.

Although these techniques were useful for delayed unions and nonunions of long bones, they are now rarely, if ever, used.

26. Enumerate modalities leading to biological enhancement of fracture healing. Mention the methods of preservation of allogenic bone grafts. Comment on mode of action, advantages and disadvantages.

Ans: Modalities for biological enhancements of bone healing written in answer above.
The different methods for preservation of allograft are:
- Cryopreservation—kindly also see Answer to Question 27 below.
  - Frozen allografts
  - Freeze-drying—lyophilization

  Disadvantages: Frozen grafts require special shipping and storage conditions, and freeze-drying requires special lyophilization equipment and procedures that may impact biomechanical integrity.
- *Glutaraldehyde preservation:* Formaldehyde has antibacterial, antifungal and antiviral properties but has slow action. A concentration of 0.5%, 6–12 hours is required to kill bacteria and 2–4 days is required to kill spores. The grafts are well-tolerated by patients and no immunological rejection has been reported. Formalin is an irritant and can cause adverse reaction in body. Also, it is a toxic agent and there are concerns of carcinogenicity so it is not a favored method now for bone preservation.
- *Glycerol preservation:* Glycerol has a low molecular weight, which allows it to replace the water molecules by filling in available space within the tissue structure. By keeping the grafts moist, glycerol allows bone allografts to be stored at room temperature without drying out. The properties of glycerol protect tissue and keep it fully hydrated, avoiding freeze-drying and associated costs and tissue alterations. This improves convenience and reduces costs associated with shipping and storage at ambient temperatures compared to frozen or refrigerated tissue.

27. Enumerate the bone bank and the role of allografts in orthopedic practice.

Ans:

Bone bank: A bone bank provides usable bone grafts (implants) on demand that serve predictable function, and are free from transmissible disease. An increase in the demand of bone grafts due to higher number of complex (spinal fusion, tumor resection reconstruction) and revision surgeries have pressed the need for developing storage and procurement facilities for allograft bone.

Bone banking protocol: Ideally a protocol should be developed by the responsible person from department of orthopedics (preferably the HOD), organ donation and retrieval unit or a bone banking administrator, operation theater nurse, hematological laboratory technician, pathologist and microbiologist in a combined effort depending on the needs and availability of resources for that center and surroundings. They also comprise the team or organizational unit of bone bank. The bone banking administrator need not be a medical personnel but should have adequate training to handle the bone bank.

Donor selection: Informed consent from the person is a must before retrieving the tissue if says he is undergoing hip arthroplasty (for obtaining femoral head). For cadaveric bone retrieval, it is ideal if the person has expressed his wish for donation premortem but deviation may be legally obtained if closest of the relatives freely and voluntarily give consent to do so (depending on state laws) postmortem.

Excision of graft bone, processing and storage: The removed graft is inspected and capsule and synovial tissue are cultured on aerobic and anaerobic bacteria. In order to exclude malignancies, autoimmune inflammatory processes, or infections, a biopsy of 1 cm^3 of representative bone and capsule is sent for histopathological examination (though histopathological examination as a routine standard procedure is debated by agencies and really not mandatory for lacking literature support of utility). The dimensions are noted and it is wrapped using double jar technique (described by Nather). The graft is washed in normal saline or biofiltered water followed by hydrogen peroxide to remove grossly visible fat and debris and dipped in 2% aqueous iodine solution for 15–30 minutes followed by a thorough repeat wash with normal saline. The excess water is then drained and the graft put in a smaller sterile glass jar with a screw-on cap. This is then put in a larger glass bottle with air seal lock, both the jars are sterile. Due labeling of the graft is done with dimensions and it is sent to storage deep-freezer within 30 minutes. The freezer has a temperature of –80°C and that has a continuous temperature registration device charting temperature changes round the clock. The ambient storage temperature range is between –90°C and –70°C to protect against temperature-induced damage to the tissue. Blood samples are collected simultaneously while harvesting the bone graft to determine blood type and routine hemogram. Serological screening for infectious diseases is reperformed 6 months after surgery to exclude infections with window period. This takes care of persons that might be recently infected.

For harvesting cadaveric bone, the donor's limbs are prepped and draped using standard surgical principles, and the tissue is recovered by trained persons. Bones are commonly retrieved from ilium, femur, humerus, tibia, ribs and vertebrae. Small bones and soft tissues are collected using the described "double jar" technique while long bones should be triple wrapped in sterile packaging. The three layers consist of inner gamma-irradiated polyethylene bag, middle layer of autoclaved linen where the bone is tied at ends with cotton tape and outer again a sterile polyethylene bag. The dimensions of bones should be measured and put on the label (to match in future with recipient). All obtained graft material is swab cultured immediately upon retrieval prior to processing. The periosteum is immediately stripped, cleaned as above and the grafts from hereon are kept frozen at –80°C for all further processing and storage (fresh-frozen graft). If gross bacterial contamination is identified or suspected, the material is kept under surveillance and newer techniques, such as bacterial extraction, are used to confirm the results.

For cadaveric donors as it is not possible to reobtain blood samples after 6 months, the blood samples are also stored with the grafts and serological tests reperformed at 6 months before release into storage facility.

Sterilization of graft: Commonly the harvested graft bone is cut and washed with biofiltered water (with or without pressurization) followed by pasteurization (shaker bath at 60°C for 3 hours) and centrifugation with alcohol (70% for 3 hours) or detergent solution. Pasteurization (not necessarily required and should be omitted if aseptic precautions are followed) removes most bacteria, fungi and viruses including human immunodeficiency virus (HIV) (heating greater than 60°C damages the healing properties of bone so should be avoided). Alternatively aqueous solution of iodine may be used to similar effect but prolonged exposure is cytotoxic. Alcohol therapy is effective against HIV, bacteria and spores.

Terminal sterilization is usually done by gamma irradiation. Gamma radiation is effective in killing bacteria, fungi, spores, and, to a lesser degree, viruses. Depending on the dose, however, gamma radiation can weaken the graft. Doses below 1.5 mrad do not adversely affect the tissue strength. A minimum dose of 2 mrad is required to kill bacteria and 4 mrad for killing viruses. A dose of 2.5 mrad is chosen for processed bone giving priority to sterilization and is given by cobalt-60 gamma generators. After processing, the grafts are sent to quarantine for final storage. Grafts are stored at the tissue bank during the quarantine period (6 months) until the second stage serologic and bacteriologic test results and autopsy reports (when required) are received and cleared. The graft is then released for human use after proper labeling and sent to definite storage.

Choice of freeze-dried versus fresh-frozen graft: The shelf life in storage depends on the method of processing and storage; commonly either freeze-drying (lyophilization—infinite) or deep-freezing (5 years) is used. Fresh-frozen grafts are obtained under strict sterile conditions and may not be processed (though most units process them with above method to minimize chances of infection). Freezing an allograft has little impact on the mechanical properties and reduces its immunogenicity; however, it does reduce viability of articular cartilage unless cryopreserved. Lyophilization removes more than 95% of the water enabling biological material (arresting the enzymatic lysis) to be stored for long periods of time even at room temperature. This process is achieved by first freezing the graft and then sublimated in vacuum; the drying is achieved by water evaporation from the specimen and condensation in the condenser.

Quality control of bone banking: As stated above as lot many procedures are involved in bone banking so a stringent protocol should be followed that needs regular monitoring most important of which are:
- Histopathological screening
- Culture swab.

Role of allograft: "Allografts, allogenic bone grafts" (better called "implant" differs from transplant as the bone is nonviable) are available in various forms. Supply in our country is limited for awareness and lack of banking facilities. A graft may be orthotopic (transplanted to the same site in the recipient that it occupied in the donor, e.g., distal femur to distal femur); heterotopic (transplanted to a different site but one occupied by the same tissue as in the donor, e.g., fibula to spine); or ectopic (transplanted to a site normally occupied by a different type of tissue, e.g., fascia lata as a tendon graft). Ectopic sites are mainly investigational for bone grafting. The various types of allografts are as follows:
- Fresh—no clinical use due to high immunogenic potential.
- Fresh-frozen—less immunogenic but needs secondary procedure for sterilization. Preserves BMP.
- Freeze-dried (lyophilized)—bone should be extracted from donor within 8–12 hours of death. The bone loses its inductive factors and BMP due to enzymatic autodigestion by intracellular and extracellular enzymes. Antigen-extracted allogeneic (AAA) bone as advised by Urist may retain inductive factors. Here, chloroform-methanol is used to extract lipids and cell membrane lipoproteins (4 hours); hydrochloric acid extracts acid-soluble proteins and demineralizes the surface in 24 hours; and neural phosphate buffer is used to remove endogenous intracellular and extracellular transplantation antigens. The bone is then frozen and freeze dried and stored at –60°C.
- *Demineralized bone matrix (DBM or bone matrix gelatin, BMG):* This is a digested source of BMP, used as bone graft extender. DBM is available in two forms, dry or injectable. DBM is mixed with a carrier. Carriers (inert with regard to bone generation) include hyaluronic acid, collagen, glycerol, gelatin, and actual derivatives of DBM itself. Second-generation DBM putties (carrier is loaded with BMP) have higher concentrations of BMP and are possibly better.
- *Osteochondral allografts:* Bony chunk with cartilage cover, used for large articular defects in osteochondroses of knee.
- *Shell allografts:* Biologic resurfacing of articular defects using devascularized osteoarticular graft with a small bony component.
- *Large composite allografts:* Usually required for excision of large tumors or reconstruction of defects in revision arthroplasty after freeze thawing.

Indications for use of allograft: Reconstruction of massive bone defects arising from trauma, infection (debridement), osteolysis or revision arthroplasty and resection of bone tumors requiring amount of bone that cannot be supplied by extended autografting procedures. The following are the typical common procedures for which allografts are used (some are common indications for bone grafting in general):
- Reconstruction of skeletal defects following tumor resection
- Reconstruction of bone defects as a result of primary joint arthroplasty osteolysis
- Reconstruction of extensor mechanism of knee
- Reconstruction of congenital or developmental bone and joint defects (protrusio acetabuli, dysplastic hip) and deformities. Acetabular plastic remodeling is required to:
  - Improve coverage of the femoral head
  - Obliteration of cystic cavities of bone
  - Repair of fresh comminuted fractures with bone loss
  - Treatment of nonunion and complicated osteoporotic fractures

- Arthrodesis of large joints
- To provide bone blocks for limiting joint motion (arthrodesis), e.g., flail joint in poliomyelitis
- Treatment of scoliosis and spinal fusion
- Repair of massive segmental bone defects
- Repair of periodontal osseous defects.

28. Describe the key principles of allograft harvest, preparation and preservation in a bone bank.

Ans: Kindly see the answer above.

29. Discuss autografts: Possible sites of harvest, advantages and limitations.

Ans: Bone autografts represent the gold standard for osseous reconstruction due to their osteogenic, osteoinductive, and osteoconductive properties. They are harvested from the patient's own skeleton and transplanted to reconstruct skeletal defects.

Harvest sites
- *Iliac crest*:
  - *Anterior*: Less morbidity, suitable for small defects
  - *Posterior*: Larger volume available but more painful
- *Fibula*:
  - Provides long cortical struts (up to 26 cm)
  - Commonly used for mandibular/long bone reconstruction
- *Rib*:
  - Curved structure useful for craniofacial reconstruction
  - Limited mechanical strength
- *Calvarium:*
  - Split-thickness grafts for craniofacial surgery
  - Low resorption rate
- *Tibia*:
  - Proximal metaphysis provides cancellous bone
  - Less commonly used due to donor site morbidity
- *Radial bone*:
  - Distal radius useful for small hand reconstructions

Advantages:
- *Osteogenic potential:*
  - Contains viable osteoblasts and mesenchymal stem cells
- *Osteoinductive properties:*
  - Contains native BMPs and growth factors
- *Perfect histocompatibility:*
  - No immune rejection or disease transmission
- *Structural integrity:*
  - Cortical grafts provide immediate load-bearing capacity
- *High fusion rates:*
  - Superior to allografts (90–95% vs. 60–80% in spinal fusion)

Limitations:
- *Donor site morbidity:*
  - Chronic pain (iliac crest: 15–30% incidence)
  - Gait disturbance (fibula harvest)
  - Herniation (iliac crest)
  - Fracture risk (fibula, tibia)

- *Limited quantity*:
  - Restricted by anatomical constraints
  - May require supplemental allograft for large defects
- *Increased surgical time:*
  - Requires additional harvesting procedure
- *Variable resorption:*
  - Cancellous grafts more prone to resorption
- *Dimensional mismatch:*
  - May not perfectly match recipient site anatomy

2.3 METABOLIC DISORDERS OF BONE (OSTEOPOROSIS AND ITS TREATMENT, CALCIUM METABOLISM AND ITS DISORDERS, FLUOROSIS, ALKAPTONURIA AND OCHRONOTIC ARTHROPATHY, RENAL OSTEODYSTROPHY) (Q30–72)

30. Explain osteoporosis.
  A. Definition.
  B. Enumerate various causes of osteoporosis.
  C. Enumerate techniques for bone mass measurement.
  D. Drug therapy available for osteoporosis.

Ans:

A. Osteoporosis is defined as a "progressive (often), systemic (commonly) and skeletal disease characterized by overall low bone mass (quantitative) predominated by microarchitectural (qualitative) deterioration of bone tissue that results in increased bone fragility, and hence susceptibility to fracture".
   WHO definition: Bone mineral density (BMD) more than or equal to 2.5 standard deviations below the peak BMD of gender and ethnicity matched 30-year-old healthy Caucasian woman.

B. *Causes:*

   Nonmodifiable:
   - Advanced age
   - Frailty
   - Parental history of fragility fracture
   - Early menopause (<45 years)
   - Primary androgen (males) and estrogen (females) deficiency
   - Hypogonadal states
   - Ethnicity
   - *Genetic factors:*
     - Cystic fibrosis
     - Ehlers-Danlos syndrome
     - Gaucher's disease
     - Glycogen storage disorders
     - Hemochromatosis
     - Homocystinuria
     - Hypophosphatasia
     - Marfan syndrome
     - Osteogenesis imperfecta
   - Small stature
   - Rheumatologic and autoimmune diseases—RA, ankylosing spondylitis
   - Gastrointestinal disorders—peptic ulcer disease, celiac disease, gastric bypass, inflammatory bowel disease, malabsorption
   - Endocrine disorders—type 1 diabetes mellitus and type 2 diabetes mellitus, Cushing's syndrome
   - Hematological disorders—hemophilia, leukemia and lymphoma, monoclonal gammopathy, multiple myeloma

- Neurological and musculoskeletal risk factor—spinal cord injury, epilepsy
- Chronic liver and renal disease.

Modifiable:
- Hyperthyroidism and hyperparathyroidism
- Body mass index (BMI) <20 kg/m² in women (<25 kg/m² in men)
- Low body weight [<127 lb (57.6 kg) in women, <154 lb (69.9 kg) in men]
- Glucocorticoid intake
- Secondary estrogen and androgen deficiency
- Smoking
- Alcohol consumption >3 units (1 unit = 5 oz spirits, 12 oz beer)
- Caffeine intake >4 cups/day
- Inadequate calcium and vitamin D intake
- Prolonged immobility.

C. *Techniques for bone mass measurement:*
   - Radiographs—Singh's index
   - Dual-energy X-ray absorptiometry
   - *Peripheral dual-energy X-ray absorptiometry*
   - Quantitative computed tomography
   - Ultrasound.

D. *Drug therapy:*
   - *Calcium, vitamin D and minerals:* Calcium alone may somewhat reduce, but not fully prevent bone loss. Calcium may be most beneficial for postmenopausal and elderly women. The current recommendation stands at supplementing 600–800 IU of vitamin D_3 per day for older adults with discrete indications. Vitamin K supplementation has been shown to improve BMD possibly due to role in carboxylation of osteocalcin.
   - *Estrogen:* Estrogen replacement therapy (ERT) improves bone mass through receptors on osteoclasts lowering bone turnover and resorption. ERT is most effective in decreasing bone loss when initiated soon after menopause and used continuously.
     - *Selective estrogen receptor modulators (SERMs):* It has been shown to lower the biochemical markers of bone remodeling and it also increases lumbar spine BMD.
   - *Calcitonin:* Minimally effective drug not used primarily for osteoporosis except to reduce osteoporotic pains.
   - *Bisphosphonates:* First-line drugs for treatment of osteoporosis. The main effect of bisphosphonates is to reduce bone resorption and bone turnover, required for treatment of osteoporosis. The secondary effects are reduction of angiogenesis by depression of blood flow and a significant reduction in vascular endothelial growth factor (VEGF). The rank order of potency for inhibiting farnesyl pyrophosphate synthase is zoledronate > risedronate > ibandronate > alendronate. Over prolonged administration, a regional paracrine effect of continuously deposited and recycled bisphosphonates may have persistent effect seen on discontinuation of medication. Bisphosphonates with higher mineral binding affinity, such as alendronate and zoledronate, are associated with greater reduction of bone turnover and have a longer duration of effect.
   - *Receptor activator of nuclear factor kappa-B ligand inhibitors:* Denosumab inhibits the RANKL/RANK formation on the osteoblast, and hence preventing the osteoblast-osteoclast interaction decreasing bone resorption. The "inhibitory effect of denosumab on RANK/RANKL interaction" results in increase in bone mass and strength in both cortical and trabecular bone primarily by antiresorptive action and minimal, if any anabolic effect (it is hence not an anabolic agent).
   - *Teriparatide:* Intermittent parathyroid hormone (PTH) is a potent anabolic agent that stimulates skeletal remodeling and improves BMD. Due to its unique efficacy profile, some even recommend the use of teriparatide as first-line treatment for postmenopausal women and for men with severe osteoporosis. Currently, the treatment with teriparatide is recommended for 2 years whereby the gains in bone mass are quite secure and significant.

(For further details on lesser used drugs, rarely used drugs and futuristic approaches kindly refer to Chapter 3 of the book Essential Orthopedics: Principles and Practice, 2nd edition.)

31. Describe diagnosis of osteoporosis.

Ans: Osteoporosis is diagnosed based on bone mineral density (BMD) measurements, clinical risk factors, and fracture history. The gold standard is dual-energy X-ray absorptiometry (DXA), but other tools and assessments also play a role.

1. *Diagnostic criteria:*

A. DXA scan (T-score classification):
- T-score compares BMD to young healthy adults (peak bone mass).
- WHO classification:
    - Normal: T-score ≥ −1.0
    - Osteopenia (Low bone mass): T-score between −1.0 and −2.5
    - Osteoporosis: T-score ≤ −2.5
    - Severe Osteoporosis: T-score ≤ −2.5 + fragility fracture

B. Z-Score (for younger patients and men < 50 years):
- Compares BMD to age-matched peers.
- Z-score ≤ −2.0 suggests secondary osteoporosis (e.g., steroid use, hyperparathyroidism).

C. FRAX score (fracture risk assessment tool):
- Estimates 10-year probability of major osteoporotic fracture (hip, spine, forearm, and humerus).
- Used when T-score is −1.0 to −2.5 (osteopenia) to guide treatment decisions.

Alternative Tests (If DXA Unavailable):
- Quantitative CT (QCT): More sensitive but higher radiation.
- Peripheral DXA (pDXA): Measures wrist/heel (less accurate).
- Ultrasound (QUS): Heel bone screening (not diagnostic).

32. A. What are risk factors for development of osteoporosis?
B. Explain prevention strategies for risk of osteoporosis.

Ans: A. Risk factors for the development of osteoporosis can be divided into nonmodifiable and modifiable factors.

1. Nonmodifiable risk factors:
These cannot be changed, but help in identifying high-risk individuals:
- Age—risk increases with advancing age.
- Sex—more common in females, especially post-menopausal.
- Genetics—family history of osteoporosis or fragility fracture (especially hip fracture in a parent).
- Ethnicity—higher risk in Caucasian and Asian populations.
- Previous fragility fracture—strongest predictor of future fractures.
- Low peak bone mass achieved in adolescence.

2. Modifiable risk factors
These can be addressed to reduce risk:
- Low calcium and vitamin D intake
- Sedentary lifestyle—lack of weight-bearing or resistance exercise.
- Low body weight/BMI < 19 kg/m^2.
- Smoking—increases bone resorption.
- Excess alcohol intake—≥3 units/day associated with increased fracture risk.
- High caffeine intake—in excess can impair calcium absorption.
- Poor nutrition/eating disorders (e.g., anorexia nervosa)

B. Reduction of risk factors and nutritional modifications: Risk reduction
Patient's education is primary mechanism to modify the environmental factors at home and elsewhere.

Measurements of BMD can be used to assess the risk of a fracture with a high degree of specificity. There is a 1.5- to threefold increase in the fracture rate for each standard deviation of decrease in BMD. The perimenopausal transition is a good opportunity to initiate discussion about risk factors for osteoporosis and to consider a BMD test. A careful history and physical examination should be performed to identify risk factors for osteoporosis. A low Z-score increases the suspicion of a secondary disease. Thorough review of the medications and necessary adjustments should be made. Identification of hypogonadal state and thyrotoxicosis by laboratory tests, orthostatic hypotension by clinical methods and treatment of visual impairment are some of the key measures. Height loss >2.5–3.8 cm (1–1.5 inch) is an indication for radiography to rule out asymptomatic vertebral fractures, as is the presence of significant kyphosis or back pain, particularly if it began after menopause.

The clinical history, physical examination and radiological evaluation/biological tests are aimed at:
- Excluding a disease that can mimic osteoporosis
- Elucidating causes of osteoporosis and contributory factors
- Assessing the severity of osteoporosis and the risk of subsequent fractures
- Selecting the most appropriate form of treatment.

Control of Risk Factors
The following are common measures initiated for most patients:
- *Lifestyle*: Walk briskly for a minimum of 1 hour, three times a week
- Smoking cessation
- Alcohol cessation.

33. Describe medical management of postmenopausal osteoporosis.
Ans: Please see the answer above.

34. Juvenile idiopathic osteoporosis.
Ans: Juvenile idiopathic osteoporosis is a rare form of self-limiting osteoporosis (bone fragility and low bone mass) of unknown cause that has been described in children aged as young as 1 year to 14 years old. It was first described by Schippers in 1938 but first recognized by Dent in 1965. Most of the available literature is in the form of case reports so generalizations of the disease have been generated from them only.

There is no genetic linkage yet recognized and no familial occurrence has been reported. One report suggests autosomal recessive inheritance without scientific support.

Pathogenesis: There appears to be a primary reduction in the number of remodeling cycles initiated in cancellous bone and additional secondary reduction in amount of bone deposited in each cycle. The bone formation rate per unit bone surface (BFR/BS) is decreased to 38% of the value found in age-matched controls. These effects are due to fewer recruitment of osteoblasts and osteoclasts producing thin mature trabeculae and reduction in secondary trabeculae in the metaphyses. The resulting weak bones are susceptible to fracture with low-energy injuries itself. Cortical bone is spared. The chief concern is that the children is in bone accumulation phase during these years but due to the osteoporosis the golden period of bone mass accumulation is lost.

Clinical and radiological presentation: Common presentations are:
- Insidious onset of pain in back and lower extremities
- Abnormal gait preceding fragility fractures
- Long bone fractures—impaction type fractures at ends of long bones —distal tibia and distal femur.
- Vertebral compression fractures
- Clinical examination is frequently normal, but some patients may show:
  1. Kyphosis
  2. Scoliosis
  3. Pectus carinatum
  4. Long bone deformity
  5. Difficult ambulation
- Cancellous areas of bone showing new, abnormal bone formed in the metaphyseal region as "neo-osseous osteoporosis" appearing as a linear radiolucent, submetaphyseal band.
- Generalized low aBMD and vBMD with more a pronounced reduction in the trabecular compartment.

Differential diagnoses: One needs to rule out all causes of secondary osteoporosis (as below) and osteopenia before the disease can be labeled juvenile idiopathic osteoporosis. In particular, osteogenesis imperfecta is a difficult differential to rule-out:
- Osteogenesis imperfecta
- Rickets
- Turner syndrome
- Malabsorption syndrome
- Acquired disorders such as celiac disease, medical diseases (hypothyroidism, diabetes mellitus, malabsorption disorders, anorexia nervosa, etc.)
- Wilson's disease
- Osteoporosis
- Pseudoglioma syndrome
- Homocystinuria
- Immobilization
- Malignancy
- Glucocorticoids

Treatment and prognosis: There are no prescribed treatments for the condition and the patients are mainly treated symptomatically. The main modalities include calcium supplements with vitamin D and antiresorptive therapy with bisphosphonates. Fall protection is included to prevent fragility fractures while muscle mass improvement is also simultaneously introduced with physical therapy and exercises. The disease has been self-limiting in most of the reports taking 2–5 years to subside and only a few reports indicate persistence into adulthood.

35. Distinguish between osteoporosis and osteopenia.

Ans: Osteopenia is a radiological diagnosis per se. While osteoporosis is a disorder affecting bone quality and mineralization with specific complications. Osteopenia is an essential radiological component of osteoporosis but osteopenia may be also seen in any disorder of bone mineralization be it metabolic, inflammatory or infective impacting bone negatively. Osteopenia may also be localized and is commonly used when bone loss is localized. The objective difference between generalized osteopenia and osteoporosis can be established by DEXA scanning (Table 2.3.1).

TABLE 2.3.1: Differentiation between osteopenia and osteoporosis based on DEXA values.

DEXA T-score	Bone mineral density (BMD)	Interpretation
Between −1 and −2.5	Between 1 and 2.5 standard deviation below that of the mean level for a young adult reference population	Low bone mass (osteopenia)
T-score ≤ −2.5 (i.e., "Numerical values" higher than 2.5 say 3 or 3.2, etc.)	BMD value ≥2.5 standard deviation below mean peak bone mass of a young adult reference population	Osteoporosis

36. Describe briefly principle and indications of pulsatile PTH therapy in orthopedics.

Ans: Continuous infusions of PTH and analogs cause persistent elevation of the serum PTH concentration and result in bone resorption, the usual effect of PTH. However, interestingly and contrary to the conventional thinking exogenously administered intermittent PTH is a potent anabolic agent that stimulates skeletal remodeling and improves BMD. RhPTH (1–34) has significant effect on reducing the risk of vertebral fractures and nonvertebral fractures in postmenopausal women. The increase in BMD is, however, noted most prominently at vertebral sites than at nonvertebral sites when given in a dose of 20 µg/day. There is an initial reduction in cortical bone density possibly due to initial increase in intracortical porosity. The appositional new bone formation is also stimulated that increases the cross-sectional area of bone and cortical bone strength. The effect of teriparatide are mediated in a multifactorial manner possibly involving Wnt pathway (stimulating Wnt10b and inhibiting sclerostin), IGF-I mediated anabolic effect, etc.

General Orthopedics

37. Enumerate various metabolic and endocrine diseases having skeletal manifestations

Ans:

Metabolic diseases:
- Rickets
- Osteomalacia
- Hypervitaminosis D
- Scurvy
- Fluorosis
- Malabsorption syndrome
- Gout
- Ochronotic arthritis

Endocrine diseases:
- Hypogonadism
- Hypopituitarism
- Hypothyroidism/hyperthyroidism
- Hyperparathyroidism/hypoparathyroidism
- Hyperadrenalism/hypoadrenalism
- Diabetes
- Gigantism/acromegaly
- Glucocorticoid excess

38. Discuss the tests that prognosticate osteoporosis.

Ans: A number of risk factors have been identified and used to predict the risk of developing osteoporosis and associated fracture. Using some of these validated risk factors and clinical assessment tools, the risk to fracture in a patient can be estimated as low (<10% chance to fracture in next 10 years), moderate (10–20% in next 10 years) or high (>20% in next 10 years). Three such tools are available developed by different agencies to give an approximate measure of chance to suffer from osteoporosis-related fracture over next 10 years (10-year fracture risk in a given patient).

1. FRAX® tool developed and available free by the World Health Organization (WHO)
2. The QFracture scores
3. CAROC tool produced by the Canadian Association of Radiologists and Osteoporosis, Canada.

Fracture risk assessment (FRAX®) tool is a web-based calculator that includes a number of clinically identified risk factors [bone mineral density (BMD) can be optionally included]. FRAX® has been developed to calculate the 10-year probability of a hip fracture taking into account the femoral neck BMD and clinical risk factors. It can also be used to calculate the 10-year probability of other major osteoporotic fractures (defined as clinical vertebral, hip, forearm, or proximal humerus fracture) using the mentioned clinical risk factors. FRAX® tool is most useful in patients with low BMD at femoral neck, when the same is included. It has been found, however, that FRAX® underestimates the fracture risk in patients with multiple osteoporosis-related fractures, recent fractures and those at increased risk for falling. Also, when FRAX® underestimates risk when applied to patients with low BMD at vertebral body but relatively normal BMD at femoral neck. The WHO algorithm is not validated for use of lumbar spine BMD. The specific applications are:

- FRAX® is intended to use in postmenopausal women and men aged 50 years or older
- FRAX® may be calculated with total hip BMD or femoral neck BMD, but the latter is preferred. Other sites are not recommended.
- FRAX® has not been validated for use in currently or previously treated patients with pharmacotherapy for osteoporosis. Patients off the pharmacotherapy for 1–2 years may be considered untreated.

QFracture scores do not require laboratory measurement. It utilizes simple parameters that are known to the individual and are easily accessible without rigorous testing such as age, sex, height, weight, previous fracture, parental history of hip fracture, current smoking, glucocorticoid treatment, RA, secondary osteoporosis, and use of alcohol (>3 units/day). It is a good tool for primary care or for individual self-assessment and has the biggest advantage of not requiring any BMD score. This tool also shows some improved discrimination and calibration compared with the FRAX algorithm but does not include the risk assessment for osteoporotic proximal humerus fracture.

Being simple, there is likelihood of its use as a systematic population-based program to identify high-risk patients. Also, QFracture has been developed and validated on a large and representative primary care population so is specifically useful in primary care population. The inclusion of risk factors such as history of falls, type 2 diabetes mellitus, cardiovascular disease, use of tricyclic antidepressants (TCA), hormone replacement therapy, and menopausal symptoms make Qfracture a more individualized tool. Unlike FRAX tool that has been adapted for international use, the current version of Qfracture is designed only for use in UK.

The CAROC tool takes into account age, sex, fracture history, and glucocorticoid use to determine a 10-year absolute risk of all osteoporotic fractures. Here, BMD is mandatory to calculate risk. Similar to this is the American Special Operations Forces (SOF) research group model that is based only on the age and BMD to predict the 10-year risk of hip and major osteoporotic fracture. Regardless of the tool used, it is important to understand that all these highlight the importance of patient's age (higher the age higher the risk), bone density (lower the density higher the risk), and previous history of osteoporosis-related fracture (higher the risk in such patients) as important determinants of possibly suffering from osteoporosis-related fracture.

Bone mineral density and dual-energy X-ray absorptiometry (DEXA): BMD has been considered the strongest predictor of sustaining a primary osteoporotic fracture (secondary and future fractures are better predicted by having a primary fracture itself). The bone strength variation is dependent on BMD, but in only 50% or less of the cases as the strongest predictor cannot be the sole measure to define osteoporosis as in the WHO definition. As a significant impact of BMD, the vertebral fracture risk is inversely correlated to bone mineral content. It is estimated that roughly for a decline of 1 standard deviation in bone mass, there is a 1.3–2.5-fold increase in risk of osteoporosis-related fracture. 1% increase in BMD decreases fracture risk by about 4%. But the expectation and relation are nonlinear and nonuniversal. The National Osteoporosis Foundation (NOF) study itself revealed that 82% of postmenopausal females that presented with a fracture within 1 year had a T-score above –2.5, and 67% had a T-score above –2.0 as measured with peripheral densitometry. Each standard deviation decrement in femoral neck BMD has been found to increase the risk of fracture 2.6-fold. BMD at the femoral neck is a better predictor of hip fracture than BMD at other places. Patient with previous fracture and current low BMD would have additive influence and is more likely to suffer with a fracture than either factor alone. The risk of fractures in women with two fractures is 75-fold greater, if their BMD currently is <–2.5 standard deviation compared to those with no fractures and normal BMD.

39. Explain FRAX and FRAX Plus score. Enumerate current evidence-based treatment guidelines for osteoporosis and sarcopenia.

Ans: FRAX (Fracture Risk Assessment Tool)

FRAX is a widely used clinical tool developed by the University of Sheffield in 2008 to estimate an individual's 10-year probability of a major osteoporotic fracture (spine, hip, forearm, or shoulder) and hip fracture specifically. It integrates clinical risk factors with or without bone mineral density (BMD) measured by dual-energy X-ray absorptiometry (DXA) at the femoral neck to assess fracture risk in men and women aged 40–90 years. FRAX is particularly useful for identifying high-risk individuals who may benefit from treatment, even if their BMD does not meet the osteoporosis threshold (T-score ≤ –2.5).

Key Components of FRAX:
- **Risk factors** (12 clinical factors):
  – Age
  – Sex
  – Weight and height (to calculate body mass index, BMI)
  – Previous fragility fracture
  – Parental history of hip fracture

- Current smoking
- Glucocorticoid use
- Rheumatoid arthritis
- Secondary causes of osteoporosis (e.g., type 1 diabetes mellitus, untreated hyperthyroidism, hypogonadism, chronic liver disease, chronic malnutrition)
- Alcohol intake (≥3 units/day)
- Femoral neck BMD (optional, improves accuracy)

Calculation:
- FRAX uses country-specific fracture and mortality data to calculate the 10-year probability of:
  - Major osteoporotic fracture (MOF): ≥20% indicates high risk.
  - Hip fracture: ≥3% indicates high risk (per National Osteoporosis Foundation, NOF).

FRAX plus: FRAX plus is an enhanced version of FRAX introduced to address some of its limitations by incorporating additional risk factors to refine fracture probability estimates. It adjusts FRAX scores based on the following:
- *Recency of fracture:* Recent fractures (within 2 years) significantly increase the risk of subsequent fractures.
- *Number of prior fractures:* Multiple prior fractures increase risk more than a single fracture
- *Glucocorticoid dose:* FRAX assumes average glucocorticoid exposure, but FRAX plus adjusts for specific doses/durations.
- *Type 2 diabetes mellitus duration:* FRAX underestimates fracture risk in type 2 diabetes mellitus
- Falls history
- *Hip axis length (HAL):* Longer HAL increases hip fracture risk, while shorter HAL reduces it.
- Lumbar spine/femoral neck BMD discordance: Significant differences between lumbar spine and femoral neck T-scores can enhance MOF risk assessment.

Evidence-based Treatment Guidelines for Osteoporosis

National Osteoporosis Foundation [NOF] (USA):
- Treat postmenopausal women and men ≥50 years with:
  - Hip or vertebral fracture (clinical or morphometric)
  - T-score ≤ -2.5 at femoral neck, total hip, or lumbar spine
  - T-score between -1.0 and -2.5 with FRAX 10-year risk of:
    - Hip fracture ≥3%.
    - Major osteoporotic fracture ≥20%

National Osteoporosis Guideline Group (NOGG) (UK):
- Treat based on FRAX risk (with or without BMD):
  - *High risk:* MOF ≥20% or hip fracture ≥3%.
  - *Very high risk:* FRAX probability exceeding intervention threshold by 60% (age-dependent).
  - *Intermediate risk:* Consider BMD if available; treat if history of fragility fracture or risk exceeds threshold.
  - *Low risk:* Offer lifestyle advice without pharmacological treatment.

Goal: Prevent fractures, improve bone mineral density (BMD), and reduce mortality.
1. Nonpharmacological Measures:
   - Calcium and vitamin D supplementation:
     - Calcium: 1,000–1,200 mg/day (diet + supplements if needed).
     - Vitamin D: 800–2,000 IU/day [maintain serum 25(OH)D ≥ 30 ng/mL].
   - Lifestyle modifications:
     - Weight-bearing exercise (walking, resistance training).
     - Fall prevention (balance training and home safety modifications).
     - Smoking cessation, alcohol moderation.

2. Pharmacological Therapy (First-line, see **Table 2.3.2**)

TABLE 2.3.2: Pharmacotherapy for osteoporosis.

Drug class	Examples	Indication	Key evidence
Bisphosphonates	Alendronate, Zoledronate	First-line for most postmenopausal women and men	↓ vertebral fractures by 40–70%, hip fractures by 40–50% (FIT trial)
RANK-ligand inhibitor	Denosumab (Prolia)	High-risk patients (prior fractures, very low BMD)	↓ vertebral (68%) and hip (40%) fractures (FREEDOM trial)
Anabolic agents	Teriparatide, Abaloparatide	Severe osteoporosis (T-score ≤–3.5 or multiple fractures)	↑ BMD by 10–15%, ↓ fractures
SERMs	Raloxifene, Bazedoxifene	Postmenopausal women (if bisphosphonates contraindicated)	↓ vertebral fractures (30–50%)
Romosozumab (anti-sclerostin)	Evenity	Very high fracture risk (short-term 1-year use)	↑ BMD 15%, ↓ vertebral fractures by 73% (ARCH trial)

Evidence-based Treatment Guidelines for Sarcopenia

Sarcopenia, characterized by age-related loss of skeletal muscle mass and function, is closely linked to osteoporosis (osteosarcopenia) and increases fracture risk.

Diagnosis
- European Working Group on Sarcopenia in Older People (EWGSOP2):
  - *Criteria:* Low-muscle strength (e.g., grip strength <27 kg men and <16 kg women) and low muscle mass (e.g., appendicular skeletal muscle mass <20 kg men, <15 kg women by DXA).
  - *Severe sarcopenia:* Add low physical performance (e.g., gait speed ≤0.8 m/s).
- FRAX as a screening tool:
  - FRAX scores (MOF ≥ 20% and hip ≥ 3%) are associated with sarcopenia in chronic liver disease (CLD) and may predict sarcopenia risk with high sensitivity.

Goal: Improve muscle mass, strength, and physical function.
1. Nonpharmacological Measures:
   - Resistance exercise training (RET):
     - 2–3 sessions/week, progressive intensity (↑ strength by 30–150%).
   - Protein supplementation:
     - 1.0–1.5 g/kg/day (higher for severe sarcopenia)
     - Leucine-rich foods (whey protein, eggs, and soy)
   - *Vitamin D*:
     - 1,000–4,000 IU/day if deficient (↓ falls/fractures)
2. Pharmacological Therapy (see **Table 2.3.3**)

TABLE 2.3.3: Pharmacotherapy for sarcopenia.

Drug/Therapy	Evidence
Testosterone (men with deficiency)	↑ muscle mass (modest effect)
Selective Androgen Receptor Modulators (SARMs)	Under investigation (Ostarine, Enobosarm)
Myostatin Inhibitors	Experimental (Bimagrumab – failed Phase 3)
Ghrelin Agonists	Improved appetite/muscle mass in cachexia

40. A. Classify osteoporosis.

B. Discuss the clinical presentation and management of senile osteoporosis.

Ans:

A. *Classification:*
  Primary:
  - Type 1 (postmenopausal)

- Type 2 (senile or involutional)
- Type 3 ("postclimacteric", it is not a part of original classification but is similar to type 1 osteoporosis but occurring in males)

Secondary:
- *Hormonal:* Hypogonadism, thyrotoxicosis, Cushing's, hyperprolactinemia and diabetes mellitus
- *Drugs:* Steroids, phenobarbital, anticonvulsants, anticoagulants, cytotoxic agents, etc.
- *Nutritional:* Calcium deficiency, vitamin C and vitamin D deficiency, malabsorption, alcohol intake and malnutrition
- *Metabolic diseases:* Osteogenesis imperfecta, homocystinuria, Marfan syndrome, etc.
- Chronic liver and renal disease
- *Miscellaneous disorders:* Multiple myeloma, RA, mastocytosis, thalassemia, Wilson's disease, hemochromatosis, etc.

B. **Clinical Presentation:**

There are no specific clinical signs or symptoms for osteoporosis. Patients generally have nonspecific, nonlocalized and mild bone pains usually in central skeletal system that slowly progress in intensity and distribution. The back pain is due to microfractures and ligament stretching and in late cases due to iliocostal impingement from kyphotic deformity. The paraspinal muscle constantly remains under strain due to altered sagittal structure of the spine getting spasm and soreness over a period of time.

Kyphosis is usually the earliest sign associated with loss of height. Loss of 2 inches in height sensitively indicates vertebral compression. The number of missing teeth has also been correlated with reduced BMD. All older persons should be evaluated for fall risk. They should be observed as they stand up from chair without using arms and walk few steps and return (get up and go test). Those who have difficulty need assessment for fall circumstances, medications, medical problems, vision, gait and balance, lower extremity evaluation (proprioception, reflexes), mobility tests, basic neurological function (cortical, pyramidal and extrapyramidal, cerebellar), mental status and cardiovascular functions.

Management: Pharmacotherapy has been described in answer above.

Principles of surgical management of osteoporotic fractures. These are:
- Manage not just the fracture, but the geriatric patient as a whole, so balance the outcome of inflicting surgical trauma on biology of body system.
- Quick and precise surgeries by expert in the field are preferable. Also one should focus on modalities that afford quickest mobilization, for example in octogenarians with even minimally fracture of femoral neck doing a quick hemiarthroplasty is beneficial over screw fixation. For relatively younger patients with osteoporosis, total hip replacement would be better.
- The rate of bone union is not affected by osteoporosis per se, but due to old age the prolongation of healing process is possibly due to age-related blunting of reactionary process. However, it is the implant holding strength that influences stabilization of fracture and union. Implants may fail as they have to maintain fracture for prolonged periods due to longer healing time and poor holding strength. Locked screw plate constructs at variable angle are preferable to dynamic compression plates. Absolute stability and lag screw techniques are not effective in osteoporotic bones. Focus should be strain reduction by utilizing relative stability techniques. Providing wide buttress to juxta-articular fractures is also a good option rather than fixing the fracture fragment.
- Plating is beneficial at juxta-articular and intra-articular fractures; however, for diaphyseal fractures, intramedullary nailing should be preferred for biology preservation, dynamic load sharing, relative stability and less invasive nature.
- Augmentation with bone cement to improve screw purchase at trabecular bone (delta bolt for hip, cannulated screws with side openings for humerus, femoral condyle and vertebrae) could be considered to improve strength of fixation. Hydroxyapatite-coated implants with deliverable growth factors like bone morphogenetic proteins (BMPs), TGF-β could provide improved fixation in future.
- Some people prefer intramedullary fibula graft to improve screw purchase, but the published literature on this method is scanty.
- Comminuted fractures at metaphyseal or periarticular regions could be better managed by arthroplasty, for example, proximal humerus and proximal femur.

41. Define peak bone mass. What factors affect attaining peak bone mass? How does it correlate with osteoporosis?

Ans: Bones are a growing tissue that continues till skeletal maturation. During this time, the bones gather mass and mineral density with collagen framework improves. After skeletal maturity, the bone mass is under maintenance mode with modeling and remodeling. Peak bone mass (PBM), which can be defined as the amount of bony tissue present at the end of the skeletal maturation. PBM is achieved in second decade (20% > in men), with age the bone mass is lost gradually in both sexes more in females (females:males = 4:1). Women tend to experience minimal change in total bone mass between age 30 and menopause but after this the bone mass rapidly reduces unless intervened. In males, there is a constant loss of mass that remains more or less constant until geriatric age or occurrence of male climacteric. Over a lifetime, a female loses 30% of cortical bone and 50% of trabecular bone; males lose two-thirds of above values. Because the loss of bone is a percentage of mass gathered during growth, it is logical to think that higher the mass gained better will be the bone strength later in life. There are a number of factors that affect PBM:

- *Genetic make-up:* This is a nonmodifiable factor but accounts for 75% of the PBM, a particular individual will gain.
- *Sex:* PBM is higher in males than females.
- *Race:* African American females have higher PBM than white females.
- *Hormonal influence:* Females that have early menarche and those taking pills containing estrogen for birth control have higher bone mass.
- *Nutrition:* Maintaining adequate calcium in diet improves bone mass during young and adolescence.
- *Physical activity:* Doing regular physical exercises improve the bone mass (Wolff's law).
- *Lifestyle:* Smoking, sedentary life, alcohol intake have been linked to reduced bone mass.

42. Discuss the management of osteoporotic spine fractures.

Ans: Osteoporotic fragility fractures are associated with significant morbidities like reduced vital capacity of lungs (thoracic vertebral compression fractures), chronic low back pain (continuous strain on back muscles due to poor posture), shift of sagittal balance, stooping posture and increased tendency to fall, chronic low back pain and further associated increased risk of vertebral fractures (19.2% increased risk in subsequent year). Overall, there is increased mortality that emanates due to variable combination of these but more related to severity of kyphosis. It is not that all of the compression fractures have a bleak outlook and indeed majority heal spontaneously and are clinically silent (silent vertebral fracture). Somewhere one-third of the fractures become painful that gradually reduces over 6–12 weeks.

Fractures that fail to heal get filled with fluid typically near the superior end plate in the anterior region. This gradually results in true intravertebral "pseudoarthrosis" formation that is associated with sclerosis of the superior end plate. The fluid is then gradually resorbed to be replaced by "air" and the surrounding bone gets necrosed with replacement of hematopoietic cells with marrow edema and fibrosis. The intravertebral pseudoarthrosis is associated with "dynamic mobility" due to the presence of cleft filled with air or fluid. On performing the supine extension radiographs, it has been noted that some 87.5% of osteoporotic vertebral fractures are mobile that could restore height by 62.6% if maintained. The intravertebral cleft is responsible for spinal instability but provides an opportunity to restore height by procedures like cement augmentation. After the diagnosis of osteoporotic vertebral fracture is made on radiographs and/or magnetic resonance imaging (MRI) scan, clinician may obtain computed tomography (CT) scan to look for posterior vertebral wall fracture or ankylosing spine both of which are contraindications for cement augmentation. Impregnation of polymethyl methacrylate (PMMA) into the vertebral body (vertebroplasty) provides improved pain relief and rehabilitation. Vertebroplasty is the direct injection of low-viscosity liquid PMMA cement into the osteoporotic vertebral body fracture. The cement then sets and provides the vertebral body with requisite strength under compressive forces.

The indications of vertebroplasty for osteoporosis include:
- Failed conservative management in symptomatic acute osteoporotic vertebral fracture
- Symptomatic osteoporotic vertebral fracture that is progressively collapsing as seen on imaging
- Symptomatic vertebral fragility fracture with dynamic mobility.

The procedure is performed in prone position under local anesthesia usually. Commonly unipedicular approach is used where the vertebral body is accessed through one pedicle or some prefer bipedicular approach where another needle is passed through the other pedicle.

Bipedicular approach is helpful where one is suspecting vascular malformation so that before injecting cement one may confirm by injecting contrast in the vertebral body flushed by normal saline before injecting cement. In case of a cavity

or cleft, there is free flow of contrast or saline from the other needle. Extrapedicular approach may be used for thoracic vertebra where the pedicles are smaller. Commonly two patterns of cement distribution are observed after vertebroplasty:
1. The trabecular or interdigitation pattern
2. The cleft or lump pattern.

Trabecular pattern represents cementation into the cancellous trabecular bone rather than void filling. Lump pattern instead represents filling of the intravertebral cleft or fluid cavity of pseudoarthrosis. Lesser amount of cement is injected in the trabecular pattern compared to the void filling pattern and on an average 4 mL of cement is needed considering all cases. One must not try to achieve complete filling of the vertebral body under pressure from end plate to another end plate which is rarely achievable and has high chances of cement leak.

The dreaded complications of vertebroplasty are extradural extravasation of bone cement that would cause neurological compromise and formation of cement emboli that may migrate in the spinal canal. Kyphoplasty (balloon kyphoplasty or balloon-assisted vertebroplasty) is considered to be a more effective procedure as it involves inflating a balloon inside the vertebra restoring vertebral height and then bone cement is injected into the balloon. This potentially ameliorates cement extravasations. Pain relief is prompt and lasting; however, there are concerns of compression fractures of adjacent vertebrae and cost with kyphoplasty.

Balloon kyphoplasty can be performed by orthopedic surgeon or interventional radiologist under general anesthesia or deep sedation. The majority of vertebral osteoporotic compression fractures occur at the thoracolumbar junction. The primary indications for balloon kyphoplasty are:
- Painful fractures with a back pain score of 4 points or more on a 0–10 scale not responding to conservative treatment for 6 weeks
- Compression fracture due to osteoporosis (primary or secondary), osteolytic metastatic tumors (D5-L5 levels), multiple myeloma
- *Junctional lesions:* "Adjacent vertebra" of a fractured and treated one at the level of D12 or L1 in severely osteoporotic patient, older than 75 years of age with good Karnofsky performance status score (>70). This is preventive treatment as it has been found that at D12-L1 level if one of the vertebrae is treated then the other one shows a fracture within 18 months.

Contraindications for balloon kyphoplasty:
- Age less than 21 years
- Previous vertebroplasty of the same vertebra
- Pedicular fracture
- Severe disease:
  - Radicular pain
  - Neurological deficit
  - Evident spinal cord compression
- Patients on uninterruptible anticoagulation therapy
- Allergy to any of kyphoplasty instrumentation
- Nonambulatory before fracture
- Fractures due to primary bone tumors, osteoblastic metastasis and high-energy trauma.

Principles of procedure: The procedure is performed as short admission of 24 hours. The success relies on regular expansion of the vertebral body that can be stabilized by intraosseous cement. Injection pressure and the cement viscosity are hence the most important parameters. It has been identified that higher viscosity and lower injection pressures are important for uniform expansion of the bone and optimal filling.

Operative Technique
These are:
- The surgery is done under anesthesia. The patient lies prone and best worked under O-arm or two C-arms to give continuous anteroposterior and lateral views
- Pedicle is localized under fluoroscopy.
- After making stab incision, 11-gauge biopsy needle is advanced into the fractured vertebral body by transpedicular approach.
- Working cannula is introduced and needle is removed.

- Inflatable balloon tamp is introduced under the collapsed end plate.
- Balloon tamps are then inflated under fluoroscopic control measuring the pressure through inbuilt manometer.
- Maximum fracture reduction is achieved and inflation is stopped when the balloon reaches the cortical wall or one obtains the "balloon kissing" position (two balloons introduced through each pedicle touching each other in the vertebral body center).
- Cement is prepared and loaded in syringes.
- At semisolid state (3–5 minutes after mixing, depends on product), the cement is introduced carefully under fluoroscopy control.
- At cement setting, the cannula is removed and wound closed.

Vertebroplasty versus Kyphoplasty: Before comparing the two procedures, it is best accepted that both the procedures are effective and safe in providing pain relief from osteoporotic fragility fractures. The improvement in quality of life and physical function is quite rapid along with reducing the disability. The comparison between procedures can be based on the following points:

- *Reduction of disability and pain relief:* Most studies and meta-analysis have demonstrated comparable pain relief and functional recovery in the patients with a slight bias toward the former in vertebroplasty and the latter in kyphoplasty.
- *Restoration of vertebral height:* It appears that by the procedure itself if pressurized balloon improves the vertebral body height then kyphoplasty must be able to restore the vertebral height better but in studies there has been quite significant evidence of finding improvement in vertebral height by vertebroplasty also.
- *Complications and sequelae:* Cement leakage is a significant complication of vertebroplasty with incidence as high as 41% (20–41%) as compared to kyphoplasty (7–9%).
- *Kyphoplasty* is comparatively much expensive than vertebroplasty and for this reason in developing countries like ours we tend to prefer vertebroplasty. Also, kyphoplasty needs general anesthesia and longer admission while vertebroplasty could be performed in local anesthesia itself as a day care procedure.

43. Explain management protocol of osteoporotic vertebral fracture with a flowchart.

Ans:

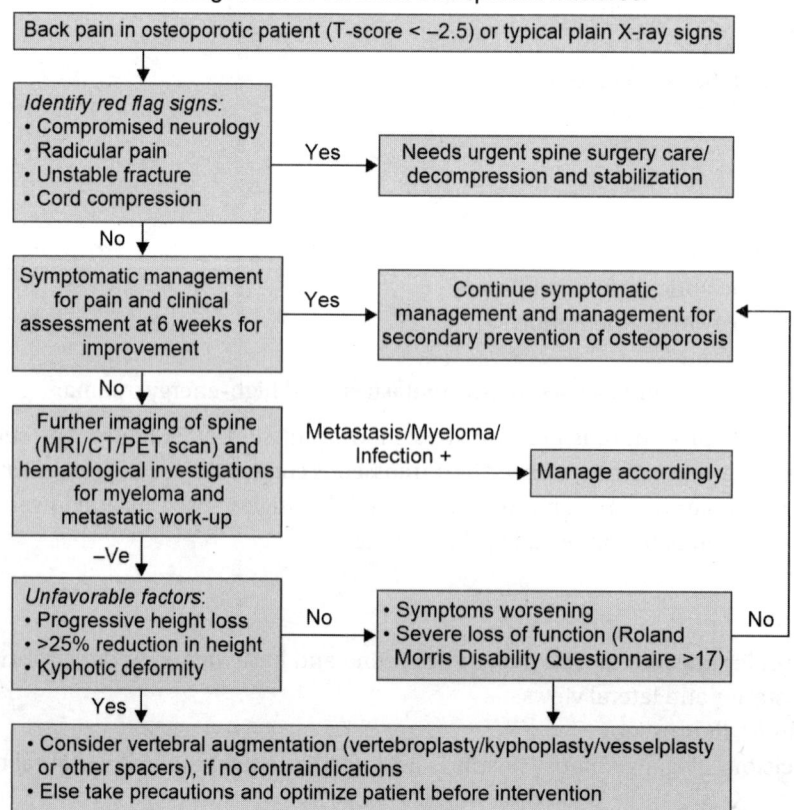

Management of vertebral osteoporotic fractures.

44. Describe the principles of management of fragility fractures of long bones.

Ans: *Following are the general principles of management of fragility fractures:*
- Manage not just the fracture, but the geriatric patient as a whole, so balance the outcome of inflicting surgical trauma on biology of body system.
- Quick and precise surgeries by expert in the field are preferable. Also, one should focus on modalities that afford quickest mobilization, for example in octogenarians with even minimally fracture of femoral neck doing a quick hemiarthroplasty is beneficial over screw fixation. For relatively younger patients with osteoporosis, total hip replacement would be better.
- The rate of bone union is not affected by osteoporosis per se, but due to old age the prolongation of healing process is possibly due to age-related blunting of reactionary process. However, it is the implant holding strength that influences stabilization of fracture and union. Implants may fail as they have to maintain fracture for prolonged periods due to longer healing time and poor holding strength. Locked screw plate constructs at variable angle are preferable to dynamic compression plates. Absolute stability and lag screw techniques are not effective in osteoporotic bones. Focus should be strain reduction by utilizing relative stability techniques. Providing wide buttress to juxta-articular fractures is also a good option rather than fixing the fracture fragment.
- Plating is beneficial at juxta-articular and intra-articular fractures; however, for diaphyseal fractures, intramedullary nailing should be preferred for biology preservation, dynamic load sharing, relative stability and less invasive nature.
- Augmentation with bone cement to improve screw purchase at trabecular bone (delta bolt for hip, cannulated screws with side openings for humerus, femoral condyle and vertebrae) could be considered to improve strength of fixation. Hydroxyapatite-coated implants with deliverable growth factors like BMPs, TGF-β could provide improved fixation in future.
- Some people prefer intramedullary fibula graft to improve screw purchase, but the published literature on this method is scanty.
- Comminuted fractures at metaphyseal or periarticular regions could be better managed by arthroplasty, for example proximal humerus and proximal femur.
- *Pharmacotherapy in surgery:* Bisphosphonates and anabolic therapy—patients on bisphosphonates can definitely undergo fracture fixation. The question is for those patients who are osteoporotic and identified with a fracture. Though bisphosphonates suppress bone resorption, and hence the coupled process of bone formation, but they have not been primarily found to alter the rate of fracture healing. Increased callus size and mineralization, reduced remodeling and improved mechanical strength have been observed in animal studies. Improved implant fixation and strength have also been observed. As regards the concern on retarding remodeling, they have not been found to have any adverse effect. Scheduling first dose is the controversy. Oral drugs can be given at any time; however, delaying by 3 weeks is considered better for compliance issues and theoretical concern of formation and organization of fracture callus. Injectable drugs should be preferably delayed for 3–4 weeks or more or withheld (oral drugs are preferable) as drugs like zoledronic acid have localizing effect so they may concentrate at the fracture site immediately after administration and systemic advantages on other bones may be lowered till next dose.
- Teriparatide has not been shown to alter fracture healing and although anabolic has also not been definitely shown to improve fracture healing, though the effect is overall positive. Sclerostin and Dickkopf-1 (DKK-1) antibodies (discussed below) have also been shown to have beneficial effect on fracture healing.

45. Write risk factors and preventive measures for the geriatric fractures for citizen's aged >65 years.

Ans: *Risk factors:*
- Older age
- Female sex
- Low bone density
- Low body weight
- History of falls and fracture
- Previous osteoporotic fracture at related (previous contralateral hip fracture) or unrelated site (vertebral fracture)
- Family history of hip fracture
- Glucocorticoid use

- Comorbidities—diabetes, atherosclerosis/cardiac disease, cerebrovascular disease, dementia, Parkinson's disease, movement disorders
- Cigarette smoking
- Heavy alcohol use

Prevention:
- Fall prevention measures—primary and secondary prevention
  - Remove small area rugs and mats
  - Avoid step-stools
  - Install nonslip mats in shower area
  - Add handrails on staircases
  - Ensure good lighting in rooms, rest-rooms and cleaning area
  - Wear foot-wear with nonslip soles
- Vitamin D supplementation + calcium supplementation
- *Promotion of weight-bearing exercises:*
  - Improves proprioception, strength and muscular balance across joints
  - Improves body balance
  - Reduces effect of sarcopenia
- Reduce caffeine intake
- Limit alcohol intake
- Control medications that cause sedation
- Primary and secondary prevention of osteoporosis.

46. **Describe the biochemical markers of bone formation and resorption. Discuss their role in the management of osteoporosis.**

Ans:

Markers of bone formation:
- Bone specific alkaline phosphatase
- Osteocalcin
- Type 1 collagen extension peptide.

Markers of bone resorption:
- Hydroxyproline
- Tartrate-resistant acid phosphatase (TRAP)
- Cross-linked N-telopeptide
- Cross-linked C-telopeptide
- Urine total free deoxypyridinoline.

Role in osteoporosis management:
- These predict quite reliably the rapidity of bone loss in untreated patients.
- Bone markers may predict fracture risk in untreated patients (independent of BMD).
- Bone markers can categorize an individual as having fast or slow bone turnover. Fracture risk is higher in the former.
- During treatment follow-up, reduction in markers of bone resorption indicates reduced bone turnover with antiresorptive therapy. This effect is considered parallel to reduced fracture risk independent of changes in BMD. Specifically, studies report that decreased urinary pyridinoline and deoxypyridinoline crosslinks after 6 months on alendronate therapy have been associated with increases in BMD at the hip and spine after 2.5 years of treatment.
- Bone markers can be used as a check mechanism on the patients on antiresorptive therapy. The compliance with antiresorptive therapies can be monitored by using these markers as minimal or no reduction in urinary N-telopeptide concentrations suggests poor compliance, though this effect may also arise with impaired drug absorption that should be considered. Urinary N-telopeptide of COL1A1 has shown the most significant association between BMD and response to hormone replacement therapy (HRT).
- Finally, they help to determine duration of "drug holiday" and also as to when the medication should be restarted.

47. Explain the merits and demerits of parathormone therapy on osteoporosis.

Ans: *Merits:*
- Only anabolic agent that consistently produces increase in bone mass
- Can improve severe osteoporosis
- Has good and established role in steroid-induced osteoporosis
- Drugs decreasing bone resorption initially increase BMD but it reaches a plateau in 2–3 years because bone formation also decreases. On the other hand, drugs promoting bone formation like teriparatide can increase BMD throughout the period of treatment.

Demerits:
- *Osteosarcoma:* In male and female rats, teriparatide caused an increase in the incidence of osteosarcoma. It should not be prescribed for patients at increased baseline risk of osteosarcoma. These include:
  - Paget's disease of bone. Unexplained elevations of alkaline phosphatase may indicate Paget's disease of bone.
  - Pediatric and young adult patients with open epiphyses.
  - Prior external beam or implant radiation therapy involving the skeleton.
- *Treatment duration:* The safety and efficacy have not been evaluated beyond 2 years of treatment.
- *Bone metastases and skeletal malignancies:* Patients with bone metastases or a history of skeletal malignancies should not be treated with it.
- *Metabolic bone diseases:* Patients with metabolic bone diseases other than osteoporosis should not be treated with it.
- *Hypercalcemia and hypercalcemic disorders:* This drug has not been studied in patients with pre-existing hypercalcemia. These patients should not be treated with it because of the possibility of exacerbating hypercalcemia. Patients known to have an underlying hypercalcemic disorder, such as primary hyperparathyroidism, should not be treated.
- *Urolithiasis or pre-existing hypercalciuria:* In clinical trials, the frequency of urolithiasis was similar in patients treated with this drug and placebo. However, this drug has not been studied in patients with active urolithiasis. If active urolithiasis or pre-existing hypercalciuria is suspected, measurement of urinary calcium excretion should be considered. It should be used with caution in patients with active or recent urolithiasis because of the potential to exacerbate this condition.
- *Orthostatic hypotension:* It should be administered initially under circumstances in which the patient can sit or lie down if symptoms of orthostatic hypotension occur. In short-term clinical pharmacology studies with teriparatide, transient episodes of symptomatic orthostatic hypotension were observed in 5% of patients. Typically, an event began within 4 hours of dosing and spontaneously resolved within a few minutes to a few hours. When transient orthostatic hypotension occurred, it happened within the first several doses, it was relieved by placing the person in a reclining position, and it did not preclude continued treatment.
- *Drug interactions:* Hypercalcemia may predispose patients to digitalis toxicity. Because it transiently increases serum calcium, patients receiving digoxin should use this drug with caution.

48. Describe the mechanism of action of teriparatide along with its potential complications.

Ans: *Mechanism of action:* It is the recombinant parathyroid hormone (PTH), the N-terminal segment rhPTH (1–34) that exerts their anabolic effect (*osteoanabolic therapy*) on bone by binding to the PTH receptor on osteoblasts. It has been noted that PTH in low and pulsatile dose stimulates bone formation whereas in excess, it causes resorption of bones. The effect of teriparatide are mediated in a multifactorial manner possibly involving Wnt pathway (stimulating Wnt10b and inhibiting sclerostin), IGF I-mediated anabolic effect, etc.

Complications:
- Tiredness and depression
- Palpitation, nausea, vomiting, and constipation or diarrhea
- Leg cramps
- Joint pains
- Osteosarcoma [therapy >2 years in rats only, not demonstrated in monkeys or humans (three cases reported, but not linked definitively)]
- Hypercalcemia

(The reader is encouraged to read the Wnt pathway and its details from the Chapter 3 of the book Essential Orthopedics: Principles and Practice)

49. What are bisphosphonates? Discuss the role of bisphosphonates in various orthopedic disorders.

Ans: These agents are used for the treatment of osteoporosis due to their inhibitory effect on osteoclast-mediated bone resorption. These drugs accelerate apoptosis of osteoclasts and also suppress differentiation of osteoclast precursors to mature osteoclasts [by inhibiting interleukin-6 (IL-6)]. This results due to reduction in cholesterol synthesis via inhibition of farnesyl pyrophosphate synthase by bisphosphonates.

Drugs in this group include:
- 1st generation—(least potent) medronate, clodronate and etidronate.
- 2nd generation—alendronate, ibandronate and pamidronate.
- 3rd generation—risedronate and zoledronate (most potent).

These are used for the treatment of:

Osteogenesis imperfecta: Quite significantly it has been demonstrated that the bone strength is improved by administration of bisphosphonates and it constitutes an important therapy in this disease irrespective of age or clinical presentation.

Osteoporosis: Second-generation bisphosphonate alendronate was the first aminobisphosphonate approved by the US Food and Drug Administration (FDA) for the treatment and prevention of osteoporosis. Alendronate inhibits bone resorption without much deleterious effects on mineralization. Spinal BMD shows continuous improvement after alendronate therapy up to 7 years of daily therapy. A once-weekly dosing is most popular, but has been randomly decided. Risedronate is a third-generation pyridinyl bisphosphonate with somewhat inferior antiresorptive effect compared to alendronate, but similar fracture reduction efficacy. Tiludronate is ineffective when administered intermittently. Zoledronate (third-generation bisphosphonate) has highest potency and very good efficacy similar to or better than alendronate.

Hypercalcemia of malignancy and antiresorptive effect in cancer patients: Bisphosphonates are the drug of choice for all patients with multiple myeloma and radiologically confirmed bone metastases from breast cancer. Bisphosphonates are to be started in these cases immediately as soon as the diagnosis is made and are continued indefinitely. Other bone metastasis should also be treated with bisphosphonates when appropriate. The effects of bisphosphonates have been twofold:
1. Reducing pain
2. Prevention of pathological fractures. It should be remembered that they are approved only for cancer with metastasis.

Paget's disease of bone: Interestingly, the antiresorptive effect of bisphosphonates was first demonstrated in Paget's disease. Use of bisphosphonates showed dose-dependent inhibition of bone resorption, and hence remodeling. As good efficacy has been established since 1980s, the treatment with bisphosphonate class of drugs for Paget's disease is currently the preferred modality. The primary drug used for the treatment of Paget's has been alendronate, intravenous. Pamidronate (preferred), oral resedronate and tiludronate usually along with calcitonin.

Pediatric uses:
- *Fibrous dysplasia and McCune-Albright syndrome:* Radiological improvement has not been demonstrated, but pain relief has been reported by most patients. Definitive role is not known.
- *Perthes disease:* Studies have been sparse, but there is a suggestion that possibly they may restrict deformation of the head and collapse similar to osteonecrosis.
- *Osteoporosis in children:* Primary osteoporosis is unknown, but secondary osteoporosis does respond to the effects of bisphosphonates. It reduces occurrence of fractures and increase BMD.

Other uses:
- *Postsurgical:* In enhancing implant fixation.
- Prevention of bone collapse in osteonecrosis at various sites, but commonly used at hip joint.
- *Bone scanning:* Bisphosphonates by virtue of their strong affinity for bone mineral get accumulated at sites of increased bone turnover acting as bone scanning agents. Also, their ability to be linked to a gamma-emitting technetium isotope serves an important advantage for detecting bone metastasis and other bone lesions.
- Prevent heterotopic ossification following hip replacement surgery.
- Treatment for calcification in renal failure and vascular disease.

50. Write a brief note on alendronate-induced fractures.

Ans: *Atypical insufficiency fractures:* These have been found to occur at sacrum, femoral shaft and proximal femur (more likely bilateral). Lot of reports have creeped up mentioning "atypical" fractures associated with the long-term use of bisphosphonates after their first description by Odvina et al. in 2005. A task force was created by American Society for Bone and Mineral Research (ASBMR) defined major and minor features of incomplete and complete atypical femoral fractures and recommended the following major features (at least four of the following five major features should be present in a fracture for classifying as atypical femoral fracture located along the femoral diaphysis from just distal to the lesser trochanter till just proximal to the supracondylar flare:

1. Localized periosteal or endosteal thickening of the lateral cortex present at the fracture site as "beaking" or "flaring"
2. Transverse or short oblique orientation
3. Minimal or no associated trauma
4. A medial spike when the fracture is complete
5. Absence of comminution

The minor features include:
- Cortical thickening
- Prodromal pain
- Bilaterality
- Delayed healing
- Comorbid conditions
- Concomitant drug use, including bisphosphonates or other antiresorptive agents, glucocorticoids and proton-pump inhibitors.

Bisphosphonate-induced subtrochanteric fractures are a serious complication. Due to the bone "freezing" effect of bisphosphonates, the microcracks keep accumulating in the bone and do not get repaired for absence of remodeling due to inhibition of osteoclasts. These are low turnover fractures due to reduction in bone remodeling induced by long-term bisphosphonate therapy. It has been found that the incidence of atypical femoral fractures is around 1–2/100,000/year in patients exposed to bisphosphonate therapy for <2 years while it increases to >100/100,000/year for those kept on bisphosphonates for >8 years.

The stress fractures develop over time on the tensile side of femur (lateral cortex). Such fractures typically accumulate in the dense cortical bone. Subtrochanteric region of femur near isthmus contains highest percentage of compact bone so it gets weakened enough to fail under repeated stress. The risk to fracture reduces rapidly as the treatment with drug is discontinued. This suggests that a process other than inhibition only of remodeling is involved as absence of remodeling would only explain the delayed healing or failure to healing of the fracture and not the inception of fracture.

Fracture without significant trauma would occur due to poor matrix and mineral properties such as reduced heterogeneity of the organic matrix, increased advanced glycation end products (AGEs like pentosidine) and reduced bone quality (alteration of pyridinoline/deoxypyridinoline ratio and collagen cross-linking reducing postyield deformation of bone and its toughness). This would suggest that the bone at the tensile surface would be unable to bear the physiological stresses and microcracks would develop which in the absence of regular fracture remodeling propagate and coalesce to form larger gaps. These gaps are high strain areas around which the osteocytes die (an effect due to high strain mechanically and reduction of angiogenesis by direct biological effect of bisphosphonates) and ultimately a stress fracture is created that gives way later.

Mechanical factors such as the geometry of femur also play a role. Bowing of femur at the upper thirds of femoral shaft is quite common in older females and may be related to the concentration of tensile stress in this region predisposing them to regular microfractures that in oversuppression of bone remodeling would give way ultimately.

A causal association between bisphosphonates and atypical fractures has not been completely established though there is a very strong correlation. However, recent observations imply that the risk rises with increasing treatment duration. Bisphosphonates are known to accumulate at the fracture site so continued dosing leads to inhibition of repair of microfractures.

The tendency to unite after fixation is also subdued having high chances of delayed or nonunion, if treatment is continued. This effect is possibly related to delayed or incomplete maturation of calcified callus into mature bone by inhibition of osteoclastic remodeling by bisphosphonates.

The atypical fractures are treated in a standard way as for shaft femur fracture with strict withholding of the drug. Role of anabolic agents in the treatment of bisphosphonate-associated atypical femoral fractures is emerging and it is considered that such patients may be put on anabolic therapy to improve the outcome (union) as reported in sporadic studies and small case series. For patients who have not developed atypical fractures but are experiencing prodrome (common in more than half of such patients), evaluate the other limb also by radiographs and if possible MRI, while the ipsilateral limb would definitely need prophylactic fixation. If a fracture is identified (marrow edema/cortical thickening), then in symptomatic patient's prophylactic fixation is recommended with or without anabolic therapy.

51. Explain the various methods of fixing severely osteoporotic fractures.

Ans: The following are some guiding principles for management of osteoporotic fractures:

- Quick and precise surgeries by expert in the field are preferable. Also, one should focus on modalities that afford quickest mobilization, for example in octogenarians with even minimally fracture of femoral neck doing a quick hemiarthroplasty is beneficial over screw fixation. For relatively younger patients with osteoporosis, total hip replacement would be better.
- The rate of bone union is not affected by osteoporosis per se, but due to old age the prolongation of healing process is possibly due to age-related blunting of reactionary process. However, it is the implant holding strength that influences stabilization of fracture and union. Implants may fail as they have to maintain fracture for prolonged periods due to longer healing time and poor holding strength. Locked screw plate constructs at variable angle are preferable to dynamic compression plates. Absolute stability and lag screw techniques are not effective in osteoporotic bones. Focus should be strain reduction by utilizing relative stability techniques. Providing wide buttress to juxta-articular fractures is also a good option rather than fixing the fracture fragment.
- Plating is beneficial at juxta-articular and intra-articular fractures; however, for diaphyseal fractures, intramedullary nailing should be preferred for biology preservation, dynamic load sharing, relative stability and less invasive nature.
- Augmentation with bone cement to improve screw purchase at trabecular bone (delta bolt for hip, cannulated screws with side openings for humerus, femoral condyle and vertebrae) could be considered to improve strength of fixation. Hydroxyapatite-coated implants with deliverable growth factors like BMPs, TGF-β could provide improved fixation in future.
- Some people prefer intramedullary fibula graft to improve screw purchase, but the published literature on this method is scanty.
- Comminuted fractures at metaphyseal or periarticular regions could be better managed by arthroplasty, for example proximal humerus and proximal femur.
- *Pharmacotherapy in surgery:* Bisphosphonates and anabolic therapy—patients on bisphosphonates can definitely undergo fracture fixation. The question is for those patients who are osteoporotic and identified with a fracture. Though bisphosphonates suppress bone resorption, and hence the coupled process of bone formation, but they have not been primarily found to alter the rate of fracture healing. Increased callus size and mineralization, reduced remodeling and improved mechanical strength have been observed in animal studies. Improved implant fixation and strength have also been observed. As regards the concern on retarding remodeling they have not been found to have any adverse effect. Scheduling first dose is the controversy. Oral drugs can be given at any time; however, delaying by 3 weeks is considered better for compliance issues and theoretical concern of formation and organization of fracture callus. Injectable drugs should be preferably delayed for 3–4 weeks or more or withheld (oral drugs are preferable) as drugs like zoledronic acid have localizing effect so they may concentrate at the fracture site immediately after administration and systemic advantages on other bones may be lowered till next dose.
- Teriparatide has not been shown to alter fracture healing and although anabolic has also not been definitely shown to improve fracture healing though the effect is overall positive. Sclerostin and DKK-1 antibodies (discussed below) have also been shown to have beneficial effect on fracture healing.

52. Describe the bone remodeling unit. Briefly describe the drugs which influence remodeling.

Ans: The remodeling is not constantly occurring throughout the skeleton at once, but it occurs in discrete packets termed bone remodeling units (BRUs) by Frost, scattered throughout the skeleton. Each packet takes 3–4 months to complete. There is, however, some quantitative bone loss with age (senile osteoporosis) as bone formation always lags temporally and quantitatively from bone resorption possibly due to decreased number of osteoblasts. The process of remodeling of bone involves three discrete steps of activation, bone resorption and bone formation that need discrete cellular and molecular components to complete. Bone remodeling is prominent at endosteal and periosteal surfaces and is also seen within Haversian canal systems that contain osteoprogenitor cells. The width of tubular bones and also the bone mass are controlled by cortical bone remodeling.

Resorption of bone is interestingly activated by stimulatory cytokines IL-1 and IL-6 produced by osteoblasts (that are ironically really meant for bone formation) and also involves modulation of the integrin RGD (Arg-Gly-Asp) sequence interaction. Bone resorption takes approximately 10 days carried out by a "cutting cone" of osteoclasts. The defect created after resorption, is filled in by fibrovascular tissue containing pericytes (later forming Haversian and Volkmann's canals), monocytes or macrophages, mesenchymal stem cells and undifferentiated osteoprogenitor cells in loose connective tissue. Histopathologically, basophilic line—the "cement" or the "reversal" line marks the outer edge of the osteon (where bone formation is initiated). The resorption front of cutting cone does not follow osteonal arrangement and progresses randomly, so that in a single go it can take down multiple osteons. With mineralization front, the osteons are partially repaired and form new interconnected channels depending on the stress pattern. The lamellae that remain as reminiscent of cutting cone activity persist as interstitial lamellae and keep accumulating over the age of person. The interstitial lamellae are less active metabolically and are, hence, unable to repair promptly. This is partly responsible for senile osteoporosis.

As BRU involves both osteoclasts and osteoblasts so the drugs affecting bone metabolism, all affect BRU like:
- Bisphosphonates
- Parathormone analog
- Vitamin D
- Calcitonin
- Strontium
- Selective estrogen receptor modulators
- Denosumab
- Statins
- Growth factors like IGF

53. Discuss rickets: pathology, types, diagnosis and treatment.

Ans: It is a defect in mineralization of osteoid matrix caused by inadequate calcium and phosphate deposition prior to closure of physis. Rickets is a disease of growing bone that occurs in children (before fusion of epiphysis) and clinical features arise from unmineralized matrix at the growth plate.

Pathology: The characteristic pathological changes in rickets arise from the inability to calcify the intercellular matrix in the deeper layers of the physis. The proliferative zone is as active as ever, but the cells, instead of arranging themselves in orderly columns, pile up irregularly; the entire physeal plate increases in thickness, the zone of calcification is poorly mineralized and bone formation is sparse in the zone of ossification. The new trabeculae are thin and weak, and with joint loading the juxta-epiphyseal metaphysis becomes broad and cup-shaped.

Types: The following are the various types/varieties of rickets **(Box 2.3.1)**.

Box 2.3.1: Etiological classification of rickets.

Vitamin D disorders:
- Nutritional deficiency of vitamin D
- Vitamin D-dependent rickets type 1
- Vitamin D-dependent rickets type 2
- Congenital vitamin D deficiency

Contd...

Contd...

- Secondary vitamin D deficiency:
  - Malabsorption
  - Decrease liver 25-hydroxylase
  - Increase degradation
- Chronic kidney disease

Renal losses:
- Autosomal dominant hypophosphatemic rickets
- Autosomal recessive hypophosphatemic rickets
- X-linked hypophosphatemic rickets
- Hereditary hypophosphatemic rickets with hypercalciuria (HHRH)
- Excess production of phosphatonin:
  - Neurofibromatosis
  - Tumor-induced rickets
  - McCune–Albright syndrome
  - Epidermal nevus
- Dent disease
- Fanconi syndrome
- Distal renal tubular acidosis

Calcium deficiency:
- Decrease intake
- Malabsorption
- Phosphorous deficiency
- Premature infants (rickets of prematurity)
- Aluminum-containing antacids

Diagnosis: A common battery of tests including serum calcium, inorganic phosphate, alkaline phosphate, vitamin-D and PTH levels along with urinary calcium and phosphate analysis is sufficient to diagnose and differentiate various types of rickets **(Table 2.3.4)**.

TABLE 2.3.4: Laboratory findings in various types of rickets.

Disorder	Ca	Pi	25-OHD	1,25-(OH)$_2$D	PTH	AlkPhos	Urinary Ca	Urine Pi
Vitamin D deficiency	N, ↓	↓	↓	↓, N, ↑	↑	↑	↓	↑
VDDR, type 1	N, ↓	↓	N	↓	↑	↑	↓	↑
VDDR, type 2	N, ↓	↓	N	↑↑	↑	↑	↓	↑
Dietary calcium deficiency	N, ↓	↓	N	↑	↑	↑	↓	↑
X-linked hypophosphatemic	N	↓	N	RD	N	↑	↓	↑
Dietary Pi deficiency	N	↓	N	↑	N, ↓	↑	↑	↓
Chronic renal failure	N, ↓	↑	N	N	↑	↑	N, ↓	↓
ADHR	N	↓	N	RD	N	↑	↓	↑
HHRH	N	↓	N	RD	N, ↓	↑	↑	↑
Tumor-induced rickets	N	↓	N	RD	N	↑	↓	↑

Treatment: Management depends on the type of rickets but mostly involves vitamin D medication along with adequate calcium and if needed phosphate supplementation.

Nutritional vitamin D deficiency: Adequate intake of vitamin D, calcium, and phosphorous is the mainstay of treatment in nutritional vitamin D deficiency rickets, which can be administered by the following methods:

- *Stoss therapy:* 300,000–600,000 IU of vitamin D is administered orally or intramuscularly as 2–4 doses over 1 day. Because the doses are observed, Stoss therapy is ideal in situations where adherence to therapy is questionable.

- *Alternate therapy:* High-dose vitamin D, with doses ranging from 2,000 to 5,000 IU/day over 4–6 weeks. Treatment of vitamin D deficiency due to malabsorption requires high doses of vitamin D. 25-D (25–50 μg/day or 5–7 μg/kg/day) is superior to vitamin D3 as it is better absorbed. Alternatively, calcitriol may be used which is better absorbed in the presence of fat malabsorption, or with parenteral vitamin D.
  Long-term treatment with calcitriol is the treatment for VDDR type I. Initial doses are 0.25–2 μg/day, with lower doses used once the rickets has healed, with adequate intake of calcium.

Renal rickets: The aim is maintaining calcium-phosphate homeostasis, avoiding aluminum toxicity and preventing heterotopic calcification. Calcitriol is the treatment of choice. This permits adequate absorption of calcium and directly suppresses the parathyroid gland. Sevelamer hydrochloride, a phosphate binder used orally, and dietary restriction of phosphate to regulate serum phosphate levels can be used individually or in combination as hyperphosphatemia is a stimulus for PTH secretion. In addition, metabolic acidosis may be corrected with alkalis. More recently a calcimimetic drug, cinacalcet, has been introduced which acts directly on the parathyroid glands increasing the sensitivity of calcium receptors and inducing a reduction in serum PTH levels.

Hypophosphatemic rickets: A combination of oral phosphorus and calcitriol is given to get an appropriate response. The daily need for phosphorus supplementation is 1–3 g of elemental phosphorus divided into 4–5 doses. Frequent dosing helps to prevent prolonged decrements in serum phosphorus because there is a rapid decline after each dose also the side effects of high dose phosphorous, such as diarrhea is avoided. Calcitriol is administered 30–70 ng/kg/day divided into two doses.

(For additional details kindly read Chapter 3 of the book Essential Orthopedics Principles and Practice, 3rd edition)

54. Describe the physiology of calcium metabolism. Explain in detail the role of PTH in calcium metabolism. Tabulate the biochemical differences between renal tubular and glomerular rickets.

Ans: *Physiology of calcium metabolism:* Calcium is essential for normal cell function and physiological processes such as blood coagulation, nerve conduction and muscle contraction. Hypocalcemia may cause tetany while hypercalcemia can lead to depressed neuromuscular transmission. The normal concentration in plasma and extracellular fluid is 8.8–10.4 mg/dL. Much of this is bound to protein; about half is ionized and effective in cell metabolism and the regulation of calcium homeostasis.

The recommended daily dosage of elemental calcium is:
- 1,200–1,500 mg/day in postmenopausal women not on HRT
- 1,000–1,200 mg/day in premenopausal women, men and postmenopausal women on HRT.

Children need less, about 200–400 mg/day. The main sources of calcium are dairy products, green vegetables and soya. About 50% of the dietary calcium is absorbed (mainly in the upper gut) but much of that is secreted back into the bowel and only about 200 mg enters the circulation.

Calcium absorption in the intestine is promoted by vitamin D metabolites, particularly $1,25(OH)_2$ vitamin D, and requires a suitable calcium/phosphate ratio. Absorption is inhibited by excessive intake of phosphates (common in soft drinks), oxalates (found in tea and coffee), phytates (*chapatti* flour) and fats, by the administration of certain drugs (including corticosteroids) and in malabsorption disorders of the bowel.

Urinary excretion varies between 100 mg and 200 mg per 24 hours. If the plasma ionized calcium concentration falls, PTH is released and causes:
- Increased renal tubular reabsorption of calcium and
- A switch to increased $1,25(OH)_2$ vitamin D production and enhanced intestinal calcium absorption.

If the calcium concentration remains low, calcium is drawn from the skeleton by increased bone resorption, which again is under the indirect influence of PTH.

Hypocalcemia: The classic feature of hypocalcemia is the development of tetany. Patients may complain of loss of sensation, paresthesiae and muscle spasms. More severe signs are convulsions and laryngeal spasm.

Hypercalcemia: Mild elevation of serum calcium concentration (up to 12.5 mg/dL) may cause no more than general lassitude, polyuria and polydipsia. With plasma levels between 12.5 mg/dL and 15 mg/dL, patients may complain of anorexia, nausea, muscle weakness and fatigue. Those with severe hypercalcemia >15 mg/dL present with severe symptoms including abdominal pain, nausea, vomiting, severe fatigue and depression. In long-standing cases, patients may develop kidney stones or nephrocalcinosis due to chronic hypercalciuria; some complain of joint symptoms, due to chondrocalcinosis. The clinical picture is aptly (though unkindly) summarized in the old adage "moans, groans, bones and stones". There may also be symptoms and signs of the underlying cause, which should always be sought (in the vast majority, this will be hyperparathyroidism, metastatic bone disease, myelomatosis, Paget's disease or renal failure).

Role of parathyroid hormone: Parathyroid hormone produced from the parathyroid gland is a polypeptide hormone synthesized from pro-PTH. PTH maintains calcium homeostasis by stimulating bone resorption. In fetal and neonatal animals, PTH is required for normal formation and development or remodeling of cancellous bone. PTH also impacts intestine and kidney function. Reduced serum calcium is the strongest stimulator of PTH release from parathyroid glands. The physiologic role of PTH includes:
- Increase in osteoclastic activity which results in calcium and phosphate release from the bony skeleton (mediated through osteoblasts and RANK and RANKL).
- In kidney, PTH reduces calcium excretion, but increases phosphate excretion. It also stimulates $1,25(OH)_2$ vitamin D production.

These measures increase serum calcium concentration which suppresses the secretion and synthesis of PTH. PTH controls the serum calcium levels on a minute-to-minute basis probably because we live in low calcium–high phosphate environment and the calcium levels are important with respect to sustaining life. Interestingly, despite being bone resorptive hormone receptors for PTH are found on preosteoblasts, osteoblasts and chondrocytes, but absent from osteoclast which supports the notion that PTH mediates osteoclastogenesis and bone resorption is osteoblast-dependent and mediated via cytokines. The ultimate effect of this action is osteoclast activation, initiation of bone resorption and maintaining adequate blood calcium levels for optimal functioning of dependent organs like contractile tissues by calcium release from bone. Simultaneous osteoblast stimulation might be a check mechanism preventing too much bone resorption and "policing" the action of osteoclasts against excessive calcium stealth. Clinical use of PTH analog has demonstrated that in certain situations PTH stimulates bone formation. It has been shown that in continuous administration of PTH there is increased osteoclastic resorption with simultaneous suppression of bone formation. The effect reverses to bone formation instead when PTH is administered in low doses, intermittently. This anabolic effect is also probably indirectly mediated via IGF-I and TGF-β. Constant high serum PTH levels, initiate osteoclast formation resulting in bone resorption that overrides the effects of activating genes that direct bone formation indicating that osteoclast function and formation requires persistently high PTH levels due to indirect action. The action on osteoblasts is more direct, but possibly the bone resorption is much more efficient process than the slower bone formation so that persistent elevated levels produce predominantly bone resorption. PTH-related protein (PTHrP) is expressed early in the osteoblast progenitor cells and regulates bone formation in a paracrine manner. This process persists longer so that pulsatile stimulation by even low doses of PTH will stimulate osteoblasts escaping bone resorption that needs high persistent levels.

Differences between renal tubular and glomerular rickets:
I am really unsure of what is exactly meant by glomerular rickets, most likely the examiner wanted to know rickets due to chronic renal failure. The differences are mentioned in **Table 2.3.5**.

TABLE 2.3.5: Biochemical differences between renal tubular acidosis and renal failure.

Criteria	Renal tubular acidosis	Renal failure
Calcium	Low	Low
Phosphorus	Low	High
Alkaline phosphatase	High	High
Parathormone	High	High
Urine phosphorus	High	Low
Urinary calcium	Low	Normal to low
Bicarbonate	Low urine pH	Low

(For a detailed understanding of the differences between different types of standard rickets causes, kindly refer to Chapter 3 of the book Essential Orthopedics: Principles and Practice, 2nd edition.)

55. Describe regulation of mineral metabolism by 1,25-(OH)2 vitamin D.

Ans: Regulation of mineral metabolism by 1,25-(OH)2 vitamin D
- Stimulates synthesis of calcium binding protein (cholecalcin—transports calcium from luminal to basal layer in intestine).
- Affects osteocalcin production.
- Osteoid mineralization
- Osteoclastic bone resorption and maintenance of blood calcium levels
- Increased active transcellular absorption of calcium from proximal part of intestine
- Increased phosphorus absorption from distal part of small intestine
- Reduced calcium and phosphorus excretion from kidney

56. Describe the anatomy of parathyroid gland. Discuss the clinical features, radiological presentation of adenoma of parathyroid gland. What is hungry bone syndrome?

Ans: *Anatomy of parathyroid gland:* Parathyroid glands (para- means near), these are commonly two pairs of small-rounded structures embedded in the posterior surface of thyroid gland **(Fig. 2.3.1)**. The glands are separated from thyroid by a thick connective tissue. Significant population has additional "ectopic" thyroid glands in neck/chest, etc. The glands contain two types of cells, the oxyphil cells function of which is unclear till date and the chief cells that secrete parathormone involved in regulation of serum calcium levels.

Superior parathyroid glands develop from fourth pharyngeal pouch and are commonly found 1 cm above the inferior thyroid artery.

Inferior parathyroid glands derive from third pharyngeal pouch and are located near the inferior poles of thyroid gland.

Vascular supply: Inferior thyroid artery supplies both the groups and veins drain into thyroid plexus of veins.

Lymphatics: Drain into deep cervical and paratracheal lymph nodes.

Nerves: Thyroid branch of cervical sympathetic ganglia.

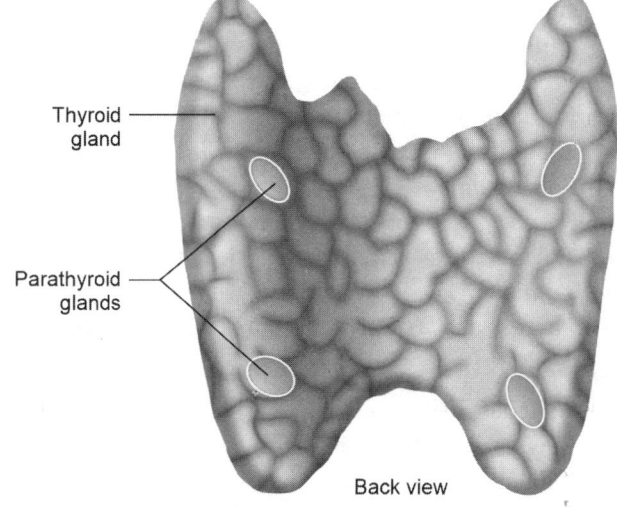

Fig. 2.3.1: Parathyroid gland.

Clinical features: Parathyroid adenoma is the most common cause of hyperparathyroidism and commonly this is idiopathic. Some conditions like chronic kidney failure or treatment with lithium may enlarge the glands. Classical patients with "stones (renal), abdominal groans, psychiatric moans, bones" are rare to find and most patients are now asymptomatic at detection. Symptoms and signs of parathyroid adenoma (benign neoplasm) are mainly due to hypercalcemia and include:

- *Renal manifestations:* Deposition of calcium in renal parenchyma (nephrocalcinosis) or recurrent nephrolithiasis, diabetes insipidus and renal failure.
- *Abdominal groans:* Constipation, vomiting, peptic ulcer disease (may be associated with Zollinger-Ellison syndrome) and acute pancreatitis.
- *Psychiatric moans:* Result from memory loss, fatigue, depression and delirium.
- *Bones:* The characteristic findings are osteitis fibrosa cystica (brown tumor), which occurs in 10–20% of patients. Histologically, there are increased giant multinucleated osteoclasts in scalloped areas on the surface of the bone (Howship's lacunae) and the normal cellular and marrow elements are replaced by fibrous tissue. Radiological changes usually include areas of subperiosteal cortical resorption which is evident radiologically replacement of the usual sharp cortical outline of the bone in the digits by an irregular outline. There is also resorption of the phalangeal tufts. Other findings include loss of lamina dura dentes, mineralization of soft tissues, development of bone cysts and an overall reduction in bone density.
- Some people add to this "thrones" referring to polyuria and constipation.

Radiological presentation: Typical X-ray features are osteoporosis (sometimes including vertebral collapse) and areas of cortical erosion. Hyperparathyroid "brown tumors" should be considered in the differential diagnosis of atypical cyst-like lesions of long bones. The classical—and almost pathognomonic—feature, which should always be sought, is subperiosteal cortical resorption of the middle phalanges. Nonspecific features of hypercalcemia are renal calculi, nephrocalcinosis and chondrocalcinosis.

Hungry bone syndrome: If hyperparathyroidism is treated by parathyroidectomy then postoperatively there is a danger of severe hypocalcemia due to brisk formation of new bone (the "hungry bone syndrome"). It may acutely result in severe hypocalcemic tetany since the half-life of PTH in plasma is approximately 20 minutes. This must be treated promptly, with one of the fast-acting vitamin D metabolites with or without intravenous calcium.

57. Discuss the role of parathyroid gland in calcium metabolism.
Ans: Kindly see answer above.

58. Describe the radiological features of scurvy and rickets.
Ans:
Scurvy:
- Generalized bone rarefaction, most marked in the long bone metaphyses.
- Cortical bone shadow is predominantly affected—"pencil thin" cortex.
- Periosteal reaction (reactionary to subperiosteal hemorrhages).
- Scorbutic rosary on chest X-rays.
- Hemarthrosis and its radiological changes in joints.
- The normal calcification in growing cartilage produces dense transverse bands at the juxta-epiphyseal zones—Frankel lines.
- *Wimberger's ring sign:* Radiodense shadow around the ossific centers of the epiphyses.
- The metaphyses may be deformed due to pathological fractures and remodeling.
- *Trummerfeld zone:* These are lucent metaphyseal band underlying the Frankel line.
- *Pelken spur:* Metaphyseal spurs due to cupping of metaphysis.

Rickets:
- Generalized osteopenia.
- Bowing deformities of the long bones, particularly the femur and tibia.
- Widening of the growth plate (secondary to deficient mineralization in the provisional zone of calcification) due to continued hypertrophy of cartilage cells.
- Cupping or flaring of the metaphysis, particularly in the proximal humerus, distal radius and ulna, and distal femur. The metaphysis is soft due to absent mineralization; hence the epiphysis is pushed into metaphysis with axial pressure causing cupping.
- Irregular calcification leads to fraying of metaphysis that instead of appearing smooth takes the form of "trees on plateau top" viewed from a distance.
- *In vitamin D-resistant rickets:* Sometimes Umbau zones (Looser's zones) are seen as sharply defined radiolucent transverse zones.
- In severe rickets, the margins of tarsal and carpal ossification centers may disappear.

Findings of healing rickets:
- Earliest finding the reappearance of the provisional zone of calcification, which gradually thickens into a transverse band.
- This is followed by recalcification of the spongiosa in the metaphysis.
- A dense line appears at the end of metaphysis.
- Epiphyseal shadow is clearly defined.
- The end of shaft and epiphysis become clearly differentiated.

59. Discuss etiopathology, clinical features, and management of scurvy.

Ans:

Etiology: Artificially fed infants between 5 and 10 months of age (vitamin C gets destroyed by heat) and also vitamin C is lacking in processed milk.

In adults, scurvy occurs in undernourished and those on restricted diet.

Pathology: Vitamin C deficiency impairs cohesive property of matrix of connective tissue and endothelium leading to capillary hemorrhages beneath mucous membranes in gums, intestines, conjunctivae, skin, bladder, kidneys, beneath the periosteum in bones. IM hemorrhage repeatedly destroys hematopoietic tissue resulting in secondary anemia results.

Osteoblasts and osteoclasts are reduced due to metaphyseal hemorrhages. The broadened layer of calcified cartilage is called white line of Frenkel due to accumulation of fragile calcified cartilage. This also weakens the epiphyseo-metaphyseal junction predisposing to fractures.

Within epiphysis, a zone of calcified cartilage accumulates about the bony centrum. This encircling dense ring is known as Wimberger line.

Clinical features: The infant is irritable, restless, febrile, and anemic. The gums may be spongy and bleeding. Subperiosteal hemorrhage causes excruciating pain and tenderness near the large joints. The child does not move the limbs due to excruciating pain from epiphyseal separations and subperiosteal hemorrhages giving clinical appearance of paralysis (pseudoparalysis).

Costochondral separations are typical. The sternum with cartilaginous portions of the ribs is displaced posteriorly, while the sharp anterior ends of the bony ribs protrude anteriorly. These form scorbutic rosary.

Management:

Diagnosis:

X-ray features already written in answer above.

Laboratory studies: Blood vitamin C level normally is 1 mg/dL. In scurvy, 0.5 or less is present. Anemia is also present.

Treatment: It consists of administration of fruit juices or tablets of vitamin C. Other vitamins are also given. Processed milk is prohibited. Fractures are immobilized without attempting reduction.

60. What are clinical features of rickets?

Ans: The following features are rarely seen in all cases; only full-blown cases with advanced deficiency that have been neglected for long present with such changes, else most patients present with a few of the features presented below.

Head:
- Craniotabes—softening of cranial bones, a sensation similar to pressing a ping pong ball on applying pressure on occiput or the parietal bones.
- Frontal bossing
- Delayed dentition and tooth caries
- Delayed closure of fontanel
- Craniosynostosis

Chest:
- Rachitic rosary—widening of osteochondral junction, feels like beads of rosary on moving finger along the osteochondral junction from rib to rib
- Harrison's groove—occurs due to pulling of softened ribs in inspiration by diaphragm. Softened ribs also predispose to atelectasis and pneumonia because of decreased air entry.
- Pectus carinatum (pigeon breast)—sternum projects forward.

Spine:
- Scoliosis (uncommon)
- Kyphosis (rachitic cat back)
- Accentuation of lumbar lordosis

Limbs and joints:
- Bone pain and tenderness
- Coxa vara
- Genu valgum or varum
- Windswept deformity
- Bowing of tibia, femur, radius, and ulna
- Widening of wrist, elbow, knee, and ankle because of enlargement of ends of long bones
- Rachitic saber shins
- Sausage-like enlargement of ends of phalanges and metacarpals, with regular constrictions corresponding of the joints string of pearls deformity
- Double malleoli sign

General:
- Failure to thrive
- Protuberant abdomen
- Apathy, listlessness, and irritability
- Proximal muscle weakness
- Ligament laxity
- Symptoms of hypocalcemia—tetany, seizures, and stridor due to laryngeal spasm
- Bilateral lamellar cataract (Vitamin D deficiency in early infancy).

61. Define osteomalacia. Describe its etiopathogenesis, clinical features, and management.

Ans: Definition: Osteomalacia is a condition of adults characterized by softening of the bones because of an accumulation of osteoid tissue, the bone matrix that fails to mineralize.

Etiology: The most common cause is vitamin D deficiency [dietary lack, malabsorption, underexposure to sunlight, decreased 25-hydroxylation (liver disease, anticonvulsants) and reduced 1α-hydroxylation (renal disease, nephrectomy, 1α-hydroxylase deficiency)].

Other causes are derangement of vitamin D and phosphate metabolism that is either hereditary or acquired.

Pathogenesis: The main theories are based on vitamin D and phosphate metabolism and the effects of chronic systemic acidosis. Less well understood are factors interfering with the synthesis and maturation of collagen fibers that produce a defective osteoid tissue within which mineralization cannot occur.

Clinical features: *Osteomalacia* has a much more insidious course and patients may complain of bone pain, backache, and muscle weakness for many years before the diagnosis is made. Vertebral collapse causes loss of height, and existing deformities such as mild kyphosis or knock knees—themselves perhaps due to childhood rickets—may increase in later life. Unexplained pain in the hip or one of the long bones may presage a stress fracture.

Management:

Diagnosis:

X-rays: The classical lesion of *osteomalacia* is the Looser zone, a thin transverse band of rarefaction in an otherwise normal-looking bone. More often, however, there is simply a slow fading of skeletal structure, resulting in biconcave vertebrae (from disk pressure) called codfish spine, lateral indentation of the acetabula ("trefoil" pelvis) and spontaneous fractures of the ribs, pubic rami, femoral neck or the metaphyses above and below the knee.

Blood values: Changes common to osteomalacia are diminished levels of serum calcium and phosphate, increased alkaline phosphatase, and diminished urinary excretion of calcium.

In vitamin D deficiency, 25-OH D levels also are low. The "calcium phosphate product" (derived by multiplying calcium and phosphorus levels expressed in mmol/L), normally about 3, is diminished in osteomalacia, and values of <2.4 are diagnostic.

Treatment:
- *Dietary lack of vitamin D* (<100 IU/day) is common in strict vegetarians, in old people who often eat very little, and even in entire populations whose traditional foods contain very little vitamin D. If there is also reduced exposure to sunlight, rickets or osteomalacia may result. Treatment with vitamin D (400–1,000 IU/day) and calcium supplements is usually effective; however, elderly people often require larger doses of vitamin D (up to 2,000 IU/day).
- *Intestinal malabsorption*—especially fat malabsorption—can cause vitamin D deficiency (fat and vitamin D absorption go hand in hand). If vitamin D supplements are administered, they have to be given in large doses (50,000 IU/day).
- *Inadequacy of hepatic 25-OHD:* Defective conversion to (or too-rapid breakdown of) 25-OHD in the liver may result from long-term administration of anticonvulsants or rifampicin, and if these drugs are prescribed, it is wise to give adequate amounts of vitamin D at the same time. Occasionally, the condition is also seen in severe liver failure. Treatment in these cases requires vitamin D in very large doses.
- *Abnormalities of 1,25-$(OH)_2D$ metabolism:* Early renal failure patients sometimes develop osteomalacia; this is thought to be due to reduced 1α-hydroxylase activity resulting in deficiency of 1,25-$(OH)_2D$. The condition can be treated with 1,25-$(OH)_2D$ (or else with very large doses of vitamin D).
- *Hypophosphatemic rickets and osteomalacia:* Chronic hypophosphatemia occurs in a number of disorders in which there is impaired renal tubular reabsorption of phosphate. Adult-onset hypophosphatemia is rare but must be remembered as a cause of unexplained bone loss and joint pains in adults. The condition responds dramatically to treatment with phosphate, vitamin D, and calcium.

62. **Describe briefly the pathology, salient clinical features and management of hypophosphatemic rickets.**

Ans: *Pathology:* Phosphorus deficiency due to:
- *Inadequate intake:* As phosphorous is present in most of the foods dietary deficiency of phosphorous is extremely rare, except in conditions of prolonged starvation or severe anorexia.
- *Malabsorption:* In malabsorption syndromes, there is decreased absorption of phosphates along with the decreased absorption of other minerals also. Rickets develop in these cases due to simultaneous malabsorption of vitamin D and/or calcium.
- *Isolated phosphorus malabsorption:* Rare cases of isolated malabsorption of phosphorus occur in patients with long-term ingestion of aluminum containing antacids. Chronic aluminum exposure results in hypophosphatemia with rickets in children and secondary osteomalacia in adults. This entity responds to discontinuation of the antacid and short-term phosphorus supplementation.
- *Role of phosphatonin in hypophosphatemic rickets:* Phosphate plays a vital role in a number of other biological processes, such as signal transduction, nucleotide metabolism and enzyme regulation, and also phosphate ions are critical for normal bone mineralization. Our understanding on role of phosphate in calcium homeostasis comes from the study of rare disorders associated with renal phosphate wasting. A number of proteins have been discovered like FGF-23, FGF-7, the secreted frizzled-related protein-4 (SFRP-4) and matrix extracellular phosphoglycoprotein that have shown to reduce renal sodium-dependent phosphate transport. Also, among the mentioned phosphatonins, FGF-23 and SFRP-4 inhibit 1, 25-dihydroxyvitamin D synthesis, which leads to a decline in absorption of phosphates from the intestine and also its retention in the body.

Clinical features:
- *Growth retardation:* Delay in walking + short stature, reduced growth rate and bone deformity.
- Bend in the lower limbs from the weight of the child:
  - Coxa vara
  - Femoral and crural bowing + tibial torsion
  - Genu varum or valgum or wind-swept deformity

Management:
Medical: Activated vitamin D (calcitriol (10–80 ng/kg/day of calcitriol) or alfacalcidol) and phosphate supplementation (1–3 g of elemental phosphorus divided in 4–5 doses) from the time of diagnosis until growth is complete. Phosphate dose need titration due to abdominal pain and diarrhea. Frequent dosing is necessary to avoid a rapid decline of the available

drug and to prevent episodes of diarrhea, which is a frequent complication of high doses of phosphorus. Increased body weight with growth needs periodic dose adjustment. Total recovery would require normalization of the serum phosphate concentration, which is not a practical goal in children with X-linked hypophosphatemic rickets as it is likely to cause hyperparathyroidism. Practically, the therapeutic endpoints are increased height, lessened severity of skeletal deformity and radiographic evidence for epiphyseal healing. Growth hormone may be used as adjunct to treatment but under expert supervision only.

Surgery: Needed for treatment of severe bowing (osteotomy + plating or *Seekh-kebab* osteotomy), tibial torsion or pathological fractures. Osteotomies are usually postponed till skeletal maturity.

63. Describe the pseudofractures.

Ans: These are also called "Looser's zones", "Milkman's syndrome". They are almost symmetrical, radiolucent bands of diminished density, resembling fractures, occur in the cortex of the bone. They represent cortical stress fractures filled with poorly mineralized callus and fibrous tissue. The "pseudofractures" are usually multiple and typically show as transverse zones of rarefaction, varying in width from 1 mm to 1 cm. Mechanical stress of the main blood vessels overlying the uncalcified cortex of osteomalacic bones is regarded as the factor determining the location of the symmetrical pseudofractures. Pseudofractures are always associated with conditions that weaken the bones or that produce unusual strains to which the bones are not adapted. So these are not specific to osteomalacia and can instead be seen in various other disorders (but may not be bilaterally symmetrical and have no site predilection as is common with osteomalacia) like:
- Osteogenesis imperfecta
- Fragilitas ossium
- Hyperparathyroidism
- Hyperthyroidism
- Paget's disease
- Adrenal-pituitary bone dystrophy
- Severe chronic acidosis or hyperglycemia
- Congenital syphilis
- Osteomyelitis
- Osteopetrosis
- States of overloading of bone
- Blood dyscrasias.

Treatment: Looser's zones usually vanish with treatment aimed to improve calcium metabolism and rest. The treatment is usually a combination of vitamin D and calcium taken orally for a prolonged period of time. For pseudofractures, in precarious zones like proximal femur, there is a concern that real fractures may occur in these areas due to high torsional and bending forces. Prophylactic fixation to improve bone strength at these areas may be done if needed.

64. Describe the fluorosis.

Ans: Skeletal fluorosis is an endemic metabolic disease of bones, widely prevalent in India and many other countries around the world. Fifty-six million people living in 200 districts are at risk of developing fluorosis. Skeletal fluorosis occurs due to excessive intake of fluoride both from drinking water and food. The optimum upper safe limit is not more than 6 mg/day. Epidemiological and experimental studies on fluorosis have greatly helped in understanding the disease and provided a rational approach of management of the menace of fluoride toxicity. States known to be endemic in various parts of India include Assam, Andhra Pradesh, Bihar, Delhi, Gujarat, Haryana, Jammu and Kashmir, Karnataka, Kerala, Maharashtra, Odisha, Punjab, Rajasthan, Tamil Nadu, Uttar Pradesh, West Bengal. The first case report of endemic skeletal fluorosis was from Prakasam district, Andhra Pradesh in 1937, a province in south India. There was also a report of neurologic manifestations of fluorosis, which usually occurs in the later stages of the disease. The fluoride levels in these areas were surprisingly low, i.e., in a range of 1–3 ppm, which is unusual as skeletal fluorosis rarely occurs at levels less than 6 ppm. The possible mechanisms through which fluorosis occurred in these areas are as follows:
- High atmospheric temperatures (115–116°F) during summer months so people drink lot of water
- Hard physical labor activity again leads to increased water intake
- Poor nutrition, deficient in calories and also vitamin C

- Impaired renal function
- Abnormal concentrations of certain trace elements, like strontium, silica, uranium, calcium, magnesium, etc. In high concentration in water and food could influence fluoride toxicity.

Clinical features: Clinical manifestations of fluoride toxicity have uniformity in the clinical presentation. Fluorosis in humans is predominantly dental and skeletal. Dental fluorosis occurs early in the disease process followed by a prolonged symptom-free period of nearly 10–30 years which is ultimately followed by a crippling skeletal fluorosis and neurologic abnormalities. During the apparent symptom-free stage, the body keeps on accumulating excess fluoride and the patient suffers from vague gastrointestinal symptoms. The neurological manifestations in skeletal fluorosis are dominated by radiculomyelopathy that arise primarily due to mechanical compression of the nerve roots and also the spinal cord from osteophytes, sclerosed vertebral column and ossified ligaments. The cervical cord is involved earlier than the dorsal cord. The lumbar spine is the first to show skeletal changes, but the involvement of cauda equina is rare.

Pathogenesis: Inorganic fluoride replaces the hydroxyl groups of calcium hydroxyapatite forming calcium fluorapatite and gets deposited in bone. Osteons become irregular in shape, size and distribution in compact bone and there is gross reduction in spongiosa. The Haversian canals get enlarged with concomitant irregular distribution of osteocytes and increased irregular interstitial lamellae. Bone marrow becomes fibrous and poor in cells, while there is secondary hyperparathyroidism due to reduced systemic calcium, producing a high bone turnover state. This may also be aided by osteoblast activation from enhanced expression of transcription factors such as activator protein-1 (AP-1) and Cbfa1, as well as upregulation of cytokines or growth factors such as bFGF, BMP-2, IGF, TGF-β, platelet-derived growth factor (PDGF) and osteoprotegerin ligand (OPGL).

Although fluoride is known to stimulate bone formation, the underlying mechanisms are not fully understood. Recent studies have implicated the Wnt/β-catenin pathway as a major signaling cascade in bone biology.

Diagnosis

Urinary and bone fluoride: Urinary fluoride levels are the best indicators of fluoride intake. Since, fluoride excretion is not constant throughout the day, 24-hour samples of urine are more reliable than random or morning samples. In normal individuals, urinary fluorides fluctuate widely between 0.1 ppm and 2.0 ppm (average 0.4 ppm) when the fluoride content of drinking water is 0.3 ppm.

Normal blood fluoride levels in nonendemic regions vary between 0.002 mg/100 mL and 0.008 mg/100 mL and in endemic regions the levels range between 0.02 mg/100 mL and 0.15 mg/100 mL, whereas in patients with skeletal fluorosis the levels vary between 0.02 mg/100 mL and 0.19 mg/100 mL. It is much less a useful reference for detecting fluoride toxicity as major portion is mineral bound.

Radiology: The radiographic findings are parallel to pathological changes. The bone tissue continues to be formed, but the trabeculae thus formed have uncalcified borders and are resistant to reabsorption by osteoclasts.

Radiological stages of skeletal fluorosis:
- *Stage I:* Axial skeleton involvement and ground glass appearance of cancellous bone.
- *Stage II:* Thick primary trabeculae merge with sclerotic secondary trabeculae to make bone homogeneously dense, bone contours become uneven and calcification of paraspinous, sacrospinous and sacrotuberous ligaments is seen.
- *Stage III:* Axial skeletal bones demonstrate the typical radiological features, marked calcification at the insertion of muscles and tendons. There may be overlap of radiological features.

Osteosclerosis (dense bone) is the typical feature of involved axial skeleton (spine, pelvis and ribs), whereas osteoporosis mainly involves the appendicular skeleton.

Imaging: The best imaging modality to appreciate bony pathology is computerized tomography.

Calcified ligaments, spinal canal stenosis and root canal stenosis are also better appreciated with CT. A fluorotic vertebra appears hypointense in both T1- and T2-weighted images.

Prevention of Fluorosis

Prevention of fluorosis is better than cure, as no cure is possible once the disease sets in.

Endemic fluorosis: Defluoridation of drinking water supplies is based on Nalgonda method (named after the village in India where the method was pioneered) of lime and alum, employs the flocculation principle and uses domestic units. The method is based on filtration of fluoride-rich water with activated alumina (PAC granules). Nutrition has a crucial role in the severity of fluorosis, and hence a balanced diet having adequate calcium and vitamins could reduce the toxicity to fluoride.

Industrial fluorosis: A monitoring of urinary fluoride levels should be done in workers in industries and mining exposed to fluorides to keep the levels below 5 ppm. It is observed that skeletal fluorosis does not occur in well-nourished individuals unless the levels exceed more than 5,000 ppm.

Spine surgery in skeletal fluorosis: Surgery in spine fluorosis is beneficial in the early stage of the disease when only a few spinal segments are involved. The neurological deficits in fluorosis are mainly mechanical.

Operative outcomes with cervical spine operation are better as compared to dorsal spine. Cord compression at the level of dorsal spine is of three types:
1. Localized posterior osteophytes spread over many vertebral levels, though technically feasible for excision, the results are not so rewarding.
2. Localized posterior osteophitic or ossified ligamentous compression, where results are likely to be excellent.
3. Diffuse, extensive where surgery is not beneficial.

65. **Describe the etiology, clinical features, diagnosis and treatment of renal osteodystrophy.**

Ans: *Etiology:* In chronic renal failure, the activity of 1α-hydroxylase in the kidney is decreased, leading to diminished production of calcitriol. Along with inadequate calcium absorption and secondary hyperparathyroidism, the rickets may be worsened by the metabolic acidosis of chronic renal failure.

In chronic renal failure, unlike the other causes of vitamin D deficiency, patients have hyperphosphatemia as a result of decreased renal excretion. The dominant picture may be that of secondary hyperparathyroidism (due to phosphate retention, hypocalcemia and diminished production of $1,25(OH)_2D$), osteoporosis, osteomalacia or—in advanced cases—a combination of these. In older patients, the effects of postmenopausal osteoporosis may be superimposed; in some, there are concomitant changes due to glucocorticoid medication; and in patients with end-stage renal failure, bone changes can be aggravated by aluminum retention or contamination of dialyzing fluids. In addition, failure to thrive and growth retardation may be accentuated because of the direct effect of chronic renal failure on the growth hormone axis.

Clinical features and radiology: Renal abnormalities usually precede the bone changes by several years.
- Children have short height; they are pasty-faced and have marked rachitic deformities associated with myopathy. X-rays show widened and irregular epiphyseal plates. In older children with long-standing disease, there may be displacement of the epiphyses (epiphyseolysis).
- Osteosclerosis is seen mainly in the axial skeleton and is more common in young patients; it may produce a "rugger jersey" appearance in lateral X-rays of the spine, due to alternating bands of increased and decreased bone density.
- In all patients, signs of secondary hyperparathyroidism may be widespread and severe.

Biochemical features are low serum calcium, high serum phosphate and elevated alkaline phosphatase levels. Urinary excretion of calcium and phosphate is diminished. Plasma PTH levels may be raised.

Treatment: Calcitriol is the treatment of choice. This permits adequate absorption of calcium and directly suppresses the parathyroid gland. Sevelamer hydrochloride, a phosphate binder used orally, and dietary restriction of phosphate to regulate serum phosphate levels, as hyperphosphatemia is a stimulus for PTH secretion. In addition, metabolic acidosis may be corrected with alkalis. More recently a calcimimetic drug, cinacalcet, has been introduced; this acts directly on the parathyroid glands increasing the sensitivity of calcium receptors and inducing a reduction in serum PTH levels.

Renal failure, if irreversible, may require hemodialysis or renal transplantation.

Epiphyseolysis may need internal fixation and residual deformities can be corrected once the disease is under control.

66. **Discuss clinical features, diagnosis and management of nutritional rickets.**

Ans: *Clinical features:* These children have an increased risk of pneumonia and muscle weakness, leading to a delay in motor development. The clinical manifestations are typical of rickets with a few presenting even with symptoms of hypercalcemia and prolonged laryngospasm is life-threatening.

Diagnosis: The diagnosis of nutritional vitamin D deficiency is based on the combination of a history of poor vitamin D intake and risk factors for decreased cutaneous synthesis, radiographic changes consistent with rickets and typical laboratory findings. A normal PTH level almost never occurs with vitamin D deficiency and suggests a primary phosphate disorder. Calcium deficiency may occur with or without vitamin D deficiency. A normal level of 25-D and a dietary history of poor calcium intake support a diagnosis of isolated calcium deficiency.

Management

Laboratory findings: Hypocalcemia is a variable as blood calcium levels are kept normal by secondary hyperparathyroidism. The hypophosphatemia is due to PTH-induced renal loss of phosphate and also decrease in intestinal absorption of phosphate. The calcitriol levels may be low, normal or high may be secondary to the upregulation of renal 1α-hydroxylase due to associated hypophosphatemia and hyperparathyroidism. The serum levels of calcitriol are normally much less than the levels of 25-D, there is still often enough 25-D present to act as a precursor for calcitriol synthesis in the presence of an upregulated 1α-hydroxylase. In severe vitamin D deficiency, the level of calcitriol may be low. There may be metabolic acidosis and generalized aminoaciduria.

Treatment: Adequate intake of vitamin D, calcium and phosphorous is the main stay of treatment in nutritional vitamin D deficiency rickets, which can be administered by the following methods:
- *Stoss therapy:* 300,000–600,000 IU of vitamin D is administered orally or intramuscularly as 2–4 doses over 1 day. Because the doses are observed, Stoss therapy is ideal in situations where adherence to therapy is questionable.
- *Alternate therapy:* High dose vitamin D, with doses ranging from 2,000–5,000 IU/day over 4–6 weeks.

Either strategy should be followed by daily vitamin D intake of 400 IU/day, typically given as a multivitamin. It is important to administer adequate dietary calcium and phosphorus; common sources for which are milk, formula diets, and other dairy products.

For the symptoms of hypocalcemia, patient may need intravenous calcium acutely, followed by oral calcium supplements, which typically can be tapered over 2–6 weeks in children receiving adequate dietary calcium. Transient use of intravenous or oral calcitriol is often helpful in reversing hypocalcemia in the acute phase by providing active vitamin D during the delay as supplemental vitamin D is converted to active vitamin D. Calcitriol doses are typically 0.05 μg/kg/day. Intravenous calcium is initially given as an acute bolus for symptomatic hypocalcemia (20 mg/kg of calcium chloride or 100 mg/kg of calcium gluconate). Alternatively, a continuous intravenous calcium drip may be tried in some patients, which is titrated to maintain the desired serum calcium level followed by conversion to oral calcium of approximately 1000 mg/day.

67. Discuss the vitamin D-dependent rickets (VDDR).

Ans: Formerly thought to be rare, it is quite common and probably is the most frequent cause of dwarfism. Compared with the usual form of rickets, it is more severe, fails to respond to usual doses, but responds to massive doses of vitamin D. There are two described types of VDDR: (1) VDDR-1 and (2) VDDR-2.

Vitamin D-dependent rickets type 1: Vitamin D-dependent rickets type 1 or pseudovitamin D deficiency is a genetic disorder with an autosomal recessive mode of inheritance. The disorder is the result of mutation in *1α-hydroxylase gene* causing reduction in the available enzyme for ultimate hydroxylation step. This prevents conversion of 25-D into calcitriol. Those patients who present within first 2 years of life, can have any of the classic features of rickets, including symptomatic hypocalcemia. Typical laboratory findings include elevated PTH levels, decreased serum calcium, low or undetectable serum concentrations of calcitriol $1,25(OH)_2D$ despite normal or increased concentrations of calcifediol $[25(OH)D]$.

Treatment: Long-term treatment with calcitriol is the treatment for VDDR type 1. Initial doses are 0.25–2 μg/day, with lower doses used once the rickets has healed, with adequate intake of calcium. The dose of calcitriol is adjusted to maintain a low normal serum calcium level, a normal serum phosphorus level and a high normal serum PTH level to prevent possible complications of hypercalciuria and nephrocalcinosis. Patient is monitored during the therapy with urinary calcium excretion, with a target of less than 4 mg/kg/day.

Vitamin D-dependent rickets type 2: This occurs due to mutations in the gene encoding the vitamin-D receptor (VDR) an autosomal recessive disorder, preventing a normal physiologic response to calcitriol because of end organ resistance. More severely affected patients present in infancy whereas less severely affected patients may not be diagnosed until adulthood. A less severe disease is associated with a partially functional VDR. In a percentage of patients, it may be associated with alopecia (ranging from alopecia areata to alopecia totalis), which tends to be associated with a more severe form of the disease. Epidermal cysts may be associated, but is a less common manifestation. Levels of calcitriol are extremely elevated and serve to differentiate type 2 from type 1 VDDR.

Treatment: A 3- to 6-month trial of high dose of vitamin D_2, 25-D or calcitriol and oral calcium is given for less severe form of disease, especially those without alopecia. This response is due to a partially functional VDR. The initial dose of calcitriol should be 2 µg/day. Oral calcium doses range from 1,000 mg/day to 3,000 mg/day. Unresponsive patients may be treated with long-term intravenous calcium with possible transition to very high dose oral calcium supplements. Patients not responding to vitamin D are difficult to treat.

68. Discuss classification of rickets?

Ans: Etiological classification of rickets has been shown in **Box 2.3.2.**

> **Box 2.3.2:** Etiological classification of rickets.
>
> - Vitamin D disorders:
>   - Nutritional deficiency of vitamin D
>   - Vitamin D dependent rickets type 1
>   - Vitamin D dependent rickets type 2
>   - Congenital vitamin D deficiency
>   - Secondary vitamin D deficiency
> - Malabsorption
> - Decrease liver 25-hydroxylase
> - Increase degradation
>   - Chronic kidney disease
> - Renal losses:
>   - Autosomal dominant hypophosphatemic rickets
>   - Autosomal recessive hypophosphatemic rickets
>   - X-linked hypophosphatemic rickets
>   - Hereditary hypophosphatemic rickets with hypercalciuria
>   - Excess production of phosphatonin:
> - Neurofibromatosis
> - Tumor-induced rickets
> - McCune-Albright syndrome
> - Epidermal nevus
> - Dent disease
> - Fanconi syndrome
> - Distal renal tubular acidosis
> - Calcium deficiency:
>   - Decrease intake
>   - Malabsorption
>   - Phosphorous deficiency:
>   - Premature infants (rickets of prematurity)
>   - Aluminum—containing antacids

69. Define vitamin D-resistant rickets (VDRR). Discuss its clinical picture, investigations and treatment. How will you differentiate it from vitamin D-dependent rickets (VDDR)?

Ans: Definition: The term VDRR (also known as familial hypophosphatemic rickets), encompasses a group of disorders in which adequate dietary intake of vitamin D is insufficient to achieve normal mineralization of the growing bone. The term "VDRR" is sometimes also loosely applied to any condition (e.g., steatorrhea, chronic renal glomerular failure, and renal tubular abnormalities) that requires amounts supranormal doses of vitamin D and phosphorus to produce healing.

Clinical picture: A familial tendency is often observed. The patient is of short stature with all the usual signs of florid rickets. Deformities are severe, particularly in the lower extremities, where bow legs, knock knees are seen marked ligamentous instability is typical. A waddling gait is due to coxa vara. These deformities are persistent and typically recur after attempted osteotomies. The skull has a characteristic appearance—anteroposterior diameter is increased and transverse diameter is decreased (dolichocephaly); frontal bossing and a marked external occipital protuberance occur. Nose is often saddle shaped.

Investigations:
- *X-rays:* Usual findings of rickets with widespread coarse trabeculae
- *Laboratory studies:* Serum phosphorus level is usually below 3 mg; calcium level is normal; and the alkaline phosphatase (ALP) level is elevated to 20 or more bodansky units.

Results of urinary qualitative sulkowitch test are negative or reveal only a trace of calcium.

Treatment: Medical treatment is with oral phosphate replacement and the administration of vitamin D and the correcting of medical abnormality present. Orthotic management to correct the lower extremity deformities has proven ineffective. Osteotomies should be done once epiphyses have closed.

Differences between VDRR and VDDR is given in **Table 2.3.6**.

TABLE 2.3.6: Differentiation between vitamin D-resistant rickets (VDRR) and vitamin D-dependent rickets (VDDR).

VDRR	VDDR
Inherited	Acquired
No muscular weakness	Muscular weakness
No hypocalcemic tetany	Hypocalcemic tetany can occur
Serum phosphorus always low before treatment; after treatment phosphorus rises a little but never returns to normal, even with prolonged treatment with large doses	Serum phosphorus low or normal; if low, return rapidly to normal with small doses
Growth rate seldom becomes normal with treatment; patient remains dwarfed	Normal growth rate is resumed with treatment

70. Discuss pathology, clinical features, laboratory findings and radiographic findings of vitamin D dependent rickets, vitamin D resistant rickets, and hypophosphatasia.

Ans: Comparison of Vitamin D-dependent rickets (VDDR), Vitamin D-resistant rickets (X-linked hypophosphatemia), and hypophosphatasia.

1. Vitamin D-Dependent Rickets (VDDR)

Types:
- VDDR Type 1 (CYP27B1 mutation → 1α-hydroxylase deficiency).
- VDDR Type 2 (VDR mutation → vitamin D receptor resistance).

Pathology:
- Defective activation of vitamin D (Type 1) or end-organ resistance (Type 2) → hypocalcemia → secondary hyperparathyroidism → rickets/osteomalacia.

Clinical features:
- Early-onset (infancy/toddler).
- Severe bone deformities: Bow legs, rachitic rosary, craniotabes.
- Muscle weakness, hypotonia.
- Type 2-specific: Alopecia (due to defective VDR in hair follicles)

Lab Findings: Summarized in **Table 2.3.7**.

TABLE 2.3.7: Various laboratory parameters for VDDR.

Parameter	VDDR Type 1	VDDR Type 2
Calcium	↓↓	↓↓
Phosphate	↓ (PTH-driven renal wasting)	↓
ALP	↑↑	↑↑
PTH	↑↑	↑↑
1,25-(OH)$_2$D	↓ (defective synthesis)	↑↑ (receptor resistance)
25-OH-D	Normal	Normal

Radiographic findings:
- *Classic rickets signs*:
  - Widened and frayed metaphyses (cupping/splaying)
  - Osteopenia and coarse trabeculae
  - Looser zones (pseudofractures) in osteomalacia

Treatment:
- Type 1: Calcitriol (1,25-$(OH)_2$D) + calcium
- Type 2: High-dose calcitriol/calcium (may need IV if resistant)

2. Vitamin D-resistant rickets (X-linked Hypophosphatemia, XLH)

Pathology:
- PHEX mutation → ↑ FGF23 → phosphate wasting (renal) → hypophosphatemia → impaired mineralization.

Clinical features:
- Short stature and bowed legs
- Dental abscesses (defective dentin)
- Enthesopathy (ligament/tendon calcification in adults)
- No muscle weakness (unlike VDDR)

Lab Findings: Summarized in **Table 2.3.8**.

TABLE 2.3.8: Various laboratory parameters for X-linked hypophosphatemia (XLH).

Parameter	XLH findings
Calcium	Normal
Phosphate	↓↓ (renal wasting)
ALP	↑
PTH	Normal/mildly ↑
1,25-$(OH)_2$D	Inappropriately normal/low
FGF23	↑↑

Radiographic findings:
- Rickets changes (metaphyseal fraying)
- Thick cortices (due to osteomalacia)
- Pseudofractures (Looser zones)

Treatment:
- Oral phosphate supplements + active vitamin D (calcitriol)
- Burosumab (anti-FGF23 monoclonal antibody)

3. Hypophosphatasia (HPP)

Pathology:
- ALPL mutation → low alkaline phosphatase (ALP) → defective mineralization + ↑ pyrophosphate (inhibits hydroxyapatite).

Clinical features:
- Perinatal lethal form: Stillbirth/severe respiratory failure.
- Childhood form: Premature tooth loss, rickets-like deformities.
- Adult form: Stress fractures, osteomalacia, pseudogout (pyrophosphate deposits).

Lab Findings: Summarized in **Table 2.3.9**.

TABLE 2.3.9: Various laboratory parameters for hypophosphatasia.

Parameter	HPP Findings
Calcium	Normal/↑ (hypercalciuria)
Phosphate	Normal
ALP	↓↓ (hallmark)
PTH	Normal
Pyridoxal-5'-P	↑ (vitamin B6 metabolite)

Radiographic findings:
- Osteopenia, metaphyseal lucencies ("tongues of radiolucency")
- Bone spurs (perinatal form)
- Pseudofractures (adult form)

Treatment:
- Enzyme replacement therapy (Asfotase alfa).
- Avoid vitamin D (worsens hypercalcemia)

71. Describe the etiopathogenesis, clinical features and management of alkaptonuria.

Ans: The term "alkaptonuria ("alkali" + "kaptein"—to suck up avidly)" was coined by Boedeker in 1859, denoting avidity for oxygen in alkaline solution. Ochronosis is a rare hereditary autosomal recessive disease with ineffective homogentisic acid oxidase in the pathway of tyrosine catabolism so that excessive homogentisic acid (ortho-meta-dihydroxyphenylacetic acid) is secreted in the urine imparting brownish black color. The kidneys rapidly clear this material and only a small amount remains in the tissues, but eventually it begins to accumulate in the cartilage of the ear, skin, intervertebral disks and sclera.

Ochronosis denotes this bluish black pigmentation (due to oxidation of pigment) of connective tissue and was coined by Virchow for microscopic appearance of the pigment ("Ochrea"—dark yellow). The relationship between alkaptonuria and ochronosis was first recognized in 1902 by Albrecht. Exogenous ochronosis has been described with the use of topical hydroquinone, phenol, picric acid and exposure to resorcinol, benzene and antimalarials but is not prominent orthopedically.

Clinical features: Alkaptonuria is asymptomatic but clinically identifiable symptoms develop with pigment deposition. By the fourth decade, these deposits begin to calcify causing the synovial joints to show chondrocalcinosis. Eventually, the patients develop secondary osteoarthritis and spondylosis related to disk degeneration caused by the deposition of homogentisic acid in cartilage. In ochronitic spondylitis, there is calcification and ossification of intervertebral disks producing rigid spine with stooped posture, loss of lumbar lordosis, knee flexed and typical stance. There are but little if any osteophytes, the sacroiliac joints are normal and spine is unaffected (no bamboo spine) differentiating this from ankylosing spondylitis. The earliest symptoms are usually localized to lumbar spine and spondylosis however with progression the dorsal and cervical spine gets involved. Radiographic calcified disks suggest but are not diagnostic of ochronosis as they can be found in pseudogout, hemochromatosis, chronic respiratory paralytic poliomyelitis, and iatrogenic (spinal fusion). Splits in disk material appear to account for radiolucencies in the disks that have been termed vacuum disks. The arthropathy is typical with brittle cartilage fragments and pigmented "shards" in the synovium. Commonly the knees, shoulders and hips are affected sparing the small joints of hands and feet. Osteochondral joint bodies are common and occasionally calcium pyrophosphate dihydrate (CPPD) crystal associated inflammation may be seen. Radiographically, the peripheral arthropathy is indistinguishable from osteoarthritis and demonstrates narrowing of the joint space, small marginal osteophytes, and eburnation. Other features include grayish black discoloration of tympanic membrane, black cerumen, systolic cardiac murmur due to stenosis of aortic and mitral valves. Prostatic calculi are seen in majority of men with ochronosis and can be digitally palpated per rectally.

Treatment: Mainly on the lines of management of osteoarthritis and spondylosis (physiotherapy, braces, analgesics, weight reduction, etc.). Patients often require arthroplasty for large joints. High-dose ascorbic acid is suggested to reduce binding of the pigment to the tissues. Protein or tyrosine-restricted diets are unpalatable. Steroids, irradiation, tyrosinase, vitamins, and phenylbutazone have been found ineffective. Nitisinone (reduces production of homogentisic acid by inhibiting 4-hydroxyphenylpyruvate dioxygenase) may be helpful (need to be studied) and is currently available for treatment of tyrosinemia type 1.

72. Define ochronotic arthropathy. Also describe its clinical features, diagnosis and management.

Ans: Alkaptonuria (that results in ochronotic arthropathy) is written above.

2.4 SYNDROMIC/GENETIC AND INFLAMMATORY DISEASES OF BONES AND JOINTS (SICKLE CELL DISEASE, ANKYLOSING SPONDYLOSIS, OSTEOGENESIS IMPERFECTA, EHLERS-DANLOS SYNDROME, MARFAN SYNDROME) (Q73–81)

73. Discuss sickle cell disease and its impact in orthopedics.

Ans: Sickle cell disease results from an abnormal hemoglobin known as Hb-S. The molecular lesion in Hb-S is the substitution of valine for glutamic acid at the sixth residue of the beta chain. By itself, this form of hemoglobin is innocuous but deoxygenation causes the red cells containing Hb-S to become rigid and deformed in the shape of an arc or crescent shape giving the red blood cells (RBCs) typical appearance of sickle-shaped cells. These changes are reversible with reoxygenation. However, the sickling may become permanent and then the red cells are called irreversibly sickled. The consequences of it are occlusion of microvascular circulation by the sickle cells leading to tissue ischemia and infarction. The orthopedic implications of the disease are many as follows:

- Sickling is a risk factor for osteoporosis.
- Sickle cell disease leads to osteonecrosis, most commonly of femoral head.
- Gastrointestinal tract organisms like *Salmonella* rarely is a cause of osseous infection, but it is characteristically associated with hemoglobinopathies like sickle cell disease. Chronic osteomyelitis (OM) may follow salmonella infection in immunocompromised subjects and in children with hemoglobinopathies like sickle cell anemia. The bacteria enter the bloodstream through the gut. In sickle cell anemia, multiple thromboses occur in the bones and may predispose to infection. Frequently affected bones include vertebrae, ribs, sternum, and calcaneum. The clinical features resemble those of subacute OM with protracted course and may be confused with tubercular infection. Surgical intervention is usually not required unless an abscess has to be evacuated or a sequestrum is to be removed.
- Acute monoarticluar septic arthritis by *Salmonella* occurs in sickle cell disease.
- Fat embolism may occur due to medical conditions causing bone infarcts, especially in sickle cell disease.
- Typing for RhD status is quite not helpful for patients with sickle cell anemia as these patients are likely to express variants of Rh "e" antigens rather than RhD antigens.
- Sickling is also a cause of protrusio acetabuli.
- There is increased frequency of revision hip replacement in these patients.
- Adequate care for tourniquet use needs to be taken in sickle cell disease (reduce application time)/intermittent inflation for prolonged surgeries—intermittent inflation should not be less than 20 minutes.

74. Ankylosing spondylitis—discuss the pathology, clinical features, diagnosis, and broad principles of management.

Ans: *Pathology*—the manifestations of ankylosing spondylitis basically emanate from:
- Synovitis of diarthrodial joints
- Inflammation at the fibro-osseous junctions of syndesmotic joints and tendons.

There is prompt involvement of the insertion of tendons and ligaments (the entheses) commonly referred to as *enthesopathy*.

Synovitis causes destruction of articular cartilage and periarticular bone and is typically seen in sacroiliac and vertebral facet joints. Similar involvement of costovertebral joints produces diminished respiratory excursion. Inflammation of the fibro-osseous junctions affects the intervertebral discs, sacroiliac ligaments, symphysis pubis, manubrium sterni, and the bony insertions of large tendons. Pathological changes proceed in three stages:

1. An inflammatory reaction with cell infiltration, granulation tissue formation, and erosion of adjacent bone.
2. Replacement of the granulation tissue by fibrous tissue.
3. Ossification of the fibrous tissue, leading to ankylosis of the joint.

Ossification across the surface of the disc gives rise to small bony bridges or syndesmophytes linking adjacent vertebral bodies. If many vertebrae are involved the spine may become absolutely rigid.

Clinical features: Patients present with back pain with prolonged morning stiffness (for greater than 1 hour) and progressive loss of motion of the axial spine. The pain should have four or more of these characteristic features (to specify as inflammatory pain):

1. Age of onset below 40 years old
2. Insidious onset
3. Improvement with exercise
4. No improvement with rest
5. Pain at night with improvement upon getting up ("gel phenomenon").

In addition to the spine, sacroiliac involvement, arthritis of the hips, peripheral arthritis, and enthesitis are common. Enthesitis is typically a principal feature, it is the fibrosis and ossification of ligament, tendon, and capsule insertions into bone (the entheses), mainly seen in the region of disks and sacroiliac joints. Typically, ankylosing spondylitis starts in the sacroiliac joints (from inferior to superior with later fusion of the joint) and slowly ascends the spine. The most specific findings involve loss of spinal mobility, with limitation of anterior and lateral flexion and extension of the lumbar spine and of chest expansion. Stress tests for sacroiliac joint (Gaenslen and FABER) are positive.

Modified Schober's test reasonably assesses the spinal flexion. As the disease progresses, increasing flexion of the neck, increased thoracic kyphosis, and loss of normal lumbar lordosis lead to a stooped posture. Disease progression can be estimated clinically from loss of height, limitation of chest expansion and spinal flexion, and occiput-to-wall distance. Onset of ankylosing spondylitis in adolescence and early hip involvement correlate with a worse prognosis. Juvenile onset disease has more frequent peripheral arthritis and delayed axial presentation. Females usually do not go to complete spinal fusion but have increased prevalence of peripheral arthritis and isolated cervical ankylosis. "Bamboo spine" develops in a few patients, but in those where it is formed, there is significant incidence of collapse of vertebral end-plate and destruction of disk-bone border. This phenomenon leads to sudden increase in pain over dorsal spine with localized tenderness and excruciating pain on movement is a dangerous sign and may represent fracture or tubercular infection or more serious "Andersson lesion", the latter is a pseudoarthrosis of thoracolumbar bamboo spine that is difficult to treat and represents instable pattern that can compromise neurology. There are various measures to measure disease activity of which Bath Ankylosing Spondylitis Disease Activity Index (BASDAI) is prominently used. Bath Ankylosing Spondylitis Functional Index (BASFI) is a measure of limitations in activities of daily living. The standardized mortality ratio is 1.5, possibly due to cardiac valve, respiratory disease, amyloidosis, and fractures so commonly associated with ankylosing spondylitis.

Mortality in ankylosing spondylitis is mainly due to spinal trauma, aortic insufficiency, respiratory failure, amyloid nephropathy, or complications of therapy such as upper gastrointestinal hemorrhage. Synovitis also occurs in larger peripheral joints (hips and knees in particular). The peripheral joint involvement has been seen in females more so than men. Nearly 50% of patients with ankylosing spondylitis will develop hip arthritis and some of them would need surgery. Ankylosing spondylitis is associated with high rates of job attrition and job changes.

Diagnosis: The Assessment of Spondyloarthritis International Society (ASAS) criteria for axial spondyloarthropathy are proposed by ASAS in 2009 for diagnosis of spondyloarthropathy **(Box 2.4.1)**. Active inflammation of the sacroiliac (SI) joints, as determined by dynamic MRI, is considered equivalent to the older criterion of definite radiographic sacroiliitis. Few clinicians however use the ASAS criteria for making the diagnosis. Modified New York criteria though not sensitive for early disease are commonly referred to by the clinicians to make a diagnosis **(Box 2.4.2)**.

Box 2.4.1: Assessment of Spondyloarthritis International Society criteria.

At least 20% improvement AND absolute improvement of ≥ 10 units in three out of the four following domains, without worsening of 20% or more AND 10 units in the remaining domain:
- Bath Ankylosing Spondylitis Functional Index (BASFI)
- Inflammation [the average of BASDAI's last two visual analog scale (VAS) concerning morning stiffness and duration]
- Patient global assessment (VAS score)
- Pain (the average of VAS score and nocturnal pain scores).

Assessment of Spondyloarthritis International Society partial remission criteria: A value below 20 units in all four domains.

> **Box 2.4.2:** New York criteria.
>
> Definitive sacroiliitis (Grade ≥ 2 bilateral or unilateral 3–4) and any one of the following (definitive ankylosing spondylitis). Probable ankylosing spondylitis, if three clinical criterion or radiological criterion present, but no signs or symptoms to satisfy clinical criteria:
> - Low back pain ≥ 3 months' duration improved by exercise not relieved by rest
> - Limitation of lumbar spine movements in sagittal and frontal planes
> - Chest expansion decreased relative to normal values for age and sex.

Principles of management: The goals of therapy for patients with ankylosing spondylitis are not only to provide symptomatic relief, but as in the treatment of RA, to prevent permanent irreversible joint damage. The baseline common factor in all therapeutic interventions include exercise program designed to maintain posture and range of motion.

Nonsteroidal anti-inflammatory drugs (NSAIDs) are the first-line pharmacologic therapy for ankylosing spondylitis and reduce pain and tenderness and increase mobility in many patients with ankylosing spondylitis. Thalidomide by virtue of inhibiting TNF-α has been found to be effective in doses of 200 mg/day but toxicity limits its use. Apremilast (phosphodiesterase-4 inhibitor) has shown improvement in initial studies.

Patients with active disease and persistent symptoms on conventional therapy are candidates for anti-TNF-α therapy. The guidelines for starting the therapy include—two different NSAID should be tested ≥3 months period, active disease for ≥4 weeks (BASDAI > 4 cm at two times, 1 months apart "or" physician global assessment ≥2 on Likert scale), patients with peripheral arthritis who failed to >1 disease-modifying antirheumatic drug (DMARD) (sulfasalazine preferred). Patients with ankylosing spondylitis treated with either infliximab (chimeric human/mouse anti-TNF-α monoclonal antibody), etanercept [soluble p75 TNF-α receptor—immunoglobulin G (IgG) fusion protein], or adalimumab or golimumab (human anti-TNF-α monoclonal antibodies) have shown effective, rapid, and sustained reductions in all clinical and laboratory measures of disease activity, other newer agents also have similar efficacy.

Surgical treatment: The indications for surgical treatment in ankylosing spondylitis are—unstable injuries, Andersson lesion with or without neurological deficit, painful spinal deformity, and functionally and/or cosmetically unacceptable deformities. For correction of lumbar and thoracolumbar deformities, a two-stage procedure is uncommonly performed with posterior and anterior osteotomies. Similarly, mobile or fixed cervicothoracic region deformities are corrected with osteotomies. For hip and knee joint disease, arthroplasty is the usual choice. Patients with ankylosing spondylitis may have an increased risk of heterotopic ossification. Indomethacin or perioperative radiation may be used to decrease this risk.

75. Discuss investigations for ankylosing spondylitis.

Ans: *X-rays:*
- The earliest—is erosion and fuzziness of the sacroiliac joints. Later there may be periarticular sclerosis, especially on the iliac side of the joint and finally bony ankylosis.
- The earliest vertebral change is flattening of the normal anterior concavity of the vertebral body (squaring). Later, ossification of the ligaments around the intervertebral discs produces delicate bridges (syndesmophytes) between adjacent vertebrae. Bridging at several levels gives the appearance of a 'bamboo spine'.
- Osteoporosis is common in longstanding cases and there may be hyperkyphosis of the thoracic spine due to wedging of the vertebral bodies.
- Peripheral joints may show erosive arthritis or progressive bony ankylosis.

MRI:
- MRI shows typical erosions and features of inflammation such as bone edema.
- Contrast enhancement may demonstrate inflammatory lesions in other areas of the spine.

Special investigations: The ESR and CRP are usually elevated during active phases of the disease. HLA-B27 is present in 95% of cases. Serological tests for rheumatoid factor are usually negative.

76. Describe clinical presentation and investigations for rheumatoid arthritis.

Ans: *Clinical presentation:* Classically RA is a symmetric, polyarthritis of small joints. Most patients of RA have weeks to months of insidious onset of fatigue and joint pains that may be transient early but later the joint inflammation becomes more persistent with warmth, effusion, tenderness, and loss of function. The DIP joints are characteristically spared.

A tenth of patients experience an acute onset of symptoms. Early morning joint stiffness lasting >60 minutes is seen in most patients that improves over next few hours and physical activity. Duration of morning stiffness usually correlates with the extent of synovial inflammation. Structural damage to the joints begin early, however, manifest usually after a year. With persistent inflammation there is damage to and weakening of ligaments, tendons and joint capsule. The unopposed physical forces and muscle imbalance leads to development of characteristic deformities in hand namely the z-deformity, swan-neck deformity and boutonniere deformity. In the feet there may be eversion at the subtalar joint, plantar subluxation of metatarsal heads, forefoot widening, and hallux valgus.

Investigations:
Lab tests: RA factor, anti-CCP, other laboratory findings that suggest but are not diagnostic of RA include presence of antiperinuclear factor, antikeratin antibodies, elevated erythrocyte sedimentation rate (ESR > 30 mm in first hour), elevated C-reactive protein (CRP) (> 0.7 pg/mL), decreased hematocrit level (normocytic normochromic anemia) and/or elevated platelet count.

Radiographic findings: In early course of disease, the radiographs are mute or show periarticular/juxta-articular osteopenia. Cartilage destruction deformities and bony erosions come later and are nonspecific. Only a clue to RA could be symmetrical involvement but much before radiologic evaluation clinical evaluation should have established diagnosis. Erosion tends to be marginal (away from the weight-bearing portion of the joint). In the hip, the femoral head tends to migrate axially or superomedially, whereas the hip tends to migrate more superolaterally in osteoarthritis. In the shoulder, the humeral head tends to be high riding. Radiographs are helpful for reconstruction planning and prognostication of patient.

77. What is osteogenesis imperfecta?

Ans: Osteogenesis imperfecta (OI) is a series of syndromes (not just a disease as previously thought) representing classes of molecular defects, each with a reasonably well-defined clinical pattern. It is the most common genetic cause of osteoporosis due to generalized disorder of connective tissue with an estimated incidence of 1:20,000. By its etymology, it simply means "imperfect development of bones".

Osteogenesis imperfecta is a hereditary condition resulting from an abnormality in type I collagen that is manifested by an increased fragility of bones and low bone mass (osteopenia). The spectrum of disorder is so broad that it ranges from perinatally lethal forms to barely recognizable disease in adulthood.

Sillence classification system as modified by Cole is the most accepted by the geneticists and researchers, but Shapiro might be more helpful from a pediatric orthopedist's point of view where one is asked the questions regarding the management and the prognosis of fractures occurring at different age. This classification has excellent practical application for the orthopedic surgeon in regard to prognosis for survival and ambulation. The distinction between the two congenita types is based on the timing of the fracture and radiographic features of the affected bones.

Patients with "congenita A" sustain fractures *in utero* or at birth, with the additional radiographic features of crumpled long bones, crumpled ribs with rib cage deformity, and a fragile skull. These features are incompatible with life, and the patients are almost always stillborn or die shortly after birth from intracranial hemorrhage or respiratory insufficiency.

Patients with "congenita B" have fractures at birth but are radiographically distinct from congenita A patients in that the long bones, as typified by the femur, are more tubular and have more normal funnelization in the metaphysis, the ribs are more normally formed, and there is no rib cage deformity. These patients are severely affected, but this type is compatible with survival.

Patients with tarda A have an onset of fractures before walking. The age at onset of fractures was not prognostic for ambulation within this group in Shapiro's study.

Patients with tarda B suffer their first fracture after walking age; all these patients were ambulatory in Shapiro's study. Older classification systems divided the disease into "congenita" and "tarda" (looser)—based on when the first fracture occurred, applying congenital only to intrauterine fractures.

Pathophysiology: Eighty to ninety percent of patients with OI can be grouped into the Sillence type I to IV categories and have mutations of one of the two type I collagen genes. The *COL1A* gene encodes the pro-1α(I) protein chain and the *COL2A* gene encodes pro-2α(I) protein chain of type I procollagen. The etiologies of the remaining 10–20% remain unclear. With further identification of more than 280 locations of disruptions in the genetic coding for type 1 collagen and finding of noncollagen mutations causing OI, the classification system is continuously expanding.

In lethal OI, a considerable increase in the concentration of types III and V and a marked variation in cross-linking are found. Other changes described in the various types of OI include:
- An increase in collagen hydroxylysine residues in bone.
- A decrease in hydroxylysinonorleucine in skin collagen.
- Abnormalities of α1- and α2-polypeptides of type I collagen in cultured skin fibroblasts.

Clinical features: In the most severe types of OI, fractures are present before birth and the infant is either stillborn or lives only for a few weeks, death being due to respiratory failure, basilar indentation or intracranial hemorrhage following injury. The clinical features of nonlethal forms of OI are osteopenia dominated by bone fragility and fractures. General features include the characteristic fragility of bone, short stature, defective dentinogenesis of deciduous or permanent teeth or both, premature middle ear deafness, laxity of ligaments, and blue tympanic membranes. Other features may include some or all of the following:
- Gracile and diffusely osteopenic bones with thin cortices and an attenuated trabecular pattern.
- *Gray-blue sclerae:* The blueness of sclerae is inversely proportional to the severity of disease with most patients with milder forms having blue or gray-blue sclerae. "Saturn ring" is caused by white sclera immediately surrounding the cornea. Embryotoxon or "arcus juvenilis" may be seen.
- Dentinogenesis imperfecta
- Kyphoscoliosis
- Many patients have misshapen skulls with wide intertemporal measurements and small triangular faces.
- Neurologic abnormalities are consequences of direct neural compression, altered cerebrospinal fluid flow, or vascular compromise.
- Inguinal, umbilical, and diaphragmatic hernias are common. The skin is thin, translucent, and easily distensible. Although increased vascular fragility is common, major arterial or aortic aneurysms are rarely encountered.
- Basilar invagination (prolapse of the upper cervical spine into the base of the skull).

X-rays: There is generalized osteopenia, thinning of the long bones, fractures in various stages of healing, vertebral compression, and spinal deformity. The type of abnormality varies with the severity of the disease. The skull may be enlarged and shows the presence of wormian bones—areas of vicarious ossification in the calvarium. After puberty, fractures occur less frequently, but in those who survive the incidence rises again after the climacteric. It is thought that very mild ("subclinical") forms of OI may account for some cases of recurrent fractures in adults.

Diagnosis: Skin biopsies and fibroblast cultures may be helpful, but are only positive in 80% of patients with type IV OI (the most commonly confused with nonaccidental trauma). Prenatal DNA (deoxyribonucleic acid) mutation analysis can be performed in pregnancies with risk of OI to analyze uncultured chorionic villus cells.

Severe OI can also be detected by level II ultrasonography as early as 16th week. Raised alkaline phosphatase in neonatal period would distinguish OI from hypophosphatasia.

Management: There is no medical treatment presently available and gene therapy is still evolving.

Conservative treatment is directed at preventing fractures—if necessary by using lightweight orthosis during physical activity—and treating fractures when they occur. However, splintage should not be overdone as this may contribute further to the prevailing osteopenia. Cyclic administration of bisphosphonates has been used to treat patients with types III and IV OI quite extensively. Bisphosphonates decrease the resorption of bone by suppressing the activity of osteoclasts. Pamidronate therapy decreases the incidence of fractures, relieves chronic bone pain, increases activity levels, decreases the reliance on mobility aids, and increases the height of the collapsed vertebral bodies. Unfortunately, there has been no decrease in the incidence of scoliosis. Radiographically, pamidronate therapy creates growth lines in the bone.

Most of the long-term orthopedic problems are encountered in types III and IV. Fractures are treated conservatively, but immobilization must be kept to a minimum. Long-bone deformities are common, due either to malunion of complete fractures or breaking of recurrent incomplete fractures; these may require operative correction, usually by 4 or 5 years of age. Principally, the orthopedic surgery is advised to decrease the risk of fracture, allow for early weight bearing, and to achieve union. The mainstay of orthopedic surgical treatment of patients with OI is realignment osteotomy. This is performed to improve the mechanical axis of appendicular bones, which in turn, also helps in balancing and reducing morbidity by reducing stress on other parts of bone and other bones. Other surgical interventions include management of basilar invagination and correction of scoliosis.

78. Describe principle, indications, advantages, disadvantages of intramedullary growth rod.

Ans: Intramedullary growth rods, also known as telescopic intramedullary rods or nails, are specialized orthopedic implants designed primarily for children with various conditions (see below). These rods are inserted into the medullary canal of long bones (e.g., femur and tibia) to stabilize fractures, correct deformities, and accommodate bone growth in pediatric patients.

Principle: Intramedullary growth rods are metal implants (typically stainless steel or titanium) designed to stabilize long bones while allowing for elongation as the child grows. They consist of two components: a *female component* (hollow sleeve) and a *male component* (inner rod) that slide relative to each other, enabling the rod to "telescope" or extend with bone growth. The rods are anchored at the proximal and distal ends of the bone, often with screws or transchondral sutures, to provide stability. The procedure involves:

- *Surgical insertion:* The rod is placed into the medullary canal through small incisions, often requiring osteotomies to correct deformities or align fracture fragments.
- *Telescoping mechanism:* As the bone grows, the rod extends, reducing the need for frequent surgical replacements compared to nontelescopic rods.
- *Load-sharing:* The rod acts as an internal splint, sharing mechanical load with the bone to promote healing and prevent re-fracture or deformity.

This approach contrasts with fixed-length rods (e.g., Rush pins), which do not accommodate growth and may require earlier replacement.

Indications

Intramedullary growth rods are primarily indicated for pediatric patients with:

1. *Osteogenesis imperfecta (OI):* To stabilize long bones (femur, tibia, and humerus) prone to frequent fractures, bowing, or shortening due to brittle bones. Telescopic rods are particularly useful in moderate to severe OI (e.g., Sillence types III and IV).
2. *Congenital bone disorders*: Conditions like congenital pseudarthrosis of the tibia or rickets, where bones are at risk of deformity or fracture throughout childhood.
3. *Long bone deformities*: To correct bowing or angulation, often through multiple osteotomies, as seen in OI or other skeletal dysplasias.
4. *Recurrent or complex fractures*: In cases where nonsurgical methods (e.g., casting) are insufficient to maintain alignment or prevent deformity, particularly in unstable or comminuted fractures.
5. *Bone lengthening or stabilization*: To support bones during lengthening procedures or after deformity correction, especially in growing children.

These rods are typically avoided in very young children with small bones or in cases where the growth plate must not be crossed to prevent growth disturbances.

Advantages:

1. *Accommodates growth:* The telescoping mechanism allows the rod to extend with bone growth, reducing the frequency of revision surgeries compared to fixed-length rods (e.g., 2–3 years for non-telescopic rods vs. longer for telescopic rods).
2. *Stabilizes fractures and deformities:* Provides robust internal fixation, promoting fracture union and correcting deformities like bowing, which is critical in OI.
3. *Load-sharing:* Shares mechanical load with the bone, enhancing stability and allowing earlier mobilization compared to external fixation or casting.
4. *Minimally invasive:* Requires smaller incisions than plating, reducing soft-tissue disruption and infection risk.
5. *Reduced re-fracture risk:* Stabilizes bones in conditions like OI, decreasing fracture frequency and discomfort.
6. *High success rates:* Studies report good outcomes, with telescopic rods like the Fassier–Duval rod achieving lower revision rates (e.g., 36% at 5 years for a novel TIR vs. 46% for Fassier–Duval).

Disadvantages:

1. *Surgical complexity:* Insertion requires precise surgical technique, often involving osteotomies, and can be challenging in small or deformed bones.

2. *Complications:*
   - *Rod migration:* Rods may loosen or displace, causing pain or loss of movement, requiring revision surgery (e.g., 9/52 cases in one study).
   - *Fracture:* Adjacent fractures can occur at unsupported bone segments (e.g., 15/52 cases in a study of OI patients).
   - *Infection:* Peri-implant infections, though rare (e.g., 2/52 cases), can necessitate rod removal or prolonged antibiotics.
   - *Mechanism failure:* The telescoping mechanism may fail to extend properly, requiring replacement.
   - *Rod bending:* Rods may bend under significant force, necessitating revision.
3. *Revision surgery:* Despite their design, telescopic rods eventually require replacement as the child grows or if complications arise (e.g., 36% revision rate at 5 years).
4. *Growth plate concerns:* Insertion may cross growth plates, potentially affecting bone length, though newer designs (e.g., interlocking telescopic nails) aim to avoid distal joint violation.
5. *Cost:* Telescopic rods are more expensive than nontelescopic options, and revision surgeries add to healthcare costs.
6. *Limited applicability:* Not suitable for all fracture types (e.g., metaphyseal fractures with short distal fragments) or in very young children with small medullary canals.

Postoperative issues: Patients may experience discomfort at insertion sites (e.g., trochanteric entry) or leg length discrepancies requiring shoe raises or further intervention.

79. Discuss Ehlers–Danlos syndrome.

Ans: Ehlers–Danlos syndrome (EDS) is a group of the most common heritable disorders of the connective tissue with considerable diversity, largely caused by extensive genetic heterogeneity. Although all heterogenic subgroups have following unifying features:
- Skin and joint hypermobility
- Easy bruisability
- Dystrophic scarring
- Increased joint mobility
- Abnormal tissue fragility.

This syndrome is named after two physicians, Edvard Ehlers (Denmark) and Henri-Alexandre Danlos (France). The combined prevalence of all types of this condition is about 1 in 5,000. The previous classification system of 11 different types has been reduced to 6 in the present Villefranche classification system (1997) on the basis of phenotypic and inheritance characteristics. EDS is presently classified based on genetic transmission, biochemical anomaly, and major and minor clinical findings. Biochemical studies have demonstrated considerable heterogeneity within individual types. Among the various heterogeneous groups, chronic joint discomfort debilitating and disabling are common orthopedically and these patients are susceptible to osteoarthritis (OA). Internal manifestations, like rupture of great vessels, diverticula of the gastrointestinal and genitourinary tracts, hiatal hernia, spontaneous rupture of the bowel, spontaneous pneumothorax, etc. tend to occur only in specific types of EDS.

The hypermobility type affects around 1 in 10,000–15,000 people, while the classic type probably involves 1 in 20,000–40,000 people.

Genetics: Mutations in the *ADAMTS2, COL1A1, COL1A2, COL3A1, COL5A1, COL5A2, PLOD1,* and *TNXB* genes cause EDS. Some of these genes *(COL1A1, COL1A2, COL3A1, COL5A1,* and *COL5A2)* provide instructions for making proteins that are used to assemble different types of collagens. Collagens are molecules that give structure and strength to connective tissues throughout the body. Mutations that cause the different forms of EDS disrupt the structure, production, or processing of collagen, preventing these molecules from being assembled properly. These defects weaken connective tissues in the skin, bones, and other parts of the body, resulting in the characteristic features of this condition.

Clinical Features
Classic:
- The classic type is characterized by hyperextensibility of joints and increased stretchability of skin along with widened atrophic scars, and joint hypermobility. Other minor criteria for identification includes the following:
  - Velvety skin

- Spheroids
- Hypotonia
- Tissue fragility.
• The patients can be identified early in life due to various manifestations of loose joints like:
  - Congenital dislocation of the hips
  - Habitual dislocation of selected joints in later life
  - Joint effusions
  - Clubfoot deformity of the feet
  - Spondylolisthesis.
• Up to 33% of patients will have aortic root dilatations (echocardiography for workup should be done).
• Nearly 30% of patients will have scoliosis (predominantly the thoracic or thoracolumbar type).
• More than 50% of these patients may have chronic musculoskeletal pain that responds to most common analgesics and better managed with physiotherapy (muscle conditioning).
• Management of the classic type include stress on prevention of trauma and great care in treating wounds.
• Most of the management resides on conservative lines and support.
  - Young athletes benefit from wearing shin guards to avoid frequent hemorrhage, unsightly scars, and absence from school.
  - Patients should be discouraged from demonstrating their joint laxity as entertainment for their friends.
  - Rigorous endurance exercises should be restricted and supervised due to fragility of tendons.

Hypermobility type:
• This is the most debilitating of all forms of EDS orthopedically, and the most likely to require orthopedic surgical intervention.
• The molecular basis is unknown, so no diagnostic test presently exists. The unifying abnormality being abnormal production of type III collagen.
• Clinically, these patients have soft skin and both small and large joint hypermobility.
  - Recurrent and/or chronic dislocations are also common. Multidirectional instability of the shoulder, patella subluxation, and chronic ankle instability are common.
• Up to 20% of patients may have aortic root anomalies.
• Surgical interventions such as capsular shift or placation should be undertaken only if physical therapy is ineffective. Results and prognosis are often reserved. Bracing is frequently used, especially of the hands because of finger instability.
• Nearly 90% of patients with hypermobility type have debilitating pain (often accompanying abnormal gait) that needs assistive devices.

Vascular:
• Though less disabling, this is the most serious type because of a propensity for spontaneous rupture of arteries and bowel. Bruisability is typically very striking and hence the term *ecchymotic type* is used as a synonym for vascular type.
• Hypermobility of the small joints is a less prominent feature.
• These patients have thin, translucent skin, and may experience spontaneous rupture of the bowel, uterus also apart from large arteries.
• Aortic root dilatation is present in more than 75% of patients. About 25% of women die during pregnancy because of complications, most often uterine rupture.
• Life expectancy is 45–50 years.

Kyphoscoliosis (Previously Type VI):
• This rare subtype is an autosomal recessive disorder with a biochemical deficiency in lysyl hydroxylase.
• In addition to the skin and joint involvement seen in EDS classic form, the hallmarks of the kyphoscoliotic form are fragility of the ocular globe and a propensity to severe scoliosis. The major diagnostic criteria include:
  - Muscle hypotonia at birth and a progressive scoliosis.
  - Scoliosis of spine (double thoracic curves common).
  - There is generalized joint laxity.
  - Ocular findings such as, scleral fragility and globe rupture are found in 50% of patients.

- Minor criteria include bruising, tissue fragility, osteopenia, and arterial rupture.
- Kyphoscoliosis EDS may be confused with Marfan syndrome as patients have scoliotic, cardiac, and ocular involvement and often a tall and thin body habitus.

Arthrochalasis:
- The patients with arthrochalasia type of EDS have predominantly loose-jointedness with congenital dislocations.
- This is extremely rare form of EDS. The basic abnormality includes an inability to convert type I procollagen to mature collagen, by cleavage of the N-propeptide.
- Patients are moderately short of stature. The children with arthrochalasis type EDS have bilateral developmental dysplasia of the hip (DDH; recalcitrant to surgical intervention).
- They may also have skin hyperextensibility, osteopenia, muscle hypotonia, and kyphoscoliosis.

Dermatosparaxis: Dermatosparaxis (tearing of skin) is a rare, autosomal recessive form of EDS notable for a deficiency of procollagen I N-terminal peptidase (defect as described above). The features are more severe in the skin for unknown reasons. This may be due to the possibility that N-propeptidase could have other molecules besides type I procollagen as substrate. Patients have redundant, severely fragile, and often sagging skin. Premature rupture of fetal membranes and large hernias can be seen.

Other forms: In addition to the six major forms of the Villefranche classification, other rare forms of EDS exist that include the previously described types V, VIII, and X. These forms are those with periodontal friability (type VIII) and the poor clotting/fibronectin deficient (type X). In addition, a form of EDS described in only one family with symptoms similar to the classic form exists that specifically has an X-linked inheritance pattern (formerly type V EDS).

80. What is Marfan syndrome? What is its orthopedic management?

Ans: Marfan syndrome is an inherited multisystem disorder of connective tissue that primarily affects the skeleton, the cardiovascular system, and the eyes, and is usually transmitted as an autosomal dominant trait. The incidence is roughly 1:10,000. There is no ethnic or gender predilection. The genetic mutation of Marfan syndrome is on the fibrillin-1 *(FBN1)* gene located on chromosome *15q21* which encodes fibrillin-1, a large extracellular matrix protein that provides stretch and elasticity to connective tissues and is also involved in regulating the bioavailability of TGF-β family members. Approximately 25% of cases arise from new mutations. More than 135 mutations in the *FBN1* gene have been identified. The genetic heterogenicity explains the pleiotropic manifestations of Marfan syndrome with variable phenotypic expression. *FBN1* is the main component of the 10–20 nm extracellular microfibrils that are important for elastogenesis, elasticity, and homeostasis of elastic fibers.

Orthopedic management:
- The success rate for bracing of spinal deformities is much lower than in adolescent idiopathic scoliosis. Curves greater than 25° in children with Risser grade II skeletal maturity will likely require surgery despite bracing. Preoperative imaging of the spine with MRI to identify dural ectasia and CT to assess fixation points are essential.
- Closure of the triradiate cartilage to treat protrusion acetabuli also has been proposed.

(Kindly read the clinical features from Chapter 26 of 2nd edition of the book Essential Orthopedics: Principles and Practice)

81. Explain the etiopathogenesis of Down syndrome. Enumerate musculoskeletal manifestations of Down syndrome. Enumerate the HLA-B27 associated rheumatologic diseases (minimum four). Explain extractable nuclear antigen test.

Ans: Down syndrome: Down syndrome is a genetic disorder caused by the presence of an extra copy of chromosome 21—also known as trisomy 21.

Etiopathogenesis:
There are three main genetic mechanisms:
1. Trisomy 21 (95%): *Nondisjunction*:
   - Failure of chromosome 21 to separate during meiosis.
   - Results in 47 chromosomes in all cells (extra 21).
   - Strongly associated with advanced maternal age.

2. Translocation (4%):
   - Part of chromosome 21 is translocated to another chromosome (usually 14 or 22).
   - Total chromosome count can be normal, but extra 21 material is present.
3. Mosaicism (1%):
   - Some cells have normal karyotype (46 chromosomes); others have trisomy 21.
   - Caused by a post-zygotic mitotic error.
   - Milder phenotype.

Molecular effects:
- Overexpression of genes on chromosome 21.
- Disruption in neuronal development, immune function, and skeletal growth.

Musculoskeletal manifestations of down syndrome
Down syndrome affects connective tissue and musculoskeletal development. Common features include:
- *Hypotonia:* Decreased muscle tone—present from birth.
- *Ligamentous laxity:* Hypermobile joints, increased risk of dislocations.
- *Atlantoaxial instability:* Excess mobility at C1–C2 joint (can cause spinal cord compression).
- *Short stature:* Due to growth retardation.
- *Delayed motor milestones:* Due to hypotonia and ligament laxity.
- *Pes planus (flat feet):* Common due to ligament laxity.
- *Genu valgum (knock knees):* May develop in early childhood.
- *Hip dislocation:* Risk increases with age.
- *Scoliosis:* Present in some cases.

HLA-B27-associated rheumatologic diseases
HLA-B27 is a class I MHC allele strongly associated with seronegative spondyloarthropathies:
1. Ankylosing spondylitis
2. Reactive arthritis (Reiter syndrome)
3. Psoriatic arthritis (especially axial form)
4. Enteropathic arthritis (associated with IBD—Crohn's, ulcerative colitis)
5. Juvenile idiopathic arthritis (enthesitis-related subtype)
6. Acute anterior uveitis (strongly associated but not a joint disease)

Extractable nuclear antigen (ENA) Test
The ENA panel detects autoantibodies against small nuclear and cytoplasmic antigens extracted from the nucleus of cells. These autoantibodies are markers of systemic autoimmune connective tissue diseases.

The following are common techniques:
- Immunoblot, ELISA, or multiplex immunoassays are commonly used.
- Performed when ANA (antinuclear antibody) is positive.

Common ENA Antigens and Associated Diseases are tabulated in **Table 2.4.1**.

TABLE 2.4.1: Common ENA antigens and associated diseases.

Antigen	Autoantibody	Associated disease
Sm	Anti-Sm	Systemic lupus erythematosus (SLE)
RNP	Anti-RNP	Mixed connective tissue disease (MCTD)
SSA (Ro)	Anti-Ro	Sjögren's syndrome, SLE, and neonatal lupus
SSB (La)	Anti-La	Sjögren syndrome
Scl-70	Anti-topoisomerase I	Diffuse systemic sclerosis
Jo-1	Anti-synthetase	Polymyositis/Dermatomyositis
Centromere	Anti-centromere	Limited scleroderma (CREST syndrome)

2.5 ORTHOPEDIC INFECTION (ACUTE/CHRONIC OSTEOMYELITIS, BIOFILMS, HIV/AIDS, SSI, LOCOREGIONAL INFECTIONS, TUBERCULAR INFECTION) (Q82–124)

82. **Explain the role of biofilm in implant-related infection in orthopedics. Describe the production, regulation, and management of biofilm.**

Ans: "Biofilm formation is a process whereby microorganisms of the same species attach to and grow on a surface and produce extracellular polymers that facilitate attachment and matrix formation, resulting in an alteration in the phenotype of the organisms with respect to growth rate and gene transcription". The body's own defense is rendered ineffective especially at the implant surfaces and within sequestrum. These being avascular, the bacteria thrive uninhibitedly here far away from the influence of antibiotics and immunity. Most bacteria and few fungi have ingenious capacity to synthesize inert glycocalyx capsule (described in 1984) that forms a "biofilm" (concept introduced in 1980) inert to host defense (see also prosthetic joint infection). The polysaccharide intercellular adhesin (PIA) is mainly responsible for formation of extracellular polysaccharide matrix that makes biofilm. Biofilm is typically, quickly, and copiously produced by *Pseudomonas aeruginosa, Staphylococcus aureus*, and *S. epidermidis*. The glycocalyx is an extracellular polysaccharide molecule that contains *host* molecules in an immunological sense. This glycocalyx (exopolysaccharide) together with environmental DNA, proteins, and lipids form the extracellular matrix commonly termed *slime* serves as protective physical barrier for microbes. The biofilm has a base layer that is near the implant and fosters adherence to target surface. The pH and local environment encourage formation of sessile variants of bacteria that collectively develop a colony. The outer layers form discrete structures such as "columns" and "mushrooms". "Streamers" can form in the outer layers that may break off to infect contiguous areas. Intercellular signaling through the extracellular matrix occurs via "quantum packets" that are transported via nanotubes formed within matrix and these nanotubes are also involved in conducting cell-to-cell electric signals.

The unique combined genetic characteristic (pangenome) prevents host from developing adaptive immune response → development of extended phenotype (the biofilm has uniquely altered host and environmental factors that cause variety of changes like altered pH, O_2 tension, and ion concentration that are favorable only to biofilm and host cells will not survive here) → surface dispersion (microbes near the surface regularly detach and are free to colonize other areas of host in remote places, also flow of biofilm due to viscoelastic nature of the slime causes streaming and spread of the biofilm to adjacent surface).

Other mechanisms involved in biofilm regulation:
- The biofilm-producing bacteria grow slowly due to highly anaerobic conditions reducing the metabolic activity so antibiotics targeting the replication process (fluoroquinolones) are rendered ineffective (see also prosthetic infections). These organisms are called "persisters" or better the "sessile" variants. The sessile variants have 103 less sensitivity to antibiotics, restricted reproduction and are difficult to culture.
- The sessile forms keep coordination among themselves by "quorum sensing" (lactone containing molecules that establish communication between intra- and interspecies that regulate metabolic activity in response to population density via signaling molecules) and slowly develop increasing resistance to administered drugs.
- Quorum-sensing is also involved in production of toxins from the microbes that cause direct lysis of host lead inflammatory response cells like the neutrophils, thus causing nearby tissue damage also. Once the local immunity falls low, the return to "planktonic form" (free-floating, virulent, reproductive form, triggering host systems) can occur accounting for clinical recurrences and acute on chronic episodes. When planktonic forms encounter a devitalized surface coated with protein, they quickly home in it.
- *Development of "pangenome":* The development of microbe diversity in biofilm causes immense changes in the genetic makeup, so much so that different organisms due to horizontal transfer of genetic material develop a similar overt genome or a de facto genome larger than that of any one strain. This genome is termed "pangenome". The pangenome gives increased survival ability to the biofilm and prevents host from mounting an effective adaptive immune response **(Flowchart 2.5.1)**.

Management of biofilm:
- *Mechanical removal:* Wherever possible the biofilm should be removed so that there is no possibility of persistent infection. It is impossible from current drug-therapies to shatter or dissolve biofilm so it has to be removed. This entails removal of all infection-associated implants from the body.

- *Drugs that can cross biofilm:* It has been tried to cross the biofilm barrier by drugs like rifampicin so that the organisms can be inhibited but only limited success has been obtained and resistance is fast to develop.
- *Prevention of biofilm formation:* This is the best approach and involves a conglomerate of best surgical practices and use of antisepsis during any open procedure. Some drugs like β-lactams have been found to prevent formation of biofilm *in situ*.

Flowchart 2.5.1: Biofilm formation and various influences on the same.

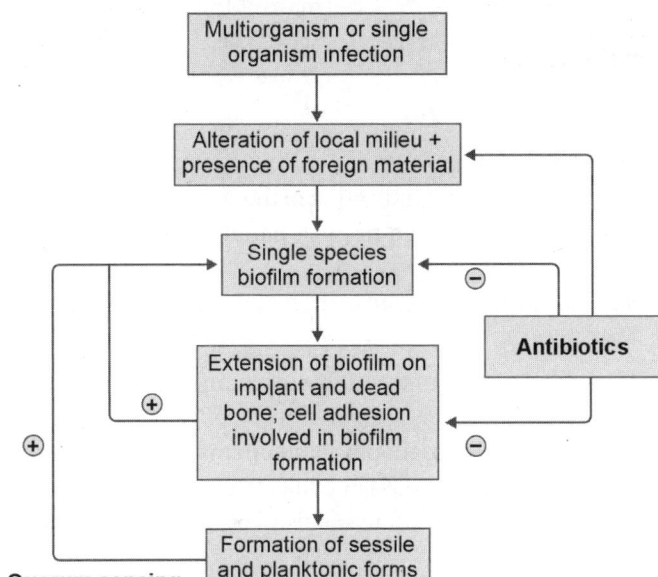

83. Describe the pathology and clinical features of acute hematogenous osteomyelitis in long bones. Give detailed management of chronic osteomyelitis of long bone.

Ans: *Pathology:* Acute hematogenous osteomyelitis is more common in males in all age groups affected. It is caused by a bacteremia, which is a common occurrence in childhood. The causes of bacteremia are many. Bacteriological seeding of bone generally is associated with other factors such as localized trauma, chronic illness, malnutrition, or an inadequate immune system. In many cases, the exact cause of the disease cannot be identified.

- *In infants and children:* The bone is thin, weak, and immature giving way easily to the pus under pressure so extensive devascularization and large sequestrum formation does not occur. Pus is however copious. Cortical damage is transient while a large involucrum forms due to high regenerating potency of periosteum.
- *In children:* The growth plate and the epiphysis are usually spared and the infection remains limited to metaphysis and proximally. The subperiosteal extension of pus and endosteal thrombosis produce extensive devascularization of the bone and large sequestrum (sometimes whole diaphysis—cylindrical sequestrum) are seen in late presentations. The cortical damage is hence extensive with prompt involucrum formation. Growth disturbance is rare seen only with extensive aggressive disease reaching the germinal layer of growth plate, else in common presentations, some growth stimulation is common due to increased vascularity.
- *In adults:* Osteomyelitis is often due to contiguous spread. Long bone involvement in hematogenous spread is rare. Infected bone is resorbed leaving behind a cavity. Whole bone involvement and chronic osteomyelitis developing is common.

Clinical features: Children with acute hematogenous osteomyelitis usually present with:
- *Bone pain of one to several days' duration:* The pain may be well-localized if the child is old enough to cooperate or difficult to discern if the child is young or if the area of involvement produces confusing findings (axial OM or osteomyelitis of the pelvis).
- Complete functiolesia of the involved extremity.
- Fever

- *Swelling of the involved extremity:* Localized to the area of the infection unless the infection has spread to involve much of the soft tissues of the extremity.
- *Later:* The overlying skin becomes red and warm—tender to touch with development of subcutaneous abscess.

Management of chronic osteomyelitis:

Diagnosis: The diagnosis of chronic osteomyelitis is based on clinical, laboratory, and imaging studies. The "gold standard" is to obtain a biopsy specimen for histological and microbiological evaluation of the infected bone.

Clinical:
- Condition of the skin and soft tissue
- Areas of tenderness
- Assess bone stability
- Evaluate the neurovascular status of the limb.

Laboratory studies—are nonspecific and give no indication of the severity of the infection. Erythrocyte sedimentation rate (ESR) and C-reactive protein (CRP) are elevated in most patients, but the white blood cell count is elevated in only 35%.

Imaging studies—should be done only to aid in confirmation of the diagnosis and to plan for surgical treatment.

Plain radiographs:
- Within a few days (some authors say 48–72 hours), soft tissue changes like muscle swelling and blurring of the soft tissue planes can be appreciated.
- Periosteal thickening, lytic lesions, endosteal scalloping, osteopenia, loss of trabecular architecture, and new bone apposition takes 5–7 days in children and 10–14 days in adults to develop.
- Periostitis, involucrum formation, sinus tracts, soft tissue fistulas, and most importantly sequestrum formation are indicative of chronic osteomyelitis.
- Sonography can be performed if a sinus track is present and can be a valuable adjunct to surgical planning.
- Isotopic bone scanning is more useful in acute osteomyelitis than in the chronic form.
- Increased uptake in areas of increased blood flow or osteoblastic activity—lack specificity (but has high negative predictive value).
- Gallium scans show increased uptake in areas where leukocytes or bacteria accumulate.
- *Indium-111:* Labeled leukocyte scans are more sensitive than technetium or gallium scans and are especially useful in differentiating chronic osteomyelitis from neuropathic arthropathy in the diabetic foot.

Computed tomography (CT) scan—detailed information and excellent definition of cortical bone and a fair evaluation of the surrounding soft tissues can be obtained.

Magnetic resonance imaging (MRI) provides a fairly accurate determination of the extent of the pathological insult by showing the margins of bone and soft-tissue edema. Especially, it is important to evaluate recurrence of infection. In chronic osteomyelitis, MRI may reveal a well-defined rim of high signal intensity surrounding the focus of active disease (*rim sign*).

The "gold standard" in the diagnosis of osteomyelitis is a biopsy with culture and sensitivity. A biopsy is not only useful in establishing a diagnosis, but also is helpful in determining the proper antibiotic regimen. Typically, staphylococcal species are identified, especially in posttraumatic infections. Anaerobes and gram-negative bacilli are commonly isolated.

Treatment: Chronic osteomyelitis generally cannot be eradicated without surgical treatment. Bacteria are able to adhere to orthopedic implants and bone matrix and evade internal immune defense. Antibiotics are usually ineffective against persisters and chronic small cell variants.

Surgery for chronic osteomyelitis consists of sequestrectomy and resection of scarred and infected bone and soft tissue and definite removal of associated surgical hardware while stabilizing the bone/fracture/nonunion utilizing alternative measures. The goal of surgery is eradication of the infection by achieving a viable and vascular environment and optimal bone healing.

Adequate debridement for excision of focus often leaves a large dead space that must be managed to prevent recurrence and significant bone loss that may result in bony instability. Appropriate reconstruction of the bone and soft-tissue defects may be needed after proper identification of the infecting organism and appropriate antibiotic therapy. Reconstruction should be undertaken only after careful planning and identification of sequestra and intraosseous abscesses by plain radiographs, sinography, CT, and MRI.

The duration of perioperative antibiotics is controversial. Traditionally, a 6-week course of intravenous antibiotics is prescribed postoperatively. The following are the commonly used strategies in management of chronic osteomyelitis but every patient has to manage individually utilizing different combinations and reductions.

- *Sequestrectomy and curettage for chronic osteomyelitis:* Sinus tracks can be injected with methylene blue 24 hours before surgery to make them easier to locate and excise the disease and focus in toto. Bony and soft-tissue defects must be filled to reduce the chance of continued infection and loss of function. Several techniques have been described below for the management of such postoperative defects:
  - Bone grafting with primary or secondary closure
  - Use of antibiotic polymethyl methacrylate (PMMA) beads as a temporary filler of the dead space before reconstruction
  - Local muscle flaps and skin grafting with or without bone grafting
  - Microvascular transfer of muscle, myocutaneous, osseous, and osteocutaneous flaps
  - The use of bone transport (Ilizarov technique).
- *Open bone grafting:* Papineau et al. described an open bone grafting technique for the treatment of chronic osteomyelitis. This procedure is based on the following principles: (1) granulation tissue markedly resists infection, (2) autogenous cancellous bone grafts are rapidly revascularized and are resistant to infection, (3) the infected area is completely excised, (4) adequate drainage is provided, (5) adequate immobilization is provided, and (6) antibiotics are used for prolonged periods.
- *Polymethyl methacrylate antibiotic bead chains:* This technique delivers high concentrations of antibiotics locally that exceed the minimal inhibitory concentrations while maintaining low serum levels and low systemic toxicity. The antibiotic is leached from the PMMA beads into the postoperative wound hematoma and secretion, which act as a transport medium. Primary wound closure is a perquisite, else the antibiotic will get washed away. If such closure cannot be performed, the wound can be covered with a water-impermeable dressing (bead pouch technique). Suction drains are not recommended. Aminoglycosides are the most commonly employed antibiotics for use with PMMA beads. Penicillins, cephalosporins, and clindamycin are eluted well from PMMA beads; vancomycin elutes much less effectively. Antibiotics such as the fluoroquinolones, tetracycline, and polymyxin B are broken down during the exothermic process of cement hardening and cannot be used with PMMA beads. Short-term, long-term, or even permanent implantation of PMMA antibiotic beads is possible. In short-term implantation, the beads are removed within 10 days, and in long-term implantation, they may be left for 80 days.

  The antibiotic bead pouch technique has been used with encouraging results for preventing infection in open fractures. It can also be used in the treatment of osteomyelitis if soft-tissue coverage is impossible after initial debridement. The bead pouch must be changed frequently, and repeated debridement should be performed until the wound is ready for a soft-tissue coverage procedure.
- *Biodegradable antibiotic delivery systems:* These have the advantage that a second procedure is not needed for removal of the beads. Some of these biodegradable substrates also contain osteoconductive and osteoinductive materials, which can be used to promote new bone formation.
- *Closed suction drains:* Using a double or triple lumen drains.
- *Soft tissue transfer:* Varies from a localized muscle flap on a vascular pedicle to microvascular free tissue transfer to fill the defect. The transfer of vascularized muscle tissue also improves the local biological environment by bringing in a blood supply that is important in the host's defense mechanisms and for antibiotic delivery and osseous and soft tissue healing.
  - Local muscle flap is commonly used in the treatment of chronic osteomyelitis of the tibia. The gastrocnemius muscle is used for defects around the proximal third of the tibia, and the soleus muscle is used for defects around the middle third. A microvascular free muscle transfer is required for defects around the distal third of the tibia.
  - A microvascular transfer of tissue may consist of muscle that is covered with a skin graft or a myocutaneous, osseous, or osteocutaneous flap. When a microvascular free muscle flap is used, and segmental bone loss has occurred, autogenous cancellous bone grafting can be done about 6 weeks after the initial free flap transfer.

- *Ilizarov technique:* Benefits patients who need extensive resection of bone and reconstruction to achieve stability as in infected nonunions. A corticotomy is performed through normal bone proximal and distal to the area of disease. The bone is transported until union is achieved.
- *Hyperbaric oxygen therapy:* The use of hyperbaric oxygen can be recommended only as an adjuvant to other treatment methods but has unsettled efficacy.

(Kindly read Chapter 4 of the book "Essential Orthopedics: Principles and Practice, 2nd edition" for further details.)

84. (A) What are the sequelae of OM in pediatric patients? (B) Describe management of each sequelae.

Ans: The following are possible sequelae of OM in pediatric patients (along with their management):

- *Lateral epiphysiodesis:* This develops due to the involvement of a part of the germinal cells in the inflammatory reaction and toxic damage leading to irreversible growth arrest in peripheral monocircumferential part of physis. Such a partial damage causes axial deviation of the limb due to eccentric epiphysiodesis.
  - *Treatment:* Removal of the physeal bar (desepiphysiodesis) is recommended in cases having <50% bone bridge of the tibial shaft surface [computed tomography or magnetic resonance imaging (CT or MRI)] and if at least 2 years of residual growth is remaining. The resection can be done either through a metaphyseal tunnel (Langenskiöld technique) or by controlled progressive distraction (Bollini technique). This is followed by interposition of a natural or synthetic inert material. The results should be guarded as failures are frequent in because the cartilage can be damaged beyond the bridge zone.
  - When the residual growth is <2 years (12 bone age years for girls and 14 bone age years for boys), epiphysiodesis and associate corrective osteotomy are recommended.
- *Limb length discrepancy:* This results from circumferential damage to the physis or extensive intraphyseal damage.
- *Lower limb length discrepancy (LLLD):* The evaluation is commonly done by stereoradiography or CT scan imaging. The younger the child, the more progressive LLLD will be. Treatment planning should hence include the child's age and prognosticate in terms of final height, and the predicted discrepancy at the end of growth. Correction is required only if expected LLLD is >2 cm.
  - *Shortening of the normal limb:* Shortening using epiphysiodesis is done when the residual growth of the shortest limb is at least equal to the limb length discrepancy.
  - In cases of greater discrepancy or those at the end of growth, progressive lengthening of the limb is the recommended option, possibly associated with epiphysiodesis of the opposite side. The principle is based on lengthening of the osseous callus (callotasis), using one of the methods—external fixator, circular or monoplanar, but the recent trend is the development of IM nails, better accepted by patients and limiting disfigurement. Orthofix intramedullary skeletal kinetic distractor (ISKD) nails have been used for >10 years and require external maneuvers to obtain lengthening.

  Upper limb length discrepancy: Classical example is damage to proximal humerus. Lengthening with an external fixator, either monoplanar or circular, is performed if the discrepancy is >5 cm. The main complications are iatrogenic fractures, elbow stiffness, varus deviations, and paralysis of the radial nerve.
- *Pandiaphyseal OM:* OM covering >75% of the diaphysis or as involvement of the opposite metaphysis. The main complications are chronic fistulization, joint stiffness, and pathological fractures, immobilized with a cast or external fixation. Treatment involves excision (which should not be overly extensive), stabilization, and then reconstruction. Masquelet technique is quite helpful as cement can be impregnated with antibiotics. The alternative methods are the Papineau technique, the Ilizarov bone transfer technique, and vascularized bone grafting.
- *Development of septic arthritis and its sequela:* The sequela of septic arthritis has been discussed in detail in Answers to Questions 80 and 82. Others are discussed here:
  - *Joint stiffness:* This often results from capsular and ligament contracture. Also important is the contracture of joint crossing musculature that frequently undergo fibrosis and shortening. Intra-articular fibrosis is managed with arthrolysis at least 1 year after clinical and biological eradication of the infection; however, results are unpredictable. Soft-tissue lengthening is simultaneously needed. In certain cases, a corrective metaphyseal osteotomy can also be envisaged to modify the joint's range of motion and make it more functional.
  - *Osteonecrosis and chondrolysis:* In these cases, therapeutic options are arthrodesis, reconstruction surgery in young patients, and arthroplasty at the end of bone growth (refer to treatment principles of sequel of septic arthritis of hip).

85. What is Caffey's disease? Outline its salient clinical and radiological features.

Ans: Infantile cortical hyperostosis, also known as Caffey's disease, is a rare disease of infants and young children. It usually starts during the first few months of life with painful swelling over the tubular bones and/or the mandible. The child may be feverish and irritable, refusing to move the affected limb. Infection may be suspected but, apart from the swelling, there are no local signs of inflammation. The ESR, though, is usually elevated.

X-rays characteristically show periosteal new bone formation resulting in thickening of the affected bone.

After a few months, the local features may resolve spontaneously, only to reappear somewhere else. Flat bones, such as the scapula and cranial vault, may also be affected.

Other causes of hyperostosis (osteomyelitis, scurvy) must be excluded. The cause of Caffey's disease is unknown but a virus infection has been suggested.

Antibiotics are sometimes employed; it is doubtful whether they have any effect.

86. Discuss local antibiotic delivery.

Ans: The delivery of local antibiotics for the treatment of musculoskeletal infection has become increasingly popular for following reasons:
- High local levels of antibiotics facilitate delivery of antibiotics by diffusion to avascular areas of wounds.
- Microbes resistant to drug concentrations achieved by systemic antibiotic are susceptible to the extremely high local drug concentrations provided by local antibiotic delivery.
- The minimum inhibitory concentration (MIC) for planktonic variant of bacteria is hundreds of order of magnitude lower than the mean-biofilm eliminating-concentrations (MBEC) needed for managing most chronic orthopedic infections. These high MBEC cannot be achieved by systemic therapy with antibiotics.
- Newer bioabsorbable agents might serve well for dead space management.
- Additional osteoconductive and osteoinductive agents can be used as delivery system helping bone healing.

The currently available systems can be divided into biodegradable and nonbiodegradable systems.

"Nonbiodegradable bone cements—antibiotic bone cement (PMMA)" is the current gold standard for local antibiotic delivery in orthopedic surgery. It is imperative here to mention and differentiate the two "modes" of using antibiotic-loaded bone cements (ALBCs). One is the very popular method amongst arthroplasty surgeons of using ALBC in each and every arthroplasty case as a "preventive" measure. This prophylactic mode is unscientific and ill-founded and gives false sense of security amongst surgeons for protection against surgical site infection (SSI) that may easily develop later. The second "mode" of using the bone cements with high dose antibiotic as a "therapeutic modality" in chronic infections and dead-space management does have rationale. The antimicrobial powder acts as a poragen in these preparations (high-dose) creating microvoids in the cement allowing fluid to penetrate but drastically reducing cement strength. In contrast, the low-dose ALBC traps most of the antibiotic and does not allow fluid penetration or elution to provide local antibiotic concentrations. The antibiotic elution from the high-dose ALBC containing greater than 10% v/v antibiotic approaches 75% at 30 days maintaining concentrations more than 100 times MIC and approaching or exceeding the MBEC concentrations. The antibiotics that have been found useful for impregnation with PMMA include (in order of preference)—aminoglycosides (gentamycin and tobramycin), vancomycin, cephalosporins, quinolones, rifampicin, linezolid, doxycycline, β-lactams, macrolides, and antifungal agents like AmBisome, amphotericin deoxycholate, voriconazole or fluconazole.

Biodegradable systems: The primary advantage of a biodegradable system is the avoidance of this second surgical procedure. A second advantage is that they can be used initially for management of dead space and eventually may also facilitate repair, if combined with newer osteoconductive and osteoinductive carriers. The biodegradable systems can also be modified to vary the magnitude and duration of antibiotic delivery.

The biodegradable systems are classified into four broad categories:
1. The bone graft and bone substitutes
2. The protein-based materials (natural polymers)
3. The synthetic polymers
4. Miscellaneous materials.

The most acceptable agents include aminoglycosides, β-lactam agents, quinolones, and vancomycin. The elution for water-soluble agents like β-lactams depends on the surface area of the carrier and on the initial concentration of the drug while for relatively insoluble agents like the quinolones porosity of the matrix decides the rate of release.

(For details kindly refer to Chapter 4 of the book Essential Orthopedics: Principles and Practice, 2nd edition.)

87. What is acute hematogenous osteomyelitis? How does it differ in different age groups?

Ans: Acute hematogenous osteomyelitis is a pyogenic infection of bone and its elements most commonly seen in children. This infection is more common in males in all age groups affected. Hematological seeding following bacteremia is the most commonly thought reason in childhood. The causes of bacteremia in childhood are many. It is truly unknown as to how bacteria lodges into the bone, but it is commonly believed that localized trauma, chronic illness, malnutrition, or an inadequate immune system are commonly associated with bacterial seeding. In children, the infection generally involves the metaphyses of rapidly growing long bones. Some pathogenic events suggested for development of acute osteomyelitis in metaphysis of long bones include:

- Acute osteomyelitis developed in the metaphysis of long bones because of "poor phagocytic activity" in metaphysis (Hobo).
- Sluggish circulation through the "hairpin bends" of arterioles at metaphysis (Trueta).
- The site of bone involvement purely depends on the occlusion of blood vessel at particular site by the "septic embolus" (Wilsenki).

Bacterial seeding leads to an inflammatory reaction, which can cause local ischemic necrosis of bone and subsequent abscess formation. The inflammatory reaction and abscess formation at metaphysis under pressure travels through Haversian and Volkmann's canals to erupt under the periosteum. The adjacent joints are protected by the tight attachment of periosteum to the growth ring. The periosteal vessels get thrombosed and intramedullary vessels are already disrupted, thus the blood supply to the cortex is lost and the part of bone becomes avascular. The pus then reenters the cortex at some other place infecting the medullary cavity setting up another focus.

Acute hematogenous osteomyelitis generally affects either children younger than 2 years or children in age group of 8–12 years. The progression and effects vary based on differences in blood supply and the anatomical structure of the bone.

- In children younger than 2 years, some blood vessels cross the physis and may allow the spread of infection into the epiphysis. This disturbs growth and causes limb shortening or angular deformity. The diaphysis rarely is involved, and extensive sequestration occurs infrequently except in the most severe cases. In severe infection, epiphyseal separation can occur in children younger than 2 years. In infants with acute hematogenous osteomyelitis, *S. aureus* is still a frequent isolate, but group B *Streptococcus* and gram-negative coliforms also are commonly found.
- In children older than 2 years, the physis effectively acts as a barrier to the spread of a metaphyseal abscess. Due to well-developed metaphysis, the pus does not rupture out subperiosteally instead spreads to the diaphysis of these patients. If the infection spreads into the diaphysis, the endosteal blood supply may be jeopardized. With extensive infection, a subperiosteal abscess also forms damaging the periosteal blood supply resulting in extensive sequestration and chronic osteomyelitis.
- After the physes are closed, acute hematogenous osteomyelitis is much less common. Hematogenous seeding of bone in adults usually is seen in a compromised host. If localized destruction of cortical bone occurs, pathological fracture can result. After the physes are closed, infection can extend directly from the metaphysis into the epiphysis and involve the joint.

Septic arthritis resulting from acute hematogenous osteomyelitis generally is seen only in infants and adults.

Staphylococcus aureus is the most common infecting organism found in older children and adults with osteomyelitis. Gram-negative bacteria have been found to cause an increasing number of vertebral body infections in adults. *Pseudomonas* is the most common infecting organism found in intravenous drug abusers with osteomyelitis. Fungal osteomyelitis is seen increasingly in chronically ill patients receiving long-term intravenous therapy or parenteral nutrition. *Salmonella* osteomyelitis has long been associated with sickle cell (SS or SC) hemoglobinopathies.

88. Discuss the anatomical classification of chronic osteomyelitis and dead space management postsurgery.

Ans:
Anatomical type of chronic osteomyelitis based on Cierny and Mader classification (**Table 2.5.1**):

TABLE 2.5.1: Anatomical classification of chronic osteomyelitis based on Cierny and Madar.

I	Medullary	Endosteal disease
II	Superficial	Cortical surface infected because of coverage defect
III	Localized	Cortical sequestrum that can be excised without compromising stability
IV	Diffuse	Features of I, II, and III plus mechanical instability before or after debridement

Dead space management: The methods described to eliminate this dead space are:

- *Bone grafting with primary or secondary closure:* Papineau et al. described an open bone grafting technique for the treatment of chronic osteomyelitis. This procedure is based on the following principles: (1) granulation tissue markedly resists infection, (2) autogenous cancellous bone grafts are rapidly revascularized and are resistant to infection, (3) the infected area is completely excised, (4) adequate drainage is provided, (5) adequate immobilization is provided, and (6) antibiotics are used for prolonged periods. The operation is divided into three stages: (1) excision of infected tissue without or with stabilization using an external fixator or an intramedullary rod, (2) cancellous autografting, and (3) skin closure.
- *Use of antibiotic PMMA beads as a temporary filler of the dead space before reconstruction:* The use of antibiotic-impregnated PMMA beads in the treatment of chronic osteomyelitis is common practice and is supported by numerous clinical studies. The rationale for this treatment is to deliver levels of antibiotics locally in concentrations that exceed the minimal inhibitory concentrations. Pharmacokinetic studies have shown that the local concentrations of antibiotic achieved are 200 times higher than levels achieved with systemic antibiotic administration. This has the advantage of obtaining very high local antibiotic concentrations, while maintaining low serum levels and low systemic toxicity. The antibiotic is leached from the PMMA beads into the postoperative wound hematoma and secretion, which act as a transport medium. High concentrations of the antibiotic can be achieved only with primary wound closure; if such closure cannot be performed, the wound can be covered with a water-impermeable dressing (bead pouch technique). Before the beads are implanted, all infected and necrotic tissue should be adequately debrided surgically, and all foreign material should be removed. Suction drains are not recommended because the concentration level of the antibiotic is diminished when they are used.
- *Local muscle flaps and skin grafting with or without bone grafting:* Soft tissue transfers to fill dead space left behind after extensive debridement may range from a localized muscle flap on a vascular pedicle to microvascular free tissue transfer. The transfer of vascularized muscle tissue improves the local biological environment by bringing in a blood supply that is important in the host's defense mechanisms and for antibiotic delivery and osseous and soft-tissue healing. The success rates for this technique reported in the literature have ranged from 66% to 100%.
- Microvascular transfer of muscle, myocutaneous, osseous, and osteocutaneous flaps.
- *Use of bone transport (Ilizarov technique):* The Ilizarov technique has been helpful in the treatment of chronic osteomyelitis and infected nonunions. This technique allows radical resection of the infected bone. A corticotomy is performed through normal bone proximal and distal to the area of disease. The bone is transported until union is achieved. Disadvantages of this technique include the time required to achieve a solid union and the high incidence of associated complications.

89. A. Describe radiological classification of chronic osteomyelitis.
   B. What is the role of this classification in management?

Ans: A. Jones et al. in 2009 described a radiological classification of chronic hematogenous osteomyelitis in children in which three main types were identified based on radiographic appearance:
1. Type A, Brodie abscess

2. Type B, sequestrum involucrum. This was the most varied type involving a spectrum of patterns of clinical importance, so it was subdivided into 4 subtypes as follows:
    i. B1, localized cortical sequestrum
    ii. B2, sequestrum with structural involucrum
    iii. B3, sequestrum with sclerotic involucrum
    iv. B4, sequestrum without structural involucrum
3. Type C, sclerotic

    Unclassifiable, inadequate X-ray/disease onset >6-months/previous surgery. Physeal damage is indicated by the addition of "P" (proximal) or "D" (distal) to the classification.

    This is a classification based on plain radiographs obviating the need of CT and MRI (difficult to obtain in underdeveloped countries). CT and MRI can definitely add more information, such as the extent of sclerosis and the presence of sequestra not visible on plain radiographs commonly altering the classification.

B. The above classification of Jones was incorporated in Beit CURE (BC) Classification of Childhood Chronic Haematogenous Osteomyelitis and its management as follows:
   - *Type A:* Drilling and curettage of abscess OR conservative treatment with 6 weeks of antibiotics.
   - *Types B1–B3:* Sequestrectomy and curettage.
   - *Type B4:* Sequestrectomy and curettage and stabilization with plaster, traction or external fixator. Reconstruction of bone defect to be performed following eradication of infection, as required (free fibula graft, ipsilateral vascularized fibula graft, nonstructural bone graft and bone transport).
   - *Type C:* Drainage and curettage of any collection and long-term antibiotics (6 weeks minimum).

90. Describe etiology, pathology, and clinical features of chronic OM.

Ans: Etiology:
- Incomplete treatment of acute OM (most common)
- Trauma (now increasing)
- Implant-related infection (probably the second most common now)
- A hematogenous type of OM
- Compound fractures
- Infection with chronic persisting type of microbes—*Mycobacterium tuberculosis, Treponema* species, fungal
- OM associated with diabetic foot, vascular disease, etc.

Pathology: Bone is destroyed or devitalized, either in a discrete area around the focus of infection or more diffusely along the surface of a foreign implant. Cavities containing pus and pieces of dead bone (sequestra) are surrounded by vascular tissue, and beyond that by areas of sclerosis—the result of chronic reactive new bone formation—which may take the form of a distinct bony sheath (involucrum). In the worst cases, a sizeable length of the diaphysis may be devitalized and encased in a thick involucrum.

Sequestra act as substrates for bacterial adhesion in much the same way as foreign implants, ensuring the persistence of infection until they are removed or discharged through perforations in the involucrum and sinuses that drain to the skin. A sinus may seal off for weeks or even months, giving the appearance of healing, only to reopen (or appear somewhere else) when the tissue tension rises. Bone destruction, and the increasingly brittle sclerosis, sometimes results in a pathological fracture.

Clinical features: Deformed bone, dusky-looking skin having scarring. Skin ulcerations may be there. Muscles are scarred with contractures. Local temperature may be raised. Sinus tracts can be seen as disease progresses with bone chips and pus discharge from tract. There are recurrent acute flare ups.

91. Describe different types of sequestrum.

Ans: The various types of sequestrum can be grouped as under:

According to shape:
- *Pencil-like:* Infants
- *Cylindrical or tubular:* Infants

- *Ring:* External fixator
- *Conical:* Amputation stump
- *Annular:* Amputation stump
- *Coralliform:* Perthes

Consistency:
- *Coke-like:* TB
- *Feathery:* Syphilis
- *Sand-like:* TB osteomyelitis in metacarpals

Colored:
- *Black:* Amputation stump and long exposure of necrotic bone to air while also attached to parent bone (formation of ferrous sulfide), fungal infection
- *Green: Pseudomonas* osteomyelitis

Miscellaneous:
Muscle: Volkmann's ischemic contracture.

92. **Write briefly the current presentation and treatment strategies in methicillin-resistant Staphylococcus aureus infection. Briefly mention about its evaluation.**

Ans: Methicillin-resistant *Staphylococcus aureus* (MRSA) is a resistant strain of *S. aureus* that is resistant to treatment with commonly prescribed drugs for management of gram-positive infections. The infections with MRSA resemble those of other staphylococcal infections only differing in the response to treatment with drugs like ethicillin, amoxicillin, penicillin, oxacillin, etc. to whom they do not respond.

The commonly affected site is skin (pustules, sores or folliculitis). If the infection spreads, then cellulitis and abscess formation readily occurs. SSIs, pneumonia, and septicemia are common presentations of hospital-acquired strains. Urinary tract infection (UTI) may also be seen presenting with dysuria, burning micturition, and increased urinary frequency. In orthopedics, *Staphylococcus* is the most common cause of osteomyelitis (acute and chronic forms), osteitis, and periostitis. Acute osteomyelitis quickly transforms into chronic form if untreated with sinus formation and pus discharge and formation of sequestrate. Sequestrate may be discharged through sinus in long-standing cases. Superimposed infection occurs in cases that do not receive treatment in chronic osteomyelitis cases.

Skin infection and SSI present with increased temperature to touch, formation of pustules, and erythematous geographic areas typically around the incision site. The area is tender and indurated with pus discharge from the site. Patient has fever and complains of general unwell-being. Pus formation is rapid and tracks into deeper tissues causing infection of the underlying structures. If implant surgery has been done, then involvement of implant is disastrous as often it needs removal and thorough debridement that may need to be repeated.

Diagnosis rests on identification of the organism from the discharge taken in aseptic manner as possible preventing contamination. Antibiogram should be ordered simultaneously to optimize the treatment.

Management: Apart from the supportive management, debridement, implant removal, etc. are needed. The choice of antibiotics can be decided based on antibiogram and consultation with infection control specialist. The patients may not be isolated but separate care should be instituted to prevent cross infection. Following are commonly used antibiotics for treatment of MRSA:
- *Vancomycin:* This glycopeptide antibiotic is the drug of choice for the management of MRSA but the concerns are slow bactericidal effect of the drug and development of VRSA variants. For patients who are sensitive to the drug, teicoplanin is a good alternative. Some use it as a primary agent for management of MRSA due to its more acceptable profile.
- *Daptomycin:* This is emerging as the drug of choice for treatment of MRSA in view of development of vancomycin-resistant *Staphylococcus aureus* (VRSA). It is a lipopeptide class antibiotic that is active against methicillin- and vancomycin-resistant staphylococci. It is commonly used for the treatment of *Staphylococcus aureus* bacteremia (SAB) and right-sided endocarditis at 6 mg/kg/day. It is the only drug that has shown noninferiority to vancomycin in trials. Historically used to salvage patients with MRSA infection, it can be used for treatment of MRSA bacteremia.

- *Linezolid:* It is an oxazolidinone bacteriostatic drug effective against MRSA. It seems to have enhanced efficacy against strains producing toxins such as Panton–Valentine leukocidin, α-hemolysin, and toxic shock syndrome toxin 1. Linezolid achieves high levels in the epithelial lining fluid of the lungs, making it a promising candidate for treatment of patients with hospital-acquired pneumonia (HAP), including MRSA.
- *Telavancin:* It is a semisynthetic lipoglycopeptide bactericidal against MRSA, vancomycin-intermediate *Staphylococcus aureus* (VISA), and VRSA. It is an alternative when other options are ineffective.
- *Tigecycline:* It belongs to new generation of tetracyclines, glycylcyclines that confers broad antibiotic coverage of drug-resistant gram-positive bacteria and certain, but not all, species of multidrug-resistant gram-negative bacteria. It may be used for the management of septicemia due to MRSA, but data is still insufficient.
- *Rifampicin:* This should not be used for MRSA as it is primary drug for tuberculosis.

93. What is chronic recurrent multifocal osteomyelitis?

Ans: It is a well-known entity with multifocal and recurrent osteomyelitic lesions characterized by subacute and chronic features. The etiology is unknown and cultures for bacteria are negative. Radiographs show osteolytic and sclerotic bone lesions with minimal or no subperiosteal bone formation. Often involved bones include spine, tibia, femur, and clavicle. Antibiotics are of no use and an episode generally subsides by 6 weeks with little or no sequelae. SAPHO (synovitis, acne, pustulosis, hyperostosis, and osteitis) syndrome (pustulotic arthro-osteitis, sternocostoclavicular hyperostosis) is a clinical variant that additionally has psoriatic-like features.

(Kindly refer to Chapter 4 of the book Essential Orthopedics: Principles and Practice, 2nd edition for details on SAPHO syndrome.)

94. Discuss pathophysiology, clinical features, and management of septic arthritis of hip in a neonate. Also discuss the sequelae of septic hip in an infant.

Ans: *Pathophysiology:* The three most important factors that lead to destruction of the hip after septic arthritis are:
1. Increased intracapsular pressure
2. *Direct destructive action of pus on the articular cartilage:* Collagen content of the cartilage which is otherwise resistant to all other enzyme (except collagenase produced by *Clostridium welchii* and *histolyicum*) undergoes destruction by proteolysis due to denaturation induced by inflammation. Similarly, proteolytic enzymes cause removal of chondromucoprotein from matrix leading to complete chondrolysis later, but is not associated with radiological changes due to inevident bone formation.
3. Thrombosis of the vessel on both sides of epiphyseal plate may result in ischemia of the plate. Ischemic damage to growth plate by infection can cause permanent damage to the plate. This may cause early closure of plate or in its complete destruction.

Clinical features: Neonatal period (Tom Smith arthritis)—the disease is most common in this age group. Classic signs of fever, chills, rigor, sweat, and prostration are not seen in this age group. Hence, disease becomes difficult to diagnose. Following clinical observation can make physician to suspect septicemia, especially with septic arthritis of the hip like:
- Refusal of feed with regurgitation
- Cyanosis during feeding
- Abdominal distension
- Presence of a focus of infection
- Edema of lower extremities/buttock/genitalia
- Crying on handling
- Child not able to use the lower limb actively
- Abnormal position of femur in flexion adduction

Management: Establishing diagnosis in infants and small children requires a high degree of suspicion with appropriate clinical findings as listed above. A raised polymorphonuclear neutrophil (PMN) leukocyte count and a raised ESR are usually present. CRP is also positive. Antistreptococcal and antistaphylococcal titers are positive if they are the causative organisms. Blood culture may also yield the infecting organism in 50% cases. Aspiration of the joint is the most valuable test. High protein and low glucose in synovial fluid are suggestive of septic infection. Radiological features in neonates and children include enlargement of the soft tissue shadows around the hip and increase in the distance and acetabulum and the visualized portion of upper end femur, lateral shift of the upper end femur due to pus under tension within the hip joint, periosteal elevation in upper and femur may be seen, and residual deformities in serial follow-up.

If pus is aspirated, hip joint must be promptly drained to prevent femoral head destruction. Delay of even few hours may result in irreparable damage to cartilaginous head and neck of femur. Anterior approach for drainage is preferred in children to avoid damage to vascular supply of head and to reduce chance of postoperative dislocation. Also, the landmarks for surgical approach are much clearer in small child in this approach. Some form of immobilization is given until infection is controlled. A long period of immobilization is often required because retarded ossification may delay the appearance of femoral head for many months. Child may become ambulatory on defective hip until a reconstruction hip procedure is planned.

Sequelae: Septic arthritis of hip (pyogenic or tubercular) results in variable destruction of hip and pathological damage ranging from nearly normal hip to destroyed joint and proximal femur. Besides, intra-articular metaphysis, hip has several other anatomical factors that make it susceptible to severe complications after a septic episode. Transepiphyseal vessels until 18 months of age may make communication of bacteria across epiphyseal plate easy. Intra-articular vessels undergo tamponade effect due to collection of pus in the capsule which results in avascular necrosis and chondrolysis. The prognosis of septic hip is directly proportional to early diagnosis and adequate treatment with arthrotomy and appropriate antibiotics. In absence of these, the treatment is suboptimal and may result in one of several sequel described for septic arthritis of the hip joint **(Fig. 2.5.1)**.

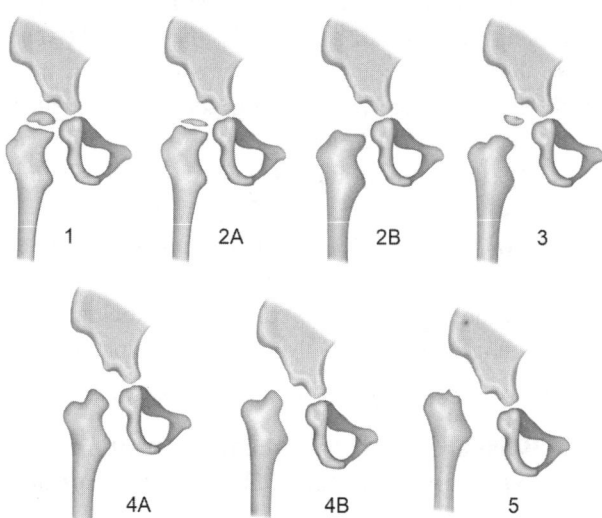

Fig. 2.5.1: Hunka classification of late sequelae of septic arthritis.

The residual deformity remains when diagnosis is not established early and proper treatment is not instituted. A severe infection and/or delay in treatment also produces this unacceptable outcome.

The spectrum of residual deformities has been included in sequel. Disability usually occurs from pain due to incongruous articular surface/pathological dislocation, stiffness during partial/complete ankylosis or abnormal angulation like coxa vara/shortening and instability resulting from bone destruction and/or pathological dislocation. Gait disturbance occurs due to shortening of the involved extremity (subluxation, dislocation, and contracture), pistoning from instability, abductor insufficiency, soft tissue contracture, and joint ankylosis.

(For a detailed discussion on late sequelae of septic arthritis of infant kindly refer to Chapter 11 of the book Essential Orthopedics: Principles and Practice, 2nd edition.)

95. **List the types and indications of each type of reconstruction of sequelae of septic hip in infancy.**
Ans: The particular procedure used in a patient depends on his age, type of deformity/deficit, residual movements or stability, amount of shortening, and previous operations done if any.
- *Loss of movements:*
  - Soft-tissue release
- *Painful joint degeneration:*
  - Interposition/cup arthroplasty—useful in young patients with ankylosed hip
  - Total hip replacement (THR) in old patients
  - Pelvic support osteotomy
  - Arthrodesis
  - Pelvic support osteotomy
  - Resection arthroplasty (in social groups where motion is desirable for work, play, and ground toilet)

- *Abductor insufficiency:*
  - Trochanteric epiphysiodesis (<7 years age)
  - Trochanteric transfer (distal, lateral, or both)
  - Pelvic support osteotomy (if there is additional joint instability)
  - Pelvic osteotomy
  - Proximal femoral osteotomy
  - Trochanteric arthroplasty with prox
  - Femoral osteotomy
  - Harmon or L-Episcopo reconstruction
- *Operation to correct deformities: They should be corrected as soon as infection has subsided:*
  - Flexion adduction contracture—treated by transferring the iliac crest
  - Hip ankylosed in flexion and adduction—treated by intertrochanteric osteotomy and fixing hip in 30° flexion, 20–30° of abduction. Various kinds of treatment for osteotomies are Gant operation (transverse open-wedge osteotomy), Whitman's operation (transverse closed-wedge osteotomy) and Bracket (ball-and-socket osteotomy).
- *Operations to equalize limb lengths:*
  - Soft-tissue release (abduction and adduction contracture of 10° cause apparent length inequality of 3 cm)
  - Osteotomy (if instability of joint exists)
  - Epiphysiodesis of other limb (for anticipated discrepancy of 2.5–5 cm)
  - Lengthening of involved limb (anticipated discrepancy >5–6 cm).

(Kindly read details from Chapter 11 of the book Essential Orthopedics: Principles and Practice)

96. What are the orthopedic manifestations of acquired immunodeficiency syndrome? Discuss guidelines to prevent the spread of human immunodeficiency virus infection during operative intervention.

Ans:

Manifestations:
- *Human immunodeficiency virus (HIV)- or acquired immunodeficiency syndrome (AIDS)-associated arthropathy:* This syndrome is a subacute oligoarticular arthritis that develops over 1–6 weeks and lasts for 6 weeks to 6 months. The large joints (knees and ankles) are predominantly affected producing only a mild inflammatory response and is nonerosive in nature. Radiographs are inconspicuous. Nonsteroidal anti-inflammatory drugs (NSAIDs) are only marginally helpful; however, intra-articular glucocorticoids give good relief.
- Osteonecrosis of distal metaphysis of femur, proximal shoulder, etc. has been associated with HIV infection seen in 4.4% of asymptomatic patients screened with MRI. Symptomatic osteonecrosis is found in 1% of cases. The cause is elusive but may be related to vasculitis, glucocorticoid or alcohol consumption. Some 10% of HIV-infected patients have been found to have symptoms of fibromyalgia.
- Painful articular syndrome is another form of arthritis thought to be secondary to HIV infection in as many as 10% of AIDS patients. Patients experience acute, severe, and sharp pain in the affected joint primarily involving the knees, elbows, and shoulders lasting 2–24 hours, and may be severe enough to require narcotic analgesics. The cause of this arthropathy is unclear; however, it is thought to result from a direct effect of HIV on the joint.
- *Other manifestations:* There have been reports of leukocytoclastic vasculitis associated with zidovudine therapy. Central nervous system (CNS) angiitis and polymyositis have also been reported in HIV-infected individuals.

Guidelines: The following are American Academy of Orthopaedic Surgeons (AAOS) recommendations regarding HIV precautions in the operating room:
- Do not hurry an operation. Excess speed results in injury. The most experienced surgeon should be responsible for the surgical procedure if the risk of injury to operating room personnel is high.
- Wear surgical garb that offers protection against contact with blood. Knee-high, waterproof, surgical shoe covers, water-impervious gowns or undergarments, and full head covers should be worn.
- Double gloves should be worn at all times.
- Surgical masks should be changed if they become moist or splattered.
- Protective eyewear (goggles or full-face shields) that covers exposed skin and mucous membranes should be used.

- To avoid inadvertent injury to surgical personnel, the surgeon should:
  - Use instrument ties and other "no-touch" suturing and sharp instrument techniques when possible.
  - Avoid tying with a suture needle in hand.
  - Avoid passing sharp instruments and needles from hand to hand; instead they should be placed on an intermediate tray.
  - Announce when sharp instruments are about to be passed.
  - Avoid having two surgeons suture the same wound.
  - Take extra care when performing digital examinations of fracture fragments or wounds containing wires or sharp instrumentation.
  - Avoid contact with osteotomes, drill bits, and saws.
  - Use space suit-type garb when splatter is inevitable, such as when irrigating large wounds or using power equipment.
  - Routinely check gowns, masks, and shoe covers of operating room personnel for contamination during the surgical procedure and change as necessary.

97. Write briefly about clinical features and management of musculoskeletal syndromes in HIV.

Ans: *(Apart from the answer above the following can be added)*
Arthralgia, myalgia and sometimes a symmetrical viral polyarthritis are common in seroconverting patients. Four musculoskeletal syndromes are commonly seen in HIV patients:
1. HIV arthritis
2. Painful articular syndrome
3. Diffuse-infiltrative lymphocytosis syndrome (DILS)
4. Immune reconstitution inflammatory syndrome (IRIS)

   Apart from above osteoporosis and osteonecrosis of bones is also commonly seen in HIV patients.

Management: Among patients taking ART reliably and with complete suppression of viral activity, use of standard rheumatological therapies appears safe and well-tolerated, particularly if the CD4+ count is above 200 cells/mm^3. Protease inhibitor ritonavir and more recently licensed boosting agent Cobicistat inhibits steroid metabolism through potent inhibition of CYP3A4 and CYP2D6 significantly increasing the risk of Cushing syndrome if administered together. There are many interactions of antiretroviral therapies with other medications. *Do not* administer intra-articular or intramuscular triamcinolone to patients taking Ritonavir or Cobicistat.

98. Describe etiopathogenesis and clinical features of post viral/post chikungunya/post-COVID musculoskeletal manifestations. Briefly describe its management.

Ans: Post-viral musculoskeletal manifestations

1. *Etiopathogenesis:*

Direct viral invasion (rare) → Some viruses enter synovium/muscle → inflammation (e.g., parvovirus B19).

   Immune-mediated (common) → Molecular mimicry → Antibodies against viral antigens cross-react with host joint proteins.
- Immune complex deposition in synovium → Complement activation.
- Cytokine storm (↑ IL-6, TNF-α, interferons) → Synovial inflammation. *Post-viral immune dysregulation:* Persistence of viral RNA fragments in tissues → Chronic inflammation.
- Altered T-cell regulation and autoantibody production. *Specific viral examples—Chikungunya virus* → α-virus family, strong tropism for joint tissues, chronic synovitis due to persistent viral antigen.
- *SARS-CoV-2 (COVID-19)* → Hyperinflammatory response, endothelial injury, microvascular thrombosis contributing to MSK pain and myalgia.

2. *Clinical Features:*

General post-viral arthritis:
- *Onset:* 1–3 weeks after viral illness
- *Joint involvement:* Usually symmetric small joints (hands, wrists, and ankles), sometimes large joints

- *Nature:* Nonerosive, transient (days–weeks) in most, but can persist.
- *Associated features:* Fever, rash, fatigue, and myalgia.

Post-Chikungunya arthritis:
- *Acute phase:* High fever, severe polyarthralgia ("bent posture" due to pain), maculopapular rash
- *Post-viral phase (after 2–3 weeks):*
  – Chronic inflammatory arthritis resembling RA
  – Morning stiffness and swelling
  – Symmetric small joint involvement (MCP, PIP, and wrists)
  – May persist for months–years
  – Positive inflammatory markers, but seronegative for RF/anti-CCP
- *Risk factors for chronicity:* Older age, pre-existing joint disease, and severe acute arthritis

Post-COVID musculoskeletal syndrome:
- Myalgia, fatigue, arthralgia—part of Long COVID
- *Onset:* During acute infection or weeks after recovery
- *Patterns:*
  – Reactive arthritis (oligoarthritis, usually lower limb)
  – Fibromyalgia-like syndrome
  – Myositis (rare)
- *Other MSK issues:* Deconditioning, steroid-induced myopathy, avascular necrosis (poststeroid use)

3. *Management:*

General principles:
- Most cases are *self-limiting;* focus on *symptom relief* and *function preservation*
- Exclude other causes (RA, SLE, septic arthritis, and crystal arthropathy)

Nonpharmacological:
- Rest during acute painful phase
- Gradual physiotherapy and joint mobilization
- *Patient's education:* Usually good prognosis, but post-chikungunya arthritis may be prolonged.
- Psychological support in post-COVID fatigue/fibromyalgia-type syndromes

Pharmacological:
- NSAIDs → First-line for pain and inflammation
- Short course corticosteroids → For severe, refractory synovitis
- DMARDs (e.g., methotrexate and hydroxychloroquine) → For persistent post-viral arthritis >3 months, especially post-chikungunya
- Analgesics (paracetamol and tramadol) → Adjunct pain control
- Antivirals → Not useful once post-viral phase starts (except in specific viruses like HIV and HBV)

99. Describe hygiene policies for prevention of viral infection in orthopedic practice. Describe the management of needle stick injuries.

Ans: There are 10 key standard infection control precautions for prevention of infections (viral or otherwise) as recommended by CDC (Centre for Disease Control):

1. *Hand hygiene:*
   a. Before touching the patient
   b. Prior to performing clean/aseptic procedure
   c. After any bodily fluid exposure risk
   d. After touching the patient
   e. After touching the patient's surroundings
2. *Placement and infection assessment—all patients must be assessed for infection risks:*
   a. Patients presenting with diarrhea, or vomiting
   b. Those with an unexplained fever

c. Patients who are known to have been previously positive with a multidrug resistant organism
d. For COVID identifiers, Public Health Agency cites, loss of taste or smell, fever, and a new persistent cough as primary symptoms
3. *Safe management and care of environment:* The environment for patients and healthcare staff must be safe for practice.
4. Safe management of equipment
5. Safe management of linen
6. *Personal protective equipment:*
   a. Stored close to the point of use in a clean area
   b. Used as single-use items unless stated differently by the manufacturer
   c. If reusable, PPE is thoroughly decontaminated after each use
   d. Within its expiration date
   e. Immediately changed after each patient
   f. Disposed of correctly (see safe disposal of waste)
   g. Disposed of if damaged or contaminated
7. *Respiratory and cough hygiene:*
   a. Cover nose and mouth with disposable tissues if coughing or blowing/wiping the nose
   b. Bin the tissue after use
   c. Ensure you wash your hands after
8. Safe management of blood and body fluids
9. Safe disposal of waste
10. *Occupational safety:* Actions taken to reduce infection risk because of occupational exposure be it biological, chemical, or physical exposure.

Management of needle-stick injuries (Flowchart 2.5.2)

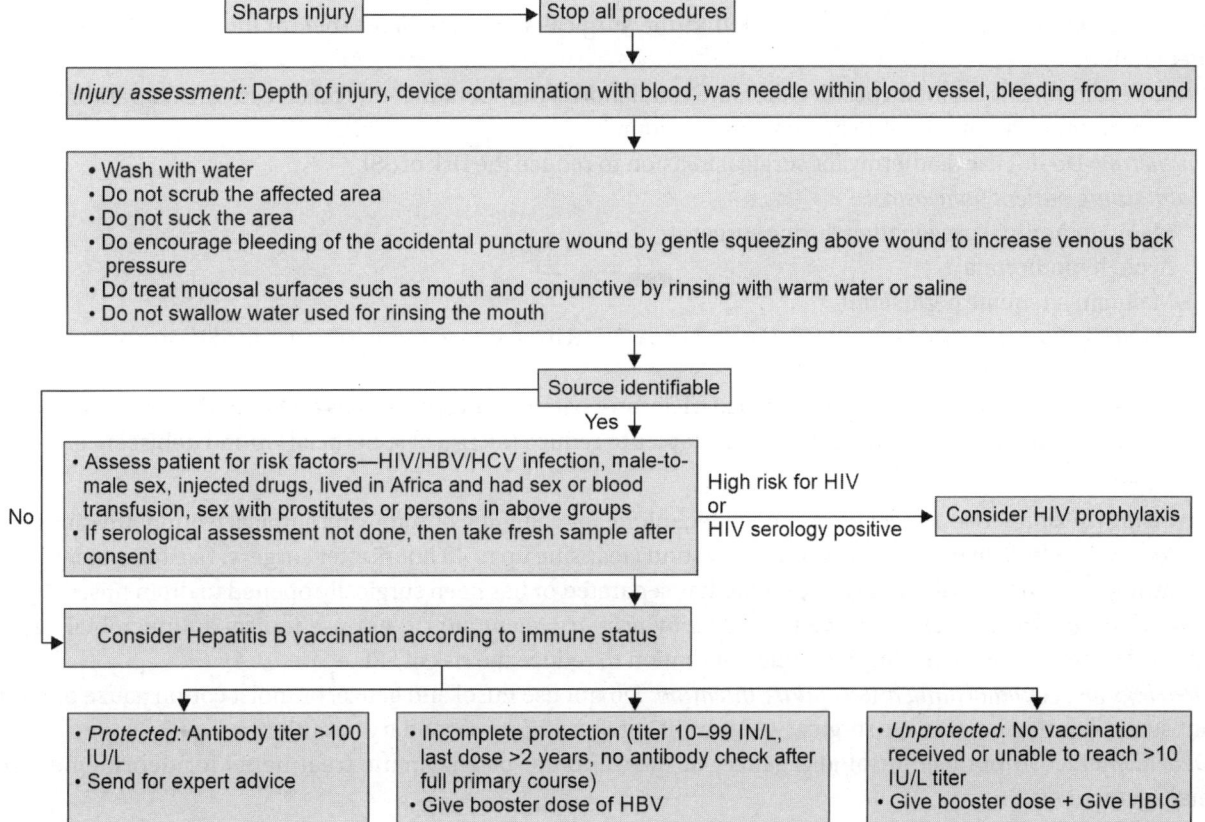

Flowchart 2.5.2: Management of needle stick injuries

100. Surgical site infection—discuss its prevention and treatment.

Ans: Prevention

Preoperative:
- *Preoperative showering:* Patients to shower or have a bath using soap, either the day before or on the day of surgery.
- *Nasal decolonization:* Nasal mupirocin in combination with a chlorhexidine body wash before procedures depending on type of procedure and individual patient risks.
- *Hair removal:* Use electric clippers with a single-use head on the day of surgery. Do not use razors for hair removal, because they increase the risk of SSI.
- *Patient theater wear:* Give patients specific theater wear that is appropriate for the procedure and clinical setting, and that provides easy access to the operative site and areas for placing devices, such as intravenous cannulas.
- *Staff theater wear:* All staff should wear specific nonsterile theater wear in all areas.
- *Staff leaving the operating area:* Staff wearing nonsterile theater wear should keep their movements in and out of the operating area to a minimum.
- *Mechanical bowel preparation:* Do not use mechanical bowel preparation routinely to reduce the risk of SSI.
- Remove hand jewelry, artificial nails, and nail polish.
- *Antibiotic prophylaxis:* Give a single dose of antibiotic prophylaxis intravenously on starting anesthesia. However, give prophylaxis earlier for operations in which a tourniquet is used. Give a repeat dose of antibiotic prophylaxis when the operation is longer than the half-life of the antibiotic given.

Intraoperative:
- *Hand decontamination:* The operating team should wash their hands prior to the first operation on the list using an aqueous antiseptic surgical solution, with a single-use brush or pick for the nails, and ensure that hands and nails are visibly clean.
- Do not use non-iodophor-impregnated incise drapes routinely for surgery as they may increase the risk of SSI.
- *Sterile gowns:* The operating team should wear sterile gowns in the operating theater during the operation.
- *Gloves:* Consider wearing two pairs of sterile gloves when there is a high risk of glove perforation and the consequences of contamination may be serious.
- *Antiseptic skin preparation:* Prepare the skin at the surgical site immediately before incision using an antiseptic preparation.
- *Theatre environment:* Maintain positive-pressure ventilation of the operating suite relative to corridors and surrounding areas. Maintain a minimum of 15 air changes per hour.
- *Diathermy:* Do not use diathermy for surgical incision to reduce the risk of SSI.
- *Maintaining patient homeostasis:*
  - Maintain optimal oxygenation during surgery
  - Avoid hypothermia
  - Maintain adequate perfusion.
- *Wound irrigation and intracavity lavage:* Do not use wound irrigation to reduce the risk of SSI. Do not use intracavity lavage to reduce the risk of SSI.
- *Closure methods:* Consider using antimicrobial triclosan-coated sutures, especially for pediatric surgery, to reduce the risk of SSI. Consider using sutures rather than staples to reduce the risk of superficial wound dehiscence.

Postoperative:
- *Changing dressings:* Use an aseptic nontouch technique for changing or removing surgical wound dressings.
- *Postoperative cleansing:* Use sterile saline for wound cleansing up to 48 hours after surgery. Use tap water for wound cleansing after 48 hours if the surgical wound has separated or has been surgically opened to drain pus.
- *Topical antimicrobial agents for wound healing by primary intention:* Do not use topical antimicrobial agents for surgical wounds that are healing by primary intention to reduce the risk of SSI.
- *Dressings for wound healing by secondary intention:* Do not use Eusol and gauze, or moist cotton gauze or mercuric antiseptic solutions to manage surgical wounds that are healing by secondary intention.
- *Debridement:* Do not use Eusol and gauze, or dextranomer or enzymatic treatments for debridement in the management of SSI.

Treatment:
- *Antibiotics:* For established infection, antibiotics should be administered based on identification of organism and antibiogram. Duration of therapy varies on the type of infection and need of additional surgical care.
- *Invasive surgical management:* Any collection should be removed by opening the wound, removing all dead necrotic tissues along with the pus. Thorough lavage is administered simultaneously. If the infection is superficial to fascia, usually the wound can be closed. If the infection is deep-to-deep fascia then additional debridement may be needed or the dead space created after removal of dead muscle and necrotic tissue needs to be managed by dead space management like rotation flap or antibiotic bead management as necessary.
- If implant has been used during surgery and it is infected then consider removal of implant to facilitate early healing of tissues, additionally consider placing antibiotic beads as infected bone may not be sterilized by single debridement and cleaning. Additional supportive measures like external immobilization are needed if the bone has not united by the time implant is removed. Surgical placement of second implant is not recommended in the same sitting.

101. A. Classify surgical site infection.

B. How will you manage surgical site infection detected on 5th postoperative day after plate osteosynthesis?

Ans: A. The SSI have been classified by CDC into superficial (subcutaneous), deep (deep soft tissue, muscle and fascia) or organ/space (bone and joints are considered organ/space). All orthopedic SSI come under the category of organ space SSI. Organ space or implant infections are essentially all biofilm based requiring removal of all surfaces and implant involved with an established infection for eradication. Few wound categories have been defined to guide the extent of preventive measures such as debridement needs to be undertaken with primary injury/procedure. Closed fractures are clean wounds, open fractures are contaminated wounds, established infections (OM, infected nonunion ± hardware) are dirty wounds, and minor break in the sterile surgical field is a clean contaminated wound.

A stab wound that gets infected is not an SSI and it may be classified as soft tissue or superficial infection depending on the extent.

B. For established infection, antibiotics should be administered based on identification of organism and antibiogram. Duration of therapy varies depending on the type of infection and need of additional surgical care. Any collection should be removed by opening the wound, removing all dead necrotic tissues along with the pus. Thorough lavage is administered simultaneously. If the infection is superficial to fascia, usually the wound can be closed. If the infection is deep-to-deep fascia, then additional debridement may be needed or the dead space created after removal of dead muscle and necrotic tissue needs to be managed by dead space management like rotation flap or antibiotic bead management as necessary. Implant removal as primary management may not be needed especially if the infection is not fulminant, and the organism is notvirulent or multidrug-resistant. Else it will be better to remove implant also and stabilize fracture using external fixator till the infection is controlled for later osteosynthesis.

102. Describe the affected tissues, pathogenesis, organism, clinical features and management of erysipelas, cellulitis, pyomyositis, necrotizing fasciitis and gas gangrene.

Ans: 1. *Erysipelas*:
- *Affected tissue:* Superficial dermis and upper subcutaneous tissue, primarily involving lymphatic vessels.
- *Pathogenesis:* Bacterial invasion through breaks in the skin → intense inflammatory response due to toxins (e.g., streptolysins).
- *Organism:*
  - Group A β-hemolytic *Streptococcus pyogenes* (most common)
  - Rarely, *Staphylococcus aureus*
- *Clinical features*:
  - Sharply demarcated, raised, erythematous, painful plaque with peau d'orange texture.
  - Fever, chills, and systemic toxicity
  - Commonly affects face (butterfly distribution) or legs
- *Management*:
  - Oral/IV penicillin (e.g., penicillin V or clindamycin if allergic)
  - Elevation, analgesia, and wound care

2. *Cellulitis:*
   - *Affected tissue:* Deeper dermis and subcutaneous fat.
   - *Pathogenesis:* Bacterial entry via skin breaks → spreading inflammation (less lymphatic involvement than erysipelas).
   - *Organisms:*
     - *Streptococcus pyogenes* and *Staphylococcus aureus* (MSSA/MRSA).
     - Gram-negatives in immunocompromised (e.g., *Pseudomonas*).
   - *Clinical features*:
     - Poorly demarcated, warm, tender, and erythematous swelling.
     - ± Fever, lymphangitis, regional lymphadenopathy.
     - *Common sites:* Lower limbs, and periorbital (preseptal cellulitis)
   - *Management*:
     - Oral/IV antibiotics (e.g., flucloxacillin, cephalexin; vancomycin for MRSA)
     - Treat predisposing factors (e.g., tinea pedis, and edema)

3. *Pyomyositis:*
   - *Affected tissue:* Skeletal muscle (purulent infection within muscle planes).
   - *Pathogenesis:* Hematogenous spread (often from bacteremia) → muscle abscess.
   - *Organisms*:
     - *Staphylococcus aureus* (90%, including MRSA).
     - *Streptococci,* Gram-negatives (e.g., *E. coli*) in tropics or immunocompromised.
   - *Clinical features*:
     - *Triad:* Fever, muscle pain, tender swelling (late: fluctuance).
     - Common in thighs, calves, gluteal muscles
     - *Risk factors:* Trauma, HIV, diabetes, and tropical regions.
   - *Management*:
     - Drainage (US/CT-guided or surgical) + IV antibiotics (e.g., vancomycin, clindamycin)
     - Empiric coverage for MRSA in endemic areas

4. *Necrotizing fasciitis:*
   - *Affected tissue:* Fascia, subcutaneous fat, and later skin/muscle (rapid necrosis).
   - *Pathogenesis:* Bacterial toxins (e.g., streptococcal exotoxins, clostridial toxins) → vascular thrombosis → tissue ischemia.
   - *Organisms:*
     - *Type I (polymicrobial):* Mixed aerobes (e.g., *E. coli, and Klebsiella*) + anaerobes (e.g., bacteroides).
     - *Type II (monomicrobial):* *S. pyogenes* (GAS) or *S. aureus* (including MRSA).
   - *Clinical features*:
     - Severe pain out of proportion to examination, edema, erythema → skin necrosis, bullae, crepitus.
     - Systemic toxicity (tachycardia, hypotension, and organ failure)
     - LRINEC score (laboratory markers: CRP > 150, WBC > 15, Na < 135).
   - *Management*:
     - Emergent surgical debridement + broad IV antibiotics (e.g., vancomycin + piperacillin-tazobactam + clindamycin).
     - ICU support for sepsis.

5. *Gas gangrene (Clostridial myonecrosis):*
   - *Affected tissue:* Muscle and soft tissue with gas production.
   - Pathogenesis: *Clostridium spp.* (e.g., *C. perfringens*) enter via wounds → alpha-toxin (lecithinase) → myonecrosis + gas (CO_2/H_2).
   - *Organisms:*
     - *Clostridium perfringens* (most common), *C. septicum* (spontaneous in malignancy).

- *Clinical features*:
  - Sudden onset severe pain, pallor → bronze/purple discoloration, crepitus, foul-smelling discharge.
  - *Systemic*: Fever, tachycardia, hemolysis, and renal failure.
- *Management*:
  - Immediate surgical debridement/amputation.
  - High-dose IV penicillin G + clindamycin (inhibits toxin production).
  - Hyperbaric oxygen (adjuvant).

103. Write about (A) antibiotic prophylaxis (B) operation theater (OT) sterilization and antisepsis.

Ans: A. Antibiotic prophylaxis in whom previously arthroplasty has been done: Patients with a total joint replacement within 2 years of the implant procedure, and some immunocompromised patients only with total joint replacements who may be at higher risk (comorbidities, immunosuppression, previous infection) for hematogenous infections, should be considered to receive antibiotic prophylaxis before undergoing invasive dental, genitourinary and gastrointestinal procedures with a higher bacteremic risk. Not all patients require antibiotic prophylaxis.

Antibiotic prophylaxis in preoperative period in routine orthopedic procedures: Following surgery in the first 2 hours, the host defense mechanism works to decrease the bacterial counts. During the next 4 hours, numbers of bacteria increasing by multiplication remain same as those being removed by host defenses. These first 6 hours are called the "golden period", after which the bacteria increase rapidly. Antibiotics increase this window by decreasing bacterial growth and reproduction. Prophylactic antibiotics are directed against the common skin pathogens. Ideally antibiotic prophylaxis therapy should be administered immediately before surgery (within 30 minutes of skin incision). The dose can be repeated every 4 hours intraoperatively or whenever the blood loss exceeds 1,000–1,500 mL. After surgery, antibiotics have a role only for first 48–72 hours. Continuing beyond this period leads to fallacious suppression of infection and development of hospital-acquired infections and superinfections.

B. OT sterilization and antisepsis: To this aspect the following points are pertinent:
- Good handwashing and surgical site skin preparation
- Postoperative dressings have not been substantiated to reduce surgical site infection (SSI).
- For hand antisepsis, some unscientific thoughts and practice prevail that must be clarified.
  - Alcohol rubs are NO superior to aqueous-based scrubs in preventing SSI and to this effect chlorhexidine as aqueous rub is more effective in removing pathogens than povidone–iodine.
- *Surgical site skin preparation:* As a time-honored recent practice, performing hair clipping in the surgical preparation area just before surgery is preferred to perform shaving with razors.
- There is no scientifically proven benefit for plastic-adhesive surgical films with or without iodophor impregnation for preventing SSI.
- Iodine solutions are no more effective than clean surgical procedure.
- There is no definite role of double surgical site preparation. One time cleaning and skin preparation are enough.
- *OT sterilization:*
  - There is no role of repeated fumigations after infected procedures.
  - Cleaning the surfaces with appropriate solution is as effective.
  - There is no role of OT sterilization before arthroplasty.

104. Discuss operation theater etiquettes.

Ans: Operation theater etiquette is crucial for ensuring patient safety, maintaining a respectful and professional environment, and promoting effective communication among surgical team members. Here are several key aspects of etiquette that should be followed in the operating room:

1. *Professional attire*:
   - *Scrubs:* All personnel should wear surgical scrubs appropriate for the procedure. These should be clean and free from contamination.
   - *Personal protective equipment (PPE):* Masks, gloves, and eye protection should be worn as required to protect both the patient and healthcare team.

- *Hair and jewelry:* Hair should be tied back or covered with a surgical cap. Jewelry, including rings and watches, should generally be removed to maintain sterility.
2. *Preparation and punctuality:*
   - *Timeliness:* Arrive on time for procedures to allow for proper setup and to honor the surgical schedule.
   - *Preoperative briefings:* Participate in preoperative checks or briefings to confirm patient identity, surgical site, and procedure details.
3. *Respect for the surgical team:*
   - *Hierarchy awareness:* Recognize the roles of each team member, from the lead surgeon to the scrub nurse, and respect their authority and responsibilities.
   - *Communication:* Use clear and concise language. Avoid interrupting others, especially when they are discussing critical patient information.
4. *Maintain a respectful environment:*
   - *No distractions:* Avoid unnecessary conversations and distractions. All focus should remain on the surgery and the well-being of the patient.
   - *Professional conduct:* Be professional in demeanor and language. Avoid jokes or comments that could be considered inappropriate, especially regarding the patient.
5. *Surgical sterility*
   - *Aseptic technique:* Adhere to sterile techniques at all times. This includes proper hand hygiene and maintaining sterile fields.
   - *Passing instruments:* Hand instruments with the working end facing the recipient and avoid reaching over sterile fields.
6. *Patient-centered focus:*
   - *Patient respect:* Always prioritize the patient's privacy and dignity. Discuss the patient's case with the utmost confidentiality.
   - *Informed consent:* Ensure that all discussions about the patient's condition and procedure have been documented and that informed consent is confirmed.
7. *During the surgery:*
   - *Stay focused:* Stay attentive and engaged throughout the procedure. Avoid unrelated discussions that might distract the surgical team.
   - *Team communication:* Use surgical counts (for instruments and sponges) and other safety checks as opportunities for team communication.
8. *Cultural sensitivity:*
   - *Diversity awareness:* Be aware of and respect diverse backgrounds and cultures among team members and patients. This includes understanding varying beliefs and practices that might affect surgical care.
9. *Mentoring and teaching:*
   - *Teaching moments*: When mentoring or teaching less experienced colleagues, do so respectfully and constructively, encouraging learning without demeaning others.

105. A. Principle of laminar airflow and its application in operation room. B. What is EUSOL?

Ans: A. Vertical laminar-airflow systems and personnel-isolator systems are recommended for orthopedic surgery. The efficacy can be improved with ultraviolet (UV) light for reducing the number of airborne bacteria. Many microscopic particles are dispersed within the OR that commonly originate from the personnel, linen, footwear, etc. serving as favorable attachment site for pathogens. The bacteria are continuously shed from external surface of the persons working there. The sum-total of bacterial load in OR can be represented by the following equation:

$$TBL = P(SRp) + [n*X(SRx)]$$

Where, TBL is total bacterial load, P = patient, SR = shedding rate, n = number of persons, X = any person. A significant fraction of this is exposed to surgical wound. So higher the mobility in the OR higher is the basal bacterial load. In between opening of doors and movements disturb the laminar flow and can be detrimental by creating eddy currents lifting the floor bacteria into air. This bacterial cloud concentration should be kept minimum by strict discipline. Continuous removal of bacteria by high efficiency particulate air (HEPA) filters is a preferable method. Use of personal OT suites with individualized airflow systems are getting more popular but clinical advantage is yet to be demonstrated.

B. EUSOL stands for Edinburgh University Solution of Lime with chemical formula of $BCaCl_2H_3O_5$. It is basically a chlorinated lime and boric acid solution containing 0.25% w/v of available chlorine. Classified as anti-infective agent—prevent infectious agents or organisms from spreading or kill infectious agents in order to prevent the spread of infection. Eusol solution protects against infection, prevents bacterial growth and can be used as a normal disinfectant. Eusol solution is only meant for external use and has better activity with freshly prepared solution. In clinical practice, Eusol solution is used for wound disinfection. Ulcers cleaning and wet dressing.

Preparation of Solution:
Take 0.25 g of sodium hypochlorite and dissolve it into 100 mL of water, then add boric acid until the pH is about 8.0 (nearly 0.65 g of boric acid is needed).

106. **Describe the current World Health Organization (WHO) guidelines for prevention of SSI.**
Ans: Perioperative patient optimization and assessment of risk factors for SSI:

It is understood that 40–60% of the SSIs can be prevented using several interventions such as carrier eradication, antimicrobial prophylaxis, and skin antisepsis. Operative environment modifications and factors have been dealt separately in joint infections. *Staphylococcus aureus* is the most common cause of orthopedic SSI and commonly originates from the native skin. In fact, skin antisepsis is considered to be the second most important factor after optimization of operating environment.

Staphylococcal colonization:
The most acceptable protocol to this regard is the use of topical intranasal mupirocin ointment for 5 days applied twice daily and giving chlorhexidine bath (for 5 days) immediately before surgery.

Operating room personnel-associated risk factors:
Mostly importantly, two factors have been found to reduce SSI—good handwashing and surgical site skin preparation. It is here important to emphasize that postoperative dressings have not been substantiated to reduce SSI. Alcohol rubs are NO superior to aqueous-based scrubs in preventing SSI and to this effect chlorhexidine as aqueous rub is more effective in removing pathogens than povidone-iodine. Surgical site skin preparation, as a time-honored recent practice, performing hair clipping in the surgical preparation area just before surgery is preferred to perform shaving with razors. There is no scientifically proven benefit for plastic-adhesive surgical films with or without iodophor impregnation for preventing SSI.

Modifiable patient risk factors:
- *Diabetes:* The American Diabetes Association recommends fasting blood glucose levels between 90 mg/dL and 130 mg/dL and postprandial levels of <180 mg/dL and HbA1c level <7%.
- *Obesity*
- *Malnutrition*
- *RA:*
  - The association is stronger for late infections rather than acute SSI. Some general recommendations appear in literature for optimization of patient with respect to the medications:
    - Corticosteroids have been traditionally associated with increased risk of SSI. There has been but no definite association proven in small studies so there is no recommendation to their use but one should delay restarting them as late as possible.
    - *Conventional disease-modifying antirheumatic drugs (DMARDs) (nonbiological agents):* There is consensus that they should not be discontinued in the perioperative period. Sulfasalazine is normally discontinued 2 days before surgery and restarted 1–3 days postoperatively (check renal and hepatic function), same holds true for leflunomide.
    - Anti-TNF agents should be discontinued at least 4 weeks before the index procedure and restarted around 1–3 weeks postoperatively or as needed, other agents are commonly discontinued 2 weeks before surgery.
- *Cigarette smoking:* It is recommended to quit smoking altogether and encourage patients for same possibly also counseling them.

- *HIV infection:* It is recommended that CD4 counts >400/mm^3 and an undetectable viral load are the appropriate measures to ward off increased SSI risk in arthroplasty surgery on such patients.
- *Dental procedures:* "Poor dental hygiene" is but associated with increased risk for SSI after arthroplasty
- *Urinary tract infection*
- *Anemia*

(Details of the headings should be read from book, Essential Orthopedics: Principles and Practice, as they have been repeated many times already and size of book does not permit multiple repetitions of answers)

107. Discuss prophylaxis to prevent SSI.

Ans: It is understood that 40–60% of the SSIs can be prevented using several interventions like carrier eradication, antimicrobial prophylaxis, and skin antisepsis. Operative environment modifications and factors have been dealt separately in joint infections. *S. aureus* is the most common cause of orthopedic SSI and commonly originates from the native skin. In fact, skin antisepsis is considered to be the second most important factor after optimization of operating environment.

Staphylococcal colonization: For *S. aureus* infections, nasal carriage is a strong marker for skin colonization and it is deemed that such patients have 2–9 times higher chances of contracting SSI. Now indeed, nasal carriage is considered an independent risk factor for SSI in orthopedic implant surgery. Whether methicillin-sensitive *Staphylococcus aureus* (MSSA) or MRSA decolonization protocols have been found to reduce the SSI by half or even less making universal decolonization an acceptable practice. The most acceptable protocol to this regard is the use of topical intranasal mupirocin ointment for 5 days applied twice daily and giving chlorhexidine bath (for 5 days) immediately before surgery.

Operating room personnel associated risk factors: Most importantly two factors have been found to reduce SSI—good hand washing and surgical site skin preparation. It is here important to emphasize that postoperative dressings have not been substantiated to reduce SSI. For hand-antisepsis, some unscientific thoughts and practices prevail that must be clarified. Alcohol rubs are no superior to aqueous-based scrubs in preventing SSI and to this effect, chlorhexidine as aqueous rub is more effective in removing pathogens than povidone-iodine. Surgical site skin preparation—as a time honored recent practice performing hair clipping in the surgical preparation area just before surgery is preferred to perform shaving with razors. There is no scientifically proven benefit for plastic adhesive surgical films with or without iodophor impregnation for preventing SSI.

Modifiable Patient Risk Factors

Diabetes mellitus: It has a strong association with SSI. Diabetes mellitus (DM) as a risk factor is not strictly modifiable but for sure blood glucose levels can be controlled. Blood glucose levels of more than 140 mg/dL in postoperative period are associated with up to three times increased risk of SSI. To be more specific in blood glucose levels, it is found that patients (diabetic or nondiabetic) with more than or equal to two readings of 200 mg/dL or a hyperglycemic index of more than 1.76 predicts SSI. To optimize patients in preoperative period, exact and universally accepted guidelines are not available but American diabetes association recommends fasting blood glucose levels between 90 mg/dL to 130 mg/dL and postprandial levels of less than 180 mg/dL and HbA1c level less than 7%.

Obesity: The association of obesity to SSI is multifactorial. Need of larger incisions, increased dissection, increased blood loss, fat necrosis, and longer surgeries are partly associated with SSI. Most of these patients also have associated comorbidities like DM and cardiac problems.

Malnutrition: Albumin level less than 3.5 g/dL, total lymphocyte counts less than 1,500/mm^3, and serum transferrin less than 200 mg/dL predict SSI.

Rheumatoid arthritis: RA association with SSI can be direct due to disease specific impairment of wound healing and immune response to pathogens or indirect due to use of various immunosuppressant medications. The association is stronger for late infections rather than acute SSI. Some general recommendations appear in literature for optimization of patient with respect to the medications.

- Corticosteroids have been traditionally associated with increased risk of SSI.
- *Conventional disease-modifying antirheumatic drugs (DMARDs) (nonbiological agents):* Despite traditional thought based on the fact that methotrexate causes immunosuppression, there is no scientific evidence that their use causes immunosuppression and its role in SSI is minimal, if any. There is consensus that they should not be discontinued

in the perioperative period. Sulfasalazine is normally discontinued 2 days before surgery and restarted 1–3 days postoperatively (check renal and hepatic function), same holds true for leflunomide.
- For biological agents, preliminary evidence suggests increased risk of SSI associated with them and is in particularly true for anti-TNF agents.

Cigarette smoking: Smoking doubles the risk of trading SSI compared to nonsmokers in implantation orthopedic surgeries. It is recommended to quit smoking altogether and encourage patients for same possibly also counseling them.

Human immunodeficiency virus infection: It is recommended that CD4 counts more than 400/mm^3 and an undetectable viral load are the appropriate measures to ward off increased SSI risk in arthroplasty surgery on such patients.

Dental procedures: There is no good clinical evidence that dental procedures would cause SSI. The bacterial load with them is 10^4 colony-forming unit (CFU)/mL which is very less compared to that needed for seeding of implanted sites in studies ($>3–5 \times 10^5$ CFU/mL). Such transient bacteremia is even associated with routine procedures like brushing teeth and chewing. "Poor dental hygiene" is but associated with increased risk for SSI after arthroplasty.

Urinary tract infection: There is no clear understanding of the relation of deep SSI with UTI though most researchers do consider it important. For asymptomatic bacteriuria, postoperative oral antibiotics would suffice.

Anemia: This is the second most common modifiable risk factor after obesity. By itself it may not be important in increasing the risk of SSI but most patients with preoperative anemia have increased requirement of postoperative blood transfusion and this allogenic transfusion has been shown to increase the risk of SSI.

108. **(A) Classify prosthetic joint infection (PJI). (B) What are the risk factors for developing infections following total hip arthroplasty (THA)? (C) Discuss the management protocol of PJI.**

Ans: (A) Classification of PJI (temporal) is given in **Table 2.5.2**.

TABLE 2.5.2: Classification of prosthetic joint infection (PJI) (temporal).

Phase	Timing after joint replacement	Clinical presentation	Mode of infection	Common pathogens
Early	<3 months	Erythema, warmth, fever, chills, joint pain, effusion, excessive perioperative drainage	Intraoperative	*Staphylococcus aureus*, gram-negative bacilli
Delayed	3–24 months	Persistent pain and/or aseptic loosening	Intraoperative	Coagulase-negative staphylococci, *Propionibacterium acnes*
Late	>24 months	Sudden-onset joint pain; fever and leukocytosis less likely	Often hematogenous	*Staphylococcus aureus*

(B) Risk factors for developing infections following THA:

Key risk factors include:
- Previous joint arthroplasty
- Noncontiguous surgical site infection (site not involving the current operative site)
- Presence of malignancy
- National nosocomial surveillance system risk score of 1 or 2
- Advanced age, diabetes mellitus, obesity, poor nutrition, skin disease
- RA
- Revision arthroplasty
- Immunocompromised
- Smoker, chronic alcoholic

(C) Management protocol of PJI:

Diagnosis: Definite diagnosis of PJI can be made as below according to the Musculoskeletal Infection Society (2011) for chronic PJI (>4 weeks from index procedure):
- A sinus tract communicating with the prosthesis

- A pathogen is isolated by culture from two separate tissue or fluid samples obtained from the affected prosthetic joint (at least three and no more than five samples should be obtained);
- Four of the following six criteria exist (probable infection if less than four criteria met):
  1. Elevated serum erythrocyte sedimentation rate (ESR) > 30 mm/1st hour, or serum c-reactive protein (CRP) concentration > 10 mg/L (these markers may also be elevated 30–60 days postoperatively)
  2. Elevated synovial white blood cell (WBC) count (>3,000/mm^3)—controversy discussed below.
  3. Elevated synovial neutrophil percentage (>80%)
  4. Presence of purulence in the affected joint
  5. Isolation of a microorganism in one culture of periprosthetic tissue or fluid (mere isolation of low-virulent pathogen such as coagulase-negative staphylococci (CoNS), *Propionibacterium acnes*, or *Corynebacterium* in the absence of other criteria is not believed to represent a definite infection. Isolation of a single virulent organism such as *S. aureus* may represent a PJI.
  6. Greater than five neutrophils per high-power field in five high-power fields observed (Feldman criteria) from histologic analysis of fresh frozen periprosthetic tissue at 400 times magnification.

(One can read other reported criteria from Essential Orthopedics: Principles and Practice)

Treatment: Options for management include no surgery (with or without antibiotic suppression), amputation, joint fusion or removal, prosthesis retention with debridement and antibiotics, and joint revision in either one or two stages.

Conservative management (no surgery): For elderly frail patient with multiple comorbidities precluding extensive surgical management (or those who refuse), a functional infected prosthesis may be retained with stoma bag over sinus to collect discharge and/or suppressive antibiotic therapy. Sinus may be deliberately created to facilitate drainage. Usually 4–6 weeks sometimes extended to 3 months is used. Rifampicin 450–600 mg can be combined for CoNS, the usual companion drugs for rifampicin are fluoroquinolones, cotrimoxazole, doxycycline, and linezolid. Rifampicin should never be used alone for emergence of resistance. Antibiotic suppression following gram-negative bacillus infection is not recommended.

Removal of prosthesis alone or with fusion (arthrodesis): Usually in patients with repeated failures to eradicate infection, failed two-stage revision and factors precluding revision surgery, the joint is preferably removed and based on discussion with patient fusion can be attempted though the failure rates are still more than native joint. Also in patients who remain wheel chair bound due to other illnesses attempting revision may be futile so that prosthesis removal for infected joint is appropriate. Prosthesis removal is relatively appropriate for hip and elbow while removal and fusion is common for knee joint.

Repeated debridement, antibiotics, and implant retention: This is indicated in the acute postoperative time frame. Criteria for this type of surgery include symptoms of <2-week duration—gram-positive organisms, no sinus tract or drainage (relative), and no loosening of the prosthesis.

Repeated debridement to remove dead infected tissue and reduce disease load is practiced along with exchange of modular liners. Cultures should be always obtained; some people locally inject antibiotics based on sensitivity pattern obtained from aspirate. Sinus tract may need flap cover for reconstruction.

Implant revision: Ideal patients for two-stage exchange strategy are patients with chronic infections with adequate bone stock, who are medically fit and willing to undergo at least two surgeries. Patients with sinus tracts or with difficult-to-treat organisms such as methicillin-resistant *S. aureus* (MRSA), enterococci, and *Candida* species would also potentially qualify for this procedure. Obtaining a prerevision sedimentation rate and CRP is recommended to assess the success of treatment prior to reimplantation. More than one two-stage exchanges can be successful if the first one fails. It involves removal of all infected prosthetic components and cement followed by debridement of infected periprosthetic tissue.

The time from resection arthroplasty to reimplantation varies significantly from 2 weeks to several months. Systemic antimicrobials are administered following resection for 4–6 weeks in many centers.

A new prosthesis is reimplanted in delayed second stage. Both cemented and noncemented prostheses are utilized depending on the technical factors. Some prefer reimplantation within 2–6 weeks while systemic antibiotics are being administered. Others prefer delayed implantation. One-stage or direct exchange strategy for the treatment of PJI may be considered in patients with a THA infection who have a good soft-tissue envelope provided that the identity of the pathogens is known preoperatively and is susceptible to oral antimicrobials. There are much fewer data for the use of this procedure for prosthetic joints other than a THA or without antibiotic-impregnated cement and with bone graft. Potential advantages of this single exchange procedure result from saving the patient and the healthcare system an additional surgery, and include lower morbidity rate and lower cost.

Amputation: It may be required in severe untreatable or unresponding infections or in patients with failed multiple surgeries and mutilated limb.

Antibiotic therapy: Teicoplanin may not be as effective as vancomycin in reducing viable MRSA counts, so can be combined with rifampicin. Linezolid is more effective in initial clearance of MRSA compared to teicoplanin but tolerance is low. In combination therapy, glycopeptide + rifampicin + fluoroquinolone have been found to generate no resistance.

109. Prosthetic joint infection:
   A. Discuss sonication.
   B. Discuss management algorithm in prosthetic joint infection in total knee arthroplasty.

Ans:

A. *Sonication:* This is the currently most reliable technique available to improve the detection of microorganisms that colonize the implant. It disrupts bacteria present within biofilms, increasing the number of culturable bacterial cells. Mostly the specimen obtained from PJI is covered with biofilms where the conventional culture modalities miserably fail or the patients have occult infection where the infecting organism is present in a very low quantity that is below threshold limit of present systems. Sonication is commonly done according to Cazanave protocol **(Flowchart 2.5.3)** as follows:

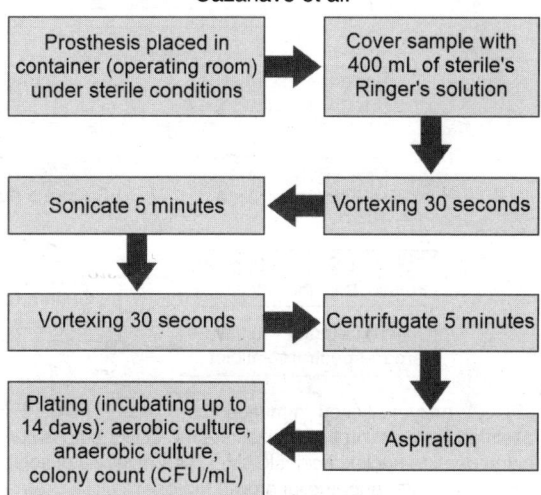

Flowchart 2.5.3: Sonication protocol of Cazanave et al.

1. Removed implant material is placed into Nalgene jars containing 400 mL lactated Ringer's solution. The jar was transferred to a degassed sonication water bath (40 ± 2 kHz, 0.22 W/cm^2) and sonicated for 5 minutes.
2. The jar is then allowed to sit for 1 minute to allow any aerosol to settle.
3. The container is then vortexed for 30 seconds and transferred to a biologic safety cabinet. Inside the cabinet, the container and lid are wiped down using a gauze square saturated with alcohol.
4. The entire volume of sonicated fluid is decanted into 50-mL conical centrifuge tubes using an irrigation syringe.
5. The tubes are now centrifuged at 4°C at 3150 × g for 5 minutes.
6. The supernatant from centrifuge tubes is decanted and discarded except for the last 1 mL of fluid in each tube. The tubes are re-vortexed to resuspend each sediment in 1 mL of supernatant and combined in a single centrifuge tube, which was again centrifuged for 5 minutes.
7. The supernatant from the single tube is now decanted except for the last 4 mL and the pellet was resuspended in this volume.
8. One-tenth milliliter volumes of the suspension were inoculated onto a blood agar plate and a chocolate agar plate, which were incubated in 5% CO_2 for 4 days. Prereduced anaerobically sterilized *Brucella* agar and phenylethyl alcohol agar are inoculated with identical volumes of specimen, which are placed in anaerobic boxes and incubated at 35°C for 14 days.
9. Organisms may be identified by standard phenotypic methods or using matrix-assisted laser desorption ionization time-of-flight mass spectrometry or multiplex PCR.

B. Management algorithm in prosthetic joint infection in total knee arthroplasty (**Flowchart 2.5.4**).

Flowchart 2.5.4: The flowchart depicting management of prosthetic joint infection in total knee replacement.

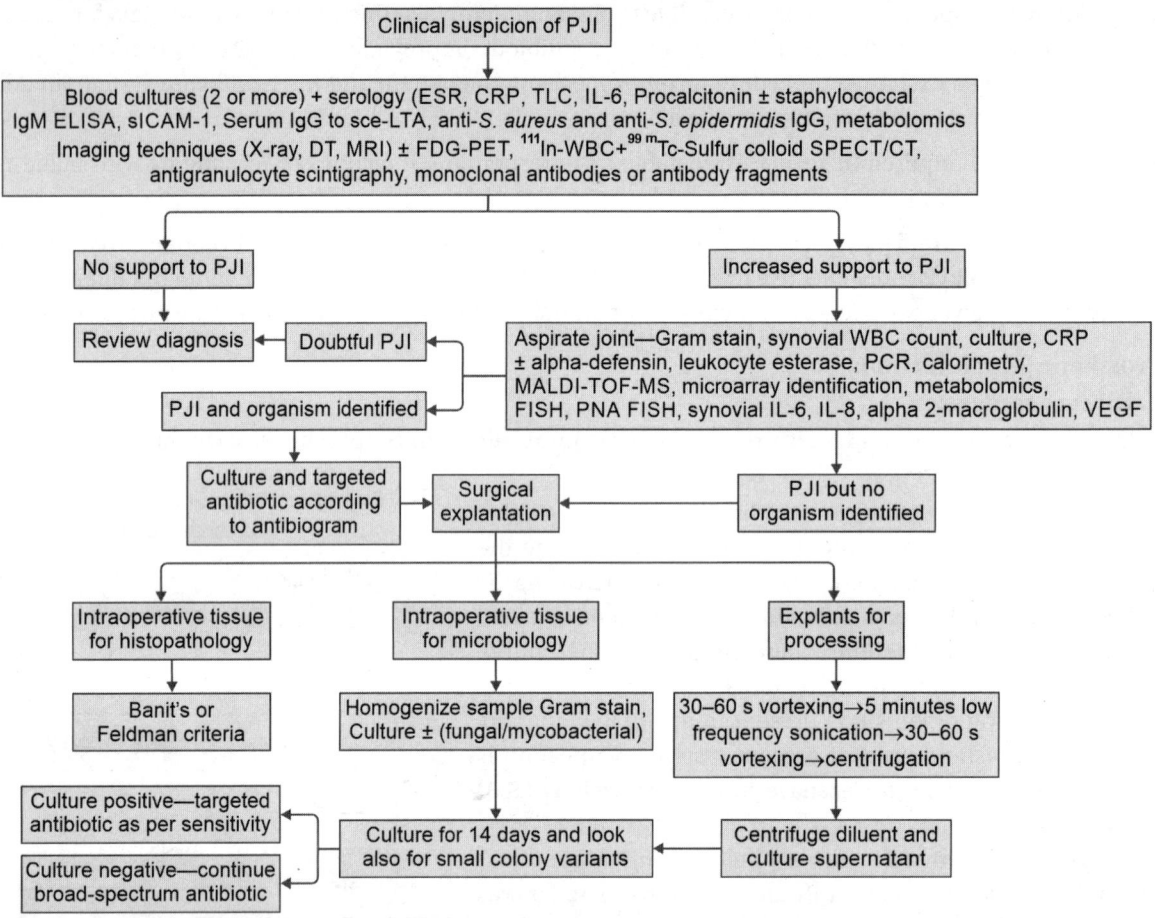

(*ELISA:* enzyme linked immunosorbent assay; *FDG-PET:* F18-fluorodeoxyglucose positron emission tomography; *MALDI-TOF-MS:* matrix-assisted laser desorption ionization-time of flight mass spectrometry; *PJI:* prosthetic joint infection; *PNA-FISH:* fluorescence in situ hybridization using peptide nucleic acid; *sICAM-1:* serum levels of soluble cell adhesion molecule-1; *SPECT:* single photon emission computed tomography; *VEGF:* vascular endothelial growth factor)

110. A. Enumerate modifiable risk factors to reduce prosthetic joint infection.

B. Briefly outline indications and principles of single stage exchange arthroplasty for prosthetic joint infection.

Ans:

A. Kindly see the answer above for risk factors (modifiable ones are 4th, 5th, 6th and last bulleted points)

B. The indications for single stage arthroplasty include:
   - The absence of severe immunocompromise state
   - No significant soft-tissue or bony compromise
   - Absence of concurrent acute sepsis
   - Infection by a drug-sensitive typical organism (unknown organism, culture negative PJI, polymicrobial infections, infection with MRSA or MRSE-resistant organisms and atypical and gram-negative organisms are associated with a higher failure rate)

Principles:
- *A multi-disciplinary approach is essential:*
  - Microbiologists—recommend appropriate systemic and local antibiotics to be delivered in the cement.
  - Plastic surgeons—to provide cover for mild-to-moderate soft tissue defects.

- *Surgical debridement:*
  - Excision of the scar and incorporating the sinus into the skin incision and excising it down to the capsule.
  - Radical total synovectomy after obtaining multiple tissue samples for microbiology and meticulous removal of any residual cement mantle.
  - Pulsatile lavage and use of antiseptic solutions such as polymeric biguanide hydrochloride (polyhexanide), hydrogen peroxide and povidone-iodine.
- All drapes, gowns, gloves, suction tip, light handles and surgical instruments are changed prior to administration of antibiotics and reimplantation.
- Antibiotics added to the cement should be bactericidal, in the powder form, based on sensitivities of the pathogens grown preoperatively and not exceed 10% of the total weight of the cement powder in order to avoid alteration of the mechanical properties of the cement.
- Build-up deficient bone stock using autogenic and allogeneic bone grafting.
- Polymethyl methacrylate (PMMA) bone cement or Tantalum augments (Trabecular Metal, Zimmer Inc, Warsaw, IN, USA) may be used if bone is not available to fill defects.
- The choice of implants may require use of semi to fully constrained implants depending on soft tissue debridement and remaining ligaments and residual bone stock.
- A drain is usually applied to avoid postoperative hematoma formation but is normally removed within 24-48 hours.
- Early mobilization is recommended.
- *Follow-up:*
  - Clinical and serological assessments
  - Repeat aspiration with analysis of the aspirate to confirm resolution of infection.

111. Discuss the management of suppurative flexor tenosynovitis of hand.

Ans: It is a bacterial infection of the digital flexor sheath. It is a painful condition and causes a cylindrical swelling of the finger, which is kept semi-flexed. If untreated, the infection promptly progress in the hand and wrist and may cause osteomyelitis of bones and involvement of hidden spaces of hand.

Treatment should be prompt and effective. The infection is treated conservatively with antibiotics if detected within first 24 hours. If this causes relief of pain, conservative treatment is continued else surgery is the treatment of choice.

Surgery: If signs and symptoms are not abating, decision to surgically drain the infection is taken. For stages 1 and 2, the incision is made classically through mid-lateral crease in case of index and little fingers where the entire sheath can be laid open. Pus is expressed from terminal part to over metacarpophalangeal joint. In case of middle or ring finger volar, a zig-zag incision (Brunner's) or a combination of mid-lateral incision in finger and a transverse incision in palm over the proximal end of the flexor tendon sheath can be made. The fibrous flexor sheath should not be completely incised along its whole length, but important pulleys should be left intact particularly A2 and A4 pulleys. After a thorough decompression, drain is put for 24 hours; hand is splinted, elevated, and treated by systemic antibiotics.

Preferred method is a two-incision approach (for middle and ring fingers) in which the A1 pulley is approached proximally through a preferred transverse incision at the level of the metacarpal head. After entering the sheath pus and debris is aspirated and a small infant feeding tube or 16-gauge suction catheter is passed up the sheath. Another palmar incision is made transversely distal to the A4 pulley in the finger and the sheath is irrigated using saline. We commonly use last wash with antibiotic before withdrawing the catheter back. Another catheter is then inserted and sutured to act as drain for next 24 hours. The radial and ulnar bursae are exposed through open technique. Horseshoe abscess is drained through both radial and ulnar bursas.

For stage 3, the treatment is more extensive with extensive debridement and patient should be counseled in advance for possible need of amputation, the decision of which is taken by two consultants after independent evaluation.

112. Define necrotizing fasciitis.

Ans: Necrotizing fasciitis is a soft tissue infection characterized by rapid spread along the fascial planes and dissolution and necrosis of fascia by enzymes released by the infecting organism. In the later stages, it involves the skin and underlying muscles. It is a potential life and limb threatening infection if not recognized and treated early.

Etiology: The infection is caused predominantly by group A *Streptococcus*, but mixed organism including *Staphylococcus* and anaerobic organisms may be present. Majority of the cases are polymicrobial.

Based on the type of organism isolated, it is classified as:
- *Type 1:* It is caused by nongroup A streptococci with anaerobic organisms
- *Type 2:* It is caused by group A streptococci alone or by group A streptococci with a species of staphylococcus
- *Type 3:* It is caused by clostridia species leading to gas gangrene or clostridial myonecrosis.

The common bacteria isolated are: Group A *Streptococcus* (*Streptococcus pyogenes*), *S. aureus*, *Bacteroides fragilis*, *Clostridium perfringens*, and others. There is initial trauma that may be trivial like lacerations, contusions, injections, and insect bites, and sometimes there is no history of trauma. Major trauma such as open fractures cutaneous abscesses, burns, frostbite or surgical procedure may also lead to necrotizing fasciitis.

Comorbid factors that reduce immunity predispose to necrotizing fasciitis like diabetes, peripheral vascular disease, alcoholism, intravenous drug abuse, multiple myeloma, HIV, and chemotherapy.

Pathophysiology: The infection is characterized by rapid spread along the fascial planes involving the whole limb and even invading the chest wall, if left untreated. This spread is facilitated by enzymes released by the bacteria which dissolve the fat and fascia and form watery gray pus known as dishwater pus. The necrotic tissue undergoes secondary aerobic and anaerobic infection leading to mixed cultures in most cases. The vascular supply to the overlying skin gets occluded leading to ischemia and necrosis of skin.

Clinical features: There is minimal redness initially which rapidly spreads. The overlying skin undergoes ischemia as its blood supply is occluded and appears bluish. Patches of gangrene appear. The underlying muscle layer usually remains red and viable but in later stages may undergo necrosis.

Patient is toxic and shows signs of sepsis even though external signs may be minimal.

Laboratory investigations: Leukocytosis raised ESR and CRP. A complete workup consists of complete blood count, serum chemistry studies, arterial blood gas analysis, urinalysis, and blood and tissue cultures.

The probability of cellulitis developing into necrotizing fasciitis can be estimated based on laboratory finding. It is called the laboratory risk indicator for necrotizing fasciitis (LRINEC) score.

The scoring is done as follows:
- C-reactive protein (mg/L):
  - More than or equal to 150: 4 points
- White blood cell count (WBC) count ($\times 10^3/mm^3$):
  - Less than 15: 0 points
  - 15–25: 1 point
  - More than 25: 2 points
- Hemoglobin (g/dL):
  - More than 13.5: 0 points
  - 11–13.5: 1 point
  - Less than 11: 2 points
- Sodium (mmol/L):
  - Less than 135: 2 points
- Creatinine (μmol/L):
  - More than 141: 2 points
- Glucose (mmol/L):
  - More than 10: 1 point

A score of equal to or greater than 6 indicates a high probability of necrotizing fasciitis.

Imaging studies like ultrasound, CT, MRI, and Doppler studies help to evaluate the extent of the disease and plan the surgical debridement. Necrotizing fasciitis is a medical and surgical emergency and the use of all the above-mentioned investigations should not delay treatment and surgical intervention if infection spreads rapidly.

Treatment: The treatment consists of general supportive measures to control sepsis, prevent organ failure and to maintain electrolytes, start of wide-spectrum antibiotic until culture reports are obtained and radical surgical debridement followed by reconstruction.

Surgical debridement is the mainstay of treatment and should be undertaken as soon as condition of patient permits and as soon as extent of disease has been determined.

The following are the certain principles of surgical debridement in necrotizing fasciitis:
- The superficial signs are usually misleading therefore proximal extension of debridement should be till fully healthy tissues are obtained.
- Finger test can be used to determine the extent of proximal spread. In this, the incision is given over skin and finger is inserted into the wound. If it can easily be passed between the skin and underlying fascia that means that the spread is till the skin can be lifted off.
- Wound should be kept open.
- Inspection and debridement should be done in the operation theater (OT) on a daily basis.
- Amputations sometimes can be lifesaving if the spread is into the deeper tissues.
- Coverage and reconstruction should be started only after complete control of infection.

113. What are the causes of postoperative fever?

Ans: *Most common causes of fever are summarized as below:*

Mnemonic: 5W's for postoperative days (POD)
- *Wind—POD 1-2:* Lungs, i.e. pneumonia, aspiration, pulmonary embolism, and atelectasis
- *Water—POD 3-5:* Urinary tract infection, catheter-induced
- *Wound—POD 5-7:* Superficial or deep surgical infection
- *Walking—POD >5:* Deep vein thrombosis
- *Wonder drugs—any POD:* Drug fever or blood products
- *Wind/Water-any POD:* Bloodstream infection, phlebitis or cellulitis due to intravenous (IV) lines.

114. Define Tom Smith arthritis and describe under the following headings: Clinical features, diagnosis, treatment, and sequelae.

Ans: Kindly see the Answer to Question 94 above.

115. What is gas gangrene?

Ans: The term *gas gangrene* (clostridial myonecrosis) implies an infection with the *Clostridium* species of anaerobic bacteria that causes life-threatening necrotizing soft-tissue infection. The infection is characterized by necrosis of muscle and production of free gas in the tissues. Several other mixed aerobic and anaerobic gram-negative and gram-positive bacteria have also been implicated to cause "gas" gangrene. Not all *Clostridium* species, however, cause myonecrosis and free gas production and most commonly *C. perfringens, C. novyi,* and *C. septicum,* cause the most dramatic infections with high mortality rates. Gas gangrene historically has been associated with war injuries, but in modern times, it has also been seen after surgery or with no antecedent trauma. During World War I, gas gangrene occurred in 6% of open fractures and 1% of all open wounds.

Clostridium perfringens (a gram-positive, obligate anaerobic, spore-forming bacillus) is responsible for 90% of gas gangrene infections and produces four major toxins: *alpha, beta, epsilon,* and *theta* of which the alpha toxin (a phospholipase) is responsible for hemolysis, platelet destruction, and widespread capillary damage.

Clinical features: Gas gangrene typically begins with the sudden appearance of pain in the region of the wound. The muscle pain is excruciating pain with edema and subsequent skin discoloration (bronze → red-purple → black) with bullae formation and gas production. Crepitus is prominent in tissues on palpation. In contrast to the pain with spreading cellulitis, the pain remains only in the infected regions and spreads with spread of infection (can progress 10 cm/h). Sweet, foul-smelling, or nonodorous discharge is indicative of anaerobic metabolism. Muscle involvement is almost always more extensive than indicated by skin changes. If left untreated, fever, sweating, and anxiety or delirium may develop with profound shock and systemic toxemia.

The diagnosis can be confirmed by local exploration (and gram-staining) of the wound and by radiographs (feathering pattern of soft tissues), CT, or MRI.

Differential diagnosis:
- Necrotizing fasciitis
- Vibrio vulnificus infection
- Group A *Streptococcus* infection

It is imperative to understand that gas gangrene is a surgical emergency and even suspicion is enough for initiating surgical treatment. Prompt surgical removal of dead, damaged, and infected tissue (debridement) is necessary. Fasciotomy may be necessary for compartment syndrome. Amputation of an arm or leg may be indicated to control the spread of infection.

Simultaneous antibiotic therapy is a must and although penicillin G is effective against clostridial species, mixed infections are common so regimen should include aminoglycosides, penicillinase-resistant penicillins, or vancomycin. Clindamycin is a preferred choice for substituting penicillin else one may also choose a third-generation cephalosporin, metronidazole, and chloramphenicol for broader coverage. Tetanus prophylaxis should be ensured.

Hyperbaric oxygen therapy may be used as an adjunct to surgery and antibiotics are debatable but may halt alpha toxin production, and necrotic tissue can be debrided more conservatively, salvaging more viable tissue than would otherwise be possible.

116. Hyperbaric oxygen therapy: its advantages and disadvantages in orthopedic practices.

Ans: This is achieved when a patient breathes pure oxygen in an environment with elevated atmospheric pressure (>1 atm absolute, UHMS recommends 2–2.5 atm). The therapy is typically given for 90–120 minutes. Based on Boyle, Dalton's and Henry's principles, there is an increase in the plasma volume fraction of transported oxygen which is available for cellular metabolism. Increased oxygenation has beneficial physiological effects in the treatment of chronic wounds.

Advantages:
- There is synergistic effect of hyperbaric oxygen and antibiotic therapy on infection control.
- It promotes better oxygenation of ischemic bone cells, irrespective of the circulating hemoglobin and without the need for the energy required for dissociation of oxygen from hemoglobin promoting bone resorption, revascularization and osteogenesis.

Disadvantages:
- It is costly, not readily available and of unproved effectiveness.
- Though transcutaneous oxygen tension at the affected extremity level is improved, but it is just one aspect of addressing the pathology.

117. Describe the molecular tests used in identification of multidrug-resistant (MDR) tuberculosis. Describe the dosage and important side effects of second-line drugs in osteoarticular tuberculosis. What is the role of positron emission tomography to assess healing in osteoarticular tuberculosis?

Ans: *Molecular diagnosis* using nucleic acid amplification test (NAAT) is gaining popularity for rapid diagnosis (few hours to less than 1 day), high sensitivity, and specificity. The specimens sent to the laboratory are directly subjected to amplification of specific *Mycobacterium tuberculosis* DNA (deoxyribonucleic acid) sequences using one of the many available techniques such as polymerase chain reaction (PCR), real-time PCR or strand displacement amplification. These are highly sensitive and specific to confirm in acid-fast bacillus (AFB) positive cases and even in AFB negative extra-pulmonary tuberculosis (EPTB) cases DNA-PCR is however unable to differentiate between viable and nonviable bacillus and cost is also a prohibiting factor. The messenger ribonucleic acid (mRNA)-based reverse transcriptase-PCR (RT-PCR) can differentiate viable from nonviable *M. tuberculosis* and is a rapid diagnostic method for EPTB too. RT-PCR has also been used to monitor drug resistance.

The GeneXpert test—Xpert MTB/RIF is a fully automated diagnostic molecular test (applied on the tissue or sputum sample) using the NAAT. It simultaneously detects TB and rifampicin drug resistance (*rpoB gene*) in less than 2 hours offering treatment opportunity the same day. World Health Organization (WHO) strongly recommends the test to be used as the initial diagnostic test in individuals suspected of multidrug-resistant tuberculosis (MDR-TB) or HIV/TB. Conditionally, it is recommended as a follow-on test to microscopy in settings where MDR-TB or HIV is of lesser concern, especially in smear-negative cases [like osteoarticular tuberculosis (OATB)]. Line probe assay (DNA strip test) for first-line drugs (approved by WHO 2008) is recommended (encouraged) for diagnosis of MDR-TB (resistance to H and/or R) and is a good supplement to diagnosis in MDR-TB regions but requires rigorous setup. Still WHO recommends conventional culture methods and drug susceptibility testing (DST) to determine extensively drug-resistant (XDR) cases in endemic regions.

Second line Drugs with dosages and side effects:
- *Thioacetazone:* 150 mg in adults—hepatitis, bone marrow suppression, and Stevens–Johnson syndrome.
- *Para-aminosalicylic acid (PAS):* 10–12 g (200 mg/kg) per day in divided doses—kidney, liver, and thyroid dysfunction.
- *Ethionamide:* 0.5–0.75 g (10–15 mg/kg) per day—hepatitis, optic neuritis, and impotence.
- *Cycloserine:* 250 mg BD, increased if tolerated up to 500 mg BD—neuropsychiatric side effects.
- *Kanamycin, capreomycin, and amikacin:* All are given in a dose of 0.75–1.0 g IM per day—aminoglyside class so have their side effects like ototoxicity, renal, and neurotoxicity.
- *Ciprofloxacin, ofloxacin, and moxifloxacin:* The generally employed doses are ciprofloxacin 1,500 mg/day and ofloxacin 800 mg/day in two divided doses—fluoroquinolone class so have their side effects.
- *Clarithromycin and azithromycin:* The dose of clarithromycin is 500 mg BD and that of azithromycin 500 mg OD—macrolide class so have that side effects.

Positron emission tomography (PET) scan in healing—18F-fluorodeoxyglucose (18F-FDG) has been found to be useful in tuberculosis for detection, assessing disease activity, staging, and monitoring response to therapy. It is considered that with chemotherapy, the tubercular lesions will reduce in activity due to diminishing viable bacteria and reducing inflammation so good response to therapy can be demonstrated. However, no change in activity of the lesions even with full dose standard chemotherapy (supplemented by persistence of immunological markers indicating disease activity) might be an early indication of failure of treatment. Thus, other intervention and further evaluation are indicated. The complex and long period required for the treatment of TB makes 18F-FDG PET particularly useful, as it is able to detect at an early point in treatment drug combinations that are ineffective and lead to a change in therapy. This is not only important to reduce morbidity and mortality in the individual, but prevents the even greater public health hazard of the individual developing resistant species of MTB and transmitting the resistant strain in the community.

118. **Define multidrug-resistant tuberculosis. Discuss the clinical features, diagnosis, and treatment of a case of MDR-TB of spine.**

Ans: "Multidrug-resistant TB"—refers to an isolate of *M. tuberculosis* that is resistant to at least isoniazid and rifampin, and possibly additional agents. The term "extensively drug-resistant TB" (XDR-TB) is defined as TB that is resistant to any fluoroquinolone, and at least one of three injectable second-line drugs (capreomycin, kanamycin, and amikacin), in addition to isoniazid and rifampin. It is estimated that 70% of XDR-TB patients die within a month of diagnosis. About 3.7% of new cases and 20% of previously treated cases were estimated to have MDR-TB. The average proportion of MDR-TB cases with XDR-TB is 9.0%.

Clinical features: Although nowadays with increased prevalence, the MDR cases present as primary but previously these patients were commonly treatment defaulters and relapsed cases most often due to lack of initiative, commitment, poverty, poor understanding of implications, and illiteracy. The patients stop responding to standard first-line therapy or there is no response to treatment from beginning. The symptoms (pain and systemic symptoms) keep worsening or suddenly begin to worsen after initial response suggesting escape from response to primary drugs. Radiologically, there is no improvement and the bones continue to show increasing destruction and developing osteopenia. Advanced imaging would show growing abscess/synovial reaction and spread of disease from previous scans. Additionally, patients may develop skip lesion(s).

Diagnosis: Drug susceptibility testing for both first- and second-line drugs (usually performed at the state laboratory or national referral center level) should be performed especially in areas with high incidence of MDR tuberculosis. Obtain material from lesion (biopsy or bus or curettings) and send for GeneXpert test and line probe assay that not only diagnose the infection but also provide DST on a rapid detection basis. At places where these tests are not available, then liquid culture is recommended.

Treatment: Multidrug-resistant TB develops due to selection of resistant mutants in the bacterial population, due to killing of susceptible bacilli by anti-TB drugs, inadequate treatment such as direct or indirect monotherapy, slow but constant mutation of *M. tuberculosis*, resulting in resistant mutant organisms and early discontinuation of treatment.

The green light committee helps nations to establish drug-resistant TB component and integrate into control program. For treatment of MDR-TB, the medications are divided into five groups according to efficacy, experience of use, and drug class. Group 1 comprises of first-line agents except streptomycin which is grouped in Group 2. Groups 2–5 are reserve drugs. The MDR-regimens are either standardized regimen or tailor-made (preferable) where DST is available, especially rapid-DST. In India, the MDR-TB patients and those with any rifampicin resistance are referred to the Revised National Tuberculosis Control Programme (RNTCP) designated directly observed treatment short-course (DOTS)-Plus site, with their DST result and request for Category IV treatment form. Under RNTCP, the MDR regimen comprises of six drugs—Km, Ofx (Lvx), Eto, Z, E, and Cs for 6–9 months of intensive phase and four drugs Ofx (Lvx), Eto, E, and Cs for 18 months in continuation phase. PAS is included in the regimen if any bactericidal drug (K, Ofl, Z and Eto) or two bacteriostatic (E and Cs) drugs are not tolerated. The general principles to design an MDR-TB regimen are as follows:

- Treatment regimens should consist of at least four drugs with either certain, or almost certain effectiveness.
- More than four drugs may be started if the susceptibility pattern is unknown or the effectiveness of one or more agents is questionable.
- Susceptibility testing for isoniazid, rifampicin, the fluoroquinolones, and the injectable agents is fairly reliable so regimen could be based on the DST pattern for these drugs. For other drugs, the clinical effectiveness of DST cannot be predicted with full surety.
- Each dose in an MDR regimen is given as DOT throughout the treatment.
- Do not use drugs for which possibility of cross-resistance exists.
- Include drugs from groups 1–5 in hierarchical order based on potency. In general, select one of the first-line drug to which add an injectable from Group 2 **(Table 2.5.3)**. Use a fluoroquinolone and then choose a drug from Group 4 to complete an effective four-drug combination. For a regimen with less than four drugs, choose two from Group 5. The total number of drugs often ranges from 5–7 depending on the degree of uncertainty.
- The duration of intensive phase for MDR-TB regimen depends on duration of treatment with injectable agent. The injectable agent should be continued for a minimum of 6 months and for at least 4 months after the patient first becomes and remains smear-negative or culture-negative. Another recommendation is to continue treatment for a minimum of 18 months following culture conversion.

TABLE 2.5.3: Various groups of drugs used in treatment of drug-susceptible and drug-resistant tuberculosis.

Group	Drugs (abbreviations)
1. First-line oral	Pyrazinamide (Z), ethambutol (E), rifabutin (Rfb), and rifapentine (Rfp)
2. Injectable drugs	Kanamycin (Km), amikacin (Am), capreomycin (Cm), and streptomycin (S)
3. Fluoroquinolones	• Levofloxacin (Lfx) and moxifloxacin (Mfx) • Ofloxacin (Ofx) is less effective and gatifloxacin is too toxic
4. Oral bacteriostatic second-line agents	• Para-aminosalicylic acid (PAS) and cycloserine (Cs) • Terizidone (Trd), ethionamide (Eto), and prothionamide (Pto)
5. Agents with unclear role	• Clofazimine (Cfz) and linezolid (Lzd) • Amoxicillin/clavulanate (Amx/Clv), thiacetazone (Thz), imipenem/cilastatin (Ipm/Cln), high-dose isoniazid (high-dose H), and clarithromycin (Clr)

119. Define drug-resistant tuberculosis. How do you suspect drug resistance in spinal tuberculosis? How will you investigate and manage a case of suspected drug resistant tuberculosis?

Ans: Kindly see the answers above.

120. What is the rationale for using metallic implants in osteoarticular tuberculosis?

Ans: Please read Chapter no 4C.

121. Discuss compound palmar ganglion.

Ans: This lesion is neither a ganglion nor compound. Chronic inflammation distends the common sheath of the flexor tendons both above and below the flexor retinaculum. RA and tuberculosis are the most common causes.

The synovial membrane becomes thick and villous. The amount of fluid is increased and it may contain fibrin particles molded by repeated movement to the shape of melon seeds.

The tendons may eventually fray and rupture.

Clinical features: Pain is unusual but paraesthesia due to median nerve compression may occur. The swelling is hourglass in shape, bulging above and below the flexor retinaculum; it is not warm or tender; fluid can be pushed from one part to the other (cross-fluctuation).

Treatment: If the condition is tuberculous, general treatment is begun. The contents of the sac are evacuated, streptomycin is instilled and the wrist rested in a splint. If these measures fail, the entire flexor sheath is dissected out. Complete excision is also the best treatment when the cause is rheumatoid disease and if the disease is recalcitrant.

122. Define spina ventosa.

Ans: Spina ventosa is a Latin expression; spina = short bone and ventosa = inflated with air. This is a typical radiological appearance of tubercular affection of small bones of hands and feet seen commonly in pediatric patients.

Pathology and pathogenesis: During childhood, these short tubular bones have a lavish blood supply through a large nutrient artery entering almost in the middle of the bone. Inoculation of the marrow cavity converts the interior of the short tubular bone into a tuberculous granuloma. With the increase in pathology and enlarging granulomatous tissue, the bone is reshaped to a spindle-shaped (spina ventosa). The blood supply is occluded either by direct pressure from enlarging tissue or arteritis causing destruction of internal lamellae (or formation of sequestra). Presence of thick periosteum and vascularized surrounding tissue causes significant subperiosteal new bone formation. Unchecked the infection might proceed subperiosteally and into surrounding tissues forming abscess (cold abscess). Over a period of time, the cortex breaks and infected tissue would get expressed out in the form of tubercular sinus that may cause secondary bacterial infection and the process would get converted to chronic osteomyelitis. In few patients, the disease heals with shortening of the involved bone and deformity of the neighboring joint.

Radiologically, the affected bone typically appears expanded with a lytic lesion in the middle and subperiosteal new bone deposited along the involved bone. The cavity may contain soft coke-like sequestra. Alternatively, the bone structure may appear honeycombed (alternate sclerotic and lytic regions) or may have diffuse uniform infiltration, or a pure cystic lesion, or rarely the involved bone may show atrophy.

123. Discuss spina ventosa: Clinical features, diagnosis, and treatment.

Ans: *Spina ventosa:* It refers to tubercular osteomyelitis of small bones of hand/feet (short tubular bones). Better and more descriptive name for this is 'tubercular dactylitis'. Children are more commonly affected than adults and are prone to multiple/consecutive bone involvement than single bone disease of adults.

Pathology: There is spindle-shaped expansion of the bone. With occlusion of the nutrient artery of the involved bone and the destruction of internal lamellae (or formation of sequestra) there is endosteal destruction and concomitant subperiosteal new bone formation; successive layers of subperiosteal new bone formation are deposited over the involved bone.

Clinical features: The patients present with swelling and skin discoloration over the affected underlying bone. Due to lack of acute inflammatory changes (fever, erythema, acute pain, etc.) the presentation is often delayed. Late abscess and sinus formation is quite common leading to secondary infection and further thickening of bone.

Diagnosis: Radiologically the affected bone shows diaphyseal lytic expansile lesion and subperiosteal new bone deposition along the involved bone. The cavity may contain soft coke-like sequestra. Alternative radiological appearances include honeycombing, diffuse uniform infiltration, or a cystic lesion, or rarely the involved bone may show atrophy.

Whenever in doubt serological, histological, and bacteriological investigations are mandatory to confirm the pathology.

Treatment: In the natural course the disease heals with shortening of the involved bone and deformity of the neighboring joint. Management is essentially by antitubercular drugs, rest to the part in functioning position and early active exercises of the involved parts or joints. In patients with unfavorable response or with recurrence of infection surgical debridement is justified. If a metacarpophalangeal, metatarsophalangeal, or interphalangeal joint is ankylosed in an awkward position excision arthroplasty or corrective osteotomy is indicated. Amputation of ray may be needed for severely deformed, scarred, finger(s) that interfers with the normal functioning.

124. Discuss madura foot: Pathology, clinical features, diagnosis and treatment.

Ans: Mycetoma or maduramycosis is a chronic infection of exogenous origin often localized to foot. "Madura foot" (term used by Colebrook in 1946) possibly originates from the modern reporting of disease from Madurai, Tamil Nadu predominantly committing to feet. Carter used the term "Mycetoma" relating it to fungal etiology. Other names for the disease include Morbus Tuberculosis pedis, fungus foot disease of India, Godfrey and Eyre's disease, endemic degeneration of the bones of the foot, fungus foot, and morbus pedis entophyticus-affection singulière. The disease has been described in "Atharva veda" referring to "pada valmikam" (literally meaning "anthill foot").

Etiopathogenesis: Literature reports some 30 and more species of bacteria and fungi causing mycetoma. The infecting agents belong to actinomycetes, eumycetes, eubacteria, and dermatophytes. The pathogenic organisms vary from region to region but most commonly *M. mycetomatis* is the infecting organism followed by *M. grisea* and *Aspergillus nidulans*. The risk factors for developing mycetoma include:
- A minor trauma or thorn prick
- Walking without protective footwear (barefoot)
- Agricultural work and farming, thorny sharp vegetable material
- Arid hot regions with prolonged hot sunshine and tropical climate predispose to maduromycosis
- *Immunocompromised patients:* HIV infection, postrenal transplant patients, and diabetic patients.

The mycetoma is classified into two groups depending on primary fungal infection (true mycetoma or eumycetoma) or actinomycotic infection.

Eumycetoma is commonly caused by:
- *Madurella mycetomati, Madurella grisea, Leptosphaeria senegalensis, Curvularia lunata*—they have "dark hard" grains. *Scedosporium apiospermum, Neotestudina rosatii,* and *Fusarium* spp. have pale soft grains.
- Actinomycotic mycetoma (bacterial infection) commonly implicated in the disease include: *Actinomadura madurae* (White grains), *Actinomadura pelletieri* (Red grains), *Streptomyces somaliensis* (Yellow grains) and Nocardia brasiliensis (small soft yellow-orange or off-white grains).

Clinical features: The disease is an exogenous infection. The disease begins as a single, small, and painless nodule. Slowly the nodule increases in size and becomes fixed to the underlying tissue. The granules grow toward skin and attach to it. The ensuing inflammatory reaction produces cavities and sinuses that discharge typical grains and pus. This process may take months to years and is faster in actinomycotic form.

Diagnosis: The clinical feature of subcutaneous swelling, subcutaneous nodule, sinus formation and pus discharge is characteristic. Attention should be given to the prolonged duration of disease, sinuses discharging grains, absence of pain and involvement of regional nodes. Culture (MacConkey agar, malt extract agar, mannitol salt agar plates aerobically incubated at 37°C for 48 hours—actinomycetes take 48–72 hours to grow so respective instruction is legible with sample) are the gold standard for any infectious disease for diagnosis but may be absent and in this instance the triad of "tumefaction", "fistulation with abscess formation", and "extrusion of colored granules" will help. Also, histopathology will help in diagnosis. FNAC demonstrates foreign body giant cells and grains with polymorphous inflammation.

Treatment: Treatment should be initiated after differentiating fungal from bacterial infection. Combination drugs are the standard modality of treatment. The therapeutic endpoint is clinical and radiological cure. For actinomycetoma trimethoprim—sulfamethoxazole (TMPSMX), dapsone (diaminodiphenyl sulfone), amoxicillin/clavulanic acid, gentamicin and cefotaxime, streptomycin, amikacin, kanamycin, etc. are used in variable combinations. Recurrences are treated with different drugs. Before initiating dapsone G6PD, deficiency should be evaluated. Welsh regimen comprises using amikacin with TMPSMX that had been effective for treating the actinomycotic infection.

Eumycetoma is a typical fungal infection that responds to standard antifungal therapy. This consists of ketoconazole 400–800 mg daily and/or itraconazole 400 mg (*P. boydii*) given for years. *Madurella mycetomatis* responds to itraconazole

400 mg daily for 3 months followed by 200 mg daily for 9 months. Other drugs effective are ketoconazole and amphotericin B. Surgery is required for complete removal or reducing the size of lesion to ease the medical treatment and deformity. Posaconazole, an investigational agent, may have a role in the treatment of eumycetoma in the future.

2.6 AMPUTATIONS AND PROSTHETICS (Q125–143)

125. Discuss the following:
   A. Indications and complications of amputation.
   B. Early management of closed above knee amputation.
   C. Principles of amputation in children and adults.

Ans:

A. *Indications:* We can group them into easy-to-remember format as follows:
   - *Dead limb:* Ischemic limb, wet and dry gangrene, and frostbite.
   - *Dying limb:* Traumatic nonreconstructable limb (crush injury), thermal trauma, electrical burns, vascular disorders like Berger's disease, and generalized atherosclerosis.
   - *Deadly limb:* Malignancy and acute spreading infections (necrotizing fasciitis and gas gangrene).
   - *Damn useless:* Congenital deficiencies and poorly reconstructed limb following trauma or malignancy that are actually functionally hindering. Here, it is deemed that the prosthetic replacement will provide better function than the useless counterpart.
   - *Damn painful:* Complex regional pain syndrome (CRPS) and neuropathic limb.
   - *Damn nuisance:* Diabetic foot and neuropathic joint (Charcot's or Syphilis). Here, the primary disease and its sequel are so dramatically unmanageable that it is better to part away the affected limb.

The only "absolute indication" for amputation is an ischemic limb where revascularization is not possible.

Complications:

Early:
- Wound hematoma
- Skin flap breakdown and wound dehiscence
- Proximal myonecrosis and wound extension, especially in peripheral vascular disease (PVD) patients
- Infection (especially in diabetics), one should be wary of clostridial infection secondary to perineal contamination
- Neuralgic pain due to excessive pulling of nerves while transecting or formation of neuroma, wound pain, phantom sensation, and phantom pain
- *Skin complications:*
  - Skin maceration
  - Blisters
  - Abrasion.

Late:
- Phantom sensation and phantom pain
- Joint contracture and instability
- Pain due to pressure of ill-fitting socket causing impingement and neuroma
- Flabby and unstable soft tissue stump due to excessive soft tissue at stump or failure to perform myodesis
- *Skin complications:*
  - Verrucous hyperplasia
  - Fungal infection
  - Skin atrophy
  - Callosities
  - Follicular hyperkeratosis
  - Allergic reactions to material of cup or liner.
- *Bone spur formation:* Due to periosteal bone formation
- Osteoporosis and fracture of bone.

B. Immediate postoperative prosthetic fitting has many advantages, especially when it is done in combined care of prosthetist, rehabilitative medicine, and physiotherapist.

This phase begins at the time of injury and continues until all wounds have successfully closed and are free of infection. The length of time spent in this phase varies depending on the extent of the patient's injury. A very important part of this rehabilitation is the fitting of "pylon prosthesis". Pylon prosthesis is also called endoskeletal prosthesis which means the internal (endo-) structure of prosthesis and has no relation to osteointegrated prosthesis. The prosthesis used initially is made of plaster and is contoured proximally but resembles a plug fit. This socket is gradually replaced by a total-contact quadrilateral socket of plaster that is hand-molded over the stump and elongated by a crutch and suspended by a waist belt and/or a shoulder strap. The initial period of standing is limited to minimal touchdown weight bearing. The patient stands on a scale to get a feel of the pressure to apply. Usually, around 20 pounds of pressure is encouraged. Pressure in excess of 40 pounds can compromise wound healing. This endoskeletal structure can be carried forward to provide or construct a definitive prosthesis. The advantages of pylon prosthesis are:

- Immediately after surgery, limb elevation prevents edema.
- Active and passive limb mobilization to prevent contractures is started as soon as pain permits.
- Immediate upright posture and ambulation with support with fitting of temporary prosthesis is encouraged for both physiological and psychological well-being of the patient. This encourages early gait training and walking.
- When managing an amputee acutely, the rehabilitation goals are to promote healing of the residual limb wound; achieve independence in self-feeding, toileting, and oral hygiene; and provide the client and family education on the rehabilitation process.
- Patients and family members are introduced to rehabilitative and prosthetic services in the early stage of this phase.
- Eases patient's and family member's fears, provides support throughout the grieving and recovery processes, and engages the patient and family with the rehabilitative team.
- *The possible other advantages are:*
  - Faster stump maturation due to edema subsidence and wound healing
  - Reduction of postoperative pain
  - May help to save knee joint in amputations done for PVD.

Immediate postoperative prosthetic fitting requires specialized cooperation between the surgeon, prosthetic specialist, and physical rehabilitation specialist. Amateur process can lead to unacceptable consequences.

C. **Principles:**

Adults:
- *Clean operative field:* The procedure should be performed through tissues that are not infected using all aseptic techniques. In case of open wounds, the surface through which the amputation plane will pass should be covered by healthy red granulation tissue or ideally should be fully healed.
- *Tourniquet:* Tourniquet should be used in all cases as it reduces surgical time, makes the surgery less traumatic and bloodless, and makes identification of muscles, nerves, and vessels easier.
- Exsanguination of limb before application of tourniquet should not be done in cases on malignancy and infection to prevent proximal dissemination.
- *Skin flap:* The greatest skin length possible should be maintained for muscle coverage and a tension-free closure. Skin should be mobile, sensate, and of adequate thickness. Scars adherent to underlying tissue and having redundant tissue and "dog ears" should be avoided. With modern day prosthesis, the location of the scar is not important, but if possible, the following principles should be used:
  - *Equal anterior posterior flaps:* Above wrist, mid-thigh, and below knee
  - *Long posterior flap (skewed flap):* Ischemic limbs, Syme amputation, and toe amputations
  - *Long anterior flap:* Below wrist and distal end femur
  - *Free vascularized or Scandinavian flaps (equal medial and lateral flaps):* Sometimes, the local tissues are insufficient to provide adequate cover and in order to preserve the length of limb and avoid a more proximal amputation, a free vascularized graft having skin, subcutaneous fat, and even muscle can be used. It is preferred for stump coverage over a split thickness graft as it is sensate and has a higher resistance to break down under the prostheses.

- *Muscles:* The muscles are divided just distal approximately 5 cm to the bone cut. Separation of muscles from overlying skin should be avoided as far as possible. Muscles are stabilized either by "myodesis" (i.e., muscle sutured through drill holes in bone) or by "myoplasty" (i.e., antagonistic muscle and fascia groups sutured together).
- *Nerves:* Nerves should be cut under tension and allowed to retract proximally to the end of the bone where there is no scar and tension. In this way, the chance of neuromas formation will be less and there will also be reduced potential for irritation and pain.
- *Blood vessels:* Separation and tying of the larger arteries and veins individually prevents the formation of arteriovenous fistulas and aneurysms.
- *Bone:* Osteophytes or bone prominences around the joint that has been disarticulated are removed and filed. The edges are beveled to reduce irritation and pressure over the stump when a prosthesis is worn or direct weight is borne on the stump end.
- *Open amputations:* The amputation in which the stump is left open is called an open amputation. It is always done in presence of established or potential infection. It is of two types—open circular amputation, also known as guillotine amputation, or it can be an open amputation with flaps designed for closure but left open. Skin traction applied postoperatively helps to prevent retraction of skin and muscles and after 6–8 weeks, the scar is excised and final closure of stump is done. Skin traction should be avoided in ischemic limbs. In these limbs, a better plan is to invert the skin margin and suture this to underlying subcutaneous fascia at the base of the flaps with nonabsorbable sutures.
- Even in case of infection it is preferred to plan the open amputation in such a way that the flaps are designed at the time of the primary procedure and then they can be closed as soon as wound condition permits without waiting for 6–8 weeks.
- *Level of amputation:* As much of the limb that is consistent with good function should be preserved. At the same time, care should be taken to perform the amputation through healthy tissue to avoid revisions which delay the rehabilitation of the patient. For above knee amputations, usually a length of 18–20 cm is left below the greater trochanter. For below knee amputation, minimum working length for prosthetic fitting is 9 cm so length more than 12 cm (ideally 15 cm) is required. Smaller stumps (<6 cm) are more of a pain due to improper prosthetic fitting and ultimately rely on hip muscles for mobilization, so should be avoided. Above elbow amputations do well with arm length of 20 cm while below elbow amputations function well with length 15–18 cm distal to olecranon. There are various proposed advantages for adequately preserved limbs with "good length" stumps:
    - Ethically preserve as much tissue as possible
    - Higher acceptability and better compliance
    - Functionality is better with less energy consumption.

Children:
- Preserve length
- Preserve important growth plates
- Perform disarticulation rather than transosseous amputation whenever possible
- Preserve the knee joint whenever possible
- Stabilize and normalize the proximal portion of the limb to deal with issues in addition to limb deficiency in children with other clinically important conditions.

126. What are the indications of amputations?
Ans: Kindly refer to answer above.

127. What is Ertl procedure of amputation osteomyoplasty and its indications and advantages?
Ans: The conventional amputation procedure produces host of issues relating to poor surgical reconstruction. Prolonged pain, nonfunctional amputation stump due to rotational instability of bone (in two bone regions like leg and forearm), loss of bone pressure, loose muscles, etc. These issues are addressed by Ertl procedure which is an amalgamation of surgical reconstructive procedures to balance the five main structures of a limb for providing as good a functional stability as

possible. This produces a pain-free, stable volume limb that resists rotation and improves end bearing. The following are incorporated in Ertl osteomyoplastic procedure:
1. *Closure of bone and making a bone bridge:* In a transtibial amputation, synostosis is created between distal tibia and fibula by way of a flexible bone graft. This re-establishes medullary canal pressure and rotationally stabilizes distal tibia and fibula. Volumetrically stabilized limb can better accept end weight bearing. At the transfemoral level (only one bone is involved), the medullary canal is covered with the flexible bone graft.
2. *Prevention of neuroma and painful stump:* Nerves are identified, placed on stretch, and transected as proximal as possible well out of the way of any traumatized tissue to eliminate neuroma formation, restoring nerve gliding and preventing nerve adhesions.
3. *Arteries and veins* are individually ligated from one another to prevent formation of any AV malformations.
4. *Motor reconstruction:* Myoplasty and osteomyoplasty is the mainstay of procedure to restablish length-tension relationship of all antagonistic group (flexor/extensor, adductor abductor, etc.) of muscles.
    a. Improve functionality of the muscle
    b. Re-establish pumping action of muscle improving venous return
    c. Reducing stump edema
5. *Skin:* Closure should be free of dog ears/invaginated skin or adhered scars. Cylindrical limbs allow improved capability for end weight bearing, minimal skin shear and better prosthetic fitting. This also prevents stump bone osteoporosis.

128. What are the levels of various foot amputations, their indications, and disadvantages?

Ans: Different foot amputations described are as follows:
- *Forefoot amputations:*
    - *Toe amputations:* Single-toe amputation is usually well accepted and minimally morbid. Amputation of the great toe does not functionally affect standing or walking at a normal pace. Amputation of the second toe frequently is followed by severe hallux valgus, so a second ray amputation and narrowing the foot are recommended. This is commonly combined with screw fixation to prevent a severe valgus deformity from occurring. Toe most commonly amputated toe is the fifth one, the usual indication being overriding on the fourth toe. Amputation of all toes causes little disturbance in ordinary slow walking but is disabling during a more rapid gait and when spring and resilience of the foot are required. It interferes with squatting and tiptoeing. All-toe amputation is commonly supplanted by shoe filler. Amputation of more than two rays often is more disabling than a transmetatarsal amputation.
    - *Amputation through the metatarsals:* The disability is proportional to the level of amputation—(the proximal the greater). Disability is in the form of loss of push-off causing gait impairment. Only shoe filler is to be provided for compensation.
- *Midfoot amputations:* Amputations through the middle of the foot include:
    - Lisfranc amputation at the tarsometatarsal joints (This commonly results in an equinus deformity that transforms into severe equinovarus deformity—so not preferred).
    - Pirogoff amputation (calcaneus is vertically sectioned and rotated forward to be fused to the tibia).
    More or less the midfoot amputations have rare definitive indications (severe trauma and in diabetic patients) and considerable uncorrectable morbidity so seldom performed. Instead more functional hindfoot/ankle level amputations are preferred. Wound healing is an issue in diabetic patients undergoing foot amputations; so, in addition to using the ankle-brachial index, toe pressures of >45 mm Hg and transcutaneous partial pressure of oxygen of >30 mm Hg are preferred for good healing of wounds. A transcutaneous partial pressure of oxygen of <20 mm Hg indicates that healing is unlikely at that level.
    To prevent equinus deformity, one or more dorsiflexors of the ankle must be transferred along with lessening the plantar flexion strength of the Achilles tendon by tenectomy (removing 2–3 cm of the tendon). The patient should be placed in a slight dorsiflexion rigid dressing for 6 weeks to prevent equinus deformity. By this simple method, skin problems, pressure irritation, and pain associated with excessive weight on the end of the stump are largely eliminated.
- *Hindfoot amputations:*
    - Syme amputation and Sarmiento modification (described below in Answer to Question 133)

- The Boyd amputation eliminates the problem of posterior migration of the heel pad. In Boyd's amputation talectomy, forward shift of the calcaneus and calcaneotibial arthrodesis are performed. The arthrodesis makes the procedure bit more difficult than the Syme amputation and results in a bulbous stump. It needs a dedicated prosthesis that is cosmetically acceptable.
- The Pirogoff amputation is technically more difficult and offers no advantage over Boyd's amputation.

129. Write short notes on:
A. Mangled extremity severity score (MESS) score
B. GANGA score.

Ans:

A. Several attempts have been made to evaluate injuries better and identify injury patterns that would best be treated by early amputation. Whether a limb should be reconstructed or amputated is decided by severity of injury, expertise of the surgeon, available resources, and socioeconomic status of the patient. Reconstruction has advantages like original limb is saved, but having disadvantages of long rehabilitation, prolonged hospital stay, economic burden, repeated operations, and difficulties to family. Amputation has advantages like early return to work, lifesaving procedure sometimes and economical relief, but having disadvantages of loss of limb and psychological trauma. It is generally decided by MESS (**Box 2.6.1**). MESS more than 7 means poor limb viability prognosis and limb should be amputated. Helfet et al. reported retrospective and prospective evaluations of the MESS and found it to be useful when combined with the experience and clinical acumen of the surgeon.

Box 2.6.1: Mangled extremity severity score.

Skeletal/soft-tissue injury:
- Low energy (stab, simple fracture, and pistol gunshot wound): 1
- Medium energy (open or multiple fractures and dislocation): 2
- High energy (high speed MVA or rifle GSW): 3
- Very high energy (high speed trauma + gross contamination): 4

Limb ischemia:
- Pulse reduced or absent but perfusion normal: 1*
- Pulseless; paresthesias and diminished capillary refill: 2
- Cool, paralyzed, insensate, and numb: 3*

Shock:
- Systolic BP always >90 mm Hg: 0
- Hypotensive transiently: 1
- Persistent hypotension: 2

Age (years):
<30: 0
30–50: 1
>50: 2

Note: *Score doubled for ischemia >6 hours
Score: >7 = correlated well with primary amputation
(MVA: motor vehicle accident; GSW: gunshot wound)

B. Please read Chapter no. 3.

130. Define mangled extremity.

Ans: A mangled extremity is defined as a limb that has sustained an injury involving at least three out of four key systems:
1. Soft tissue
2. Bone
3. Nerves
4. Vessels

This type of injury is often caused by severe trauma such as motor vehicle crashes, industrial accidents, or combat injuries, and can result in significant damage to the limb, potentially threatening its viability. The management of a mangled extremity requires prompt and coordinated care from multiple specialties, including trauma, orthopedic, vascular, and plastic surgery, to determine whether the limb can be salvaged or if amputation is necessary.

131. **How will you transport organ after amputation to a sterilized center for reimplantation? What is the order of implantation in a below elbow amputation?**

Ans: (poorly framed question—center needs to be sterilized?, rather it should be transportation to center in a sterile manner). The amputated part should be transported to the destined center in a sterile manner with the injured person. In general, the amputated part should be wrapped in a clean cloth (ideal is a sterile gauge or mop), covered fully all around. This wrapping should be placed in an air-sealed clean polybag (sterile ideally) or a waterproof container. Now place the polybag in an ice cold water solution. Do not place it directly in contact with ice. If the journey is long, exchanges of cold water can be done in between taking care that the water does not enter into polybag or container. In ideal situations if possible, clean the amputated part by washing thoroughly with sterile saline solution to remove gross contamination of soil/dirt and foreign bodies before packing. Packing should be done in as aseptic manner as possible.

Order of implantation:
Mnemonic: BE FAN of VS (Virender Sehwag)
B—bone
E—extensor tendons
F—flexor tendons
A—artery
N—nerve
V—vein
S—skin

132. **A. Describe the principles and steps of "Post traumatic Thumb Reimplantation surgery".**
  B. Explain the correct method of transport of the "amputated part" to the reimplantation center.
  C. What are the contraindications for such reimplantation?

Ans: A. Principles and Steps of Post-Traumatic Thumb Reimplantation Surgery **Principles:** Thumb reimplantation is a microsurgical procedure to restore a traumatically amputated thumb, critical for hand function due to the thumb's role in grip and opposition. The principles include:

- *Restoration of function:* Reattach the thumb to restore length, sensation, and mobility.
- *Microvascular repair:* Reestablish blood flow via arterial and venous anastomosis to ensure viability.
- *Structural integrity:* Stabilize bones, tendons, and nerves to optimize functional recovery.
- *Minimize ischemia:* Limit warm ischemia time (<6 hours ideal, up to 12 hours viable) to prevent tissue necrosis.
- *Infection prevention:* Thorough debridement and antibiotic prophylaxis to reduce infection risk.
- *Rehabilitation:* Early motion and therapy to prevent stiffness and maximize function.

Indications:
- Clean or moderately contaminated thumb amputations [distal to metacarpophalangeal joint (MCPJ) or proximal].
- Young, healthy patients with good rehabilitation potential.
- Amputated part in viable condition (not crushed or severely mangled).

Contraindications:
- Severe crush or avulsion injuries with extensive tissue damage
- Prolonged ischemia (>12 hours warm and >24 hours cold)
- Comorbidities (e.g., uncontrolled diabetes, vascular disease) or poor patient compliance

Steps of thumb reimplantation surgery:
1. *Preoperative preparation:*
   - *Assessment:* Evaluate amputation level (distal/proximal to MCPJ), injury mechanism, and condition of the amputated part (stored in saline-soaked gauze, cooled at 4°C, not frozen).
   - *Imaging:* X-rays of stump and amputated part to assess bone damage.

- *Patient optimization:* Administer IV antibiotics (e.g., cefazolin), tetanus prophylaxis, and ensure hemodynamic stability.
- *Consent:* Discuss risks (failure, infection, and stiffness) and need for rehabilitation.

2. *Debridement and preparation:*
   - Under general or regional anesthesia, clean and debride the proximal stump and amputated thumb to remove devitalized tissue.
   - Identify and tag key structures (arteries, veins, nerves, and tendons) under loupe magnification or microscope.
   - Shorten bone ends minimally to ensure clean, viable surfaces for fixation.
3. *Bone fixation*:
   - Stabilize the proximal and distal phalanges using:
     - Kirschner wires (K-wires) for simple fixation
     - Mini-plates/screws for complex fractures or proximal amputations
   - Ensure proper length and alignment to restore thumb anatomy.
   - Avoid excessive shortening to preserve function.
4. *Microvascular repair:*
   - *Arterial anastomosis:* Repair one or both digital arteries (usually radial or ulnar digital artery) using microsutures (8-0/9-0 nylon) under an operating microscope.
     - Ensure patent flow; vein grafts may be needed for vessel defects.
   - *Venous anastomosis:* Repair 1–2 dorsal veins to prevent congestion; critical for graft survival.
   - Confirm perfusion (pink color, capillary refill <2 seconds) after anastomosis.
5. *Nerve repair:*
   - Coapt digital nerves (radial and ulnar) using epineural microsutures (9-0/10-0 nylon) to restore sensation.
   - Nerve grafts (e.g., sural nerve) may be used for gaps >1 cm.
   - Prioritize sensory restoration for functional recovery.
6. *Tendon repair:*
   - Repair flexor pollicis longus (FPL) and extensor pollicis longus (EPL) using strong core sutures (e.g., 4-0 nonabsorbable and Kessler technique).
   - Ensure proper tension to allow early motion without gap formation.
7. *Soft-tissue and skin closure:*
   - Reapproximate soft tissues (muscle, fascia) to cover repaired structures.
   - Close skin loosely to avoid tension; use skin grafts or flaps if needed for coverage.
   - Ensure no compression on vascular repairs.
8. *Postoperative care*:
   - *Monitoring:* Observe for perfusion (color, warmth, and pulse oximetry) every 1–2 hours for 48 hours.
   - *Anticoagulation:* Aspirin (75–150 mg/day) or heparin (low-dose) to prevent thrombosis.
   - *Antibiotics:* Continue IV antibiotics (e.g., cefazolin) for 5–7 days.
   - *Immobilization:* Splint in functional position (thumb abducted, MCPJ flexed) for 3–4 weeks.
   - *Rehabilitation:* Begin gentle active motion at 1–2 weeks, guided by hand therapy to prevent stiffness; full rehabilitation over 3–6 months.

B. The correct method of transport of an amputated part for reimplantation:

Principles:
- The goal is to prevent desiccation, minimize contamination, and slow tissue metabolism to prolong ischemia tolerance.
- Cooling is essential — but direct contact with ice must be avoided to prevent frostbite injury.

Step-by-step method:
1. *Gentle handling:*
   - Pick up the amputated part carefully, holding only skin or soft tissue edges — avoid crushing.
2. *Rinse:*
   - Rinse briefly with sterile saline to remove gross contaminants (do not scrub).

3. *Wrap:*
   - Wrap the part in saline-moistened sterile gauze to maintain humidity.
4. *Seal:*
   - Place the wrapped part in a sterile, watertight plastic bag.
5. *Cold environment:*
   - Place the sealed bag inside a second container (e.g., another plastic bag or box) filled with a mixture of ice and water — or in a cool box.
   - Important: The amputated tissue must not directly touch ice — indirect cooling prevents ice-burn.
6. *Transport:*
   - Send with the patient to the reimplantation center as quickly as possible.
   - Maintain temperature at 4°C (refrigerator temperature).
   - Do not freeze the part.

C. Contraindications for Reimplantation of an Amputated Part:
1. *General contraindications:*
   - Life-threatening injuries requiring urgent stabilization (patient survival takes priority over limb salvage)
   - Severe systemic disease or unstable medical condition (e.g., uncontrolled diabetes, severe cardiac disease)
   - Advanced age with poor functional prognosis
   - Psychiatric illness or poor compliance likely to affect rehabilitation
2. *Absolute local contraindications:*
   - Prolonged warm ischemia time beyond tolerance:
     – Muscle-containing segments: >6 hours
     – Digits: >12 hours (warm), >24 hours (cold)
   - Severe crush injury with extensive soft tissue, vessel, and nerve destruction
   - Segmental amputation with multiple tissue level injuries (poor viability)
   - Massive contamination with high infection risk (e.g., farm machinery injuries)
   - Avulsion injuries with long nerve gap and poor reinnervation potential
3. *Relative contraindications:*
   - Multiple level injuries in the same extremity
   - Severe associated injuries in the ipsilateral limb (may compromise rehabilitation)
   - Poor tissue quality (elderly, vascular disease, chronic smoker)
   - Lack of microsurgical expertise or facility within ischemia time limit

133. What is Syme amputation? Describe indications and complications. What is the prosthesis suitable for Syme amputation?

Ans: *Syme amputation:* This involves disarticulation at the ankle joint. It is the amputation of choice in children as it leaves the distal tibial epiphysis intact. The anterior incision is at the level of the ankle joint and the posterior flap is kept longer so that the heel pad is mobilized anteriorly to the distal tibia. Anterior tibial vessels are ligated and care is taken not to damage the posterior tibial vessels. Calcaneum is removed by sharp dissection from the heel pad. The blood supply to the heel pad must be carefully preserved. Both the malleoli are resected at the level of the dome of talus. This cut must be taken parallel to the ground and not at 90° to the tibial plane. The heel pad is mobilized over distal stump of tibia and can be stabilized by one of the following methods:
- By attaching the extensor tendons to the flap
- By tying the flap to the bone by drilling holes
- By fixing the pad by K-wires
- By leaving a sliver of calcaneum attached which fuses to the tibia.

Skin tags left after the procedure should not be removed as it compromises the supply of the heel pad. They disappear as the stump matures. A special bulky prosthesis needs to be worn to accommodate the distal tibial flare. Though this prosthesis is not aesthetic, it provides a better ambulation than a transtibial amputation.

"Sarmiento's modification" of Syme amputation partially reduces this complication by trimming tibia 1.3 cm from the ankle joint, thus reducing the distal radial flare.

Indications:
- Unsalvageable foot trauma
- Infections of foot
- Tumors
- Limb deformities when foot cannot be saved as in children, e.g., paraxial fibular hemimelia.

Prosthesis: The chief objection to this amputation is cosmetic. The prosthesis used must accommodate the flare of the distal tibial metaphysis that is covered with heavy plantar skin and is large and bulky. For this reason, the amputation usually is not recommended for women. The prosthesis used for a classic Syme amputation consists of a molded plastic socket, with a removable medial window to allow passage of the bulbous end of the stump through its narrow shank, and a solid-ankle, cushioned-heel (SACH) foot prosthesis.

In the past, most surgeons did not use the Syme amputation for ischemic limbs because the failure rate of wound healing was unacceptably high. More recently, preoperative determination of local tissue perfusion and oxygenation by such techniques as Doppler ultrasound measurement of segmental blood pressures, radioactive xenon clearance tests, and transcutaneous oxygen measurements has significantly increased the success rate of the Syme amputation in these limbs.

134. Discuss principle of Syme amputation.

Ans: *Principles:*
- Preservation of adequate length of residual limb and distal tibial physeal plate to retain growth and limb-lengthening potential in children.
- Bone must be divided where its cross-section area is as great as possible to provide greatest area of support—this is achieved by retaining as much of the subarticular cancellous bone as possible.
- Providing end-bearing durable stump and preserved proprioception in the prosthesis by heel pad preservation.
- Prevention of heel pad by firm anchoring to soft tissue and bone.
- *General principles (as applied to all amputations):*
  - Prompt uncomplicated wound healing—disarticulations are better for infected limbs
  - Control of edema
  - Postoperative pain control
  - Prevention of joint contractures
  - Rapid rehabilitation

135. What are the merits and demerits of Syme amputation?

Ans: Merits:
- Full lower leg segment allows for greater quad triceps leverage
- Minimal prosthetic training
- Lower energy cost
- Higher velocity
- Greater stride length
- If done meticulously, it is the best amputation to be done at this level.

Demerits:
- Technically more difficult than below knee amputation
- Potential for delayed wound healing in patients with marginal blood flow at ankle level
- Potential for heel dislocation, but minimized by securing heel pad
- Cosmetic appearance, if large, redundant bulbous stump made
- Heel pain
- Neuroma formation
- Hypermobility of stump
- Has to be done in two stages in diabetic patients and patients with infection of heel pad.

136. What are biomechanics and clinical uses of floor reaction orthosis?

Ans: Floor reaction orthosis is a polyvinyl chloride (PVC)/plastic-molded assistive device that is customized for use in patients with weak ankle plantiflexors commonly. The device usually covers foot and ankle completely with extension partly up the calf (ankle foot orthosis).

The unique principle of its working is utilization of reaction force developed from contact with floor transmitted through toe aspect of foot plate to prevent forward tibial progression and subsequent knee collapse. The floor-reaction principle was initially used in patellar tendon-bearing, knee-locking ankle-foot orthosis for paralytic disability in children with cerebral palsy (CP) developing crouch deformity/gait.

Indications: Calf muscle and ankle plantar flexion weakness due to any cause with knee buckling during walk. Most commonly, it is used in neurological conditions like:
- Spina bifida
- Cerebral palsy
- Brain injury
- Spinal cord injury
- Postpolio paralysis.

The floor reaction ankle foot orthosis (FRAFO) maintains the affected joints in proper alignment and forces knee extension at midstance phase of gait, along with compensating for weak or absent gastrocsoleus (calf) muscles.

Presently, there are several designs of FRAFOs:
- *One piece:* Encloses the back of the lower calf, the shin, and bottom of the foot.
- *Two piece:* Same as the one piece but has a removable anterior (front) panel.
- *Rear opening:* Encloses the front of the leg and top of the foot. It may be articulated.

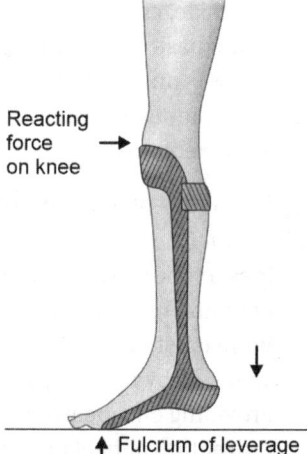

Fig. 2.6.1: Ground reaction force on knee.

Principle of action of a floor reaction orthosis:
- Based on Newton's third law of motion—during stance, the sum of the body weight and the acceleration of the center of mass acting downward create an equal and opposite reaction force acting upward. This is known as the ground reaction force (GRF) **(Fig. 2.6.1)**.
- *The GRF has three components:* Vertical, lateral, and progressional shear GRF. The latter two are small compared to vertical GRF.
- If the GRF passes at a distance from the center of a joint, it creates a turning effect known as an external moment. The size of this moment (m) depends on the magnitude of the force (f) and its perpendicular distance from the joint (d), i.e., $m = f \times d$. Normally, the external moment caused by knee flexion is well resisted by opposing extension moment created by the quadriceps. If quadriceps fails or is weak then knee buckles.
- To partly also compensate for quadriceps weakness (power >1/5 less than 5/5), if the GRF is far anterior from the joint (i.e., 'd' in the equation is large), the external moment it creates will be large creating posterior push at the knee while the brace maintains plantar flexion at the ankle. Thus, a stable extended leg is created provided the posterior capsule at knee is competent.
- *Floor reaction ankle foot orthoses in children with spastic diplegic CP:* FRAFO use produces significant kinematic gait improvements including a reduction of abnormal ankle dorsiflexion and knee flexion motion.

Wearing schedule:
Begin with a wearing time of 1 hour for initial check that the orthosis fit is good and no undue pressure points are there that would later cause pressure sores/ulcers. If the orthosis fits well, keep increasing the wear time daily so that by 7–10 days it can be worn throughout the day. Keep inspecting the skin after every use so that the orthosis fits well and needs no changes for causing excessive pressure sores.

Functions:
- To maintain the affected joints in proper alignment
- To accentuate knee extension at midstance
- Compensate for weak or absent gastrocsoleus (calf) muscles

- Limiting the ankle dorsiflexion in the single support and consequently improving knee extension.
- Floor reaction ankle foot orthosis limits the second rocker, improves knee extension, and consequently increases knee external extension moment.
- Effective to improve the extension of the knees and ankle in the stance of children with spastic CP. The FRAFO is commonly prescribed in the attempt to decrease knee flexion during the stance phase in the CP gait.

Limitations:
- Floor reaction ankle foot orthosis will not improve kinematics if knee or hip flexion is a fixed deformity. Whenever possible, fixed deformities should be corrected prior to bracing for the principle of coupling to be effective.
- Quadriceps power <2/3.
- Angular deformities of foot ankle and tibia.

Advantages over other above knee orthosis:
- Light weight
- Swing phase is not labored
- Floor reaction prevents knee from buckling
- Small training time
- Stabilizes knee without muscle action
- Ground clearance is easier
- Good patient compliance
- Cosmetically acceptable—can be worn under shoe.

137. What is Jaipur foot?

Ans: It is an indigenous transtibial prosthesis created in 1968 by Dr PK Sethi and Ram Chandra Sharma at the Department of Orthopedics at Sawai Man Singh Medical College in Jaipur, Rajasthan. It was created as a substitute for the solid ankle cushion heel (SACH) foot to suit certain local requirements and to reduce cost. The objectives were to create a low-cost, low-maintenance prosthesis that was durable, waterproof, could be used without foot wear, could be made from locally available material and allow squatting and walking on uneven terrain.

The Jaipur foot is a nonarticulated foot-ankle assembly. It consists of three structural blocks. The forefoot and hind foot are made of rubber and the ankle block is of light wood. These three blocks along with the toes are bound together and encapsulated in skin-colored compound.

It permits the following range of motion:
- Dorsiflexion: 20–35°
- Heel compression: 8–2.8 mm
- Pronation: 26–29°
- Supination: 15–22°
- Axial internal rotation: 11–12°
- Axial external rotation: 4–8°

The socket was initially a plug fit design made from aluminum, but now it is made using a molded total contact sockets. Though it is widely used in India and in other developing and underdeveloped countries, it has not found wide acceptance in the developed world because of the following disadvantages:
- It is not available in international standard sizes.
- It is not compatible with designs of western limbs.
- It is heavier than the set international standards.
- It does not come with quality assurance and standard certification.

138. Describe features and use of SACH foot.

Ans: Features of the SACH Foot: The SACH (Solid Ankle Cushion Heel) foot is a type of nonenergy-returning prosthetic foot designed for individuals with lower limb amputations. Its construction and characteristics include:
- *No true ankle joint:* The SACH foot does not have a functional ankle joint but includes a simulated joint achieved through a compressed, wedge-shaped rubber heel.

- *Solid keel:* It comprises a solid wooden keel that provides stability and support during ambulation.
- *Rubber composition:*
  - High-density rubber at the dorsum (upper surface) for durability.
  - Low-density rubber for the toes and plantar aspect (bottom surface), facilitating a smooth transition from toe-off to heel strike.
  - Variable density rubber is used in the heel to provide cushioning.
- *Impact absorption:* The design absorbs the impact during heel strike, reducing stress on the limb.
- *Vertical excursion control:* It minimizes vertical excursion of the center of gravity, which contributes to more stable walking patterns.
- *Simulated metatarsal movement:* The design allows for some simulated movement of the metatarsal heads, enhancing walking dynamics.
- *Rigidity:* The forefoot remains rigid, which provides an anterior lever arm for effective propulsion during gait as well as proprioceptive feedback.
- *Low-cost and low-maintenance:* The SACH foot is economical and requires minimal upkeep, making it an ideal choice for many users.
- *Energy consumption:* Though it is effective for smooth gait, it consumes more energy in comparison to energy-returning prosthetic feet, which may limit its use in more active individuals.
- *Terrain limitations:* The SACH foot can be challenging to use on uneven surfaces due to its rigid forefoot and lack of flexibility.

Uses of the SACH foot: The SACH foot is predominantly used in the following contexts—
1. *Common prosthetic foot:* It is widely utilized with hip prostheses, especially for individuals with limited mobility or those who are sedentary, due to its stability and user-friendly design.
2. *Rehabilitation:* The SACH foot is often recommended during the initial stages of rehabilitation because of its simplicity and ease of use.
3. *Everyday activities:* Suitable for low-impact activities and daily tasks, making it a practical choice for non-active users.

139. A. Differentiate between SACH foot and Jaipur foot.
   B. Write note on bionic hand.

Ans:

A. Difference has been shown in **Table 2.6.1**.

TABLE 2.6.1: Difference between SACH foot and Jaipur foot.

S. no.	Jaipur foot	SACH foot
1.	Appearance similar to normal foot	Dissimilar to normal foot
2.	It can be worn without shoe but if someone wishes to wear one, he can use a flat heel shoe	It requires a closed shoe to protect and hide it
3.	No restriction of movements at ankle as the metallic keel (carriage bolt) is confined to ankle only and all movements take place at natural site	Solid ankle consisting of long wooden keel restricts movements in nearly all directions
4.	Squatting possible (dorsiflexion adequate)	Not possible
5.	Cross-legged sitting is possible (adequate forefoot adduction and internal rotation possible)	Not possible
6.	Walking on uneven ground possible (good inversion and eversion)	Suitable for walking only on level ground
7.	Barefoot walking possible (cosmetic skin color, and no heel and toe height difference)	Not possible

(SACH: solid-ankle and cushioned-heel)

B. *Bionic hand:* These are externally powered prostheses. Motors and batteries can be used to operate these prostheses and they provide better proximal function and better grip. Their disadvantages are that they are heavy, expensive, and difficult to maintain. Also, they have minimal sensory feedback.

These prostheses can be controlled by either "myoelectric or switch control". In myoelectric control muscle contractions are used as a signal to move the prosthesis. Surface electrodes are used to detect the electrical activity generated by muscle without gross movement taking place in the muscle.

Different switch systems exist:
- The two-site/two-function (dual-site) system has separate electrodes for separate prosthetic activity, such as flexion/extension or pronation/supination, and is easier to control.
- But when limited control sites are available on the residual limb, a one-site/two-function (single-site) device may be used. This system uses one electrode to control two functions of a paired activity (e.g., flexion and extension); the patient uses contractions of different strengths to differentiate between flexion and extension (e.g., a strong contraction opens the device and a weak contraction closes it).
- Sometimes multiple powered components on a single prosthesis must be controlled by a single switch, (e.g., terminal device and elbow activation) using sequential or multistate controller. The electrode function can be switched from one to another either by an external switch or by a brief contraction of the muscle.
- In "switch-controlled" prostheses, there are switches in the socket or in the suspension harness of the prosthesis. These switches are activated by the movement of a remnant part or by pull on harness. They are used in those patients who are unable to control myoelectric points or if such points are not available.
- The speed or force generated in the prosthesis can be varied by changing the intensity of muscle contraction.

140. **A. Enumerate different designs of prosthetic feet in a below knee prosthesis.**
B. Describe their advantages, disadvantages and indications.

Ans: Prosthetic foot designs for below-knee (transtibial) amputees

1. *SACH Foot (Solid Ankle Cushioned Heel)*

Design:
- Solid ankle with a cushioned heel wedge (usually rubber)
- No moving parts

Advantages:
- Simple and durable
- Low cost
- Good shock absorption at heel strike
- Low maintenance

Disadvantages:
- No energy return or dynamic response
- Limited adaptability to uneven terrain
- Stiff during push-off

Indications:
- Low-activity users (elderly and limited ambulators)
- Temporary prostheses
- Developing countries with budget constraints

2. *Single-Axis Foot*

Design:
- Mechanical ankle joint allowing plantarflexion/dorsiflexion
- Often includes bumper for shock absorption

Advantages:
- Better stability than SACH during stance phase
- Controlled motion reduces knee strain
- Moderate energy absorption

Disadvantages:
- Heavier than SACH
- Limited transverse plane motion
- Requires periodic bumper replacement

Indications:
- Users needing enhanced stability (e.g., peripheral neuropathy)
- Early rehabilitation phases

3. *Multi-Axis Foot*

Design:
- Allows motion in three planes (sagittal, frontal, and transverse)
- Often uses elastomeric bumpers or hydraulic mechanisms

Advantages:
- Excellent shock absorption
- Adapts to uneven terrain
- Reduces torque on residual limb

Disadvantages:
- Higher cost than SACH/single-axis
- Increased maintenance
- Slightly heavier

Indications:
- Active users walking on varied terrain
- Amputees with joint degeneration (reduces proximal joint stress)

4. *Energy-Storing/Return (ESR) Feet*

Design:
- Carbon fiber or composite keel stores/releases energy
- Examples: Seattle Foot®, Carbon Copy®, Össur Flex-Foot®

Advantages:
- Excellent energy return (improves gait efficiency)
- Lightweight
- Dynamic response for active users

Disadvantages:
- Expensive
- Requires proper alignment for optimal function
- May feel unstable for new users

Indications:
- Active adults and younger amputees
- Sports participation (running, jumping)

5. *Microprocessor-Controlled Feet*

Design:
- Computerized ankle with sensors and actuators
- *Examples:* Össur Pro-Flex® and Ottobock Empower®

Advantages:
- Real-time adaptation to slopes/stairs
- Reduces stumble risk
- Optimizes energy efficiency

Disadvantages:
- Very high cost
- Requires charging/maintenance
- Heavier than ESR feet

Indications:
- K3-K4 ambulators (community walkers)
- Users with variable activity demands

6. *Waterproof/Specialty Feet*

Design:
- Corrosion-resistant materials (stainless steel and special coatings)

Advantages:
- Can be submerged in water
- Resists sand/salt damage

Disadvantages:
- Often heavier
- Limited dynamic features

Indications:
- Aquatic activities
- Military/harsh environments

7. *Sports-Specific Feet*

Design:
- Specialized for running (blades) or high-impact activities
- *Examples:* Össur Cheetah®, and Fillauer All-Pro®

Advantages:
- Maximum energy return for sports
- Lightweight

Disadvantages:
- Not suitable for daily walking
- Very expensive

Indications:
- Competitive athletes
- Recreational sports participation

141. What is myoelectric prosthesis? What are its components? Enumerate the applications and advantages.

Ans: Kindly refer Answer to Question 139 of part "B" above.

142. Write disadvantages of myoelectric prosthesis.

Ans: The following are some disadvantages of myoelectric prosthesis:
- Heaviest
- Slower response time
- Expensive
- Frequent maintenance
- Battery dependent
- Less durable and nonwaterproof
- Longer training period

143. Principle of myoelectric prosthesis in upper limb.

Ans: Kindly see the Answers to Questions above.

2.7 SURGICAL APPROACHES IN ORTHOPEDICS (Q144–152)

144. Discuss surgical anatomy of Ganz approach to the hip with indications.

Ans: By definition, Ganz approach preserves blood supply to the femoral head maximally while also allowing repair of the hip joint pathology. It allows safe dislocation of the joint without jeopardizing blood supply and completing joint reconstruction or preservation procedures with minimal morbidity.

Superficial dissection:
- The posterior border of gluteus medius is only identified but neither mobilized nor retracted to view the piriformis.
- The trochanteric fine vascular plexus is cauterized superficially to minimize bleeding.
- Small length incision is made along the posterosuperior edge of greater trochanter that extends distally to the posterior border of the vastus ridge to expose the trochanter and identify landmarks for trochanteric osteotomy.

Deep tissue dissection:
- Mark the tip of greater trochanter, region of piriformis fossa, and vastus ridge.
- A trochanteric flip osteotomy is done (see osteotomies around the hip) protecting the profundus branch of the medial circumflex femoral artery (MCFA) at the soft spot where it becomes intracapsular to supply the ascending lateral retinacular vessels at the level of the superior gemellus muscle.
- The greater trochanteric fragment is translated anteriorly after releasing at posterior border the tendon of gluteus maximus and inserting posterior fibers of gluteus medius.
- To ease external rotation at hip the vastus lateralis and intermedius muscles are elevated from the lateral and anterior aspects of the proximal femur.
- Next, the inferior border of gluteus minimus is separated from the relaxed piriformis.
- One should protect and retract the sciatic nerve from getting injured as the piriformis is mobilized.
- After anterior flip of the fragment with attached medius and vastus lateralis, the gluteus minimus is retracted anteriorly and superiorly to expose the superior capsule.
- To further enhance exposure to anterior, superior, and posterosuperior capsule, the leg can be further flexed and externally rotated.
- Hip joint capsule is then incised in a straight line along the long axis of the femoral neck anterolaterally as this zone is relatively watershed/avascular and avoids the deep branch of the MCFA. The incision is extended distally in the anteroinferior capsular along the base of femoral neck.
- It is important that this vertical limb of osteotomy remains anterior to the lesser trochanter to avoid damaging the main branch of the MCFA. The artery lies here just superior and posterior to lesser trochanter.
- The anterior and inferior half of the labrum can be well visualized, once the anteroinferior flap of capsule is reflected.
- After completing capsulotomy, the hip joint is dislocated by flexion, externally rotating the leg and bringing it over the front of the operating table. The leg can be placed in a sterile bag allowing inspection of most of the acetabulum.
- After completion of the procedure, greater trochanter is reattached using two or three cancellous screws or better cerclage wire.

Indications:
- Femoral head fractures (Pipkin fractures)
  - *Complex femoroacetabular impingement (FAI) deformities:*
  - Repairing of acetabular labrum
  - Reshaping the bony acetabular rim (acetabuloplasty)
  - Removing bony bumps (cam lesions) on femoral head (femoral osteoplasty)
- *Correction of major structural abnormalities of the hip joint:*
  - Reduction osteotomy (intraosseous and head splitting) of femoral head in Perthes
  - A deformed femoral head as seen in Perthes disease (cheilectomy)
  - Slipped upper femoral epiphysis (SUFE)—intra-articular osteotomy of femoral neck.
- *Articular cartilage defect reconstruction:* Autologous cartilage implantation (ACI) and matrix autologous chondrocyte implantation (MACI)

- Loose body removal in fracture dislocation of hip
- Posttraumatic hip deformities
- Hip arthrodesis
- *Other conditions:* Includes
    - Rheumatoid synovitis
    - Synovial chondromatosis
    - Pigmented villonodular synovitis.

145. Describe arthrography. Discuss the various approaches to aspirate the hip joint.

Ans: Arthrography is a particularly useful form of contrast radiography. Intra-articular loose bodies will produce filling defects in the opaque contrast medium. In the knee, torn menisci, ligament tears, and capsular ruptures can be shown. In children's hips, arthrography is a useful method of outlining the cartilaginous (and therefore radiolucent) femoral head. In adults with avascular necrosis of the femoral head, arthrography may show up torn flaps of cartilage. After hip replacement, loosening of a prosthesis may be revealed by seepage of the contrast medium into the cement/bone interface. In the hip, ankle, wrist, and shoulder, the injected contrast medium may disclose labral tears or defects in the capsular structures.

Various approaches:
A lateral, anterior, or medial approach can be used to aspirate the hip joint.

- *Lateral:* Insert the needle at a 45° angle with the surface of the thigh just inferior and anterior to the greater trochanter. Advance the needle medially and proximally close to the bone for 5–10 cm, depending on the size of the patient and into the joint.
- *Anterior:* Palpate the femoral artery in line with the inguinal ligament. Insert the needle 2.5 cm lateral and 2.5 cm distal to this point at a 45° angle to the skin surface. Advance the needle 5–7.5 cm medially and proximally into the joint.
- *Medial:* Flex and abduct the leg; this is usually a more comfortable position for patients with septic arthritis. Place the needle inferior to the adductor longus tendon, and using image intensification, advance it in a plane below the palpated femoral artery until the femoral head or neck is reached and aspirate the joint.

146. Discuss Bryan–Morrey approach (triceps reflecting approach) to elbow.

Ans: Bryan–Morrey developed a modified posterior approach to the elbow joint that provides excellent exposure and preserves the continuity of the triceps mechanism, which allows easy repair and rapid rehabilitation.

- Place the patient in the lateral decubitus position. Place the limb across the chest.
- Make a straight posterior incision in the midline of the limb extending from 7 cm distal to the tip of the olecranon to 9 cm proximal to it.
- Identify the ulnar nerve proximally and dissect it free from its tunnel distally to its first motor branch.
- Elevate the medial aspect of the triceps from the humerus, along the intermuscular septum, to the level of the posterior capsule.
- Incise the superficial fascia of the forearm distally for about 6 cm to the periosteum of the medial aspect of the olecranon.
- Carefully reflect as a single unit the periosteum and fascia medially to laterally. The medial part of the junction between the triceps insertion and the superficial fascia and the periosteum of the ulna is the weakest portion of the reflected tissue.
- Carefully dissect the triceps tendon from the olecranon when the elbow is extended to 20–30° to relieve tension on the tissues, and then reflect the remaining portion of the triceps mechanism. Modification has been suggested to take sliver of bone along with this flap from olecranon.
- To expose the radial head, reflect the anconeus subperiosteally from the proximal ulna; the entire joint is now widely exposed.
- The posterior capsule usually is reflected with the triceps mechanism, and the tip of the olecranon may be resected to expose the trochlea clearly.
- To attain joint retraction in total joint arthroplasty, release the medial collateral ligament from the humerus, if necessary.
- Return the triceps to its anatomical position and suture it directly to the bone through holes drilled in the proximal aspect of the ulna.

- Suture the periosteum to the superficial forearm fascia, as far as the margin of the flexor carpi ulnaris.
- Close the wound in layers, and leave a drain in the wound. In total joint arthroplasty, dress the elbow with the joint flexed about 60° to avoid direct pressure on the wound by the olecranon tip.

147. Describe the modified Stoppa approach for acetabulum fractures. Describe the classification of brachial plexus injuries.

Ans: *Modified Stoppa approach:*

Initially described as Cole and Bolhofner (for limited approach through a transverse midline Pfannenstiel incision in the hernia repair as an anterior intrapelvic approach).

Now modified into limited intrapelvic approach or as an extension to the traditional ilioinguinal. For acetabular fractures, this approach offers good visualization of:
- True pelvic rim
- Quadrilateral plate
- Management and reduction of significant protrusion.

General description of approach:
- The Stoppa modification requires the hemipelvis and hind limb on the affected side to be draped free.
- The standard ilioinguinal approach, which is 2 cm proximal to the pubic symphysis at the midline, is extended across the midline in slight cephalad curve (3 cm across midline) as it proceeds toward the contralateral hip.
- Medial to the third window of the ilioinguinal approach is to identify rectus insertion on the pubic tubercle and split it vertically along the linea alba up to 5 cm above the pubic symphysis (taking care to remain extraperitoneal at the proximal extension). Tag the medial and lateral edges of this hemirectus insertion. Rectus insertion is then divided, with a small cuff tissue left to facilitate repair.
- Malleable retractor is used to protect the bladder.
- Inspecting the fracture from opposite side allows the surgeon to "look back" inside the true pelvis from the contralateral side.
- Along the lateral border of the rectus, inferior epigastric or external iliac vessels are identified and must be ligated.
- Any anastomotic connection (corona mortis) between inferior epigastric or external iliac and obturator vessels, if present, must also be ligated.
- Flexion of the hip on ipsilateral side reduces tension on the iliopsoas, femoral nerve, and external iliac vessels to allow better access to the upper pelvis and iliac wing.
- Being exclusively extra-articular, no direct visualization of the joint can be accomplished.

Advantage: Further exposure of the iliopectineal (pelvic brim) and obturator fascia and the quadrilateral plate are afforded by this modification, especially in obese patients.

Precautions:
- Dissection of the external vessels must be undertaken with care.
- Obturator nerve must be visualized and respected.
- Care must be taken not to extend too proximal or to become intraperitoneal with the approach.
- Posterior retraction must also be careful to avoid the lumbosacral trunk.

Closure is performed over drains. A drain is placed in the space of Retzius as with a standard ilioinguinal approach. Large diameter nonabsorbable sutures are used to repair the medial and lateral aspects of the rectus origin from the affected side. Interrupted figure of eight nonabsorbable sutures are used to repair the midline split of the linea alba.

Classification of brachial plexus injury: Many classifications of brachial plexus injuries exist, with the most familiar distinguishing between upper plexus injuries (Erb) and lower plexus injuries (Klumpke). Leffert classified brachial plexus injuries according to mechanism and level of injury.

The *upper trunk* of the brachial plexus (C5 and C6) is most frequently injured, resulting in Erb palsy, which is characterized by the "waiter's tip" posture. It has following components:
- Weak abductors and external rotators of the shoulder + weak flexors and supinators of the elbow + weak radial extensors

- Good power in internal rotators and adductors of shoulder + elbow extensors and wrist flexors (all supplied by the middle trunk and C7)
- Sensory loss occurs over the outer aspect of the arm and forearm.

Pure lower plexus injuries: Klumpke palsy (C8 to T1), involving only the lower trunk.

These injuries may cause claw hands, drop wrists, and severe loss of hand function. Sensation is lost in the ulnar forearm and hand. There may be unilateral Horner's syndrome.

148. Discuss the approaches to radius.

Ans: The various approaches to radius are as follows:
- *Approach to the radial head and neck:* Kocher approach (posterolateral approach, plane between anconeus and extensor carpi ulnaris), Kaplan approach (interval between the extensor carpi radialis brevis and extensor digitorum communis), and Wrightington approach (modified posterior approach, osteotomy through the supinator tuberosity to detach the fragment attached to annular ligament).
- *Anterior approach to access bicipital tuberosity*/radial neck/metaphysis.
- *Approach to the proximal and middle thirds of the posterior surface:* Thompson approach.
- *Anterolateral approach to the proximal shaft and elbow joint:* Henry approach.
- *Anterior approach to the distal half of the radius:* Modified Henry approach (plane between flexor carpi radialis tendon and the radial artery), Henry approach (between brachioradialis and the radial artery), and more ulnar extensile approach to simultaneously decompress median nerve or for high energy fractures.
- *Dorsal approach to distal radius:* This can be made through various extensor compartments depending on the need for specific fractures.

149. Define bikini incision.

Ans: This is the colloquial name for incision used in direct anterior approach (DAA) to hip joint for surgical treating disorders like developmental dysplasia of the hip (DDH) and now got popular for performing total hip arthroplasty (THA). The incision is named so as it follows the bikini line in groin region and can be hidden by it for cosmesis conscious persons. The DAA for THA was first described by Hueter and was popularized in France by Judet as early as since 1947. The incision has various advantages over prevailing approaches for hip joint:
- It is an internervous and intervascular plane incision.
- No muscle detachment is needed.
- It does not violate the integrity of lateral hip structures like iliotibial band, greater trochanter, and hip abductors.
- Less postoperative pain and early recovery to function.

Disadvantages/limitations:
- Scar widening
- Injury to lateral femoral cutaneous nerve (LFCN)
- Inability to approach posterior acetabular wall/column, if need of reconstruction arises to them.

Anterior approach steps:
- Position—supine on regular operating table.
- The bikini incision starts approximately 2 cm laterally and distally from the anterosuperior iliac spine (ASIS) and is extended toward the fibular head. The oblique incision is centered in the inguinal skinfold and extended approximately two-thirds laterally and one-third medially of the ASIS.
- Tensor fasciae latae (TFL) with fascia is identified and incised longitudinally taking care to protect LFCN.
- Plane between TFL and rectus femoris is developed.
- Ascending branches of lateral femoral circumflex vessels are identified and secured.
- Exposure to hip capsule is enhanced by mobilizing gluteus minimus and TFL anterolaterally and iliopsoas and rectus femoris medially.
- Capsule is incised in L-shaped fashion and procedure performed.

150. What are indications of anterior approach to hip?

Ans: Kindly see the answer above.

151. Discuss anatomy and blood supply of proximal end femur and its importance in safe surgical dislocation of hip.

Ans: *Anatomy:* The head of the femur forms approximately two-thirds of a sphere and is covered by articular hyaline cartilage in approximately 60–70% of a sphere also the fovea centralis is devoid of cartilage. The hyaline cartilage is thickest in the superior, medial, and posterior surface that contacts with the acetabular surface.

The neck of the femur is approximately 5 cm long. The proximal metaphysic and neck are anteverted by approximately 14°. The angle between the femoral shaft and the neck is approximately 125°. In most hips, the center of the femoral head is at the level of the tip of the greater trochanter. As the neck-shaft angle increases, the center of the head comes to lie above the level of the trochanter (resulting in coxa valga).

A decreased neck-shaft angle results in coxa vara. Also, the distance between the center of the femoral head and the lateral aspect of the trochanter can vary independent of the neck-shaft angle.

Blood supply **(Fig. 2.7.1):** The blood supply to *femoral head* is derived from three primary sources (as described by Crock), the metaphyseal system, retinacular system, and the foveolar system as follows:

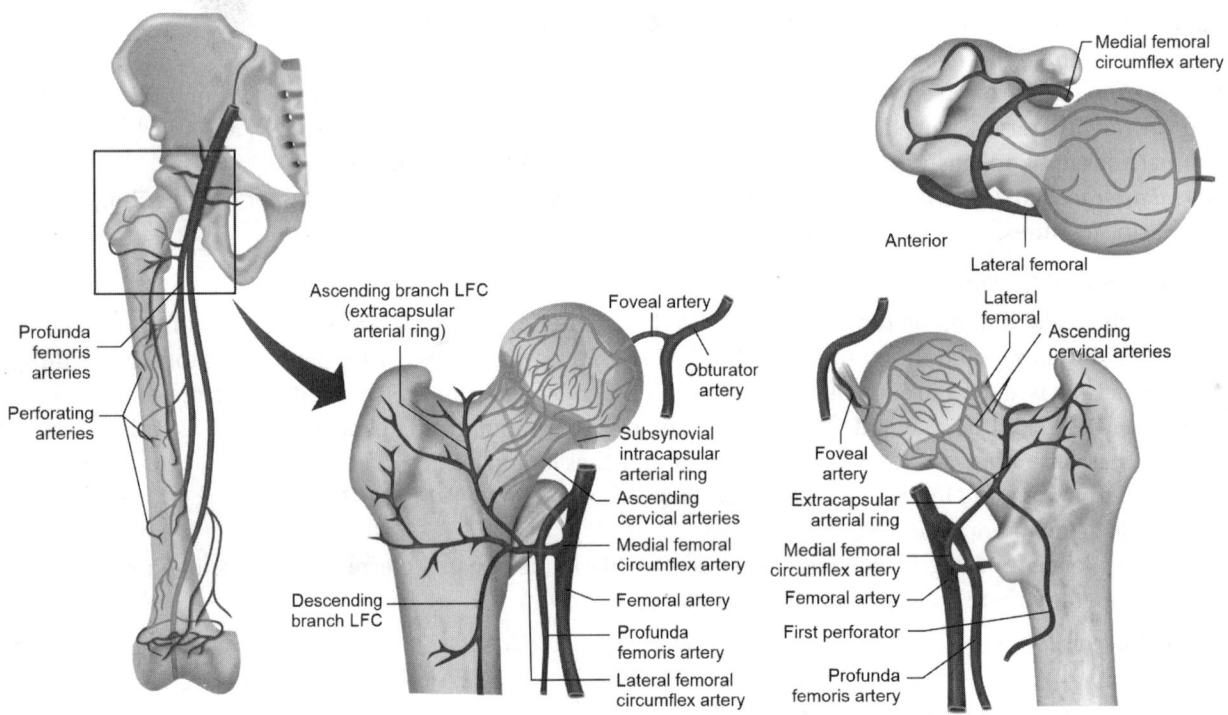

Fig. 2.7.1: Vascular anatomy of femoral head.
(LFC: lateral femoral circumflex)

1. *Extracapsular arterial ring (ECA):* This is the chief system giving rise to both intramedullary and extramedullary arterial systems. The ECA gives less prominent metaphyseal branches to intertrochanteric region which also supply the head through neck (intramedullary metaphyseal system). It is located at the base of femoral neck and is formed:
   - Posteriorly by branch of MCFA
   - Anteriorly by branch of lateral circumflex femoral artery more often a branch of profunda femoris artery (main branch of femoral artery)
   - Ascending cervical branches of ECA (also known as epiphyseal arteries of Trueta or retinacular arteries) that arise from ECA (more prominent system) and ascend up the neck partly also supplying the neck in due course:
     - Divided into anterior, posterior, medial, and lateral groups.
     - Anteriorly, these vessels penetrate the capsule at intertrochanteric line while, posteriorly they pass underneath the orbicularis fibers of the capsule.
     - Lateral group (*lateral ascending cervical vessels*) is the most important group carrying major portion of blood supply to head and neck of femur.

2. *Subsynovial intra-articular arterial ring of Chung (Circulus articuli vasculosus of Hunter)* is formed from lateral ascending cervical vessels:
   - It is located at the margins of articular cartilage on surface of neck of femur.
   - It is either a complete or incomplete ring.
   - It provides epiphyseal vessels (that penetrate the head just outside the articular cartilage to supply major portion of head).
3. *Artery of ligamentum teres:*
   - Branch of obturator artery (more often) or MCFA
   - Variable supply in adults
   - Supply head around the region of fovea.

The metaphyseal *femoral neck* is well vascularized in comparison and is supplied by a cruciate-shaped anastomosis between:
   - Branches from ascending cervical arteries
   - Branches from subsynovial intra-articular arterial ring
   - Intramedullary branches of superior nutrient artery system
   - Metaphyseal vessels from intertrochanteric region.

Importance: Deep branch of the MCFA primarily supplies the femoral head that should be protected during most surgical procedures. The vessel crosses the intact obturator externus muscle from below and is violated during standard posterior approaches to hip. The main idea of surgical dislocation of the hip is to protect this vessel.

152. Describe steps of Lobenhoffer approach.

Ans: The Lobenhoffer approach first described in 1977 provides access to the posteromedial and posterior aspects of the proximal tibia. This has gained importance for reduction and fixation of sagittal tibial plateau fractures with displaced posteromedial fragment. The following are the surgical steps of the approach:
1. Incision—between the medial collateral ligament and posterior oblique ligament.
2. Reflect the ligamentous borders to allow open reduction of the fragment.
3. Fix the fragment using antiglide plate or a similar implant taking care of the thin, soft tissue envelope.
4. To access the proximal medial tibial wall small transverse cut in the medial collateral ligament may be made and it may be subperiosteally stripped to expose fracture lines or area for implant fixation.
5. The MCL is later sutured back.
6. The above method would suffice in simple fractures, but in comminuted large, displaced fractures in step 2 detach the entire fascial-periosteal layer from anterior to posterior, including the insertions of the pes tendons of the medial collateral ligament. Medial meniscus is retained with this layer and retracted out of the joint. After osteosynthesis, resuture the fascial-periosteal layer as a single unit back to bone.
7. Standard wound closure.

2.8 WOUND MANAGEMENT (Q153–162)

153. What are the characteristic changes in the blood supply of femoral head in various age groups?

Ans: Characteristic changes in the blood supply of femoral head in children are:
- Children <3 years have two major arteries supplying the head—the metaphyseal and retinacular system.
- From 4 years to 8 years—the metaphyseal supply is obliterated with development of capital physis so only the retinacular system is the predominant blood supply that enters the head as lateral epiphyseal artery. The lateral epiphyseal system is divided into posterosuperior and posterior inferior systems. Obliteration of the former is responsible for osteonecrosis of anterolateral aspect of femoral head.
- After 8 years, the development of foveolar system gives the head a dual supply again (foveolar and retinacular).
- From 16 years to 18 years as the growth plate disappears, all three groups become re-established to supply the femoral head.

*(Mnemonic: MRF where **M** is **m**etaphyseal, **R** is **r**etinacular, and **F** is **f**oveal.*

So as per age group,
- <4: MR
- 4–8: R
- 8–16: RF
- >16: MRF

154. What is negative-pressure wound therapy?

Ans: Negative-pressure wound therapy (NPWT) or vacuum-assisted closure (VAC) incorporates the use of negative pressure to optimize conditions for wound healing and has been found to reduce the need for frequent dressing changes, improve patient comfort, and reduce associated costs.

Vacuum-assisted closure is recommended to be used as a comprehensive treatment plan in indicated acute or chronic wounds, especially those that fail (or show delay) to heal normally and are challenging. A polyurethane ether sponge is placed/packed into the wound cavity and sealed under an adhesive drape. Controlled negative pressure (50–125 mm Hg) is applied by an adjustable vacuum pump which reduces interstitial fluid accumulation and edema formation helping minimize bacterial colonization of the wound and increase proliferation of the granulation tissue by arteriolar dilation in negative pressure. Commercial dressings are very costly so one can improvise in-house materials for producing a NPWT system also. The noted benefits of VAC therapy are:

- Removal of exudate from the wound and reduction in interstitial edema
- Increased local microvascular flow and improved vascularity (arteriolar dilation)
- Increased controlled production of granulation tissue formation by reduction in the exposure to proteolytic enzymes. Vacuum also puts shear force producing cellular hyperplasia
- Reduce the complexity of wound
- Wound shrinkage
- Optimization of wound bed reducing the complexity of future surgical procedures
- Reduction in the need of antibiotics.

Indications for VAC therapy (or NPWT): The following are some of the common indications of NPWT:
- Chronic wounds such as diabetic ulcers, neuropathic ulcers, and pressure sores
- The best indication for NPWT/VAC in orthopedics is a large wound that is not considered suitable for skin grafting due to exposed tendons or bone
- Open abdominal wounds (including burst abdomen)
- Large and deep burn wounds
- Postflap surgery or skin grafting
- Sternotomy defects.

Contraindications for the use of NPWT:
- Local malignancy
- Untreated underlying osteomyelitis or implant-related infection
- Presence of fistulas
- Copious necrotic tissue in the bed
- Active soft tissue infection
- Exposed viscera (as in abdominal wounds)
- Naked unsupported blood vessel or graft in the wound.

(For details on technique and NPWT, kindly refer to Chapter 129 of the book *Essential Orthopedics: Principles and Practice*, 2nd edition.)

155. What is VAC?

Ans: *Vacuum-assisted closure (VAC® and NPWT):* This is a versatile way of managing chronic wounds, especially in the elderly. VAC has improved patient outcomes significantly with respect to the wound care over past 10–15 years. VAC is recommended to be used as a comprehensive treatment plan in indicated acute or chronic wounds, especially those that fail (or show delay) to heal normally and are challenging. A polyurethane ether sponge is placed/packed into the wound cavity and sealed under an adhesive drape. Controlled negative pressure (50–125 mm Hg) is applied by an adjustable

vacuum pump which reduces interstitial fluid accumulation and edema formation helping minimize bacterial colonization of the wound and increase proliferation of the granulation tissue by arteriolar dilation in negative pressure. The noted benefits of VAC therapy are:
- Removal of exudate from the wound and reduction in interstitial edema
- Increased local microvascular flow and improved vascularity (arteriolar dilation)
- Increased controlled production of granulation tissue formation by reduction in the exposure to proteolytic enzymes. Vacuum also puts shear force producing cellular hyperplasia.
- Reduce the complexity of wound
- Wound shrinkage
- Optimization of wound bed reducing the complexity of future surgical procedures
- Reduction in the need of antibiotics.

Indications for VAC® therapy (or NPWT):
- Chronic wounds such as diabetic ulcers, neuropathic ulcers, and pressure sores
- *Traumatic wounds:* There is a recommendation that if it is deemed useful to use NPWT for traumatic wounds, then it should be applied as early as possible rather than waiting for some improvement in the condition
- The best indication for NPWT/VAC® in orthopedics is a large wound that is not considered suitable for skin grafting due to exposed tendons or bone
- Postflap surgery or skin grafting.

Contraindications for the use of NPWT:
- Local malignancy
- Untreated underlying osteomyelitis or implant-related infection
- Presence of fistulas
- Copious necrotic tissue in the bed
- Active soft tissue infection
- Exposed viscera (as in abdominal wounds)
- Naked unsupported blood vessel or graft in the wound.

Technique of applying NPWT: For an adequate wound, perform adequate debridement so that healthy and clean bed and margins are obtained. Clean the surrounding skin and dry it. Cut a polyurethane sponge of size just smaller than the size of wound and cover with an adhesive dressing that seals the wound. Normally, the adhesive dressing overlaps 6 cm of the normal skin to achieve a hermetic seal. Make a puncture in the center and connect a suction tube to this assembly.

156. What are the principles of wound debridement?

Ans: Wound debridement is the essential first step in management of open injuries and proper soft tissue management to hasten healing and prevent infective complications. Exact extent of debridement necessary is guided by patient characteristics, nature of injury, and vascularity/viability of tissues.

Skin: The skin should be debrided until there is a bleeding edge (outside tourniquet control). In projectile wounds with high velocity, the internal injury may be more than is evident on surface. Longitudinal incisions of the skin and underlying fascia to relieve pressure (wound toileting), remove hematoma and debris, and expose the underlying muscle should be done. Surgical removal of skin is rarely indicated for the initial surgery, other than trimming irregular edges.

Muscle debridement—should remove all nonviable muscle that is noncontractile or grossly contaminated. Completely severed tendon ends that are highly contaminated also may require excision. Removal of contamination with preservation of the tendon in cases of intact musculotendinous units may be possible. Tendon are highly prone to desiccation so maintain moisture around as if the tendon becomes dried it is dead and needs excision. Early flap placement or a sealed dressing is helpful in preventing desiccation.

When dealing with muscles, the four "C's" must be observed:
- *Consistency:* Muscle should be of normal consistency, not waxy or stewed.
- *Color:* Meat color and pinkish muscle indicate good vascularity and deepening of color indicates loss of blood supply. Muscle that looks like hamburger should be excised, and muscle that looks like steak should stay.
- *Contractility:* Normal muscle contraction should be seen when the muscle is pinched or electrically stimulated.
- *Circulation:* Pinkish muscle with controlled blood ooze indicates good vascularity.

Lavage: The current consensus seems to lean toward high-volume, low-pressure lavage, repeated an adequate number of times to effect the best healing and prevention of infection. The amount of fluid used varies with the method of application. The protocol has been to use 9 L of pulsed irrigation. Additives to the irrigation solution are questionable.

If debridement does not result in a surgically clean wound, closure should not be done. In addition, the skin should not be closed under tension because this may result in further skin necrosis and ischemia. The proper tension has been described as a wound that can be closed with 2-0 nylon without breaking. Structures should be kept moist with occlusive dressings.

Dead space management: The use of a "bead pouch" technique has been shown to be very cost effective in control of deep infection. Early closure of the wound has been shown to decrease the incidence of infection, malunion, and nonunion. A variety of other methods can be used like direct suturing, split-thickness skin grafting, and free or local muscle flaps.

Vacuum-assisted closure may be used for wounds that cannot be covered due to extensive loss and poor wound bed.

157. Describe the various myocutaneous flaps used to cover tibia in different levels.

Ans: (*Term myocutaneous is not completely correct so it will be essentially both muscle and skin coverage—as conceptually asked*). Below is a comprehensive list of soft tissue coverage for leg (tibia).
(*The details can be read from Chapter 129 "wound healing and principles of wound care—Essential Orthopedics: Principles and Practice, 2nd edition".*)

- *Proximal third tibia*:
    - Muscle flaps—gastrocnemius
    - Myocutaneous flaps—gastrocnemius
    - Fasciocutaneous flaps:
        - Saphenous flap
        - Sural flap.
- *Middle third tibia*:
    - Muscle flaps:
        - Soleus flap
        - Extensor digitorum longus (EDL)
        - Tibialis anterior.
    - Fasciocutaneous flaps:
        - Lower leg septocutaneous perforator flaps
        - "Ponten flap".
- *Distal third tibia*:
    - *Muscle flaps:* Limitation of all muscle flaps in this region is of providing only a limited small area reconstruction.
        - Soleus flap
        - Extensor digitorum longus
        - Tibialis anterior
        - Peroneus brevis.
    - *Fasciocutaneous flap:*
        - *Reverse flow flaps based on:*
            - Anterior tibial artery
            - Posterior tibial artery
            - Peroneal artery.
        - Lateral leg fasciocutaneous flap.

158. Discuss flap reconstruction and its classification.

Ans: In few circumstances, it is not possible to close the defect primarily as the skin is either not pliable or the defect is irregular and large. Other indications include:
- Suturing/skin grafting not possible
- Flap over a bare bone may make the difference between viability and sequestration of bone.

The principles or creating local flaps include:
- Carefully map the area on donor tissue with an allowance of 25% excess to compensate for shrinkage of skin after transfer. Circular defects may be closed by creating tangential cuts in the skin making double opposing semicircular flaps or making petal-shaped flaps.
- Should not be from a weight-bearing area, also it should not result into an unsightly conspicuous scar.

Distant skin flaps

Cross-leg flap (Hamilton, 1854): The cross-leg flap is obtained from the other leg (well-leg) and can be of following types:
- Calf-leg flap (preferred)
- Thigh-leg flap indicated in:
  - Female patients wishing to avoid a visible secondary defect
  - Large defects that cannot be closed by opposite calf skin.

Principles of cross-leg flap:
- Cover defect in every direction.
- Design in a way that the lymphatics are oriented in a direction same as of defect.
- Delay is indicated if length-to-width ratio exceeds 1½ to 1.
- Should not undergo even slightest degree of traction.

Donor site:
- Best-medial calf and anterior aspect of lower one-third of thigh
- *Alternate sites:* Anterior thigh, posteromedial calf, and cross foot flap

Coverage of raw surface of donor site can be achieved by:
- Skin grafting the donor site
- *Hinge technique:* A hinge is created at the recipient site for proper coverage of the donor site.

Postoperative: As there is propensity for movement, the two limbs are fixed by either applying plaster cast or by using an external fixator. One must give deep vein thrombosis (DVT) prophylaxis to these patients.

The "tube flap": These are usually removed from anterolateral aspect of abdomen and transferred via wrist or caterpillar technique.
- *Indication:* Mainly in a female who cannot tolerate position in cross-leg flap or in whom it is not possible due to amputated or disfigured limb.
- *Shortcomings:*
  - Although unlimited in length, but its width is dependent on looseness of tissues to form a tube
  - Flaps are usually bulky
  - Excess of fat may constrict circulation
  - Minimum of fat causes shrinkage.
- *Disadvantage:* Multiple procedures required.

The jump flap: It is typically indicated for coverage of large defects.
- Flap carried from abdominal wall to forearm as an intermediary host and then to fill the defect.
- Success depends upon maintenance of short broad pedicle throughout all stages of transfer.
- Sufficient mobility of leg, shoulder, body is essential
- *Limitations:*
  - Limited to children and young adults
  - Excess of at least one-third of size of defect needed for shrinkage compensation.

Rotational Myocutaneous Flaps

As with rotational skin local flaps, muscle can also be incorporated into the cutaneous flaps.

General principles:
- Pedicled muscle flaps are workhorse for reconstruction.
- Proceed by classifying wounds as acute, subacute, and chronic, and by dividing leg into proximal, middle, and distal third.

- Raised flap should be slightly larger than the defect.
- Necessary to have adequate pedicle length.
- Choose donor site as per size of flap and its arc of rotation.
- Donor site should be out of injury site.
- Prefer free-tissue transfer techniques for complex wounds.

Goals:
- Close the defect with durable tissue
- Aesthetically acceptable result
- Minimal donor site morbidity
- Functional result.

Contraindications:
- Wounds resulting from high energy injuries
- Treatment resulting in functional deficit
- Concomitant radiation injury.

159. **A. What are fasciocutaneous flaps and musculocutaneous flaps?**
    B. What are free flaps?

Ans: A. Fasciocutaneous flaps:

A fasciocutaneous flap is classified as:
- *Type A:* Multiple perforators at base (Cross-leg flap, medial thigh flap)
- *Type B:* Single vascular pedicle (medial arm flap, antecubital forearm flap, scapular flap)
- *Type C:* Segmental vascular pedicle (radial forearm flap)
- *Type D:* Single vascular pedicle (radial forearm flap with bone, fibular osseocutaneous flap).

For a fasciocutaneous flap, the feasibility of flap is determined by extent of periosteal damage, location of defect and availability of soft tissue. Usually, the tissue over anteromedial tibia is unsuitable so that mostly the flap is based on lateral intermuscular septum or posterior tibial artery to base flap on fascial perforators. These commonly limit their usefulness in all cases so muscular flaps are preferred over them.

Muscle flap is better than a fasciocutaneous flap which is prone to undergo secondary necrosis.

Musculocutaneous flaps: Rotational myocutaneous flap already written above.

B. Free flaps:

These flaps require meticulous preoperative evaluation. Evaluate the needed coverage for size, thickness, durability, and cosmetic appearance of the area to be covered. Ascertain that the recipient site has good availability of and accessibility to adequate size and length of recipient vessels. It should be possible to place anastomoses away from recipient defect, if possible. Ideally, the site should free from infection. Every effort should be made to place the anastomoses away from infection.

Examples include:
- *Gracilis muscle free flap:*
    - Based on medial femoral circumflex vessels
    - Motor innervation from obturator nerve (L4-5)
    - Can be used as either muscle flap or a myocutaneous flap
    - Ideal for small soft-tissue defects
    Advantages:
    - No significant functional deficit
    - Donor site scar minimal
    - Atrophies over a time period of 3–4 months—so good cosmetic result
- *Rectus abdominis free flap (Type III muscle):*
    - Based on deep inferior epigastric vessels
    - Ideal for intermediate-sized defect

- Extraordinary geometric versatility due to:
  - Long length of muscle and
  - Long pedicle
- *Types:* Vertical, transverse rectus abdominis (TRAM), bipedicled, superiorly based, inferiorly based

Advantages of a TRAM flap:
- Suprapubic horizontal donor site scar is quite acceptable.
- Simultaneous abdominoplasty
- Quality of skin better than LD flap

- *LD free flap:*
  - Ideal for covering large soft-tissue defects
  - Flap can be based electively on different vessels depending upon required diameter and length of vessels:
    - Usually based on thoracodorsal artery
    - For the need of a small bridging graft—subscapular and medial circumflex scapular artery can be used.
    - Also, subscapular artery can be used as an interposition graft in lower limb injuries with thoracodorsal artery supplying the flap.

  Advantages:
  - LD is a relatively thin muscle.
  - It can also be used in arteriosclerotic vessels when end-to-side anastomoses are not possible.
  - Muscle atrophies over time to give a pleasing contour

- *Tensor fascia lata (TFL) flap:*
  - Provides abundant skin and subcutaneous tissue
  - Based on lateral femoral circumflex artery
  - Neural innervation—inferior branch of superior gluteal nerve (L4-5, S1)
  - Now abandoned due to formidable donor site morbidity.

- *Groin flap:*

  The groin flap is a *fasciocutaneous type A* flap supplied by the *superficial circumflex iliac* system that has a variable anatomy. The skin is innervated from T12 segment. The flap can be used either as a rotational flap for coverage of the abdominal or perineal wounds or as a free flap based on its vascular pedicle or even for soft-tissue coverage of hand as a parasite flap (like a cross-leg flap, the defect in hand is covered with the harvested flap and kept in place for 3–4 weeks). The flap is then detached to provide skin coverage.

  The *advantages* of the flap are as under:
  - Versatile and readily available
  - Can be designed into large dimensions
  - Texture and quality of skin are excellent.
  - Donor site can be primarily closed.
  - Residual defect can be easily concealed.
  - Now status is relegated to "last resort" flap.

  Disadvantages:
  - Variable arterial anatomy
  - Short pedicle
  - Unsuitable in obese patient

- **Dorsalis pedis flap:**
  - Based on dorsalis pedis artery:
    - Accompanies deep peroneal nerve
    - Supplies a mean of 3.8 vertical branches
  - Venous drainage:
    - Superficial dorsal venous arch medially into great saphenous vein and laterally into short saphenous vein
  - Sensory supply—superficial peroneal nerve

Advantages:
- Thin pliable skin
- Large pedicle

Disadvantages:
- Donor site morbidity
- Simple spilt skin grafting (SSG) and long-term care are required.
- Chronic aching foot—obvious disadvantage for footwear

- **Fasciocutaneous free flaps:**
  - Lateral arm free flap
  - Parascapular free flap

Osteocutaneous free flaps:
- Iliac crest with overlying skin.

Osteofasciocutaneous free flaps:
- For coverage of large osseous and skin defects
- Based on fibula with intact lateral septum as vascular supply and variable skin island.

160. What are skin grafts?

Ans: This is one of the most basic of reconstructive procedures performed for reconstituting the continuity of integument. In simplest terms, the skin or a portion of it is transplanted to a defect for reconstitution of integument integrity. Though appearing innocuous and simple, it is prone to failures and complications if not performed well and in a defined manner, so should not be taken lightly anyways.

There are three basic modes in which a skin grafting can be done.

1. *Primary skin grafting:* This is done primarily while wound management; it is also done to cover the rotational muscle flaps to seal the skin cover primarily.
2. *Delayed skin grafting:* If the wound is unhealthy with doubtful vascularity of the bed, one should let the wound granulate and then skin grafting is done (usually 2–5 days later), it is the most common mode of management for open wound in orthopedics. The other indication is if the hemostasis at the site is incomplete, then one should wait for the wound to stabilize before grafting.
3. *Dermal over grafting (Webster 1958):*
   - For coverage of defects, weight-bearing surfaces and unstable scars of leg are required.
   - Multiple grafting is done at 3-week interval to provide a thick laminated layer of dermis.

Skin grafts are harvested from a donor site and transferred to the recipient site without carrying its own blood supply. Based on the thickness of the obtained (required), the grafts are classified into:

- *Full-thickness skin grafts (FTSG):* These consist of entire epidermis and dermis. These grafts leave no dermal appendages that can reproduce epidermis, so the donor site has to be primarily closed. Commonly, they are obtained using a knife free-hand to create a plain between dermis and subcutaneous fat. Due to requirement of high vascularity and good supply of nutrients, these grafts are contraindicated in beds with poor vascularity.

Indications of FTSG are as follows:
- Defects in which the adjacent tissues are immobile or scarce
- Adjacent tissue has premalignant or malignant lesion precluding the use of flap.
- When multi-staged procedures are precluded
- Punch grafting for hair transplantation

- *Split-thickness skin grafts (STSGs):* STSG comprises epidermis and variable thickness of the underlying dermis. Depending on the thickness of the dermis, they can be classified as thin, intermediate-thickness, and thick STSGs. The STSG leaves skin adnexa at the donor site (hair follicles/sweat glands) that allow repopulation of epidermis. The STSGs are used to resurface larger defects and when cosmesis is not of much concern.

Skin graft survival and adherence to the recipient site: A variety of mechanisms are proposed for graft attachment at the grafted defect that vary with the aging of graft and should occur in a sequence to help in graft survival and complete uptake:

- *Plasma imbibition:* As soon as the graft is applied, it is an avascular structure and gains its nutrition from the nutrients in the wound bed that reach it via diffusion. This requires a healthy wound bed with healthy granulation tissue.
- *Inosculation:* By day 3, under appropriate environment, the cut ends of the vessels in the underside of dermis begin to form connections with those of wound bed, a process called inosculation.
- *Angiogenesis:* This is the process of growth of blood vessels from the wound bed into the graft and occurs by 5th day to a week.
- *Development of lymphatics and bridge vascularity:* After a week, lymphatics develop in the transplanted skin.

Complications of skin grafting:
- *Graft failure:* The skin grafts fail primarily by one of the following four mechanisms:
  1. *Poor wound condition:* Graft put on avascular structures on the wound bed or structures that are relatively avascular will not let the graft uptake to happen. Tendons, ligaments, slough, or bare bone will not let graft uptake. Fat is relatively avascular and only very thin grafts on a thin fat layer may survive.
  2. *Shearing movements at graft-bed interface:* Shear forces separate the graft from wound bed preventing necessary contact and stability for above uptake processes to complete successfully.
  3. *Formation of seroma or hematoma that lifts graft above the bed:* If found or any doubt exists, one should drain them by 3 days else complete failure of graft would occur.
  4. *Infection:* Bacteria produce proteolytic enzymes and the pus accumulation lifts the graft off the bed.
- *Injury to deeper structures at the donor site:* Underlying neural and vascular structures are at risk of damage at the donor site, if they are penetrated by an inexperienced person.

161. Classify decubitus ulcers. Describe its etiopathogenesis and management.

Ans: The terms decubitus ulcer (from Latin decumbere, "to lie down"), pressure sore, pressure ulcer and bedsores are often used interchangeably.

Classification: This is Shea's modification of pressure sore classification
- *Stage I:* Nonblanchable erythema (skin intact)
- *Stage II:* Epidermis ulcerated and most of the dermis also eroded or nonviable
- *Stage III:* Dermis ulcerated completely with visible deeper subcutaneous tissue
- *Stage IV:* Ulceration extends to underlying bone (usually superficial OM)
- *Stage V:* Gross infection with closed large cavities and a small sinus opening.

Etiopathogenesis: Pressure ulcers result from constant pressure sufficient to impair local blood flow to soft tissue for an extended period. This external pressure must be greater than the arterial capillary pressure (32 mm Hg) to impair inflow and greater than the venous capillary closing pressure (8–12 mm Hg) to impede the return of flow for an extended time. If a patient cannot move for a protracted length of time because of immobilizing medical conditions, paralysis, general anesthesia, or physical restraints, the externally applied pressure on prominent body surfaces may exceed the capillary pressure within the tissue, with ensuing interruption of circulation, hypoxic tissue damage, and finally, necrosis. The critical duration of ischemia that can cause pressure injury varies greatly among individuals; as a rule of thumb, it lies somewhere between 30 and 240 minutes. The superficial dermis can tolerate ischemia for 2–8 hours before breakdown occurs. Deeper muscle, connective tissue, and fat tissues tolerate pressures for 2 hours or less. Peripheral arterial occlusive disease puts patients at higher risk of developing decubitus ulcers.

Other physical influences that can damage the skin include friction at the skin surface, shearing forces (i.e., lateral displacement of the skin, whose layers are of differing firmness), and moisture. Moisture does not cause a pressure injury per se, but it can promote the generation of chronic wounds by softening the upper layers of the skin (maceration) and changing the cutaneous chemical environment (altered pH).

- Immobility is the main risk factor for decubitus ulcers as described above. Risk factors can be classified as intrinsic (patient-related) or extrinsic [related to the patient's environment (see adjoining **Flowchart 2.8.1**)].
- *Friction:* Friction may make fragile skin more vulnerable to injury due to constant rubbing.
- *Shear:* Shear occurs when two surfaces move in the opposite direction such as when the skin stays still and is stretched or pinched as muscles or bones move.
- *Moisture:* Makes the skin soft and vulnerable to damage
- *Increased temperature:* This increases the oxygen demand reducing the critical duration of ischemia.

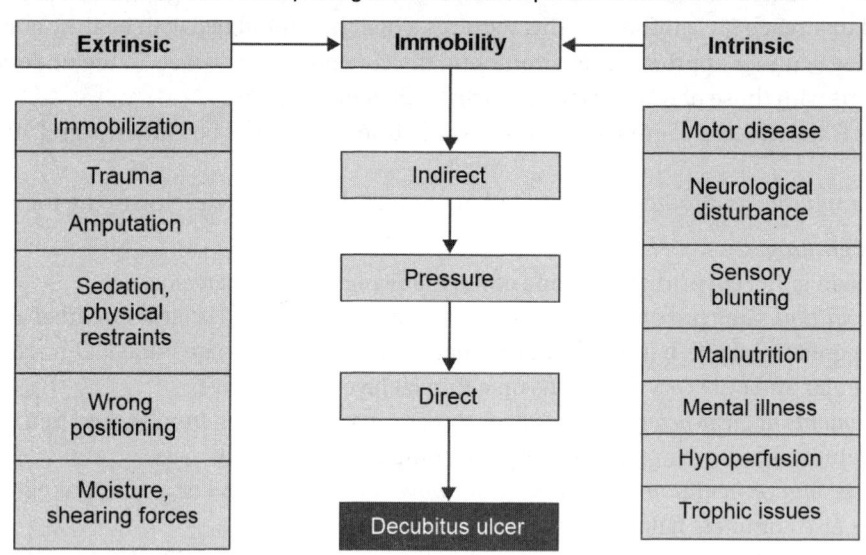

Flowchart 2.8.1: Etiopathogenesis of development of decubitus ulcers.

Management:

Conservative management:

Strategies for conservative management of pressure sores:
- *Pressure-relieving strategies:* Frequent turning, low air-loss beds, water mattress, are commonly employed but turning in bed is the most important measure. For heel ulcers, special pressure-relieving boots are important. Patients using wheel chairs should be provided with soft cushions.
- *Dressings and debriding agents:* These are the cheapest measures deployed commonly as first line of treatment for ulcer higher than stage 1. Gauze dressings are applied after debriding an eschar. Commonly moist dressings are deployed and repeatedly changed to limit infection and enhance granulation tissue formation. Stage-1 ulcers may be managed by transparent film dressings. For stage-2 ulcer, a moist dressing is best; hydrogels may also be employed. Stage-3 and 4 ulcers need wet-to-dry dressings after a thorough debridement. The dressings dry within the wound and also in turn debride the tissue. The dressing is changed three to four times a day. If the wound has a foul smell, then use 0.25% Dakin's bleach to wet the dressing. Other enzymatic debriding agents may also be used. If the ulcers are slow to heal or are very large, then primary flap coverage may be considered.
- *Negative-pressure wound therapy:* This is a faster way of granulating the wound and healing it.
- *Hydrotherapy:* This is more commonly employed for debridement of the venous stasis ulcer in the lower extremity. Pulsed lavage has now replaced hydrotherapy and provides faster granulation tissue formation and reducing infection.

Surgical management:

Debridement: All necrotic ulcers with slough or eschar are to be debrided for formation of granulation tissue and allow healing. Attempt should be made to preserve as much of bone as possible. The procedure of complete ischiectomy should only be reserved for excessive destruction of bone.

Flap coverage: Most large and deep ulcers will ultimately need a flap coverage. Muscle flaps should be used to fill deep spaces. Commonly, the following flaps are used for coverage of a pressure sore:
- Gluteal posterior flap or posterior thigh flap for covering ischial pressure sore
- V-Y advancement gluteal flap for covering sacral pressure sore
- TFL or posterior thigh flap for covering trochanteric pressure sores

Adequate debridement of the ulcer base to reach the viable tissue and healthy bleeding is a must. The skin margins at the defect should also be viable and bleeding.

For all flap surgeries, one must protect the site from shear forces postoperatively, else the flap will fail. Drains should be used to eliminate dead spaces and use of antibiotics is variable with longer course needed for underlying OM.

General Orthopedics

162. Explain the role of gluteus maximus flap in management of decubitus ulcer.

Ans: Ger in 1971 first reported using gluteus maximus muscle transposition for coverage of sacral decubitus ulcers, while later it was used as rotational musculocutaneous flap by Minami, et al. The muscle can be used either with superior gluteal artery as pedicle or the inferior gluteal artery as pedicle so the designing of flap is essential.

Anatomy:
The gluteus maximum is one of the largest muscle in terms of cross-sectional area and forms major part of buttock contour. Muscle originates from gluteal line of ilium and sacrum inserting on iliotibial band and fascia lata gluteal ridge of femur. The muscle is supplied by inferior gluteal nerve. The superior and inferior gluteal vessels supplying the muscle belly emerge from the greater sciatic notch that passes around the upper and lower margins of the piriformis muscle, respectively providing suspension for the muscle, if hung freely. The overlying skin and subcutaneous tissues of the buttock are supplied by perforating vessels through the fascia of the gluteal muscle.

Various methods of reconstruction utilizing the gluteus maximus muscle are:
- V-Y advancement using superior half of muscle supplied by superior gluteal vessels
- Inferior half muscle—rotation flap supplied by inferior gluteal vessels
- Whole muscle—rotational flap.

Procedure for rotational flap:
- Prone position on operating table
- Excise the decubitus ulcer to healthy margins
- Usually for rotation flap, the pedicle is based along a line joining the greater trochanter and anterior superior iliac spine (ASIS).
- The skin is incised and the muscle is freed from medius below by blunt dissection.
- Vascular pedicle is protected and muscle is lifted from attachment as a composite musculocutaneous flap to cover the defect.
- Bleeding is secured before closure of defect before closure over drains.
- Donor defect less than 8 cm can be closed primarily else cover with split-thickness skin graft (STSG).

2.9 GAIT (Q163–170)

163. Define gait.

Ans: Gait is the process of locomotion using lower limbs. It is a rhythmic sequential movement of the lower limbs that moves the body along the required line and maintains stability and conserves energy.

164. What are the phases of gait cycle? Enumerate various pathological gaits with their causes and detail on Trendelenburg gait. Why a patient with hip pain walks with a stick in the opposite hand? Illustrate your answer with suitable diagrams.

Ans:

Phases:
- *Stance phase is divided into:*
  - Heel strike
  - Foot flat
  - Midstance
  - Heel off
  - Toe off.
- *Swing phase is divided into:*
  - Preswing or initial swing
  - Midswing
  - Late swing or terminal swing.

Various gaits:
- *Quadriceps weakness:* In quadriceps weakness, forces tend to flex the knee.

- *Pretibial muscle weakness:* Ipsilateral high stepping gait (*steppage* or *equine gait*)—weakness of the pretibial muscles causes slapping of the foot during the stance phase at the time of loading response.
- *Antalgic gait:* The patient tries to reduce the weight borne by the painful limb.
- *Lateral trunk bending:* In the stance phase, it is seen toward involved side in Trendelenburg, bilaterally in waddling gait. In the swing phase, it is toward unaffected side. Causes include hip abductor weakness, hip dislocation, coxa vara, hip pain, short limb, fixed flexion deformity, skeletal shortening, and discomfort between thigh band and perineum.
- *Hip hiking:* In the swing phase, there is elevation of pelvis by quadratus lumborum and abductors to clear the foot.
- *Circumduction gait*
- *Internal hip rotation/In-toe stance*
- *External hip rotation*
- *Wide base gait*
- *Narrow base*
- *Inverted foot stance*
- *Everted foot stance*
- *Anterior trunk bending*
- *Posterior trunk bending*
- *Hemiplegic gait*
- *Diplegic gait*
- *Parkinsonian gait*
- *Choreiform (hyperkinetic) gait*
- *Ataxic (cerebellar) gait*
- Sensory gait
- Psoatic gait
- Gluteus maximus gait or rocking horse gait
- Hamstring gait
- Unequal leg length gait
- *Gluteus medius weakness or trendelenburg gait:* The Trendelenburg gait is caused by a unilateral weakness of the hip abductors, mostly the gluteal musculature. In normal gait during single stance phase when weight of body is on one limb, the sag of pelvis to the opposite side is prevented by the ipsilateral gluteus medius. When this muscle is weak, the pelvis tilts downward instead of upward on the nonweight-bearing extremity. In an attempt to lessen this effect, the person compensates by lateral tilt of the trunk away from the affected hip, thus center of gravity is mostly on the stance limb causing a reduction of the pelvic drop. If this is bilateral, it is known as *waddling gait* or *duck gait or chorus girl swing gait*.

Antalgic gait and hip pain: Canes may be used to reduce hip pain by reducing the joint contact force. A cane held in the contralateral hand reduces joint reactive forces through the affected hip approximately 30–40% by reducing hip abductor muscle pull **(Fig. 2.9.1)**. A cane creates an additional force that keeps the pelvis level in the face of gravity's tendency to adduct the hip during unilateral stance. The cane's force must substitute for the hip abductors of the affected hip and creates a moment arm that is relatively long and originates on the side opposite the hip whose abductor muscles are weak. Additionally, the person needs adequate strength in the muscles of the wrist, elbow, shoulder girdle, and trunk.

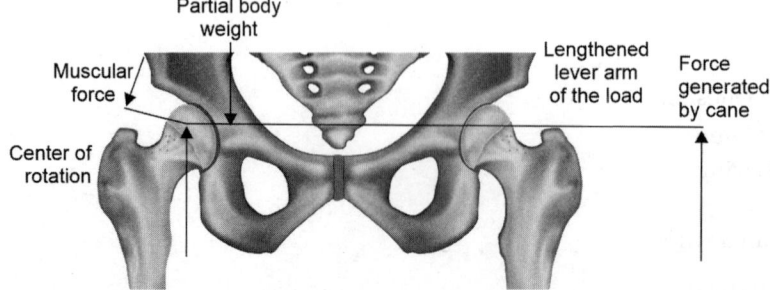

Fig. 2.9.1: The efficacy of force transmitted though cane. The cane has longer lever arm acting through the handle of cane this produces higher moment (product of distance to force) despite smaller force transmitted through it.

165. Explain pseudo-Trendelenburg test.

Ans: The students can describe the mechanism of Trendelenburg test (Fig. 2.9.2) as described above in Question 164 (Gluteus medius weakness) and supplant with figure. The patient is asked to stand on one leg for 30 seconds without leaning to one side. The examiner observes the patient to see if the pelvis stays level during single-leg stance. The test is positive if pelvis on the unaffected/unsupported side (contralateral side) dips/drops during unilateral weight-bearing (or sustained elevation of iliac crest is not obtained or the iliac crest fails to elevated, i.e., remains parallel to ground). However, if the hip remains level and does not drop, then test is negative (abductor mechanism of tested side is strong/healthy). Negative test is not just affected by healthy abductor mechanism but also depends on healthy and strong 'quadratus lumborum' muscle. If the quadratus lumborum muscle is weak (as in myopathy or poliomyelitis), then also the unsupported hip may drop producing a 'positive test' despite patient having healthy abductor mechanism. This will be a false-positive test also called pseudo-positive Trendelenburg test.

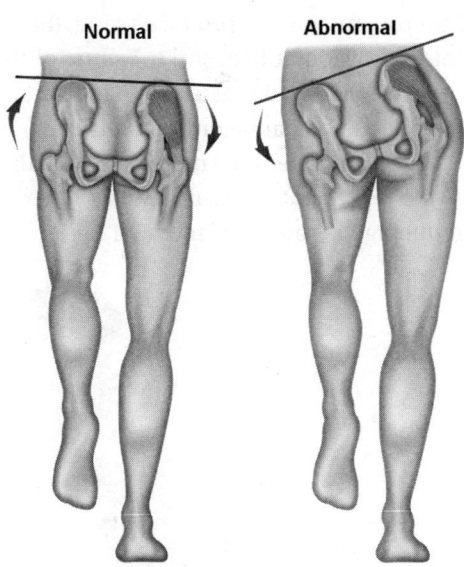

Fig. 2.9.2: The Trendelenburg test.

166. Discuss concentric and eccentric contraction during gait cycle. How will paralysis of tibialis anterior affect gait?

Ans:

Types of contractions:
- Concentric contraction also called shortening contraction occurs when the force generated by the contraction is greater than the resisting load and produces muscle shortening.
- Eccentric contraction occurs when the resisting load is greater than the amount of tension being produced. In this case, there will be a muscle lengthening with contraction.

Muscles acting during various phases of gait cycle are:
- *Heel strike:* Eccentric contraction of quadriceps.
- *Foot flat:* Concentric contraction of quadriceps.
- *Midstance:* Both the quadriceps and hamstrings are inactive and knee is extended passively.
- *Heel off:* An active gastrocnemius prevents hyperextension.
- *Push off:* Vastus intermedius and rectus femoris become active toward end to prevent hyperflexion.
- *Toe off to late swing:* The quadriceps is active during this phase and just before heel strike, the hamstrings act to prevent forward swing of the leg and to decelerate it.

Paralysis of tibialis anterior—causes slapping of the foot during the stance phase at the time of loading response. The compensatory mechanisms that prevent this foot slapping are:
- Ipsilateral circumduction of the limb
- Ipsilateral high stepping gait (*steppage* or *equine gait*)
- Contralateral hip hiking
- Instead of normal heel strike, there is slapping of whole foot.

167. What are the features of antalgic and Trendelenburg gait?

Ans: Kindly see Answer to Question 142 above.

168. What is crouch gait? How will you evaluate such a patient? Discuss the management.

Ans: Please read Chapter no. 4B.

169. What is the etiopathogenesis of hand to knee gait? Give biomechanical features of floor reaction orthosis.

Ans: Hand to knee gait—in quadriceps weakness, forces tend to flex the knee causing buckling and patient would fall. Hand to knee gait is when patient physically pushes anterior thigh backward to prevent knee from buckling. In normal gait, there is a torsional moment force at the knee during toe off that causes knee flexion and pushes forward the knee into progression. To produce swing, the quadriceps must be strong and counter the moment force to bring knee again into extension at heel strike. Failure of this mechanism would let the knee persist in flexion at heel strike that would increase the rotational moment and reaction of floor to further produce knee flexion. In such a case, the patient would fall due to weak antagonist (quadriceps). To prevent fall, patient uses hand on knee to push it back countering the floor reaction and rotational moment so that the knee is in extension during heel strike or the knee does not flex further at heel strike **(Fig. 2.9.3)**. This also causes anterior trunk bending to bring the center of gravity forward in front of knee further reducing the rotational moment.

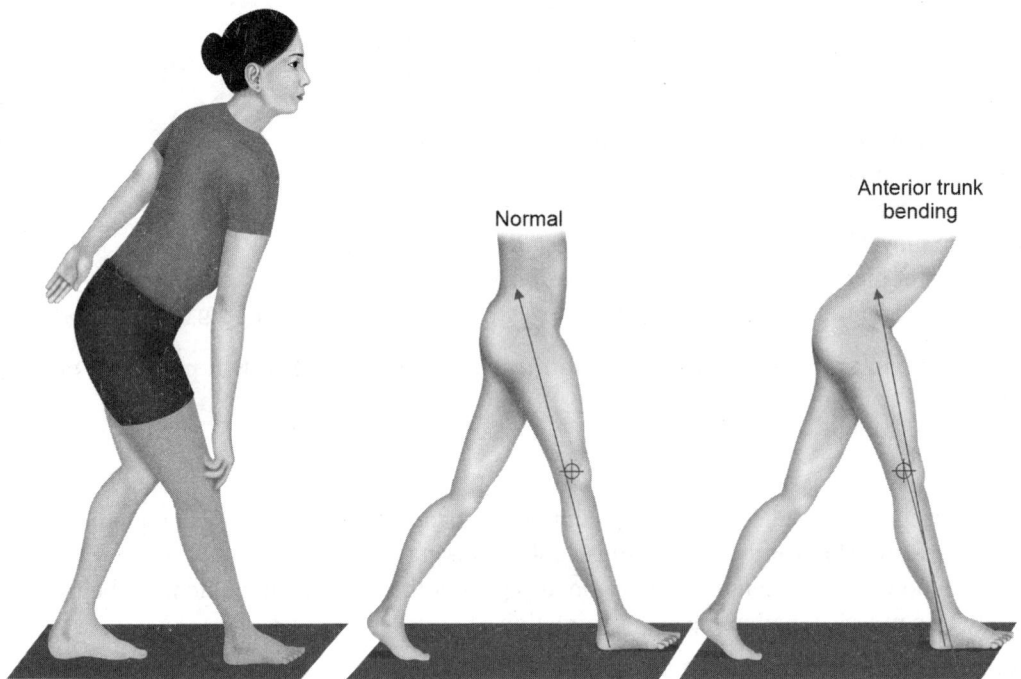

Fig. 2.9.3: Pathophysiology of hand-to-knee gait.

(Floor reaction orthosis has been described well in Answer to Question 136 above.)

170. Discuss crutch walking gait and its importance.

Ans: *There are four main walks or "gaits" when using crutches:*
1. *Four-point gait:* The patient can bear some weight on both lower extremities. The following sequence is then followed: Move the right crutch forward → move the left foot forward → move the left crutch forward → move the right foot forward → repeat the crutch-foot-crutch-foot sequence.
2. *Three-point gait:*
   - *Partial weight-bearing three-point gait:* Here the injured foot is allowed some weight bearing. The following sequence is used: Put both crutches forward → step with bad foot up to the crutches → step with good foot past the crutches → repeat sequence.
   - *Three-point nonweight-bearing gait:* The patient should not bear any weight on the affected leg. The following sequence is adopted: Move the affected (nonweight-bearing) leg and both crutches forward together → move the unaffected (weight-bearing) leg forward → repeat sequence.
3. *Two-point gait:* The patient is allowed to bear some weight on both lower extremities. The following sequence is followed: Move the right leg and left crutch forward together → move the left leg and the right crutch forward together → repeat sequence.
4. *Swing-through gait:* It is used for patients with lower extremities that are paralyzed and/or in braces. The following sequence is followed: Place the patient in tripod position → move both crutches forward together about 6 inches → move both legs forward together about 6 inches → repeat sequence.

2.10 MYOSITIS OSSIFICANS (Q171–172)

171. Define myositis ossificans and its diagnosis and management.

Ans: The term specifically refers to the presence of bone formation (ossification) at a place where it should not be present (heterotopic) that is usually the soft tissue.

Diagnosis and management: The extent of lesion is evident on radiographs in late stages, or computed tomography (CT) scan in earlier stages or magnetic resonance imaging (MRI) in earliest stages. Hip being the most common site for development of heterotopic ossification (HO) has received most attention and few classification systems exist. Metabolic activity of the lesion is evident by scintigraphic scanning that supplements the radiographs if the combination is resorted to instead of complicated investigations. In the early stages, the scintigraphic scan reveals intense uptake at the site of lesion that reduces in intermediate stages and finally becomes cold in late stages. Approximately 2.5 weeks after injury, flow studies and blood pool images can detect development of incipient HO. The typical findings on delayed scintigrams however become positive nearly 1 week later. The bone scans are sensitive enough that they can be performed serially to identify metabolically silent lesions that can then be excised.

Laboratory investigations: The levels of alkaline phosphatase (ALP) are elevated early and are abnormal approximately 2 weeks after injury. The ALP levels have been shown to increase to approximately 3.5 times the normal value after 10 weeks of the inciting trauma and they return to normal by nearly 18 weeks in a typical case due to maturation of mass. These, however, do not reflect the true metabolic activity of the lesion and cannot guide the timing of surgical removal. Also, in many cases with limited disease or small lesions, the levels may remain normal. Serum creatine kinase levels correlate with the muscle involvement; with a higher level correlating to severe form of HO. Similar to any inflammatory event rise in C-reactive protein (CRP) early has been reported but is nonspecific. The only value of this marker could be to evaluate the treatment response of nonsteroidal anti-inflammatory drugs (NSAIDs), in which case the levels fall with favorable response. Measurement of the 24-hour urinary excretion of prostaglandin E2 (PGE2) has been recommended to identify HO early in predisposed cases. A rise in levels indicates qualifying the lesion metabolism with bone scan.

Treatment: Because the treatment of a well-developed lesion is not very effective (recurrence common) or easy (undefined planes of involvement and possible secondary deficits after excision), it is considered that preventing the development of HO by appropriate prophylaxis or its early treatment would be the best strategy. The first step to management once the diagnosis of early HO is confirmed is to initiate passive joint range of motion (ROM) exercises to maintain mobility. Early active mobilization versus aggressive delayed mobilization is debated, however, we feel that movements should begin early that may be intensified later as the lesion matures. The following agents have been recommended for prophylaxis of HO:

- Bisphosphonates (etidronate) and specific NSAIDs (such as indomethacin > ibuprofen > diclofenac) have been used for prophylaxis against development of HO or its treatment. Drug dosing, type of drug, timing of dosing, and length of treatment are undefined and surgeons often devise their own protocol. It is logical and recommended to start bisphosphonates as soon as serum ALP or urinary PGE2 levels are noted or imaging studies demonstrate the presence of incipient HO.
- Heterotopic ossification can be successfully prevented and treated by radiation therapy. A single irradiation of 7 Gy has been used successfully in patients who developed HO previously after a surgery. The modality is especially useful in patients having contraindications to receiving indomethacin. Considering the complications of radiation therapy including secondary sarcoma development, the treatment should be reserved only to these high-risk patients.
- *Thalidomide:* Thalidomide has been found to reduce the progression of ossification of soft tissues and may serve to improve functional status. The action may be related to reduction of tumor necrosis factor alpha (TNF-α) during flare-ups.

Surgical resection of HO should be delayed until when it has matured. This is done with the aim of reducing both the intraoperative complications like identification problem and hemorrhage, and minimizing postoperative HO recurrence. The ideal candidate for surgical resection of HO will hence be one who has clinically silent lesion (no joint pain or swelling), a normal ALP level, and a three-phase bone scan not showing any uptake in flow or blood pool images suggesting maturation of HO. Variously recommended measures like serial bone scans, evaluating ALP, creatine kinase or recently urinary PGE2 levels can be followed or developed on institutional basis and should be strictly followed if found adequate.

Garland proposed an approach independent of bone scintigraphy, serving as only a rough guide to management. In this approach, surgery is delayed as long as possible depending on the etiology underlying the development of HO. In general, a period of 6 months is recommended after direct trauma to musculoskeletal system, a period of 1 year after spinal cord injury, and 1.5 years after head injury has been proposed. It is imperative here to note that such prolonged delay in managing the patient leaves them at risk of the development of complete joint ankylosis and resulting intra-articular secondary damage or other complications of HO. This approach is hence not very popular due to lack of objective measures for initiation of treatment in this modern world of evidence-based medicine and protocol-followed management. This has encouraged attempts to stage and identify the maturity of HO using various imaging studies. Quite unfortunately, however, still accurate indicators of maturity have remained elusive.

Radiographic findings, ALP levels and bone scans are at best, an approximation to balance appropriately delayed intervention without the mentioned complications.

172. Discuss the pathophysiology, clinical features, and differential diagnosis of HO.

Ans: *Per se* in newer nomenclature HO refers to heterotopic ossificans circumscripta and not traumatic HO.

Pathophysiology: It is a localized, non-neoplastic HO, predominantly seen in extremities. Majority of the cases have been described in quadriceps and brachialis muscles. Due to lack of clarity on the pathogenesis, it has been variably thought to occur idiopathically, associated with certain systemic disorders [tetanus, hemophilia, and disseminated idiopathic skeletal hyperostosis (DISH)] or due to trauma (minor injuries as in sports person). Huge amount of controversy exists over trauma as inciting event. There is a possibility that injured muscle (e.g., sports injury) heals with fibrous tissue that degenerates to undergo ossification as for endochondral ossification possibly related to alteration in local growth factors. HO however develops in 7–8 weeks but bone formation takes a bit longer so this could be an argument against this hypothesis. Once the lesion is matured (usually 2 months), spontaneous regression is seen in significant number of patients (30%).

Clinical features: The fever, swelling, erythema, and joint stiffness typically seen in early HO.
- *Early disease (inflammatory phase):* Early there is swelling and pain similar to an infection or soft tissue aggressive tumor.
- *Intermediate stage (consolidation phase):* The lesion becomes clinically firm with constant pain. There may be limitation of movements at adjacent joints if the lesion is large.
- *Late stage (maturation phase):* The mass becomes bony hard and easily discernable from its surrounding tissue. The pain reduces dramatically but the swelling and deformity is a concern for most patients. The mass may merge with the adjacent bone resembling osteochondroma. The movements at the associated joints may be limited in a large mass.

Differential diagnosis: Osteomyelitis, osteochondroma, osteosarcoma, myositis, pentazocine-induced myopathy, hematoma formation, intramuscular parasitic cysts, rhabdomyosarcoma, and synovial sarcoma.

(In case one is interested to read details of traumatic HO and otherwise for better understanding, kindly refer to Chapter 5 of the book Essential Orthopedics: Principles and Practice, 2nd edition.)

2.11 DIAGNOSTIC MODALITIES IN ORTHOPEDICS (Q173–189)

173. Discuss:
    A. Role of ultrasonography in orthopedics.
    B. Robotics in orthopedic surgery.

Ans:
A. Ultrasonography has various diagnostic and therapeutic implications in orthopedics as follows:

Diagnostic:
- *Tendons:*
    - Tears
    - Tendinosis, tendinitis, and tenosynovitis
    - Peritendinitis.
- Cysts.

Therapeutic low-intensity pulsed ultrasound (LIPUS):
- Application of ultrasonography for different tissues and their associated conditions:
  - Enthesopathy
  - Bursitis
  - Postoperative
  - Interventional
  - Aspiration of cysts, abscess and hematoma, etc.
  - Injection of sclerosant into cysts.

Diagnostic Uses

Antenatal diagnosis of musculoskeletal disorders: Various disorders can be readily identified in the prenatal period at various stages of development:
- Osteochondrodysplasia
- Club foot
- Arthrogryposis
- Limb abnormalities associated with syndromes.

Joints and tendon disorders: "Tendon tears" like that of biceps, triceps, rotator cuff, adductor, quadriceps, and posterior tibial tendon can be readily evaluated. The following are the typical findings:

Discontinuity of fibers (complete or incomplete) or focal thinning of tendon (partial tendon tears): Confirmed by tenography (injecting radiopaque dye in tendon sheath and visualizing radiologically).
- *Hematoma of variable size:* Hematoma develops around the whole tendon.
- *In case of bone avulsion:* The bone fragments are seen as bright echogenic foci with acoustic shadowing.
- Nonvisualization of tendon commonly indicates retracted tendon (in case of complete tear, e.g., biceps brachii, rotator cuff, and flexor tendons of finger)
- For Achilles tendon tears, ultrasonography is a good modality if there is pain around the region and no clinical tendon tear.

Tendinosis:
- Degenerative changes in a tendon (no signs of inflammation within the tendon or paratenon).
- *Mostly associated with painful focal or diffuse nodular thickening of tendon:* Mainly described with patellar tendon and Achilles tendon (achillodynia).
- Hypervascularity is seen on Doppler imaging, if performed concomitantly.
- There is decreased echogenicity of enlarged tendon.

Tendinitis:
- Thickening of tendon with inflammatory features (edema and blurred margins)
- Decreased echogenicity
- Increased vascularity on Doppler imaging
- Calcification (patellar tendon and rotator cuff predominantly) can be detected in chronic tendinitis.

Tenosynovitis:
- Acute tenosynovitis shows fluid in the sheath.
- Suppurative tenosynovitis depicts fluid with internal echoes representing debris.
- Chronic tenosynovitis reveals hypoechoic thickening of synovial sheath, with little or no fluid.
- Rheumatoid tenosynovitis is peculiar as the fluid may be absent and the tendon sheath is involved by pannus that is hypoechoic.
- Ultrasonography can also be used for tenography.

Ganglia and cysts around joints: Ganglia around joints and cysts like popliteal and meniscal cysts are readily identified. They are composed of low echogenic, oval mass adjacent to joint space or anechoic material which surrounds the tendon echo complex; percutaneous drainage can be readily guided. Chronic cysts may have internal echoes mimicking hypoechoic solid tumor.

Bursitis:
- Acute bursitis shows sonolucent and fluid-filled collection, with ill-defined margins.
- Chronic bursitis depicts a complex sonographic appearance with internal echogenic debris resulting from granulomatous tissue, precipitated fibrin, and calcification.

Enthesopathy: Sonographically, the tendon at insertion appears swollen and hypoechoic, with calcification developing in longstanding cases.

Rotator cuff tear: This is one of the emerging methods in diagnosis that also reveals dynamic motions in the tendon region. Persons need to be thoroughly trained and being highly observer-based, the technique is mastered with a steep curve.

Major criteria for diagnosis of rotator cuff tear are:
- Nonvisualization of the cuff
- Focal nonvisualization or discontinuity
- Abnormal echogenicity.

Assessment of muscle and osseous structure: Thoroughly performed assessment of the bone and muscle structure helps in assessment of various disorders.
- Quantitative and qualitative assessment of bone can be performed that helps in diagnosing and classifying osteoporosis. Quantitative ultrasound is capable of providing information about the qualities of bone, such as trabecular microarchitecture. Trabecular microarchitecture accounts for up to 50% of total bone strength and is a valid indicator for the risk of pathological fractures.
- Quantitative assessment of structural muscle abnormalities can be easily done.
- Ultrasonography also helps in diagnosis and assessment of fractures, especially stress fractures.
- Ultrasonography has also been utilized to evaluate the progress of healing callus formation and consolidation. Some centers use it to monitor the progress of regenerate formation and adjust the distraction rate according to the quality and quantity of regenerate.

Vascular complications: It can never be forgotten that ultrasonography Doppler is indispensable in diagnosing *deep vein thrombosis* (DVT) which is a frequent complication of many orthopedic surgeries and a frequent cause of otherwise unaccounted for mortality. Other lesions that can be identified are soft tissue hemangiomas (especially differentiating them from ganglion), hemangioendotheliomas and bone vascular lesions like intraosseous hemangiomas.

Neonatal Conditions

Developmental dysplasia of hip (DDH): Clinical assessment of the neonatal hip is performed routinely in the first day of life, and it has become diagnostic modality of choice for DDH due to its ability to evaluate cartilaginous structures. It is a good idea to perform an ultrasonography assessment for doubtful cases before the appearance of femoral head ossification center (4–6 months of age) after which radiographs can be equally useful. Graf (1980) described a static nonstress ultrasound measurement technique utilizing the nonossified head as a transmitting material. This is a morphological assessment relying on anatomic landmarks. The transducer is placed on the greater trochanter allowing visualization of the deeper structures. Measure the alpha (angle between the roof and baseline) and beta (angle between the inclination line and baseline) angles. The acetabular angles are carefully measured on a coronal view of the hip and subcategorized depending on labral echogenicity.

It is also now a preferred modality for evaluation of children on treatment with Pavlik harness.

A good use of ultrasonography could be to evaluate infants with risk factors for DDH like breech position, family history, torticollis, etc.

Observations for DDH:
- Morphologic evaluation of the location of the femoral head and the degree of acetabulum development.
- Dynamic evaluation of the location of femoral head and degree of hip instability with stress.
- The depth of acetabulum and displacement of femoral head are measured by alpha and beta angles.
- Alpha angle is between body weight baseline and acetabular baseline.
- Beta angle is measured between body weight baseline and acetabular labrum line.

- *Disadvantages of X-ray:* These include—
  - The exposure to ionizing radiation
  - Lack of ossification of the femoral head in early infancy.
- *Spinal lesions:* Various conditions of spine can be readily identified using sonography as it has the advantage of being performed in mild sedation. Investigations like magnetic resonance imaging (MRI) need anesthesia for examination. The conditions that can be identified are:
  - Tethered cord syndrome
  - Low lying conus medullaris below the l2/l3 level
  - Subcutaneous and epidural masses of the spine
  - Spinal neoplasms like sacrococcygeal teratoma with characterization into cystic, solid (commonly malignant) or mixed types.

Femoral anteversion: Ultrasonography is also emerging as a good screening tool for evaluation of femoral anteversion.

Joint effusions: Plain radiographic films are normal in presence of small joint effusions. In such cases, ultrasonography can be used to determine, if effusion is present. Ultrasonography has been called "orthopedist's stethoscope" very aptly, especially in children. As little as 1 mL of fluid can be detected in the hip and ultrasound can also guide needle aspiration simultaneously. To guide arthrocentesis, saline lavage can be used if fluid cannot be withdrawn. Ultrasonography can determine the nature of fluid collection—anechoic or hypoechoic fluid is seen in transient synovitis and more echogenic fluid in septic arthritis.

Hematomas and masses: Calcification in the soft tissues, particularly in myositis ossificans, is seen more readily and earlier by ultrasound than by radiography, computed tomography (CT) or MRI. The differentiation between myositis ossificans and a calcified tumor is based on the combination of the ultrasound findings of a mass with highly reflective internal echoes and a characteristic centripetal pattern of development with time.

- Ultrasonography can differentiate tumor mass from hematoma or muscle rupture. Also the tissue can be characterized like fat has high echogenicity, but distinction is poor to differentiate benign from malignant lesion. Benign lesions are often indirectly identified. They have a well-defined margin and have tendency to displace the surrounding tissue rather than invading it. Color Doppler may help evaluate the vascularity that is raised in malignant lesions. Ultrasonography can also help in guided biopsy of the lesion.

Septic arthritis: May arise *de novo* or may occur secondary to infection in adjacent soft tissue or bone:
- Fluid is seen as anechoic or hypoechoic areas
- Ultrasonography-guided, joint fluid aspiration can be done simultaneously.

Infection of soft tissues: Ultrasonography can be used to evaluate infection of soft tissues:
- *Cellulitis:* Heterogeneous soft tissue thickening increase echogenicity in affected area
- Polymyositis
- *Abscess:* Usually, hypoechoic can be isoechoic/hyperechoic.

Osteomyelitis: Early sign–deep soft tissue swelling.

Late sign:
- Fluid along cortex of the bone or subperiosteally
- Fluid in adjacent joint (sterile or aseptic).

Trauma: Brachial plexus injury from birth trauma can be identified by identifying avulsed nerve roots.

Interventional procedures:
- Localized aspiration of fluid/abscess
- Injection of drugs into subtle spaces like tenosynovial sheath injection of steroids
- Localization of masses and guided biopsy
- Localization of foreign body for placing incision for extraction. Also, the size, site, and nature of foreign body can be identified.

Therapeutic
- Aid in fracture healing in fresh fractures or nonunions. Act by upregulating the receptor activity of neurotransmitters at the fracture site like the nitric oxide pathways and the prostaglandin pathways. Reports suggest that the effect of application of LIPUS (low-intensity pulsed ultrasound of 0.03 W cm at 1.5 MHz, up to a maximum of 0.1 W cm^2) on stress fractures, delayed or nonunion or postsurgical intervention is positive.
- Low-intensity pulsed ultrasonography has been used for improving regenerate consolidation in distraction osteogenesis, postspinal fusion, and improving the osteogenesis with the use of porous implants.
- Low-intensity ultrasound has a heating effect that prevails superficially and has been utilized in controlling tendinopathies like the tennis elbow, plantar fasciitis tendoachilles inflammation, etc.

B. **ROBOT** is a term used for a machine that automatically carries out various tasks, requires little or no assistance from outside and can be programmable. "Robot" word is derived from Polish word "*robota*" which means *forced labor*. Robotic systems can be classified into two categories:
1. Haptic (or tactile or surgeon-guided)
2. Autonomous system.

Haptic system requires surgeon's continuous input for efficiently performing and completing surgery. The surgeon uses or drives the robot to perform an operation.

Autonomous systems differ from the above by having more independency. After the operative site is approached by the surgeon, he sets up the machine and then engages the robot, which completes the remaining task, without the help of a surgeon.

Proposed advantages of robotic surgery include:
- Minimal invasive surgery (MIS) is possible
- Implants can be placed more accurately
- Radiologically, improved alignment of extremities.

Haptic Robotic Systems

Robotic arm interactive orthopedic system (RIO®): It is commercially available tactile system for unicondylar knee replacement (other more popular systems for total knee and hip is MAKO system and for spine surgery is the Spine Assist system). As it is tactile system, surgeon's participation is must to complete unicompartmental knee replacement (UKR). Three-dimensional (3D) computer model of the knee is prepared with the use of CT scans preoperatively, which forms the basis of preoperative planning. Based on this, surgeon will mark the bony surfaces of femur and tibia during operation. He merges the preoperative model into active anatomy of the knee. After taking the knee through a full range of motion, the flexion-extension gaps assessed, component size and implant placement finalized, and a cutting zone is created for the robot. Preoperative planning and templating process forms the base for the system's algorithm. By viewing the 3D model of the knee on the monitor, the surgeon accurately manipulates the burr and resects the bone.

Forced controlled tip of the rotating burr cannot resect the bone outside the predefined cutting space. The safety system automatically stops the burr when the surgeon goes beyond the cutting zone. This feature also engages if the computer determines that the surgeon is resecting more bone than necessary.

Examples: These include:
- Robot-assisted unicompartmental knee replacement (UKR) systems
- Acrobot systems.

They have proposed advantages like smaller incisions, short recovery and rehabilitation time, hence can be performed as an outpatient procedure, better American Knee Society (AKS) scores need large study for confirmation, improved tibiofemoral alignment, and implant positioning within 2° of preoperative plan. The disadvantage is obviously the increased operating time.

Autonomous robotic systems: They differ from the tactile system by their independency. Autonomous robotic systems do not require surgeon's assistance. They can carry on and complete the surgery on their own, defined on the preset program. It is worth mentioned that a surgeon can immediately shut off the process with the help of the emergency switch. Currently, autonomous systems are still under investigation for use in orthopedic surgery.

ROBODOC (California): It is an autonomous robotic system, developed in 1980s and taken into surgical practice in 1992 for total hip arthroplasty (THA). Though it became popular for a while in Germany due to its ability of good component positioning, it fell into disrepute because of safety concerns.

Other examples: These include:
- Mini bone-attached robotic system (MBARS) (Pittsburgh, Pennsylvania)—a hybrid semiautonomous robotic system which mounts on to the femur and completes the bony resection in total knee replacement (TKR).
- Praxiteles (France)—another similar robotic system developed in France.

Pitfalls and limitations of robotic surgery:
- An alternative of robotic surgery in place of a conventional one is a costly option, unless the institute has large volumes of surgery being performed routinely. Also, it constantly requires software upgradations and calibrations, making the option more expensive.
- Superiority and cost efficiency of robotic surgery in routine practice are yet to be demonstrated by long-term outcomes studies. Though some advantages like short hospital stay, less blood loss, greater accuracy are proposed.
- As per dictum, total knee arthroplasty (TKA) is a soft tissue operation where the bony cuts are supplementary. Bony anatomy can be well identified by the robots, but the same is yet to be identified by soft tissue dissection by a robot.
- Because of increased risk of infection, blood loss, neurological damage and perhaps an increased rate of litigation, the autonomous robotic system, the ROBODOC, fell into disrepute.
- Currently, high quality level I studies including randomized control trials are not available for the use of robotic surgery in clinical practice. The robotic surgery systems have promising short-term improvements at present, compared to their conventional counterpart. But, due to economic barriers and the lack of prospective, long-term, clinical outcome data, widespread adaptation of robotic surgery has still not occurred.

However, there is a hope for robotic surgery to become more accessible as the technology continues to improve and let the world know how the ideal surgery should be performed.

174. Outcome measures of robotics in trauma and orthopedics.

Ans: Outcome measures of robotics in trauma and orthopedics
1. *Clinical effectiveness:*
   - *Precision:* Robotic systems (e.g., MAKO and NAVIO) reduce alignment errors in TKA/THA (↓2–3° deviation vs. manual techniques).
   - *Revision rates:* Fewer revisions due to malpositioned implants (e.g., 1.5% vs. 4% in conventional TKA at 5 years).
   - *Operative efficiency:* Shorter OR times for complex cases (e.g., pelvic fractures) with preoperative 3D planning.
2. *Safety metrics:*
   - *Complications:* ↓50% intraoperative soft-tissue/nerve injuries (robotic haptic boundaries).
   - *Blood loss:* ↓30% in robotic-assisted spine/stabilization surgeries.
   - *Infection rates:* Comparable to conventional methods but with potential ↓ due to reduced instrument manipulation.
3. *Patient-reported outcomes (PROs):*
   - *Functional scores:* Higher postoperative KSS (85 vs. 78) and OKS (40 vs. 35) in robotic TKA cohorts.
   - *Recovery:* Faster return to ADLs (6 vs. 8 weeks) and ↓ opioid use (20% reduction).
   - *Satisfaction:* 90% patient satisfaction vs. 75% with manual techniques (PROSPECT trial data).
4. *Economic impact:*
   - *Costs:* Higher upfront investment ($500K–$1M/system) but ↓ long-term costs:
     – Fewer revisions ($20K savings per avoided revision)
     – Shorter hospital stays (↓0.5 days average)
   - *Value-based care:* Cost-effective for high-volume centers (ICER: $45K/QALY for robotic THA).
5. *Emerging evidence:*
   - *Trauma:* Robotics improve accuracy in percutaneous screw fixation (e.g., pelvic fractures—98% accuracy vs. 85% manual).
   - *Customization:* Patient-specific implants with AI-driven planning (↓ implant overhang/undersizing).

175. **Robotic surgery in orthopedics:**
- **Discuss present role, usage, and indications.**
- **Comment on cost to benefit ratio of robotic surgery in orthopedics in developing countries.**

Ans:
- Kindly see the answer above
- *Cost-effectiveness:* In various western reported analysis, the robotic-assisted total knee arthroplasty (TKA) has been found to be as cost-effective as a manually performed TKA provided higher volumes are performed in the hospital. The volumes reportedly producing this cost-effectiveness vary from 49/year to 250/year. Also, the difference in surgical outcomes for robotic and manual TKA in terms of survival and functional scores are not startling (QALY of 6.18 in robotic vs 6.17 in manual TKA!). I would certainly differ from this scenario in developing counties like India where there is a huge pressure now for performing surgeries under affordable medical care schemes sponsored by government. This is based on two premises—one the schemes do not cover the cost of disposables used with robotic systems that on an average cost somewhere around 30,000 INR if not reused or not obtained from grey market. Also, the pay-out from government schemes will not recover the cost of robot in surgeons life-time so in a way the surgeon will remain in debt throughout his remaining life. Private insurers in the country have recently started to bear the cost of robotic surgery disposables but it is still growing and the reach of private insurance is mostly limited to metro and tier-2 cities. Patients getting surgery done under direct cash payments are not very keen to bear the extra cost of robotic surgeries. Finally, the cost-effectiveness demonstrated in western studies is based on various assumed variables that is not applicable to Indian population like willingness to pay $50000/QALY = 40 lakh INR/QALY, this is whopping and out of reach assumption even for richest population of the country! In my honest opinion in India centers doing >200 TKA/year with cash/insurance packages ranging around 2 lakh per knee (including implant cost) may be able to make the surgery cost effective over a duration of 3–4 years provided they are able to prove that robotic surgery outcomes are fairly superior to manual TKA in terms of survival and functional scores. Otherwise the extra-cost borne by the patient or insurer is just a waste.

176. **Discuss the principles of ultrasonography. What are their usage in orthopedic practice?**

Ans: Ultrasound is sound above the audibly perceptible range of frequencies (20 Hz–20 kHz). Ultrasound waves are produced by piezoelectric crystals. They pass through various interphases and are reflected back based on the variable acoustic impedance produced at tissue interphases. The ultrasonography identifies changes in tissue based on physical characteristics rather than MRI scan that discriminates on the basis of changes in chemical structure. Depending on the density of tissue and other variables, the reflected waves when correctly interpreted gives information regarding various characteristics of the tissue like the size, shape, and internal structure, and hence the same can be studied for normal and pathological tissues. The waves in the form of electric energy are converted into mechanical energy. Such transfer of energy can be utilized in imparting therapeutic abilities to the modality. The frequency used for therapeutic ultrasound is usually 0.5 MHz (LIPUS) while those for diagnostic ultrasound range between 2 MHz and 10 MHz. Higher the frequency used, the greater the spatial resolution but the shallower the depth of tissue that can be reached. Higher frequency probes (5–7.5 MHz) are mainly used in pediatric scans and scans of small parts or superficial structures. For adult scans and for deeper structures, the lower frequency probes are preferable (3–5 MHz).

"Piezoelectric effect" was described by Pierre and Jacques Curie in 1880. It is defined as change in physical dimensions of certain materials, when subjected to an electric field. Such materials are made of innumerable dipoles arranged in a geometric pattern. An electric dipole is a distorted molecule that has a positive charge on one end and a negative charge on other end (much like an ordinary magnet). Positive and negative ends are so arranged that an electric field will cause them to realign, thus changing the dimension of crystal. Sudden burst or pulse of high frequency *alternating current* (AC) voltage causes crystal to vibrate and emit ultrasound waves. Waves travel through the medium and get reflected back from different interphases. The reflected waves carry energy that causes physical compression of the crystal in turn. The dipoles do not get reoriented and the reverse phenomenon occurs, i.e. compression produces voltage. This voltage difference between electrodes is amplified producing—ultrasonic signal for display. This compression force and associated voltage are responsible for the name piezoelectricity also called "pressure electricity". In "A" (amplitude) type scanning, the returning echo is displayed as a spike and used to measure the depth of objects in the beam. If there are no returning signals, then it indicates a fluid medium. In "B" (brightness) type scanning, the returning echo is seen as a dot which is deciphered on the cathode-ray screen according to the position and impedance of the reflecting tissue. The "hypoechoic" tissues appear black/dark gray while the "hyperechoic" (dense) tissues appear white/light gray.

For usage kindly see Answer to Question above.

177. **A. Describe the concept, advantages, and disadvantages of FAST/e-FAST and CT angiography of abdomen to evaluate abdominal injury in a polytrauma victim (with or without pelvic fracture).**
B. What does a positive-FAST indicate in a case of pelvic fracture?
C. Compare e-FAST with diagnostic peritoneal aspiration.

Ans: A. Focused Assessment with Sonography for Trauma (FAST) and extended FAST (e-FAST)

Concept: FAST is a rapid, noninvasive bedside ultrasound used in trauma to detect free intraperitoneal fluid (blood) and guide management. e-FAST extends this to include thoracic assessment for pneumothorax, hemothorax, and pericardial effusion. It targets four key areas (pericardial, perihepatic, perisplenic, and pelvic) in FAST, plus lungs and pleural spaces in e-FAST, to identify life-threatening injuries in the acute setting.

- *Indications:* Blunt or penetrating trauma, suspected hemoperitoneum, hemothorax, pneumothorax, or pericardial tamponade.
- *Procedure:* Performed with a portable ultrasound (3–5 MHz probe) in 3–5 minutes, typically in the emergency department during primary survey (ATLS protocol).

Advantages:
- *Speed:* Rapid (3–5 minutes), performed at bedside, no patient transport required.
- *Noninvasive:* No radiation, safe for pregnant patients and children.
- *Repeatable:* Can be repeated to monitor dynamic changes (e.g., increasing fluid).
- *Cost-effective:* Low cost, widely available in trauma centers.
- *Sensitivity for fluid:* Detects as little as 100–200 mL of intraperitoneal blood; e-FAST adds high sensitivity for pneumothorax (lung sliding absence).

Disadvantages:
- *Operator-dependent:* Accuracy relies on user expertise; sensitivity varies (70–90% for hemoperitoneum).
- *Limited specificity:* Cannot differentiate blood from other fluids (e.g., ascites) or identify solid organ injuries (e.g., liver laceration without free fluid).
- *Poor visualization:* Suboptimal in obese patients, gas-filled abdomen, or subcutaneous emphysema.
- *Misses retroperitoneal injuries:* Limited for retroperitoneal bleeding or vascular injuries (e.g., aortic dissection).
- *e-FAST limitation:* Less sensitive for small hemothorax or subtle pneumothorax compared to CT.

CT Angiography (CTA)

Concept: CTA is a contrast-enhanced computed tomography technique that visualizes blood vessels and surrounding tissues to detect vascular injuries, bleeding, or organ damage. In trauma, it is used to assess for active bleeding, pseudoaneurysms, vessel occlusion, or solid organ injuries, particularly in stable patients. It involves IV contrast (e.g., iodinated) and multi-detector CT scanners for high-resolution imaging.

- *Indications:* Suspected vascular injury (e.g., aortic dissection and extremity vessel trauma), solid organ injury, or complex fractures in hemodynamically stable patients.
- *Procedure:* Performed in a radiology suite with IV contrast injection, timed to capture arterial and/or venous phases (5–10 min total).

Advantages:
- *High sensitivity/specificity:* >95% for vascular injuries, organ damage, and active bleeding; gold standard for trauma imaging.
- *Comprehensive:* Detects visceral, vascular, and skeletal injuries, including retroperitoneal bleeding missed by FAST.
- *Detailed anatomy:* Provides 3D reconstructions for precise surgical planning (e.g., vessel repair and embolization).
- *Rapid acquisition:* Modern multi-detector CT scanners complete scans in seconds.

Disadvantages:
- *Radiation exposure:* Significant risk, especially in young patients or repeated scans (5–10 mSv per scan).
- *Contrast risks:* Nephrotoxicity, allergic reactions, or extravasation with iodinated contrast; contraindicated in renal failure or severe allergies.
- *Requires stability:* Not suitable for hemodynamically unstable patients due to transport to CT suite.
- *Cost/Time:* More expensive and time-consuming than FAST; requires radiology infrastructure.
- *False negatives:* Rare for small vessel injuries or early bleeds without contrast extravasation.

B. Positive FAST in the context of pelvic fracture

A positive focused assessment with sonography for trauma (FAST) in a patient with a pelvic fracture indicates the presence of free intraperitoneal fluid, most likely hemoperitoneum (blood in the peritoneal cavity). In the pelvic view of FAST (suprapubic window), free fluid appears as an anechoic (dark) area in the pelvis, typically in the pouch of Douglas (rectouterine or rectovesical space).

Clinical significance in pelvic fracture
- *Implication:* Suggests intra-abdominal bleeding, often from associated visceral injuries (e.g., bladder, bowel, or spleen) rather than the pelvic fracture itself, as most pelvic fracture bleeding is retroperitoneal and not detected by FAST.
- *Common sources:*
    - Bladder or urethral injury (common in anterior pelvic fractures)
    - Mesenteric or bowel injury
    - Concomitant abdominal organ injury (e.g., liver and spleen) due to high-energy trauma.
- *Urgency:* Indicates potential need for urgent laparotomy or further imaging (e.g., CT angiography in stable patients) to identify and control bleeding sources.
- *Limitations:*
    - FAST does not detect retroperitoneal bleeding (common in pelvic fractures).
    - Cannot differentiate blood from other fluids (e.g., urine from bladder rupture).
    - Sensitivity for hemoperitoneum is 70–90%, operator-dependent.

Management implications:
- *Unstable patient:* Positive FAST with hemodynamic instability warrants immediate surgical exploration (e.g., laparotomy) to address intra-abdominal hemorrhage.
- *Stable patient:* Proceed to CT angiography for detailed assessment of bleeding source and associated injuries.
- *Pelvic stabilization:* Regardless of FAST, stabilize pelvic fractures with a binder or external fixation to control retroperitoneal bleeding, as FAST-negative does not rule out pelvic hemorrhage.

C. Comparison of e-FAST and diagnostic peritoneal aspiration (DPA) in trauma assessment (Table 2.11.1)

TABLE 2.11.1: Comparison of e-FAST to DPA in trauma.		
Feature	*e-FAST*	*DPA*
Invasiveness	Noninvasive (ultrasound)	Invasive (catheter insertion)
Speed	3–5 minutes, bedside	5–10 minutes, sterile setup
Sensitivity	70–90% for hemoperitoneum	>95% for hemoperitoneum
Specificity	Moderate (cannot identify fluid type)	High (gross blood/enteric contents)
Scope	Abdomen, thorax, and pericardium	Intraperitoneal fluid only
Repeatability	Highly repeatable	Limited due to invasiveness
Safety	Safe, no radiation	Risk of bowel/vessel injury
Availability	Widely available and portable	Requires surgical setup/expertise
Pelvic fracture utility	Detects associated intraperitoneal bleeding; misses retroperitoneal	Detects intraperitoneal bleeding only
Contraindications	Few (obesity, emphysema limit view)	Previous surgery, pregnancy, coagulopathy

178. Define MRI scan. Discuss its principles and applications.

Ans: Magnetic resonance images are created by placing the patient in a strong magnetic field ranging from 5 Tesla in low resolution machines to up to 3 Tesla in high resolution machines. When the tissues are subjected to a strong magnetic field, protons align themselves with respect to the field. This is called the steady state or equilibrium. In this steady state, a radiofrequency (RF) pulse is applied, which excites the magnetized protons in the field. After application of this pulse, the magnetized protons return back to their steady state and in this process, emit a RF signal. This RF signal is captured a receiver coil or antenna and processed to create the magnetic resonance image. For imaging large areas like chest, abdomen, pelvis, hip, thigh or legs, a main large coil shaped like a hollow tube is used in which the patient lies during the study. For smaller areas like wrist, rotator cuff or meniscus special surface coils are used. For adequate MRI, surface coils are necessary because they provide improved spatial resolution.

Most surface coils are designed specifically for different areas of the body, such as knee, shoulder, and wrist. Closed magnetic resonance scanners are also being replaced by open varieties that are more patient friendly. The method and timing of excitation and acquisition of the RF signal can be varied to affect the contrast of the various tissues and thus, create various types of magnetic resonance images. Most musculoskeletal MRI examinations use the spin-echo technique, which produces T1-weighted, proton (spin) density, and T2-weighted images. T1 signal is captured when the protons return to their steady or equilibrium state whereas T2 images are captured immediately after the application of the exciting RF. T1 and T2 are tissue-specific characteristics. Fat has a high signal (bright) on T1-weighted images and fluid has a high signal on T2-weighted images. Structures with little water or fat, such as cortical bone, tendons, and ligaments, remain dark in all types of sequences.

Applications:

Knee:
- Meniscal tears
- Degenerative conditions of meniscus
- Ligament tears [anterior cruciate ligament (ACL) and posterior cruciate ligament (PCL) collateral ligaments]
- Patellar or quadriceps tendon tears
- Tendinitis
- Cysts
- Synovial pathology
- Avascular necrosis (AVN)
- Osseous contusion
- Occult fractures
- Popliteal mass
- Physeal injuries in children
- Osteochondritis dissecans
- Evaluation of articular cartilage.

Shoulder:
- Rotator cuff tear
- Impingement syndromes
- Instability
- Evaluation of the labroligamentous complex
- Occult fractures
- Osteonecrosis
- Pathological conditions of the tendon of the long head of the biceps, including rupture, dislocation or tendinitis
- Suprascapular nerve entrapment.

Spine:
- Evaluation of intervertebral disk disease
- Evaluation of nerve roots, posterior longitudinal ligament, and intervertebral foramen
- Postoperative back pain (failed-back surgery)

- Discitis
- Pyogenic and tuberculous infections
- Epidural hematoma or abscess
- Primary and metastatic tumors of the vertebral column
- Spinal cord injury
- Spinal cord tumors (extradural and intradural)
- Abnormalities of thecal sac
- Developmental deformities of the spinal cord and vertebral column.

Foot and ankle:
- Tendinopathy
- Articular disorders
- Osseous pathological conditions
- Avascular necrosis
- Fracture
- Osteochondral injuries
- Osteomyelitis
- Tendon injury
- Ligament injury.

Hip:
- Avascular necrosis
- Transient osteoporosis of the hip
- Occult fractures
- Evaluation of the acetabular labrum.

Wrist: The most common indication for MRI is evaluation of the intrinsic carpal ligaments and injuries to the triangular fibrocartilaginous complex. Tears in the triangular fibrocartilage (TFC) are seen as linear defects or gaps filled with hyperintense fluid on coronal gradient-echo or T2-weighted pulse sequences. MRI can show masses within the confines of the carpal tunnel as well as edema and swelling of the median nerve. MRI is used to detect marrow abnormalities seen in AVN, of lunate in Kienböck's disease or in the scaphoid after fracture. Like ankle, tenosynovitis and tendon injuries in the wrist and hand can be assessed.

Tumor imaging: Good soft tissue contrast combined with detailed anatomy and multiplanar capability has placed MRI at the forefront of musculoskeletal tumor-imaging methods. MRI is most helpful in defining tumor extent and planning surgical and radiation therapy. It helps in defining aggressive versus indolent processes.

Magnetic resonance imaging examinations are performed after roentgenographic or clinical detection of a lesion. For small lesions (<20 cm), surface coil is used and for larger masses or lesions in the pelvis or thigh body coil or phased-array torso coil is used. The relation of the mass to the surrounding tissue like muscles and neurovascular structures and also the extraosseous extension of bone tumors is best visualized in the axial plane as this plane best shows the anatomy of various compartments. To assess the proximal and distal extent of the lesion, the sagittal or coronal images are used. The extent of bone involvement is seen as bone marrow edema on T1-weighted images. In T2-weighted images, most tumors appear hyperintense when compared to surrounding soft tissue like muscle and fat. Fat suppression techniques further define smaller foci of tumor or edema. Differentiation between solid and cystic tumors and between active and necrotic tumors is done by contrast enhanced T1-weighted images. With contrast active tumor, tumor edema and granulation tissue all become enhanced and cannot be differentiated. To help separate tumor from surrounding edema, dynamic contrast enhancement is used. Routine use of contrast like gadolinium in the initial evaluation of neoplasm is not done. It is more useful in a patient who has undergone surgery to distinguish surgical scar from residual or recurrent tumor nodules. Vascular lesions can be studied with contrast using MRI angiography technique.

The differential diagnosis of bone tumors is derived from routine roentgenograms and later by biopsy and the role of MRI is to define the extent of disease. MRI has replaced CT for the assessment of skeletal tumors, except for densely sclerotic lesions, such as osteoid osteoma.

Most bone tumors are seen as areas of low or intermediate signal intensity on T1-weighted sequences and high-signal intensity on T2-weighted sequences. MRI reliably identifies the spatial boundaries of tumor masses, encasement, and displacement of major neurovascular bundles and the extent of joint involvement. T1-weighted spin-echo images enhance tumor-contrast with bone, bone marrow, and fatty tissue and T2-weighted spin-echo images enhance tumor contrast with muscle and accentuate peritumoral edema.

For most soft tissue lesions, MRI is not diagnostic for any specific histology. Most soft tissue lesions present a nonspecific MRI appearance, typically isointense to muscle on T1-weighted images and hyperintense to muscle and fat on T2-weighted images. The diagnosis of soft-tissue masses is more dependent on history, physical examination, and histopathology.

Certain lesions do exhibit specific signal patterns.
- Lipomas that arise from soft tissue have a homogeneous fat signal on all sequences. The subcutaneous fat makes lipomas in this plane difficult to see. Liposarcomas sometimes show areas of fat and nonfat signal.
- The presence of fat and flowing blood in hemangiomas make them exhibit bright signal on both T1-weighted and T2-weighted studies.
- Hemosiderin present in pigmented villonodular synovitis shows up as a T2-weighted hypointensity.

179. Describe principle, advantages, indications of contrast-enhanced MRI in orthopedics.

Ans: Gadolinium-based contrast agents are mostly used in orthopedic MRI studies. They are principled on:
- Being highly water-soluble gadolinium chelates are extracellularly distributed and eliminated rapidly through renal glomerular filtration.
- Gadolinium-based contrast agents are paramagnetic, that is, these atoms act like ferromagnetic and superparamagnetic substances, and have a positive magnetic susceptibility.
- Enhancement in-vivo is achieved by an increase in the tissues signal intensity (SI), but a decrease in longitudinal relaxation time (T1) and transverse relaxation time (T2)
- They produce an increased signal (positive contrast) on T1-weighted images (the effect on T2-weighted images is generally negligible).

Advantages:
- Improves the sensitivity and specificity of diagnostic images by altering the intrinsic properties of tissues, which influence the fundamental mechanisms of contrast.
- Strategic localization of the agent can regionally change the tissue properties and resulting preferential enhancement helps in disease localization.

Indications:
1. Better localization and visualization of metastatic or infective lesions—improved sensitivity and characterization.
2. Differentiation between neoplastic and inflammatory/infective lesion—infection and demyelination have a much less impressive signature than tumor with respect to blood volume, blood flow, and permeability.
3. Diffusion imaging is helpful in the detection of spine tumor; assisting in determining whether an intraspinal mass is intramedullary or outside the spinal cord.
4. Differentiation between lymphoma (less striking permeability signature) from metastasis
5. Perfusion and permeability scanning helps differentiate treatment-related enhancement from recurrent tumor.
6. Addition of fat-suppressed imaging helps evaluation of metastasis in and around spine.

180. Explain the role of positron emission tomography (PET) scan in orthopedics.

Ans: It is a state-of-the-art hybrid imaging technique which combines the strengths of structural and functional imaging namely PET coupled with CT (PET-CT). The following are the common uses of PET scan in orthopedics:

Infections:
- *Spinal infections:* Fluorodeoxyglucose-PET (FDG-PET) is superior to MRI for detecting low-grade spondylitis or discitis and is used in association with MRI for differentiating degenerative changes from infections. PET clearly outperforms technetium-99m (Tc-99m) bone and gallium-67 (Ga-67) imaging. Limitations of FDG-PET are differentiation between infection and tumor.

- *Diabetic foot infections:* Uninfected neuropathic joints show relatively low maximum standardized uptake value. FDG-PET can differentiate osteomyelitis and soft tissue infection from neuropathic disease.
- *Prosthetic joint infections:* Differentiating aseptic loosening from infection is possible with FDG-PET. The correct diagnosis depends on location, pattern, and intensity of periprosthetic uptake.

Tumors: Fluorodeoxyglucose-PET has an overwhelming role in the evaluation of skeletal metastasis disease. FDG accumulation in skeletal lesions detects direct uptake by the tumor (increased activity on conventional bone scans reflects new bone formation in response to destruction of bone by tumor).

- Successful treatment assessment on FDG-PET is reflected by decrease in or disappearance of the abnormal uptake. "Burnt out" malignant bone lesion may remain abnormal on CT component of PET-CT but will not demonstrate increased FDG accumulation.
- Advantage of detecting extraskeletal disease remains with PET-CT. PET-CT is more sensitive for detecting bone marrow and lytic lesions than sclerotic lesions.
- Fluorodeoxyglucose-PET is more sensitive than conventional bone scintigraphy for detection of bone metastasis of breast carcinoma, non-small-cell lung carcinoma, and lymphoma.
- It is useful for monitoring response to neoadjuvant chemotherapy.

Limitations:
- Fluorodeoxyglucose-PET has a limited role in patients with prostatic carcinoma where F-18 choline may be preferred.
- Role of FDG-PET in imaging algorithm of primary musculoskeletal malignancies is also limited. It is also not possible to differentiate between benign and malignant lesion.
- Accuracy of FDG-PET is affected by therapy. Performing the study within less than 2 weeks after chemotherapy may result in decreased sensitivity because of metabolic shutdown of tumor cells. Irradiated bone behaves variably and may show increased, normal or decrease in activity depending on the time interval between therapy and imaging.
- Treatment with CSFs may induce increase in FDG uptake in the bone marrow which can mask malignant infiltration or can be misinterpreted as disease.

181. Describe briefly principle of FDG-PET scan in orthopedic practice.

Ans: A radiolabeled biological compound F-18 FDG (fluorodeoxyglucose) is injected intravenously. Uptake of this compound followed by further breakdown occurs in the cells. Tumor cells have a high metabolic rate, and hence they also metabolize this compound. FDG is metabolized to FDG-6-phosphate which cannot be further metabolized by tumor cells. So, its gets accumulated and concentrates there. This is detected and quantified using a scanner.

182. A. Describe the pathophysiologic basis of whole-body PET-CT.
B. Elaborate on the nononcologic role of PET-CT in orthopedics.

Ans: For part (A) see above answers.

B. PET-CT has several nononcologic applications in orthopedics:
1. *Infection imaging*
   - *Osteomyelitis*:
     - PET-CT (especially with 18F-FDG) is highly sensitive and specific for detecting chronic osteomyelitis, particularly in complex cases (e.g., postsurgical or diabetic foot infections).
     - Helps to differentiate between soft-tissue infection and bone involvement.
   - *Prosthetic joint infection (PJI)*:
     - Differentiates aseptic loosening from infection in joint replacements.
     - 18F-FDG PET-CT shows increased uptake at the bone-prosthesis interface in infections.
   - *Spinal infections (spondylodiscitis)*:
     - Detects early vertebral osteomyelitis before structural changes appear on CT/MRI.
2. *Inflammatory and autoimmune diseases:*
   - *Rheumatoid arthritis and psoriatic arthritis*:
     - Assesses disease activity, synovitis, and bone erosion progression.
     - Helps to monitor treatment response (e.g., biologics).

- *Spondyloarthropathies (e.g., ankylosing spondylitis)*:
  - Detects active inflammation in sacroiliac joints and spine.
3. *Fracture healing and nonunion assessment*:
   - Evaluates metabolic activity in delayed unions or nonunions.
   - Helps to distinguish viable versus nonviable bone in complex fractures (e.g., scaphoid or femoral neck fractures).
   - May predict healing potential before structural changes are visible.
4. *Metabolic bone disease*:
   - *Paget's disease*:
     - Detects active disease phases (increased FDG uptake).
     - Monitors treatment response (e.g., bisphosphonates).
   - *Fibrous dysplasia*:
     - Differentiates active lesions from quiescent ones.
5. *Bone marrow evaluation*:
   - Detects bone marrow edema (e.g., in complex regional pain syndrome, CRPS).
   - Helps to assess avascular necrosis (AVN) by identifying metabolically active vs. necrotic regions.
6. *Soft tissue and muscle disorders*:
   - Myositis and polymyalgia rheumatica:
     - Identifies inflammatory muscle involvement.
   - *Sarcoidosis*:
     - Detects musculoskeletal granulomatous lesions.

183. A. What is brachytherapy?
B. Explain the role of embolization in orthopedics.

Ans:

A. *Brachytherapy* is primarily a method of administering the radiation therapy.
Brachytherapy is delivered by implantation of radioactive source in tumor tissue (e.g., through catheters) filled with substance or by implanted beads or needles. The advantage is direct delivery to the involved region, minimal wastage of radiation as the radiation is primarily absorbed in the affected region, relative sparing of comparatively distant normal tissue (the radiation intensity falls according to inverse square law for distance). The technique though interesting and quite logical is less often used, as it is invasive and requires association between surgeon and radiation oncologist.

B. *Embolization* has a unique and definitive role in orthopedic neoplastic and traumatic bleeding disorders. While in neoplasia embolization can reduce the vascularity of the lesion, thus aiding surgical treatment and improving response to chemoradiotherapy, in trauma it can be lifesaving by stopping blood loss from surgically inaccessible sites during emergency. The main purpose of embolization is to achieve thrombus formation and occlusion by administrating embolizing materials through a selective catheter placed in an arterial or venous vessel. The following are the indications for embolization:

- Vascular embolization in bone tumors (selective or superselective embolization):
  - Definitive treatment of benign lesions
  - Reducing the risk of bleeding prior to biopsy or surgery
  - Palliation of pain, bleeding, fever, and hypercalcemia-like symptoms in inoperable tumors
  - Preventing further dissemination of a tumor
  - Increasing the response to chemotherapy and radiotherapy
  - Retention of selectively delivered antimitotic agents or monoclonal antibodies deep into the tumor substance
  - Chemo- and radioembolization have not been very popular in orthopedic oncology, however, some dedicated centers have been using them for advanced selective tumor management.
- Uncontrolled bleeding in trauma (generally pelvic trauma)—can be done by a selective embolotherapy or shotgun embolotherapy:
  - Embolization of bleeding arterial vessels—transcatheter embolization
  - Bleeding from:
    - Presacral venous plexus

- Fractured cancellous bone
- Vessels like arteria corona mortis.

184. Write briefly about principle, interpretation and indications of Technetium-99 scan in orthopedics.
Ans:

Principle: Bone scan is used to study reactive bone formation. The radioisotope tracer is incorporated in the hydroxyapatite crystals that make identification of the lesion much ahead of the conventional radiography. The bone scan will however identify any lesion that involves active new bone formation—fracture/infection/infarction/bone forming neoplasia/metastasis, etc. Tracer uptake is also affected by the age of patients (physis have very high uptake), blood flow alterations (myelofibrosis), renal clearance and temperature. Lesions that have minimal bone formation like metastasis from thyroid neoplasms or reticulum cell sarcoma will be bone scan silent while they may demonstrate radiographic lesions (false-negative bone scans).

Interpretation: The standard technique of technetium-99m phosphate imaging is to perform a three-phase study. The three-phase bone scan consists of images taken in:
1. The flow phase
2. The immediate or equilibrium phase
3. The delayed phase

The flow-phase image is similar to a radionuclide angiogram in that it shows blood flow. The equilibrium or blood pool image shows relative vascular flow and distribution of the radioisotope into the extracellular space. The delayed-phase image generally is obtained 2–4 hours after injection when renal excretion has eliminated most of the isotope except that taken up by osteoblastic activity. This image shows osteoblastic activity and is positive in numerous disease states, including osteomyelitis, tumors, degenerative joint disease, trauma, and postsurgical changes. Usually, a focus of osteomyelitis appears as an area of increased tracer uptake on delayed images. To have a "hotspot" on bone scan, the vasculature to the involved bone must be intact. If blood flow to the involved area is decreased by subperiosteal pus, necrosis (i.e., sequestrum), joint effusion, vasospasm, or soft-tissue swelling, a "cold" scan may result.

Indications (most are superseded by PET scan now):
- Patients with known (to know extent) or suspected (to identify) malignant disease.
- Revealing metastasis of an evident primary locating suitable biopsy site
- Evaluating areas difficult to read on roentgenogram
- Differentiating pathological from traumatic fracture
- Reviewing X-ray interpretation (X-rays are false negative in 30% cases)
- Planning radiation therapy portals
- Identification of most active metastasis
- Follow-up evaluation of therapy
- Differentiating bone islands from metastasis
- Patients with meningioma—to study the extent of bone involvement
- Detecting soft tissue metastasis in osteosarcoma
- Multiple myeloma—increased long bone or vertebral activity indicates impending fracture
- Staging of lymphoma or Hodgkin's disease
- Predicting response to ^{32}P therapy in patients with bone metastasis.

185. Explain bone scan: Types and limitations in musculoskeletal conditions.
Ans: *Types of bone scans*
1. *Conventional bone scintigraphy (planar imaging):*
    - Standard whole-body scan in 2D (anterior and posterior views).
    - Used for detecting metastases, stress fractures, and infections.
2. *Single-photon emission computed tomography (SPECT):*
    - Provides 3D imaging with better localization.
    - Useful for spine, pelvis, and complex joint pathologies (e.g., spondylolysis and osteoid osteoma).

3. *SPECT/CT (hybrid imaging)*:
   - Combines functional (SPECT) and anatomical (CT) imaging.
   - Improves diagnostic accuracy in tumors, infections, and trauma.
4. *Three-phase bone scan*:
   - Assesses blood flow (angiographic phase), blood pool (soft-tissue phase), and delayed (bone phase).
   - Helps to differentiate osteomyelitis (all phases positive) from cellulitis (only early phases positive).

Limitations of bone scans in musculoskeletal conditions
1. *Limited specificity:*
   - Detects increased osteoblastic activity but does not distinguish between tumors, infections, fractures, or arthritis.
   - *False positives in*:
     - Degenerative joint disease (OA)
     - Healing fractures
     - Paget's disease
     - Heterotopic ossification
2. *Poor soft-tissue resolution:*
   - Cannot evaluate soft-tissue tumors or muscle injuries effectively.
3. *Radiation exposure:*
   - Uses ionizing radiation (~4–6 mSv, higher than X-rays but less than CT).
4. *Time-consuming:*
   - Requires 2–4 hours between tracer injection and imaging.
5. *False negatives in certain conditions:*
   - *Purely lytic lesions* (e.g., multiple myeloma, aggressive metastases) may not show uptake.
   - *Early osteomyelitis* (first 24–48 hours) may be missed.
6. *Limited use in pediatric patients:*
   - High sensitivity but often requires additional MRI for precise diagnosis.

186. Explain the role of nuclear scan studies in orthopedic practice.

Ans: Nuclear medicine plays a crucial role to provide sensitive functional information in a variety of clinical settings. *Isotope bone scan or "bone scintigraphy"* is an investigative modality which uses radioisotope-tagged tracers which are specifically taken up by the bone. These tracers are taken up in areas of increased bone turnover. The detected abnormality may consist of decreased uptake (e.g., early stage of osteonecrosis) or increased uptake (e.g., fracture, neoplasm, and focus of osteomyelitis).

Scintigraphy is a sensitive imaging modality, but it lacks specificity. It is not possible to differentiate between various processes that can cause increased or decreased uptake.

However, in some lesions, the bone scan may yield very specific information and even suggest the diagnosis.
- In cases of myeloma, there is no significant increase in the uptake of the radiopharmaceutical, but in skeletal metastases, the uptake of the tracer is significantly elevated.
- In osteoid osteoma, there is more increased uptake in the center, due to the nidus and less increased uptake at the periphery, due to the reactive sclerosis surrounding the nidus.
- A three-phase technique can be used to differentiate soft-tissue infection (cellulitis) and osseous infection (osteomyelitis).

Hybrid scanning techniques: In hybrid scanning, an imaging modality like MRI or CT is combined with a nuclear scan to provide information on both anatomy and function. Some examples of such hybrid scan would be single-photon emission computed tomography (SPECT)/CT and PET/CT.

Indications:
- Bone tumors both malignant and nonmalignant
- For diagnosing metastatic bone disease in cases of primary form breast, lung or prostate
- *Avascular necrosis* of femoral head
- Infections

- Diagnosis of stress fracture
- Diseases of bone metabolism like Paget's, osteomalacia, etc.
- Fracture of the spine to rule out pathological fracture
- Legg–Perthes disease and sacroiliitis.

Commonly used tracers in orthopedics:
- *Technetium methylene diphosphonate (MDP):* Technetium 99 MDP is the most commonly used scan. After injection of the tracer, the scan is performed in three stages (triphasic bone scan).
- *Thallium-201:* Thalium-201 is a potassium analog, and as it is selectively taken up by active tumor cells, its main use is in identifying tumor recurrence and metastatic lesions.
- *Gallium-67:* 67 Gallium citrate is used to diagnose infectious processes in bone and joints.
- *Indium-labeled leukocyte scan:* This technique is specific in the detection of abscesses or acute infectious processes, including osteomyelitis and septic arthritis with high specificity and sensitivity. False-positive results are seen in patients with inflammatory process without infection (e.g., RA mistaken for septic arthritis).

Clinical Indications in Orthopedics
Infections:
- *Spinal infections:* FDG-PET is superior to MRI for detecting low-grade spondylitis or discitis and is used in association with MRI for differentiating degenerative changes from infections. PET clearly outperforms Tc-99m bone and Ga67 imaging. Limitations of FDG-PET are differentiation between infection and tumor.
- *Diabetic foot infections:* Uninfected neuropathic joints show relatively low maximum standardized uptake value. FDG-PET can differentiate osteomyelitis and soft tissue infection from neuropathic disease.
- *Prosthetic joint infections:* Differentiating aseptic loosening from infection is possible with FDG-PET. The correct diagnosis depends on location, pattern, and intensity of periprosthetic uptake.

Tumors: Fluorodeoxyglucose-PET has an overwhelming role in the evaluation of skeletal metastasis disease. FDG accumulation in skeletal lesions detects direct uptake by the tumor (increased activity on conventional bone scans reflects new bone formation in response to destruction of bone by tumor).
- Successful treatment assessment on FDG-PET is reflected by decrease in or disappearance of the abnormal uptake. "Burnt out" malignant bone lesion may remain abnormal on CT component of PET-CT but will not demonstrate increased FDG accumulation.
- Advantage of detecting extraskeletal disease remains with PET-CT. PET-CT is more sensitive for detecting bone marrow and lytic lesions than sclerotic lesions.
- Fluorodeoxyglucose-PET is more sensitive than conventional bone scintigraphy for detection of bone metastasis of breast carcinoma, non-small-cell lung carcinoma, and lymphoma.
- Fluorodeoxyglucose-PET has a limited role in patients with prostatic carcinoma where F-18 choline may be preferred.
- Role of FDG-PET in imaging algorithm of primary musculoskeletal malignancies is also limited. It is also not possible to differentiate between benign and malignant lesion. It is useful for monitoring response to neoadjuvant chemotherapy. Accuracy of FDG-PET is affected by therapy. Performing the study within less than 2 weeks after chemotherapy may result in decreased sensitivity because of metabolic shutdown of tumor cells. Irradiated bone behaves variably and may show increased, normal or decrease in activity depending on the time interval between therapy and imaging.
- Treatment with CSFs may induce increase in FDG uptake in the bone marrow which can mask malignant infiltration or can be misinterpreted as disease.

(Details of FDG-PET can be obtained from Answer to Question 180 above)

187. Discuss nuclear medicine and its application in orthopedics.
Ans: Kindly refer to Answer to Question 186 above.

188. Discuss bone scan in musculoskeletal disorders.
Ans: Kindly see the Answer to Question 186 above.

189. Describe dual-energy X-ray absorptiometry (DEXA) scan.

Ans: DEXA involves very limited radiation exposure. It affords fast, reliable, and accurate measurement of bone mass, so is commonly used in screening population and also defining osteoporosis according to the WHO criteria. DEXA has replaced dual-photon and single X-ray absorptiometry and is now the most widely used bone mass measurement tool sort of becoming the currently gold standard for diagnosis, evaluation, and follow-up of osteoporosis patients (discussed above in indications of DEXA). Soft-tissue radiation exposure and attenuation is compensated in DEXA by using a combination of high and low X-ray energies. Both pencil-beam and fan-beam (cone beam, C-arm) devices are currently in use. Pencil beam has less scatter, require less dose (≈ 1 μSv), and reduces operator or patient radiation compared to cone pencil-beam or fan-beam systems, where the required dose is around 18 μSv.

However, the fan-beam systems improve image quality and possibly the accuracy of measurement also. DEXA gives a two-dimensional (2D) measure of BMD. It does not, however, measure true volume density as with quantitative CT. Bone mass is reported as an absolute value in grams per square centimeter in DEXA and is then presented as T-score and Z-score as defined below.

- Z-score compares patient's value to an age-matched and sex-matched reference range. The Z-score is of less clinical value and is used in young adults and postmenopausal females <50 years of age, Z-scores significantly deviating from normal may indicate an alternative cause of a metabolic bone disease.
- T-score is a comparison to mean bone mass of young adult normal individuals defined as healthy women population 20–40 years of age. Thus, T-score may be called young adult Z-score. Women are chosen specifically as they represent the lower normal values of healthy population (without any increased risk of fracture, while reference from male population will fallaciously put even some of normal females into osteoporotic category). T-scores are used to both predict fracture risk and classify disease status as in the WHO definition. This score was suggested to avoid confusion between different BMD measurement technologies. The score is calculated by the formula:

$$\text{T-score} = \frac{\text{mBMD} - \text{YN}}{\text{SD}}$$

Where, mBMD is the measured bone density, YN is the normal value from young population (reference) and SD is the standard deviation of young adult population.

Quantitatively, a change of 1 standard deviation in either the T-score or Z-score corresponds to a change of approximately 0.06 g/cm^2 (about 10% BMD). DEXA can be used to measure bone mass at central (vertebral and proximal femur) and peripheral sites, the choice of site(s) being primarily guided by the anticipated or expected rates of change in bone mass within these skeletal locations. The choice is also influenced by precision of the testing device at these discrete sites. The central DEXA sites of the hip and spine are commonly preferred because it has:

- Higher precision
- The quantity of trabecular bone at central sites is usually indicative of the osteoporosis burden, and hence the fracture risk.
- Bone loss begins early in the trabecular bone as it is highly metabolically active compared to cortical bone and is predominant in central skeleton.
- Ward's triangle has lowest BMD, but is much less predictive or reproducible, so BMD at other locations such as the femoral neck (preferred), trochanter, or total hip should be measured.

Regular follow-up with serial DEXA scan to monitor therapy is controversial. One school of thought recommends yearly scan, while others site benefits of osteoporosis therapy beyond change in BMD and inability to discern true change by relative insensitivity of DEXA as precluding factors to its use. This is substantiated by the fact that minimum 2.77% change in BMD is required between two successive DEXA studies to reach statistical significance for estimating difference with 95% confidence ($p < 0.05$). Not only this, but the measured changed value needs to be multiplied by the "precision error" of the measuring device. If the device has a 2% precision error, a change in BMD of about 5.6% is needed to substantiate BMD change not by chance. Any clinician would know that no currently available modality would achieve this improvement by 1 year of treatment making repeat estimation futile.

Pitfalls in DEXA measurement:
Osteoporosis though systemic occurs inhomogeneously across the body with significant discordance between sites, especially in the elderly. Imaging only one site may thus be misleading. Osteophytes due to high prevalence of facet and posterior element spinal osteoarthritis in elderly may yield a falsely elevated bone mass in anteroposterior projection. This is circumvented by measurement of the spine BMD in lateral projection or measuring hip DEXA. Lateral spine scan is still limited in accuracy by soft-tissue attenuation due to greater thickness and nonuniformity of soft tissues in this projection.

2.12 MATERIALS AND IMPLANTS IN ORTHOPEDICS (Q190–211)

190. Describe the use of plaster of Paris (POP) in orthopedics and precautions in applying hip spica. Detail the principles of functional cast bracing.

Ans:

Use of POP in orthopedics:
- To support fractured bones, controlling movement of the fragments and resting the damaged soft tissues
- To stabilize and rest joints where there has been ligamentous injury
- To support and immobilize joints and limbs postoperatively until healing has occurred, e.g., repair of nerve and tendons
- To correct a deformity by wedging the cast or the application of serial or turnbuckle casts
- To ensure rest of infected tissues
- To make a removable splint to aid mobilization or prevent deformity
- To render it difficult for a patient to remove dressings or tamper with a wound
- To make a negative mold of a part of the body, as a preliminary step in the accurate construction of orthotic or prosthetic appliances.

Precautions:
- To prevent abdominal compartment syndrome and anterior impingement place a folded towel or two cotton bandage rolls and apply padding cast over it. Remove it at end of procedure
- Better use goretex soft wrap instead of cotton as it can be cleaned if soiled
- Use a thick belt of felt across the chest just below the nipple line to prevent pressure sores
- Cover bony points like sacrum, posterior superior iliac spine (PSIS) and anterior superior iliac spine (ASIS) with Felt or similar padding to prevent pressure sores
- Reduce the joint/fracture well under fluoroscopy before applying the cast—cast cannot be expected to produce reduction.
- It is helpful to put minimal casting material over the injured area while adequately casting the other regions. Once the cast is set use fluoroscopy and if needed then reduction can be done by rotation of extremity after cutting the thin shell and reapplying this segment.
- Apply a broom-stick between the thigh to strengthen cast and prevent its breakdown at hip joint
- Similarly reinforce the groin folds of the cast by hard materials like small sticks taking care that they do not penetrate inside or cause sores themselves.

Functional cast bracing: Kindly see answer below.

191. What is PTB cast?

Ans: PTB cast (patellar tendon bearing cast) is a type of functional bracing that is used to promote healing in minimally displaced fractures or where operative treatment is deemed unnecessary or risky. Functional bracing enables nonoperative method of treating fractures that allows continuing function during fracture union encourages osteogenesis and promotes healing of tissues. It prevents the development of joint stiffness, thus accelerating rehabilitation. The core belief of functional cast bracing is that the loss of the anatomical reduction of a fracture is a small price to pay for the rapid healing and the restoration of function, without compromising the appearance of the limb by operating scars.

The principle: As detailed by Sarmiento, functional cast bracing promotes formation of external bridging callus which is situated at a distance from the axis of potential movement (fracture). This has a greater mechanical advantage than medullary callus, and therefore makes a much stronger early repair. Sarmiento asserts that rigid immobilization (produces only intramedullary callus) is detrimental to fracture healing and that the intermittent loading of the fracture area, by muscle activity and weight bearing, promotes local blood flow and the development of electrical fields which are beneficial for healing.

The muscle compartments act as a fluid mass surrounded by an elastic container, the deep fascia. Fluid is not compressible and the fascia cannot be stretched beyond the confines of the cast. Pressure and load is transmitted without further deformation. Elastic recoil takes place when the load is reduced. When muscles contract, they bulge. When this occurs within a rigid constrained cylinder, the muscles are forced inwards away from the rigid walls and to oppose displacement of fracture fragments from displacing. The hydraulic forces control the fragments and resist overlap and angulation until callus forms and takes over that function. Rotation is resisted usually by components of the brace and/or the tendency of the muscle contraction and joint movement to align the fragments.

Timing: Initially conventional casts, which immobilize the joints above and below the fracture, are applied to correct any angular or rotational deformity as the position following the cast bracing of a fracture is basically dependent upon the position of the fragments before the brace is applied. PTB cast is then applied within 6 weeks of the fracture occurring.

Application methods:
- The patient is seated on a couch with his legs dangling over the edge and the thigh supported on a sand bag.
- Roll the cast sock or stockinette onto the limb from the toes to above the knee
- Apply minimal orthopedic wool padding over the heel, tendo-calcaneus, malleoli, common peroneal nerve and tibial condyles and crest.
- Apply POP bandage from the toes to 2 inches above the ankle, keeping ankle at 90°.
- Apply further POP from the toes to the tibial tuberosity and mold it over the medial proximal half of the soft tissues of the calf.
- Flex the knee to 40° and rest the patient's heel on your lap.
- Apply further POP from the top of the cast to 1 inch above the proximal pole of patella.
- Firmly mold the plaster cast over the medial flare of the tibia and the patellar tendon. At the same time apply firm pressure in the popliteal fossa and the back of the calf with the flat of the hand, to produce a triangular cross-section in this area to help to control rotation.
- Mark out and trim the upper end of the cast, keeping the ears as long as possible on both sides of the knee. Posteriorly the upper edge of the cast is level with the tibial tuberosity. Inferiorly the toes must be free to flex and extend fully.

192. What is cast syndrome? Explain its clinical symptoms and management.

Ans: Cast syndrome (better known as body cast syndrome) refers to symptoms arising mostly from mechanical compression causing gastric dilatation with intestinal obstruction (3rd part of duodenal obstruction that can be complete or incomplete). It is also known as superior mesenteric artery syndrome.

Pathophysiology: Superior mesenteric artery arises as a branch from aorta and sharply turns down at an angle of 45° in front of duodenum. The duodenum is obstructed between superior mesenteric artery anteriorly and aorta and spinal column posteriorly that can occur within days or weeks following the procedure. Same compression can occur if the angle of mesenteric artery increases as in rapid growth of children or in chronic anorexia.

Causes: The syndrome is seen following tight spica (hip/shoulder) or body casts in children and in patients following spine scoliosis surgical correction. Other uncommon causes are rapid growth in children, anorexia, trauma, etc.

Symptoms: Patient experiences bloating, intermittent to pernicious vomiting which is often sudden, unexpected, and copious. Patient may go into metabolic alkalosis. If not promptly treated by removal of cast then patient may aspirate causing complete airway obstruction, and cardiac arrest or gastric perforation with peritonitis may occur if the cast is not promptly removed.

Radiographs: X-rays demonstrate gastric distension. Contrast studies might reveal duodenal obstruction.

Management: Removal of the cause of obstruction. Nil by mouth and suction aspiration of gastric contents. Maintaining homeostasis by intravenous fluids and correction of acid-base imbalance. Position the patient toward left side or semi prone may pull the mesenteric pedicle away from duodenum. If measures fail and patient is deteriorating, then duodenojejunostomy or gastrojejunostomy is indicated.

193. Describe the biomaterials used in orthopedics. Discuss their characteristic features.

Ans: Biomaterials are those materials that are implanted in the body to replace or treat tissues. In orthopedics, they are called implants and used for fracture fixation, as anchors and for replacing articular surfaces. An ideal biomaterial should have the following properties. The various biomaterials in use are described here.

Metals and their Alloys

Steel: It is one of the most commonly used biomaterials in orthopedics. Most often 316L alloy is used which contains chromium, nickel, molybdenum. It is the chromium which forms an oxide layer on the outside of the implant that acts as a corrosion resistant layer.

Advantages:
- Strong material
- Cheap and easy to manufacture

Disadvantages:
- Stiff material leads to stress shielding **(Table 2.12.1)**
- Not as inert as titanium
- Undergoes stress and crevice corrosion
- Nickel and chromium allergy

Uses: Fracture fixation in form of screws, nails, and plates. Femoral prosthetic stem in hip replacement.

Titanium: Commercially pure titanium (CP Ti) and titanium alloy with aluminum and vanadium (Ti-6Al-4V) are the two most commonly used alloys. Ti-6Al-4V has twice the tensile and yield strength as compared to CP Ti **(Table 2.12.1)** and is the major titanium alloy currently in use in orthopedics. The vanadium component in Ti-6Al-4V has the potential to be cytotoxic therefore vanadium free alloys like Ti6Al7Nb and Ti5Al2.5Fe with similar mechanical characteristic to Ti-6Al-4V are under investigation but are not yet available commercially. By using special forging techniques the strength of CP Ti can be improved. The excellent corrosion resistance of Ti and Ti alloys is due to the formation of an adhesive TiO_2 oxide layer at their surface.

TABLE 2.12.1: Comparison of various properties of commonly used implant materials with respect to bone.

Material	Elastic modulus	Yield strength	Ultimate strength
Steel (316 L)	205–210	170–750	465–950
Titanium	105–110	850–900	960–970
Cobalt	220–230	275–1585	600–1785
Bone	125–184	75–85	110–130

Advantages:
- Increased flexibility
- Less stiffness causing less stress shielding
- Light weight
- Greater strength when compared to stainless steel
- Better ability to withstand cyclic loads
- More inert and resistant to corrosion
- Spontaneous formation of a strong passivating oxide layer
- Reduced crevice corrosion at the contact point between screw heads and plates
- Smaller diameter implants can be manufactured because of greater strength.

Disadvantages:
- Increased cost
- Difficult manufacturing technique
- More brittle as compared to steel, therefore, cracks occurring from notches in the metal to propagate easily, this limits implant design and makes manufacturing process more exacting.
- Poor resistance to erosion making it unacceptable for bearing surfaces.

Tantalum: Tantalum is a metal which can be fabricated in a highly porous form making it an excellent material to promote bone ingrowth. It acts as a scaffold for bony ingrowth. It is also inert and resistant to corrosion and has modulus of elasticity close to that of bone making it a good material for implants like stem of uncemented prosthesis.

Polymers

Ultrahigh molecular weight polyethylene (UHMWPE): It has low coefficient of friction with metal and this makes it ideal for use as a bearing surface in joints. But the commonly used gamma-ray sterilization increases the rate of production of particles produced during the wear process. These particles produce an inflammatory reaction in the surrounding tissues. These problems are overcome by new processing and sterilization techniques like ETO, by reducing the fraction of low molecular weight chains in the polymer and by changing the orientation and compaction of the polymer chains.

Advantages:
- High abrasion resistance
- Low friction and high strength
- Toughness and low density
- Ease of fabrication
- Biocompatibility

Disadvantages:
Wear particles released lead to inflammatory reaction in the surrounding tissues, osteolysis, and bone resorption.

Bone Cement
Kindly see Answer to Question 210.

Bioabsorbable Biomaterials
Kindly see Answer to Question 215C for Bioabsorbable Biomaterials *in orthopedics.*

Ceramics: Ceramics are a group of polycrystalline materials that have metallic as well as nonmetallic elements. They are extremely hard and brittle and have good resistance to compressive forces and erosion but have poor tensile strength and poor ductility. They have low friction and wear coefficient and therefore used mainly in joint replacement. Their microstructure is dependent on the applied manufacturing process and it has an effect on both the mechanical and biological properties. Generally, a manufacturing process which increases porosity leads to greater bone in growth and osteointegration but reduces strength. Therefore, high density ceramics are used on weight bearing surfaces and porous ceramics like hydroxylapatite are used to coat femoral stem to promote osteoinduction.

The main ceramics used in orthopedic surgery are alumina (Al_2O_3) and zirconia (ZrO_2) for acetabular and femoral components. Hydroxyapatite [$Ca_{10}(PO_4)_6(OH)_2$] for coating stem femoral components.

Advantages:
- Good wear rates
- High corrosion resistance
- Biocompatibility
- High strength

Disadvantages:
- Low fracture toughness
- Stress shielding, due to a very high elastic modulus
- Brittle nature
- Exacting manufacturing process as hip prosthesis components must be perfectly spherical and congruent, making surface finish crucial.

194. **A. Describe biomaterials and their role in THR.**
   B. Explain biocomposite materials.

Ans: A. See Answer to Question 193
Please read Chapter no. 6
B. This is a wrong question—There is nothing called 'biocomposite materials'—there are either biodegradable composite materials or there are biomaterials. The commonly used materials include metals, bioceramics, and polymers (both

synthetic and natural). Metals like titanium that have high biocompatibility which are used mostly for implant synthesis due to favorable mechanical properties. Bioceramics like hydroxyapatite, bioglass, and calcium phosphate are good for bone restoration and substitution, as they are osteogenic, porous, maintain shape, and promote cell proliferation on surface. Bioceramics have an important limitation of poor mechanical properties due to which they are unsuitable for load-bearing. Tissue engineering has been utilized to produce composite materials like HA-TCP (hydroxyapatite with tricalcium phosphate), PCL-HA (polycaprolactone with hydroxyapatite) amalgamated to carbon nanotubes, PCL-PLGA (polycaprolactone with polylactic-co-glycolic acid), PLGA-TCP (polylactic-co-glycolic acid with tricalcium phosphate), etc. These composites are utilized to prepare scaffolds with optimized architecture, biocompatibility, and manufacturing properties such as sintering conditions. Hydrogels have now been the most successful tissue-engineered products commonly used as cell carriers providing a 3D environment to grow. Hydrogels are essentially "water-swellable" but "water-insoluble" crosslinked networks that can provide multiple advantages in tissue engineering by incorporating cells, encouraging their growth and proliferation (by retaining water-simulating biological tissues), and acting as carrier system. Polymers like collagen, chitosan, hyaluronic acid (HA), silk proteins, gelatins, and alginates are all used as hydrogels. These commonly have a common property of inducing a phase change from liquid to semisolid by crosslinking. Crosslinking can be induced by various means, viz., chemicals (calcium to crosslink alginate), thermally or using ultraviolet or visible light. The composite of hydrogel with cells (mature derived cells or stem cells) can act as a bioink to deposit cells or growth factors in a scaffold supported basically by hydrogel. One major issue with hydrogels is their inability to maintain uniform 3D structure for long, and hence they have to be commonly coupled with synthetic biomaterials such as polyglycolic acid (PGA), hydroxyapatite (HA), polycaprolactone (PCL), methacrylate, etc. Bioink can be, for example, made by combining an alginate-gelatin hydrogel with HA, to which cells (say stem cells) can be added. HA is nowadays the most commonly used in building block for creating biomaterials due to its properties that allow cellular signaling, wound repair, and morphogenesis (alginates commonly restrict the cellular signaling).

195. Use of biological adhesives in orthopedics.

Ans: Adhesive biomaterials are emerging new tools for repairing bone and tissue in surgical applications. The currently used adhesive biomaterials include fibrin, collagen, polyurethane, epoxy resin, cyanoacrylates, polyesters, and polymethylmethacrylate. Orthopedic applications mostly fall into their use as scaffolds, filler materials to treat bone defects and as carrier materials to deposit other bioactive materials to a site. These materials can be better studied on the basis of 'base' material used for synthesis of final usable product:

Fibrin-based biomaterials: Fibrin is a viscoelastic biomaterial with great flexibility and extensibility. Primarily fibrin is used as a soft tissue engineering scaffold in orthopedics. Some applications where it has been tried and is under development include:

- Creation of new cartilage using a fibrin film.
- Use of fibrin microbeads to implant into a scaffold to preserve the seeding cell types more effectively. The stem cells were seeded and applied into a bone scaffold.
- Another use of fibrin is as a bone glue. It is commonly mixed with hydroxyapatite to create fibrin-ceramic composite having a high potential for being an osteoinductive bone graft adhesive.
- Now fibrin is also being used as a platelet rich fibrin (PRF) matrix to treat bone defects. The fibrin scaffold is used with impregnated mesenchymal stem cells that differentiate into bone lineage.
  Advantages of fibrin include that its hemostatic properties and excellent biodegradability. Disadvantage is that it is difficult to standardize the product and that it is easily coated with plasma proteins making pure fibrin difficult to maintain. Also, it can cause thrombus formation if one is not careful.

Collagen-based biomaterial: The most deliberate use of collagen has been in burn and wound repair, bone fillings, antithrombogenic surface creation and as an immobilizer of enzymes.

- Collagen has also been used to deliver drugs in the form of a collagen film.
- Collagen matrix scaffold has been used to hold bone morphogenetic protein for promotion of osteogenesis and induce direct osteoinduction.

- Collagen powder has been used as self-setting collagen cement where the collagen powder is mixed to composite of tetracalcium phosphate and anhydrous dicalcium phosphate to form a paste with distilled water and fill bone defects.
- Similarly, collagen scaffold composite material impregnated with β-tricalcium phosphate was used to treat critically sized bone defects.
- Collagen microspheres have been used to encapsulate mesenchymal stem cells that would then differentiate with respect to bone lineage.

Advantages of using collagen as a biomaterial include excellent biodegradability, biocompatibility and versatility. Combined with many other bioactive compounds and serve as a delivery vehicle.

Use of epoxy resins: Composite bone models are increasingly utilized in orthopedic biomechanics research and surgical education applications. Fourth generation resin composites provide reproduction of human bone biomechanical properties when placed under bending, axial, and torsional loads. Shape memory polymers (SMPs) are being increasingly developed that can adopt one (dual-shaped), two (triple-shaped) or several (multi-shaped) stable temporary shapes and recover to their original, permanent, version upon external stimulus. External stimulus could be changes in temperature, pH, light wavelength, and mechanical load.

Polyesters: Polyesters in orthopedics are mostly used as a bone tissue repair scaffold.
- PLLA [poly (L-lactide)] scaffolds result in increased human osteoblast like cells deposition around the implant suggesting positive osteoinductive activity.
- Polycaprolactone (PCL) was used to create a scaffold membrane for treatment of oral and maxillofacial deficiencies.
- Poly (L-lactide) injectable pins were developed into biodegradable implants but withdrawn due to inconsistent tissue reaction.

Polymethylmethacrylate: Kindly see Answer to Question 210.

Other adhesive biomaterials in pipeline include Polyethylene glycol (PEG), chitosan, and albumin.

196. Explain stress, strain, and Young's modulus of elasticity in relation to orthopedic implants.

Ans: The mechanical properties of orthopedic biomaterials can be studied under the following heads:
- *Stress:* This is the force to which the implant is subjected per unit area. It can be normal stress perpendicular to the surface of the implant or shear stress parallel to the surface of implant. Its unit is Newton/m^2.
- *Strain:* It is the change in dimension that the implant undergoes when it is subjected to stress and is expressed as:

$$\text{Strain} = \frac{\text{Final length} - \text{original length}}{\text{original length}}$$

- *Young's modulus of elasticity:* It is the linear slope of the materials elastic stress-strain curve before the material undergoes irreversible plastic deformity. It is an intrinsic property of the material and does not vary with thermal or mechanical history.

197. Describe biodegradable implants.

Ans: Kindly see Answer to Question 215C.

198. Describe biodegradable implants and their chemical composition. Mention the indications of their use, advantage, and disadvantage of their use.

Ans: Kindly see Answer to Question 215C.

199. Discuss evolution of plate osteosynthesis starting from *Sherman* plates to present day locking plates. What are the principles of locked plate osteosynthesis including their advantages and disadvantages?

Ans: This answer includes developers even before Sherman as who knows next time the question starts at Lane's or Danis!!

The inception and trial and error reign: Dissatisfied with the limited stability provided by external immobilization methods, researchers and developers started looking at methods to internally stabilize the bone for improved and sustained alignment. Plating of fractures began with Lane's crude metal plate introduced in 1895 to stabilize fractures, but was immediately abandoned due to corrosion of the plate. Attention was shifted to improve the corrosion resistance of implants without any study of implant bone mechanics and mechanical properties of metal implants. This produced two different versions of plating introduced by Lambotte and Sherman in 1909 and 1912, respectively. As expected the implants started failing due to poor fatigue strength. The initial fixation was too rigid but there occurred resorption at the fracture ends producing instability that lead to implant failure due to poor fatigue strength to bear this increased instability. This new development encouraged Egger to introduce a plate with oblong holes that permitted screws to slide within the holes compensating for fracture resorption gap. The plate was a success initially and used by many but lack of knowledge of creating construct and understanding of different requirements for separate bones and force caused failures in hands of many.

The era of compression plating and principle of "absolute stability": Eggers plate was a static construct that presumed that instability due to fracture end resorption would be compensated by slide of screw within holes, however there were failures as the expected slide to cover the gap did not occur. It was hence thought that compression should be achieved at index surgery itself so that fractures would not become unstable and construct stay long enough for union to occur. Danis in 1949 introduced the concept of compression plating and a new mode of healing that he called soudure autogène (autogenous welding), a process now known as primary bone healing. He named his plate "coapteur" that had a transverse screw mechanism to compress the fracture site reducing interfragmentary motion. This concept revolutionized the plating systems and all following designs incorporated some element of compression at fracture to improve stability. In 1958, Bagby and Janes described a plate with specially designed oval holes to provide interfragmentary compression during screw tightening. This construct has a finite element of achievable compression due to design limitations. Muller in 1965 hence introduced a tensioner device that would produce desirable compression at fracture site before finite fixation. This plate was also thicker than Egger's or Danis's plate. This construct became popular and introduced concepts of primary healing of fractures without formation of callus using compression plating. Presence of callus implied some degree of instability. To further improve the compression Bagby and Muller designs were combined to produce the popular "DCP" (dynamic compression plates) although we know that the compression was actually static and noting dynamic as it was a single event. The advantages of the DCP included low incidence of malunion, stable internal fixation, and no need for external immobilization, thus allowing immediate movement of neighboring joints. These advantages further improved with introduction of AO principles of osteosynthesis now aimed at preserving soft tissues and vascularity. With widespread usage few disadvantages were identified including delayed union as well as persistence of a microscopically detectable fracture gap that acted as a stress riser after plate removal. Cortical bone loss under the plate was another disadvantage. It was difficult to identify fracture union with implant *in situ.* It was proposed by Perren that porosis and refractures are due to cortical necrosis that is secondary to excessive plate-bone contact interfering with cortical perfusion.

Perren's guidelines thus indicated reduction of pressure on bone by the implant—so LCDCP (Limited contact DCP) were introduced with slots on the undersurface to reduce bone contact. The design was further bettered by PC-FIX (point contact fixator) that reduced the implant bone contact to just point making it essentially negligible. Field, however, found no difference in DCP and LCDCP plate fixation constructs in view of contact area stress and reduction of cortical blood flow. This led to new research for cause of bone loss. It was found that "stress shielding" appears to have a major role in producing osteoporosis of the underlying bone and any mode of rigid fixation that takes away stress would cause bone to develop osteoporosis whether it is implant or space travel—challenging the Perren hypothesis. Similar to LCDCP, raled plates were also introduced to limit the bone implant surface contact however stress-shielding being the dominant cause still produced osteoporosis. The osteoporosis is on the endosteal part widening the canal and follows the Wolffe's law. PC-FIX was considered more "biological" but no difference between PC-FIX or LCDCP fixation had been documented, further strengthening the fact that stress shielding causes porosis. The real biological concept was introduction of bridge plate osteosynthesis but that still did not solve the problem of stress shielding. The learnings from all above evolutionary processes can be put down as:

- To remain strong, bone must be dynamically loaded.
- To heal a fracture, nature must sense the absence of bony continuity.
- Primary bone healing is a slow process and especially with stress shielding it produces a weak bone.
- A construct that allows micromotion through the fracture site in axial direction while resisting bending, torsional, and shear moments is needed for optimal healing.

The era and principles of locked plate osteosynthesis: The primary design of screw compressing plate against the bone to achieve rigidity and fixation was given a rethought to counter stress shielding. Also it was learnt that external fixators do lead to production of callus sometimes profuse but lack the stability. The stability can be increased by bringing the rods as close to the body as possible. This meant if plate can be applied at a distance locked to screws away from bone would improve the results of external fixators. This anchorage point change produced the locked plates we commonly use now. Now achieving compression was an issue and was primarily not considered to be a part of this concept. The Less Invasive Stabilization System (LISS) for distal femur was designed. However, surgeons still considered fracture site compression a good mode in achieving union so "çombi-hole" technology was introduced where locked holes and compression slots were combined. The following are other principles of LCP design and mode of fixation:

- The most important conceptual difference is that it becomes unnecessary for the plate to intimately contact the underlying bone in all areas. As the screws are tightened, they "lock" to the plate, thus stabilizing the segments without the need to compress the bone to the plate. Locking plate/screw systems do not disrupt the underlying cortical bone perfusion as much as conventional plates, which compress the undersurface of the plate to the cortical bone.
- *Selection of plates of appropriate length:* Longer plates can be selected without associated traumatization of the soft tissues, and the length selected needs to take account only of the biomechanical situation in the fracture. In the case of LCP, the ideal plate length can be determined by the plate span width and the plate screw density—the plate span width is the quotient of plate length divided by overall fracture length. This quotient should generally be more than 2–3 for comminuted fractures and higher than 8–10 in the case of simple fractures.
- *Screw density (quotient of screws inserted divided by number of plate holes):* This value should be under 0.4–0.5. In contrast to conventional plate osteosynthesis, when LCP are used it is no longer possible to recommend a definite number of screws or cortices to be used in each fragment. It is much more important that the number of screws inserted is as small as is consistent with the provision of high plate leverage so that screw loading is kept low. Two monocortical screws should be the minimum for each main fragment, to keep the construct stable. An increase from 4.5 mm (conventional cortical screw) to 5.0 mm (locking head screw) provides already 70% holding force in a monocortical locking head screw (LHS) compared to a 100% of the holding force of a conventional bicortical 4.5 mm screw.
- In cases where both conventional screw and locking head screws are applied, it is necessary to apply the LHS after the conventional screw. If the conventional screw would be applied after the LHS, the screw–bone interface would be overloaded and the screw would be worthless.
- The screws should be in the correct orientation so one should use the jig unless it is a variable angle construct.
- In osteoporotic bones the plates can be bent to change the direction of fixation of screws to reduce the failure. Different direction of screws increases pull-out strength further.
- Another advantage to the use of locking plate/screw systems is that the screws are unlikely to loosen from the plate. This means that even if a screw is inserted into a fracture gap, loosening of the screw will not occur. Similarly, if a bone graft is screwed to the plate, a locking screw will not loosen during the phase of graft incorporation and healing.

200. Discuss locking compression plate—indications
Ans:
Indications:
1. Pathological bones including osteoporotic patients
2. Complex periarticular fractures
3. Intra-articular fractures
4. Periprosthetic fractures
5. Fixation of corrective osteotomies
6. Malunion, nonunion and failed fixation

201. What are the principles of volar locking plate?
Ans: The goal of operative treatment of unstable intra-articular distal radial fractures is anatomical reduction of the scaphoid facet, lunate facet, and sigmoid notch of the distal radioulnar joint.

There are two types of plates available for fractures of the distal radius: Conventional and fixed angle locking plates. When using conventional plates and screws, comminution must be minimal. Axial forces across the wrist and toggle of the screws in the distal holes of the plate lead to settling and loss of reduction.

Plates with fixed-angle locking distal screws or pegs have a distinct advantage over conventional plates. Fixed-angle locking screws or pegs support subchondral bone and resist axial forces across the wrist that lead to settling and loss of reduction. Stability is achieved through the fixed angle design. Comminution or segmental bone loss does not lead to settling and loss of reduction. With a conventional plate and screws, stability is achieved by compression of the plate to bone with bicortical screws. Compression of a locking plate to bone is unnecessary for stability, and periosteal blood supply is maintained under the plate. These plates are applied to the volar surface of the distal radius and are strong enough to be used in the presence of severe comminution of the dorsal cortex.

(Additionally, one can write column concept of distal radius)

202. Describe static compression and dynamic compression.

Ans: To improve fracture fixation, compression is given across the fracture site to facilitate healing. Adequately compressed fractures across an anatomically reduced fracture would result in primary healing by cutting cones. Intermittent compression would result in molecular and electrical changes where newly formed tissue like callus or regenerate would get ossified. So, two types of compression are used, static compression and dynamic compression:

1. *Static compression:* There is fixed, uniform compression across the fracture site achieved by hardware that are designed to fix and produce compression simultaneously. Such devices include compression plates and lag screws. Static compression aims to provide fracture healing with minimal or no callus formation so that there is primary bone healing. This entails that the gap should be completely closed between the fracture fragments else hardware failure would result.
2. *Dynamic compression:* Here the primary role of hardware is to provide fixation maintaining acceptable alignment across the fracture whilst the compressive force is provided by the patient's weight and muscular contraction. The implant devices that exploit such modality to enhance fracture healing include the dynamic hip screw, tension band wiring, and a dynamized nail. Dynamic compression facilitates healing by callus formation.

203. What are the pitfalls in using locking compression plate?

Ans:
- Locking screw insertion in a fixed direction (unless variable angle plates used).
- Overly rigid construct → implant failure as the fracture often goes to delayed/nonunion and stress is placed on the implant. The plates have larger holes to accommodate large diameter screws so implants have lesser fatigue tolerance.
- Screw jamming and cold welding makes implant removal challenging if need arises.
- The fracture needs to be optimally reduced before plate application as plate acts as a fixator only.
- Indirect reduction through plate is not possible and also the compression across fracture if needed is not that effective as is with the use of conventional plates.

204. Describe in brief lag screw principle with appropriate diagram and example. What is osteoinduction?

Ans: Lag screw principle is a technique for interfragmentary compression **(Fig. 2.12.1)**

Application of a fully threaded screw as a lag screw: A fully threaded screw can be used as a lag screw, provided that the thread does not engage the cortex close to the screw head (near cortex). This principal technique is achieved by drilling a glide hole into the near cortex with a diameter slightly larger than the outer diameter of the screw thread. In the opposite or far cortex, a smaller hole is drilled using a drill guide that inserts into the glide hole. This is called the pilot hole. It is the same diameter as the core of the screw to be inserted. A self-tapping screw may be introduced to the pilot hole or a tap can be used to cut a channel for the threads of a screw. It is then called a threaded hole. When a fully threaded cortex lag screw is applied, it only has purchase in the thread hole

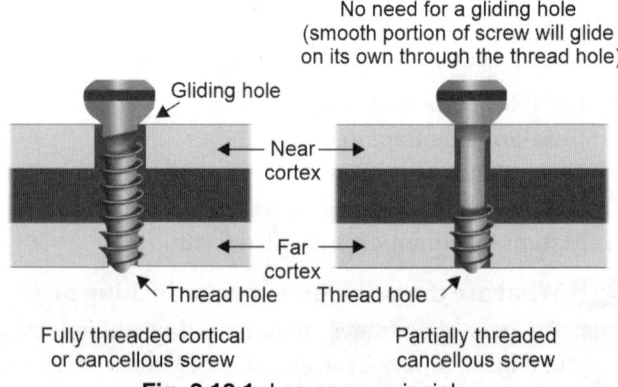

Fig. 2.12.1: Lag screw principle.

and does not engage in the glide hole. As the head of the screw is pressed against the cortex, preload is created. The bone fragments are compressed as the screw is tightened, producing interfragmentary compression.
- *Application of a partially threaded screw as a lag screw:* This principal technique is indicated in cancellous bone. It is achieved by drilling a pilot hole into the near cortex, across the fracture and into the far cortex. The smooth shaft of the partially threaded cancellous screw serves as the gliding hole, the threaded part engages the far cancellous and cortical bone and, as the head is compressed against the near cortex; preload is created which results in interfragmentary compression

Osteoinduction (Table 2.12.2):

Osteoinduction (term introduced by Marshall R Urist) is a process that supports the mitogenesis of undifferentiated mesenchymal cells, leading to the formation of osteoprogenitor cells that form new bone.

In bone grafting, it is the property by which the graft causes stimulation of osteoprogenitor cells to differentiate into osteoblasts that then begin new bone formation. Demineralized bone matrix, bone morphogenic proteins, growth factors, and gene therapy are typical examples. Autogenous bone, especially cancellous bone, carries with it the factors and cellular elements that can act for "osteoinduction" in paracrine manner. These grafts serve as a scaffold for currently existing osteoblasts and also trigger the formation of new osteoblasts promoting faster integration of the graft. Bone reamings are example of pure osteoinductive grafts.

TABLE 2.12.2: The osteoinduction property of various types of bone grafts.

Graft type	Osteoinduction
Cancellous autograft	+ +
Cortical autograft	+
Allograft	+
Calcium phosphate	–
Demineralized bone matrix	+ +
Xenograft	–
Bone marrow	–

205. Describe Herbert's screw.

Ans: Herbert screw is a headless compression device that has a smooth thin shaft and threads at the two ends. The pitch of distal threads is more while the proximal thicker portion has threads with much smaller pitch. This differential thread pitch (variable pitch) produces fracture site compression when tightened as the distal threaded portion tends to advance faster thus pushing the distal portion back into proximal portion. Being headless the screw gets fully countersunk in bone wherever used. It is a noncannulated screw while its modification Herbert-Whipple screw is cannulated version. Due to cannulation this screw has a thicker cross-section than Herbert screw.

Uses:
- Scaphoid fracture fixation
- Inter phalangeal arthrodesis
- Distal humerus intra-articular fractures
- Radial head fractures
- Femoral head fractures
- Condylar fractures of distal humerus
- Osteochondral fractures of the knee
- Large osteochondritis dissecans (>2.5 cm).

206. Explain machine screw and AO-ASIF screw.

Ans:

Machine screws: Machine screws are threaded their whole length and can be self-tapping or require threads to be cut before insertion. Most are self-tapping; the end has a cutting flute that cuts the screw threads as the screw is inserted.

Machine screws are used primarily to fasten hip compression screw devices to the shaft of the femur. The size of the hole drilled for machine screws is crucial. A hole that is too large results in an insecure purchase by the threads, and a hole that is too small can result in inability to insert the screw or fragmentation of the bone as it is inserted. The drill point selected should be slightly smaller than the shank of the screw minus its thread. For a self-tapping screw, the drill point used for a hole in cortical bone should be 0.3 mm larger than that used for a hole in soft bone. Screws and drill points should be checked for proper size before surgery.

AO-ASIF screws: Screws designed for the techniques and principles of osteosynthesis developed by the ASIF group in Switzerland are widely used. There are three basic alterations from machine screws that were incorporated to suit osseous fixation:
1. Alteration of thread diameter to core diameter from 4:3 in machine screws to 3:2
2. Reduction of thread surface area to one-sixth that of machine screws
3. Buttress thread design instead of V-shaped thread to increase pull out strength. The threads are more horizontal than those of machine screws.

For screws that are not self-tapping, the drill hole must be tapped with a cutting tapper before the screw is inserted. Cortical, cancellous, and malleolar designs are available in ASIF screws. Miniscrews for fixation of small fragments and small bones and the standard cancellous and cortical screws come in multiple lengths and diameters. The heads of the standard cancellous and cortical screws have a hexagonal recess for a special screwdriver, whereas the smaller screws have a Phillips head.

207. Describe the importance of polyethylene in orthopedics. Explain the role of fibrin gel in orthopedics.
Ans:

Polyethylene: Polyethylene (PE) is a polymer of ethylene. The surgical grade PE is UHMPE, also known as high-modulus polyethylene or high-performance polyethylene. The older name for ultra-high-molecular-weight polyethylene (UHMWPE) was high-density polyethylene (HDPE) or polythene. Clear distinction has been laid now and HDPE refers only to a material with a molecular weight of 100–250,000 Daltons that suits domestic usage in kitchens for water or milk jugs and not joint arthroplasty bearings at all. UHMWPE has been used in orthopedic hip and knee applications from the times of Sir John Charnley since 1962. It has a molecular weight from 2 million Daltons to 6 million Daltons. It has the goodness of wear and impact resistance combined with ductility and toughness desirable in a being surface. The UHMWPEs are fabricated resin using one of three distinct methods:
1. *Ram extrusion process:* Polyethylene powder/resin is driven by a ram through heated nozzle. This high temperature-pressure process fuses the flakes into a continuous bar. The bar can be then machined into specific products.
2. *Compression molding:* The resin is placed in a large mold and heated under pressure. This produces a block or sheet from which the final components can be machined.
3. *Net-shape molding:* This process is a modification of compression molding in the sense that the resin is molded into the desired shape of the implant itself and no final machining is required.

Fibrin gel:
- Hyaluronic acid and fibrin gel with bone marrow derived mesenchymal stem cells (MSCs) and monoolein-water gels have been used as an alternative treatment for bone and soft tissue infections.
- Scaffold like fibrin gel have been used to reproduce the tendon structure. The scaffolds provide matrix for even distribution of the MSCs that can then be used at repair sites typically the tendon-bone interfaces and also be injected into bone tunnels. These techniques currently are meant for improving the tendon to bone healing and not suitable for tendon only reformation. The problem with gel constructs is the issue of stability as most of these tend to wear away quickly over time.

208. What is highly cross-linked polyethylene? How is it manufactured? How has it affected modern total hip arthroplasty?
Ans: Cross-linking is the most talked about and flaunted characteristic (by different manufacturers) of all modern PE total hip bearings that are marketed under the banner term "highly cross-linked poly", even they have variations of crosslinking quantity. Cross-linking per se refers to the joining of two independent polymer molecules by a chemical covalent bond. In modern practice, radiation cross-linking is the recommended and most practiced method. Other methods, not commonly

used for cross-linking, include chemical-induced cross-linking by free-radical-generating chemical and by use of silane compound cross-linking whereby silane compound is grafted onto the polymer.

Manufacturing "Highly Cross-linked" Polyethylene

Annealing or remelting (thermal processing): This is the step to produce a highly cross-linked UHMWPE. We know that increasing radiation dose will produce trapped free radicals in the new crystalline state as amorphous areas continuously decrease with radiation. The cross-linked material is hence subjected to a thermal treatment step for reducing the level of free radicals that induces further crosslinking reactions. Higher temperature increases the mobility of molecules by energy transfer that is true also of UHMPE. This increases the probability of unsettled free radicals on adjacent chains to get excited and hence react with each other forming cross-links. In order to eliminate all free radicals however the material must be heated above the melting temperature normally 150°C. This induces another problem that at such high temperatures, the crystallinity is jeopardized and the mechanical properties are lost. A compromise solution commonly followed commercially is to heat the poly to 130–135°C (just below the melting temperature). This method though fails to eliminate "all" free radicals, preserves the original crystal structure and retains mechanical properties while most of the free radicals still get cross-linked. The number of free radicals is substantially reduced. Some manufacturers have, however, resorted to remelting the poly by heating it above melting temperature (Altrx®, Depuy-Synthes) where the base resin is itself different as persistence of free radicals increases oxidative degradation and reduces shelf-life. Annealing refers to thermal treatment done below the melt transition of 135°C while remelting is done above the melt transition. The former increases crystallinity while the latter decreases it. The other way out to reduce free radicals is by introducing antioxidants like vitamin E in the poly.

Effects: Ultra-high-molecular-weight polyethylene has low friction and dampening properties but has high adhesive and abrasive wear. The thickness of conventional PE should not be less than 6–8 mm otherwise accelerated wear and poly failure occurs. This causes osteolysis in the short time. Highly cross-linked PE has reduced PE wear rate of 42–100% compared to conventional PE. The newer highly cross-linked PE show annual linear wear at 45% of conventional UHMPE in prosthesis implanted for 5 years. This indicates that osteolysis may not possibly occur at all. The optimum value of cross-linking is debatable and still undecided, for simple arguments that follow:

- Higher cross-linking reduces some mechanical properties quite significantly the most important of which are mechanical strength parameters like ductility and fracture toughness and fatigue strength.
- Noncross-linked poly will have best values for ultimate strength, elongation and fracture toughness but will have worst values of linear and volumetric wear values.
- At the other extreme is to irradiate poly with higher (9.5–11 mrad) than recommended doses to gain additional 5–10% of wear resistance that might avoid osteolysis even in the most active patient but resulting in increased chances of mechanical failure of the poly.
- Moderate doses of 5 mrad used commonly in various products maintain the benefits of reduction in wear at 85% or below that of a noncross-linked UHMPE while maintaining the mechanical properties.

209. Explain highly cross-linked polyethylene.
Ans: Kindly see Answers to Questions 207 and 208.

210. Describe bone cement.
Ans: Bone cement is provided as biphasic module (2–3 parts powder and 1 part monomer liquid). The solid phase comprises powder form microbeads (1–100 μm) of polymerized component (PMMA) with opacifier (barium sulfate or zirconium oxide) and initiator (benzoyl peroxide). The liquid phase consists of monomer methyl methacrylate and coinitiator (also known as activator—dimethyl-p- toluidine, DMPT) along with stabilizers to prevent autopolymerization (hydroquinone and/or ascorbic acid). The coloring agents like chlorophyllin can be added to any phase while antibiotics are added only to solid (powder) phase.

Mnemonic: (P for powder and P for polymer)

Types:
- *High viscosity cements:* Standard arthroplasty procedures now not preferred
- *Low viscosity cements:* The most commonly used cement, surface replacement and vertebroplasty (very low viscosity cement)

- *Antibiotic impregnated cements:* Revision and infection in arthroplasty, spacer, and cement beads for defect management in chronic osteomyelitis
- Cold curing cements (Mjoberg) using butyl methacrylate
- Biodegradable aqueous gel phase cement.

Antibiotics are often mixed to the cement. The most commonly used are aminoglycosides, vancomycin.

However, the β-lactams, cephalosporins, macrolides, quinolones, and doxycycline can all be used. Basically, the antibiotic should be heat stable, water soluble, hypoallergic, bactericidal, and available as a powder.

Phases of polymerization:
- *Mixing phase:* Wetting
- *Waiting phase:* Swelling + polymerization, ↓viscosity, sticky dough
- *Working phase:* Chain propagation, ↓movability, ↑viscosity
- *Setting phase:* Chain growth finished, no movability, high temperature.

There is shrinkage of the mix finally and the whole process is exothermic (heat of polymerization = 43–46°C).

Uses:
- Arthroplasty procedures
- Infection control as cemented beads and masquelets procedure
- Filling defects after fracture fixation as in tibial plateau fractures, balloon kyphoplasty
- Bone tumors-filling defects.

211. Explain properties of bone cement.

Ans: *Properties of bone cement*
- *Compressive strength:* Measured according to standards ISO 5833 and ASTM F 451, this refers to the maximum stress a material can withstand before failing in compression. PMMA cement requires a minimum compressive strength of 70 MPa.
- *Bending strength:* Assessed through a four-point bending test per standard ISO 5833, the minimum bending strength is 50 MPa, and the bending modulus is 1,800 MPa. All commercial cements meet these standards. The elastic modulus should match the prosthesis and bone, and changes with temperature and additives, but current cements comply with regulations.
- *Tensile strength:* Evaluated using standards ISO 527-1 or ASTM D 638, it defines the maximum stress before failing in tension. Most manufacturers achieve a tensile strength of 50–60 MPa, mostly unaffected by additives.
- *Shear strength:* Tested according to ASTM standards D732, shear strength at the stem-cement interface is vital for preventing failure. The surface finish of the implant significantly affects this strength, and increased roughness can enhance it but may also lead to wear due to micromotion.
    - *Fracture toughness:* Measured by ASTM E399 and ISO 13,586, this property decreases significantly with gamma irradiation, making ethylene oxide the preferred sterilization method.
    - *Impact strength:* This measures the energy required to induce fractures. The impact strength of PMMA decreases with radiopacifiers and antibiotics. The hierarchy of strength is: compressive > flexural > tensile. Bending tests are the most realistic for evaluating material stress.
- *Fatigue behavior:* Fatigue determines PMMA's capacity to withstand varying loads. It can be tested through four-point bending, uniaxial tensile tests, and compression-tension tests. Sinusoidal cyclic loading is typically used until failure. Irradiation and porosity can decrease fatigue strength.
- *Water uptake:* Water absorption negatively affects the modulus of elasticity, lowering stiffness, which may enhance fracture resistance. Plain cements have a water uptake of 1–2%, while antibiotic cements have higher absorption. Water saturation occurs within 4–8 weeks and can lower the glass transition temperature, contributing to implant loosening.
- *Cement creep behavior:* PMMA exhibits viscoelasticity, experiencing immediate elastic deformation and time-dependent continuous deformation under load, with the latter being partially recoverable. Practically for prosthesis the creep is not very significant. The creep behavior is explained by two properties of cement polymer:
    1. *Stress relaxation:* This is the change in stress (reducing) with time under constant strain (deformation). The stress relaxation is caused by a change in structure of polymerized cement. Temporal changes in stress are observed by reduction in stress at night that reduces load allowing stress relaxation.

2. *Hysteresis*: The loading and unloading curves for PMMA are not identical. Not all the energy applied to the specimen during loading is recovered on unloading so some energy is lost/stored in the PMMA possibly responsible for the secondary creep.

2.13 TECHNIQUES AND PROCEDURES IN ORTHOPEDICS (Q212–248)

212. Describe tension band wiring.

Ans: *Biomechanical principle:* A curved, tubular structure under axial load always has a compression side as well as a tension side. From these observations the principle of tension band fixation evolved.

"A tension band converts tensile force into compression force at the opposite cortex. This is achieved by applying a device eccentrically, on the convex side of a curved bone". If a fracture is to unite, it requires mechanical stability, which is obtained by compression of the fracture fragments. Conversely, distraction or tension interferes with fracture healing. Therefore, tension forces on a bone must be at least neutralized or, more ideally, converted into compression forces to promote fracture healing. This is especially important in articular fractures, where stability is essential for early motion and a good functional outcome.

In fractures where muscle pull tends to distract the fragments, such as fractures of the patella or the olecranon, the application of a tension band will neutralize these forces and even convert them into compression when the joint is flexed. The method can also be applied to places where a bone fragment can be avulsed at the insertion of a tendon or ligament. Examples include the greater tuberosity of the humerus, the greater trochanter of the femur, or the medial malleolus. Here, too, a tension band can reattach the avulsed fragment, convert tensile force into compression force allowing immediate motion of the joint.

- Tension band principle applied to a fracture of the patella. The figure-of-eight wire loop lies anterior to the patella and fracture. Upon knee flexion, the tensile force (between the quadriceps muscle and the tibial tuberosity) is converted into compression at the articular surface.
- In the olecranon fracture, the figure-of-eight wire loop acts as a tension band during flexion of the elbow. This is an example of a dynamic tension band.
- Application of the tension band principle at the proximal humerus for an avulsion of the greater tubercle. The wire loop is anchored to the humerus by a 3.5 mm cortex screw.
- Application of the tension band principle to the medial malleolus. The wire loop may be anchored to the tibia by a 3.5 mm cortex screw. This is an example of a static tension band.

Complications: The most common complication is implant failure. A wire under tension only is very strong. However, if bending forces are added, it will break quite rapidly due to fatigue.

213. Explain tension band principle in fracture surgery.
Ans: Kindly see answer above.

214. Explain the concept of TBW with help of diagram.
Ans: The concept of tension band principle (**Fig. 2.13.1**) is written in Answer to Question 212 above.

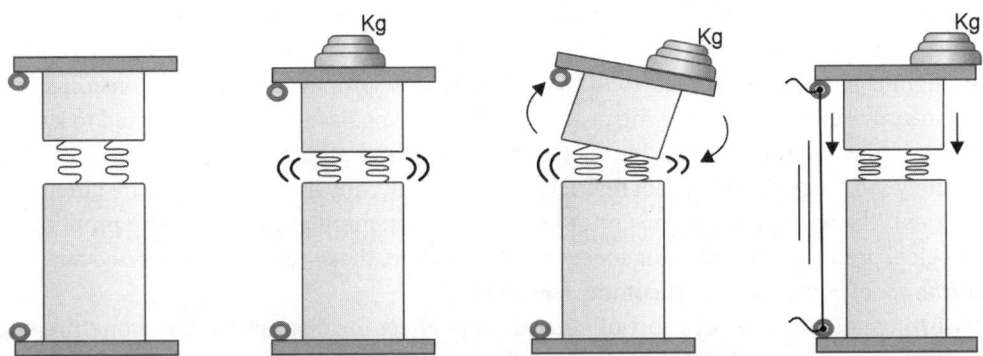

Fig. 2.13.1: Illustration of tension band principle.

215. Write notes on:
A. MIPPO
B. Distraction histiogenesis
C. Bioabsorbable implants.

Ans:

A. **MIPPO**—With emergence and popularity of minimally invasive surgery following increasing use of locked implants and anatomical plates unique techniques have evolved. Minimally invasive plate osteosynthesis (MIPO) or minimally invasive percutaneous plate osteosynthesis (MIPPO) is one such method. The core principle of MIPO/MIPPO is to reduce the trauma to the soft tissue and to the bone by specific reduction techniques.

- Minimally invasive percutaneous plate osteosynthesis for intra- and periarticular fractures requires precise anatomical reduction through a small soft tissue window. The plate is then applied to achieve absolute stability using the compression method. Anatomical reduction often requires direct reduction maneuvers that is best achieved using tools having small footprints like pointed reduction clamp, collinear reduction forceps or reduction handles/joysticks that can be applied close to fracture percutaneously.
- Minimally invasive plate osteosynthesis for shaft fractures involve making a soft tissue window away from the fracture site, large enough for implant insertion and place it centrally over bone. The reduction is obtained through indirect closed or percutaneous direct methods. For diaphyseal fractures the restoration of the length, axis, and rotation is needed. Small individual fracture fragments need not to be anatomically reduced, however alignment needs to be exact. Some reduction maneuvers applied to achieve this are manual traction, traction table, large distractor, external fixator, push–pull forceps.

Fixation: Multifragmentary fractures of the diaphyseal or metaphysical zone are fixed by the locked splinting method where the fracture zone is bridged the chosen locked implant. This construct acts like an internal fixator. Additional compression can be applied to simple fractures.

Disadvantages of MIPO:
- Difficulties in indirect closed reduction
- Increased C-arm exposure
- Malunion
- Pseudoarthrosis through diastases
- Delayed union with flexible fixation in simple fractures.

Advantages of MIPO:
- Faster bone healing
- Reduced infection rate, no or less need for bone graft
- Less postoperative pain (small incisions)
- Faster rehabilitation (less soft tissue trauma)
- More aesthetic result.

B. **Distraction osteogenesis (DO)** is a surgical technique in which the intrinsic capacity of bone to regenerate is being harnessed for various purposes. Controlled stress to a biologically created bone defect is utilized to this effect. The method emanated from the observation that hypertrophic callus when subjected to "tension-stress" ossifies and forms new bone. The principle was highlighted by Professor Gavril Abramovich Ilizarov (propagated as law of tension-stress) from Kurgan in western Siberia in early 1950s. The underlying principle is that "living tissues when subjected to slow, steady traction (distortional strain), under appropriate conditions (of vascularity and alignment) become metabolically active and regenerate indefinitely". So, this principle is not restricted to bone only, any living tissue can be indefinitely regenerated (including soft tissues). The term "appropriate conditions" in the statement above should be properly understood as it underlies the biological principles essential for success of the method, these can be summarized as:

- *Minimal disturbance of bone:* Use of corticotomy (see below).
- *Delay before distraction:* This provides sort of conditioning effect for distraction. The bone prepares healing and osteogenesis (or new bone formation) begins that can then be utilized for progressively increasing bone formation in the form of "regenerate". This new tissue is just a regenerative tissue (so better called "distraction neohistogenesis") that

under adequate conditions will form bone so the term "regenerate" was originally chosen instead of callus. Duration of delay varies (5 days in a child to 7 days, and in adult and even more in elderly—nearly 10 days).

- *Regenerate:* Regenerate and bone formation is basically a physiological process closely resembling fracture healing. Hematoma formation followed by fibrous and fibrocartilaginous tissue formation in a longitudinal pattern along the direction of distraction is seen with progressive distraction. New bone is formed from periosteum, cortex and spongiosa that proceeds from the osteotomy cuts toward the center supported by a fibrous "radiolucent interzone" located at the center of regenerate. As one proceeds from center of regenerate to cut bone ends the bone maturation increases. A process of mechanotransduction underplays at the regenerate—mechanical tension-stress forces due to distraction of the bony segments stimulate molecular signals and cytokines [bone morphogenetic protein (BMP), FGF, IGF, platelet-derived growth factor (PDGF), TGF-β, vascular endothelial growth factor (VEGF)] that activate cellular events like differentiation and proliferation forming bone ultimately.
- *Rate of distraction:* Ilizarov recommended a rate of distraction of 1 mm/day by his various experiments and he proposed motorized distraction for continuous distraction throughout the day. However, for sake of convenience, it is divided into four equal periods as 6 hourly intervals where 0.25 mm distraction is done at each sitting (0.25 × 4 = 1 mm).

C. Bioabsorbable materials:

Polyglycolic acid (PGA), polydioxanone (PDS), polylevolactic acid (PLLA), and racemic poly (d,l-lactic acid) (PDLLA) are currently the commonly used polymers that are used to make bioabsorbable orthopedic implants. They cannot be contoured intraoperatively and their physical and chemical properties can be modified by changing their chemical composition, manufacturing process and by addition of reinforcing fibers. They undergo biodegradability mainly by hydrolysis of the polymer chain.

- Polyglycolic acid is degraded by hydrolysis primarily to pyruvic acid and is excreted as carbon dioxide and water.
- Poly (d,l-lactic acid) is similarly hydrolyzed via the tricarboxylic acid cycle to carbon dioxide and water and excreted by respiration.
- Polydioxanone also is hydrolyzed, but it primarily is excreted in the urine.

Common indications for use of bioabsorbable implants are:
- Fracture fixation like forearm and malleolar fractures
- Fusions
- Osteochondritis dissecans
- Osteotomy staples
- As screws and pins for ligament repair and reconstruction
- Fixation of osteochondral lesions
- Cell transplantation
- Nerve reconstruction
- Prevention of adhesion.

Advantages:
- Gradual load transfer and less stress shielding
- Avoidance of second surgery for hardware removal
- Radiolucency.

Drawbacks:
- Rapid loss of strength after implantation
- Uneven rate of absorption in different individuals
- Formation of sinus
- Inflammatory reaction to the degradation products
- Synovitis.

216. Describe cardinal principles and complications of distraction histiogenesis in brief.

Ans: Distraction osteogenesis is a surgical technique in which the intrinsic capacity of bone to regenerate is being harnessed for various purposes. Controlled stress to a biologically created bone defect is utilized to this effect. The method emanated from the observation that hypertrophic callus when subjected to "tension-stress" ossifies and forms new bone. The principle was highlighted by Professor Gavriil Abramovich Ilizarov (propagated as law of tension-stress) from Kurgan in Western Siberia in early 1950s.

Cardinal principles:
- Minimal disturbance of bone—use of corticotomy
- Delay before distraction
- Rate of distraction—distraction of 1 mm/day
- Rhythm of distraction—higher the frequency of distraction the better is the quality of regenerate
- Site of the osteotomy—metaphyseal corticotomy is the best place for optimal result

Complications:
- Pin site infection
- Pain at the corticotomy site and during lengthening procedure (usually initial period only)
- Vascular complication—direct arterial/venous injury by the Ilizarov wires. Aneurysm formation is a reported complication that commonly occurs with partial damage to the arterial walls, as may occur when the Ilizarov wire brushes the artery. The weakened wall then gradually distends forming aneurysm.
- Neurological damage—usually direct injury to nerves while passing wires. Traction injury is less common, can be reduced or minimized by reducing the rate of distraction and early identification by clinical examination during follow-up.
- Soft tissue contractures and joint stiffness—when the frame spans joints—common in knee, elbow, and ankle (Achilles tendon contracture is common). One should hence incorporate foot plate in cases of frame fixation near to ankle joint else equinus deformity develops.
- Osteoporosis
- Reflex sympathetic dystrophy (RSD)
- Progression of angular deformity or creation of new one after fixator is removed. Pathological fracture may also ensue if the regenerate is not strong enough.
- Swelling of limb—usually due to immobilization, the venous tone is reduced causing edema and may progress to lymphedema—manage with passive mobilization, massage and physiotherapy.
- Lengthening site—nonunion and premature consolidation

217. Describe antiglide plate with appropriate diagnosis and example.

Ans: If the fracture of the lateral malleolus is not transverse or the bone is osteoporotic and does not lend itself to stabilization with lag screws, a one-third tubular plate can be placed posteriorly on the fibula as a buttress, counteracting the posterior displacement and known as antiglide plate. This technique is highly desirable for fractures in which the distal fragment has a spike extending posteriorly and there is posterior angulation (apical posterior fractures with a distal fragment spike). Occasionally, a lag screw can also be incorporated through the plate in such cases.

For antiglide plating, the incision should be placed more posteriorly to allow access to the posterior edge of the fibula. Usually, a five-hole or six-hole one-third tubular plate is applied to the posterolateral aspect of the fibula so that it covers the proximal apex of the distal fragment. The plate is straight and either clamped to the fibula proximally or attached with a screw through the most proximal hole. The screw just proximal to the fracture is now inserted and this forces the straight plate to push the distal fragment along the oblique fracture surface, effecting a reduction and stability. Placing reduction forceps on the tip of the fibula is helpful in controlling rotation during plate application. The remaining screws are then inserted and a lag screw can be placed through the plate.

This technique is also useful in patients, such as those with diabetes, where fracture union is likely to be delayed.

218. What is corticotomy? Discuss reamer/irrigator/aspirator (RIA) system.

Ans: To lengthen a bone, a special type of percutaneous osteotomy, corticotomy, is required. Paley et al. described an effective method of corticotomy in which a 5-mm osteotome is used to cut the medial and lateral cortices, extending subperiosteally into the posteromedial and posterolateral corners. The osteotome is turned 90° to wedge open the incomplete osteotomy and to crack the remaining posterior cortex. This maneuver is repeated with the osteotome in the posteromedial and posterolateral cortices. The fixator rings above and below can be rotated to complete the osteoclasis. The corticotomy preserves the soft tissue inside and outside the bone (the periosteal and endosteal circulation). On radiograph, the corticotomy should appear as a nondisplaced osteotomy.

RIA system: The harvest of femoral bone marrow using the techniques of femoral nailing and a specialized RIA (Synthes) is a more recent method for obtaining significant amounts of marrow from the femur. The RIA was developed to decrease IM pressure and fat embolism during reaming, and significant decreases in IM pressure and femoral vein fat have been documented with its use.

In the process of doing this, the reamings and effluent are captured, and a sizable amount of marrow may be aspirated for bone grafting. Depending on the patient and the source bone, 25–90 mL of bone marrow may be captured. These bony fragments are rich in mesenchymal stem cells. Additionally, the supernatant is rich in FGF-2, IGF-β1, and latent TGF-β1 but not bone morphogenetic protein-2 (BMP2). As a result, the RIA is a potential source for autologous bone, mesenchymal stem cells, and bone growth factors. When used as a spinal graft, however, this technique may require obtaining the graft before the spinal procedure with a different position and draping.

Complications:
- Fractures of the donor bone
- Perforation of the cortex of the reamed bone
- Blood loss:
  - Preoperative radiographs of the donor bone should be evaluated for deformity, and the isthmus should be measured to determine the limits of reaming.
  - Blood should be available to replace aspirated blood and marrow.

Preventing complications:
- Turn-off aspirator when reaming is not being performed.
- Check donor bone after reaming to look for perforations.
- Protected postoperative ambulation
- Avoid in patients with known metabolic bone disease such as osteoporosis.

219. Describe surgical reduction of fractures.

Ans: Reduction of fracture means restoring the correct relation and position of fragments. This includes the process of reconstruction of impacted cancellous bone and articular fragments.

Reduction reverses the process which created fracture displacement during the injury and calls for forces in opposite directions to those which produced the fracture. So, one should analyze the impacting force, displacement, and deformation, with good knowledge of muscle-deforming forces, to plan the steps needed to achieve reduction.

Aim of reduction:
In the diaphysis and metaphysis, the aim of fracture reduction is to restore length, alignment, and rotation, regardless of geometry of fracture and number of fragments. Every fragment need not be fitted into the puzzle. For articular fractures, the aim of reduction is perfect restoration of the joint surface to provide a congruent and stable joint. Anatomical reduction of the joint surface, as well as restoring axial alignment, especially in the lower extremity are important to reduce the risk of post-traumatic osteoarthritis.

Reduction techniques:
Reduction techniques must be gentle, must preserve the vascularity of the soft-tissue envelope and fracture fragments, and create as little additional damage as possible. There are two fundamental techniques for fracture reduction: (1) Direct and (2) indirect reduction:
1. Direct reduction means that hands or instruments are in contact with fracture fragments for manipulation under vision. In simple diaphyseal forearm bone fractures, direct reduction is used to produce coaptation of the two main fragments restoring anatomical length, alignment, and rotation. Surgical exposure should not add vascular damage to the bone or soft tissues and should maintain biology. In multifragmentary and unstable fractures, the repeated use of bone forceps and other reduction tools and tendency to exactly reduce each fragment may completely devitalize the fragments. This may lead to delayed union, nonunion, infection, and implant failure. Only by understanding and

respecting the biology of bone, periosteum, and soft tissues can the surgeon avoid failure after open reduction and internal fixation.
2. Indirect reduction means that fragments are not exposed and are manipulated by applying corrective force at a distance from the fracture. Intraoperative radiological imaging is required to ensure appropriate positioning of the fracture. It requires understanding of the fracture pattern, anatomy (muscle pull), and meticulous preoperative planning. If correctly applied, indirect reduction causes minimal surgical damage to tissues. All reduction tools are applied away from the fracture focus so that any local damage from the instruments themselves will not affect fracture healing.

220. **Describe the following:**
A. Types of frames and methods to increase the stability of external fixator.
B. How will you prevent complications of external fixator?

Ans:

A. *Types of frames:*
- *Pin fixators:*
  - Unilateral
  - V-shaped
  - Bilateral frame
  - Triangular.
- *Ring (wire fixators):*
  - Hybrid fixators (wire and pin)
  - Pinless external fixator
  - Mefisto.

Methods to increase stability:
- Distance of pins/Schanz screws:
  - *From the fracture line:* The closer the better
  - Within each main fragment, the further apart the better
  - *Distance of longitudinal connecting tube/bar from bone:* The closer the better.
- *Number of bars/tubes:* Two are better than one
- *Configuration:* unilateral → V-shaped → bilateral → triangular frame—ascending order of stability
- Combination of limited internal fixation (lag screw) with external fixation.

B. **Preventing loosening of pins:**
- Use bicortical pins
- Use cancellous Shanz screws in mataphyseal regions or in cancellous bones (ilium)
- *For longer term fixator use:* Hydroxyapatite-coated pins may improve osteointegration, silver coated pins may prevent florid pinsite infection.

Use a stable frame for better outcome—vide above for improving stability.

Preventing pin site infection:
- Stable frame for need specific bone/fracture/duration of application
- Low energy pin insertion and as atraumatic as possible
- Sterile technique
- Minimum soft tissue damage
- Perform adequate debridement for open injuries
- Pins should pass through viable and healthy tissue
- Predrill holes before pin insertion
- Avoid very hard cortical bones like anterior tibial crest
- Irrigate the drill during hole preparation
- Irrigation of drill holes
- Follow no-touch technique

- Pin site dressing immediately after pin insertion
- Dressing should not increase pressure on site else skin necrosis and infection would ensue
- Regular inspection of the pin site and dressing to enhance pin site healing
- Replacing the loosened pins as early as possible.

221. Outline (A) Principles of external fixators, (B) Modular and hybrid external fixators, Taylor spatial frame®.

Ans: A. Biomechanical principles of external fixators:
- At least two pins must be inserted into each main fragment through an anatomical safe zone.
- Pins should be spread as wide apart as possible:
  - If the soft-tissue situation allows, pins are inserted as close to the fracture focus as possible but should not enter the fracture hematoma or degloved areas. If delayed internal fixation is planned, the pins should avoid potential incisions and surgical approaches (the zone of surgery).

  Also see answer above to see methods to increase stability of frame.

Pin insertion technique: When inserting a Steinmann pin or Schanz screw, the following is important:
- Know the anatomy and avoid nerves, vessels, and tendons—these will indicate the safe zones of pin insertion.
- Do not place pins or screws into a joint.
- Avoid the fracture focus and hematoma.
- Avoid degloved and contused skin.
- Predrill the cortex to avoid burning the bone (ring sequestrum is produced).
- Insert a Schanz screw of the correct length to allow appropriate frame construction.

In diaphyseal cortical bone, it is essential to avoid thermal damage to the bone when inserting a pin or Schanz screw. Use sharper drill bits or screws and avoid burning the bone by using correct speed of insertion. Get a bicortical purchase but do not protrude too far. For metaphysis, heat generation is not such a problem. Prefer self-drilling screws since it is easy to miss the predrilled hole. Joint penetration must be avoided.

B. Modular and hybrid external fixators, Taylor spatial frame®:

Modular external fixator: This is a versatile tool used both as an indirect reduction tool and fixation device.

Conventional procedure for applying modular fixator:
Schanz screws are inserted into each main fragment with the pin close to the fracture placed in slightly different plane or, in the case of joint-bridging configurations, into each of the two bones supporting the bridge (in some cases possibly more than two). Using single pin clamps, the position and orientation of the Schanz screws can be adjusted in all plains. On either side of fracture, these Schanz pins are connected to tube creating partial frame and these two partial frames are then joined using tube-to-tube clamps. Fracture reduction can still be performed in all planes till the tube-to-tube connections are open. Once satisfactory reduction is achieved, the tube-to-tube clamps are tightened.

Modifications:
Schanz screws in any one main fragment can be initially connected to double pin or multipin clamps and partial frames can be constructed on each side of the fracture. The partial frame can also be formed by a ring or a partial ring system (hybrid fixator).

Advantages:
The principal advantage of modular external fixation is increased freedom in reduction, bridging, and stabilizing the fractures and joints. The Schanz screws can be positioned freely, which allows the most favorable, anatomical insertion site for the Schanz screws and the most favorable zone for the fracture pattern or soft-tissue injury. Manipulation of the main fragments is facilitated by leverage and indirect reduction techniques which preserve bone and soft-tissue vascularity. Primary and secondary adjustments to the reduction can be performed at any time with this technique.

Hybrid external fixator: The hybrid external fixator is used in fractures close to a joint. It is called "hybrid" because it combines tensioned fine-wire fixation and an external ring at the joint with pin fixation in the diaphysis. It requires tensioned K-wires for the ring and conventional Schanz screws for the shaft. Generally, three-fourths circumference rings are used. Hybrid ring fixators have mainly been used in proximal and distal tibial fractures

Taylor spatial frame®: The Taylor spatial frame® (Smith and Nephew, Memphis) is a unique ring and wire fixator consisting of two rings connected by six oblique struts. Its application is similar to that of the Ilizarov, except that FastFx® struts are used, and reduction is performed manually under image intensification until the best possible reduction is obtained in the anteroposterior and lateral planes. The struts are then locked in place. Additional rings can be added as necessary. With the aid of computer programs, the struts can be adjusted as an outpatient procedure to effect anatomical reduction at the fracture site. Radiographic parameters are entered into a computer to help calculate strut and frame adjustments for fracture reduction, compression, or distraction. Length, rotation, translation, and coronal and sagittal alignment, all can be corrected by changing the lengths of the six struts as dictated by the computer program. This fixator is primarily used to correct malunions, but it can be useful in treating acute fractures as well as infected and noninfected nonunions.

The Taylor spatial frame® also has been used for deformity correction and lengthening. This frame uses the slow correction principles of the Ilizarov system but adds a six-axis deformity analysis incorporated in a computer program. The Taylor spatial frame® has been shown to have a steep learning curve and has a high cost. In addition, no differences between the Taylor and Ilizarov frames have been noted in terms of lengthening index and complication rate, although rotational, translational, and residual deformity correction is easier with the Taylor frame.

222. **Describe clinical application of distraction osteogenesis in orthopedic practice.**
Ans: The clinical applications of distraction osteogenesis include:
- *Nonunion:* The Ilizarov external fixator is a labor-intensive, but very effective, tool in the treatment of nonunions. It is especially useful in nonunions associated with defects, shortening, and deformities. More traditional pin external fixators, using the Ilizarov principles, also can be used in the management of nonunions, especially when complicated by infection. External fixation can be used for temporary or definitive stabilization. One advantage of external fixation is that it is relatively noninvasive and does not disturb soft tissues surrounding the nonunion. Other advantages are its ability to correct deformity and provide stable fixation.
- *Limb lengthening:* Lengthening by callotasis (or low-energy corticotomy followed by gradual distraction of the bone fragments with a mechanical apparatus) has been the basic procedure for limb lengthening. Osteotomy and fixation techniques have been modified by several authors, but the principles remain the same. The corticotomy should be made by low-energy methods, usual multiple percutaneous drill holes connected by an osteotome, with care taken to avoid significant disruption of the surrounding soft tissues. Distraction should begin after a brief latent period of 1–3 weeks to allow for early callus formation. The rate of distraction should be approximately 1 mm per day divided over four 0.25-mm increments. The formation of the distraction regenerate should be closely monitored with frequent radiographic assessment, and the rate of distraction should be altered accordingly to avoid premature consolidation or poor regenerate formation. No matter what type of external apparatus is used, the device should remain in place for 1 month for every 1 cm of length achieved. Despite careful technique and excellent patient cooperation, high complication rates are reported with all methods, including deep infection, nonunion, fracture after device removal, malunion, joint stiffness, and nerve palsy. The Ilizarov device is extremely modular and can be adapted with extensions and hinges to lengthen and correct angular and translational deformities simultaneously. Rotational deformities can be corrected either at the time of fixator application or later by applying outriggers to the rings.
- *Deformity correction:* Deformity correction had been one of the primary applications of Ilizarov technique. To achieve deformity correction, special frame using hinges on the connecting rods is prepared but this requires very accurate frame construction to avoid simultaneous lengthening, compression, or translation (reason for popularity of Taylor frame). Deformity assessment requires a thorough knowledge of normal anatomical alignment and rotation that is individual to each patient. Usually, the contralateral limb can be used as a reference, and full-length, standing, anteroposterior radiograph of both lower limbs are taken. The normal mechanical axis is identified and measure of deformity (deviation) from this normal is taken. The site of the deformity must be identified and mid-diaphyseal lines can be drawn on a radiograph on either side of a deformity. The point at which these lines bisect is the center of rotation and angulation (CORA), and the angle between these lines is the magnitude of the deformity. A corrective osteotomy at this site will allow angular correction without translation. In cases where there is length discrepancy and angular deformity, correction can be made at one level, the CORA, if bone regeneration potential is good. Alternatively,

a double-level osteotomy may be performed, one at CORA for deformity correction and one at the advised level for lengthening. Common applications are:
- Correction of angular deformities of tibia and femur (genu varum/valgum)
- Congenital lower limb angular deformities
- Malunions

223. Define tribology.

Ans: Tribology (Greek word, "tribos", meaning "rubbing" or "to rub", coined by H Peter Jost in England) is defined as the science and technology of interacting surfaces in relative motion and all practices related thereto and includes the study of wear, friction, and lubrication.
- *Friction:* Friction is the resistance to relative motion between two bodies in contact. Friction arises from the interaction between moving surfaces in contact.
- *Wear:* Wear is defined as removal (or displacement) of material from one body when subjected to contact and relative motion with another body.
- *Lubrication:* Lubrication interposes a material between two contacting solids to minimize usual interaction between them so that if the interaction was predominantly of friction then it will be reduced.

(For a detailed understanding kindly refer to Chapter 60 of the book Essential Orthopedics: Principles and Practice, 2nd edition.)

224. Describe various cementing techniques. Discuss their differences in brief.

Ans: Over a time, refinements in the way cement was applied to the components have led to developments into generations in cementing:
- *First generation:* Finger packing, no distal plug
- *Second generation:* Distal plug of canal, "preparation" of canal with pulsed lavage, distal centralizer and use of cement gun to insert the cement in a retrograde fashion
- *Third generation:* Precooling of cement, vacuum mixing and centrifugation, pressurization of cement by use of proximal seal
- *Fourth generation:* In addition, this uses a proximal centralizer to ensure symmetric cement mantle.

(Kindly also see the answer above for writing the basic cementing technique preparation and method.)

225. Explain increasing role of minimal invasive techniques in orthopedics.

Ans: Most of the orthopedics surgeries are dreadful for producing stiffness in the nearby joints if infection is excluded as a complication. This is due to violation of soft tissues and tissue planes during exposure of the deeper bones and joints. Also, healing tissues usually undergo contraction further restricting the postoperative mobilization. Attempts have been made to improve the outcome by minimizing tissue trauma thus helping rehabilitation. This led to emergence of minimally invasive surgeries in orthopedics that aim to minimize the trauma to soft tissues and manipulation. The following are some of the indications of this technique:
- *Minimally invasive fracture repair:* This is aimed to minimize damage to the soft tissue attachments of the bones and fragments and also preserve the periosteal blood supply as much as possible for optimal fracture repair. Various techniques have evolved to this end like:
    - Minimally invasive percutaneous plate osteosynthesis (MIPPO) has been made successful by introduction of anatomical locked compression plating systems. The implant is introduced percutaneously in an aligned fracture and locked in place using jigs. This avoids opening large fractures and also preserves fracture hematoma. The method is quite popular to stabilize periarticular and metaphyseal fractures at the proximal humerus, distal femur and both ends of tibia.
    - *Nailing of long bone fractures:* Closed nailing involves distant site insertion of implant that provides relative stability to implant under good alignment. Open fractures can also be managed using nails and this prevents additional trauma to soft tissues around the fracture. TENS nailing also helps in managing pediatric fractures and some open fractures in a percutaneous manner.
    - Computer-guided navigation or fixation under CT guidance is also getting increasingly popular especially for pelvic bone injuries.

- *Minimally invasive spine surgery:*
  - Minimally invasive spine surgery techniques are being increasingly applied for removal of prolapsed disk. Endoscopic and microscopic disk removal are the examples.
  - Kyphoplasty and vertebroplasty are commonly deployed for management for osteoporotic collapse of vertebrae.
  - Percutaneous reduction and fixation of listhesis has become a common place for management of reducible listhesis. Fusion can then be done with a small incision.
- *Arthroscopic surgery:*
  - This is by far the best demonstrable example of minimally invasive surgery whether it be ACL/PCL reconstruction, meniscal repair or balancing, shoulder Bankart repair or rotator cuff repair. The indications have also advanced to smaller joints like TFCC repair in wrist and management of talus osteochondritis dissecans at ankle.
  - Tendinoscopy has been increasingly used for management of recalcitrant tenosynovitis not responsive to conservative management.
  - Carpal tunnel release is also being increasingly performed using endoscope.
- *Minimally invasive joint replacement surgery:*
  - For knee arthroplasty quadriceps sparing approaches with small incision has been used but complication rates have been a bit higher.
  - Hip arthroplasty is being increasingly performed in a minimally invasive manner and single very small incision or two small incisions. Also, this has been enhanced by availability of robotic arm.

226. **Describe the method to prepare PRP? What are the indications of PRP in orthopedic lesions. How does it work? Compare the role of local injection of steroid versus PRP in plantar fasciitis.**

Ans: *Platelet-rich plasma (PRP, platelet-enriched plasma, platelet-rich concentrate, or autologous platelet gel):* The basis of using the platelet concentrate obtained as autologous plasma fraction by centrifuging anticoagulated human blood is to capture the goodness of alpha-granules of platelet that are a rich source of numerous growth factors not limited to—PDGF, IGF, platelet factor-4 (PF4), IL, epidermal growth factor (EGF), vascular endothelial growth factor (VEGF), TGF superfamily, platelet-derived endothelial growth factor (PDEGF), etc. The platelets are usually obtained by centrifugation into the inactive leukocyte-rich concentrate that can be further processed to deplete leukocytes by filtration and/or activate platelets by adding calcium chloride. Activated platelets are usually applied with thrombin in gel form at the desired site of action. Leukocyte rich or depleted makes no difference in the clinical results for orthobiological application. The platelet concentrate has been used for (indications):

- Lateral epicondylitis—can be considered as alternative to corticosteroid injections.
- Rotator cuff repair—can be considered as adjuvant for surgical cuff repair—unclear efficacy.
- *Knee osteoarthritis:* The results show no substantial benefit in late osteoarthritis of knee and have no logical reason for use also. Early osteoarthritis (Ahlback-1) may improve symptomatically with PRP injection—unknown value.
- *Nonunion of long bones:* Some initial encouraging results fizzled out in uncertainty over study criteria and equivocal benefits. May be preferred to or added to bone marrow injections.
- *Achilles tendinopathy:* It may be considered as a failure to use of PRP, dismal results as only very few low-level supportive studies with no substantial benefit on record.
- *Patellar tendinopathy:* Not many studies to provide recommendation but some benefit reported in Jumper's knee.
- *Plantar fasciitis:* Equivocal results may consider alternative to steroid injections.
- *Shoulder osteoarthritis:* Unsubstantiated evidence suggests early improvement but long-term efficacy unknown.

How to prepare? Platelet-rich plasma is volume of plasma that contains a concentrate of platelets above (usually 4–5 times) that of baseline blood levels (150,000–200,000/μL). In a special container the patient's own blood (20–60 mL) is centrifuged after mixing it with anticoagulants (hard spin). The RBCs are separated and remaining contents are recentrifuged (soft spin) to get PRP. Separated PRP (3–7 mL) is injected in the indicated areas. Sometime platelets activators (bovine thrombin or 10% calcium chloride) are also mixed to activate the platelets before injection.

How it works in osteoarthritis: PRP augments tissue healing through the natural healing cascade. Growth factors are released from the granules of platelets and induce chemotaxis, cell migration, angiogenesis, proliferation, differentiation and matrix production. PRP also enhances hyaluronic acid secretion and increases release of angiogenic growth factors.

This biological therapy uses the patient's own platelets and plasma, which mainly convey fibrin and growth factors as effectors. These growth factors act on the entire joint. They promote restoration of joint homeostasis, have inductive and protective effects on chondrocytes and stimulate the production of hyaluronic acid by synoviocytes. All these properties help to promote a generative biological environment and to slow down joint and cartilage degeneration, thereby relieving symptoms.

Comparison of role of local steroid versus PRP injection: Though good results have been demonstrated for the use of PRP in various chronic enthesopathies, however no significant longer term benefits over other modalities have been reported. Good early response is seen with the use of local steroid preparations while PRP seems to have good role in intermediate term but over longer time periods no difference is seen with their use in dedicated comparisons.

227. What is PRP? Describe various types of PRP, their advantages and disadvantages.

Ans: Platelet-rich plasma (PRP) is a form of regenerative medicine that involves using a patient's own blood to create a concentrated solution of platelets and plasma. PRP is an *ultraconcentrate of centrifuged blood t*hat is composed of leukocytes and platelets. This solution contains growth factors and other cytokines that can stimulate healing in damaged tissues, including muscles, tendons, ligaments, and joints. Platelet-rich plasma is volume of plasma that contains a concentrate of platelets above (usually 4–5 times) that of baseline blood levels (150,000–200,000/µL). In a special container the patient's own blood (20–60 mL) is centrifuged after mixing it with anticoagulants (Hard spin). The RBCs are separated and remaining contents are recentrifuged (soft spin) to get PRP.

1. *Types of PRP:* There are primarily two types of PRP based on the concentration of white blood cells (leukocytes):
   a. *Leukocyte-rich PRP (LR-PRP):* Contains a higher-than-normal level of leukocytes, which can potentially enhance the inflammatory response and promote healing.
   b. *Leukocyte-poor PRP (LP-PRP):* Contains a lower-than-normal level of leukocytes, which may be used to minimize inflammation and optimize tissue repair in certain conditions.
2. *Advantages:*
   - *Autologous origin:* PRP is derived from the patient's own blood, reducing the risk of adverse reactions.
   - *Healing stimulation:* PRP injections can promote tissue repair and regeneration by delivering growth factors directly to the injury site.
   - *Reduced medication use:* PRP therapy can decrease the need for pain medications and anti-inflammatory drugs.
   - *Versatile applications:* PRP is used in various medical fields, including orthopedics, dermatology, and sports medicine.
3. *Disadvantages:*
   - *Varied efficacy:* The effectiveness of PRP can vary depending on the condition being treated, with mixed evidence in some cases.
   - *Multiple sessions:* Often require multiple treatments to achieve desired outcomes.
   - *Cost:* PRP therapy can be expensive compared to traditional treatments.

Limited standardization: Different preparation protocols and variability in platelet concentration can affect outcomes.

228. What is the role of bone marrow aspirate in orthopedic trauma?

Ans: Bone marrow aspirate (BMA) from "red active marrow (RAM)" (typically posterior iliac crest) contains mesenchymal stem cell (MSC) in the strength of 1:100,000. Volumes ranging from 15 to 150 mL have all been used. Aspiration is done in volumes of <4 mL (ideally 2 mL) from every 2–3 mm depths in a fan-like fashion to capture as many MSCs without dilution. It is estimated that typical BMA from RAM contains 70 million marrow cells of which 700 would be MSCs. It is postulated that MSCs act synergistically with BMP to produce effective fracture repair response (osteoinductive and osteogenic) and can also be used for delayed and nonunions. Transpedicular harvest from vertebral bodies has also been described. For optimum clinical efficacy, it is recommended that a high-degree open-pore scaffold with interconnected geometry is used to deliver the BMA. Ceramic hydroxyapatite (HA), β-tricalcium phosphate (TCP), and ultraporous β-TCP have been studied to be effective. The BMA can be ultracentrifuged to yield high concentration of stem cells in a lower volume that can be incorporated with scaffolds to produce similar effects. Composite grafting of BMA with BMP is found to yield better results. Recently, the isolated MSCs have been induced by dexamethasone in vitro to enhance the ability of BMP-2-modified MSCs in osteogenic conversion as part of stem cell therapy.

229. What are the types of epiphysis?
Ans:
1. Pressure epiphysis—helps in transmission of body weight and protection of epiphyseal cartilage.
   Type—articular ends.
   Example— head of femur, lower end of radius, condyles of humerus and tibia, head of humerus.
   5 paired bones having pressure epiphysis at both ends: humerus, radius, femur, tibia, fibula.
2. Traction epiphysis—caused by pull of muscles to withstand pull, i.e., muscle tendons attach here.
   Type—nonarticular.
   Example—trochanters of femur, greater and lesser tuberosity of humerus, mastoid process.
3. Aberrant epiphysis—when a bone has one epiphysis, an occasional separate epiphysis may be present.
   Type—not always present.
   Example—epiphysis at the head of 1st metacarpal, base of other metacarpals.
4. Atavistic epiphysis—separated in evolutionary process.
   Type—phylogenetically an independent bone, in humans it is fused to another bone.
   Example—posterior tubercle of talus (os trigonum), coracoid process of scapula.

230. A. Enumerate common orthopedic conditions related to disorders of physis.
B. Management of post-traumatic unilateral physeal bar in a growing child.
Ans: A. The following are common orthopedic conditions related to physeal disorders according to the zone involved:
- *Reserve zone:*
  - Gaucher's disease
  - Diastrophic dwarfism
  - Pseudo-achondroplasia
  - Kniest syndrome
- *Proliferative zone:*
  - Achondroplasia
  - Gigantism
- *Hypertrophic zone:*
  - Mucopolysaccharidoses
  - Rickets
  - Osteomalacia
  - SUFE (Slipped Upper Femoral Epiphysis)

B. A central physeal bar disrupts longitudinal growth causing limb length discrepancy (LLD). A peripheral physeal bar produces both a limb length discrepancy and angular deformity. These are more common with types III and IV Salter-Harris fractures because they involve the reserve zone. This results from injury to the germinal cells of the physis → physeal bar formation, ultimately tethering the epiphysis to the metaphysis.

Evaluation: Radiography in several planes of the involved part is prerequisite but CT and MRI elucidate more information concerning size, location, and shape of associated physeal bars. MRI (especially the fat-suppressed 3D spoiled gradient echo-weighted sequence) has the added benefit for providing additional information concerning abnormalities in cartilage (nonossified cartilage bar) and surrounding soft tissue injury and is radiation exposure free. Three-dimensional MRI allows for accurate anatomical assessment of the physeal bar. Centers equipped with computer-assisted navigation have added advantage of accurate identification of the bony bar intraoperatively.

Management proper: 'Goals' of treatment are: (1) restore limb length and mechanical alignment, (2) mobilize adjacent joints, and (3) correct deformity without subsequent cosmetic or functional deficiency. Available surgical options to achieve them include:
a. Physeal bar excision
b. Epiphysiodesis
c. Chondrodiastasis
d. Limb lengthening and deformity correction
e. Combination of above

Physeal bar excision: Physeal bar resection is primarily used when it can restore normal growth of the epiphysis. The physeal arrest should be detected early and ensuing deformity should be minimal or not developed. Goal of treatment is to remove the bony/fibrous bar and to fill the defect with a material that prevents recurrence taking care to cause least trauma to surrounding tissues as possible.

Indications:
- Documented existing or developing deformity with at least 2 years of growth remaining (calculate the bone age by X-ray of left hand).
- 25–40% of the physis is affected.
- Add corrective osteotomy if there is additional angular deformity of 10–25°.

Prerequisite: For infected physeal bars—at least 1-year free from pus drainage

Salient features of surgical technique:
- CT images allow for highly accurate real-time 3D monitoring of the bony bridge when combined with computer navigation (as against fluoroscopic visualization)
- Peripheral bridges are approached directly.
- Central bridges can be approached either through a metaphyseal window or through a metaphyseal osteotomy.
- Completeness of resection assessed by arthroscopic visualization/dental mirror in association with radiological guidance—fluoroscope/navigation.
- Interpositional material is legible (use fat graft or fascia or heterogeneous cartilage transplant or bone wax or artificial duramater or PMMA cement)
- Use metallic markers to monitor growth resumption (titanium wires)

Epiphysiodesis: This is preferred in following conditions:
- Physeal bar >50%
- Expected limb length discrepancy between 2 and 5 cm (use Anderson growth remaining charts or Paley multiplier method)

If a central physeal bar causes growth arrest and LLD; contralateral epiphysiodesis (other limb) is done else for peripheral physeal arrest producing angular deformities, ipsilateral epiphysiodesis for correction of angular deformity with contralateral epiphysiodesis for correction of growth abnormality is done. Permanent methods include open Phemister technique or percutaneous ablation of the physis with drilling and curettage. Temporary methods of epiphysiodesis include—stapling, guided growth plate method (8-plate, peanut plate, pediplate, etc.) or transphyseal screw.

Chondrodiastasis: This method is opposite to epiphysiodesis, here physeal distraction is done using external fixator facilitating bone formation. This helps in correcting angular deformities while also correcting limb length discrepancy. The distraction is done in a gradual progressive manner to correct the deformity/limb length. Both unilateral and Ilizarov type circular fixator apparatuses may be used to correct peripheral or central physeal arrest. Ilizarov type fixators are preferred for better control of angular distractions. Osteotomies are not needed and vascular supply to regenerate tissue is fully retained, physeal bar excision is not particularly needed.

Deformity correction: This may be combination of angular deformity correction + limb lengthening or may involve only single component. The deformity correction may be done acutely or may be done gradually. The various methods include—unilateral external fixator distraction, Ilizarov type circular fixators for complex deformities, mechanical motorized intramedullary nails, rail-road lengthening using external fixator and intramedullary nail, Taylor spatial frame.

231. Discuss principles of surgical correction of angular deformity in an 8-year-old child.
Ans: The following are the stepwise principles practiced for correction of angular deformities:
- Record a good, detailed history to know the cause of malunion.
- Ascertain the level of functional deficit/limitation.
- Correlate the functional disability with radiological findings.
- Measure coronal and sagittal plane deviations, viz., varus/valgus angulations, adduction/abduction deformity, procurvatum, and recurvatum deformity

- Evaluate nearby joints for movements/stiffness, limitation in mobility, deformity, and ligament laxity. Contractures across joints have significant bearing on the correction of deformity planning.
- Record leg length inequality
- *Assess mechanical axis deviation (MAD):* This is the frontal/coronal plane deviation of current limb axis from standard measures. For example, for the lower limb the line joining the center of femoral head to center of ankle joint passes within 6–7 mm medial to center of tibial spines (the correct reference is 4.1 mm ± 4 mm). If it deviates by any measure more than this on compensated measurements (for magnification, etc.) then MAD is said to be present.
- *Drawing AA is the next step:* AA is drawn for all fragments of deformity in coronal and sagittal planes. Intersection of these AA lines reveal the angular deformity and CORA. Oblique plane of complex deformities can be calculated by trigonometric or graphical method.
- *Joint orientation angle:* This is created by drawing a line tangential to subchondral shadow of the joint surface.
- Angular deformity correction is usually done by oblique osteotomy or wedge osteotomy.
- For closed wedge osteotomy, pass a K-wire transversely across the femoral shaft just proximal to the deformity. Place another K-wire distally at the desired angle of correction from first wire. Intraoperatively this angle is difficult to draw so preoperatively prepare a template by bending K-wire and send it for autoclave with the instrumentation the day before. Alternatively, a thin metal sheet or foil can be cut in the shape of a triangle with desired corrective angle that can be used intraoperatively.
- *In open wedge osteotomies:* There should be cortical contact at the apex of the wedge for pure angular corrections. The void is overfilled with prepared bone graft and bone graft obtained from reamings. If lengthening is desired to correct additional shortening, then distraction at osteotomy is maintained using femoral distractor.

232. Write notes on:
   A. Epiphysiodesis
   B. Callotasis.

Ans:
A. Epiphysiodesis is better called physiodesis. This is a popular method and considered treatment of choice for:
- The surgical correction of limb length discrepancy (LLD)
- Secondary choice for correction of angular deformities of limb.

The major limitations are:
- Need for early capture of patient and consistent follow-up so that enough data is available for accuracy of the procedure. It is only suitable for children who have sufficient growth remaining and have sufficient leg-length data to enable a confident prediction of the discrepancy at maturity.
- Also, corrections of 2–6 cm are favored with these methods and not more.

The methods used for physiodesis can be either temporary or permanent, the latter being preferred for correction of LLD often.

Temporary physiodesis: This was proposed by Blount to control the growth of physis temporarily so that:
- It can be done any time before achieving a particular age for permanent procedure.
- There is no need for accurate predictions of future growth from the charts.
- Growth would resume following later removal of the staples and both limbs would proportionately grow.

However, the method went into disfavor due to:
- Permanent fusion of the physis (due to ensuing physeal damage from the operative procedure itself)
- Extrusion or intra-articular migration of staples and superficial bursitis caused by the staples commonly
- Asymmetrical growth arrest by the procedure
- Compensatory overgrowth occurred after removal of staples recurring the limb-length discrepancy.

The arrest of physis was done by placing three staples on each side till equalization of limb length is achieved (one staple breaks, two bend or extrude). The staples are then removed requiring another surgery. Modification is to place the staples extraperiosteally so that intraoperative injury to physis does not occur and growth resumes after removing the staples, though other complications still can occur. Also, the staples have changed from steel to vitallium for better strength and fixation so that they do not break or extrude.

Permanent physiodesis: It is the preferred method by most surgeons. The prerequisite for performing the procedure is accurate determination of remaining growth and hence the gain from the procedure if done. Permanent method is an all-or-nothing procedure that completely and permanently arrests physeal growth. Performing the operation too late results in undercorrection otherwise performing it too early results in overcorrection. Slight discrepancies are well tolerated in population so commonly undercorrection of 0.5–1.0 cm is aimed for (commonly done by delaying surgery a bit). In general, the following points should be realized:
- The loss from proximal tibial physiodesis is 27%.
- Loss of growth from distal femur physeal arrest is 38%.
- If both the plates are fused, then there is 65% loss of remaining growth.

Tibial epiphysiodesis should be accompanied by concomitant proximal fibular physeal arrest, if the tibial shortening is greater than 2.5 cm. Permanent fusion can be achieved in many ways.
- *Conventional physiodesis:* Done through open method on both sides of growth plate. A block of bone from both sides is removed and plate extirpated (curette or burr). The block is then replaced distorting the disposition of growth plate. This produces a bony bridge precluding the growth. Phemister removed a rectangular block, two-thirds on the metaphyseal side and one-third on the epiphyseal side of the plate, and reversed it while replacing. White and Stubbins used a special chisel to remove a square block that is rotated 90° at replacement. Blount used a circular trephine to remove a cylindrical block that is also rotated 90° before replacing.
- Physiodesis using Blount's staples.
- *Percutaneous physiodesis:* Due to cosmetic dissidence of the open procedure, percutaneous methods were proposed. Percutaneous physeal ablation is done with a drill or burr, through small medial and lateral incisions, under image intensifier control. This technique has become popular and accepted well and now most of the surgeons use percutaneous method for physiodesis, especially in tibia; femoral side procedure is more technically demanding. Approximately 50% of the area of the plate should be removed.
- *Physiodesis using 8-plate:* This method is more appropriate for correcting angular deformities rather than doing growth arrest.

The disadvantages of physiodesis in general include:
- Unsightly scar is the primary concern with the open procedure.
- As such it is a compensatory, and not a corrective operation. Well leg is being disturbed rather than correcting the affected leg; it makes the normal leg abnormal.
- Infection causing local growth disturbances and hypertrophic bone formation.
- Compared to lengthening, it results in a decrease in the patient's stature that may be undesirable.

B. *Callotasis* as a concept was introduced by DeBastiani in 1980s. This depends on increasingly organization of callus tissue for reliable bone formation. As callus takes minimum 2 weeks so here the delay or priming period was kept at 2 weeks. Distraction is gradually achieved with a distractor. The construct can be modified to achieve angular correction or lengthening or shortening as the case may be.

Callotasis for correcting genu varus: This is distraction of the callus and done with the help of external fixator. Osteotomy is done at the desired site (CORA) and the fixator distracts the healing tissue formed at the site. It differs from Ilizarov as callus forms and not "regenerate", and osteotomy is done rather than corticotomy.

233. Compare and contrast ankylosis and arthrodesis.

Ans: The comparison between ankylosis and arthrodesis is described in **Table 2.13.1**.

TABLE 2.13.1: Comparison between ankylosis and arthrodesis.

Arthrodesis	Ankylosis
Merging together of similar or different elements of bone	Growing together of bones to form a single mass
Achieved surgically	Natural occurrence—either physiological or pathological (say after infection)
Commonly needs bone grafting at the site	Requires milieu of cytological soup for successful ankylosis
Commonly compression has to be given at the site	Not needed
Stabilization is achieved with surgical metallic implant or external immobilization with fixator/cast	Not needed. In pathological cases the muscles act as splint

234. General principles of arthrodesis.

Ans: The following are the common principles for doing arthrodesis modified from Glissan:
- Adequate debridement to remove all cartilages and fibrous tissue
- Preserving the blood supply to the involved surfaces for fusion
- Large opposing surfaces that are congruently placed for good interlocking and minimum dead space between them for optimal bone filling/union
- Obtaining anatomic reduction and optimal positioning of the joint to be fused for best functional results later
- Clearing away infection by meticulous excision of focus
- No necrotic bone in the region as it hampers new bone formation and union
- Providing stable spanning fixation with compression across the fusion site
- Bone grafting the defects
- Proper soft tissue cover to provide surrounding vascularity and avoiding dead spaces
- Immobilization till stable union is obtained.

235. Explain free vascularized bone transplant. Describe its principles of technique and applications in orthopedic practice.

Ans: Vascularized bone grafts are procured with their vascularity intact and placed at their intended place of use with vascular anastomosis keeping them viable. Commonly vascularized fibular bone transplant has been described in most of the orthopedic literature and use. Sporadic use of vascularized rib and vascularized ilium has also been reported however. Currently it is the vascularized fibula that is most popular.

Free vascularized fibula graft (Judet and Gilbert, Brunelli and Brunelli) is a remotely transplanted microvascular bone graft that maintains viability, strength and has theoretically improved incorporation by bypassing the stages of creeping substitution and regaining vascularity.

Surgical Technique

Exposure of the fibula:
- The fibula is harvested using a straight incision from middle third of leg.
- After reflecting the peronei anteriorly, the fibula is dissected free extraperiosteally and anterior intermuscular septum divided. The periosteum is preserved fully reflecting the anterior musculature and exposing interosseous membrane.
- Posterior intermuscular septum is divided and muscles are exposed and dissected free.
- The fibula cuts are made 15 cm apart protecting the peroneal vessels and separating from interosseous membrane close to fibula.
- Quite often the modern surgeons take a "buoy skin flap" as a marker for sustained vascularity of the graft for postoperative and follow-up assessment, this is taken along with the vascularized fibular graft as its extension. The first use of this "buoy flap" was done by Yoshimura et al. for sentinel surveillance of the vascularized fibular graft.
- The vessels are flushed with heparin saline and graft prepared.
- Prepared graft is passed through generously spacious femoral core and anastomosis done.

Postoperative course: The patients are kept nonweight-bearing for 6 weeks followed by mobilization of the hip joint and static exercises. For patients with preoperative collapse the protected weight bearing is done for 6 months.

Modification: The above extra-articular technique is most popular and commonly used at dedicated centers. Zhang's technique requires an anterior arthrotomy, with the creation of an anterior cortical trough in the femoral neck. This technique has advantage of requiring shorter fibular pedicle, and hence less dissection at the donor site. The disadvantage is, however, creating a stress riser in the neck of femur and possible hip stiffness due to anterior arthrotomy.

Complications:
- Postoperative bleeding (fall of up to 4 g/dL is seen after this surgery not uncommonly)
- Postoperative infection
- Subtrochanteric fracture
- Neurapraxia of peroneal nerve
- Flexor hallucis longus (FHL) induced toe contracture (use a below knee cast with foot platform extension for 2 weeks as preventive measure)

- Ankle pain
- Leg length discrepancies
- Accelerated head collapse
- Transient foot drop.

Indications:
- Osteonecrosis of femoral head
- Bone reconstruction in traumatic bone loss (>6 cm) following trauma
- Diaphyseal bone reconstruction following tumor surgery
- Congenital ulnar pseudoarthrosis
- Treatment of long bone nonunions (usually failed cases)
- Management of congenital pseudoarthrosis of tibia
- Failed spinal fusions
- Complex arthrodesis.

236. Describe autologous chondrocyte implantation.

Ans: Autologous cartilage implantation (ACI) is a first-generation cell-based therapy that involves transplantation of autogenous cells into articular cartilage defects. The ACI procedures, first introduced by Brittberg and coworkers, have become the most competent surgical procedure for treatment of cartilage defects. The specific advantage is that it promises to provide complete hyaline repair tissues for articular cartilage repair. In ACI cells are taken from nonweight-bearing regions of joint typically the lateral trochlear ridge. The chondrocytes then are enzymatically isolated from the ECM and cultured in monolayer for 3–4 weeks. This increases the volume of cells available for implantation 30-fold. The defect is prepared into a circular or oval shape by debriding all damaged and unstable tissue down to subchondral bone with a rim of stable healthy cartilage. The walls of the defect are kept as vertical as possible to allow for suture fixation of the graft. Periosteum harvested from proximal tibia is used to seal the defect. The cambium layer containing multipotent stem cells is sutured facing the defect. The chondrocyte containing solution is injected into the prepared partially sealed cavity and suturing of periosteum completed.

The main drawbacks of ACI are:
- Need for large open arthrotomy
- The two-stage procedure (one for cell harvesting and the other for implantation)
- The prolonged period of time required to expand sufficient numbers of chondrocytes *in vitro*
- High cost of cell culture system
- Poor retention and dedifferentiation of cells following implantation
- Ablation and loss of implanted cells from the defect site
- Prolonged nonweight-bearing
- Periosteal hypertrophy and other problems with the use of periosteal patch (discussed below).

237. Describe gene therapy in orthopedics.

Ans: In genetic diseases of primarily orthopedic interest such as osteogenesis imperfecta (OI) or Duchenne muscular dystrophy (DMD), today's treatment options are purely symptomatic. Even in conditions that have been classically treated operatively like osteoarthrosis, bone tumors, ligament and tendon regeneration, osteoporosis, etc.; role of genetics is fast emerging. The direct application of proteins (growth factors or cytokines) though potentially beneficial is limited by very short half-life and requirement of high doses. Gene therapy could be the potential answer to overcome these problems. The healing response can be improved by the local targeted application of growth factors into the injury site but they have their own shortcomings. Gene therapy successfully applied provides these growth factors in a sustained manner locally. The following are the potential applications of gene therapy as relevant to orthopedics:
- *Fracture healing:*
    - Nonunion
    - Delayed-union
    - Compound fractures

– Grade 3 open fractures.
- *Ligament healing:*
  – Regeneration of ligaments like patellar tendon (extensor mechanism), ACL or improved fixation and incorporation of grafts
  – Meniscal tears.
- Chondral (articular cartilage) healing and regeneration
- *Muscular diseases:*
  – Muscular dystrophies
  – Muscle strain
  – Utilization of muscle cells as *ex vivo* delivery vehicles
- *Osteoarthritis (OA):*
  – Primarily chondral regeneration
  – Alteration of joint milieu to retard joint degeneration.
- *Rheumatoid arthritis:*
  – Altering or remitting the inflammatory process.

Gene therapy cannot only be used for management of genetic defects but also to introduce therapeutic agents directly into somatic tissue cells. This somatic gene therapy (as distinct from germline gene therapy) opens up immense possibilities beyond the single gene defect disorders. Somatic gene therapy can be performed locally or systemically, whereas the latter may be advantageous in cardiac or vascular diseases former is more amenable to orthopedic diseases.

Thus, a local gene delivery into the diseased or injured tissue is desirable. Gene therapy is the excellent application to transfer growth factors and to produce them at cell level in a continuous manner. For example, poor strength local tissue scar with reduced mechanical strength can be modified with the application of the growth factors. A gene for a specific growth factor can be transferred to the injured tissue either directly or indirectly. In direct approach, vector with gene is directly injected into the injured tissue. Indirect approach utilizes cells taken by biopsy from the injured tissue, cultured *in vitro* and vector is injected into the stabilized cells. This vector can be nonviral (transfection) or viral (transduction) **(Flowchart 2.13.1)**.

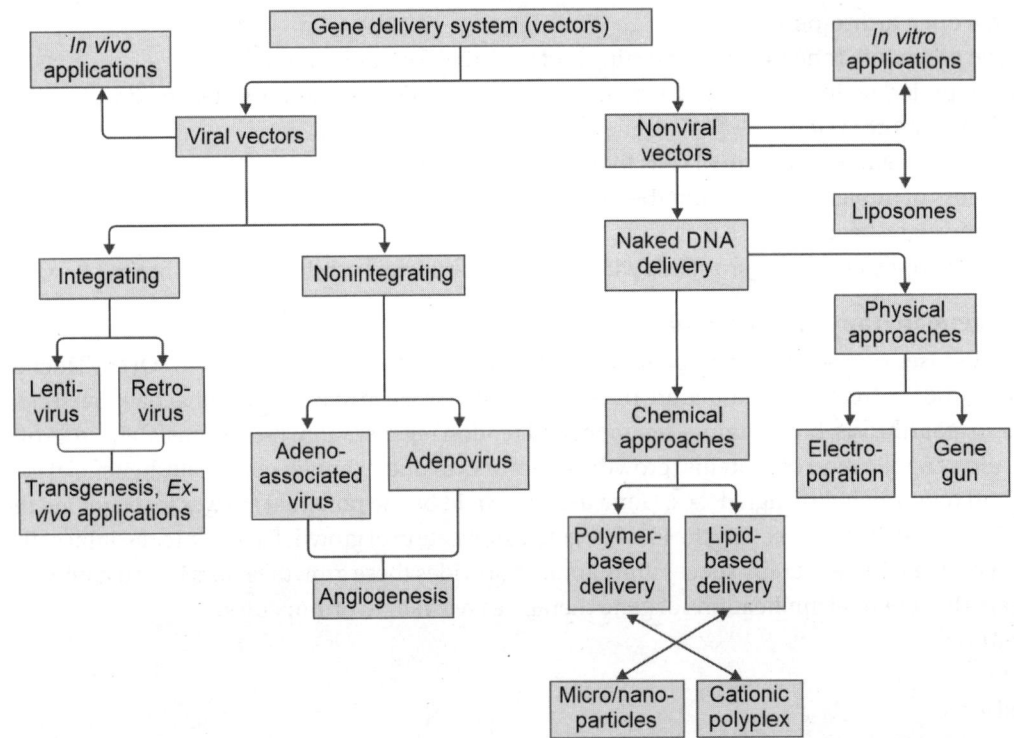

Flowchart 2.13.1: Main methods of gene delivery systems.

238. Explain induced membrane formation to cover bone defects.

Ans: *Induced membrane technique (Masquelet technique):* Masquelet (2000) reported on a series of 35 cases of large diaphyseal bone defects reconstructed by autologous bone grafting. The technique is aimed at helping solve the problems of bone graft containment around the bone defect and the commonly desired need for growth supplementation using proteins. They successfully repaired wide diaphyseal defects (≤25 cm) with concurrent severe soft tissue loss using fresh autologous cancellous bone grafts in two-step (first step is more or less mechanical while second step is biological) surgical procedure. In the first step (membrane induction), a PMMA cement spacer is inserted into the defect (after repeated debridement and obtaining clean bed) inducing formation of an encapsulation membrane. The bone is stabilized using external fixator or intramedullary nail. After 4–6 weeks, the spacer is removed and the cavity filled with autologous cancellous graft from iliac crest. Morselized cancellous autograft harvested from the iliac crests is preferred but if this amount is not sufficient then demineralized allograft can be added to the autograft in a ratio that does not exceed 1 part of allograft: three parts of autograft. Bone formation and union occurs in approximately 8–9 months.

The advantages of this technique are:
- Prevention of encroachment by adjacent soft tissues into the bone defect
- Stable placement of the graft in place
- Prevention of resorption of graft material by or local production of osteoinductive substances maintains graft volume and helps in augmenting the bone formation (Masquelet).

Biology of induced membrane technique: Nearly 4–5 weeks are needed for development and maturation of a biologically active membrane around the cement filled nidus that slowly becomes strong enough for bone grafting later. The cement spacer also maintains the defect and inhibits fibrous ingrowth. Masquelet and Begue proposed that this membrane prevents bone graft resorption (but this has not been found always true for filling large bone defects) and improves vascularity and corticalization. Biomembrane formed around PMMA is actually a pseudosynovial membrane that can be 0.5–1 mm thick and has microscopic characteristics of being both hypervascular and impermeable. Deeper into the membrane the fibroblastic cells derived from mesenchymal tissue are arranged in a random fashion. They play an important role in the laying down of extracellular matrix forming the organized pseudosynovial membrane that has been found to express bone morphogenic protein 2 (BMP2), TGF-β, vascular endothelial growth factor (VEGF), von Willebrand factor (vWF), IL-6, and IL-8. While VEGF is crucial for angiogenesis the vWF has been implicated in the regulation and normal formation of blood vessels and in the membrane, it assists in new tissue growth.

The overall construct produces a combination of intramembranous and endochondral ossification histologically producing a progressive healing response. It must be remembered that the membrane alone has been found inadequate to heal a defect greater than critical bone defect. But when autologous bone graft was placed within the membrane nearly all the defects would heal (few defects more than 15 cm would show premature bone graft resorption). Reconstruction of the femur seems to be specifically associated with a risk of graft resorption. It has also been demonstrated that the 1-month-old membrane has higher osteogenesis-improving capabilities compared to 2-month-old membrane so some have recommended that optimal time for performing second-stage surgery may be within a month after PMMA implantation. Large amount of graft and sometimes repeated surgery are needed in some patients.

239. What is chondrocyte culture?

Ans: Chondrocytes are extremely difficult to culture and proliferate and require strict conditions. The requirements have increased for the current use of these cells in ACI and similar cartilage reconstruction techniques. Chondrocyte give us good insight to investigate intracellular and molecular events associated with chondrocyte differentiation and activation.

The main problem during culture is the tedious procedure and that the cultured chondrocytes tend to dedifferentiate into fibroblasts, especially during monoclonal expansion phase. This dedifferentiation during culture can be detected when chondrocytes start synthesizing collagen types I and III instead of collagen type II (articular chondrocytes) or type X (epiphyseal chondrocytes). The dedifferentiated cells also switch synthesis from high molecular weight proteoglycans (aggrecan) to low molecular weight proteoglycans (biglycan and decorin). Various factors have been identified for this untoward process like low-density plating, monolayer culturing, extraction from human adult cartilage, extraction from chondrosarcoma or immortalization, etc. To minimize conversion to fibroblasts extensive use of cells from young animals such as rabbits or cattle which are more stable than human adult chondrocytes is being promoted.

Several immortalized chondrocyte cell lines have been shown to express a chondrocyte specific phenotype with a high proliferation rate. The problem with these is that the phenotypic stability is lost more quickly during expansion in serial monolayer cultures, compared with primary cultures of cells from juvenile animals. Recently, efforts to obtain a better phenotype than that of 2D cultured chondrocytes have evolved. These include embedding the cells in an artificial matrix commonly made of stabilizers like alginate, agarose, or collagens. The chondrocyte phenotype is improved with their use, but on the flip side cellular growth is slowed making less number of cells available in the same time.

Procedure of human chondrocyte culture:
1. For human primary articular chondrocytes complete culture medium consists of Dulbecco's modified Eagle's medium (high glucose) supplemented with 4 mM L-glutamine, 100 U/mL penicillin and 0.1 mg/mL streptomycin and with 10% (v/v) fetal calf serum.
2. Place the specimen in collection medium at 4°C. Mince all collected cartilage slices into about 1–3 mm in three pieces.
3. Rinse the cartilage once with sterile Dulbecco's phosphate-buffered Ca^{2+} and Mg^{2+} free saline (PBS).
4. Add these to 10 mL of 0.2% trypsin solution. Stir the mixture, rinse and transfer to 0.2% collagenase solution and centrifuge.
5. Wash the cartilage pieces in adding 10 mL serum-free culture medium.
6. Incubate for 90 minutes at 37°C in a CO_2 incubator while shaking.
7. Centrifuge for 5 minutes at 200 g and discard the supernatant.
8. Resuspend the pellet in 10 mL of complete culture medium and count the cells in a hemocytometer. Bring up to volume with complete culture medium and seed the suspended chondrocytes onto tissue culture plates or dishes at a density of 1×10^5 cells/cm^2.
9. Incubate the culture plates or dishes for 2 days undisturbed at 37°C under humidified conditions and 5% CO_2/95% air to ensure strong attachment.
10. Change the medium on the day before harvest.

The most recent advancement in cartilage reconstruction is the development of *coculture systems*. These systems are emerging as novel methods that are a step ahead to the use of MSCs. They enhance the differentiation and chondrogenesis potential of MSCs. The major drawback of using MSCs only in the reconstruction is possibility of potential mineralization that occur with their use in chondrogenic conditions *in vitro*. This produces conditions similar to an endochondral ossification pathway. Such misrepresentation of differentiation pattern can be checked by the use of coculture systems by controlling the "crosstalk" between cells. The tendency to hypertrophy of the MSCs is inhibited by chondrocytes that secrete parathyroid hormone-related protein (PTHrP) in coculture (chondrocytes + MSCs) systems. The other interesting advantage of these systems is that MSCs have enhanced the proliferation of chondrocytes and stabilized their phenotype by secreting trophic factors. The chondrocyte-related gene expression and production of cartilage-like matrix *in vitro* have been seen in these coculture systems by upregulation of the specific pathways. These advantages (that nullify the disadvantages of either cell culture system individually) make coculture systems current favorites though these are also not without limitations.

240. (A) What is limb length discrepancy? (B) Classify limb length discrepancy. (C) Discuss management of limb length discrepancy due to congenital pseudoarthrosis tibia in children.

Ans:
A. Limb length discrepancy, also known as anisomelia, is defined as a condition in which paired lower extremity limbs have a noticeably unequal length.
B. **Classification of limb length discrepancy:**
   - Leg length discrepancy (LLD) can be divided into "congenital-syndromic" and "acquired" causes that may both include inhibition or stimulation of growth.
   - McCaw and Bates (1991) gave a classification as per inequality:
     - Mild is <3cm
     - Moderate is 3–6 cm
     - Severe is >6 cm

C. **Management of limb length discrepancy due to congenital pseudoarthrosis tibia in children:**
   - IM nailing with iliac crest bone graft and transfixation of ankle (Charnley). It involves extraperiosteal pseudoarthrosis excision and IM stabilization of the tibia and fibula. An autogenous bone graft, with or without iliac crest periosteum, is used at the resection site. The success rate for IM nailing and bone grafting approaches 80–90%, although the pseudoarthrosis may recur and necessitate repeated bone grafting, with or without bone stimulation units.
     - IM nailing with two-part solid Peter Williams rod—pseudoarthrosis excision and iliac crest bone grafting. The rod is advanced into the talus and calcaneus correcting the calcaneovalgus deformity of the foot simultaneously and then the rod is advanced retrograde into the proximal fragment. The gap at osteotomy site is filled with bone graft obtained from iliac crest. Another osteotomy may be required proximally in case of extensive deformity and tibial bow.
- *Ilizarov method:* The method is versatile in producing consolidation at the fracture site and simultaneous correction of the deformity. It can be applied in various forms including compression only, compression plus tibial lengthening, compression followed by distraction, and distraction alone for hypertrophic nonunion. This method can also be used in children who were not successfully treated using the previous method or those who are older or in patients with atrophic bone ends at the fracture site. The pseudoarthrosis is resected, and the two bone ends are impacted. A proximal corticotomy allows for bone transport to make up for the tibial shortening. The bone is compressed distally. As in other techniques, autogenous bone graft and bone morphogenetic protein are used to facilitate union at the distal site.

241. **Describe the principles and devices of limb length equalization.**

Ans: Principles: The decision to treat limb-length discrepancy depends on the predicted discrepancy at skeletal maturity.
- A patient with a predicted discrepancy of less than 2 cm requires no treatment, although a 1–2 cm shoe-lift can be used inside the shoe; sometimes a wedge is placed on the bottom of the shoe.
- *For LLD between 2 cm and 6 cm, the reasonable treatment options are:*
  - A shoe-lift
  - Epiphysiodesis
  - Skeletal shortening.

  Lengthening is socially favored over shortening for advantages of height. Hence, shortening procedures are usually not appropriate for correction of greater than 6 cm, because a disproportionate appearance results (smaller lower limbs compared to the body height) which may not be pleasing to the patient. It is better to leave the decision of shortening versus lengthening on the patient at LLD of 5–6 cm as this is a gray zone.
- Limb-lengthening should be performed for a patient with a predicted discrepancy between 6 cm and 17 cm at skeletal maturity. This is commonly performed by osteotomy of the short bone and gradual lengthening with internal or external devices.
- A predicted discrepancy greater than 17 cm often requires amputation and prosthetic fitting (see below). Though intriguing one major limitation to limb lengthening is the long period of external fixator required for the bone to consolidate. Two recent methods developed to circumvent this problem include:
  1. Bone-lengthening using external fixation over an IM nail
  2. Bone-lengthening from within, using IM nails. The use of lengthening IM nails offers the benefit of decreased pin tract complications and elimination of exposed hardware. These newer methods are particularly useful for patients with minimal growth potential or closed growth plates.

Devices: Four types of treatment are available for limb-length equalization—shoe lift or prosthetic conversion, epiphysiodesis of the long leg, shortening of the long leg (in patients too old for epiphysiodesis), and lengthening of the short leg.

Shoe-lift: Shoe-lift is the best option for those patients who do not agree or are not good candidates for surgical correction. The shoe-lift is given only for walking patients for logical reasons. Cosmetically, up to 2 cm of the lift can be put inside the shoe to hide it and the remainder on the outside. It should be borne in mind that infinite shoe-lift is not possible and lifts higher than 5 cm result in frequent ankle sprains, you see ladies walking with high heels have unstable gaits and is not recommended; this is only one of the drawbacks of high heels! This is due to the fact that muscles controlling the subtalar joint are not strong enough to resist inversion stress. For higher lift, an orthotic extension up the posterior is added for stability.

Prosthetic fitting: This is considered a treatment of last resort but is useful for patients with very large discrepancies (PFFD) and those with deformed and functionally useless feet (tibial, fibular hemimelia).

Epiphysiodesis: Better called physiodesis (as it is done to control the growth of physis and not epiphysis). This is a popular method and considered treatment of choice for the surgical correction of LLD. The major limitation is needed for early capture of patient and consistent follow-up so that enough data is available for accuracy of the procedure. It is only suitable for children who have sufficient growth remaining and have sufficient leg-length data to enable a confident prediction of the discrepancy at maturity. Also, corrections of 2–6 cm are favored with these methods and not more. One should recollect that distal femur and tibia contribute for 65% of the growth of lower extremity. The average contribution for distal femur is nearly 9 mm/year accounting for 37% while that of tibia is nearly 6 mm/year accounting for 28%. Also, one should remember that males would typically grow till 16 years of age and females till around 14 years of age, so if there is 3 years of remaining growth then some 4.5 cm of correction can be achieved by combined physiodesis of distal femur and proximal tibia. The methods used for physiodesis can be either temporary or permanent, the latter being preferred for correction of LLD often.

Limb shortening: Shortening usually is reserved for skeletally mature patients who can accept the loss of stature necessary to equalize limb lengths. When planning surgery, ultimate length and alignment should be considered. Wagner outlined the standard approach to limb shortening, but improvements have been made in femoral shortening techniques, such as a closed technique for diaphyseal shortening described by Winquist, Hansen, and Pearson. In the femur, 5–6 cm is the maximal length that can be removed without seriously affecting muscle function; in the tibia, the maximum probably is 2–3 cm.

Limb lengthening: A limb-lengthening program requires a patient and family fully committed to maximal participation in an extended project. The success of limb lengthening depends largely on the patient's efforts in physical therapy and the care of the external fixator. Although technical improvements have reduced the frequency with which major complications associated with limb lengthening occur, the process remains difficult and should be performed by surgeons with appropriate experience.

Shortening procedures are preferable for many patients who are candidates for limb lengthening. Patients who are unable to participate in frequent follow-up or who do not have the support to care for the fixator properly and to undergo vigorous physical therapy are best treated by means other than lengthening. Candidates for limb lengthening and their parents benefit from meeting other patients in various stages of the lengthening process. Acute long bone lengthening seldom is indicated.

Lengthening by slow distraction: Osteotomy followed by gradual distraction of the bone fragments with a mechanical apparatus has been the basic procedure for limb lengthening since Putti's report of the technique in 1921. Osteotomy and fixation techniques have been modified by several authors, but high complication rates were reported with all methods, including deep infection, nonunion, fracture after plate removal, malunion, and nerve palsy. Wagner introduced a low-profile, mobile, monolateral fixator that improved results, and DeBastiani designed a similar but more versatile fixator (Orthofix). In the early 1950s, Ilizarov devised a thin-wire, circular external fixator for fracture fixation and found that slow distraction with the device caused regeneration of bone in the distraction gap. Also, introduced were lengthening over an intramedullary nail.

242. **Discuss briefly the technique of bone lengthening by various external fixation devices. Mention the role of other devices and its advantages.**

Ans: Various external fixation devices have been used for bone lengthening, as follows:
- *Wagner's device:* Lengthening using Wagner frame is a three-step surgical procedure. The first involves osteotomy, releasing soft tissues and applying the device. Lengthening is then continued. At the end of the lengthening phase, a second procedure involves bone-grafting the lengthening gap, and fixator removal is done. Plating the bone at this stage is advised by and performed by Wagner. Later when the bone has achieved sufficient strength, a third procedure

is done to remove the plate. The plating is not recommended following fixator removal due to contaminated pin tracts, so newer methods that involve neither plating nor grafting were searched.

- *Orthofix technique (Monorail fixator):* De Bastiani and colleagues developed the Orthofix device applied to bone with two sets of conical screws. The pin blocks move along a rail placed beside the pins. It is technically similar in operation to the Wagner device, but it offers more stability. The disadvantage is that it has a more cumbersome method of elongation and is not easily adjustable once in place.
- *Ilizarov technique using ring fixators:* They are technically more complex than the Wagner and Orthofix devices but are highly versatile. Ilizarov method can not only lengthen limb but also correct the deformity in coronal, sagittal and axial planes if required simultaneously including translation of fragments. They allow intermediate adjustments and have been consistent in success. Also, they can be fixed in trifocal manner controlling more than two segments and can extend across joints. Frame assembly is applied to the bone using the tensioned through- and through wires attached to rings. Rancho modification evolved to provide unilateral fixation possibility using half-pins.

Other devices:

- *Taylor spatial frame:* This is a versatile device where multiplanar deformity can be corrected along with limb lengthening based on computerized assessment and precise planning. This device is better used for deformity correction than limb lengthening.
- *Limb lengthening over intramedullary rod:* This method is considered more effective than using Wagner or orthofix external fixation alone for bone lengthening with regard to time of external fixation, index of external fixation and complication rate. This is due to better control of the fragments at the osteotomy site and minimal chances of them migrating away from desired alignment.

243. Discuss principle, indications, advantages and disadvantages of motorized intramedullary bone lengthening in adults.

Ans: *Principles:*

- The device is capable of both bone fragment stabilization and lengthening, which obviates the need for external fixation altogether.
- The nails require intermittent axial rotation of the limb to affect distraction. Motorized nails have magnetic motor imbedded in the telescopic rod that is activated by intermittent transcutaneous transmission of radiofrequency waves to an implanted antenna/receiver that converts these waves into an electrical impulse that is discharged via a connecting cable.
- In the newer PRECICE® nail, the telescopic rod has a magnetic actuator drive mechanism that is activated by a handheld external electromagnetic activator and does not require cable or subcutaneously imbedded antenna/receiver and it can be both lengthened or shortened.

Indications: The antegrade nail can be used for:
1. Patients with a femoral LLD who have an open IM canal with a diameter large enough to fit the IM nail.
2. Deformity in the region of proximal meta-diaphyseal to mid-diaphyseal region
3. Correction of rotational deformity
4. Tibial lengthening with a telescopic nail is ideal for the skeletally mature patient with a 1.5- to 6-cm LLD, a straight bone with no deformity, an open medullary canal, and adequate bone size to accommodate an IM nail. Smaller deformity of ≤10° can be acutely corrected and fixed with nail.

The retrograde femoral nail is used for:
1. Patients with arthrodesis or deformity of the hip or proximal femur that precludes the use of antegrade femoral nailing.
2. Distal deformity that will be corrected with osteotomy.

Advantages:

- Maintaining stability and alignment during distraction
- No external implants that preclude hygiene and mobilization
- Controlled smooth rate and rhythm of distraction minimizing chances of failure/nonunion, etc.

Disadvantages:
- Mechanically activated nails may get activated too fast or too slow so magnetic/electromagnetic nails are better.
- The nails do not fit well in expanded medullary canal portions—distal femur and proximal or distal tibia so additional stability is needed in the form of polar/blocking screw.
- Deformities in expanded medullary portions need planning so that the site of osteotomy does not get deformed while distraction.
- Nails slide proximally with distraction so lose mechanical stability limiting the magnitude of lengthening that can be done.
- Mechanical failure and failure of mechanisms need revision surgery for implanting another device.

244. A. Discuss method and principle of Ilizarov hip.
B. What are the indications, advantages and shortcomings of Ilizarov hip reconstruction?

Ans: *Principle:* Ilizarov hip reconstruction is a well-accepted but complication-prone operative salvage procedure. According to the Ilizarov method, the use of external fixation was an inherent part of this procedure, which was named "Ilizarov hip reconstruction". Painful hip instability acquired as a result of trauma, septic/tuberculous arthritis, or developmental dysplasia is difficult to treat in the young population. The aim of treatment are to achieve a functional, stable and pain-free hip joint. Although total hip replacement is amenable to such goals but it is limited by life-span of prosthesis, it can offer and need for revision surgeries. So pelvic-support osteotomies are the best possibilities in these patients fixed using various systems—Ilizarov is one of them.

Indications:
- Salvage of damaged hips is needed, where arthrodesis and total hip arthroplasty are not indicated.
- Infantile/early septic arthritis or proximal femur osteomyelitis (Hunka types 4 and 5)
- Girdle stone due to failed previous reconstructive surgery or arthroplasty
- Congenital hip dislocation
- Femoral neck pseudoarthrosis
- Traumatic hip dislocation with instability

Method (steps only):
- *Preoperative planning:*
  - Physical examination and local examination with particular emphasis on ROM, LLD, and Trendelenburg's sign and gait.
  - X-ray pelvis AP in neutral and maximum adduction cross-legged position—to determine the level of proximal femoral osteotomy and amount of acute abduction to be created in the proximal osteotomy.
  - Scanogram to calculate the limb-length discrepancy and deformities in femur/tibia can be identified and calculated.
  - Level of the second compensatory osteotomy was determined on a tracing paper of the pelvis and femur with the proximal femoral segment maximally adducted.
- *Surgical technique:*
  - Supine position
  - Preparation of parts and draping as standard
  - Identification of proximal osteotomy site under fluoroscopy under maximum adduction of the femoral shaft at the level of ischium
  - Assembly of external fixator—pelvic arch for holding proximal femur segment, 5/8 ring for middle segment and 2 rings for distal segment. Hinges are placed between the distal and middle segments of assembly
  - Insert three 6-mm Schanz pins into proximal femur obliquely so that with adduction they become parallel to horizontal line.
  - Connect pins to arch and adjust extension by tilting arch
  - Insert three Schanz pins in different planes into the middle fragment and connect to full-ring and 5/8th ring.
  - Use Ilizarov wires in distal fragment and connect to the distal full ring parallel to the knee joint.
  - Perform the osteotomies and tighten the frame with pins/wires and rings/arch appropriately placed.

Advantages:
- Osteotomy stabilization and lengthening simultaneously
- Once established—lasts for lifetime

Disadvantages:
- Pin tract infection
- Knee stiffness
- Nonunion
- Fracture in regenerate
- Premature consolidation
- Delayed consolidation
- Residual leg-length discrepancies

245. Explain the principles and applications of interlocking nail.

Ans: Interlocked intramedullary nails gradually evolved from 1950s. Modny and Bambara introduced the transfixation intramedullary nail in 1953. Nailing of tibia is introduced by Herzog in 1950. Livingston bar introduced a short I-beam pattern pointed nail at both ends that had short slots for cross-pinning with screws. Locking screws were introduced with second generation nailing to provide rotational stability to fracture fixation/splinting.

Principles of interlocked nailing:
- *Choosing implant and nail:*
    - The nail should be strong enough and provide sufficient stability to maintain alignment and position, including prevention of rotation—choose interlocking nail.
    - Adequate preoperative planning is required to ensure that the fracture can be adequately stabilized within the working zone of the nail.
        - Consider bone morphology (nailing not good for irregular canal), canal dimensions (nail should be 1–1.5 mm greater than narrowest canal diameter), comminution and fracture extensions before choosing implant.
    - The patient should be able to tolerate a major surgical procedure. Special consideration should be given to patients with severe pulmonary injury because the added fat emboli from the procedure may intensify pulmonary problems.
    - Suitable instruments (along with nails of all sizes of the chosen type), trained assistants, and optimal hospital conditions are necessary for successful insertion of intramedullary nails.
- *Principles of surgical technique:*
    - Closed nailing techniques should be used whenever possible. Higher union rates and fewer infections have been reported with the use of these techniques.
    - The entry portal is critical for all nails and should be in the region that would minimize insertional forces. In the femur, this is at the piriformis fossa in line with the medullary canal. For the tibia starting the nail at the level of the fibular head minimizes forces of insertion.
    - Sufficient diameter and continuity of the medullary canal should be ensured.
    - Reaming is recommended to maximize the nail diameter for improved stability. Excessive reaming, however, should be avoided because it significantly weakens the bone and increases the risk of thermal necrosis.
    - Nail-fracture construct should allow good contact-compression forces that can impact the fracture surfaces.
    - If the medullary canal is much larger in one fragment than in the other, poor control of rotational forces frequently results in these situations, interlocking techniques and the use of blocking (Poller) screws are required.
    - Generally, the interlocking screws should be positioned at least 2 cm from the fracture to provide sufficient stability to allow functional activity postoperatively. Axially unstable fractures are best treated with static or double-locked nails.
    - Locked intramedullary nailing techniques should allow nailing of fractures to within 2–4 cm of the joint.
    - It should be placed so that it is accessible for easy removal; attachments are provided to facilitate removal.

Applications of interlocking nails: They are one of the most popular orthopedic implants. The following are common indications:
- *Managing the fractures of:*
    - Femoral shaft, proximal femur (intertrochanteric, subtrochanteric), and distal extra-articular fractures of femur
    - Tibial shaft fractures and proximal fractures at metaphyseodiaphyseal junction

- Humerus shaft fractures
- Forearm fractures.
• Managing nonunion following plate fixation of diaphyseal long bones
• Exchange nailing for treatment of diaphyseal nonunion
• Fixation of bones following corrective osteotomy in shaft region
• Masquelet technique for management of long bone gap nonunion
• Arthrodesis of knee, ankle joints.

246. What is dynamization? Describe its role in orthopedics using various implants.

Ans: *Dynamization:* Dynamic stimulation of the fracture ends occurs when the implant permits only axial displacement while bending and torsional stiffness is maintained. The fracture ends are under uniform axial compression on weight-bearing and remain in contact even when the weight-bearing load is removed. Such stimulation is also called dynamization. For various implants, the process of dynamization can be explained as follows:

• *Interlocking nail:* A standard practice is to dynamize (weaken) the interlocked nail assembly by removing the locking screws. If healing is progressing normally, then there is no need to dynamize. If consolidation is continuing well, the removal of the static screw will not improve the quality of the callus. Dynamization is indicated when there is a risk of development of nonunion or in established pseudoarthrosis. The screws are then removed from the longer fragment, maintaining adequate control of the shorter fragment. Premature removal of locking screws may cause shortening, instability, and nonunion.

• *External fixator:* Dynamization is affected by increasing the load placed upon the fracture, by encouraging patient activity and by one of the following methods:
  1. The use of an elastic frame with overall low rigidity
  2. Progressive dismantling of the frame
  3. Increased weight bearing in a low-axial-stiffness frame
  4. *Biocompression:* The method uses a unilateral frame which allows free sliding. Weight-bearing controls the axial strain on the fracture and it is believed that the patient's natural feedback mechanism ensures the most appropriate strain for healing.

In practice, one of the easiest ways to "dynamize" the fixation as healing progresses is to loosen the pin clamps and slide them away from the skin, providing a longer pin span. In addition, or by itself, a reduction in the number of planes of fixation achieves greater flexibility in the fixation.

  - *Medoff plate for peritrochanteric fractures:* The biaxial compression plate (Medoff) permits biaxial sliding, along both the femoral neck and the femoral shaft. A lag screw similar to sliding hip screw assembly allows compression along the axis of the femoral neck. The femoral side plate, however, utilizes a coupled pair of sliding components that enable the fracture to impact parallel to the longitudinal axis of the femur. For most intertrochanteric fractures, biaxial dynamization is recommended. A locking set screw prevents independent sliding of the lag screw within the plate barrel; when the locking set screw is applied, the plate slides only axially on the femoral shaft. Uniaxial dynamization is suggested for a plain subtrochanteric fracture. When opting for biaxial dynamization, it is necessary to distally enlarge the lag screw entry site by approximately 2.5 cm to prevent the impingement of the barrel on the lateral cortex of the distal fragment and obstructing dynamic axial compression.

247. What are the effects of reaming of bone?

Ans: Reaming for nailing is done to make the canal more uniformly circular that would accept the interlocking nail. This involves incrementally reaming the canal till a snugly fitting nail can be passed through. The advantage of reaming is that a larger diameter nail can be passed through the canal improving stability but reaming has various positive and negative physiological effects on bone and body as follows:

• Embolization of bone marrow fat to the lungs adversely affects pulmonary function.
• Reaming damages the endosteum and decreases the torsion strength of the femoral fragments.
• Winquist and others have shown that elevation in intramedullary pressures and thermal damage caused by reaming can be decreased by using sharp reamers with deep cutting flutes and narrow shafts and by using minimal force during reamer insertion.
• Insertion of reamed nails disturbs cortical blood flow to a greater extent than does insertion of unreamed nails.

Advantages:
- Providing bone graft (autograft) from reaming at the endosteal side
- Stimulation of bone formation by reaming process that alters blood flow making it centripetal from the usual centrifugal one. There is increased vascularity at the periosteal side and surrounding soft tissue that enhance the migration and maturation of multipotent cells in the cambium layer of periosteum.
- The nonunion site is grossly untouched surgically so preventing additional loss of vascularity from periosteal stripping or soft tissue trauma.
- The reaming process also debrides the fibrous tissue formed at the nonunion site giving way to formation of newer callus and fibrocartilaginous tissue capable of healing the bone.
- Sometimes, for a distracted fracture, compression can be achieved by backslapping the nail.

248. What is the difference between reamed and unreamed nail?

Ans: Kindly see answers above.

The differences between reamed and unreamed nail are given in **Table 2.13.2**.

TABLE 2.13.2: Differences between reamed and unreamed nail.

Characteristic	Reamed nail	Unreamed nail
Canal reaming	Done	Not done
Cannulation	Nails are cannulated	Noncannulated nails
Nail diameter	Larger usually	Thinner nails usually
Biomechanical stability	Higher due to larger diameter nail	Lower
Secondary surgeries (bone grafting/implant exchange)	Lower requirement	Higher incidence of secondary procedures needed for bone union
Rate of bone union	Higher and faster	Lower and slower
Operative time	More time needed	Less time needed
Blood loss	Higher	Lower
Embolism	Higher incidence	Lower
Presence of local bone graft	Available from reaming	None
Utility	Universally preferred for shaft fractures of long bones	Preferred only for high grade open injuries where soft tissue envelop has also damaged vascularity
Intraoperative complications	More—embolism, reamer problems, bone necrosis, intraoperative fractures	Less
Late complications	Less	More—higher delayed and nonunion and need for secondary procedures

2.14 ORTHOTICS (Q249–256)

249. What is Knuckle bender splint?

Ans: Knuckle stands for metacarpophalangeal (MCP) joint of hands. In conditions like ulnar nerve palsy the individuals are unable to bend the MCP joint that produced disability of inability for form fist. For making fist or lifting any object there should be smooth transition of flexion movements that occur from MCP joints to interphalangeal (IP) joints in a rhythm. Inability to flex the MCP joints pushes the object rather than grasping it. The Knuckle Bender Splint is a finger flexion splint designed for use by individuals with disabilities of the fingers. This splint simultaneously flexes the MCP joints of 2nd to 4th digits while simultaneously extending the IP joint without blocking or wrist motion. The splint has following two active components that achieve flexion across MCP joint:

1. *Palm component:* This is usually a stabilization unit that has dorsal padded support that stabilizes 2nd to 4th metacarpal together while counterforce is provided from the volar palmar component.
2. *Phalangeal component:* This is placed on the dorsal aspect of proximal phalanx of the 2nd to 4th fingers providing flexion moment. The flexion moment is rendered through a spring that is connected to the volar palmar component so that the metacarpals remain in extension as the fingers are bending by providing a counter force.

The splint has a dynamic function to assist the MCP flexion. For claw hand deformity from ulnar nerve palsy, the splint also prevents extensor contracture formation while also supporting the lumbrical function is static manner. The splint can be used to reduce disability from Hansen's disease in patients who do not want surgical correction.

The splint is also used following reconstruction of motor for claw hand from ulnar nerve palsy.

250. Write short notes on Volkmann splint.

Ans: *Volkmann splint* is also called Volkmann turnbuckle splint. This splint is a dynamic splint that permits application of incremental low-load force to the wrist joint to gradually reduce contracture while hand is aligned in a functional position. The typical application of the splint finds its use in treating contractures of uniplanar joints such as wrist, elbow (modification), and ankle (modification). The classical example and possibly the first use of splint was correction of Volkmann ischemic contractures so the splint got its name. The splint has following parts:

- *Hand plate/shell:* This holds the hand in functional position and is provided with soft-to-firm padding to prevent development of pressure sores. There may be additionally a support for thumb and stretching the 1st web space. The dorsal straps at the wrist provide primary counter to correction of contracture. These counters are always placed at the convex side of deformity usually at the apex. However, they should be adequately packed to prevent pressure sores.
- *Forearm plate/shell:* This holds the forearm and provides secondary counter for movement of the hand plate/shell. It is also adequately packed. The shell has to be customized to fit the different forearm girths remaining in the patients after established contractures.
- *Screw-rod mechanism:* This is the turnbuckle mechanism that can be lengthened slowly to correct the contracture. The screw-rod mechanism is placed on the volar aspect and usually they are always placed at the concavity of deformity. It uses a screw mechanism where the screw is rotated at frequent fixed intervals to provide the lengthening effect indirectly producing derotation torque at the centered joint. For this reason, the hand and forearm plate should be connected with a stable hinge centered at the targeted joint. This mechanism provides low-load stretch to the joint to gradually correct contracture.

Alternatives:
- Regular application of corrective casts—cumbersome method to correct contracture of wrist
- Wedge correction of applied casts to the upper limb—cumbersome
- Continuous passive motion—needs visit to facility

Advantages:
- Home-based correction of contractures
- Minimal need of supervision
- Can be adjusted based on individual needs
- Does not need heavy or big parts that cannot be assembled

251. Describe SOMI brace.

Ans: *SOMI (sterno-occipito-mandibular immobilizer):* It consists of a metal chest section, shoulder bands and upright bars that connect to the pads at the back of the head and under the chin. It is held in place by the shoulder straps that cross at the back and fasten to the chest chapter.
- Has no back plate, hence allows patients to lie down comfortably
- 3 uprights (2 occipital, 1 anterior)
- Most effective in controlling forward flexion C1-C4 especially at AA joint, also rotations.
- Not so effective in controlling lateral flexion and extension.

SOMI brace is commonly used in various traumatic and nontraumatic pathologies for immobilization of cervical spine like:
- Cervical spondylosis
- Acute cervical strain
- Postsurgical immobilization of cervical spine
- Transportation of patient with suspected cervical spine injury
- Polytrauma patient.

252. Describe halo-pelvic device.

Ans: The halo-pelvic device is a static traction apparatus (unless modified) used to correct or treat spinal deformities/injuries. The device has two components:
- *The "halo":* This consists of a metal ring that is usually secured to the outer table of skull bone using four (sometimes 6) screws
- *Pelvic portion:* This comprises of a hoop that is attached to the pelvic bone of the patient using threaded pins (4–6) inserted into the ilium bone. (For cervical spine nowadays instead of pelvis portion, a chest vest is devised that can provide countertraction well to the cervical ring—the "halo-chest/vest" traction device.)
- Four extension bars connecting the pelvic hoop to halo
- Force measuring system
- Backwinder.

History of development: The concept of halo-pelvic traction was developed by Dr William Green. The skull halo was developed by Perry and Nickel in the 1970s for prolonged cervical traction in place of the old-fashioned, two-screw skull tongs used in cervical fractures. Initially the halo device was provided by countertraction through femoral pins that complicated soon to pin-tract infection and also the patient had to be bedridden. Soon the concept was changed to pelvic traction to provide ambulatory care and also the pelvis width compares to skull width thus the ring diameter. Perry and Nickel proposed use of skull halo directly to pelvis but caused skin necrosis. After several failed attempts worldover Professor A Hodgson, Professor A Yau, and Dr J O'Brien developed the pelvic attachment of the halo-pelvic traction (HPT) device. The pelvic ring is secured to the two halves of the pelvis by two threaded pins that traverse the whole length of the two halves of the pelvis. Extension bars fitted to the halo and pelvic rings provide fixation and traction when the bars are gradually elongated. This was a successful device that could provide good traction for months. Modifications were proposed to measure the distraction force by including gauges attached to extension device that were either mechanical or electrically operated.

Indications: Following are common indications for the apparatus:
- Treatment of severe and rigid spinal deformities such as healed tuberculous kyphosis. The device allowed osteotomies of the rigid deformity to be staged and simultaneously allowed distraction forces to be gradually applied between stages of surgery without fear of instability or spinal cord compression.
- Correction of various types of severe scoliosis such as that due to neurofibromatosis and poliomyelitis. Spinal fusions are performed after preliminary correction of the deformities.
- Immobilization of unstable spine in tuberculosis, surgically inaccessible/untreatable trauma.
- Upper cervical spine trauma (not good for lower cervical spine injuries due to poor lateral bending control producing "snaking" phenomenon):
  - Occipital condyle fracture
  - Occipitocervical dissociation
  - Stable type II atlas fracture
  - Type II Hangman's fracture
  - Type II odontoid fracture
  - C1-C2 dissociation in pediatric patients
  - Subaxial cervical spine trauma in pediatric patients.

Contraindications:
- Cranial fractures
- Active infection at pin insertion sites
- Soft tissue loss at pin insertion sites
- Severe chest trauma
- Morbid obesity
- Elderly patients.

Application of device: Though the skull halo can be applied in local anesthesia, the pelvic device requires general anesthesia. The pelvic pins are applied in lateral position. Site of pin placement is on the iliac crest at the tubercle of the crest which is 5 cm posterior to ASIS and is the thickest part of the iliac crest. Posteriorly the pins exit through posterior superior iliac spine.

Perquisites:
- MRI scan is a must to identify any intraspinal pathology, diastematomyelia, intrathecal lipoma, etc. and any internal gibbus that compresses the spinal cord.
- *Respiratory function test:* To assess baseline pulmonary function
- CT scan in all trauma cases.

Complications:
- Pin site infection
- Palsy of 6th, 10th, 11th, and 12th cranial nerves with traction
- Supraorbital and supratrochlear nerve palsy due to faulty pin insertion
- Dural puncture
- Compression of spinal cord by internal kyphus in severely kyphoyic patients
- *Excessive stretching and distraction of cervical spine (due to higher mobility):* This may also produce medullary coning (indicated early by suddenly developed swinging temperatures and fluctuating rises in blood pressure).
- Osteonecrosis of odontoid
- *Snaking phenomenon:* In lower cervical spine injuries as the patient lies down the cervical spine undergoes focal kyphosis while the lordosis is maintained in radiographs taken in upright position.
- Pneumonia, ARDS and arrhythmia.

253. Discuss the principles of application of Milwaukee brace.
Ans: Please read Chapter no. 4C.

254. Write brief notes on orthosis in club foot.
Ans: Currently three major groups of braces are available:
1. Ankle foot orthosis
2. Wheaton brace or Wheaton's type brace
3. Foot abduction bar.

Ankle-foot orthosis: It is similar to historically used tin rectangular night shoe covering the ankle and foot fully with neutral position at ankle. There is correction of plantarflexion only while abduction is not provided by the brace so metatarsus adductus may not be corrected. This brace does not allow movements at the ankle joint so atrophy of calf muscles is often seen, so it is not preferred for congenital talipes equinovarus (CTEV) management that well. In cases of arthrogryposis or peroneal nerve palsy this brace may be used as an adjunct to the abduction orthosis.

Wheaton's type braces (knee-ankle-foot orthosis): They provide reasonable abduction to the foot and medial stretching force pushing the forefoot in abduction if applied properly. Velcro strap is tightened against the apex of deformity to provide direct force for correction of deformity. The brace comes in two forms one in plantigrade position (foot in 15° dorsiflexion) and the other with ankle in neutral position (0° plantar flexion). The brace being tied to the thigh may produce thigh muscle atrophy also along with the calf atrophy.

Adjustable length foot abduction brace: Ponseti advised abduction and dorsiflexion of the foot for proper maintenance of the correction. Both these are optimally met with the use of foot abduction brace (also called though wrongly Denis-Browne shoe/bar/splint or "wobbly shoes"). The brace comprises of two shoes connected by an abduction bar, the length of bar being guided by the distance between shoulders and changed with the growth of child. Feet are typically placed in 60–70° of external rotation or in case of unilateral deformity the normal foot is placed in 30–40° of external rotation.

The Denis Browne Split utilizes an L-shaped bracket to hold the foot in significant dorsiflexion and is connected to open-toe boots. For concerns of cost Steenbeek braces (developed in Uganda by Michiel Steenbeek and David Okello)

have been developed that can be made from locally available cheap material while following the recommendations of Dr Ponseti. Various modifications have been added to the standard brace for improving the comfort and pliability of use:
- Flexible connecting bar (Kessler brace)—this facilitates the dorsiflexion twist provided by child's kicking action.
- Horton's click brace—here the shoe can be easily changed by just attaching the shoe through a clicking mechanism. The shoe size changes fast in a growing infant and need frequent changes. This is facilitated by the brace.
- Dobb's dynamic clubfoot brace—to improve compliance this brace allows independent movement of the legs and thus allows movements at knee and hips.
- ALFA-Flex shoe produced in Europe has nontoxic biocompatible materials and has "intelligent' foam (having both viscous and elastic components) allowing close fit to the child's foot and equidistribution of pressure.

255. Describe orthotic management of insensate foot particularly in reference to leprosy.

Ans: The neuropathic foot in leprosy arises due to the involvement of both sensory and motor components. This makes the foot susceptible to trauma and infection along with later development of Charcot's foot. Despite wearing a footwear there could be inadvertent trauma to the foot due to abnormal pressure distribution causing pressure sores and ulcers. The role of orthotics, hence, lies in preventing traumatic events to the foot directly and providing good cushioned support to the foot so that pressure is distributed equally throughout. Four general types of footwear have been in vogue to achieve above goals:

Sandals: Sandals are prescribed to be worn immediately following the healing of plantar ulcers or postoperative wounds while the patient is waiting for shoes being fabricated or for the delivery of purchased shoes. Sandals can be either a simple "quickie" or a modified "clog". The "quickie" sandal consists of a soft, flat insole of expanded polyethylene foam backed with a 6 mm-thick microcellular rubber, which is attached directly to an outer sole of neoprene crepe rubber. The patient stands on the heated foam before it is attached to allow the foam to conform to the contour of the foot.

The "clog" sandal has a thick base consisting of a polyethylene insole fully molded in its entire extent, and is supported by a neoprene crepe sole with a mixture of wood flour and latex placed between the soles to maintain the molding of the insole.

The healing shoe: The "healing shoe" was developed as a compromise when the patient refuses absolute bed rest or will not tolerate a plaster cast. It is made over a recently made plaster model of the foot and ankle and the insole can be removed for adjustment or replacement.

The modified regular shoe: This comes with regular or extra depth. Alterations are made mainly of the insole and outer sole, for the purpose of relieving high pressure points by distributing weight-bearing forces evenly to the plantar surface of the foot while standing and during propulsion. The extra-depth shoe is designed so that the insole can be removed and a custom-made insole (of closed cell polyethylene foam material and microcellular rubber) can be substituted.

Custom fabricated shoes: The outer sole of footwear may be made of leather or resilient neoprene crepe sole. Two modifications are made to alleviate plantar pressure as the foot "rolls" or "rocks" forward during propulsion. One is placement of the metatarsal bar under the metatarsal shafts to receive some of the weight ordinarily transmitted to the metatarsal heads and another one is the "rocker sole" which is used when the foot is short.

Based on the type of deficit in patient shoe can be provided in a customized manner as follows:
- *Category I:* The foot is grossly normal but possesses loss of plantar sensation: soft insole within a proper fitting shoe, with the addition of a Spenco insole worn on a prophylactic basis.
- *Category II:* The grossly normal foot possesses loss of plantar sensation and plantar scarring, commonly affecting the ball of the foot: molded insole, which is preferably made of Plastazote. Should Plastazote alone be inadequate to relieve the plantar high-pressure points, the Plastazote insole is complemented by the addition of either Pelite or microcellular rubber (in extra-depth shoe).
- *Category III:* The foot is deformed with loss of plantar sensation and plantar scarring; however, the length and width of the foot is not affected appreciably: molded Plastazote insole alone or supplemented by a layer of microcellular rubber. For rigid claw toes provide extra-depth shoe with wide box.
- *Category IV:* The pathologic short and/or narrowed foot is due to metatarsal phalangeal or lateral ray absorption or to amputation: custom fabricated shoe.

256. What are thermoplastic splints?

Ans: A thermoplastic (thermos—heat; plastic—moldable) splint is a device made of specific materials that allow easy molding by application of temperature to fit the body part. These splints are commonly used to immobilize, protect, and support injuries such as fractures, sprains, and strains. The splints have largely replaced POP materials being easier to use and apply. Thermoplastic splints are lighter, easily molded to fit the body of the individual patient, and can be removed for cleaning and patient bathing. There are the two basic types of thermoplastic splints:

1. *Low temperature thermoplastic splints:* These can be softened in hot water and placed directly on the skin for rapid molding and are most appropriate for temporary splintage of limbs. These splints have found good usage in accident and emergency for quick immobilization of upper limb fractures or injuries.
2. *High temperature thermoplastic splints:* These are made from a cast and require higher temperatures and a longer curing time to harden. Splints made from them are commonly prefabricated and cannot be modified at point usage but they provide good, light-weight support to injured limb. Such splints are commonly advised for immobilization of lower limb or back injuries that would require a longer healing period.

In addition to above:
- These splints can also be used to stabilize limb prior to surgery as well as in rehabilitation for corrective surgeries, flaps or soft tissue transfers, and repair/reconstruction of tendon injuries.
- Thermoplastic splinting is done to maintain range of movement and prevent joint stiffness commonly used in individuals who cannot move the limb independently like in neurological condition/injury.

2.15 COMPARTMENT SYNDROME (Q257–267)

257. Describe compartment syndrome.

Ans: Compartment syndrome is the emergency condition in which the pressure within an osteofascial compartment rises to a level that exceeds the intramuscular arteriolar pressure, resulting in decreased blood flow to capillaries, reduced oxygen diffusion to the tissues and ultimately cell death. Compartment syndromes may be acute or chronic (exertional), based on cause and reversibility.

Etiology: Fractures are the most common cause followed by blunt trauma to soft tissues. The following can cause compartment syndrome due either to fluid accumulation and tissue expansion within the confines of a closed, noncompliant, impermeable osteofascial compartment or from decrease in the space available for tissues **(Table 2.15.1)**.

TABLE 2.15.1: Etiology of compartment syndrome.

Increased compartment contents	*Decreased compartment volume*
- Bleeding (fractures, hemangioma, etc.) - Major vascular injury - Coagulation defect - Anticoagulant therapy - Reperfusion after ischemia - Trauma - Contusion - Seizures - Burns - Fluid extravasation - Venous obstruction - Reimplantation - High-pressure injections - Intraosseous fluid transfusion in children - Reaming in intramedullary nailing - Use of fluid pumps in arthroscopy	- Tight casts, dressings, or air splints - Military antishock garments - Tourniquet - Lying on limb (e.g., well leg in lithotomy position) - Entrapment under collapsed weights - Tight closure of facial defects - Excessive traction to fractured limbs - Limb lengthening - Thermal injuries, burn eschar - Intramedullary nailing for long neglected fractures or deformity correction stretching individual muscles

Pathogenesis: Excessive pressure beyond a critical limit prevents perfusion of tissues from capillaries (Starling's law) and results in tissue anoxia and death. With cellular anoxia and death, there is increased intracellular calcium concentration drawing in water into the cells and tissue swells. The cellular toxicity raises capillary permeability further and "leaking capillaries" adds to further increase in the compartment pressure setting vicious "edema-ischemia" cycle. Matsen's unified concept suggests that compartment syndrome, Volkmann's ischemic contracture and crush syndrome are a continuum of sequel to raised intracompartmental pressure and a temporal function of the same (develop over time).

Chronic compartment syndrome (CCS) occurs most probably due to increased muscle mass in a closed fascial space occurring during exercise or exertion. Muscle volume can increase up to 20% of its resting size during exercise. Increased muscle volume causes an increase in the internal pressure within the fascial compartment.

Diagnosis: Diagnosing the compartment syndrome has been traditionally only on clinical suspicion, however, a lot of interest and debate has always occurred regarding some quantitative measure to diagnose compartment syndrome. Physical signs of acute compartment syndrome include tightness of the involved compartment, pain with passive motion of the muscles passing through the compartment, and weakness of the muscles. Hypoesthesia or paresthesia should be evaluated by testing with pinprick, light touch, and 2-point discrimination. The most important sign is pain out of proportion to that expected with the injury. Objectively a pressure of 30 mm Hg (critical pressure) was reported to be maximum pressure above which muscle necrosis would ensue. Currently, however, absolute intracompartmental pressure is thought to convey no meaning and a pressure gradient is considered better reference.

One or more of the following criteria are diagnostic of CCS:
- Rest pressure more than or equal to 15 mm Hg.
- 1-minute and 5-minute postexercise pressure more than 30 mm Hg and more than 20 mm Hg, respectively. An elevated pressure after 15 minutes is a more reliable cutoff. Often in patients with CCS, the pressure is more than 25 mm Hg for 30 minutes after exercise.
- There is also a prolonged period for return to pre-exercise levels.
- One should keep the ankle and knee joint in uniform position commonly the resting positions.

Management: Immediately provide oxygen by mask, correct any hypotension, and remove the circumferential bandages. Splitting of cast reduces pressure by 30% that increases to 65% if the cast is split and spread. Complete splitting and padding the cast adds 10% to relieve pressure, and complete removal adds another 15%. There could be total of 85–90% reduction if cast is fully removed. Limb should not be elevated as this reduces the mean pressure but not the compartment pressure. Maintain hydration to decrease chances of renal damage from "crush syndrome".

Patients suspected of having acute compartment syndrome by an expert should have emergent fasciotomy. Compartment syndrome associated with a fracture of the lower extremity should be treated at the time of fracture stabilization. Nonreamed intramedullary nailing is preferred for fracture stabilization because animal studies have shown an increased propensity for the development of compartment syndrome when reamed tibial nailing is used.

Nonoperative treatment (older concept) of this emergency is debatable and is reserved only for patients presenting too late or missed (>24–48 hours) such that the compartment syndrome has fully set in and a fasciotomy will not provide any improvement to the present condition of patient.

(For details on measuring compartment pressures and surgical details kindly refer to Chapter 16 of the book Essential Orthopedics: Principles and Practice, 2nd edition.)

258. Describe the pathophysiology of acute compartment syndrome.

Ans: Why a compartment syndrome develops is still unclear and researchers have not been able to pin-point the microvascular changes/physiology behind compartment syndrome. There are a few explanations, though, for development of acute compartment syndrome:
- *The venous hypertension theory*: The impermeable fascia prevents fluid from leaking out elevating intracompartmental pressure. Elevated pressures beyond a critical limit prevent perfusion of tissues from capillaries (Starling's law) and results in tissue anoxia and death. This is clarified by Rowland and supported by Matsen equating the local blood flow (LBF) and the arteriovenous pressure gradient expressed by following equation:

$$LBF = (Pa - Pv)/R$$

Where, (Pa − Pv) is the arteriovenous pressure gradient and "R" is the vascular resistance. Raised interstitial pressure proportionately increases venous pressure (Pv) producing local venous hypertension. The gradient (Pa − Pv), thus, reduces and finally LBF = 0, so no capillary perfusion occurs. So, it is clear that perfusion within a compartment is only present when the diastolic blood pressure exceeds the intracompartmental pressure. During vasoconstriction or hypotension, perfusion ceases at even lower pressures.
- The other theory suggests *occurrence of arterial spasm* after increased compartment pressure.
- Matsen's unified concept suggests that compartment syndrome, Volkmann's ischemic contracture and crush syndrome are a continuum of sequel to raised intracompartmental pressure and a temporal function of the same (develop over time).

With cellular anoxia and death, there is increased intracellular calcium concentration drawing in water into the cells and tissue swells. The cellular toxicity raises capillary permeability further and "leaking capillaries" adds to further increase in the compartment pressure setting vicious "edema-ischemia" cycle.

259. Management of compartment syndrome in proximal tibia fractures briefly.

Ans: Kindly see the answer above.

260. What are the clinical features of compartment syndrome of leg? What is Whiteside's technique?

Ans: The typical symptoms and signs in a patient are classically briefed into six "p"; four of which (pain, paresthesia, paresis, pain with stretch) were described by Griffiths in 1948; pallor and pulselessness were added later.

1. *Pain:* It is the most sensitive and earliest sign, especially if the pain is out of proportion for the injury (symptom) and increases with passive stretch of muscles (sign). Bony injury may cause tremendous pain in a sensitive patient (false positive), or the pain may be absent if compartment syndrome has already set in injuring the nerves or patient has received efficient analgesia/anesthesia (postoperative). Patient's underepidural anesthesia is four times more likely to develop compartment syndrome as it blocks the sympathetic system increasing local blood flow (LBF). Also, patients under local anesthesia and receiving narcotics are at a higher risk. Other difficult patients to evaluate for pain are those with head injuries, those under influence of ethanol or drugs, those intubated or sedated or any other circumstance that alters patient's ability to accurately sense and communicate pain levels. In pediatric patients, pain is particularly difficult to evaluate as are other signs mentioned below; so instead clinical signs such as anxiety, agitation, and analgesic requirement take prominence.
2. *Paresthesia:* Nerve conduction is altered within few minutes of ischemia. Paresthesia develops early within 2 hours due to early involvement of sensory nerves. Decreased light touch is suggested as the best and first indicator for compartment syndrome as it comes early. It may be better than two-point discrimination as the former represents change in ability of nerves to detect pressure while latter tells the density of nerves in the region that may remain unaltered.
3. *Pulselessness:* Not a reliable sign of compartment syndrome.
4. *Pallor:* Reflects loss of arterial flow and is rarely present ever.
5. *Paralysis* is difficult to interpret and may be caused by ischemia, guarding, pain or a combination of the above. True paralysis develops late (being a function of thicker motor nerves), and till then lot of damage has already occurred.
6. *Pressure:* Just feeling for tight compartments is not enough though they give good indication. Objective pressure recording is better though not an absolute requirement for considering fasciotomy, which is commonly judged clinically. The indication for pressure evaluation is presence of one or more signs or symptoms in a suspected patient with confounding factor (anesthesia, sedation, head injury), unreliable examination with firmness of limb, prolonged hypotension in a swollen extremity and spontaneous increase in pain after adequate analgesia.

Whiteside's technique: It is a method of pressure measurement known as Whiteside infusion technique. If commercial instruments are not available, then Whiteside's technique can be used and every orthopedic surgeon should have an idea of it. A simple arterial line setup (16–18-gauge needle) and a mercury manometer are set up to record intracompartmental pressures, but it is important to recognize that this method is considered the least accurate. The values obtained are consistently higher, by an average of 5–19 mm Hg, than those obtained with the other methods.

261. Write a note on reperfusion injury.

Ans: This is a lately recognized complication. Initially only ischemia was considered to be the cause of tissue damage. Ischemic injury is understood well in the form of deprivation of cellular energy to maintain ionic gradients and homeostasis, enzymatic failure and death. Reperfusion injury occurs by the interaction of free radicals (hydroxyl radical), endothelial factors, and neutrophils. These damage proteins, DNA, and lipids. Lipid peroxidation disrupts cell membranes especially the endothelial system, which are composed of polyunsaturated fatty acids and phospholipids. The endothelial disruption induces neutrophil chemotaxis, adherence, and migration inducing systemic injury and local tissue destruction.

- Accumulation of lactic acid, sodium (associated with water ingress into cell), and calcium (causes mitochondrial disruption) are basic alterations of anaerobic metabolism. The potassium leaks out causing hyperkalemia.
- Reperfusion removes the accumulated toxic components and replenishes the energy supply to cells. But these produce simultaneously collateral damage by causing systemic toxicity and sensitive organs show depressed function under influence, reoxygenation causes formation of reactive oxygen species.
- Formation of superoxide radical—this is converted into hydrogen peroxide by superoxide dismutases (SOD) which in turn is destroyed by catalase into water as follows:

  $2O_2 + 2H^+ \rightarrow H_2O_2 + O_2$ [SOD]

  $2H_2O_2 \rightarrow 2H_2O + O_2$ [catalase]

  The enzymes are dysfunctional often due to ischemia, so instead the superoxide ions form hydroxyl radicals that are highly reactive as follows:

  $O_2 + H_2O_2 \rightarrow 2OH. + O_2$ (Haber-Weiss reaction—catalyzed by ferrous ions and xanthine oxidase). These radicals are not scavenged and cause extensive damage at the site of formation itself. These free radicals produce the thiobarbituric acid reactive substances and diene conjugates causing extensive myocyte damage.
- Neutrophils release proteolytic enzymes and peroxidases into the circulation
- Pharmacological modification of reperfusion injury
- Allopurinol–xanthine oxidase inhibitor may modify the generation of peroxide radical though relevant clinical effect has not been demonstrated
- Deferoxamine chelates iron and may limit the production of toxic hydroxyl free radicals
- Mannitol has been used to systemically scavenge hydroxyl free radicals
- Dantrolene controls the release of calcium, limiting the mitochondrial and muscular damage
- High dose ascorbic acid and corticosteroids have also not shown much of clinical effect
- Hypothermia has shown to benefit from reperfusion injury possibly by reducing the metabolic demand and oxygen requirement itself. This also actually prolongs the ischemia time.

262. Describe crush syndrome.

Ans: Crush syndrome is a sequelae of muscle necrosis (creatine phosphokinase >20,000 IU) and manifests as nonoliguric renal failure, myoglobinuria, and later oliguria, shock, acidosis, hyperkalemia and cardiac arrhythmias and may need dialysis. Crush syndrome is a part of reperfusion injury that results from a limb compressed for extended periods producing prolonged ischemia, e.g., following entrapment in a vehicle or rubble. The syndrome has also been observed after prolonged use of a pneumatic antishock garment. The crushed limb is underperfused resulting in anaerobic metabolism and myonecrosis follows, leading to the release of toxic metabolites when the limb is freed and so generating a *reperfusion injury*. Reactive oxygen metabolites create further tissue injury. Membrane damage and capillary fluid reabsorption failure result in swelling that may lead to a compartment syndrome, thus creating more tissue damage from escalating ischemia. Tissue necrosis also causes systemic problems such as renal failure from free myoglobin, which is precipitated in the renal glomeruli. Myonecrosis may cause a metabolic acidosis with hyperkalemia and hypocalcemia.

Clinical features and treatment: The compromised limb is pulseless and becomes red, swollen, and blistered; sensation and muscle power may be lost. Prevention of complications is best achieved by adequate hydration and maintaining good urine output to flush myoglobin. Alkalization of the urine with sodium bicarbonate also prevents myoglobin precipitating in the renal tubules. If oliguria or renal failure occurs, then dialysis is needed. If a compartment syndrome develops, and is confirmed by pressure measurements, then emergent fasciotomy is indicated. Excision of dead muscle must be radical to avoid sepsis.

263. Explain the etiopathogenesis of crush syndrome. Describe its clinical features and management.

Ans: *Definition:* Systemic manifestation of muscle necrosis caused by prolonged crushing of skeletal muscle, leading to the release of toxic intracellular contents (e.g., myoglobin, potassium, and phosphate) into circulation.

Etiopathogenesis

1. *Mechanism of Injury:*
- *Direct trauma:* Prolonged compression (e.g., earthquakes, building collapses, prolonged immobilization, coma).
- *Ischemia-reperfusion injury:*
  - Compression → muscle ischemia → cell death.
  - Reperfusion upon relief of pressure → influx of calcium, free radicals, and inflammatory mediators → further muscle necrosis.

2. *Pathophysiological Effects:*

(A) *Myoglobin release:*
- Rhabdomyolysis → myoglobin leaks into blood → filtered by kidneys → myoglobinuria (red-brown urine).
- Renal toxicity:
  - Myoglobin precipitates in acidic urine → tubular obstruction.
  - Ferrihemate (from myoglobin) causes oxidative damage → acute tubular necrosis (ATN).

(B) *Electrolyte abnormalities:*
- Hyperkalemia (K^+ release from damaged cells) → life-threatening arrhythmias.
- Hyperphosphatemia → binds calcium → hypocalcemia (can cause tetany, QT prolongation).
- Metabolic acidosis (lactic acid from muscle ischemia).

(C) *Hypovolemia and shock:*
- Third-spacing of fluid into damaged muscles → hypotension, reduced renal perfusion → acute kidney injury (AKI).

(D) *Disseminated intravascular coagulation (DIC):*
- Thromboplastin release from muscle → activates coagulation cascade → microthrombi, bleeding.

Clinical Features

1. *Local manifestations:*
   - Swollen, tense, and painful muscles (compartment syndrome may develop)
   - Skin bruising, blistering, or necrosis over affected area
2. *Systemic manifestations:*
   - Dark (cola-colored) urine (myoglobinuria)
   - Oliguria/anuria (AKI)
   - Cardiac: Arrhythmias (from hyperkalemia) and hypotension.
   - Neurological: Confusion and seizures (due to hypocalcemia, uremia)
   - DIC: Bleeding, petechiae, and ecchymoses
3. *Laboratory findings:*
   - ↑ Creatine kinase (CK) (>5,000 U/L, often >100,000 U/L)
   - ↑ Serum myoglobin (earliest marker)
   - ↑ Potassium, phosphate, uric acid
   - ↓ Calcium (early; late hypercalcemia may occur during recovery)
   - ↑ BUN/Cr, metabolic acidosis
   - *Urinalysis*: Dipstick (+) for blood (but no RBCs on microscopy → myoglobinuria)

Management

1. *Prehospital and early management:*
   - Remove compression ASAP (but beware of reperfusion injury).
   - IV fluids (0.9% saline or LR) even before extrication to prevent AKI.
   - Avoid tourniquets unless bleeding is life-threatening (worsens ischemia).

2. *Aggressive fluid resuscitation:*
   - *Goal*: Urine output ≥300 mL/hour (adults)
   - Isotonic saline (0.9% NaCl): 1–2 L bolus, then 500–1,000 mL/hour
   - *Alkalinization of urine (controversial):*
     - Sodium bicarbonate (if pH < 6.5) to prevent myoglobin precipitation.
     - Mannitol (osmotic diuretic) may be used but risks worsening AKI if oliguric.
3. *Electrolyte management:*
   - Hyperkalemia:
     - Calcium gluconate (10%) (stabilizes myocardium)
     - Insulin + glucose, salbutamol, sodium bicarbonate
     - Kayexalate or dialysis if severe
   - *Hypocalcemia:* Avoid routine calcium unless symptomatic (risk of metastatic calcification).
4. *Renal protection and dialysis:*
   - Indications for dialysis:
     - Refractory hyperkalemia, severe acidosis, volume overload, and uremia
     - Early dialysis improves survival.
5. *Compartment syndrome management:*
   - Fasciotomy if compartment pressures >30–40 mm Hg.
6. *Monitoring:*
   - CK levels (trend until declining)
   - ECG (for hyperkalemia: peaked T waves, QRS widening, sine wave)
   - Urine output (catheterize if oliguric)

264. Crush syndrome: Pathophysiology and complications.

Ans: *Definition:* Crush syndrome (also called traumatic rhabdomyolysis) is a life-threatening systemic complication caused by prolonged muscle compression.

Pathophysiology
1. *Muscle compression and ischemia:*
   - Mechanical pressure (≥1 hour) → muscle cell membrane damage.
   - I*schemia-reperfusion injury* occurs when circulation is restored, generating *oxygen-free radicals* that worsen tissue damage.
2. *Rhabdomyolysis and Toxic Release*
   - Necrotic muscle cells release:
     - *Myoglobin* → Clogs kidney tubules → *acute kidney injury (AKI).*
     - *Potassium (K^+)* → *Hyperkalemia* → Cardiac arrhythmias (peaked T waves, V-fib).
     - *Creatine kinase (CK)* → Levels >5,000 U/L confirm diagnosis.
     - *Phosphate (PO_4^{3-})* → Binds calcium → *Hypocalcemia* (muscle spasms, QT prolongation).
     - *Uric acid* → Contributes to renal injury.
3. *Systemic effects:*
   - *Hyperkalemia* → Cardiac arrest (main cause of early death)
   - *Hypocalcemia* → Tetany, seizures, hypotension
   - *Metabolic acidosis* (due to lactic acid and impaired renal function)
   - *Disseminated intravascular coagulation (DIC)* (from thromboplastin release)
4. *Acute kidney injury (AKI):*
   - *Mechanisms*:
     - *Myoglobinuria* → Tubular obstruction and direct toxicity
     - *Renal vasoconstriction* (from hypovolemia and acidosis)
     - Intrarenal calcium-phosphate deposition

Complications:
1. *Renal*:
   - Acute tubular necrosis (ATN) → Oliguria/anuria
   - Chronic kidney disease (CKD) if recovery is incomplete.
2. *Cardiac*:
   - Hyperkalemia-induced arrhythmias (e.g., ventricular fibrillation)
   - Hypocalcemia → Prolonged QT interval and cardiac depression.
3. *Metabolic*:
   - Severe acidosis (pH < 7.2) → Coma and respiratory failure
   - Compartment syndrome (swollen muscles → ischemia → necrosis)
4. *Hematologic*:
   - DIC → Bleeding/clotting disorders
5. *Infectious*
   - Necrotic tissue infection → Sepsis.

265. Describe chronic compartment syndrome.

Ans: The importance of an accurate history cannot be overemphasized in the evaluation of patients with lower extremity pain. A typical patient with chronic exertional compartment syndrome (CECS) is a competitive runner, 20–30 years old, who describes exercise-induced pain and a feeling of tightness that begins after 20–30 minutes of running. The pain usually resolves within 15–30 minutes of cessation of exercise. Paresthesias of the nerves running through the involved compartment often are reported. Physical examination may reveal tenderness over the musculature of the involved compartment.

Differential diagnosis of anterior compartment syndrome includes periostitis (medial tibial syndrome) and entrapment of the superficial peroneal nerve. Deep posterior compartment syndrome must be differentiated from periostitis, tendinitis of the posterior tibial tendon, stress fracture of the tibia, and intermittent claudication caused by anomalous insertion of the medial head of the gastrocnemius-soleus, causing compression of the popliteal artery.

If physical examination is not diagnostic, other studies can be instituted. Periostitis is easily seen on bone scan, with diffuse uptake often covering one-third of the bone. Stress fractures show a more localized, intense uptake of the radioactive isotope, although 90% of stress fractures can be diagnosed with plain radiographs. Entrapment of the peroneal nerve can be determined by provocative tests, as described by Styf, in which pressure over the point at which the superficial peroneal nerve emerges from the deep fascia produces pain during active, resisted dorsiflexion and eversion of the ankle. Tinel sign also may be positive in the same area. Nerve conduction studies can be helpful. Rorabeck et al. reported promising results with MRI as a noninvasive diagnostic tool.

Several authors have attempted to establish objective guidelines for the diagnosis of CECS by compartment pressure measurements, and various pressures have been reported as the upper limits of normal, but the pressures reported by Pedowitz et al. seem to be good baseline measurements on which to base the diagnosis of CCS. They considered one or more of the following as diagnostic: (1) preexercise, resting pressure of 15 mm Hg or more; (2) pressure of 30 mm Hg or more 1 minute after exercise; and (3) pressure of 20 mm Hg or more 5 minutes after exercise.

Treatment of CCS usually is operative. Conservative therapy with anti-inflammatory medication can be successful if the patient is willing to reduce significantly or stop completely athletic activities. Most patients prefer to continue their present activity level, however, and require surgical release of the involved compartment.

Fronek et al. described a single-incision technique for release of the anterior and lateral compartments, but the two-incision technique described by Rorabeck can be used for all compartments of the leg. Mouhsine et al. described the use of a "minimal" two-incision technique for release of anterior and lateral compartments. The authors emphasized that fasciotomy should be done without the use of a tourniquet to allow control of hemostasis and prevent postoperative hematoma formation.

Some authors have recommended combining partial fasciectomy with fasciotomy, particularly in patients in whom fasciotomy alone is unsuccessful. In this technique, the involved compartment is released in the usual fashion, and then a window of fascia is removed to ensure that scar tissue cannot form between the split fascial ends.

266. Describe exertional compartment syndrome.
Ans: Kindly see answer above.

267. What are different compartments of leg?
Ans: The compartments of leg are divided into anterior, lateral, and posterior osseofascial compartments. The posterior is further divided into superficial and deep components. The compartments usually have distinct neurovascular anatomy making them isolated units for pathology development in initial stages such as tumor progression, movement, and accumulation of pus, progression of ischemia, etc.

Muscles of anterior compartment: Tibialis anterior, extensor hallucis longus, extensor digitorum longus, and peroneus tertius. This compartment additionally has neurovascular structures—deep peroneal nerve and anterior tibial vessels.

Muscles of *lateral* compartment—peroneus brevis and longus. This has superficial peroneal nerve and fibular vessels (absent in many).

Muscles of posterior compartment:
- *Superficial:* Gastrocnemius, soleus, and plantaris. Sural nerve lies lateral to Achilles tendon.
- *Deep:* Popliteus, flexor hallucis longus, flexor digitorum longus, tibialis posterior. Posterior tibial nerve and vessels along with peroneal vessels are prominent in this compartment.

(For further details, kindly refer to Chapter 16 of the book Essential Orthopedics: Principles and Practice).

2.16 MODALITIES IN PHYSIOTHERAPY AND PAIN MANAGEMENT (Q268–275)

268. What are various types of exercises? Discus the benefits and indications of isometric exercises.
Ans: Exercises are an important component of orthopedic rehabilitation. It is to ensure enough strength in muscles to produce effective movement at joint with stability. Muscle strength is the maximum voluntary force produced in a single muscular effort. In general, three broad categories of muscle strength rehabilitation are deployed to improve muscular effort, which include isometric, isotonic, isokinetic exercises. These can be applied in closed or open chain mode for specific needs.
- *Isometric (same length) training:* Here the muscle length and joint angle does not change. Contraction of muscle does not produce any shortening and the tension never exceeds opposing force. The strength training is done in static position unassisted. The muscles are made to contract repetitively for endurance.
    - Isometric exercises are indicated where there is muscle mass loss due to inhibition either because of pain from disease or due to immobilization. Such conditions include degenerative arthritic condition of joints, spondylosis, and rehabilitation post-immobilization of surgery. The exercises can also be applied to patients of trauma where there is often muscle inhibition due to pain. The exercises also improve stability around the joint.
    - The benefit of this training is that it is easy, improves muscle strength and muscle mass, and does not need any special equipment completing the session in a small amount of time. Common exercises that fall into this group include quadriceps and hamstring strengthening, yoga exercises, hand presses, etc.
- *Isotonic (same tension) training:* Here the tension generated in the muscle remains constant though the length changes and hence consequently the angle of joint also alters. The exercises are aimed at improving joint mobility while so also strengthening muscles by continuous and sustained movement of arms and legs. Devices are commonly deployed to assist the patient in performing the exercises. Some of these devices include—weight lifting machines, medicine balls, free weights, dumb bells, etc. apart from orthopedic benefits these exercises are also beneficial to heart endurance by increasing the heart rate and improving circulation to other parts of body.
- *Isokinetic (same motion) exercises:* In this training the muscles contracts at constant rate throughout the motion against variable resistance. These have been generally considered good for postoperative muscle rehabilitation, but recently they have been shown to perform inferior to isotonic exercises. Also, these are considered best to prevent injuries by optimizing response and customization of activities to body's momentum. Postinjury the exercises help the enduring muscle to hypertrophy and adjust to the developing need of the joint during recovery. Usually assistive devices are deployed to perform the isotonic exercises that include—elastic bands, stationary bike, exertubes, ankle/wrist circles, etc.

Comparison of various forms of exercises: Isometric training is not as good as isotonic training in increasing functional performance. Because isometric training is performed at a particular angle so it improves muscle performance only at the joint angle at which the training takes place but person may experience decrease in speed and functional performance at all other positions of joint in contrast with the dynamic movements performed in dynamic training which is more functional.

Isokinetic training is also not as effective as isotonic training in improving functional performance, because although having dynamic nature, isokinetic movements are always performed with same speed while the velocity of limb movement during many daily living and sport-related activities far exceeds the maximum velocity settings available on isokinetic equipment. Also most functional tasks occur at multiple velocities, not at a constant velocity, depending on the conditions of the task. Isokinetic training usually isolates a single muscle or opposite muscle groups, involves movement of a single joint, is uniplanar, and does not involve weight-bearing.

Isokinetic testing is the best way of strength testing and it can improve the strength maximally, so it is the best way of training as well. Isotonic strength training is the best way of increasing functional performance that is needed in rehabilitation.

269. Describe the following:
  A. Isokinetic exercises.
  B. Steenbeek brace.

Ans: A. Kindly see answer above.
B. Kindly see Answer to Question 254.

270. What is isotonic contraction?
Ans: Kindly see answer above.

271. Describe interferential therapy.
Ans: Interferential therapy (IFT) involves use of low frequency (<250 pps) electrical stimulation of nerves. Delivering current at depth produces strong discomfort to the overlying tissues like skin whose impedance is inversely proportional to frequency of current (so low frequency means high impedance). This causes increasing discomfort at attempts are made to deliver lower frequency currents to deeper tissue across the skin barrier. Thus, only higher frequency currents can be used to easily permeate the skin barriers. Conventionally currents of approximately 4,000 Hz are used (called moderate frequency as they fall between 1 kHz-100 kHz bandwidth). These, however, preclude the purpose of delivering low frequency current to the tissues. Thus, interferential mode is used where another lower frequency current is simultaneously applied in opposing path that cancels out the first current resulting in a beat frequency. So, for example, 4,000 Hz and 3,850 Hz current are applied in different path; a beat frequency of 150 Hz would result. This current stimulates the deeper structures.

There is another problem, however, the nerves quickly adapt to the passing current frequency by phenomenon of neural adaptation so to produce a sustained stimulation frequency sweep has to be applied that changes the applied frequency over time (usually 1–6 seconds). The sweep patterns are applied in various forms like triangular, rectangular, trapezoidal sweep to achieve this goal of producing sustained neural stimulation.

Method of application: The IFT is usually applied either by one or two (bipolar) electrical pad electrodes for a period of 15 minutes to produce the desirable effects. The therapy is usually instituted daily for 10–15 sittings or more depending on the disorder.

Indications: The IFT basically acts by stimulation of peripheral nerves though some also say that muscle stimulation also occurs without demonstrable twitch. Currently, the IFT is generally prescribed ancillary modality for:
- *Pain relief:* Usually for chronic painful conditions. The effect is possibly due to endogenous production of opioids like endorphins and enkephalins at spinal level.
- Muscle stimulation and counter relief by reduction in the spasm of muscles
- Increased local blood flow
- Improved healing of tissues as in joint stiffness, better healing may restore pliability of tissues
- Reduction of edema

- *Other indications:*
  - Stress and urge incontinence
  - Spasticity following cerebrovascular accident.

Contraindications:
- Pregnancy
- Active skin infection
- Deep infection
- Patients with pacemakers
- Underlying metallic implant in the vicinity
- Infants and children below 12 years of age
- Some patients on treatment with opioids may experience excessive sedation, loss of alertness, nausea, etc. due to potentiation of the drug effect from endogenous endorphin production.

272. Explain transcutaneous nerve stimulation.

Ans: Transcutaneous electric nerve stimulation (TENS) is a modality used to reduce pain and possibly spasm of the muscles in a noninvasive way utilizing the pain gateway theory of pain perception. In this technique a low-voltage electric current is passed through skin surface that overwhelms the pain receptors and blocks pain perception. The electrodes are applied to intact skin surface that may be delivered through epidermal needles or better by adhesive electrodes secured by Velcro straps. The amplitude, frequency, pattern, and duration of the pulsed electrical current are varied depending on pain of origin and individual patient need for nociceptive, neuropathic, and musculoskeletal pain. Conventional TENS (low intensity, high frequency) alleviates pain through selective activation of non-noxious, low threshold, large diameter Aβ fibers which in turn inhibit ongoing central nociceptive cell activity and reduce central sensitization in the spinal cord (spinal mechanism resulting in segmental effects). Acupuncture-like TENS (high intensity, low frequency) alleviates pain through selective activation of small diameter, (skin and muscles) high threshold Aδ peripheral afferents which in turn activates descending pain inhibitory pathways arising in the midbrain periaqueductal grey and the rostral ventromedial medulla (supraspinal mechanism resulting in segmental and extrasegmental effects). Intense-TENS (high intensity, high frequency) alleviates pain by stimulating high threshold small diameter cutaneous afferents leading to inhibition of central nociceptive transmission via spinal and supraspinal mechanisms.

The most common conditions that TENS therapy is used to treat are:
- Osteoporosis-related joint, bone, or muscle problems
- Fibromyalgia-related joint, bone, or muscle problems
- Tendinitis (muscle tissue inflammation)
- Bursitis (inflammation of the fluid-filled pads that cushion the joints)
- Neck pain
- Labor pain
- Cancer pain
- *Unlabeled indications:*
  - Dementia
  - Postoperative nausea, vomiting
  - Wound healing enhancement.

Common indicates areas and sites for TENS application include:
- *Painful area:* Cervical/Lumbar spasm. Trapezius, quadriceps muscle, etc.
- Painful neural pain like superficial radial nerve irritation, etc.
- Spinal nerve root-induced pain
- Specific dermatomes/myotomes affected by nerve irritation/stimulation.

Contraindications of TENS therapy:
- Patients with pacemakers
- Patients with neurological illness—epilepsy/poststroke
- Pregnancy
- Anterior neck and transorbital areas should be avoided.

273. What is paraffin wax? How is it useful in treatment of orthopedic conditions? What are its indications and contraindications of wax bath therapy?

Ans: For medical usage the hard paraffin wax has to be mixed with mineral oil so that its melting heat is reduced and does not burn tissues. The wax has better specific heat than water which is adjusted by mixing mineral oil for better conductive heat gains. Commonly used paraffin wax for therapeutic purpose is a mixture of 7 units of wax and 1 unit of mineral oil, this way the wax can be kept at a lower temperature (40–44° celsius instead of melting point of 55°) while maintaining its state.

Wax therapy involves bathing/immersing the limb or application of wax on the affected part to deliver heat for reducing pain through irritation of skin and there is also some soothing action on deeper tissues making them bit more pliable for mobilization and stretching purpose. The heat penetrates to a depth of 1 cm and rate of heat transfer is much slower (6 times slower) than water at same temperature. Also, specific heat of water is higher so water at same temperature transfers heat much faster causing burns.

Benefits of wax therapy:
- *Provides moist heat:* As the wax is applied for a prolonged period of time so the sweat accumulates between wax and skin that gets heated and provides heat. The water also does not evaporate due to insulator effect of paraffin wax.
- Pain relief by irritating the skin and closing the pain pathways.
- Soothing effect on muscles and subcutaneous tissues due to heating effect.
- Reflex vasodilatation of superficial capillaries and arterioles also produces heating of joint.
- Increased pliability of soft tissues for improving range of motion (ROM).

Contraindications:
- Sensory impairment
- *Dermatological disorders:* Eczema, dermatitis
- *Vascular disorders:* Varicose veins, deep vein thrombosis, etc.
- Infection and open wounds
- Neoplastic conditions and tuberculosis of the region
- Radiation therapy to area
- External/internal metal implants to the region applied recently.

274. Describe shortwave diathermy.

Ans: Shortwave diathermy (SWD) uses high-frequency (10–100 MHz) electromagnetic radio waves to convert energy into heat. The modality improves physiology by thermal and nonthermal processes, including:
- Vibration induction of tissue molecules—increase activity of cells, reduce edema, increase collagen deposition, improve hematoma resorption, possible improvement in nerve growth, and repair
- Increasing blood flow
- Relieving pain
- Improving the mobility of tissues as they heal.

The SWD produces heat within tissues through application of high-frequency electrical (condenser shortwave diathermy) or magnetic fields (induction shortwave diathermy). It may be applied in pulsed or continuous energy waves.
- Continuous SWD is applied to tissues either inductively (metal cable, covered in insulating rubber, which is wrapped around the part to be treated) or capacitively (plate or malleable electrodes placed next to the area to be treated), usually for 20–30 minutes. It increases skin temperature by 3–7°C, muscle temperature by 2–6°C.
- Pulsed shortwave diathermy is an intermittent oscillating high frequency (27.12 MHz) output. Heat generation is not the prominent effect here, instead tissue and cellular vibration is thought to result in physiological effects (see above).

It is commonly applied for 5–20 minutes depending on indications and dosage. Treatments can be done on daily or every other day. The common indications for SWD are:
- Chronic arthritis
- Back pains
- Neuralgia/neuropathy

- Sprains
- Strains
- Bursitis
- Tenosynovitis
- Chronic sinusitis/otitis/laryngitis
- Bronchial asthma/chronic obstructive pulmonary disease
- Chronic colitis
- Chronic pyelonephritis, etc.

The SWD should be avoided around metal devices such as bone pins, dental fillings, metal sutures as this can produce extreme heat causing burns in the tissue near the implant. Diathermy should also be avoided over open growth plates in children and over certain areas like eyes, brain, ears, spinal cord, heart, reproductive organs, and genitalia.

Contraindications for use of SWD:
- *Implanted devices like:*
  - Pacemaker
  - Prosthesis
  - Intrauterine device.
- Cancer
- Reduced skin sensation
- Peripheral vascular disease
- Tissue with restricted blood supply (ischemia)
- Infections
- Fractured bone
- Bleeding disorders
- Severe heart, liver or kidney conditions
- Low skin sensation
- Pregnancy.

275. **What are the various modalities of pain management? Discuss recent advances in pain management in orthopedics.**

Ans: The various modalities of pain management include:
- Multimodal analgesia
- Preemptive analgesia
- Preventive analgesia
- Locoregional analgesia for postoperative pain management:
  - Local wound infiltration
  - Epidural analgesia
  - Peripheral nerve blocks
- Patient-controlled analgesia (PCA)
  - Intravenous
  - Epidural
  - Nasal
  - Transcutaneous
  - Oral
  - Inhalational
- Patient-controlled regional analgesia

[For recent advances, one can write detailed discussion on PCA and nerve blocks (like femoral nerve block for knee arthroplasty) as given in Chapter 114 of the book, Essential Orthopedics: Principles and Practice, 2nd edition]

2.17 MISCELLANEOUS QUESTIONS (Q276–313)

A. Postoperative Infection (Q276)

276. Enumerate various diagnostic tests with their relative merit for postoperative infection. Outline the treatment of postoperative infection after internal fixation.

Ans: *The various diagnostic tests in a case suspected of having postoperative infection are:*

Hematological investigations: Total leukocyte counts, erythrocyte sedimentation rate (ESR), and C-reactive protein (CRP) are elevated and sensitive but nonspecific. CRP could be a better measure and a value of greater than 100 mg/L should prompt physician to aspirate the pathological site.

Bacteriological evaluation: The most definitive evidence for infection is isolation and culture of the pathogenic organism (rest all investigations tell probability). Needle aspiration from the lesion under aseptic precautions is the most recommended method.

Molecular markers: Typically, two types of molecular methods are used: (1) amplified and (2) nonamplified. Amplification methods include: polymerase chain reaction (PCR), reverse transcriptase polymerase chain reaction (RT-PCR), ligase chain reaction, and branched chain reaction. Monoclonal antibodies, direct detection of ribosomal ribonucleic acid (rRNA), and hybridization of rRNA are nonamplified techniques. The molecular methods target specific macromolecules unique to infecting pathogens (like *Mycobacterium tuberculosis*) and can provide rapid results with high accuracy.

Imaging: These are easy, sensitive, noninvasive, specific, and patient friendly screening test for infection. The following are used in variable sequence often beginning with the simplest first. Morphological imaging using X-rays, CT-scan, MRI, and USG provide anatomical localization. Functional imaging enables visualization of pathological process.

These mainly involve the use of radiopharmaceuticals that trace the physiological changes. Plain scintigraphy, single-photon emission computed tomography (SPECT), and positron emission tomography (PET) are the modalities used. No investigation is absolutely perfect or specific for diagnosis of infection and their use vary depending on evolution of disease and planning.

Treatment of postoperative infection is written in Answer to Question 85.

B. Cerebral Palsy (Q277–283)

277. Classify cerebral palsy. Describe crouched gait and its management in a 10-year-old child.

Ans: Cerebral palsy (CP) is most often classified as either spastic, dyskinetic or ataxic. Although spasticity is often the dominant disorder, many children with CP have mixed spasticity and dystonia. When more than 1 type of movement disorder is present in patients, experts recommend classifying patients by the predominant disorder.

- Hypertonia is defined as "abnormally increased resistance to externally imposed movement about a joint". Hypertonicity can be caused by spasticity, dystonia or rigidity (though rigidity is rare in children and not associated with CP).
- Spasticity is hypertonia in which resistance to passive movement increases with increasing velocity of movement (or exhibits a spastic catch), and "varies with direction of the movement, and/or rises rapidly above a threshold speed or joint angle". Spasticity is often a component of upper motor neuron syndrome. Spasticity is caused by a hyperactive stretch reflex mechanism.
- Dystonia is defined as "a movement disorder in which involuntary sustained or intermittent muscle contractions cause twisting and repetitive movements, abnormal postures or both". Dystonic hypertonia is present in cases where the resistance to passive movement does not change with changes in speed of passive movement or joint angle, may be associated with simultaneous agonist and antagonist contraction (equal resistance when the direction of passive movement is reversed). Dystonia is not associated with hyperreflexia and often disappears when the child is asleep. Dystonia is associated with disruption of the basal ganglia and therefore is not improved by selective dorsal rhizotomy. It is generally accepted that tendon lengthening and transfer procedures are contraindicated in cases of dystonia, because of the risk for recurrence of deformity or development of reverse deformities. Dystonic hypertonia is responsive to botulinum toxin as well as intrathecal baclofen, which generally weaken overactive muscles or muscle groups.

- Hyperkinetic movements are defined as "any unwanted excess movement" that is performed voluntarily or involuntarily by the patient, and represent what have traditionally been referred to as extrapyramidal symptoms. The hyperkinetic movements most commonly seen in CP include dystonia, chorea, athetosis, and tremors. Hyperkinetic dystonia is characterized by "abnormal postures that are superimposed upon or substitute for voluntary movements". Orthopedic surgery in cases of predominantly hyperkinetic movement disorders associated with CP is most often limited to bony procedures, as fixed contractures are rare because of the often nearly continuous movements of the extremities and joints. Such patients should be referred to a movement disorders specialist for management. Tendon lengthening in patients with hyperkinetic movement disorders is unreliable and may result in a reverse deformity. It should be remembered that split tendon transfers are more successful in patients with dystonia than are whole tendon transfers.
- Chorea is defined as "an ongoing random appearing sequence of one or more discrete involuntary movements or movement fragments". Choreiform movements are also random, can appear continuous and jerky, and can be difficult for patients to relax. Athetosis is defined as "a slow, continuous, involuntary writhing movement that prevents maintenance of a stable posture". It usually involves the hands or feet and perioral muscles. Athetosis is not common as an isolated movement disorder in CP and is most often found in combination with chorea.

Geographical classification:
- *Monoplegia:* It is very rare and usually occurs after meningitis. Most patients diagnosed with monoplegia actually have hemiplegia with one extremity only very mildly affected.
- *Hemiplegia:* These account for approximately 30% of patients with CP. In hemiplegia, one side of the body is involved. The upper extremity is usually more affected than the lower extremity. The patients with hemiplegia also have sensory changes in the affected extremities and may have leg-length discrepancy. Severe sensory changes are a predictor of poor functional outcome after reconstructive surgery.
- *Diplegia:* This is the most common anatomical type of CP representing half of all the cases. The patients have motor abnormalities in all four extremities where the lower extremities are more affected than the upper. This type is most common in premature infants; intelligence usually is normal. Most children with diplegia walk eventually by 4 years.
- *Quadriplegia:* Here all four extremities are equally involved and patients commonly have significant cognitive deficiencies. Head and neck control is usually present, which helps with communication, education, and seating. Treatment is aimed to keep straight spine and level pelvis while maintaining hips stable to maintain 90° of flexion and 30° of extension ROM. It is also good to have plantigrade feet that can fit in shoes.
- *Total Body:* In addition to quadriplegics, these patients have profound cognitive deficits and loss of head and neck control. These severely crippled patients require full-time assistance for activities of daily living and specialized systems to assist with head positioning. Drooling, dysarthria, and dysphagia are also common and complicate care.
- *Other types:* Some patients have a double hemiplegia pattern as a result of bleeding in both hemispheres of the brain. It is often difficult to differentiate this from diplegia or quadriplegia, but the upper extremities typically are more involved than the lower (*compare from*-diplegia).
- *Paraplegia:* It is very rare where bilateral lower extremity is involved with complete sparing of motor skills in the upper extremity. Many patients diagnosed with paraplegia actually are diplegic. Triplegia does not exist.

For crouch gait, please read Chapter no. 4B.

278. Differentiate between spasticity and rigidity.
Ans:
The **Table 2.17.1** tabulates the differences between spasticity and rigidity.

TABLE 2.17.1: Comparison of spasticity from rigidity.

	Spasticity	*Rigidity*
Lesion in	Pyramidal tracts	Basal ganglia
Muscles involved	Either agonists or antagonists	Both are involved
Hypertonia	Clasp knife type	Lead pipe or cog wheel
Characteristic posture	Present	Absent
Velocity dependent	Yes	No

279. What are the principles of dorsal root rhizotomy in management of static cerebral palsy?

Ans: Principles:

It is done in patients with:
- Spastic diplegia
- Mainly spastic with no or minimal dyskinesia, ataxia, or rigidity
- History of prematurity
- Spasticity-limiting function
- Absence of profound weakness
- No spinal or joint deformity
- Some forward locomotion and adequate truncal balance
- Adequate cognitive and motivational ability
- *Age:* 3–8 years.

About 40–60% dorsal abnormal rootlets from T12 to S1 are sacrificed. Extensive physiotherapy is required afterward to treat the weakness. Selective dorsal rhizotomy (SDR) should not be done with underlying dystonia, spastic quadriplegia, and spastic hemiplegia.

280. Role and mode of action of pharmacological treatment in cerebral palsy.

Ans: Spasticity may also be treated by oral medications. Benzodiazepines (e.g., diazepam), baclofen, dantrolene sodium, and tizanidine have been used in the past. Benzodiazepines act by facilitating transmission at the inhibitory synopsis in the central nervous system called the γ-aminobutyric acid type A gamma-aminobutyric acid (GABA) receptors. Facilitated transmission reduces monosynaptic and poly-synaptic reflexes resulting in increased inhibition, thereby reducing spasticity. Benzodiazepines can act in the brain as well as spinal cord. Sedation is one of the most common side effects. In addition, there is a risk of developing tolerance or dependence. The pediatric dose ranges from 0.12 to 0.8 mg/kg/day. The drug should never be stopped abruptly as withdrawal symptoms may include agitation, irritability, tremor, muscle fasciculation, nausea, hyperreflexia, and seizures.

- Baclofen is a structural analog of GABA and binds to GABAB receptors resulting in inhibition of mono and poly-synaptic reflexes. It also reduces release of excitatory neurotransmitters and substance peptide (P). It primarily acts at the spinal cord, thus offering an excellent treatment for patients with CP. It reduces spasticity, hyperreflexia and clonus. It can often cause sedation. The pediatric dosing starts between 2.5 and 10 mg/day and may increase up to 40 mg a day in divided doses. Withdrawal symptoms can occur when the drug is stopped suddenly after an extended period. These include intense spasticity, hallucination, compression, and seizures.
- Dantrolene sodium acts at the site of skeletal muscle as opposed to other drugs which act on the neurotransmitter system. It acts by inhibiting the release of calcium ions from sarcoplasmic reticulum during muscle contraction. The drug reduces clonus and muscle spasm. It is usually preferred in hemiplegia, traumatic brain injury, spinal cord injury, and spasticity due to CP. The pediatric dose is 6–8 mg/day is divided doses. The most important side effect is hepatotoxicity for which regular monitoring with liver function test is required.
- Tizanidine has also been used for treatment of spasticity. It is an α2-adrenergic agent which reduces the tone through hyperpolarization of motor neurons. The drug has not been used extensively for the pediatric patient and common side effects include hepatotoxicity, sedation, dizziness, and dry mouth.
- Neuromuscular/chemodenervation with extramuscular injection is an extremely effective method of controlling spasticity selectively in a single muscle/joint. Injection of phenol and ethyl alcohol perineurally results in decrease of spasticity by axonal degeneration. However, the effect is reversible with reinnervation occurring over months to years. The side effects include muscle necrosis and vascular complications. The advantage is their cost-effectiveness and their use in spasticity in large powerful muscles which cannot be treated with recommended dose of botulinum toxin.
- Botulinum toxin is an effective synaptic blocker which acts by inhibiting the release of acetylcholine at the presynaptic junction. This toxin is produced by *Clostridium botulinum*. Effects are reversible; hence the injection is required every

3–4 months. Dosing is usually 10–12 U/kg but should never exceed 400 units in a single sitting. Two serotypes are available in the international market—A and B. Botulinum toxin type A is commonly marked at BOTOX®. Type B is generally available as MYOBLOC®. The most appropriate candidate for botulinum toxin is a patient where reduction of spasticity in a limited number of muscles can provide a meaningful benefit in care, comfort and activity of the child. It acts by reducing spasticity in focally affected muscles. Thus, the affected muscles can be stretched, antagonists can be rebuilding by physiotherapy helping improve balance around joints and also surgeon can assess the possible effects of surgery if needed. It can also be used in conjunction with orthopedic surgery or in combination with serial casting and splinting.

- Neurosurgical treatment of spasticity includes selective dorsal rhinotomy (SDR) and intrathecal baclofen therapy (IBT). SDR, first started by Warrick Peacock, is performed through laminoplasty. The dura is opened and dorsal rootlets are identified from T12 through S1. Each rootlet is stimulated and the response is recorded electromyographically. Those with abnormal or generalized response are severed. About 40–60% of nerve rootlets are sacrificed. The procedure helps by cutting of the aberrant afferent activity from muscle spindles which are normally conveyed by dorsal nerves. This reduces the spasticity profoundly, so that the patient has significant amount of weakness postoperatively. Extensive physiotherapy is required afterward to treat the weakness. SDR should not be done with underlying dystonia.
- Intrathecal baclofen pump uses just 1% of the dose that is required orally to produce reduction of spasticity. It is an excellent method for patients with multisegmental/extensive spasticity with limited side effects. The pump placement is done subcutaneously or intramuscularly and the catheter is inserted intrathecally at the levels of T11–T12. Dose adjustments are done through telemetry with a remote. Refills which are required every 2–6 months are usually delivered through needle which passes through the skin into the part of the pump. Refills should not be missed to avoid dangerous withdrawal symptoms like itching, paresthesia, rebound spasticity, seizures, and change in mental status.

The drug treatment and neurosurgical treatment of dystonia are limited. Dystonia due to CP may be dopamine (DOPA)-responsive or DOPA-resistant. The carbidopa/levodopa is highly effective in the former. In the latter, anticholinergic drugs can be tried. Trihexyphenidyl is usually given in such cases. The limiting factors being side effects like confusion, memory loss, dry mouth, blurred vision, and urinary retention. Intramuscular injection with botulinum toxin may be successful in focal dystonia. Those refractory to above treatments may benefit by intrathecal baclofen pump or deep brain stimulation (pallidal stimulation).

281. A. Classify cerebral palsy in relation to its musculoskeletal manifestations (physiologic, anatomic, and functional classification).
B. Write a note on treatment of spasticity.
C. Describe gait disorders and its treatment in cerebral palsy.

Ans: The following answer is a concise form of discussions and answers written above just for sake of rapid revision.

1. Physiologic classification **(Table 2.17.2)**
(Based on type of muscle tone and movement abnormality)

TABLE 2.17.2: Physiological classification of cerebral palsy.

Type	Features	Common musculoskeletal effects
Spastic (most common, ~70–80%)	↑ tone, hyperreflexia, velocity-dependent resistance	Contractures, scissoring gait, equinus deformity
Dyskinetic (athetoid/choreoathetoid/dystonic)	Involuntary writhing or twisting movements, fluctuating tone	Joint instability, scoliosis, involuntary posturing
Ataxic	Poor coordination, tremor, wide-based gait	Balance problems, falls, delayed motor milestones
Hypotonic	Low tone, floppy posture	Ligamentous laxity, delayed weight-bearing
Mixed	Features of more than one type	Combination of above deformities

2. Anatomic classification **(Table 2.17.3)**
(Based on limb distribution)

TABLE 2.17.3: Anatomical classification of cerebral palsy.

Type	Limbs involved	Musculoskeletal manifestations
Monoplegia	One limb	Minimal deformity, mild weakness
Hemiplegia	One side of body (arm > leg)	Limb length discrepancy, equinus, fixed flexion deformity
Diplegia	Both lower limbs (arms less affected)	Crouch gait, scissoring, hip subluxation
Triplegia	Three limbs	Asymmetric gait, multiple contractures
Quadriplegia	All four limbs	Severe contractures, scoliosis, hip dislocation
Double hemiplegia	Both sides but upper limbs more affected	Upper limb spasticity > lower limb involvement

3. Functional classification **(Table 2.17.4)**
(Based on mobility and self-care abilities—often using GMFCS: Gross motor function classification system)

TABLE 2.17.4: Gross motor function classification system (GMFCS) of cerebral palsy.

Level	Description	Musculoskeletal implications
Level I	Walks without limitations	May have mild stiffness or weakness
Level II	Walks with limitations	Minor contractures, reduced endurance
Level III	Walks using a hand-held mobility device	Moderate lower limb deformities
Level IV	Self-mobility with limitations; powered mobility outdoors	Significant contractures, hip/knee deformities
Level V	Transported in manual wheelchair	Severe deformities, dislocations, scoliosis

Treatment of spasticity
1. *Goals of treatment*:
    - Improve functional abilities (mobility, self-care, and communication).
    - Reduce pain and discomfort.
    - Prevent secondary complications (contractures, deformities, and skin breakdown).
    - Facilitate care (ease of dressing, hygiene, and positioning).
2. *General principles*:
    - Identify and treat underlying cause (e.g., brain/spinal injury, MS, and CP).
    - *Multidisciplinary approach:* Neurology, orthopedics, physiotherapy, and occupational therapy.
    - Combination of nonpharmacological + pharmacological + surgical options.
3. *Nonpharmacological measures*:
    a. *Physical and occupational therapy:*
        - Stretching exercises (reduce muscle tightness)
        - Strengthening of antagonist muscles
        - Range of motion (ROM) exercises
        - Weight-bearing activities
        - Orthotic devices (splints and braces) to prevent contractures
    b. *Positioning and casting:*
        - Serial casting for contracture prevention
        - Standing frames for postural control
4. *Pharmacological treatment*:
    a. *Oral agents*:
        - *Baclofen*: GABA-B agonist; reduces excitatory neurotransmission.
        - *Tizanidine*: α2 adrenergic agonist; reduces muscle tone.

- *Diazepam*: GABA-A agonist; useful but sedating.
- *Dantrolene sodium*: Acts peripherally on muscle (reduces Ca^{2+} release).
  b. *Focal injections:*
  - Botulinum toxin type A/B—local chemodenervation; best for focal spasticity.
  - Phenol/alcohol nerve blocks—longer lasting but destructive.
  c. *Intrathecal therapy*:
  - Intrathecal baclofen pump—for severe generalized spasticity; adjustable dosing.
5. *Surgical treatment:*
   - *Orthopedic surgery:*
     - Tendon lengthening (e.g., Achilles and hamstrings)
     - Osteotomies to correct deformities
   - *Neurosurgical:*
     - Selective dorsal rhizotomy (SDR) – cutting selected sensory rootlets to reduce reflex arc hyperactivity.
6. *Algorithmic approach:*
   - Mild focal spasticity → PT + Botulinum toxin
   - Moderate generalized spasticity → Oral drugs ± PT
   - Severe refractory cases → Intrathecal baclofen/SDR/orthopedic surgery.

Common gait disorders in CP
1. *Spastic hemiplegic gait:*
   - *Presentation:*
     - Unilateral involvement (one side affected)
     - *Circumduction:* The affected leg swings outward due to spasticity in the calf muscles.
     - *Equinus gait:* Toe-walking due to spasticity in the gastrocnemius/soleus.
     - *Arm posture:* Flexed elbow, wrist, and fingers on the affected side.
2. *Spastic diplegic gait:*
   - *Presentation:*
     - Bilateral lower limb spasticity (legs more affected than arms)
     - *Scissoring gait:* Thighs cross due to adductor spasticity.
     - *Crouch gait:* Excessive knee and hip flexion with ankle dorsiflexion (common after Achilles tendon lengthening without addressing hamstring tightness).
     - *Toe-walking:* Due to spastic plantar flexors.
3. *Spastic quadriplegic gait:*
   - *Presentation:*
     - Severe involvement of all four limbs.
     - Poor trunk control, significant crouch posture, and limited ambulation (may require assistive devices or wheelchair).
4. *Dyskinetic/ataxic gait:*
   - Dyskinetic (athetoid/dystonic):
     - Involuntary movements, fluctuating tone, unstable gait.
   - Ataxic:
     - Wide-based gait, poor balance, and incoordination.

Treatment of gait disorders in CP
1. *Physical therapy and gait training:*
   - *Strengthening and stretching:* Focus on spastic muscles (hamstrings, hip adductors, and gastrocnemius).
   - *Balance and coordination training:* For ataxic/dyskinetic CP.
   - *Treadmill training:* With or without body-weight support.
   - Orthotic management.

2. *Orthotics and assistive devices:*
   - *Ankle-foot orthoses (AFOs):* Control equinus, prevent crouch gait.
   - *Supramalleolar orthoses (SMOs):* For mild instability.
   - *Hip-knee-ankle-foot orthoses (HKAFOs):* For severe weakness.
   - *Walkers, crutches, canes:* For stability.
3. *Pharmacological management:*
   - *Oral medications:* Baclofen and diazepam (reduce spasticity).
   - *Botulinum toxin (Botox):* Focal spasticity management (e.g., gastrocnemius and hamstrings).
   - *Intrathecal baclofen pump:* For severe generalized spasticity.
4. *Surgical interventions:*
   - *Soft-tissue surgeries:*
     – Achilles tendon lengthening (for equinus)
     – Hamstring lengthening (for crouch gait)
     – Adductor release (for scissoring gait)
   - *Bone surgeries:*
     – Femoral derotation osteotomy (for excessive hip internal rotation)
     – Foot osteotomies (for severe deformities)
   - *Selective dorsal rhizotomy (SDR):* Cutting sensory nerves to reduce spasticity (careful patient selection required).
5. *Emerging therapies:*
   - Robotic-assisted gait training (e.g., Lokomat)
   - Functional electrical stimulation (FES)
   - Stem cell therapy (experimental)

282. **Describe spastic diplegia in paediatric cases: presentation, nonoperative and operative management.**

Ans: *Definition:* Spastic diplegia is a form of cerebral palsy (CP) characterized by bilateral spasticity (stiffness) and motor impairment, predominantly affecting the lower limbs more than the upper limbs. It is commonly caused by periventricular leukomalacia (PVL) due to preterm birth or perinatal hypoxia.

Clinical presentation
1. *Motor symptoms:*
   - *Spasticity* in legs > arms (may have mild upper limb involvement)
   - *Scissoring gait* (hips and knees flexed and legs cross midline)
   - *Toe-walking* due to tight Achilles tendons.
   - *Delayed motor milestones* (late sitting, crawling, and walking)
2. *Musculoskeletal complications:*
   - *Contractures* (Achilles tendon, hamstrings, and hip adductors)
   - *Hip dysplasia/subluxation* (due to muscle imbalance)
   - *Foot deformities* (equinus, valgus/varus)
3. *Associated conditions:*
   - *Mild intellectual disability* (varies; some have normal cognition).
   - *Seizures, strabismus, and speech delays.*

Nonoperative management
1. *Physiotherapy:*
   - Stretching, strengthening, balance training.
   - *Gait training* (walkers, orthotics-assisted walking).
2. *Orthotics (braces and splints):*
   - *Ankle-foot orthoses (AFOs)* to prevent toe-walking.
   - *Knee-ankle-foot orthoses (KAFOs)* for severe weakness.
3. *Medical management:*
   - *Oral antispasmodics* (baclofen and diazepam).

- *Botulinum toxin (Botox) injections* for focal spasticity.
- *Intrathecal baclofen pump* (for severe spasticity).
4. *Assistive devices:*
   - Walkers, crutches, or wheelchairs (if non-ambulatory).

Operative management
1. *Neurosurgical interventions:*
   - *Selective dorsal rhizotomy (SDR):*
     – Cuts overactive sensory nerves to reduce spasticity (best in *ambulatory children with pure spasticity*).
2. *Orthopedic surgeries:*
   - *Tendon Lengthening:*
     – *Achilles tendon* (for equinus deformity)
     – *Hamstring lengthening* (for crouched gait)
   - *Hip reconstruction:*
     – For *hip subluxation/dislocation* (osteotomy and adductor release).
   - *Bony corrections:*
     – *Femoral derotation osteotomy* (for inward hip rotation)
     – *Foot stabilization* (triple arthrodesis for severe deformities)
3. *Spinal Surgery (if needed):* Scoliosis correction (if severe spinal curvature develops).

283. Guiding principles of removal of orthopedic implants after fracture union. What are the current recommendations for removal of implant in commonly encountered fractures?

Ans: *Guiding principles for removal and timing:* In general implant removal may be indicated because of:
- Patient preference
- To restore skeletal strength
- For complications that may develop after surgery—nonunion/infection/implant failure, etc.
- Need of MRI for the part for related/unrelated cause.

The AO-ASIF published general guidelines for implant removal are shown in **Table 2.17.5**.

TABLE 2.17.5: AO-ASIF guidelines for implant removal.

Bone fracture	Time after implantation (months)
Malleolar fractures	8–12
Tibial pilon	12–18
Tibial shaft	
Plate	12–18
Intramedullary nail	18–24
Tibial head	12–18
Patella, tension band	8–12
Femoral condyles	12–24
Femoral shaft	
Single plate	24–36
Double plates	From months 18, in two steps (interval, 6 months)
Intramedullary nail	24–36
Peritrochanteric and femoral neck fractures	12–18
Pelvis (only in case of complaints)	From months 10
Upper extremity (optional)	12–18

C. Sexual Dimorphism (Q284)

284. What is the sexual dimorphism in orthopedics?

Ans: This does not refer to any disorder. It's a term to understand the subtle and gross differences in the body's anatomy and physiological response due to differential sexual make-up. Males and females respond differently to physiological and pathological stimuli thus "one size fits all" theory does not apply. We should evaluate and manage the patient discretely taking into consideration the physiology of sexual dimorphism. Sexual dimorphism refers to differences in biological response that is inherent in one's sex or chromosomal make-up that arises from differences in hormone responsive genes located on X and Y chromosomes. In general, the prominent difference lies in higher muscle mass of males and consequent larger bones. Also, effect of testosterone and no cessation of estrogen stimulation produce delayed bone loss in males. The specific effect of sexual dimorphism in various conditions is briefed below:

- *Osteoporosis:* Males are affected nearly 10 years later than females. Estrogen produces early epiphyseal closure.
- *Osteoarthritis:* Females are more commonly affected than males especially this difference is significant in obese females. This difference may be accounted by higher leptin levels that is a produce of adipose tissue.
  - Higher incidence of 1st carpometacarpal joint arthritis in females is supposed to be due to relaxin receptors in this joint that upregulates matrix metalloproteinase (MMP)-1 and 3.
- AMBRI type shoulder instability is more common in females that may be related to reduced proprioception at shoulder in females.
- Males have higher incidence of Dupuytren's contracture 9:1 while females have higher incidence of adhesive capsulitis 3:1.
- Scoliotic curves are seen commonly in females [curves >30° (F:M) = (3:1)].
- Females have higher incidence of spinal symptoms due to instability.
- Hip arthritis and pincer type impingement are more common in females may be latter is a consequence of former.
- Developmental dysplasia of the hip has higher occurrence in females.
- Males have higher morbidity following hip fracture and has higher incidence of secondary hip fracture.
- Following sacral fracture (or its treatment) and urethral injury males have high rate of sexual dysfunction than females.
- Females have higher incidence of anterior cruciate ligament (ACL) injury and possibly rerupture rates.
- Total knee arthroplasty is more commonly advised for males at a lower grade than females.
- Females have higher q-angle (higher incidence of chondromalacia), higher anteversion, patella alta, sider forefoot, shorter arch, and lesser cartilage thickness.
- Females have higher incidence of bunion and posterior tibial tendon dysfunction causing flatfoot.
- Females are more sensitive to pain stimuli and less tolerant to pain while more sensitive to adverse effects of opioids.
- Most of osseous neoplasia are more common in males (3:2) except giant cell tumor, surface osteogenic sarcoma, desmoid tumor that are more common in females.
- Females experience more toxicity of chemotherapy drugs.

D. Humeral Head Blood Supply (Q285)

285. What is the relevance of blood supply of humeral head in planning management of fracture of proximal humerus?

Ans: Blood supply to proximal humerus is partly derived from anterior circumflex humeral artery through anterolateral ascending branch (along with biceps tendon in the groove) and arcuate artery. The anterolateral ascending branch runs medially and crosses the subscapularis tendon anteriorly running along with two venae communicantes along the intertubercular groove. The arcuate artery is a continuation of the ascending branch of the anterior humeral circumflex. It enters the bicipital groove and supplies 34% of the head. This is the reason why osteonecrosis is not very frequent despite disruption of anterior blood supply in 80% of fractures. The other major group enters the greater tubercle after originating from extensive anastomoses between circumflex (anterior and posterior circumflex) and rotator cuff vascular supply, so it receives its own blood supply despite being separated from humeral head in a fracture. Similarly, lesser tubercle is supplied through vascular supply to subscapularis.

The posterior circumflex humeral artery is now considered to be the main supply for humeral head—64% of the superior, posterior and inferior aspects of humeral head.

Fragments of a proximal humeral fracture usually have an independent blood supply. The medial vessels to the head gain high importance in fractures of the anatomical neck. The nutrient artery lies regularly medial to the humeral midshaft and is at risk at open reduction of this region. Fractures of the anatomic neck have a poor prognosis because of the precarious vascular supply.

E. Orthobiologics (286–295)

286. What are orthobiologics? How will you diagnose gout? Discuss newer drugs in gout and its specific indications.

Ans: Orthobiologics encompasses use of biological substances to help musculoskeletal injuries to heal more quickly. Initially restricted to improvement of fracture healing; the term has now been extended to finding its use in enhancing the healing of injured cartilage, muscles tendons, and ligaments with identified substances that can do so. The effectors used in orthobiologics are made from substances that naturally occur in the body. The strategy is to harness cells and proteins naturally found in the human biology (usually in higher than physiological concentration) help to support efficient/enhanced regrowth of injured tissues. It is interesting to note that most of these [like bone grafts, platelet-rich plasma, bone morphogenetic protein (BMP), etc.] were already in vogue for decades but only recently they have been grouped into fancy term "orthobiologics" by improvement in understanding the human biochemistry and biology.

Orthobiologics use both cell-based therapies and biomaterials to enhance healing for improved repair and regeneration. The expected benefits of using orthobiologics in orthopedics are:
- Less invasive and possibly more effective at restoring function than large surgeries
- Improving the long-term health of patients suffering from disabling disorders and injuries
- Biological and natural alternatives to repair instead of artificial device implantation
- Reducing hospital visits and shortening stays
- Minimizing impact of degenerative diseases
- Most are outpatient day-care procedure requiring no overnight admission
- Recovery is more rapid
- Much less financial liability.

Following are currently considered orthobiologics that would soon expand with continued search:
- *Bone grafts:* Both autologous and synthetic.
- *Autologous blood:* This involves simply injecting the venous blood at the desired site like that for chronic tendinopathies (tennis elbow, Achilles insertional tendinosis, etc.) or to improve the strength of repair as in rotator cuff repair or Bankart repair.
- *Autologous conditioned serum:* It is a process to improve the concentration of interleukin-1 (IL-1) receptor antagonist in blood. The preparation involves incubation of 50 mL venous blood for 24 hours in 5% CO_2 in pH-neutralized environment with small glass beads.
- *Platelet-rich plasma (PRP, platelet-enriched plasma, platelet-rich concentrate, or autologous platelet gel):* The platelet concentrate has been used for—
  - Lateral epicondylitis
  - Rotator cuff repair
  - Knee osteoarthritis
  - Nonunion of long bones
  - Achilles tendinopathy
  - Patellar tendinopathy
  - Plantar fasciitis
  - Shoulder osteoarthritis.

- *Growth factors:* This is an emerging field in targeted drug delivery system which also utilizes the modalities like genetic engineering, stem cell therapy, and tissue bioprinting to deliver the required growth factors at a site considered deficient in them.
- Stem cells.

(For details on orthobiologics kindly refer to Chapter 132 of the book Essential Orthopedics: Principles and Practice, 2nd edition.)

GOUT: The American College of Rheumatology has 11 criteria and the presence of six or more suggests that gout is present.
1. More than one attack of active arthritis
2. Maximum inflammation develops within one day
3. Oligoarthritis attack
4. Redness observed over joint
5. First metatarsophalangeal joint painful or swollen
6. Unilateral first metatarsophalangeal joint attack
7. Unilateral tarsal joint attack
8. Tophus (proven or suspect)
9. Hyperuricemia
10. Asymmetrical swelling within a joint on radiography
11. Complete termination of an attack.

Newer drugs for treatment of gout: Febuxostat (TMX-67) is a new class of uric acid lowering drug. It is a nonpurine, selective inhibitor of xanthine oxidase distinguishing it from allopurinol and oxypurinol (purine analogs) that are nonselective inhibitors and inhibit at least five enzymes in the purine and pyrimidine pathway other than xanthine oxidase. Febuxostat is also not reincorporated into nucleotides and does not regulate pyrimidine metabolism. It has been found superior in reducing serum urate levels in stage 2 or 3 chronic kidney disease patients compared to allopurinol. There is recently a labeled warning concerning cardiovascular safety with the use of febuxostat. Febuxostat could be considered primarily in patients with compromised renal function (stage >2 CKD), urolithiasis, inability to increase hydration or identified uric acid production; however, allopurinol remains drug of choice for cardiac patients and otherwise. Tophus size is reduced by 50–80% after 1 year of either febuxostat or allopurinol treatment, with the greatest tophus and gout flare reduction linked to the greatest degree of serum urate-lowering irrespective of drug. All xanthine oxidase inhibitors should be used with great precaution for major interactions in patients receiving azathioprine, 6-mercaptopurine and theophylline.

Uricase therapy has been tried and is still evolving. Expression of uricase enzyme ceased in human during evolution. The therapy is based on premises that the enzyme converts uric acid to allantoin (along with one hydrogen peroxide molecule) which is much more soluble and the fact that rodents that express uricase have uric acid levels less than 1 mg/dL. Rasburicase (the non-PEGylated recombinant fungal enzyme) has gone out of favor due to high antigenicity and plasma halflife of 18–24 hours. The recombinant porcine-baboon uricase (pegloticase) has less antigenicity and longer plasma half-life so that intravenous administration has shown good relief in refractory hyperuricemia and debulking of tophi in weeks to months (compared to years on allopurinol therapy).

(For further details kindly refer to Chapter 11 of the book Essential Orthopedics: Principles and Practice, 2nd edition.)

287. **Biological therapies in tendon regeneration for chronic tendinopathies.**
Ans: Kindly see the Answer to Question above.

F. Miscellaneous Combination Questions (Q288–295)

288. **Discuss in detail:**
   A. The watershed zone of spinal cord.
   B. Draw a cross-section of spinal cord in dorsal region.
   C. Stages of Pott's paraplegia in a typical paravertebral lesion based on anatomy of tracts.

Ans:

A. The blood supply to the spinal cord is rich, but the spinal canal is the narrowest and the blood supply is the poorest at T4–9. T4–9 should be considered the critical vascular zone of the spinal cord, a zone in which interference with the circulation is most likely to result in paraplegia.

B. Cross-section of spinal cord at dorsal region is illustrated in **Figure 2.17.1**.

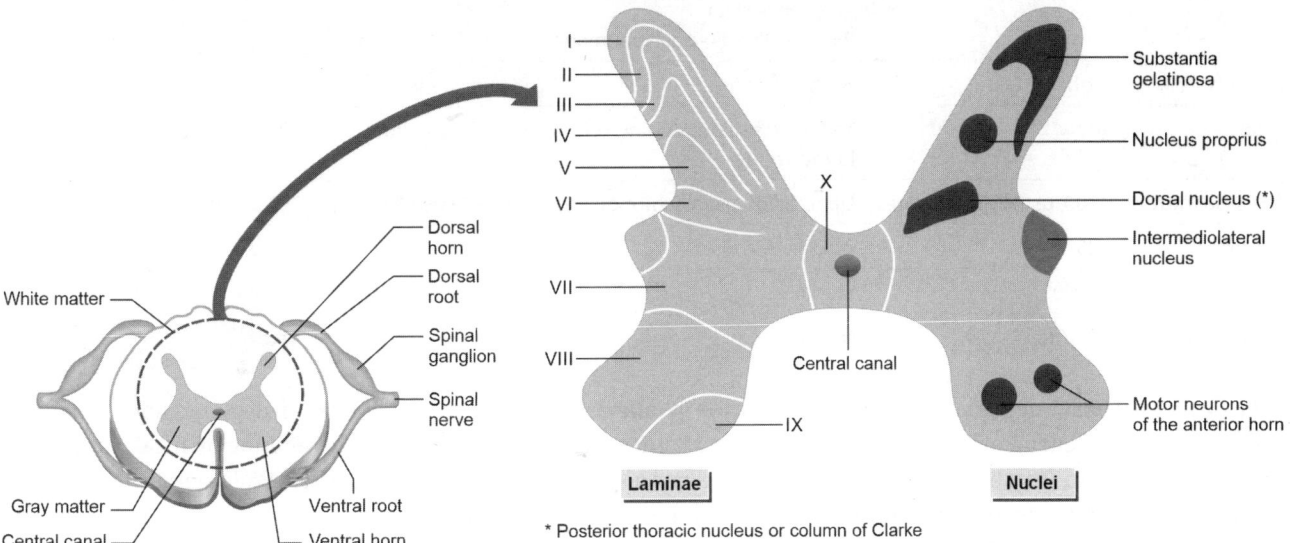

Fig. 2.17.1: Spinal cord in dorsal region.

C. Please read Chapter no. 4C.

289. Write notes on:
  A. Synovial fluid analysis.
  B. Wallerian degeneration.
  C. Nerve conduction velocity.

Ans:

A. Synovial fluid analysis can differentiate between noninflammatory, inflammatory, and traumatic conditions (**Tables 2.17.6 and 2.17.7**). Systematic examination includes macroscopic and microscopic, and biochemical analysis.
- *Microscopic examination:* Differential white blood cell count, total white and red blood cells, evaluation for crystals is done.
- *Physical characteristics:* The fluid volume, color, clarity, viscosity of the joint fluid is seen.

TABLE 2.17.6: Differing leukocyte count and neutrophil cell variation in various synovial joint pathologies.		
Disease	Leukocytes	Neutrophils (%)
Normal	<200	<25
Traumatic	<5,000	<25
Toxic synovitis	5,000–15,000	<25
Acute rheumatic fever	10,000–15,000	50
Juvenile rheumatoid arthritis	15,000–80,000	75
Septic arthritis	>80,000	>75

TABLE 2.17.7: Differentiating features of synovial fluid analysis in various pathologies.

Gross	Normal fluid composition	Noninflammatory (like traumatic, reactive, degenerative)	Septic arthritis	Inflammatory arthropathies (like rheumatoid)
Appearance	Clear, oil like	Reactive and degenerative effusion—clear Blood stained—post-traumatic	Turbid	Cloudy
Viscosity	High	High	Inconsistent	Low
Color	Straw	Yellow to red depending on hemorrhage	Cloudy to yellow	Cloudy yellow
WBCs per mm^3	<100, usually monocytes	Up to 2,000 usually monocytes	>80,000 usually poly	2,000–50,000 (poly and mono)
Neutrophil	<25%	<25%	>75%	≥50
Culture	Sterile	Sterile	±	Sterile
Protein	<2 g/dL	N to ↓	↑↑↑	N to ↑↑

B. **The process of nerve degeneration and regeneration (Wallerian degeneration)**—Wallerian degeneration (WD) is also called anterograde degeneration, named after Augustus Volney Waller to describe the degeneration of distal nerve stump after injury to neuron. This process is *not* apoptosis and has a specifically conserved pathway. Wallerian degeneration is also seen in CNS and in neurodegenerative and demyelinating diseases.

The sequence of events can be summarized as follows:
- The lag between injury and degeneration may range from 24 hours to few days.
- *Phase of granular disintegration:* Just a few hours after injury axons become swollen and their axoplasm is filled with an amorphous matrix (24–72 hours). During this period, the major cytoskeleton proteins (microtubules and neurofilaments) are being degraded. This phase is triggered by large influx of Ca^{++} ions that cause:
    - Disruption of mitochondrial oxidative phosphorylation
    - Excessive formation of free radicals
    - Activation of calpains, calcium-activated neutral cysteine proteases—causing cytoskeletal breakdown.
- By 72–96 hours, the myelin lamellae are disrupted into small fragments known as myelin ovoids. Visualization of these is the basic criterion used by investigators to define Wallerian degeneration.
- Within 96 hours after the injury, the Schwann cells from neurolemma synthesize growth factors which attract axonal sprouts to the distal end of the severed axon. These axonal sprouts originate at the proximal end of the severed axon.
- Myelin and axonal debris are removed by resident and newly recruited inflammatory cells (monocytes/macrophages) and microglia (in the CNS) and by Schwann cells (in PNS). This is important as without clearance the new axonal sprouts will not grow. The process is undertaken by:
    - *Immune cells:* Monocytes/macrophages, T and B lymphocytes, dendritic cells, and neutrophils. The monocyte-macrophage system (both resident and recruited) works a great deal to remove myelin by "opsonization".
    - *Resident non-neuronal cells:* Astrocytes and microglia in the central nervous system and Schwann cells in the PNS.
- The neurolemma of axons (the outermost layer of the neuron made of Schwann cells) does not degenerate and remains as a hollow tube. Immediately after axonal degeneration and fragmentation, Schwann cells in the PNS enter continuous cell division, degrade their own membrane and phagocytose myelin and axonal debris.
- If an axon sprout reaches the tube, it grows into it and advances about 1 mm/day (3 cm/month, Steindler). The tubes provide pathways for the sprouting (regenerating) axons to follow to muscles and skin (topographic sensitivity, discussed below in role of Schwann cells). The Schwann cells then remyelinate, the newly formed axons which eventually reach and innervate the target tissue.

The first responder (Role of Schwann cells)—immediately after injury, the process of regeneration is dependent on Schwann cell that is the first responder. This also processes the initial degeneration to clean up the area for regeneration.

C. Please read Chapter no. 4A.

290. Describe intraosseous therapy in orthopedics?

Ans: Intraosseous therapy in orthopedics:

Definition and purpose:
Intraosseous (IO) therapy involves infusion of fluids/medications directly into bone marrow, serving as an alternative when IV access is difficult (e.g., trauma, shock, or pediatric cases). In orthopedics, it provides rapid vascular access during emergencies like hemorrhagic shock or sepsis.

Key applications:
- Trauma resuscitation
- Rapid delivery of blood products, antibiotics, or analgesics in polytrauma patients with compromised IV access.

Preferred sites:
- Proximal tibia, distal femur, or humeral head (avoiding fracture sites).

Perioperative use:
- Administering emergency drugs during surgery if IV lines fail.

Pediatric orthopedics:
- Critical for small children with fragile veins during emergencies (e.g., septic arthritis).

Advantages:
- *Speed:* Achieves vascular access in <60 seconds.
- *Efficacy:* Marrow absorption parallels IV route for most medications.
- *Safety:* Lower complication rates versus central lines in emergencies.

Technique:
1. *Device options:* Battery-powered drills (e.g., EZ-IO) or manual needles.
2. Insertion:
   - Sterilize site, insert needle at 90° angle until "pop" (cortical breach).
   - Confirm placement by aspiration of marrow/blood or flush without resistance.

Complications:
- *Rare:* Osteomyelitis, compartment syndrome, or extravasation.

Contraindications:
- Fracture at insertion site, osteopetrosis, or prior IO in same bone.

291. A. Describe with diagram the extensor expansion of finger.
B. Explain pathological anatomy of boutonnière and swan neck deformities in rheumatoid arthritis.
C. Discuss biological and pharmacological agents used in treatment of rheumatoid arthritis.

Ans:

A. This is an interesting apparatus and probably the most intricate mechanism to be reproduced mechanically. We can actively extend the proximal interphalangeal (PIP) and distal interphalangeal (DIP) joints without extending the MCP joints, but we cannot extend the PIP joint without extending the DIP joint at the same time. Also flexing only, the DIP joint without flexing the PIP joint is difficult (actively). Full (active or passive) flexion of the PIP joint prevents active extension of the DIP joint. All these phenomena are made possible by intricate disposition of various components of the extensor apparatus **(Fig. 2.17.2)**.

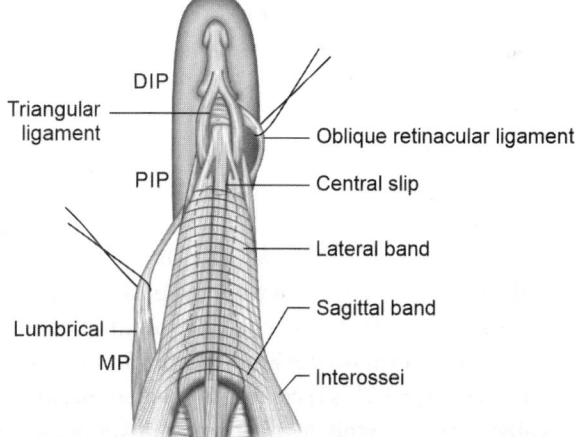

Fig. 2.17.2: Extensor expansion of finger.

Structures that comprise the extensor mechanism:
- The extensor digitorum communis *tendon* attaches by a tendinous slip to the proximal phalanx, through which it extends the MCP joint.

- The *central tendon* (or "slip") proceeds dorsally to attach to base of middle phalanx, where tension can extend the PIP joint.
- The *lateral bands* proceed on either side of dorsal midline and rejoin before attaching to the distal phalanx. Tension in the lateral bands extends the DIP joint.
- The *extensor hood* surrounds the MCP joint laterally, medially, and dorsally, and receives tendinous fibers from the lumbricals and interossei.

All the tendinous attachments transmit forces imparted to them by respective muscles.

Force develops in the extensor mechanism mainly in two ways:
1. Active tension—produced and transmitted by muscular contractions (hand intrinsics).
2. Passive tension—the extensor mechanism develops *passive tension* whenever it is elongated. This is generated by the reciprocal movements.

The extensor mechanism's fibers have lines of application that are always dorsal to the lateral axes of the PIP and DIP joints. Therefore:
- Activity in the intrinsic muscles that attach to the extensor mechanism always produces DIP and PIP extension.
- Passive flexion of the MCP joint elongates the extensor mechanism and extends the PIP and DIP joints.

B. *Pathoanatomy of Boutonnière deformity:* The deformity is produced by a progressive involvement of IP joints and extensor mechanism and pathological changes in the following manner:
- *Synovial proliferation due to RA in the PIP stretches and weakens the extensor mechanism:* Full extension cannot be achieved.
- Also, the effusion and distended joint due to the synovitis forces joint to go into partial flexion (position of maximum capsular volume).
- Over time, the lateral bands are displaced volarly and the SORL are shortened. SORL shortening causes DIP hyperextension.
- The MP joint, hence, hyperextends to compensate increasing PIP joint flexion.

Swan neck deformity: Zancolli has emphasized the fact that the two constituent deformities (PIP recurvatum and DIP flexion) are interrelated. Any hyperextension of the PIP for any reason will secondarily produce flexion of the DIP. Conversely, a DIP flexion deformity produces hyperextension at PIP due to alteration of forces. The deformities also tend to vary equally in severity.

Mechanisms that contribute to the secondary DIP flexion from a primary PIP hyperextension.
- *Proximal interphalangeal* recurvatum relaxes the normal tension on the lateral extensor bands. These hence move centrally and dorsally. In such a lax position the bands lose ability to extend the DIP, which hence drops into flexion.
- The flexor digitorum profundus (FDP) is pulled by recurvatum of the PIP causing prominent flexion of DIP by the law of maintaining constant length.
- The mechanical advantage of FDP flexion at DIP produces equivalent mechanical disadvantage of the spiral oblique retinacular ligament (SORL) in extending the DIP.
- The last possible factor producing PIP recurvatum is the stretching of the capsule secondary to active synovitis or ruptured flexor digitorum superficialis (FDS) tendon, removing the restraint to PIP joint hyperextension (commonly seen in RA).

Only for the sake of completion, it should be mentioned here that the extensive work of Zancolli divides the causes of PIP hyperextension (commoner cause of SND in RA) into three types based on action of intrinsic and extrinsic hand muscle activity:
1. *Extrinsic type (not seen with RA):* Due to excess traction of the extrinsic extensor tendons (say with CP, etc.) the central slip is tightened that inserts at the base of the middle phalanx.
2. *Intrinsic type:* Due to overactivity of intrinsic muscles (intrinsic plus hand as in ischemic contracture, spasticity or tendon adhesions as in RA). The test for intrinsic plus deformities are positive here.
3. *Articular type:* This is commonly seen in RA and is due secondary to weakening or destruction of normal stabilizing mechanisms of the PIP that prevent hyperextension.

The latter two are the pathogenic mechanisms in RA that produce a primary hyperextension at the PIP followed by DIP flexion and hence complete SND.

C. Pharmacotherapy for RA:

Pain relief: Nonsteroidal anti-inflammatory drugs (NSAIDs) are the mainstay for providing acute pain relief and cover for the time taking effect of disease-modifying antirheumatic drugs (DMARDs) to develop. If a satisfactory clinical response is not achieved after 2–3 weeks, another NSAID should be tried. None is superior and usually conventional NSAIDs are started reserving COX-2 specific inhibitors to patients not tolerating the former.

Corticosteroids: They were used as anti-inflammatory agents but have shown good disease modifying activity. Clear decision as to how and when to start them should be the concern instead of their bad reputation. They are rapidly acting drugs and relieve joint inflammation; improve symptoms of stiffness, fatigue, and loss of appetite; reduce ESR and CRP levels; and increase hemoglobin values. They also have protective influence on joint destruction. The improvement in the rate of disease progression appears to be greatest in the first 6 months of treatment with low-dose prednisolone. Restrict the dose of prednisolone to 10 mg/day in men and 7.5 mg/day in females. Women who take more than 7.5 mg/day for longer than 3 months risk bone loss. Abrupt withdrawal often induces an acute flare-up of the arthritis, and rarely, a systemic rheumatoid disease with necrotizing vasculitis and mononeuropathy develops in patients with rheumatoid nodules and strongly positive serum RF tests.

Single joint effusions can be well managed with intra-articular crystalloid preparation of steroid that gives lasting relief for months.

Doxycycline: Tetracyclines inhibit MMPs and are immunomodulatory. Classically suspicion on mycoplasma as a causative agent leads to the use of tetracyclines. It is now evident that tetracyclines are useful in RA because of their anti-inflammatory effects and not for antimicrobial effects. Studies reveal mixed results.

Statins: These drugs also seem to have anti-inflammatory properties. Statins have been reported to inhibit interactions between leukocytes and endothelial cells, to reduce the production of inflammatory cytokines, and to decrease T-cell activation. Current data on efficacy of statins for treatment of RA are mixed and still preliminary.

Disease modifying antirheumatic drugs: They are now the first line agents and in new terminology they are called "synthetic" DMARDS in view of availability of biological agents.

Treatment with synthetic DMARDs should be started as soon as the diagnosis of RA is made. There are usually three approaches to initiate treatment: (1) the sequential approach (the ineffective DMARD is dropped and new one added—abandoned nowadays), (2) step-up approach (in case of less than desired response add another DMARD and continue doing so till desired response gained), and (3) induction approach (add a combination of DMARDs till remission and then may step down).

Methotrexate: The "anchor" drug for isolated or commonly combination therapies. MTX therapy should always be a part of the first-line treatment strategy (other drugs may be combined) in patients with active RA (low disease activity patients may not need MTX) and in relapse or difficult cases (patients who did not receive MTX initially should receive this).

The beginning dose is usually 7.5 mg (three tablets) taken together on 1 day each week. Incremental increases of 2.5 mg/week are made every 4 weeks until either maximum control of joint inflammation or symptoms of toxicity appear. Higher weekly doses (20–30 mg) are more effective than lower doses and take 3–4 weeks for full effect to develop. The efficacy has not been surpassed by any of the available synthetic DMARDs or anti-TNF monotherapy. Stomatitis, anorexia, nausea or diarrhea often limits increase in dosage that can be partially controlled by twice weekly dosage or injectable preparations. Folic acid should be combined with the dose. Disease suppression is lost within 4 weeks of stopping the drug, but control is regained after restarting the medication within 3–4 weeks. It is recommended to do regular blood counts and liver function tests (LFTs) every month for first 3 months and 2-monthly thereafter. Bone marrow suppression can result from renal insufficiency, serious systemic infection, and concomitant administration of trimethoprim-sulfamethoxazole. There might be an increase in opportunistic infections in RA patients treated with MTX. Rheumatoid nodules can appear or enlarge in patients taking MTX and it has been suggested that concomitant hydroxychloroquine (HCQ) can control this complication.

Hydroxychloroquine: Hydroxychloroquine is a very slow-acting (around 3–9 months) low efficacy drug. It is commonly prescribed in combination therapy (empirically only) for low toxicity profile and infrequent drug interactions, but the additive efficacy for RA is undocumented. The most common side effects are maculopapular rashes, gastrointestinal disturbances, and nonspecific neurologic complaints; however, the major concern is ocular toxicity due to drug deposition in retinal pigment. Toxicity is reversible if recognized early, however, blindness may result if ignored. Sulfasalazine is a preferable drug compared to HCQ.

Sulfasalazine: It has rapid onset of action (within 3 weeks) and low incidence of serious side effects. It can be used as monotherapy in low disease activity patients. Usually, 500 mg twice daily is starting dose increased to 1 g twice daily in the absence of nausea, vomiting, photosensitivity, or skin rash. Because of the rare complications of myelosuppression or hemolytic anemia in individuals with glucose-6-phosphate dehydrogenase enzyme deficiency, monthly blood counts are recommended for first 3 months then 3 monthly.

Leflunomide: It is a pyrimidine inhibitor with good efficacy for RA. The drug has a long half-life hence a loading dose of 80–100 mg is given followed by 20 mg daily. Drug takes 6–8 weeks to take full effect improving arthritis activity and functional status. Diarrhea (managed with reducing dose) and hepatotoxicity (additive with MTX) are the usual side effects. Severe toxicity can be managed by cholestyramine as it enhances leflunomide excretion. This can be used as a primary drug in patients contraindicated for MTX therapy (rare).

Several older drugs like gold compounds (painful intramuscular injections), D-penicillamine (proteinuria, nephrotic syndrome), cyclosporine-A (hypertension and renal insufficiency), cyclophosphamide, chlorambucil (bone marrow suppression, neoplasms), and azathioprine have either low efficacy or severe side effects or low benefit to risk ratio so they are seldom prescribed anymore. Azathioprine, however, has a mild side effects profile, and is favored by some rheumatologists, especially for lowering the prednisone dose in patients with corticosteroid dependency.

Biological agents: These can be broadly divided into:
- anti-TNF (etanercept, adalimumab, infliximab, golimumab, and certolizumab pegol)
- non-TNF groups (abatacept, rituximab, and tocilizumab).

Biologic agents refer to complex protein molecules produced by using molecular biology methods in prokaryotic or eukaryotic cell cultures. Molecular 3D structure is more important rather than molecular weight and molecules with same molecular weight can have different function so it involves complex assessment methods. Their biological activities can be predefined and are usually directed toward a specific cytokine or cell surface molecule, making it possible to predict a range of activities both in terms of efficacy and toxicity. It is imperative to screen for latent tuberculosis infection (LTBI) in all RA patients being considered for therapy with biologic agents, regardless of the presence of risk factors for LTBI. Clinicians should assess the patient's medical history to identify risk factors for TB. The tuberculin skin test (TST) or interferon-γ–release assays (IGRAs) should be done as the initial test in all RA patients starting biologic agents, regardless of risk factors for LTBI, the latter is preferred in patients who have received BCG vaccination. A positive test mandates chest radiograph and sputum examination to detect active tuberculosis. Screening tests may be negative in RA patients due to immunosuppression. With a negative screening, repeat test should be done in high-risk patients after 1–3 weeks. Biological agents should be started in patients with active TB after completion of antitubercular treatment and after 1 month of latent TB treatment in patients with latent infection.

Anti-TNF agents improve symptoms while reducing radiographic progression of joint erosions. Five TNF blocking agents are available and approved for use in RA.

Etanercept, adalimumab, and certolizumab have been approved as monotherapy for RA but infliximab and golimumab have been approved only with concomitant use of MTX. MTX in combination has been shown to improve efficiency for prevention of joint structural damage. Etanercept was first agent approved for use in 1998 and bears lower efficacy then infliximab but good response has been demonstrated clinically. It is approved for use in DMARD-naïve patients also. Other approved uses of etanercept are in treatment of PsA and juvenile idiopathic arthritis. Infliximab being a chimeric protein induces antibody response against murine component that is successfully suppressed with MTX. Adalimumab has high specificity for TNF-α and is indicated in patients with moderate to severe RA and persistent disease despite DMARD therapy. Certolizumab pegol is a novel agent containing Fab domain of humanized monoclonal anti-TNF antibody bound to polyethylene glycol. It does not contain the Fc portion so does not activate complement or form immune complexes with TNF.

Seven types of side effects are encountered in different patients: (1) serious infections, including disseminated tuberculosis, (2) hematologic disorders, such as pancytopenia, (3) demyelinating disorders, (4) exacerbation of congestive heart failure, (5) systemic lupus erythematosus-related autoantibodies and clinical features, (6) hypersensitivity infusion or injection site reactions, and (7) severe liver disease. The increased risk of serious infections particularly tuberculosis especially with anti-TNF agents can be seen with all biological agents.

Other significant infections that have been found include *Pneumocystis carinii*, candidiasis, histoplasmosis, listeriosis, nocardiosis, aspergillosis, *cytomegalovirus*, cryptococcosis, and coccidioidomycosis. No cause has been identified though. Higher risk of heart failure has been found so it is better to avoid these agents in risk patients. Malignancy is a matter of debate and no concrete evidence has emerged till now. The presence of demyelinating disease in patients receiving these agents is cause for concern because its incidence seems to be higher than in the general population.

(For a detailed specific description of the drugs used, kindly refer to Chapter 11 of the book Essential Orthopedics: Principles and Practice, 2nd edition.)

292. Describe DMARD's in rheumatoid arthritis.

Ans: *Kindly see answer above (New modified classification is described for biological agents in updated 3rd edition of Essential Orthopedics: Principles and Practice).*

293. Factors affecting regeneration after peripheral nerve repair.

Ans: *Factors affecting the success of nerve repair:* Technical errors are the most common cause of failure of nerve repairs. The other causes are:

- *Type of nerve:* Pure motor or sensory has the best chance of recovery compared to mixed nerves.
- Younger patients have better recovery in least time.
- Proximal nerve injuries have poor chances of recovery as percentage cell death is quite high due to high metabolic demands.
- Gap defect in nerve have poor chances of recovery compared to direct repair.
- Clean vascular beds and absence of infection improves chances of recovery.
- *Delay between injury and repair:* Motor recovery has been reported for delay in nerve as long as 12 months (Suntherland). For sensory nerve this time delay is not known. In any case earlier the suture faster is the recovery.
- Associated injuries (like deep wounds/polytrauma) reduce chances of successful healing.
- *Condition of the nerve ends:* Lacerated ends may indicate tractional injury that may have occurred along the course of nerve unidentified. Clean cut ends are liable to recover much better.
- Neurogenic atrophy, fibrosis of denervated muscle, scar formation and wound contraction all lead to poor results.

294. Discuss etiopathogenesis of RA.

Ans: Etiology: Infections, genetic susceptibility, and environmental factors have been implicated in etiology. The concordance rate in monozygotic twins is high (12–15%) compared to a prevalence of 1% in the general population. Major histocompatibility complex class II loci are the prime culprit that hosts the DR4β chains (*DRB*0401* and *DRB*0404*) having greatest association with RA. Other loci that may have a role include the major histocompatibility complex class III genes for TNF-α, heat shock protein 70 (*HSP70*), and complement C4.

Although there is no consistent evidence of any specific microorganism in RA synovium, there may be a subclinical infectious trigger outside the synovium. *Mycoplasma*, Epstein–Barr virus, cytomegalovirus, parvovirus, and rubella virus have all been suggested, but mechanism is undefined. Cigarette smoking is considered the strongest known environmental risk factor for RA and is associated with anti-cyclic citrullinated peptide (anti-CCP) and rheumatoid factor (RF)-positive RA. Alcohol consumption may lower the risk of developing RF and anti-CCP-positive RA. Nulliparity and early menopause are associated with increased risk of developing RA while breastfeeding seems to have protective effect.

Pathogenesis: There is an imbalance in the T-helper (Th)17 and T-regulatory (Treg) cells where the former cells are increased while the latter get reduced in patients with active disease. It is a well-known fact that the Th1, Th2, and Th17 cells specialize in immunity against viral, parasitic, and other infections while Treg cells control the immune response and mediate tolerance against harmless self- and non-self-antigens. Differentiation and function of Treg cells require transcription factor forkhead box p3 (Foxp3) and also inducible Treg can be generated in periphery from CD4+ T-cell. The primary imbalance between ↑Th17/↓Treg cells is primarily responsible for progression of RA and in fact, cell-based therapy with Treg cells has been shown to produce durable disease remission in RA patients.

Inflammatory cytokines and chemokines are at the heart of development of RA. Classically it was thought that RA arises due to imbalance between Th1/Th2 imbalance, but this is an incomplete story. Within the synovium T-cell expansion and differentiation is dependent on the presence of proinflammatory cytokines. The balance of cytokines produced by Th1/Th2 subsets of Th cells determine what distinct Th subpopulation will develop. So in the presence of IL-1β, IL-6, and IL-23 differentiation into Th17 is promoted but presence of TGF-β will inhibit the same and favor differentiation into CD4+CD25+Foxp3+Tregs. Balance to Th17 differentiation will further lead to production of proinflammatory cytokines such as IL-2, TNF-α, IFN-γ, IL-17A, MIP (macrophage inflammatory protein)-1, MCP (monocyte chemotactic protein)-1, and IL-1β-continuing inflammation and progression of RA. Even the expression of IL-17 has been linked to the severity of RA. Expansion of Treg cells leads to production of IL-4 and IL-10 that are mainly anti-inflammatory and control and downregulate inflammation. Treg cells also secrete TGF-β1 that suppresses T cell, B cell proliferation and cytokine [interferon-gamma (IFN-γ)] production. It also reduces multiorgan inflammation and excessive lymphocytic infiltration.

Antigen-mediated activation of T-cell (especially the Th17) initiates a cascade activation of endothelial cells, proliferation of types A and B synoviocytes, and recruitment of additional inflammatory cells from the bone marrow. TNF-α and IL-1 stimulate inflammatory cells to release oncostatin M into synovial fluid. TNF-α and oncostatin M work together to induce production of collagenases called MMPs by the diseased synoviocytes and chondrocytes resulting in excessive collagen degradation and cartilage matrix collapse. When the immune response is triggered by the antigen, additional antigens may be created and recognized by the T-cell to create an ongoing immune response. The major population of T-cells in the rheumatoid synovium is composed of CD4+ memory T-cells. Although, the T-cells outnumber the B-cells, there are active plasma cells in the synovium and the expanded B lymphocyte pool, which suggest a significant humoral component to inflammation that is manifest in the synovial fluid. The antibody, a gamma globulin (rheumatoid factor), is produced in lymph nodes and coats the cell membranes of lymphocytes and plasma cells, which travel to the synovium where they react with the antigen causing acute inflammatory reaction. The synovium is transformed to pannus of synoviocytes, T-cells, and macrophages. This vascular granulation tissue is composed of proliferating fibroblasts, small blood vessels, and a variable number of mononuclear cells and produces a large amount collagenase and stromelysin-producing tissue damage. The cytokines IL-1 and TNF play key role. The synovitis and vascular proliferation invade adjacent cartilage and bone. These further degrade cartilage and stimulate osteoclasts to promote periarticular bony erosion and osteopenia.

295. A. Describe masquelet technique—indications and steps in an infected nonunion.
B. Explain evolution of different generations of cementing techniques in arthroplasty.

Ans: A. *Masquelet Technique*

Indications:
- Bone defects 5–25 cm
- Acute traumatic bone defects
- Septic as well as aseptic nonunions
- Pseudoarthrosis
- Post-tumor defects
- Chronic osteomyelitis.

Steps: Bone defects are reconstructed by autologous bone grafting. The technique is aimed at helping solve the problems of bone graft containment around the bone defect and the commonly desired need for growth supplementation using proteins. Repairing of wide diaphyseal defects (≤25 cm) with concurrent severe soft tissue loss using fresh autologous cancellous bone grafts in two-step (first step is more or less mechanical while second step is biological) surgical procedure.

In the first step (membrane induction), a PMMA cement spacer is inserted into the defect (after repeated debridement and obtaining clean bed) inducing formation of an encapsulation membrane. The bone is stabilized using external fixator or intramedullary nail. Surgeons have also used internal fixators (locked plates) for smaller bones of forearm, hand. After 4–6 weeks, the spacer is removed and the cavity filled with autologous cancellous graft from iliac crest. Morselized cancellous autograft harvested from the iliac crests is preferred but if this amount is not sufficient then demineralized allograft can be added to the autograft in a ratio that does not exceed 1 part of allograft: 3 parts of autograft. Bone formation and union occurs in approximately 8–9 months. *(Kindly also see Answer to Question 238 above)*

B. *Evolution of Different Generations of Bone Cementing*
   Over a time, refinements in the way cement was applied to the components have led to developments into generations in cementing:
- *First generation:* Finger packing, no distal plug
- *Second generation:* Distal plug of canal, "preparation" of canal with pulsed lavage, distal centralizer and use of cement gun to insert the cement in a retrograde fashion
- *Third generation:* Precooling of cement, vacuum mixing and centrifugation, pressurization of cement by use of proximal seal
- *Fourth generation:* In addition, this uses a proximal centralizer to ensure symmetric cement mantle.

During the same periods there were some "implant characteristics" that improved, however they are not grouped into generations. In the first generation, the implants had "sharp" borders that used to split the mantle and were prone to "midstem pivot effect" whereby there was excessive medial pressure in the proximal portion and lateral pressure distally. In the second generation, the implants were made of superalloys and sharp corners were removed. During third generation, the surface characteristics were improved to increase bonding.

G. Zone 2 Flexor Tendon Injury (Q296)
296. Treatment of cut flexor tendons in no man's land in hand.

Ans: Zone II flexor tendon is classically called Bunnell's "no man's land". This region when repaired with less than adequate skills cause scar and adhesion formation. The technique and suture materials have both improved to reasonably allow primary repair with good success. The most common mode of injury is cut injury of the tendon. If both tendons are cut at the same level, there are high chances of stuffing of the repair as well as increased volume due to ensuing edema. Also, there are high chances of cross-union and intertendinous adhesion formation between FDS and FDP. If only one of the tendons is injured, it may be left unrepaired with proper patient explanation and counseling. This especially holds true for FDS injury. Cut FDP is better repaired. Partial lacerations up to even 90% of the tendon width heal spontaneously but if the torn ends cause triggering then they may be trimmed. The injury must be repaired immediately, if associated with neurovascular damage is there, else elective repair scheduled within 2–3 days is also appropriate. Use Brunner's incisions and assess the status of A2 and A4 pulley. Open a flap through pulley to retrieve the cut ends of FDP tendon and perform a four-strand repair using cruciate repair. For FDS slips, perform modified Kessler repair taking care not to narrow the Camper's chiasm. If only one slip of FDS is damaged, leave it alone. If FDS is cut proximal to chiasm, try to do up both the tendons in an ideal sitting, but if the repair is getting too bulky then only repair the FDP. FDP tendon is then closed with epitendinous 6-0 nylon stitch in Lin-locking fashion. Look for the integrity of pulley system. If A2 pulley is damaged, then reconstruct it using dorsal retinaculum or palmaris longus tendon.
- For delayed cases (>3 weeks), there is a high chance that the repair is not possible as the cut ends would have retracted, contracted and hypertrophied. Tendon grafting is the best possible option in this scenario. This can be done as single stage or a double-stage technique. If the peritendinous tissue is healthy (not scarred and provide gliding) then I will do a single stage tendon grafting else do a two-stage grafting. Mostly for acute cases with intact pulley system single stage tendon graft using palmaris longus tendon or plantaris tendon if the former is absent suffices. There are a few prerequisites that must be fulfilled before tendon grafting procedure:
    - There should be no extensive scarring and hand should be supple. Passive joint movements should be nearly normal.
    - Circulation should be adequate.
    - At least one digital nerve of the finger should be intact.
    - Cooperative patient.

Tubiana recommended some principles for a successful tendon grafting that hold true for both primary procedure and two-staged one but especially true for the former.
- Only one tendon for one finger.
- Do not sacrifice intact superficialis tendon.
- Ends of tendon graft should be fixed away from tendon sheath.
- Save as much pulleys as possible.

Two-stage tendon grafting: If the tendon bed and peritendinous tissue are badly disrupted so that the gliding sheath for tendon is not available and/or pulley system is damaged, place a silicone sheath in place (as spacer) so that pseudosheath develops around it which will act as tendon sheath for the future graft preserving or reconstructing A2 and A4 pulley. It is often difficult for the surgeon to know beforehand the condition of flexor sheath (which is deemed normal in fresh cases). But if one finds excessive fibrosis, poor tendon bed or incompetent pulley, then it is better to do a two-staged procedure.

H. Limping Child (Q297–301)

297. **Management of painful limp with high grade fever in a 5-year-old child.**

Ans: *The differential diagnosis for a limping child with high grade fever includes:*
- Septic arthritis
- Osteomyelitis
- Pyomyositis
- Kawasaki disease
- Diskitis
- Meningitis
- Synovitis usually has only low-grade fever but if the child has additional viral infection, say of respiratory tract or urinary tract, then there may be accompanied high grade fever also.

Evaluation:

Laboratory studies: Investigations should be used to exclude or confirm suspected diagnoses based on history and physical examination. CBC count and ESR or C-reactive protein (CRP) level are the most initial investigations. A WBC count greater than 12,000 cells/mm and ESR greater than 40 mm/h in combination with an inability to bear weight and history of fever, commonly known as the Kocher criteria, have been suggested as diagnostic criteria to distinguish septic arthritis from transient synovitis in patients with acute hip pain and guide arthrocentesis.

A blood culture should be considered for patients with limp and fever.

Plain radiographs should include views of the entire limb, bearing weight when possible. Consider obtaining films of the contralateral, unaffected side for comparison and detailing subtle changes. Spine films may be indicated with back pain, midline tenderness, or any neurologic complaints.

Bone scan: Technetium 99m–labeled methylene diphosphonate 3-phase scan consisting of a blood flow, blood pool, and delayed imaging phases is the current recommended protocol to detect early osteomyelitis, diskitis, stress fractures, and osteoid osteomas. Scintigraphy is 84–100% sensitive and 70–96% specific for osteomyelitis. Scanning too early may be reported as false-negative as results may not become positive until 48–72 hours into an inflammatory process. Joint aspiration should be done after scanning, else it may cause false-positive scintigraphy results.

Ultrasonography is useful for diagnosing soft tissue and joint pathology with evaluation possible both statically and dynamically. It is particularly useful in younger children in whom the skeleton is incompletely ossified. Ultrasonography can confirm the presence of a joint effusion and can guide diagnostic or therapeutic aspiration.

Magnetic resonance imaging: It has the advantage of multiplanar imaging capabilities and no radiation exposure. MRI is the imaging modality of choice for evaluating internal joint derangement, soft tissue or bony infection, tumors, and osteonecrosis. It is also helpful for imaging the brain and spinal cord.

Cerebrospinal fluid: Meningitis has been associated with limping, probably due to meningismus. A cerebrospinal fluid (CSF) analysis should be obtained if meningitis is strongly suspected (i.e., symptoms including fever, headache, and meningismus).

Arthrocentesis: Aspiration of synovial fluid from the hip, knee, ankle, metatarsophalangeal, or interphalangeal joints should be performed as clinically indicated. Ultrasound-guided aspiration can be performed by the bedside by trained orthopedic surgeons, and serial aspiration is a treatment modality that can obviate the need for hip arthrotomy.

Treatment: Emergency care of the limping patient with fever should be directed to relief of acute pain, identification of the cause, and initiation of therapy for the source of the limping. In cases of suspected osteomyelitis, diskitis, or septic joint, intravenous antibiotics should be initiated as soon as diagnosis is confirmed.

After diagnosis, treatment is directed to identified pathology.
- For osteomyelitis, kindly see Answers to Questions 87 and 88.
- For septic arthritis, kindly see Answer to Question 94.
- Diskitis and meningitis are managed in high dependency unit in consultation with infection care personnel and experts.

298. Enumerate the differential diagnosis of limping child (10 years old). Differentiate between a case of septic arthritis and transient synovitis.

Ans:

Differential diagnosis: [of acute painful limp (kindly see answer below also)]
- Septic arthritis
- Transient synovitis
- Tuberculosis of hip joint
- Legg-Calve-Perthes disease (LCPD)
- Slipped capital femoral epiphysis (SCFE)
- Osteomyelitis
- Juvenile RA.

Differences: **Table 2.17.8** shows the difference between septic arthritis and transient synovitis.

TABLE 2.17.8: Difference between septic arthritis and transient synovitis.

Characteristic	Septic arthritis	Transient synovitis
Fever	+	–
Limitation of movements	+++	+
Failure to thrive	+	–
Local raised temperature	+++	+
Constancy of symptoms	Pain and fever increases, if no treatment done	Symptoms remain more or less constant
Preceding ailments	Usually none or pyogenic focus may be present	Viral diseases like common cold or diarrhea
CRP levels	More than 20 mg/L	Raised but mild
MRI	Reduced perfusion of the femoral epiphysis	–
Radiographs	Osteopenia is marked	Mild osteopenia
Spontaneous resolution	Occasional	Often
Residual changes	Often if untreated (see squeal of septic arthritis)	Never (as of now, some authors consider this to be a prelude to Perthes, etc., but need substantiation)

299. Discuss differential diagnosis and investigation in an 8-year-old child with persistent limp.

Ans: Differential diagnosis

Limb length discrepancy

Neoplasia:
- Osteoblastoma
- Osteoid osteoma
- Malignant bone neoplasia—osteosarcoma, Ewing's, and leukemia.

Congenital condition:
- Clubfoot

- Proximal focal femoral deficiency
- Developmental dysplasia of hip
- Congenital dislocation of knee
- Anterolateral tibial deformity
- Coxa vara.

Developmental conditions:
- Perthes disease
- Slipped upper femoral epiphysis
- Genu varum/valgum.
- Infection—cellulitis, pyomyositis, osteomyelitis, viral myositis, and soft tissue abscess.

Trauma:
- Child abuse
- Fracture.

Intra-articular conditions:
- Discoid meniscus
- Hemophilia
- Lyme disease
- Septic arthritis or its sequel
- TB hip
- Acute rheumatic fever
- Juvenile RA
- Reactive arthritis
- Transient synovitis.

Neuromuscular conditions:
- Cerebral palsy
- Poliomyelitis
- Meningitis
- Muscular dystrophy
- Myelomeningocele.

Spinal conditions:
- Diskitis
- Spinal cord tumors
- Pott's spine.

General:
- Chondromalacia patellae
- Osgood-Schlatter disease
- Sever disease and other osteochondrosis
- Jumper's knee
- Psoas abscess
- Appendicitis
- Neuroblastoma
- Stress fracture
- Sickle cell disease.

Approach to diagnosis: A detailed history and physical examination, in addition to appropriate laboratory tests and imaging, are essential for making a correct diagnosis. Kindly vide **Flowcharts 2.17.1 and 2.17.2**.

Flowchart 2.17.1: Approach to differential diagnoses in a patient with painless gait.

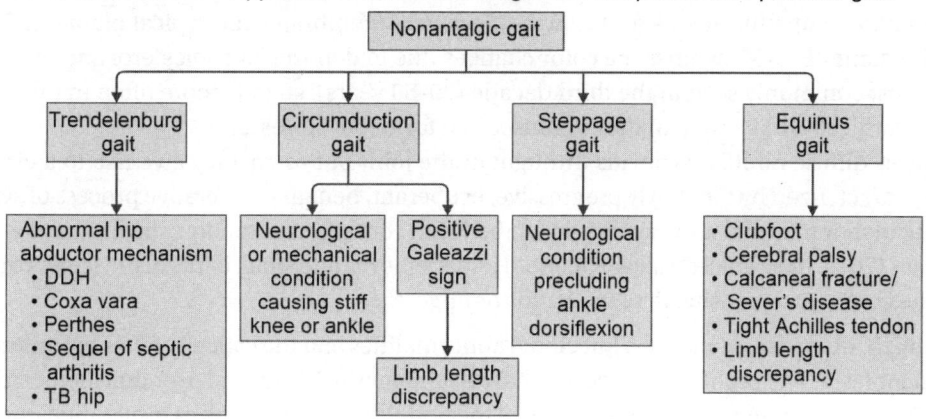

Flowchart 2.17.2: Approach to differential diagnoses in a patient with antalgic gait.

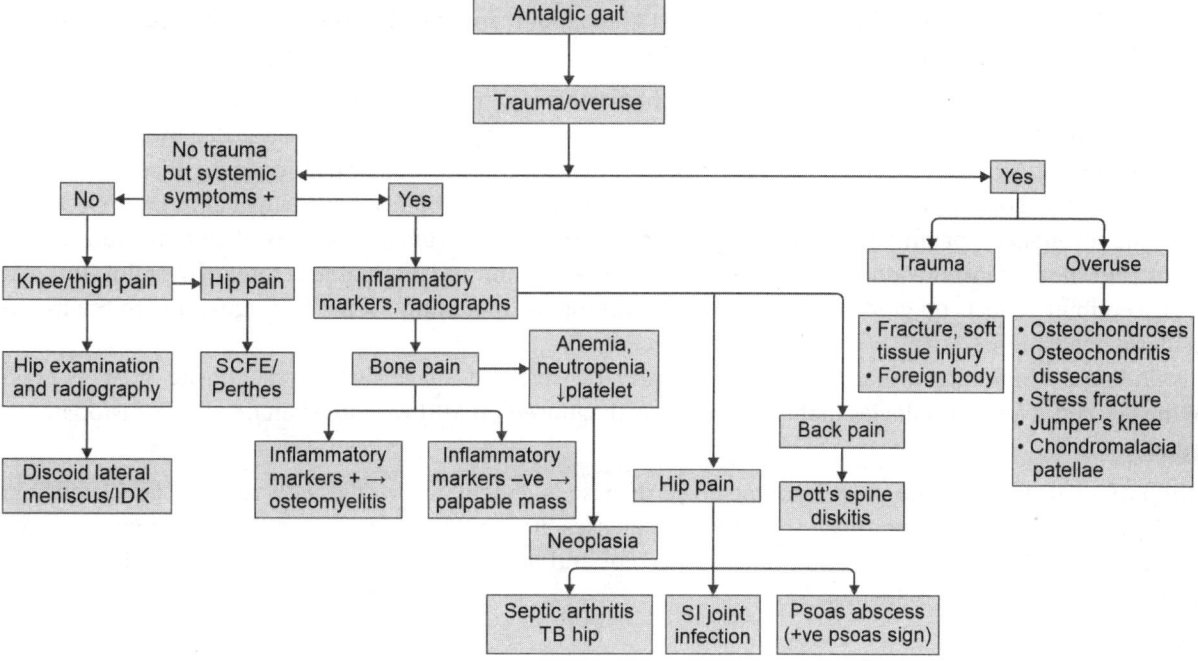

300. Pathology, clinical features and management of synovial chondromatosis.

Ans: Please read Chapter no. 5.

301. Orthopedic manifestations of neurofibromatosis.

Ans: Please read Chapter no. 5.

I. PVNS (Q302–304)

302. Explain PVNS.

Ans: Pigmented villonodular synovitis (PVNS) is an intra-articular locally destructive fibrohistiocytic proliferation that is considered to be a diffuse counterpart of GCT of tendon sheath. It is an uncommon and benign proliferative disease of the synovial joint, synovial bursa, and tendon sheath seen within 3–8 cases per million per year general population.

Of the described two forms—*diffuse* form affecting often the synovium and the *localized* form affecting the tendon sheaths and bursae, the former is far more common in joints and now described as PVNS while the latter is far more common at extra-articular sites and described as giant cell tumor (GCT) tendon sheath or bursa. The term PVNS was used by Jaffe to describe idiopathic villous overgrowth of synovial membrane and typical pigmentation usually found in a single joint. The name "PVNS" signifies the color changes due to deposits of cholesterol and hemosiderin on gross examination. It is most commonly seen in the third decade (20–50 years), slightly more often in men. The diffuse form tends to occur a bit early (20–40 years) than the circumscribed form (30–50 years).

Typically, it causes diffuse nodular synovitis throughout the joint but *rarely* may give rise to a circumscribed focal nodular form. It is characterized by the slowly progressive, exuberant, benign proliferative process of synovial tissue and is usually monoarticular. It may affect the synovium of the joints, bursae, and tendon sheaths, and is most commonly observed in the knees (76%), hips, ankles, calcaneocuboid joints, elbows, and small joints of the fingers or toes. The disease may also involve the common flexor sheath of the hands or fingers.

Pathogenesis: Although, the cause is unknown but clonal abnormalities and the capacity for autonomous growth suggest PVNS to be a true neoplasm. The proliferative nodules have a tendency to bleed, and over time hemosiderin is deposited in the joint giving rise to the characteristic pigmentation of the nodules and the "crank case oil" appearance of the affected joint fluid.

Currently, autogenous proliferation is considered to be the primary (i.e., a neoplasm) event rather than ascribing other causes. A breakpoint in the CSF-1 gene at the 1p13 breakpoint and translocation at the *COL6A3* gene at 2q35 are the current contenders found in the development of PVNS.

Radiology: The nodules cause appearance of recurrent hemarthroses (hyperdense effusion), smooth cortical saucerized erosions, and subchondral cysts on X-ray. The joint space is initially preserved but later degenerative changes of osteoarthritis appear. MRI has proven very useful to make the diagnosis because of the paramagnetic effects of hemosiderin (dark on T1 and T2). Localized PVNS of knee is commonly seen near the Hoffa's fat pad lying behind it.

Magnetic resonance imaging easily demonstrates a globular mass artifact with frond-like appearance of folded synovium. MRI shows joint effusion with dark signal lining the synovium and internal structures of the joint. This material shows susceptibility effects on gradient echo imaging resulting in "blooming" of the low signal due to the iron in the hemosiderin deposition.

This finding of "blooming artifact" and a low T1- and T2-weighted image signal is diagnostic of PVNS making it one of the few soft tissue pathologies that can be directly diagnosed on MRI without even needing a histopathological confirmation.

Surgical pathology: Grossly, the mass from localized disease is chocolate-colored with rubbery consistency and is encapsulated lacking any villonodular structure. The masses are nodular and may be large or small, soft or hard. The synovium in diffuse variant is red to brownish in color and has numerous large, finger-like villi that fuse to form pedunculated nodules (often more than 5 cm).

Microscopically:
- *Villi stroma:* Cellular, diffuse, expansile, and somewhat infiltrative sheets of small ovoid, polyhedral or spindle-like synovial cells admixed with larger cells
- The proliferative synovium invades adjacent cartilage and bone. Cleft-like and blood-filled spaces are relatively prominent. In the diffuse form usually two types of mononuclear cells are seen—the small histiocyte-like cells and larger cells.
- Hemosiderin granules and lipids are prominent in macrophages. Multinucleated giant cells may be present.
- The smaller cells are histiocyte like and often display grooved nuclei. Sheets of foam cells can also be observed.
- Mitoses can be quite frequent in rare malignant cases, showing more than 20 mitoses per 10 high-power fields (HPF) and necrosis. The mitosis, however, is not correlated with metastatic potential.
- Chromosomal studies show that translocations involving chromosome 1p11–13 are common in PVNS and GCT of tendon sheath.

Clinical course: Pigmented villonodular synovitis is considered a benign disease. Localized PVNS occurs most often in the hands, but is also seen in knee and ankle where the diagnosis is usually made while ruling out other causes for swelling. Symptoms may be mild and intermittent and may be present for years before the patient seeks medical attention. Diffuse

form is much more aggressive to present with, although patient may still present after 9–12 months of onset of swelling that commonly precedes pain.
- Clinically, PVNS presents with insidious onset of swelling and pain in one joint, most commonly the knee.
  - Limp usually arises later due to advancement of disease.
  - Often the joint as a whole is swollen by the swelling and effusion.
  - On examination, a firm to hard swelling that fills the joint is clinically palpable.
  - Tenderness as a whole is mild to moderate with minimal localized inflammatory signs.
  - Radiographs may show joint space narrowing, erosions, and subchondral cysts.
- Mechanical symptoms in the form of locking, snapping or limitation of movement (usually extension) are more often seen with the rare localized variety of disease.
  - Localized disease may present as a small intra-articular tumor.
  - Less common than the diffuse form.
  - Does not show similar destructive joint changes.
  - Aspirate may be normal color due to less frequent hemarthrosis.

Diagnosis: Ultrasound-guided biopsy is recommended for histopathological diagnosis else percutaneous biopsy from suprapatellar pouch may be taken.

Treatment: Patient's anxiety and satisfaction after complete excision of the localized lesion makes this the most commonly used approach. Extra-articular lesions are rationally treated by open excision of the lesion while for intra-articular lesion open or arthroscopic approach needs to be decided by the access of the lesion by arthroscopy and experience of the surgeon and his comfort. Lesions behind the ACL and far posterior lesions may be treated by open arthrotomy while for posterior approach posterolateral/medial approaches may be still used. The treatment for diffuse form usually consists of complete synovectomy. Partial synovectomy is liable to recur with vengeance.

The disease has a tendency to recur (around 20–30%), sometimes requiring extensive synovectomy and total joint arthroplasty (for aggressive end-stage disease). Complete macroscopic resection, female gender, and fresh cases were associated with better local control of the disease while incomplete excision, mitotic activity, bone involvement and knee location versus hip is associated with increased incidence of disease recurrence.

External beam radiation may be used to control recurrent disease but is not a favorable option for primary treatment due to intractable complications like joint stiffness, skin necrosis, and permanent changes and development of secondary sarcoma. Doses of 30–35 Gy in 15 divided fractions have been used (higher doses of 50 Gy in 25 fractions is possibly overcure) either as primary treatment or adjuvant to surgical management with recurrence rates much below surgical management. Complications, typically the risk of secondary sarcoma that develops at mean 7 years are the major limitations to its use. Intra-articular yttrium-90 has been also used but is associated with serious complications of skin necrosis and draining sinus.

Monoclonal antibodies [imatinib, nilotinib, emactuzumab (RG7155), and pexidartinib] targeting the CSF-1/CSF-1R axis for treatment is underway. Emactuzumab had good response within a few weeks but with significant adverse effects. Till date none of the systemic treatments have been approved for treatment of PVNS but if future favorable response is seen, they may serve as important adjuvant (to surgery) or even first-line treatment for this disorder either for treatment of primary advanced disease or recurrent/intractable cases.

Amputation is mutilating but is last resort for severe intractable disease.

303. Wound ballistics.
Ans: Please read Chapter no. 4C.

304. Discuss the pathoanatomy of wound ballistics.
Ans:
- The *skin* around wounding site exhibits vasospasm, which produces blanching; this area usually do not get revascularize for several hours after injury. An impact velocity of only 150–170 feet per second is required to penetrate skin. Cherry-hue appearance is a clue to close-range injury of underlying muscle due to carboxyhemoglobin, formed by carbon

monoxide release during combustion. If the loss of blood supply is a criterion for excision, the transitory nature of the blanching shows that viable tissue would be sacrificed in this area if evaluated soon after wounding.
- *Muscle* that is touched by the projectile in the permanent tract has a microscopic rim of tissue that is actually necrotic. If the blood supply to the muscle remains intact, it can heal overtime without surgical intervention. The area of cell death sloughs and, as long as the wound can drain, will heal up spontaneously. Microscopically, there are disrupted skeletal muscle fibers and capillaries. After a period, there is leukocyte infiltration followed by inflammation and healing.
- *Bony injury:* Gunshot injuries to the extremities are usually associated with bony injuries (fracture). There are two mechanisms of fractures occurring, first and commonly when the projectile strikes bone directly or, rarely, indirectly by the temporary cavitation:
    1. Direct fractures occur when a projectile strikes the bone. Because of the density and relative inelastic behavior of bone, fracture line propagation may occur well beyond the area crushed by the projectile itself, leading to bone comminution and the production of secondary missiles from the bone itself. Because the secondary missiles of bone disrupt tissue before it is stretched by the temporary cavity, this has the effect of increasing comminution around the bullet path, and might even cause increased soft-tissue disruption, reminiscent of the previously mentioned synergism between bullet fragmentation and temporary cavity stretch.
    2. Indirect fractures may occur when a projectile passes close to the bone in soft tissue and a strain occurs to such a degree as to cause a fracture. Indirect fractures are almost always simple. Clinically, indirect fractures to bone are rare compared with those formed when bone is struck directly by the projectile. They may be of further two types:
        a. *Divot fractures:* These are eccentric perforations of a diaphyseal long bone; they may be occult complete fractures.
        b. *Drill hole:* It occurs when a bullet or its fragment completely pierces both the cortices, with minimal comminution around the bullet tract. More extensive injury may be present than apparent on plain radiographs, such fractures may be treated as complete fractures unless confirmed by CT.

The possible sources of contamination of wound include:
- Combination of soil, clothing, etc., carried by the projectile. High-energy fragments tend to shred the clothes that are then carried into wound by temporary cavitation.
- Skin
- The bullet shell
- The barrel of the gun
- Peripheral material in contact with the wound—although less common, from the exit wound, the vacuum in the temporary cavity pulls foreign material into the wound.

J. Tourniquet (Q305)

305. What is pneumatic tourniquet? Discuss its uses, complications, and safety guidelines.

Ans: *Pneumatic tourniquet and its uses:* Operations on the extremities are made easier by the use of a tourniquet as they provide good control over blood spillage and oozing into the surgical wound. The following types of tourniquets are in common usage:
- *Pneumatic tourniquet:*
    - Automatic continuous pressure controlled and regulated
    - Hand pump with pressure gauge.
- Esmarch bandage
- Martin rubber sheet.

Complications:
- *Asymptomatic/symptomatic pulmonary embolism:* The embolus after migration remains static till tourniquet deflation and then quickly travels to lungs causing embolism within 1 minute after tourniquet release.
- *Chemical burn* from solutions seeping underneath the tourniquet.
- *Superficial slough/abrasion* of the skin usually occurs at the upper margin of the tourniquet near the gluteal fold.

- *Tourniquet paralysis* (from mechanical effect of tourniquet pressure) is caused by insufficient oxygenation of the tissues and nerves. It may result from one of the following scenarios:
  - Excessive pressure used for inflation
  - Insufficient pressure causing passive congestion of the limb
  - Prolonged inflation of tourniquet on (>3 hours)
  - Tourniquet application without considering local anatomy.
- *Post-tourniquet syndrome* is a common reaction to prolonged ischemia seen over too long periods of tourniquet usages. The limb develops edema, joint stiffness, pallor, motor weakness, and subjective numbness without objective anesthesia. This complication is specifically related to duration of ischemia and not to the mechanical effect.
- *Compartment syndrome* from microvascular occlusion is seen more in previously compromised limbs that go unrecognized.
- *Rhabdomyolysis* from use of tourniquet is extremely rare and few reports exist.
- Vascular complications after tourniquet use occur in predisposed patients like those with severe arteriosclerosis or prosthetic vascular grafts.
- *Intraoperative bleeding:* This develops from venous congestion resulting from poorly fitting tourniquet.
- *Reperfusion syndrome:* This is a lately recognized complication. Initially only ischemia was considered to be the cause of tissue damage. Reperfusion injury occurs by the interaction of free radicals (hydroxyl radical), endothelial factors, and neutrophils. These damage proteins, DNA, and lipids.
  - Accumulation of lactic acid, sodium (associated with water ingress into cell), and calcium (causes mitochondrial disruption) are basic alterations of anaerobic metabolism.
  - Reperfusion removes the accumulated toxic components and replenishes the energy supply to cells. But these produce simultaneously collateral damage by causing systemic toxicity and sensitive organs show depressed function under influence, reoxygenation causes formation of reactive oxygen species.
  - *Formation of superoxide radical:* This is converted into hydrogen peroxide by superoxide dismutases (SOD) which in turn is destroyed by catalase into water. These free radicals produce the thiobarbituric acid reactive substances and diene conjugates causing extensive myocyte damage. Neutrophils release proteolytic enzymes and peroxidases into the circulation.

Safety Guidelines:

Before applying a tourniquet:
- Regular maintenance checks and marking the date last checked (preferably weekly).
- Aneroid pressure gauges for hand held tourniquets should be checked against calibration devices monthly.
- Check cuff, pipes, and connection for air leaks and do a thorough visual inspection.
- Pressure should remain constant over time.
- Cuff length should exceed the limb circumference by 7–15 cm and be properly chosen for equidistribution of pressure.
- Cuff width should be matched appropriately to the patient's age/size (discussed below).
- *Use caution while tourniquet application in following patients as they are at high risk at exsanguination:*
  - Morbidly obese patients (high pressure causes subcutaneous fat amputation).
  - Prolonged immobilization prior to surgery—weak osteoporotic bones may fracture during Esmarch application.
  - Patients with deep vein thrombosis (DVT)—embolus may dislodge during exsanguination.
  - Isolated limb malignancies and infections—infection/pus may migrate and go into circulation.
  - Patients with left ventricular dysfunction—may load the cardiovascular system excessively.

During use:
- Monitor the pressure gauges continuously to check variations.
- Cuffs should be positioned at the level of maximum limb circumference.
- The tourniquet should be adequately padded using cotton or soft foam sheet; newer silicone sheets may also be used.
- After application do not rotate the cuff.
- Apply an adhesive tape on the distal edge of tourniquet to prevent liquid solutions from seeping under the cuff.

- Regulate the tourniquet inflation time and pressure according to patient's age and comorbidities.
- Surgeons should be kept informed of the inflation times.
- Document the duration and use of tourniquet in patient's notes.

After tourniquet use:
- Thoroughly clean the reusable cuffs to prevent cross infection.
- The limb should be thoroughly inspected for signs of prolonged usage and inadequate pressure transmission in the form of developing blisters at the site of application of tourniquet, distal vascularity should be restored before shifting patient.
- Gently massage the site of application of tourniquet. For tourniquet application on fingers and toes, rubber ring tourniquet or a tourniquet made from a glove finger that is rolled onto the digit is not recommended. Instances have been noted when it had been inadvertently left in place under a dressing, resulting in loss of the digit. The alternative is application of glove finger or Penrose drain that can be looped around the proximal portion of the digit, stretched, and secured with a hemostat. This is a much safer method for surgery on hand, especially for digits.

K. Orthopedic Sutures (Q306)

306. What are the commonly used absorbable sutures in orthopedics? Compare their properties.

Ans: Commonly used absorbable sutures in orthopedics have been given in **Table 2.17.9**.

TABLE 2.17.9: Absorbable sutures in orthopedics.		
Plain catgut	Sheep/cattle intestine	This absorbs within a week so that it is useful only for securing fast healing areas like mucous membranes. The tissue reactivity is very high and knot security is poor
Chromic catgut	This is treated plain catgut	The suture has high tissue reactivity but less than plain catgut and has higher knot security. The suture absorbs in around 3–4 weeks
Vicryl	Polyglactin 910	This braided suture has average reactivity and knot security. The suture usually absorbs in 3 weeks (50% reduction in strength)
Vicryl-OS	Treated Vicryl with antibacterial coating (blue stained usually)	This is specially used in orthopedic surgery and has average tissue reactivity. The average half-life of strength in tissue is 3 weeks
Monocryl	Poliglecaprone 25 and Irgacare MP	It has good knot security and low tissue reactivity. It is a monofilament suture that absorbs in 1–2 weeks
Dexon	Polyglycolic acid	It has good knot security and low tissue reactivity. It is a braided suture that absorbs in 2–3 weeks
Maxon	Polyglyconate	This suture absorbs in around 2–3 weeks and has average knot security and tissue reactivity
PDS or PDS-II (Orthocord®)	Polydioxanone	This has low to minimal tissue reactivity but the knot security is also low. The suture absorbs in nearly 2–3 months

L. Anatomy-based Questions (Q307–310)

307. Discuss iliotibial band.

Ans: *Anatomy:* The fascia lata is thickened laterally where it forms a 5 cm long band called the iliotibial tract/band. Superiorly the tract splits into 2 layers. The superficial lamina is attached to tubercle of iliac crest, and deep lamina to the capsule of hip joint. Inferiorly, the tract is attached to a smooth area on anterior surface of the lateral condyle of tibia.

The importance of iliotibial tract is as follows:
- Two important muscles are inserted into its upper part, between the superficial and deep laminae. These are the three-fourths part of the gluteus maximus, and the tensor fascia lata.
- The iliotibial tract stabilizes the knee both in extension and in partial flexion; and is therefore used constantly during walking and running. In leaning forward with slightly flexed knees, the tract is the main support of the knee against gravity.

- It is frequently involved in polio leading to contracture of band that in turn causes triple deformity of knee and FABER deformity at hip. Surgical procedures (Yount's release at knee.) are done to incise band to correct deformity.

Clinical test for evaluation of iliotibial band (ITB) contracture—Ober's test.

(Lateral decubitus position; knee flexion to 90° → hip abduction 40° → hip extension as permitted → gentle hip adduction; inability to adduct hip indicates tight ITB.)

308. Discuss ITB contracture in polio.

Ans: Kindly see answer above.

309. Anatomy of ITB and its effect of contracture on the lower limb. How do you clinically detect its contracture?

Ans: Kindly see the answer above.

310. Discuss extensor mechanism of knee.

Ans:

The extensor mechanism is formed by the following components:

- Patellofemoral articulation
- Quadriceps apparatus—muscle and quadriceps tendon
- Knee capsule with retinaculum and ligaments of extensor mechanism
- Patellar tendon.

The patellofemoral articulation is a part of the larger extensor mechanism of knee **(Fig. 2.17.3)**. It is formed by femoral trochlea and patella gliding in it. Trochlear groove consists of a shallow depression (5-6 mm) bound by the medial and the lateral femoral articular surfaces. The patella develops in the retinacular layer of the extensor mechanism and serves as insertion to vastus intermedius proximally and as origin of the deeper layer of the patellar tendon distally. The articular surface of the patella contains a broader lateral facet (larger), a medial facet (smaller) and a still smaller, more medial "odd" facet (far medial) separated by a vertical central ridge.

Quadriceps mechanism: The quadriceps muscle group consists of seven discrete heads that is responsible not only for extension at the knee but also stabilizing the patellofemoral joint dynamically:

- Articularis genu (deepest head) is the only muscle that does not insert directly into the patella. The muscle prevents impingement of the superior synovial plica between patella and femoral sulcus by dynamically raising it.
- The vastus intermedius originates through a broad origin on the anterior femoral shaft and inserts into the superior pole of the patella.
- The rectus femoris (two heads) parallel originates on the anteroinferior iliac spine (AIIS) and blends into the central tendon of the quadriceps.
    - The rectus femoris tendon is 8–10 cm in length, triangular in shape with insertion 3–5 cm in width at the superior pole of patella. A bursa separates the rectus tendon from the intermedius tendon along the entire length. It crosses two joints and causes flexion at hip while extension at the knee.
- *The vastus lateralis originates from the anterolateral aspect of the femur and lateral intermuscular septum:*
    - It makes up approximately 50% of the bulk of the entire quadriceps muscle group. Its angle of insertion is approximately 22–45° laterally off the axis of the femur (producing lateral displacing moment at patella).
- The vastus medialis originates from the anteromedial aspect of the femur and medial intermuscular septum. Its angle of insertion is approximately 50° medially off the axis of the femur (producing medial displacing moment at patella, balancing lateral displacement partially). It is responsible for last 10–15° of knee extension.
- The VMO originates from the adductor tubercle and distal medial intermuscular septum. Its angle of insertion at superomedial border of patella is oriented obliquely 55–70° medially off the axis of the femur (producing medial displacing moment at patella—its primary function is in balancing patella dynamically against the force of vastus lateralis).

- The rectus femoris, along with the VMO, vastus medialis, and vastus lateralis terminates in an aponeurosis that merges into the anterior-third joint capsule forming the retinacular layer:
  - The retinacular layer is a continuous layer on the superficial aspect of patella. Distally it extends to the tibial periosteum and invests the superficial portion of the patellar tendon.

  Knee capsule and ligaments: The capsular ligaments spanning patellofemoral joint are studied by dividing them into thirds:

  The anterior-third capsular ligaments are formed by the medial and lateral retinacular ligaments of the extensor mechanism that form a sling action. They also attach to the anterior horns of the menisci but are devoid of femoral attachments.

  The extensor mechanism, tendinous and capsular structures also provide dynamic stability to the patellofemoral joint and are organized into following layers:
- A thin peritendinous membrane, the arciform layer (superficial) spans from the sartorial fascia medially and the biceps fascia laterally and embrace along the patella and patellar tendon anteriorly. They serve a proprioceptive role.
- *The retinacular (intermediate) layer is made up of:*
  - Anterior-third capsule and its condensations.
  - Iliopatellar ligament laterally is a condensation of retinaculum lying on the anterolateral aspect of the knee. It has surgical significance in stabilizing the patella.
- Patellofemoral ligaments course along the distal and deep border of the VMO and vastus lateralis obliquus. The muscles have a dynamic role in stabilizing patella in the region. The patellofemoral ligaments originate from medial or lateral isometric points on femur and insert on the corresponding superior poles of the patella.

Patellar tendon:
- The patellar tendon extends from the inferior pole of the patella and inserts on the tibial tubercle.
- The infrapatellar tendon bursa and fat pad separate the patellar tendon from the underlying tibia.
- The patellar tendon comprises of a superficial layer (continuous with the retinacular layer) and a deeper layer—the deep layer of the extensor mechanism. While operating on patella these layers are more or less confluent and inseparable.
- The infrapatellar fat pad (IFP) (Hoffa's fat pad) is attached to ligamentum mucosum (a persistent plica—discussed below). The pad is often inflamed by mechanical misalignment (females), injury, microtrauma (Hoffa's disease) and may also undergo ankylosis causing extension block and secondary contracture of the patellar tendon producing limitation in flexion.

M. Psoas Abscess (Q311–313)
311. Discuss psoas abscess.

Ans: Tubercular affection of lumbar or dorsolumbar spine typically produces psoas abscess (though primary infection with other aerobic/anaerobic infections may also produce infection but is very rare). The tubercular cold abscess may track to form paravertebral abscess palpable posteriorly on one side of spine or may travel along the intercostal, ilioinguinal, and iliohypogastric nerves.
- It may go to Petit's triangle along the flat muscles of abdominal wall or in the ischiorectal fossa along the internal pudendal nerve.
- Posteriorly it may track to buttock along the gluteal nerve.
- Anteriorly it may form typical psoas abscess that may point anywhere from abdomen to groin to thigh to even popliteal region.
- If it develops a connection in the inferior abdominal wall, it may form an inverted horseshoe abscess also (uncommon presentation).

Psoas abscess is as a rule associated with detectable tuberculous disease of the vertebral column from dorsal 10th vertebra to the sacrum, or disease of sacroiliac joint, pelvic bones, and hip joint. Psoas abscesses can lead to pitfalls in diagnosis; they can give rise to "hip flexion deformity" the so-called "pseudo-hip" flexion deformity. The flexion deformity of the hip joint due to spasm of iliopsoas muscle does not show any limitation of external and internal rotations of the hip joint when tested in the position of flexion deformity.

Radiological manifestation of psoas abscess is unilateral or infrequently bilateral widening of the psoas shadow. However, it needs an excellent quality X-rays to detect any bulging of the lateral border of the psoas. MRI and CT scan may demonstrate an abscess contained within the psoas sheath much before it can be clinically palpated as an iliopsoas abscess in the iliac fossa.

A "psoas abscess" can be aspirated through the Petit's triangle whereas the iliopsoas abscess is aspirable through the Petit's triangle as well as through the iliac fossa. Diagnosis of an abscess only on roentgenographic findings is less accurate as many of the densities giving a radiological diagnosis of an abscess may be only absorbed abscesses replaced by fibrous tissue, calcified inspissated matter or granulation tissue.

Psoas abscess can be drained along the pointing regions or along the anterolateral region of iliac crest.

312. Discuss (A) three-dimensional (3D) and four-dimensional (4D) printing.

Ans: 3D printing: It was developed initially by Charles W Hull in 1986 based on techniques of topography assessment and photosculpture. The objects are build layer-by-layer based on the digital drawings obtained through special imaging tools (usually a 3D scanner) and software, by a process called "additive manufacturing." A computer-controlled robotic system is used commonly to create 3D objects through layer-by-layer addition of material.

The technique is principally utilized currently in medical field to print *in vivo* abnormal objects *in vitro*, so that independent detailed study can be done to formulate surgical plans and understand how to best deal with the problems encountered. For example, using images from echocardiography for abnormal cardiac valves (say aortic or mitral), one can draw the valves *in vitro* with a pliable material that can be studied in detail by a cardiac surgeon and planned for further treatment. Steps are being made to develop custom-made orthopedic implants (replacing the diseased or absent tissue!). This process is termed biofabrication—"process involving automated generation of biologically functional products with structural organization from living cells, bioactive molecules, biomaterials, cell aggregates such as microtissues, or hybrid cell material constructs, through bioprinting or bioassembly and subsequent tissue maturation processes." One can synthesize complex tissues by depositing bioinks to couture tissue to be repaired. "Bioprinting" or printing of biological tissues has been made possible by advances in automation, miniaturization, and computer-aided designing along with the development of bioinks and cell systems that can survive in there.

Perspectives: Four-step process—
1. *Imaging and data processing:* To obtain high-resolution images for better accuracy; so pertinent X-rays, CT scans, and MRI are sought for.
2. *Selection of printing technique:*
   - Fused deposition modeling
   - Selective laser sintering
   - Pneumatic extrusion printing
   - Inkjet printing
   - Stereolithography
3. *Identifying the biomaterials and components:* The commonly used materials include metals, bioceramics, and polymers (both synthetic and natural). Metals such as titanium that have high biocompatibility which are used mostly for implant synthesis due to favorable mechanical properties. Bioceramics such as hydroxyapatite, bioglass, and calcium phosphate are good for bone restoration and substitution, as they are osteogenic, porous, maintain shape, and promote cell proliferation on surface. Polymers such as collagen, chitosan, hyaluronic acid (HA), silk proteins, gelatins, and alginates are all used as hydrogels.
4. Bioprinting

Applications in orthopedics:
- Modeling of pathological bone
- Patient-specific surgical instruments
- Patient-specific implants
- Cartilage regeneration
- Bone regeneration

- Coverage of open wounds
- Meniscus substitution
- Connective tissue, tendon, and muscle
- Regeneration
- Synthesis of prosthetics and orthoses

4D printing: Also known as 4D-bioprinting, shape-morphing systems, functional printing, active origami. Simply speaking 4D printing is 3D printing that transforms over time when removed from printer. The stimulus for the transformation can come from various sources such as light, heat, and electricity/magnetic field. The printed objects change their shape dynamically based on needs and demands of the situation. It is like printing function into the material that will execute once activated. The meta-material structure is created by combining different materials that provide structural responses when activated by external stimuli.

Differences between 3D and 4D printing is given in **Table 2.17.10**.

TABLE 2.17.10: Differences between 3D and 4D printing.

Characteristic	3D printing	4D printing
Dynamic shape change	Not a feature	Changes color, shape, function, etc.
Materials used	Thermoplastic, metals and alloys, biomaterials, nanoparticles	Smart materials—shape-memory alloys and shape memory polymers, hydrophilic polymers, biomaterials and plant oil
Printing requirements	3D printer, fused deposition modeling, selective laser sintering	3D printer and multimaterial 3D printers

Applications of 4D printing:
- *Medical and healthcare:* 4D-printed splints that can automatically expand up to double the size with the need—pediatric splints and prosthesis. Development futuristic splints that can be applied on the lib directly and they self-assemble into casts/slabs. Development of foldable molecules that can release drugs as needed (say releasing antipyretics if fever occurs). Development of artificial tissues that can expand or contract or self-assemble on implantation. Targeted drug delivery that would discharge the drug on encountering the target molecule.
- *Aerospace:* Shield for spacecraft antennas and spacesuits
- *Apparels:* Developing a shoe that can self-assemble—avoiding cumbersome process
- *Automotive:* Expandable materials in response to air pulses

313. Discuss the (A) radiation hazards in orthopedics and (B) their preventive measures in orthopedics.

Ans: Radiation hazard in inherent to orthopedic surgeries as the use of fluoroscopy has become a common place. Most of the osteosyntheses for trauma and some planned reconstructions need fluoroscopy assistance to better implant placement and improve anatomy. Fluoroscopy uses X-rays, so radiation exposure for the surgeon and staff will be imperative. Certain orthopedic procedures are associated with higher radiation doses; these include open reduction and internal fixation (ORIF) of hip fractures, femoral and tibial intramedullary nailing, and spinal cases. The X-rays passing through the patient interact with bone and soft tissue within the patient resulting in different patterns of X-ray distribution. X-rays are also deflected during the penetration and continue on with lower energy. This pattern of deflection, or scatter, produces a field of radiation, that is, responsible for the incidental radiation exposure to the surrounding staff.

Radiation hazards:
Radiation damage occurs at the cellular level in living tissues. Rapidly replicating cell components such as DNA and cell membranes are the most susceptible to damage from radiation. This may occur by both direct and indirect mechanisms. Direct damage occurs as energy is absorbed and molecular bonds are broken resulting in cell death or mutations which are the initial step in radiation-induced carcinogenesis. Indirect damage results from ionization of water molecules generating free radicals that disrupt bonds and commonly result into long-term effects of radiation. The thyroid, eyes, hands, and gonads are among the most sensitive organs to radiation exposure. The eyes may exhibit the first effects of chronic radiation exposure in the form of cataracts. 85% of papillary carcinomas of the thyroid are thought to be radiation induced. A surgeon's hands have the greatest exposure risk due to their constant proximity to the radiation beam. Due to

these risks, the International Commission on Radiological Protection established dosage limits for radiation exposure. The maximum annual dose limit is 20 mSv for the body, 150 mSv for the thyroid and eyes, and 500 mSv for the hands.

Radiation damage can have deterministic and stochastic effects. Deterministic effects of radiation have a clear relationship between the exposure and the effect. These typically result when very large dosages are received in a short amount of time. The effects are characterized by nonlinear dose responses, with a threshold dose below which the effect is not observed. These effects arise within a few days and may manifest over years. Examples of deterministic effects include erythema, skin and tissue burns, cataract formation, sterility, radiation sickness, and death. Below a certain threshold of exposure, there is no increased risk of radiation-induced effects such as cancer or genetic mutation. The deterministic effects can be avoided if the limits are not exceeded. Stochastic effects are those that are expected to occur in populations exposed to ionizing radiation. These effects have no threshold dose and often show up years after exposure, the assumption being that damage from radiation is cumulative over a lifetime.

As the thickness of an area being imaged increases, more X-ray beams will be required in order to achieve an image of similar quality. Therefore, as the size of a patient increases, the dose to the patient's skin and amount of scatter increases as well. Continuous or live fluoroscopy obtains about 30 images per second, which increases the amount of radiation exposure. Pulsed fluoroscopy obtains 1–6 images per second, which lowers the amount of radiation exposure.

Magnification of the image also greatly increases the dose to both the patient and surgeon, and should be used only when necessary.

Methods to reduce radiation exposure:

Principles:
- The benefit of obtaining imaging must exceed all risks to the patient and operating room personnel, including radiation exposure.
- The three basic factors that determine the safety are the time, distance, and shielding. In simple terms; these factors reduce the exposure time, increase the distance from the source and use appropriate shielding.
- The ALARA (as low as reasonably achievable) principle refers to reducing the amount of radiation delivered without compromising the integrity of imaging.
- Radiation should be limited to the permissible radiation exposure limits as prescribed (see above).
- *Personal protective equipment (PPE):* PPE contains lead or similar lightweight materials that attenuate scattered X-rays. There are multiple designs of PPE that may be worn by operating room personnel. Aprons may be one-piece front shielding or offer 360° coverage. A lead-equivalent thickness of at least 0.5 mm is typically required, which attenuates over 95% of scattered X-rays that strike it. Lead aprons must be inspected annually for damage that may cause X-rays to pass through. This may include cracks from improper folding or storage. Another important piece of PPE is thyroid shields.

Image intensifier:
- Keep it as close as possible to reduce the scattering, to reduce the patient dosage, and to obtain a larger field of view.
- Personnel should stand on the side of image intensifier to reduce exposure to scatter rays. Laser targeting, floor and draping landmarks, adjusting the size of the aperture, and manipulation of the X-ray beam, all reduce the radiation exposure.
- The mini C-arm substantially reduces overall radiation exposure to the surgeon but may increase dosage to the hands as they can be in the direct path of the X-ray beam.
- An understanding of the terminology used and the ability to effectively communicate with the c-arm technician must be present in order to decrease exposure, reduce frustration and conflict, and avoid wasting valuable operating room time.

Technique:
- Use the lowest mA and as large a kVp as possible. Larger kVp increases the penetrability of beam allowing the use of a lower mA.
- Reduce the exposure time to the minimum.
- Use pulse mode rather than continuous mode.
- When using pulse mode, use a lowest frequency possible.
- Reduce the magnification to the minimum. Dose increases at the rate of square of magnification.

Personnel and PPE:
- *Use protective aprons, thyroid shields, and lead goggles:* Protective eyewear is commonly used in interventional radiology and is becoming more commonplace in Orthopedics. The lens of the eye is a radiosensitive anatomic structure and must be protected from scatter. Leaded eyewear should include lateral protection, as the eyes are susceptible to backscatter from the head and direct scatter when the head is turned. The hands have the greatest exposure to direct radiation during surgical procedures and are the most difficult to protect. Sterile protective gloves are available; however, they do not offer nearly as much protection as aprons or thyroid shields. Hands should not be placed directly in the beam when at all possible. The use of a Kocher forceps or other surgical tool to aid with positioning may help reduce exposure of the hands when obtaining images. Protective gloves should have at least a 0.25 mm Pb equivalency but remember that these gloves do not protect the hands if placed within the primary beam.
- Exposure from a radiation source decreases by the inverse of the distance squared. Hence stay as far away as possible from the X-ray source—the X-ray source should be kept as far away from the patient as possible. This is also the reason for keeping the gun beneath the patient to increase the distance from radiosensitive parts.
- Stand on the side of image intensifier as far as possible.
- Use dose monitors.

CHAPTER 3

Orthopedic Trauma

3.1 GENERAL ASPECTS OF ORTHOPEDIC TRAUMA, TENS, CAST, ROLE OF LIGAMENTOTAXIS, ARTHROSCOPY, CT IN FRACTURES, SPINAL SHOCKS, AND SCIWORA (Q1–15)

1. What are ATLS guidelines?

Ans: *(Please read Chapter no. 1 for additional information)*

- Preparation and triage—an effective trauma system needs the teamwork of emergency medical services (EMS), emergency medicine, trauma surgery, and surgery subspecialists.
- *Primary survey*:
  - Patients are assessed and treatment priorities established based on their injuries, vital signs, and injury mechanisms. ABCDEs of trauma care:
    - A: Airway and C-spine protection
    - B: Breathing and ventilation
    - C: Circulation with hemorrhage control
    - D: Disability/neurologic status
    - E: Exposure/environmental control.
- Resuscitation—oxygenation and ventilation, shock management, intravenous lines, and warmed Ringer's lactate solution [normal saline (NS), hydroxyethyl starch (HES), etc.]. Management of life-threatening problems identified in the primary survey is continued.
- Adjuncts to primary survey and resuscitation—blood pressure, pulse oximetry, electrocardiography (ECG), X-rays and other diagnostic studies, trauma series X-rays (chest, cervical spine, and pelvis), FAST (focused abdominal sonography in trauma), urinary catheters, arterial blood gas (ABG)/lactate analysis (metabolic and respiratory acidosis), and respiratory rate.
- Secondary survey—does not begin until the primary survey (ABCDEs) is completed, resuscitative effort is well-established and the patient is demonstrating normalization of vital signs.
- Adjuncts to secondary survey—hemodynamic status, contrast computed tomography (CT) scan/magnetic resonance imaging (MRI) scan, extremity X-rays, endoscopy, and ultrasonography (USG).
- Postresuscitation monitoring and reevaluation—reevaluation for new findings or overlooked ones, continuous monitoring of vital signs, urinary output - 0.5–1 mL/kg/h, ABG, ECG, pulse oximetry, and effective analgesia: avoid IM injections.
- Definitive care—only done after identifying the patient's injuries and managing life-threatening problems.

2. Describe the salient features of TENS.

Ans: TENS stands for titanium elastic nailing system. It is commonly used in the treatment of pediatric femoral, tibial, and forearm fractures.

- It is a minimally invasive method of surgical stabilization that tends to minimally disrupt fracture biology.
- Nails can be inserted in retrograde or antegrade fashion.

- The immobilization is based on three points of fixation (two at the ends and one at the site of nail bending in middle). The biomechanical principle of titanium elastic nail is based on the symmetrical bracing action of two elastic nails inserted into the metaphysis, each of which bears against the inner bone at three points. This produces the following four properties essential for achieving optimal results:
  1. Flexural stability
  2. Axial stability
  3. Translational stability
  4. Rotational stability
- The nails are usually "stacked" with multiple nails at the fracture to prevent angulation.
- Usually, medial and lateral insertion sites are used, but a single insertion site, either medial or lateral, can be used in the distal femoral metaphysis.
- It is a load-sharing device and as such if used properly, it allows rapid rehabilitation of patients and much earlier weight bearing than conservative methods.
- It leads to rapid healing with low incidence of malunion allowing early return to function.
- Two divergent C-configuration nails or one C-configuration and one S-configuration nail (bent by the surgeon). [No significant difference between the mechanical properties of three different retrograde nail constructions (two C-shaped, two S-shaped, and two straight flexible nails) has been demonstrated.]
- Special expertise is needed to stabilize subtrochanteric fractures and fractures of the distal third of the femur; antegrade insertion commonly is used for the latter. Fixation of some proximal and distal long spiral fractures may lack stability as far as rotation, and angulation and testing for stability after nailing at surgery is indicated. If instability is present, a long leg cast with a pelvic band is additionally used.

3. Fracture fixation using shape memory (NITINOL) staples.

Ans: NITINOL stands for Nickel Titanium–Naval Ordnance Laboratory that is a novel alloy obtained by mixing equal quantities of nickel and titanium bearing characteristic properties of shape memory and pseudoelasticity (super-elasticity). Pseudoelasticity is an elastic response to an applied stress that is caused by a phase transformation absorbing large strain before undergoing plastic deformation. Shape memory is the ability to undergo reversible deformation with changes in temperature. Being a biphasic alloy Nitinol exhibits super-elastic properties below transition temperature while maintaining martensite state. Above transition temperature, it exhibits austenite phase making it more stable and rigid. Most nitinol implants are manufactured to have transition temperature just below human body temperature. A fixed shape implant is manufactured and is cooled to its martensitic phase which makes it flexible. The staple is opened without plastically deformation, and then it is loaded onto and retained by the insertion tool and the open, active position. The tines of the staple are perpendicular to the transverse limb of the staple after loading, facilitating insertion. Because the transition temperature is below body temperature the implant returns to its original, stable configuration after fixation causing the tines to close toward the center of implant. This produces continuous interfragmentary compression. This property is utilized in fracture fixation and osteosynthesis.

Proposed indications: It is used primarily for transverse fracture fixation with static compression of clavicle, scapula, long bones of the upper and lower extremity, patella, olecranon, wrist, and metacarpal/phalanges as well as the pelvis and acetabulum. It has also been used for metatarsophalangeal joint arthrodesis, scaphoid fractures, and intercarpal fusion.

Advantages: Generates continuous interfragmentary compression, small foot-print instrumentation needed, small exposures, strong provisional fixation, can be combined with conventional plating technique.

Contraindications for staple fixation—severely osteoporotic bone, absent or poor cortical bone quality, and fractures with significant comminution.

4. Discuss the general principles and techniques of plaster cast. Describe technique of resin cast also.

Ans: Principles: The primary principle of cast immobilization is external support to fracture and maintaining reduction using three-point relationship.
- Using splints or casts means using an external force. Stabilizing only two points, distally and proximally of the fracture, will not be sufficient or control of angulation. A third point is needed in order to counteract the forces on the various

fragments once the muscle pulls. The three-point fixation technique is necessary in order to stabilize or immobilize a fracture as this will achieve a new balance between the different fragments.

For example, the three-point principle, using the example of a traction and reduction cast for the distal radius using POP. This fracture presents with typical dorsal displacement and angulation of the distal fragment:
- *Point one*: Dorsal molded rim
- *Point two*: Palmar aspect, where the surgeon's palm is situated
- *Point three*: Proximal shaft of the cast where the four fingers are kept.

Technique of applying POP:

Stockinette is applied first and then padding. Padding should be adequate, especially over bony prominences. POP should not be too tight or loose. Check neurovascular status after cast application.

Before beginning the casting procedure, prepare a container of water at room temperature (at or around 20°C). The correct water temperature is important to avoid allow sufficient time for cast application, and to excessive heat and due to the normal exothermic reaction of the setting cast. A higher temperature of the dipping water will accelerate setting, and shorten molding working time. Increased heat within the cast might result in burn injuries. Furthermore, in hot water, plaster will detach from the fabric layer or dissolve into the water, a process that will result in reduced stability. It must also be remembered that cast thickness also contributes to heating of a setting cast. Thus, the more cast layers that are used **(Table 3.1.1)**, the higher the temperature during the setting. Water used in the cast basin or sink should be clean and changed routinely several times during the day.

Rolled plaster bandages will become wet rapidly if submerged into water in the correct way. The best way is to hold the POP roll between thumb and fingers during the dipping process, with the axis of the roll more or less vertical in the water (or slightly oblique to a minimum of 45°). The POP bandage roll lies in the palm of the hand, the thumb rests on the roll without much pressure, while the free end of the bandage is supported by the long fingers. This way "the eyes can look into the bandage" as it is unrolled onto the patient's limb. Dipping the plaster roll without leaving the first layer free causes the cast layers to stick together, and interferes with identifying the free end.

When dipping plaster rolls, the depth of the water should be at least 20–30 cm. When rolls are dipped as described above, air bubbles will escape through the core of the roll, allowing the water to saturate all layers of plaster uniformly. After a few seconds, when the bubbling ceases, the plaster is adequately wet. A gentle squeeze eliminates excess water. Then, the free end is applied to the patient's limb and the roll material is wrapped onto the limb while the roll itself remains in contact with the cast padding. Plaster of Paris rolls are applied using the half overlapping technique so that at least half of each preceding wrap is covered by the following turn. When the rolling plaster is held over an angled region, or, e.g., the ankle joint, plaster overlaps halfway over the heel while much greater overlapping is seen anteriorly.

POP slab:

Adequate padding is done first with extra care over bony prominences. POP splints (longuettes) are folded and dipped into water at an angle of 45° in order to let the air bubbles escape. A water column of 20–30 cm produces enough pressure to expel air bubbles. The immersion time is approximately 3 seconds or until bubbling ceases. The excess water is then squeezed out as it is with plaster rolls. Hold each end separately, so that they can readily be separated to preserve correct alignment of the splint layers.

The layers of the splint (longuette) are now stuck together by manual longitudinal compression "massage" on a fat, easily cleanable surface of a counter or the cast cart **(Table 3.1.2)**.

Dry spots or dry POP layers reduce the quality and strength of the cast. Insufficiently soaked plaster will result in delaminated, uncompounded plaster, resulting in so-called puff pastry plaster.

After having smoothed the plaster splints (longuettes), they are applied where desired, and the smoothing process is repeated manually on the extremity, rubbing them into previously applied plaster, or onto the padding if an end product splint rather than a circumferential cast is intended. This smoothing process should result in wrinkleless POP cast material, positioned as chosen on the extremity, which remains in the desired functional position without wrinkles or weak spots in the plaster, and without irregularities in the padding. While the plaster is still soft, it is molded to the extremity, with smooth broad appropriately located pressure surfaces to maintain fracture reduction and limb alignment. During the application and molding of POP, avoid creating finger-tip pressure points (indentations) by using only the heel and flat surface of the hand (flat hand technique).

Technique for resin cast:
Both dry and wet methods for resin cast application have been described in standard books and documentation but the dry method is most commonly used. Stockinette is applied first and then padding with soft cotton roll is done. Padding should be adequate, especially over bony prominences. POP should not be too tight or loose. Check neurovascular status after cast application.

Synthetic material when applied dry (without previous dipping into water) increases the working time, before the cast can no longer accept molding. This application technique is recommended or inexperienced users or in complex cases where more time is needed, as well as on occasions when an assistant is not available. After dry application of synthetic cast material, polymerization can be accelerated by wrapping the cast temporarily with a wet elastic cloth bandage. Like POP, synthetic cast rolls are applied using the half—overlapping technique.

TABLE 3.1.1: Layers for cast.

Body part	POP	Synthetic resin cast
Upper limb	8–10 layers	4–6 layers
Lower limb	8–10 layers	6–8 layers

TABLE 3.1.2: Layers for slab/splint.

Body part	POP	Synthetic resin cast
Upper limb	8–10 layers	6–8 layers
Lower limb	12–16 layers	9–12 layers

5. What are the advantages and disadvantages of POP cast?
Ans:

Advantages:
- No need for surgical resources and logistics
- Normally, no danger of surgically induced or implant-related infection or complications
- Reduced risk from general anesthesia
- No need for subsequent implant removal by surgery.

Disadvantages:
- Casts require intensive surveillance for loss of reduction (at least once a week under normal circumstances), and a cooperative patient
- Full-functional recovery can at times be delayed, also depending on the age of the patient
- There is the possibility of developing "fracture disease" with contracture, loss of muscle and/or bone (demineralization), accompanied by pain and swelling, which can lead to a disastrous loss of function, the so-called complex regional pain syndrome (Sudeck's atrophy)
- Significantly weakened construct if patient starts mobilization in a wet cast before complete drying
- Messy application method.

6. What is a hanging cast?
Ans: Hanging casts have been used for many decades for the management of humeral shaft fractures, especially in cases with shortening and displacement. By virtue of gravity, the fracture is maintained in traction reducing the fracture if a good snug fit is provided by the cast. Most frequently, these casts are applied for simple, oblique, or spiral fractures in the middle third region of the humerus. In cases of transverse fractures with shortening, a hanging cast can be applied to reduce the humerus to the proper length and alignment (but overdoing may produce distraction at fracture and delayed or nonunion).

The hanging cast technique requires a full arm cast, with the plaster extending from above the fracture to the wrist, with the elbow flexed to 90°, and the forearm in the neutral position. The patient should be instructed to keep the arm in a "hanging" position for as long as possible to allow gravity to restore humeral length and alignment. Most surgeons use hanging casts routinely for 1 week to 10 days to achieve fracture reduction and then continue with Sarmiento-type functional bracing.

Indications:
Acute/closed/isolated fracture in a cooperative and ambulatory patient.

Relative indications:
- Type A fracture (AO classification)
- Proximal third and long oblique fracture
- Segmental fracture
- Open fracture without neurovascular injury
- Noncompliant patient.

Relative contraindications:
- Multiple injuries
- Vascular injury
- Additional injuries to the ipsilateral arm
- Persisting or increasing nerve dysfunction
- Bilateral fractures
- Pathologic fracture
- Nonunited fracture.

7. What is stress fracture? Discuss etiopathogenesis and its diagnosis.

Ans: A stress fracture is the accumulation of microtrauma that ultimately leads to the macrofracture of bone.
The common high-risk lower extremity fractures (in order of their potential to displace) include:
- Femoral neck—superolateral (tension side)
- Patella
- Anterior tibial diaphysis
- Talus
- Tarsal navicular
- Fifth metatarsal
- Medial malleolus
- Femoral neck—inferomedial
- Sesamoids.

Etiopathogenesis:
Fatigue/stress fractures occur when normal bone is subjected to abnormal stress. The accrual of microfractures then lead to development of a discontinuity in bone and becomes symptomatic. The radiologically barely discernible discontinuity may become complete to a full-blown fracture.

The most common mechanism *is repetitive injury* due to continuous excessive activity. *Other mechanisms* that result in higher strain could be:
- Fatigue of muscles around the joints that result in diminished shielding effect and transmittance of all of the compressive and tensile forces across bones. Muscle contraction converts tensile forces into compressive forces; a phenomenon referred to as stress shielding.
- This protects the bone and prevents injury. This mechanism fails with muscle fatigue.
- Also, muscle fatigue results in gait alteration and instability which may also alter the forces on bone.
- In nonweight-bearing bones, repetitive pull of overworked contracting muscles can produce microfractures that propagate to produce stress fracture.

Risk factors:
- Pronated feet—tarsal and tibial stress fractures
- Talocalcaneal and calcaneonavicular coalitions—stress fracture of neck of talus
- Leg-length inequality and excessive forefoot varus
- Rigid cavus foot.

Diagnosis
History:
- Insidious onset of pain that persist from weeks to months in a localized area. Onset could be related to changes in distance, intensity or frequency of workout. There may also be change in the running surface or shoes. Inadequate footwear can contribute to development of stress fractures.
- The pain is exacerbated by repetitive activity and relieved by rest.
- As the injury progresses, the pain will occur earlier and with greater intensity during activity.

Examination:
Point tenderness over the affected bone along with some subtle soft tissue swelling. No signs of inflammation (osteomyelitis/periostitis). Joints and surrounding muscles are normal. Neurovascular examination is also normal.

Imaging:
- Classically, the radiographs will initially be negative. After several weeks, long bones such as the metatarsals or tibia will show periosteal new bone formation or frank but incomplete cortical break.
- Cancellous bones such as the calcaneus show medullary sclerosis.
- A Tc-99m bone scan is the investigation of choice, and it will be positive as early as 3 days after injury. The bone scan will be positive in all three phases with a focal intense area of uptake, even in the setting of normal X-ray findings. The bone scan is virtually 100% sensitive in diagnosing stress fractures, but its specificity is less than X-ray. Bone scan also cannot distinguish stress fracture from neoplasm or infection.
- Ultrasonography is an important tool that can be used in case of normal radiology; for metatarsal fractures, the USG scan has been found to have 83% sensitivity, 76% specificity; 59% positive predictive value, and 92% negative predictive value.
- Computed tomography scans may be ordered for strongly suspected navicular, calcaneal, tibial, and pediatric fatigue fractures.
- Magnetic resonance imaging can be a useful adjunct in cases with negative radiographs and equivocal bone scan. It can now be considered investigation of choice as it has marked specificity and is able to differentiate other lesions remarkably well.

8. Differentiate intracapsular fractures between children and adults.

Ans: Generally, a child's hip differs from an adult's because the physis can contribute to a type I transepiphyseal separation in which the capital femoral epiphysis may stay within the acetabulum or may be dislocated. The blood vessels to the femoral head are easily damaged, and a high incidence of osteonecrosis occurs in cervical and transepiphyseal fractures in children, even higher than in adults. Growth arrest in the physis can cause shortening of 15% of the total extremity. Varus or valgus angulation of the femoral neck can also occur from arrest of only one side of the physis.

Hip fractures in children also differ from fractures in adults because a child can tolerate immobilization much more readily than an adult, and more choices for treatment are available, including traction, a spica cast, and bed rest, in addition to operative treatment. Internal fixation with threaded pins often is used in adult hip fractures and can be used through the capital femoral physis in a child to secure firm fixation of the femoral neck. In an infant, however, this can cause premature physeal closure and significant leg-length inequality.

9. Explain the role of ligamentotaxis in acute trauma.

Ans: The term *ligamentotaxis,* common in the European literature, literally means traction (pull) applied through ligaments. But for this to be effective, the pulling force needs to be counterbalanced by soft tissues and ligaments surrounding the bone. Certain intra-articular fractures can be treated by external fixation/distractor where traction gives the pulling force while countertraction is provided by the fixator on the capsular and ligamentous structures around the joint. In primary fracture, care setting reduction is commonly achieved manually by pulling along the long axis of bone perpendicular to the main fracture alignment where the surrounding soft tissues form an unyielding cylinder compressing the fragment(s) and ligament pull aligns the fragment in position. The counter traction is usually given by assistant. This alignment may be achieved by plaster of Paris (POP) cast (usually fails overtime) or by percutaneous pinning (needs anesthesia).

The muscle envelope under distraction exerts a concentric pressure on the shaft, easing fragments into place. This also holds true for metaphyseal and epiphyseal bone, although the distraction required to align fragments is transferred not so much via muscular attachments as through capsular tissues, ligaments, and less often tendons. This phenomenon regularly seen as a part of conservative fracture management is described by the term ligamentotaxis coined by Vidal.

The joints/fractures where ligamentotaxis is useful are:
- Distal radius fractures
- Tibial plateau fractures
- Distal tibial fractures.

It must be remembered that there is a tendency for loss of fracture reduction over time due to counter pull of muscles and tendons persistently so some type of distractor or external fixation is imperative.

10. Define ligamentotaxis.
Ans: Kindly vide Answer to Question 9.

11. Discuss arthroscopy in managing intra-articular fractures.
Ans: Arthroscopically-assisted reduction and fixation techniques are being used with increased frequency for the treatment of intra-articular fracture of tibial plateau (Schatzker type I, type II, and type III), distal radius fractures, and tibial plafond fractures as it is nearly impossible to ascertain the articular reduction by two-dimensional image intensification (also cartilage is radiolucent). Arthroscopic techniques require minimal soft tissue dissection, afford excellent exposure of the articular surface, and can be used to diagnose and treat concomitant meniscal injury in case of tibial plateau fracture and distal radioulnar joint (DRUJ) pathologies can be addressed in distal radius fractures.

Technique for tibial plateau fracture reduction:
- Patient is placed supine and tourniquet is inflated
- Standard arthroscopy portals (anterolateral and anteromedial) are placed approximately to inspect the tibial plateau and articular surface. A complete diagnostic assessment is performed. It is recommended not to use pump as it predisposes to compartment syndrome, especially in extracapsular fractures (Schatzker type I, type III, and type IV). One may additionally expose the metaphyseal portion of the fracture site in these cases to prevent extravasation of irrigation fluid into the soft tissues. This incision can be used later to create a bony window for reduction and bone grafting.
- Schatzker type III fractures usually are intra-articular, and extravasation is less of a concern. The joint should be thoroughly lavaged to evacuate the hemarthrosis and remove loose bony and chondral fragments.
- When the diagnostic evaluation has been completed, the reduction can be performed with probe or dental pick. If the lateral meniscus is entrapped in the fracture site, it can be lifted out with a hook.
- Meniscal tears usually can be repaired and should be treated accordingly. *Techniques for meniscal repair are described in detail in the book Essential Orthopedics: Principles and Practice, 2nd edition, Chapter 34.*
- Depressed fragments are elevated through a small cortical window from below to provide support. The depressed fragment can be localized by using an anterior cruciate ligament tibial guide to place a Kirschner wire into the displaced fragment. The fragment can be elevated using a cannulated impactor. The reduction can be evaluated accurately through the arthroscope.
- For further support and the resulting defect in metaphyseal, bone window can be filled with autogenous bone graft or hydroxyapatite.
- Fixation is achieved with percutaneously placed 6.5 mm cancellous screws. Because buttress plating may be necessary in patients with osteoporotic bone (in general arthroscopically assisted reduction is less suitable for this patient population as future demands are low and often joint is already arthritic).

12. Explain the role of whole body CT in trauma.
Ans: Whole body computed tomography (WBCT) scan is a highly useful investigation in polytrauma patients, especially in whom multiple injury evaluation would otherwise consume lots of "golden" time. WBCT provides detailed information on known and occult injuries and has been implemented since mid-90s as a routine procedure in the Swedish health care system. Sweden was an early adopter of WBCT in trauma care. Now, the use of WBCT as an adjunct has been well-established for 20 years in severely injured patients. It has two prominent advantages:

1. WBCT has much higher accuracy in describing the extent of injuries compared to other conventional investigations.
2. WBCT is also used to exclude occult injuries in the seemingly not injured high energy trauma patients.

A typical order of WBCT includes:
- Noncontrast CT of head and cervical spine
- Intravenous (IV) contrast-enhanced imaging of chest, abdomen, and pelvis
- Three-dimensional (3D) reconstruction of cervical, thoracic, and lumbar spine.

Drawback:
There is high exposure to ionizing radiation in a WBCT, usually totaling to cumulative dosage of >20 mSv. Such high dose in patients 40 years or younger may induce cancer in 1/1,000 patients.

Indications:
- Penetrating trauma—gunshot wound (including air rifle) and blast injury (bomb/explosion)
- Blunt trauma—combined velocity ≥50 km/h, motor vehicle crash with ejection, motorcyclist or pedestrian hit by a vehicle >30 km/h, fall >3 meter, fatality in the same vehicle, entrapment >30 minutes, and crush injury to thorax/abdomen.

13. Describe autonomic dysreflexia in spinal cord injuries.

Ans: This is a worrisome complication occurring in patients with lesions above T6. A painful or noxious stimulus below the level of the lesion causes sudden fall in blood pressure (BP) by triggering the autonomic nervous system. This, if untreated, can lead to convulsions, hemorrhage, and death. These patients can be identified by a cluster of symptoms of high BP, severe headache, blurring of vision, presence of a stuffy nose, sweating, presence of goose bumps below, and vasodilation (flushing) above the level of the injury.

Some conditions that can precipitate these catastrophic events are a distended or full bladder caused by blockage in the catheter, any bladder infection, pressure ulcers or ingrown toe nail, sudden and extreme temperature change or tight clothing. The treatment is resuscitation and identification, and treatment of the noxious stimulus. Sitting position is recommended as lying will further elevate the BP.

14. Discuss spinal shock.

Ans: The term spinal shock was introduced by Marshall Hall in 1841 to indicate the state of transient inexcitability or hypoexcitability of the isolated spinal cord below the level of a transection of the cord. Spinal shock may be due to the loss of facilitation from descending tracts, to persisting inhibition from below the transection acting upon extensor reflexes, or to the axonal degeneration of interneurons. The following are common features of spinal shock that may variably last several hours to days:

- There is a transient reflex reduction in cord function below the level of injury
- Initially hypertension due to release of catecholamines → followed by hypotension
- *Flaccid paralysis*: The initial paralysis is always flaccid even if the injury is of upper motor neuron (UMN) type.
- All cutaneous and tendon reflexes are depressed though bulbocavernosus and anal reflexes may persist.
- Bowel and bladder involved
- Sometimes, priapism develops.

The intensity and duration of shock varies on the evolution ladder of the vertebrate, the higher the degree of cerebral development, the greater the shock.

- *Motor paralysis or paresis*: There is either complete or partial loss of muscle function below the level of the lesion.
- *Sensory loss*: Impaired or absent sensation below the level of the lesion due to disruption of the ascending sensory fibers.
- *Respiratory dysfunction*: Depends on level of injury, premorbid status of respiratory system, and additional injury. Cervical injury commonly is associated with respiratory dysfunction. The impairments include decreased chest expansion and lowered inspiratory volume.
- *Impaired temperature control*: The connection with hypothalamus is lost so there is no temperature regulation through control of cutaneous blood flow or sweating. The person loses ability to shiver and there is absence of thermoregulatory sweating below the level of lesion. This lack of sweating is associated with compensatory diaphoresis above the lesion.

- *Spasticity*: Characterized by hypertonicity, hyperactive stretch reflexes, and clonus. It typically occurs below the level of the lesion after spinal shock subsides. The spasticity gradually increases during first 6 months and plateaus by 1 year. Spasticity is increased by internal and external stimuli [position changes, cutaneous stimuli, environmental temperature, tight clothing, bladder or kidney stones, fecal impaction, catheter blockage, urinary tract infection (UTI), decubitus ulcers, and emotional stress].
- *Bowel and bladder dysfunction*: Neurogenic bladder.
- *Sexual dysfunction*: Sexual function is a vital part of the rehabilitation process as is providing other information to enable the patient to better understand and adapt to his medical condition. Male erection and ejaculation are possible depending on the level of the lesion and complete/incomplete injury.

Reversal of shock: When the shock subsides, the reflexes return back. In humans, the duration of the areflexia varies, with reflex activity sometimes appearing within a period of 3 or 4 days in children or after 3-6 weeks in adults. The first reflexes to return are the anal and bulbocavernosus reflexes and as a rule further, reflex return is in the cranial direction (the exception is probably the early return of knee reflex than ankle reflex).

15. Define SCIWORA.

Ans: SCIWORA (spinal cord injury without radiographic abnormality), as a syndrome unique to children, was first described by Pang and Wilberger, though the first report in literature was made by Burke in 1974. This condition is defined as a spinal cord injury (as diagnosed by clinical symptoms of traumatic myelopathy) in a patient with no visible fracture or dislocation on plain radiographs, tomograms, or CT scans. The lesion is usually seen in cervical cord region but rare lesions in thoracic or lumbar region have also been described. SCIWORA is also seen in adults but underlying degeneration is an associated factor in them. So, in adults, the differentiation of traumatic from nontraumatic degenerative form becomes difficult/impossible. For this reason, better term for adults will be SCIWORET (spinal cord injury without radiographic evidence of trauma) or spinal cord injury without computed tomography evidence of trauma (SCIWOCTET).

Pathomechanics and pathophysiology of SCIWORA: The spinal cord injury may be complete or incomplete, and the injury is commonly believed to result from severe flexion or distraction of the cervical spine. SCIWORA occurs because the spinal column (vertebrae and disk space) in children is more elastic than the spinal cord and can undergo considerable deformation without being disrupted. The spinal column can elongate up to 2 inches in them without disruption, whereas the spinal cord ruptures with only a quarter-inch of elongation.

SCIWORA also may represent an ischemic injury in some patients (mostly adult patients—due to venous congestion), although most are believed to be due to a distraction type injury resulting from hyperextension forces in which the spinal cord has not tolerated the degree of distraction but the bony ligamentous elements have not failed. Posttraumatic SCIWORA may also arise in children from a fracture through a pediatric vertebral endplate that reduces spontaneously (Salter–Harris type I fracture), giving a normal radiographic appearance, although the initial displacement could have caused spinal cord injury. SCIWORET in adults mostly results from low energy injury like falls from standing height, but in them, degenerative changes in the spinal column are prominent. This is also the reason for development of central cord syndrome in adult patients with simple hyperextension injuries.

Epidemiology and presentation: SCIWORA abnormalities are more common in children under 8 years of age than in older children, perhaps because of predisposing factors such as cervical spine hypermobility, ligamentous laxity, and an immature vascular supply to the spinal cord. The reported incidence of this condition varies from 7 to 66% of patients with cervical spine injuries. Recorded neurological deficit has been very broad ranging from paresthesia in limbs to complete quadriplegia. Weakness is usually more severe in the upper extremities than in the lower extremities and is the most typical clinical presentation in patients with SCIWORA. Delayed onset of neurologic symptoms has been reported in as many as 52% of patients in some series that actually suggests ischemia due to vascular injury/venous congestion as predisposing factor or may represent repeated microinsults to the spinal cord from striking against the unstable column. Pang and Pollack reported 15 patients who had delayed paralysis after their injuries. Nine had transient warning signs such as paresthesia or subjective paralysis. In all patients with delayed onset of paralysis, the spine had not been immobilized after the initial trauma, and all were neurologically normal before the second event. This underlines the importance of diligent immobilization of a suspected spinal cord injury in a child. Approximately, half of the young children with SCIWORA in reported series had complete spinal cord injuries, whereas the older children usually had incomplete neurologic deficit injuries that involved the subaxial cervical spine.

Investigations: Plain X-ray has sensitivity of over 90% if full trauma series is done (AP, lateral, oblique, and open mouth views) to rule-out SCIWORA. Flexion extension and dynamic views are usually not ordered but may reveal instability. CT scan is the best diagnostic modality to identify bony pathology. MRI is most useful in evaluating patients with SCIWORA for spinal cord pathology. The preferred imaging involves use of spin-echo T1 (T1 SE), gradient-echo T2 (T2-weighted GRE) and short tau inversion recovery (STIR)-weighted MRI pulse sequences. Spinal cord edema, hematoma, cord transection, and disc pathologies are well demonstrated. Ischemia with increased concentration of deoxygenated hemoglobin is revealed in T2-weighted images, while edema is best seen on STIR images. Prognostication is also good based on MRI where small hematomas (< one-third of spinal cord diameter) have good prognosis while cord transection has bad prognosis.

Differential diagnosis: Vertebral artery embolism, arteritis or bleeding disorders.

Treatment: Immobilization of spine for 12 weeks is the primary treatment. Precautions are followed for further 6 months and contact sports are not allowed to prevent any further injury.

3.2 GENERAL ASPECTS OF PEDIATRIC FRACTURES (Q16–18)

16. What are torus fractures?

Ans: Compression fractures are found most commonly at the metaphyseal-diaphyseal junction and are referred to as "buckle fractures" or "torus fractures". They occur due to thick periosteal sleeve and greater elasticity. Complete fractures are therefore rare in children. Torus fractures rarely cause physeal injury, but they may result in acute angular deformity. Because torus fractures are impacted, they are stable and rarely require manipulative reduction. It commonly occurs in distal radius in children but also occurs in tibia. If only one cortex is involved, then the injury is stable and may be treated with protected immobilization for pain relief. Bicortical injuries should be treated in a long arm cast in radius torus.

17. Discuss the relevance of Salter-Harris classification to skeletal growth.

Ans: The most commonly used classification is that of Salter and Harris, which is based on the radiographic appearance of the fracture. This classification depicts the amount of involvement of the physis, the epiphysis, and the joint. The higher the classification, the more likely is physeal arrest or joint incongruity to occur.

Routine use of the Salter–Harris classification shows that any physeal injury may result in growth disturbance, although it is more common after Salter–Harris types III, IV, and V fractures.

Most types I and II fractures can be treated by closed reduction. Types III and IV fractures often require open reduction and internal fixation to reposition the fragments anatomically and to fix them securely, so that growth in the physis may continue and the joint may be congruous. An example is a type IV injury of the lateral humeral condyle, which is a "fracture of necessity" and almost always requires reduction and internal fixation. If not treated adequately, this fracture does not unite, causing joint incongruity and angular deformity. In type V fractures, the cartilage cells of the physis are crushed, and regardless of the form of treatment, growth disturbance can occur. A type V fracture usually is diagnosed only in retrospect, when a growth disturbance develops.

Although the Salter–Harris classification has been an excellent one, some fractures do not behave as predicted, in that not all types I and II fractures do well after closed reduction, and not all types III and IV fractures do well after open reduction. A type II distal femoral physeal fracture that is significantly displaced often results in growth arrest and angular deformity. A gentle closed anatomical reduction of this fracture is required to avoid crushing or otherwise injuring the germinal cells in the physis in the proximal fragment; even so, the physis may close prematurely.

(To learn about the detailed structure of physis and impact of various conditions on it refer to Chapter 1 of the book Essential Orthopedics: Principles and Practice, 2nd edition.)

18. Define and classify epiphyseal injuries. Discuss the management of Salter–Harris type IV epiphyseal injury.

Ans: *Definition*: Osseous injuries that involve epiphysis as their component wholly or partially are called epiphyseal injuries.

Classification:
Salter–Harris classification:
- Type I fractures are epiphyseal separations through the physis only, with or without displacement. Stress radiographs are useful in determining whether this fracture is present.
- Type II fractures have a metaphyseal spike attached to the separated epiphysis (Thurston–Holland sign) with the separation also through the physis.
- Type III fracture is a physeal separation with a fracture through the epiphysis into the joint with joint incongruity when the fracture is displaced.
- Type IV fracture is a fracture through the metaphysis, through the physis, through the epiphysis, and into the joint, and also with possible joint incongruity.
- Type V fracture, which can be diagnosed only in retrospect, is a compression fracture of the physis, producing permanent damage.

Rang modified the Salter–Harris classification, describing a "bruise" or contusion to the periphery of the physis. This seemingly minor injury can cause scarring, tethering, and arrest of the periphery of the physis, that may produce angular deformity.

Ogden classification:
His first five classes are basically the same as those of Salter and Harris, except for subclasses used for peculiar fracture patterns in special joints, such as the hip, and for certain traction epiphyses. His type VI fracture is similar to that described by Rang. The type VII fracture is an intra-articular osteochondral fracture. Types VIII and IX fractures are not epiphyseal or physeal fractures, but seem to stimulate the physes and contribute to longitudinal bone growth.

Peterson described two previously unclassified physeal fractures. The first is a fracture completely across the metaphysis with a linear longitudinal extension to the physis. The fracture usually does not extend along the physis. In the second fracture, a portion of the physis is missing.

Management of type IV Salter-Harris injury: Type IV fractures often require open reduction and internal fixation to reposition the fragments anatomically and to fix them securely so that growth in the physis may continue and the joint may be congruous.

An example is a type IV injury of the lateral humeral condyle, which is a "fracture of necessity" and almost always requires reduction and internal fixation. If not treated adequately, this fracture does not unite, causing joint incongruity and angular deformity. Some basic requirements of treating this injury are:
- The pins should cross the epiphysis in the fractured areas.
- The pins should cross the metaphysis rather than the physis, if possible.

3.3 UPPER LIMB INJURIES FROM SHOULDER GIRDLE TO HAND (Q19–62)

19. Classify acromioclavicular (AC) joint injuries. Discuss its diagnosis and management.

Ans: *Tossy-Rockwood AC joint dislocation classification* (**Fig. 3.3.1**):
- *Type I*: A mild force to the point of the shoulder produces a minor strain to the fiber of the AC ligaments. The ligaments remain intact, and the AC joint remains stable.
- *Type II*: A moderate force to the point of the shoulder produces ruptured ligaments of the AC joint. The distal end of the clavicle is unstable anteroposteriorly, but vertical stability is preserved by virtue of the intact coracoclavicular ligament. Medial rotation of scapula produces widening of the AC joint. There may be a slight, relative upward displacement of the distal end of the clavicle secondary to stretching of the coracoclavicular ligaments.
- *Type III*: A severe force is applied to the point of the shoulder, which tears the AC and coracoclavicular ligaments resulting in a complete AC dislocation. The scapula and shoulder complex droop inferomedially making distal clavicle prominent. Radiographic findings include a 25–100% increase in the coracoclavicular space in comparison to the normal shoulder.

- *Type IV*: AC dislocation involves posterior dislocation of the distal end of the clavicle. The clavicle is displaced into or through the trapezius muscle as the force applied to the acromion drives the scapula anteriorly and inferiorly. Some refer to this injury as a "posterior dislocation of the clavicle," and others prefer the term "anterior dislocation of the AC joint".
- *Type V*: This is a markedly severe version of the type II injury. The distal clavicle has been stripped of all its soft tissue attachments (i.e. AC ligaments, coracoclavicular ligament, and the deltotrapezial muscle attachments) and lies subcutaneously. When combined with superior displacement of the clavicle owing to unopposed pull of the sternocleidomastoid muscle, the severe downward drop of the extremity produces a marked disfiguration of the shoulder. The coracoclavicular space is increased greater than 100% in comparison to the opposite, normal shoulder.
- *Type VI*: Inferior dislocation of the distal clavicle results from severe trauma and is frequently accompanied by multiple injuries. The mechanism of dislocation is thought to be severe hyperabduction and external rotation of the arm, combined with retraction of the scapula. The distal clavicle occupies either a subacromial or a subcoracoid location.

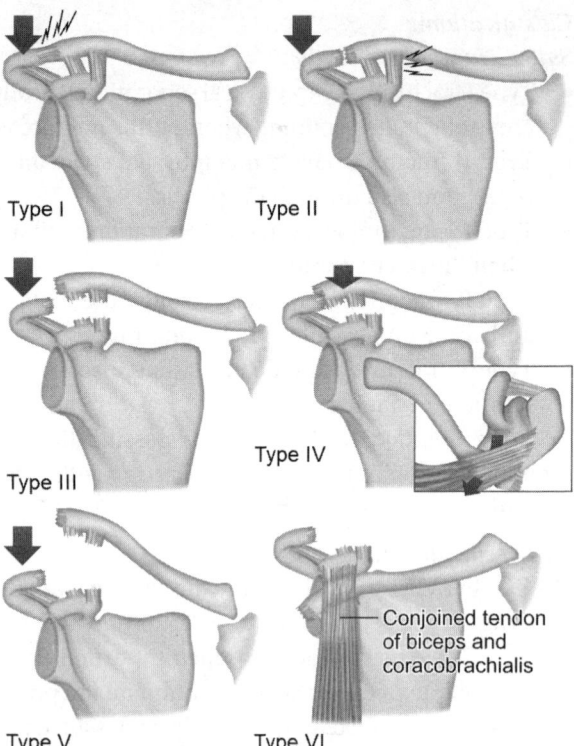

Fig. 3.3.1: Tossy–Rockwood classification.

Diagnosis

Physical examination:
- Diffuse shoulder pain
- Point tenderness at AC joint
- Deformity
- Positive crossarm adduction test (arm flexed 90°, adducted across chest) produces compression pain localized to AC joint
- O'Brien's active compression test—localizes pain over AC joint
- Paxinos test (thumb pressure directed anteriorly at the posterior AC joint)
- Diagnostic analgesic injection—provides relief in pain/symptoms.

Radiology:
- Zanca view determines displacement with comparison to contralateral AC joint and CC distance. The beam is placed 10–15° cephalad and using 50% of the AP penetration strength
- Axillary view—determines anterior/posterior position of distal clavicle in relation to acromion
- Cross arm stress view—Basmania view (AP with arm adducted).

Management

Nonoperative: This is recommended for pseudodislocations, type I and II injuries, and most type III injuries. Modalities include nonsteroidal anti-inflammatory drugs (NSAIDs), ice therapy, activity modification, and complete rest (one week for type-I, longer for type II and III). Simple sling or elbow support in brace would help. Physical therapy should then be started with both passive and active shoulder motion; and contact sports and weightlifting are only allowed once the patient is completely pain free and range of motion (ROM) is similar to uninjured shoulder. Warn patients that pain may persist for 6 months at AC joint and a significant minority (33%) may experience it till 6 years. For type III injury, the management is still controversial but significantly tilted to nonoperative having equivalent results as for type I or II injury. Cosmetic deformity, however, persists and functional improvement is nonlimiting (reduced power only of extreme activities like bench press). To maximize function in high-demand athletes and overhead activity-requiring jobs, some authors have advocated surgery for acute type-III AC joint injuries in young patients.

Operative treatment: It is indicated for patients with type-III AC joint injuries for which nonsurgical treatment is unacceptable or had been unsuccessful, as well as for medically stable patients with type-IV to VI AC joint injuries. A number of methods and modifications had been proposed but common to them are—anatomic reduction of the AC joint correcting superior displacement and anterior-posterior translation, direct repair (acute injury) or reconstruction (chronic injury) of the CC ligament, supplementation or protection of the CC ligament repair or reconstruction with synthetic material, rigid implant may be used to maintain AC joint stability during initial healing, repair of dynamic stabilizers (deltoid and trapezius), and distal clavicular resection in patients with chronic acromioclavicular injuries where AC joint arthritis is present.

(Details of operative treatment can be fetched from Annexure 1 of the book Essential Orthopedics: Principles and Practice, 2nd edition.)

20. **Explain AC joint dislocations—relevance of its classification in management.**

Ans: AC Joint Dislocations: Relevance of Classification in Management—the Rockwood classification (6 types) guides treatment by correlating injury severity with ligament damage and joint instability.

Classification and Management:
- Type I: (AC ligament sprain) → Conservative [rest, sling, and nonsteroidal anti-inflammatory drugs (NSAIDs)]
- Type II: (AC tear, CC ligament intact) → Conservative (sling ± rehabilitation)
- Type III: (AC + CC tear) → Controversial:
  - Nonsurgical (rehab first; surgery if chronic pain)
  - Surgical (for laborers/athletes)
- Types IV-VI: (Severe displacement ± muscle/trapezius detachment) → Surgical (open reduction, CC ligament reconstruction)

21. **Acromioclavicular joint injuries:**
   A. Discuss pathoanatomy and clinical assessment.
   B. Describe in short management of chronic injuries.

Ans:

A. *Pathoanatomy*: AC joint is a diarthrodial joint between lateral end of clavicle and acromion, with the bony ends covered by fibrocartilage. It is stabilized by four articular and two extra-articular ligaments (coracoacromial ligament is redundant for stability) and a meniscus inside along with the dynamic muscular support. The joint may be inclined vertically or medially 50° making the joint both horizontally and vertically vulnerable. The horizontal stability of the AC joint is conferred by the AC ligaments (anterior, posterior, superior, and inferior) that strengthen capsule, whereas the vertical stability is maintained by the CC ligaments. The superior AC ligament confers 56% stability while posterior confers 25% resistance to posterior displacement. CC ligament has two parts—conoid and trapezoid, while the latter inserts 3 cm from end of clavicle and the former inserts 4.5 cm from end of clavicle in the posterior border. The conoid (medial) gives primary restraint to anterior and superior forces/displacement, while the trapezoid (lateral) provides restraint to posterior displacement at the AC joint. Overall AC ligaments are the primary restraints to posterior instability (89%) and the posterior translation (68%). With increasing deformation, conoid ligament becomes primary restraint (62%) while AC ligaments still maintain posterior stability. Trapezoid provides primary restraint to AC joint compression. The average CC distance is 1.1-1.3 cm that may be maintained in base of coracoid fractures but still mimic AC separation due to (pseudo-) CC disruption. The superior shoulder suspensory complex (SSSC) is a ligamento-osseous ring composed of the upper part of glenoid, the coracoid process, the CC ligament, the distal clavicle, the AC joint, and the acromial process. The displacement resulting in subcutaneous superior bony strut comprises the mid-shaft clavicle and the inferior bony strut is made by the junction of the lateral scapular body and the medial glenoid neck.

Types III, IV, V, and VI AC separations comprise double disruptions of this complex where both the CC and AC ligaments are injured needing combined assessment and stabilization preferably.

Inherently, the AC joint has minimal mobility and the fibrocartilaginous intra-articular disk demonstrates an age-related degeneration until it is essentially nonfunctional beyond the 4th decade.

Pediatric AC joint: Here, the clavicle is encased in thick periosteum that also encompasses CC ligament while AC ligaments are separate, so it gets damaged more frequently.

Clinical assessment: The characteristic presenting feature is a downward sag of the shoulder and upper extremity with prominent lateral clavicle end and tenting of skin. Local tenderness can be elicited. Deformity can be pronounced by placing the upper extremity in a dependent position and even giving a downward pull to it. Range of shoulder motion may be limited by pain. In standing or sitting position, stress the AC joint horizontally for AC ligament assessment and stress vertically for CC ligament assessment. Assess neurovascular status and possible associated other upper extremity injuries.

Paxinos test is performed by placing thumb pressure at the posterior AC joint to elicit tenderness and instability.

Cross-arm adduction test: The arm is elevated to 90° and then adducted across the chest with the elbow bent at approximately 90° to rest the hand on other shoulder. This cross-arm adduction produces pain specifically at the AC joint.

O'Brien's active compression test: It helps to differentiate symptoms of AC joint arthrosis from intra-articular superior glenoid labrum (SLAP lesion). The test is performed with the arm elevated to 90°, elbow in extension, adduction of 10–15°, and a maximum pronation of the forearm with obligate internal rotation of the arm. The examiner applies a downward force resisted by the patient. Symptoms referred to the top of the shoulder indicate AC joint lesion. This can be confirmed by palpation of the AC joint. Symptoms referred to the anterior glenohumeral joint suggest labral or biceps injury.

B. A number of methods and modifications had been proposed but common to them are—anatomic reduction of the AC joint correcting superior displacement and anterior-posterior translation reconstruction (chronic injury) of the CC ligament, supplementation or protection of the CC ligament repair or reconstruction with synthetic material, rigid implant may be used to maintain AC joint stability during initial healing; distal clavicular resection in patients with chronic acromioclavicular injuries where AC joint arthritis is present.

Resection of the distal end of the clavicle (Mumford procedure) is indicated for symptomatic grade I or II unreduced dislocations in which the coracoclavicular ligaments are intact. With improvements in techniques and instrumentation, arthroscopic distal clavicular resection has become more widely used, with results equal to or better than those of open techniques.

In chronic unreduced acromioclavicular dislocations of grades III, IV, and V, the coracoclavicular ligaments should be reconstructed.

CC ligament reconstruction: These are the most preferred method(s) and so many modifications exist that it is difficult to list all here. Few of these are:

- *Weaver-Dunn procedure*: Transfer of coracoacromial ligament to the distal clavicle to recreate CC ligament. Distal clavicle excision is needed. Added internal fixation needed as reconstruction has only 20% strength of native CC ligament. Arthroscopic modification is described. Augmentation with tendon or fascia auto-/allograft has also been described. CC ligament reconstruction with biological tissue: Figure of eight or rectangular reconstruction of CC ligament using palmaris longus or other tendon or fascia lata. Reinforce with internal fixation. The reconstruction may be done only for conoid component or for both conoid and trapezoid components (anatomical).
- *CC reconstruction with sutures/tapes*: This first commonly preferred for anatomical ligament reconstruction using endobutton and Mersilene tape. Suture/tapes are placed either around or through (preferred) clavicle and around the base of the coracoid, suture anchors may also be used. To prevent excess anterior translation of clavicle, the drill hole should be made in anterior thirds of bone for conoid portion. Simple cerclage around clavicle with suture or wire loops has chances of slippage and fracture of clavicle from attrition.

Rockwood described transfer of the coracoacromial ligament from the acromion to the clavicle while the clavicle is held reduced with a Bosworth screw.

22. Classify proximal humerus fractures. Discuss management of four-part fracture in an elderly man.

Ans: *Classification*:

Neer classification (Fig. 3.3.2): Classification is based on the four-part anatomy of the proximal humerus—the humeral head, the lesser and greater tuberosities, and the proximal humeral shaft. The criterion for displacement is greater than 1 cm of separation of part or angulation of 45°.

In each two-part pattern, segment named is the one displaced. Two-part surgical neck fractures can be impacted, unimpacted, and comminuted. All three-part patterns have displacement of shaft segment, and displaced tuberosity identifies type of three-part fracture. In four-part pattern, all segments are displaced. Fracture-dislocations are identified by anterior or posterior position of articular segment.

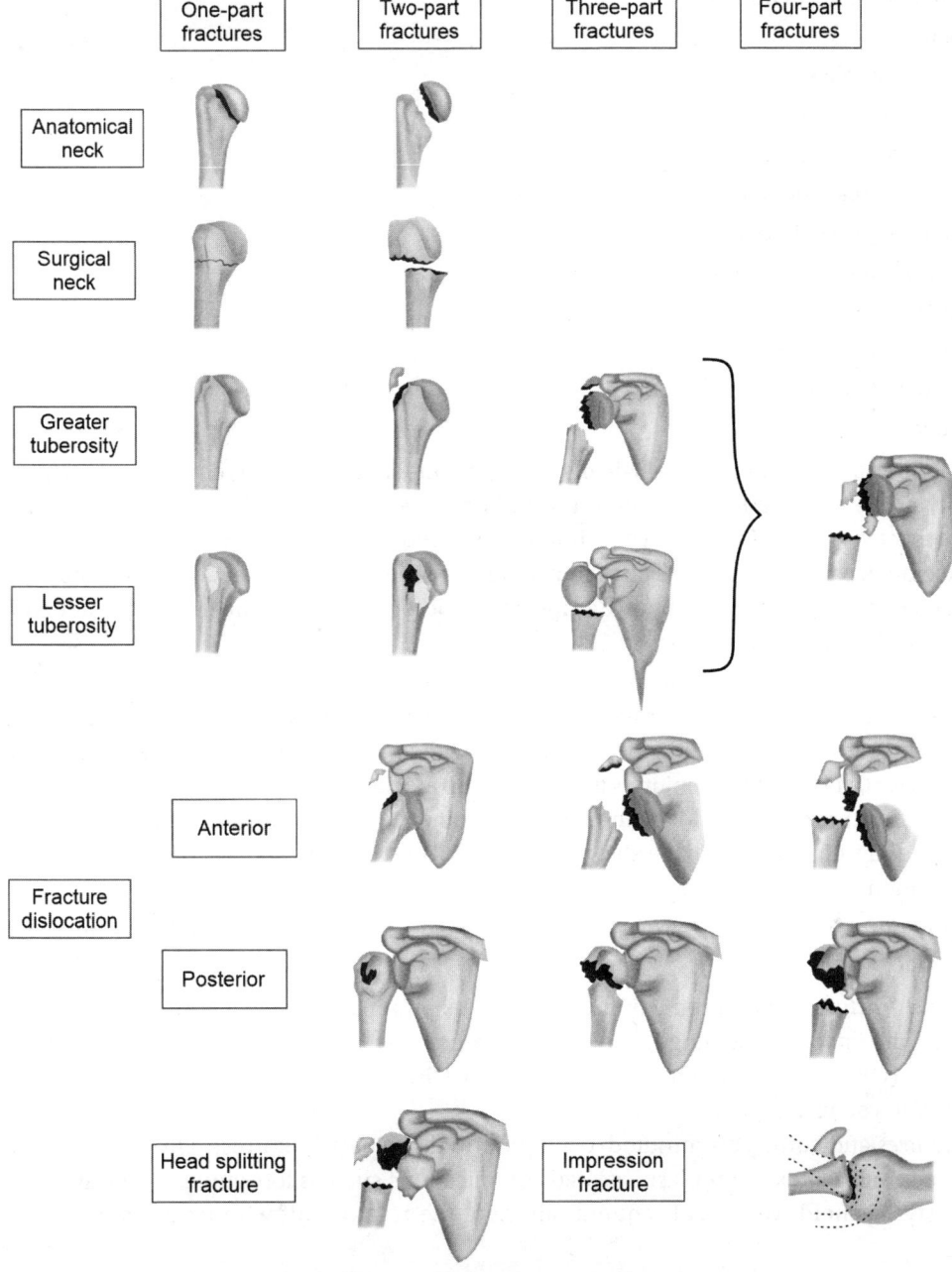

Fig. 3.3.2: Neer's classification.

- *One-part fractures*: No displaced fragments regardless of number of fracture lines/fragments.
- *Two-part fractures*: Any number of fractures/lines but one is displaced, viz., displaced anatomic neck or surgical neck or greater tuberosity or lesser tuberosity.
- *Three-part fractures*: 3–4 parts with displaced two parts relative to third (usually shaft). Surgical (commonly)/anatomical (unlikely) neck with greater lesser tuberosity.
- *Four-part fractures*: Fracture line involves four parts but three are displaced related to fourth.
- Fracture dislocation.
- *Articular surface fracture*: Head splitting/articular impression fractures like the Hill–Sachs lesion.

AO classification:
- 11-A extra-articular unifocal fracture
- 11-A1 tuberosity
- 11-A2 impacted metaphyseal
- 11-A3 nonimpacted metaphyseal
- 11-B extra-articular bifocal fracture
- 11-B1 with metaphyseal impaction
- 11-B2 without metaphyseal impaction
- 11-B3 with glenohumeral dislocation
- 11-C articular fracture
- 11-C1 with slight displacement
- 11-C2 impacted with marked displacement
- 11-C3 dislocated.

Management: Fractures that occur in physiologically older patients should be treated nonoperatively, if there is residual cortical continuity of the humeral head fragment on the shaft, the tuberosities are not too widely displaced, and the humeral head appears viable. Stable fractures (minimal comminution, three or less fragments, absence of significant tuberosity displacement, cortical contact, relative impaction of the stem into the head, and no history of dislocation) are a good candidate for conservative management. Complications of conservative management include stiffness, nonunion, loss of function, and osteonecrosis.

Operative treatment is offered to physiologically younger patients, where it is thought that the risk of nonunion, cuff dysfunction, or osteonecrosis is high or where operative treatment is likely to provide a significant improvement in shoulder function over nonoperative treatment. General indications for surgical management are open fractures, significant displacement, and segmental injuries in patients who are healthy enough for surgery. The risk of osteonecrosis is determined by the fracture configuration with wide displacement of the head from the shaft with probable loss of the medial periosteal and capsular hinge, and the absence of a medial metaphyseal spike particularly associated with a higher risk of this complication.

Isolated GT fractures: Prefer osteo-suturing/transosseous-equivalent suturing or perform else tension-band fixation or figure eight construct.

Two- and three-part fractures: Closed reduction percutaneous pinning (displaced surgical neck fractures and valgus impacted fractures with intact medial hinge). Pinning contraindicated in medial comminution—prefer open reduction and internal fixation (ORIF) with locked plate osteosynthesis. ORIF preferred for displaced two-, three-, and four-part fractures, especially in younger patients.

Four-part fractures and some comminuted/osteoporotic three-part fractures—ORIF versus arthroplasty. ORIF preserves bone stock and avoids arthroplasty-related complications such as loosening and wear. Other complications of hemiarthroplasty—glenoid wear + subsequent failure of the rotator cuff with proximal humeral migration and pseudoparalysis. The patient is always preoperatively counselled that if the fracture is deemed to be unreconstructable, an arthroplasty will be performed. In young patients, a cemented humeral head replacement will be performed, while a reverse total shoulder arthroplasty will be performed in the older patients. Indications of reverse total shoulder arthroplasty are controversial and possibly include three- or four-part fractures in patients older than 70 years, nonconstructible tuberosities, presence of rotator cuff tear, preexisting arthritis, and symptomatic malunion/nonunion.

23. Discuss management of fracture shaft of humerus with radial nerve palsy. What is Holstein–Lewis lesion and its management?

Ans: Classically, the occurrence of the nerve injury during an attempt at reduction of a distal third spiral oblique humerus fracture has been termed a *Holstein-Lewis injury*. The features that make radial nerve susceptible to injury during midshaft and distal one-third fractures of the humerus include:

- Its location in the spiral groove on the posterior aspect of the midshaft of the humerus close to bone
- Tethering of the nerve as it pierces the lateral intramuscular septum to enter the anterior compartment
- The factors are more pronounced when traction is applied or fracture angulates with a sharp lateral spike compressing the nerve.

Management: The incidence of radial nerve palsies has been reported to be as high as 18% but in 90% of these injuries, nerve function returns by 4–5 months. Usually, the radial nerve injury is a neurapraxia, with recovery rates of 100% in low-energy injuries and 33% in high-energy injuries. This time for waiting to return of function is logically derived. According to Steindler's formula, the nerve usually regenerates 1 mm/day or 3 cm in a month. Radial nerve injury often occurs 90–110 mm above the lateral condyle. Innervation of brachioradialis that originates 2 cm above the lateral condyle thus requires 70–90 mm of nerve regeneration. Considering the delay at neuromuscular junction of 1 month and a week delay at the nerve injury site for regeneration to begin, it will take 4–5 months' time for clinically detectable functional recovery of muscle. This implies that most radial nerve palsies are secondary to stretch or contusion. Treat the fractured humeral shaft in the usual nonoperative manner, support the wrist and fingers with a dynamic splint, and reserve exploration of the nerve, for instances, when function has not returned in 3–4 months and the fracture has healed. Routine exploration of all the nerve injuries (irrespective of pathological status) would subject many patients to an unnecessary operation and might increase the frequency of complications. Although it is possible for the nerve to be severed by the sharp edge of a bone fragment, this rarely occurs. Laceration rate of 12% has been reported in the literature, but considering the fact that there is hardly any discernible difference between early and late repairs (functional outcome), it is better to wait for the recovery than explore the nerve. This saves many patients of unnecessary exploration. Acute nerve exploration is, however, indicated when:

- The palsy is associated with open humeral fractures.
- The palsy is associated with fractures requiring open reduction and internal fixation (displaced and nonreducible fractures). The fracture may be nonreducible due to nerve interposition itself.
- Fracture associated with vascular injury
- The palsy occurs following an attempted reduction of the humerus shaft fracture.

While the surgeon is awaiting neurological recovery, the patient is encouraged to passively mobilize the joints of hand and wrist. Additionally, to maintain the wrist in extension for preventing any flexion contracture, he can be given dynamic or static cock-up splint.

In open fracture of the humeral shaft with radial nerve palsy, explore the radial nerve and if found impaled on bone or is caught between the fragments, then formal exploration is needed else just wait for recovery. Ultrasonography by an experienced observer may be helpful for identifying entrapped nerve.

In patients with radial nerve palsy for whom operative treatment of a humeral shaft fracture is indicated, the nerve should be explored at the time of fracture fixation. Complete transection of the radial nerve usually occurs with open fractures of the humerus and requires nerve repair or grafting; most nerve palsies that occur with a closed fracture recover without treatment.

Holstein–Lewis lesion is managed conservatively, if the fracture is closed and radial nerve palsy usually resolves. If fracture is compound or conservative, measures fail over reasonable period of time (see above), then only surgery is undertaken.

24. Discuss algorithm for management of radial nerve palsy.

Ans: The **Flowchart 3.3.1** is a comprehensive algorithm depicting the decision making and management of radial nerve palsy.

Flowchart 3.3.1: Management of radial nerve palsy.

```
Closed Injury                                                    Open Injury
     │                                                                │
     ├──────────────┐                                                  ▼
     ▼              ▼           NCV vs. ultrasound for        Nerve exploration
Injection-related  Observe ──► documenting continuity ──No──►         │
nerve palsy                    and conduction                         ▼
     │                         (medicolegal implication)    Cut/severely thinned out/visibly
     ▼                              │         │              so damaged that recovery
>3 months/no                        ▼         ▼              impossible/delayed cases
improvement                    Intact/      Entrapped        with neuroma formation
     │                         contused        │
     ▼                            │            ▼
Neurolysis/Excision              ▼         Extricate
(partial vs complete)         Observe         │
and repair/grafting              │            ▼
     │                           │         Surgical    Injury extent   Surgical repair
     │                           ▼         repair      not definite    impossible
     │                    Calculate waiting time           │                │
     │                           │                         ▼                │
     │              ┌────────────┼──────────┐       Re-exploration          │
     ▼              ▼            ▼          │       after 2–3 months        │
             Improved      No improvement ──vs.──►              ──► Tendon transfer
```

25. Enumerate injuries due to FOOSH (fall on outstretched hand).

Ans: *In adults*:
- Distal radius fractures like Colles, Smith, Barton and Chauffeur fracture.
- Carpal fractures like scaphoid, triquetrum and hamate fracture
- Forearm fractures like Galeazzi, Monteggia, Essex Lopresti, radial head fracture.
- Dislocation of shoulder— commonly anterior others are rare, acromion fracture.
- A-C joint dislocation

In children:
- Torus fractures
- Salter-Harris fractures of distal forearm
- Supracondylar fracture
- Lateral condyle Salter-Harris types 2 and 4 fracture of distal humerus
- Proximal humerus S-H types 1 and 2 injury to physis
- Scaphoid fracture.

26. Classify fractures around the elbow in a 6-year-old.

Ans: Pediatric elbow fractures include various fractures important of which are fractures of distal humerus and proximal radius, and monteggia injuries.

Descriptive classification describes the involved anatomical region. Commonly following fractures are described:
- *Supracondylar fractures*:
  - Extension-type
  - Flexion-type.
- Transcondylar fractures
- Intercondylar fractures
- Capitellum fractures
- Lateral condylar fractures
- Medial epicondylar fractures
- Radial neck fractures
- Monteggia fractures
- Olecranon fracture/epiphyseal injury.

Supracondylar fractures of distal humerus:
- *Type I*: Nondisplaced fractures
- *Type II*: Displaced with angulation but intact posterior cortex
- *Type IIA*: Angulation only
- *Type IIB*: With rotation
- *Type III*: Completely displaced with no cortical contact. Some add two subtypes as A without rotation and B with rotation of the fragment.

  Modified Gartland classification divides type III into two subtypes and adds a fourth type as follows:
- *Type IIIA*: Completely displaced posteromedially
- *Type IIIB*: Completely displaced posterolaterally
- *Type IV*: Multidirectional instability with circumferential periosteal disruption.

Pediatric lateral condyle humerus fracture: Milch classification divides the fracture based on the fracture line extension, but is less useful in guiding treatment.
- *Type I (uncommon)*: Fracture line lateral to trochlear groove (elbow is stable and less common fracture type). Salter-Harris type IV physeal injury.
- *Type II*: Fracture line extends into trochlear groove (more common and unstable fracture pattern). Salter-Harris type II pattern fracture.

Song classification: This is a recent classification that also incorporates the medial and lateral fracture gaps to better guide treatment.
- *Stage 1*: ≤2 mm having limited fracture line within metaphysis in all views—stable fracture
- *Stage 2*: ≤2 mm with lateral gap in all views—doubtful stability
- *Stage 3*: ≤2 mm with lateral gap as wide as medial one—unstable
- *Stage 4*: >2 mm without fragment rotation on all views—unstable
- *Stage 5*: >2 mm with fragment rotation—unstable

Pediatric radial neck fracture classification: Judet classification:
- *Type I*: Undisplaced
- *Type II*: <30° angulation
- *Type III*: 30–60°
- *Type IVa*: 60–80°
- *Type IVb*: >80°.

Pediatric medial epicondyle fracture: No standard classification. The fractures can be classified as follows:
- Nondisplaced fractures—≤5 mm displacement

- Displaced fractures—>5 mm displacement
- Medial epicondyle fracture associated with dislocation of the elbow joint.

Monteggia fracture dislocation: Bado classification with modifications fracture of proximal or middle third ulna with anterior radial head dislocation.
- *Type 1*: Anteriorly angulated fracture of proximal or middle third ulna with anterior radial head dislocation.
- *Type 2*: Posteriorly angulated fracture of proximal or middle third ulna with posterior/posterolateral radial head dislocation.
- *Type 3*: Fracture ulnar metaphysis distal to coronoid with lateral/anterolateral radial head dislocation.
- *Type 4*: Fracture of proximal or middle third ulna and radius with dislocation of radial head in any direction (commonly anterior).

Jupiter sub-classification of type 2 Bado:
- *Type 2A*: Coronoid level
- *Type 2B*: Metadiaphyseal junction
- *Type 2C*: Distal to coronoid
- *Type 2D*: Fracture extending to distal half of ulna.

27. Functional and surgical anatomy of distal humerus.

Ans: Functional anatomy:

The distal humerus is triangular in shape formed of two curved columns interconnected by an articular region forming base of the triangle. The articular part includes the following:
1. The capitulum is a rounded projection rotated 30° anteriorly which articulates with the concavity of head of the radius.
2. The trochlea is a pulley-shaped surface. It articulates with the trochlear notch of the ulna. The axis of rotation is angulated 6–8° anteriorly in coronal plane projecting distally on medial side contributing to the valgus and the formation of the carrying angle. This is lost in flexion, so the valgus is lost in flexion.

The nonarticular part includes the following **(Fig. 3.3.3)**:
- The medial epicondyle—serves as attachment to superficial flexor muscles of the forearm (the common flexor origin).
- The lateral epicondyle—gives attachment to superficial extensor muscles of the forearm, supinator and anconeus.
- The lateral supracondylar ridge—gives attachment to brachioradialis, extensor carpi radialis longus.
- The medial supracondylar ridge—gives attachment to pronator teres.
- The coronoid fossa
- The radial fossa
- The olecranon fossa

Ligamentous attachments at distal humerus:
- *Ulnar collateral ligament*: It has three parts **(Table 3.3.1)**
- *Lateral collateral ligament*: It has 4 parts **(Table 3.3.2)**

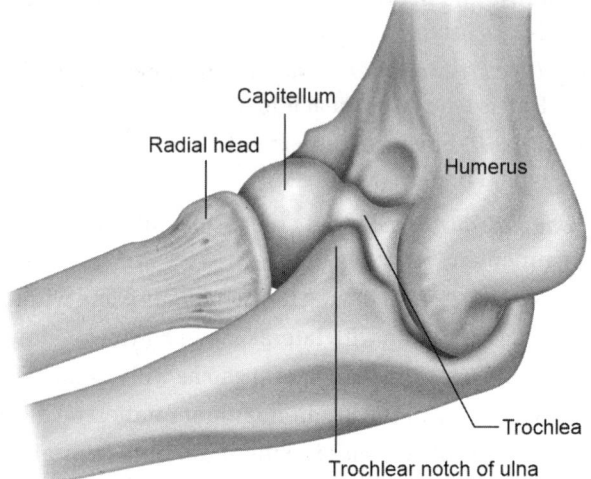

Fig. 3.3.3: The bony anatomy of elbow joint.

TABLE 3.3.1: Ulnar collateral ligament.

Part	Origin	Insertion
Anterior	Medial epicondyle anteroinferior aspect	Sublime tubercle
Posterior	Medial epicondyle anteroinferior aspect	Greater sigmoid notch
Transverse band (ligament of cooper)	Traverses the medial border of greater sigmoid notch	

TABLE 3.3.2: Lateral collateral ligament.

Part	Origin	Insertion
Radial collateral ligament	Lateral epicondyle	Lateral aspect of annular ligament
Annular ligament	Anterior margin of sigmoid notch	Posterior margin of sigmoid notch
Lateral ulnar collateral ligament	Lateral epicondyle	Supinator crest of ulna
Accessory radial collateral ligament	Distal margin of annular ligament	• Type I—bilobed • Type II—broad • Distal to lateral *ulnar collateral ligament*

Movements at elbow as conferred by distal humerus:
Elbow is a hinge joint in 5° axial rotation. It is a highly conformed joint with very small locus of rotation.

- *Range of motion (normal joint)*:
  - Flexion = 0–140°
  - Pronation = 75°
  - Supination = 80°
- *Range of motion needed for activities of daily living*:
  - Flexion range = 100° (30–130°)
  - Rotation range = 100° (50° pronation and 50° supination)
- The elbow is a slightly loose hinge with small amounts of varus, valgus and rotational laxity throughout its range of motion.
- The center of the arc formed by the trochlea and capitellum is on a line that is coplanar to the anterior distal cortex. Therefore, 5–7° of internal rotation is observed at the distal humeral articular surface with respect to midline.
- In a frontal plane, there is about 6° of the valgus tilt of the condyles with respect to the longitudinal axis of the humerus. Articular surface accounts for more than 50% of elbow stability in extension and more than 70% of elbow stability when the elbow is flexed 90°.

Constraints of elbow:
- *Valgus stress*:
  - *Primary*:
    - *Medial collateral ligament*:
      - *Anterior bundle*: Principle-stabilizer in 30–120° flexion
      - *Posterior bundle*: Co-restraint
  - *Secondary*: Radial head
    - *Tertiary*: Flexor-pronator muscle groups (flex carpi radialis, flexor digitorum superficialis)
- *Varus stress*:
  - *Primary*: Lateral collateral ligament and annular ligament complex
  - *Secondary*:
    - Extensor muscles with fascial band
    - Intermuscular septa

Surgical anatomy:
Critical neurovascular structures pass all around distal humerus nerves.

Ulnar nerve: Highly variable course. The ulnar nerve runs initially in the anterior compartment of the arm and goes posteriorly through the medial intermuscular septum at an average distance of about 6–8 cm proximal to the medial epicondyle. In some cases, a band of fibrous tissue is present at the level of passage of ulnar nerve through intermuscular septum—arcade of Struthers which serve as a potential site of nerve compression. In vicinity of distal humerus, the ulnar nerve engages in the cubital tunnel, which is comprised proximally by the Osborne ligament (a fibrous structure stretched between the two heads of the FCU) and is formed distally by the deep flexor/pronator aponeurosis (approximately 5 cm distal to the medial epicondyle).

The radial nerve: After crossing the back of the humerus and giving off branches to the lateral head and the lateral part of the medial head of the triceps, the radial nerve pierces the lateral intermuscular septum, entering the anterior compartment. At this point, the nerve may be vulnerable to distal locking bolts inserted from the lateral side of the arm. The nerve lies between the brachioradialis and brachialis muscles as it crosses the elbow joint.

The median nerve remains in the anterior compartment, anteromedial to the humerus. It runs with the brachial artery, lateral to it in the upper arm and medial to it in the cubital fossa.

Vessels:

The brachial artery: At the elbow, it curves laterally to lie over the anterior surface of the bone, where it may be damaged in supracondylar fractures of the humerus.

The profunda brachii artery runs with the radial nerve, supplying the triceps brachii muscle.

The ulnar collateral artery runs with the ulnar nerve. The three arteries anastomose freely with one another around the elbow joint.

28. Complications of lateral condyle fracture elbow in children.

Ans: Complications of lateral condyle fracture of distal humerus in children:
- Physeal arrest
- Physeal stimulation
- Osteonecrosis
- Nonunion and proximal migration of the fragment—cubitus valgus deformity
- Cubitus varus deformity—transient stimulation resulting in lateral condylar overgrowth, radial prominence, and variation in the carrying angle of the elbow have been described. Osteonecrosis of the capitellum
- "Fishtail" deformity (deepening of the trochlear groove)
- Tardy ulnar nerve palsy.

29. Classify distal humerus fractures in adults. Describe the surgical approaches used for internal fixation of these fractures.

Ans: *Mehne and Matta classification*:
- *Type A*: High T-fractures
- *Type B*: Low T-fractures
- *Type C*: Y-fractures
- *Type D*: H-fractures
- *Type E*: Medial lambda
- *Type F*: Lateral lambda.

AO classification:
- 13-A extra-articular fracture
- 13-A1 apophyseal avulsion
- 13-A2 metaphyseal simple
- 13-A3 metaphyseal multifragmentary
- 13-B partial articular fracture
- 13-B1 sagittal lateral condyle
- 13-B2 sagittal medial condyle
- 13-B3 coronal

- 13-C complete articular fracture
- 13-C1 articular simple and metaphyseal simple
- 13-C2 articular simple and metaphyseal multifragmentary
- 13-C3 articular multifragmentary

Surgical approaches:
- Alonso-Llames triceps sparing approach—medial and lateral windows are developed by side of triceps and triceps erased subperiosteally from humerus. Done for limited extra-articular fractures.
- Campbell triceps splitting approach—triceps is split in the midline but approach is limited proximally by radial nerve.
- Van Gordner approach—distal tongue of triceps fascia is prepared in an inverted-V and rest as for triceps splitting approach. Better repairs extensor mechanism.
- Bryan-Morrey approach—medial approach raising triceps and extensor mechanism as a full subperiosteal sleeve off posterior humerus and ulna.
- Triceps-reflecting and anconeus pedicle (TRAP) approach of O'Driscoll—the extensor mechanism is raised with vascularized anconeus pedicle to act as dynamic stabilizer. The approach begins laterally in Kocher's interval [between extensor carpi ulnaris (ECU) and anconeus] raising anconeus from ulna preserving lateral collateral ligament (LCL) and flap is continued with extensor mechanism and triceps. Medially ulnar nerve is preserved. The tongue—this raised contains triceps, extensor mechanism, and anconeus.
- Olecranon osteotomy—preferred by many. Site of osteotomy is decided by either raising anconeus off laterally or medial capsular dissection to visualize trochlea. Chevron osteotomy is preferred as this enters in area relatively devoid of articular cartilage. Incomplete osteotomy is completed by hand allowing interdigitation during replacement. Reflect the olecranon and triceps together to expose distal humerus.

30. **What is terrible triad of elbow and how will you manage it? Outline principles of management of intercondylar fracture.**

Ans: The "terrible triad" consists of an elbow dislocation in conjunction with fractures of the radial head and coronoid (Fig. 3.3.4).

Principles of managing terrible triad injuries:
- Restore coronoid stability—fracture fixation in type II or III fractures versus anterior capsular repair for type I.
- Restore radial head stability ORIF versus radial head replacement.
- Restore lateral elbow stability (repair of the LCL complex ± secondary constraints—the common extensor origin, posterolateral capsule).
- Repair medial collateral ligament (usually needed in patients with residual posterior instability).
- Use hinged external fixator when sufficient joint stability cannot be restored with above methods.

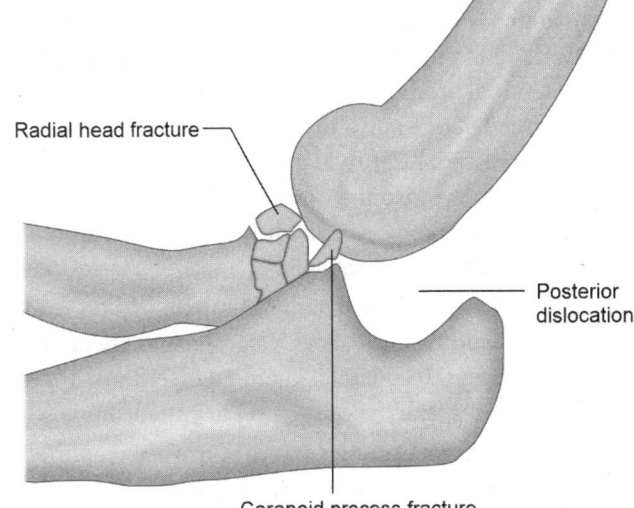

Fig. 3.3.4: Illustration of terrible triad injury to elbow.

Treatment: The choice of approach depends primarily on fracture pattern, type of instability, soft tissue injury, and surgeon experience. A direct lateral approach or a midline incision with subcutaneous flaps to the Kocher interval usually is used; the latter allows a second interval medially, if necessary. Every effort should be made to operate through the traumatized planes and minimize surgical dissection. The fixation strategy usually is from deep to superficial as seen from the lateral approach (coronoid to anterior capsule to radial head to lateral collateral ligament to common extensor origin).

Coronoid fixation depends on the size of the fragment. Small tip avulsions usually are reduced and fixed with sutures through holes drilled in the posterior olecranon. This effectively anchors the anterior capsule to the coronoid. Larger fragments are stabilized with lag screws from the posterior olecranon.

Management of the radial head fracture depends on comminution, quality of the bone and existing joint condition. If the fracture cannot be reduced and stabilized adequately or the joint is arthritic, replacement with a metal prosthesis is indicated. Usually, radial head replacement is kept at the end of operative procedure as the fixation of coronoid fracture is facilitated by removal of the radial head giving adequate exposure of the coronoid fragment.

After coronoid and radial head stabilization or replacement, the lateral collateral ligament is reattached to its origin, as is the common extensor origin.

Principles of managing intercondylar fracture of elbow:
- Every screw should pass through a plate.
- Each screw should engage a fragment on the opposite side that is also fixed to a plate (now not needed with newer anatomical locking plates and screws).
- As many screws as possible should be placed in the distal fragments.
- Each screw should be as long as possible.
- Each screw should engage as many articular fragments as possible.
- Plates should be applied such that compression is achieved at the supracondylar level for both columns [now with locking compression plate (LCP) is not necessary instead anatomical reduction and alignment is of utmost importance].
- Plates used must be strong enough and stiff enough to resist breaking or bending before union occurs at the supracondylar level.
- Medial and lateral column should be restored separately with implants.
- The medial and lateral column plates should not end at same level in the shaft region, else a stress riser is created predisposing to fracture of the shaft.

31. Discuss clinical presentation of terrible triad elbow. What are its short- and long-term complications of terrible triad elbow?

Ans: Clinical presentation:
Because this is a circumferential injury with associated subluxations and dislocations, there is extensive ecchymosis and swelling of the elbow. The typical presentation is of dislocated elbow—loss of three-point relationship, prominent triceps tendon, prominent olecranon and fullness in anterior elbow region. A detailed neurovascular examination must be performed before and after reduction of a dislocated elbow. Soft-tissue status and the condition of the skin should be carefully assessed. After reduction, the elbow is unstable in varus and valgus stress test indicating ligament injury and loss of lateral bony restraint from radial head. Movements at elbow may be restricted if there is interposed bony fragment and elbow may spontaneously dislocate in extension if the coronoid fragment is large and there is complete injury of collateral ligaments and capsule.

In chronic/old cases, patients complain of pain, and clicking and locking with elbow in extension. Range of motion is decreased and painful. Varus/valgus instability patterns are also observed. The elbow should be palpated for signs of tenderness over the collateral ligament insertions. The shoulder, wrist, and distal radioulnar joint should be examined. Radiographic signs of these fractures are often subtle stressing the importance of detailed physical examination.

Ipsilateral upper extremity injuries have been reported in 10–20% of patients with fracture dislocations of the elbow with the majority involving fractures of the wrist. Associated injuries of the head, chest, abdomen, pelvis, or lower extremities are seen in patients with higher-energy trauma.

Complications:

Early:
- Nerve palsy
- Residual instability/subluxation
- Redislocation
- Failure of internal fixation

Late:
- Elbow stiffness and heterotopic ossification
- Post-traumatic arthritis

32. Explain management of supracondylar fracture with pink pulseless hand.

Ans: An absent radial pulse is not in itself an emergency, as collateral circulation may keep the limb well perfused in the short term and potentially even in long term. However, in the presence of an associated nerve injury, there is higher risk of a compartment syndrome and more cautious close observation until surgery is indicated. In the case of a pulseless, perfused hand, urgent, but nonemergent, reduction with pinning in the operating room is indicated. Further course of action depends on the condition of limb in post-reduction/fixation period. There are following scenarios that may arise and respective common recommendation after closed pinning is done (**Flowchart 3.3.2**):

Flowchart 3.3.2: Management of supracondylar fracture.

```
Pediatric supracondylar fracture
with absent distal pulses
          │
          ▼
Gentle traction and flexion
       to 35–40°
          │
          ▼
Closed/open reduction
     and pinning
   ┌──────┼──────┐
   ▼      ▼      ▼
Perfusion +  Perfusion present;  Perfusion doubtful;
Pulses +     Pulses absent       Pulses absent
   │           │                    │
   ▼           ▼                    ▼
Standard    Admit and          Exploration and
operative   observation        repair as needed
care
```

- Limb remains perfused with good capillary refill pulses present—standard postoperative care to be followed
- Limb remains perfused with adequate capillary refill but no pulses—observe closely under admission for progression/deterioration
- Perfusion of limb is jeopardized, no pulses and poor capillary refill—take immediate vascular consult and consider exploration.

33. Describe supracondylar fracture humerus in pediatric age group:
   A. Management of the poorly perfused white hand.
   B. Management of a supracondylar fracture with associated nerve injury.

Ans:

A. Following a fracture reduction, the presence of a poorly perfused, pulseless hand necessitates immediate and decisive intervention. If a pulse was detected prior to the reduction, one must infer that the arterial supply or associated soft tissues may be compromised or entrapped at the fracture site. In such cases, the appropriate course of action involves the removal of any fixation devices, such as pins, and a thorough exploration of the affected artery. Conversely, if the hand exhibited inadequate perfusion prior to the fracture reduction and continues to demonstrate poor perfusion postprocedure, urgent arterial exploration becomes imperative.

Utilizing an anterior approach for exploration serves to elucidate any potential kinking of the artery caused by entrapped adjacent soft tissues or the incarceration of the artery between fracture fragments. Upon successful liberation of the artery from the fracture site, it is crucial to address any resultant arterial spasms. This can be achieved through the application of lidocaine, gentle warming of the area, and a subsequent observation period of 10–15 minutes to assess for improvement in perfusion.

Should the clinical situation necessitate, following anatomic reduction of the fracture and adequate decompression of the neurovascular bundle in the pulseless limb, and if perfusion remains compromised, vascular reconstruction by a qualified specialist must be urgently indicated. Timely and thorough assessment, along with prompt surgical intervention, is essential to preserve limb viability and optimize patient outcomes.

B. The management of nerve injuries associated with closed fractures requires a nuanced understanding of the potential for neural recovery and the necessity for surgical intervention. Open reduction and direct exploration of the injured nerve is not universally warranted in these cases. Empirical evidence indicates that, irrespective of the specific nerve affected, neural recovery is typically observed within a timeframe of 2–2.5 months, although in certain circumstances, full recovery may extend up to 6 months.

In the context of supracondylar fractures, it is critical to recognize that nerve compression, coupled with the development of perineural fibrosis, is frequently implicated as a principal cause of prolonged neurologic deficits. Thus, careful monitoring following injury is imperative, as the degree of fracture displacement does not always correlate with the presence of nerve injury; even minimally displaced fractures can give rise to significant neural deficits.

A comprehensive neurologic examination is essential prior to initiating any therapeutic interventions, even in cases classified as mild injuries. The assessment should aim to elucidate the extent of neural involvement and guide subsequent management strategies. In scenarios where a fracture is irreducible and simultaneously presents with a nerve deficit, open reduction becomes an imperative procedure. This intervention serves a dual purpose: to realign the fracture and to ensure that there is no nerve entrapment contributing to the deficit.

Moreover, it is important to acknowledge that chronic nerve entrapment within a healed callus can mimic a radiographic phenomenon known as Metev's sign, which manifests as an apparent osseous defect or "hole" in the bone. This sign underscores the necessity for clinicians to maintain a high index of suspicion for underlying nerve pathologies in the setting of healed fractures, thereby ensuring that appropriate diagnostic and therapeutic measures are taken. In summary, while nerve exploration may not be required in all cases, diligent observation and assessment remain cornerstone components of the management protocol for nerve injuries associated with closed fractures.

34. Discuss management and complications of pediatric supracondylar humerus fractures.

Ans:

Management:
- Closed reduction and casting is reserved for stable, nondisplaced fractures (type I).
- Closed reduction with percutaneous pinning for all unstable, displaced fractures (types II and III). This is the most common operative treatment of supracondylar fractures. An initial attempt at closed reduction is indicated in almost all displaced supracondylar fractures that are not open fractures. Under general anesthesia, the fracture is first reduced in the frontal plane with fluoroscopic verification. The elbow is then flexed while pushing the olecranon anteriorly to correct the sagittal deformity and reduce the fracture. Criteria for an acceptable reduction include restoration of Baumann's angle (which is generally <10°) on the AP view, intact medial and lateral columns on oblique views, and the *anterior humeral line* passes through the middle third of the capitellum on the lateral view.
  The two main issues with crossed-pin versus lateral entry pinning of these fractures are: (1) Risk of ulnar nerve injury and (2) risk of loss of reduction. Iatrogenic injury to the ulnar nerve with use of crossed pins has been reported.
- *Open reduction*: Open reduction is indicated in cases of failed closed reduction, a loss of pulse or poorly perfused hand following reduction, and open fractures.

Complications:

Early complications:
- Neurological compromise—usually a neurapraxia—is reported to occur in 3–22% of patients with supracondylar fractures. Any of the peripheral nerves—median, anterior interosseous, radial, or ulnar—may be damaged, and mixed nerve lesions have been reported.
- Injury to the brachial artery occurs in 10% of patients with supracondylar fractures. Often the problem is corrected after the fracture has been reduced and circulation returns to normal.
- Compartment syndrome is an uncommon but serious complication of supracondylar fractures. Compartment syndromes occur as the result of hypoxic damage caused by interruption of the circulation to the muscles. Any evidence of compartment syndrome requires vascular consultation, compartment pressure measurements, and possibly fasciotomy.

Late complications:
- *Malunion*: Cubitus varus is the most common angular deformity that results from supracondylar fractures in children. Cubitus valgus, although mentioned in the literature as causing tardy ulnar nerve palsy, rarely occurs and is more often caused by nonunion of lateral condylar fractures.
- *Myositis ossificans*: It is an ectopic new bone formation around the elbow resulting in stiffness. Massaging after injury leads to this complication.
- *Volkmann ischemic contracture*: It is a sequel to Volkmann ischemia. The ischemic muscles are gradually replaced by fibrous tissue that contract and produce deformity of wrist and fingers.

35. Discuss outcomes of a supracondylar fracture of humerus in children.
Ans: Kindly see the answer above.

36. Describe management of brachial artery injury in association with supracondylar fracture of humerus.
Ans: Vide answer above.

37. Discuss the following procedure—Modified French osteotomy.
Ans: *French, Modified by Bellemore et al.*
- The surgical procedure initiates with a posterolateral incision, which provides access to the underlying anatomical structures. Upon exposing the triceps muscle, it is imperative to carefully split the muscle and detach it from its insertion at the olecranon. The next step involves reflecting the triceps proximally, which allows for unhindered access to the humerus.
- Attention must then be directed toward the subperiosteal elevation of the middle two-thirds of the triceps from the surface of the humerus. It is crucial to protect the neurovascular bundle during this dissection to avoid any potential vascular or nerve injury.
- A laterally based wedge is subsequently outlined on the humeral bone, ensuring that the incision does not extend into the medial cortex. Following this delineation, a screw is inserted into the lateral cortex in the proximal region, positioned above the proposed osteotomy. A second screw is placed distally, below the intended osteotomy, at an angle that closely approximates that of the wedge intended for resection.
- Utilizing an oscillating saw, the wedge is then resected while the apex remains attached to the medial cortex. Upon resection, the elbow is extended, facilitating the closure of the wedge by fracturing the medial cortex. It is essential to retain a periosteal hinge during this maneuver to preserve the viability of the surrounding tissue.
- With the forearm placed in a supinated position, it is necessary to assess the carrying angle to determine its adequacy. Should the carrying angle meet the desired criteria, a wire loop is tightened around the heads of the screws. This action will appose the cut surfaces securely. In the event that any rotational deformities are observed, corrective measures must be implemented at this stage by adjusting the position of the distal screw. This involves derotating the distal fragment, addressing any identified deformity, and ensuring proper alignment with the superior screw. Finally, the wires around the screw heads are tightened to ensure stable fixation and alignment of the osteotomy site.

38. Classify fractures of capitellum and discuss management of each type.
Ans: *Classification*: Bryan and Morrey with Mckee modification—
- The Hahn–Steinthal or conventional type 1 fracture involves the capitellar articular surface along with the subchondral bone.
- The Kocher–Lorenz or conventional type 2 fracture is rare and consists of the capitellar articular surface along with a thin shell of subchondral bone.
- Type 3 fractures which are comminuted capitellar fractures.
- Type 4—type 1 fracture with medial extension to include the lateral half of the trochlea.

Management
Nonoperative treatment of partial articular fractures: Closed reduction and casting is a described method for the treatment of displaced capitellar fractures. The reduction maneuver involves placing the elbow into full extension and forearm

supination, which usually results in the capitellum spontaneously reducing. If still displaced, manual pressure over the capitellum and a slight varus force to the elbow may assist with the reduction. If successful, the elbow is flexed so the radial head captures the capitellar fragment and then fluoroscopy is used to confirm the reduction. The elbow is immobilized in an above-elbow plaster for 3 weeks with weekly radiographs to confirm maintenance of the reduction. If this technique is used, recommended is postoperative CT imaging to confirm an anatomic reduction.

Operative: Goal is anatomic restoration.

Open reduction and internal fixation is the technique of choice.

This technique is indicated for displaced type I fractures.

Via a posterolateral or posterior approach, screws may be placed from a posterior to anterior direction; alternatively, headless screws may be placed from anterior to posterior.

Fixation should be stable enough to allow early range of elbow motion. Fixation modalities include headless compression screws (Herbert or mini-Acutrak type) or mini fragment screws sunk well below the articular cartilage.

Type IV fractures—these are better exposed by extensile lateral approach to address medial trochlear fragment and any associated radial head/neck fracture. Supplemental medial exposure may be also necessary to preserve the collateral ligaments.

Excision: This is rarely indicated for severely comminuted type I fractures and most type II fractures. Care must be taken in the elderly, as these are often type IV fractures, which if excised, will lead to elbow instability.

This may be the recommended treatment in chronic missed fractures with limited range of elbow motion.

39. Discuss mechanism of injury of radial head fractures along with its classification and management.

Ans: *Mechanism*: Most radial head fractures occur as the result of low-energy mechanisms such as a trip and fall on an outstretched hand. Sporting activities as well as motor vehicle collisions cause higher-energy fractures typically with greater displacement and a higher incidence of concomitant injuries. Mechanisms of fracture vary but include three common patterns:

1. A valgus load causes impaction of the radial head into the capitellum, commonly with rupture of the medial collateral ligament (MCL).
2. Posterolateral rotatory subluxation of the radial head with respect to the capitellum causes a partial articular shear fracture of the anterior portion of the radial head often with rupture of the LCL.
3. An axial forearm load causes impaction of the radial head into the capitellum with more severe trauma producing a fracture of the coronoid or rupture of the interosseous membrane and distal radioulnar joint ligaments; the so-called Essex–Lopresti injury.

Classification: Mason classification **(Fig. 3.3.5)**:

- *Type I*: Undisplaced segmental (marginal) fracture
- *Type II*: Displaced segmental fracture
- *Type III*: Comminuted fracture
- *Type IV*: Fracture associated with posterior dislocation of the elbow

Management: Radial head fractures are common, however, the majority is minimally displaced or undisplaced, and can be treated successfully nonoperatively.

Management of type II isolated, displaced, stable, and partial articular fracture is highly debated with equivalent results from operative and conservative management.

Mason type III: It is recommended to reconstruct the radial head by ORIF if up to three simple fragments are present and fixable. The osteosynthesis is done in the safe zone identified by either the Smith and Hotchkiss method or Caputo et al. method. For more than three fragments, the results of osteosynthesis are not very favorable and should be replaced by arthroplasty.

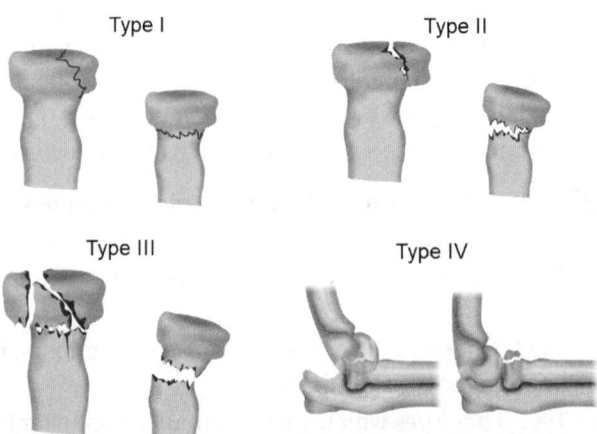

Fig. 3.3.5: Mason classification.

Radial head excision is uncommonly performed for acute radial head fractures due to a significant incidence of concomitant ligament injuries and the advent of reliable prosthetic arthroplasty.

Type IV Mason and terrible triad injuries: These need thorough evaluation of associated ligament and bony injuries. Restoration of ulnohumeral articulation is a priority along with elbow stability. So, fix olecranon/coronoid, repair/reconstruct LCL/MCL, and if osteosynthesis is possible, then perform ORIF for radial head, else replace the same.

40. Define and classify Monteggia fracture dislocation. Discuss the treatment principles of neglected Monteggia fracture dislocation in a 10-year-old child.

Ans: *Definition*: Monteggia fracture-dislocations are a rare but a complex injury usually involving a fracture of the ulna associated with proximal radioulnar joint dissociation and radiocapitellar dislocation.

Classification: Bado classification

Bado Type I: A Bado type I lesion is an anterior dislocation of the radial head associated with an apex anterior ulnar diaphyseal fracture at any level. This is the most common Monteggia lesion in children and represents approximately 70–75% of all injuries.

Bado Type II: A Bado type II lesion is a posterior or posterolateral dislocation of the radial head associated with an apex posterior ulnar diaphyseal or metaphyseal fracture. This pattern is the most common Monteggia lesion in adults, but is relatively rare in children.

Bado Type III: A Bado type III lesion is a lateral dislocation of the radial head associated with a varus (apex lateral) fracture of the proximal ulna.

Bado Type IV: A Bado type IV lesion is an anterior dislocation of the radial head associated with fractures of both the ulna and the radius.

Letts classification: Letts types A, B, and C are analogous to Bado type I lesions and are characterized by anterior dislocation of the radial head with an associated ulnar fracture.
- *Type A lesion*: There is plastic deformation of the ulna.
- *Type B lesion*: There is an incomplete or greenstick ulnar fracture.
- *Type C lesion*: There is a complete ulnar fracture.
- *Type D lesion*: Equivalent to Bado type II injuries and are characterized by posterior radial head dislocation.
- *Letts type E lesion*: Equivalent to Bado type III injuries and are characterized by lateral radial head dislocation.

Treatment principles in neglected case: Surgical reconstruction of a chronic Monteggia is needed when—
- The diagnosis is made early.
- There is preservation of the normal concave radial head and convex capitellum.
- Especially when there is progressive deformity (i.e. valgus), loss of motion and pain.
- The patient and family are well aware of the concerns with operative reconstruction.

In patients younger than 12 years of age with delayed diagnosis of a Monteggia lesion, reduction and stabilization of the radial head to its anatomic relationship with the capitellum is done, if the radial head is still concave centrally. Even though the child may do well in the short term without reduction of the radial head, problems usually develop in adolescence or adulthood when progressive instability, pain, weakness of the forearm, and restriction of motion are likely. There is also a risk of tardy radial or ulnar nerve palsies. The concavity of the radial head and convexity of the capitellum are assessed preoperatively, usually by MRI scan. Appropriate discussion with the patient and family regarding the risks and complications of surgery is performed. This is not an operation for the inexperienced surgeon or uninformed patient and family.

41. Discuss management of Monteggia fracture dislocation in children. Describe management of a 3-month-old neglected Monteggia fracture dislocation in a 6-year-old child.

Ans: *In general, the management of different types of Monteggia fracture dislocations is as follows*:
- *Type 1*: An anatomic, stable reduction of the ulnar fracture almost always leads to a stable reduction of the radiocapitellar joint. Failure to obtain and maintain ulnar fracture and radiocapitellar reduction will lead to a chronic Monteggia lesion, which is a complex clinical and surgical problem with risk of a suboptimum outcome. Transverse and short

oblique ulna fractures can be managed by percutaneous intramedullary fixation. Open reduction internal fixation (ORIF) with plate and screws is recommended for uncommon long oblique and comminuted fractures. Mostly the radiocapitellar joint reduces itself following management of the ulnar fracture, if not then open reduction is needed that usually entails replacing the interposed annular ligament. This aggressive approach avoids late complications.
- *Type 2*: For incomplete ulnar fractures, ulnar length is re-established by applying longitudinal traction and straightening the angular deformity. The radial head commonly reduces spontaneously or may be done so by gentle, anteriorly directed force over the radial head. This position can be maintained by holding the elbow in extension and applying a cast for stable ulnar fractures. If there is any doubt, percutaneous intramedullary fixation is preferred. Comminuted or very proximal fractures may require ORIF with plate and screws or tension band fixation. For nonreduced radial head dislocations, Boyd approach is used for open reduction. Associated compression fractures of the radial head require early detection to avoid late loss of alignment. ORIF may be required to maintain radiocapitellar joint stability.
- *Type 3*: Treatment is primarily aimed at obtaining and maintaining reduction of the radial head, either by an open or closed technique. This is usually performed by anatomic, stable, closed reduction of the ulnar fracture that in turn leads to a stable reduction of the proximal radioulnar and radiocapitellar joints.
- *Type 4*: Percutaneous intramedullary fixation of ulna is frequently necessary because of inherent fracture instability. Radial head reduction is done and maintained as for type I injuries.

Management of a 3-month-old neglected Monteggia fracture dislocation in a 6-year-old child:
{No specific type of Monteggia lesion is given here in question – strange poor framing of question?}
Assuming anterior or posterior angulation of ulna, it is imperative to correct the angular deformity of ulna as a prerequisite to managing the Monteggia lesions. According to reports in the literature, the radial head can be reduced satisfactorily 6 months or even longer after traumatic dislocation. This generally requires osteotomy of the angulated ulna. If the ulna has malunited, regardless of how little or how much remodeling has occurred, an osteotomy usually is necessary to "lengthen" the ulna and produce a stable radial head reduction. The radial head may reduce spontaneously. If the head does not reduce, then in increasing order of necessity open reduction of the radial head, reconstruction of the annular ligament with fascia or other soft tissue, and stabilization of the radial head in normal position against the capitellum would be needed depending on step-wise assessment of the radial head stability and reduction. Annular ligament reconstruction can be done with:
- Slip of fascia from the extensor aponeurosis (Boyd)
- Central slip of the triceps fascia (Bell-Tawse)
- Lateral aspect of the triceps fascia attached distally (Lloyd-Roberts)
  Oblique pin fixation from the radial neck to the olecranon and proximal ulna can be used if the reduction is unstable.

42. **Discuss current concepts in management of fractured neck and head of radius in children and adults.**
Ans: Obtain standard AP and lateral views of elbow and Greenspan views to diagnose and classify radial head fractures. Obtain CT scan for complicated injuries. MRI is needed for identification and management of associated ligament injuries. Classify radial head fractures with Mason classification (Vide Answer to Question 91).

Management in adults:
Aims: Regaining the movements by removing block, stabilizing elbow, and limiting the development of arthrosis later.

Conservative management: Mason type I fractures are amenable to nonoperative treatment with symptomatic immobilization in a posterior elbow splint in relative flexion until pain free, followed by range of motion, and strengthening exercises. Aspiration of joint hematoma does not make much of a difference. It is recommended that mobilization be started early by 3 weeks or even earlier if pain free.

Management of type II isolated, displaced, stable and partial articular fracture is highly debated. Currently, the literature reports equivalent results for both conservative and operative management of stable/unstable type II Mason–Johnston radial head fractures. Block to range of motion (ROM) is an indication of fixation.

Mason type III: It is recommended to reconstruct the radial head by ORIF if up to three simple fragments are present and fixable. The osteosynthesis is done in the safe zone identified by either the Smith and Hotchkiss method or Caputo et al. method. Placement of implant beyond this zone would result in articular attrition arthritis of ulnar sigmoid notch and pain. For more than three fragments, the results of osteosynthesis are not very favorable and should be replaced by arthroplasty. It is difficult to comment on use of monopolar/bipolar, monoblock/modular, cemented/uncemented or material (pyrocarbon versus metallic versus poly) in view of evolving data.

Fragment excision is usually not advisable as it anyway causes instability; unless it cannot be fixed despite best of efforts. So concepts of small free fragments <30% of articular surface to be excised and others to be preserved possibly does not hold true.

Radial head resection—a nonanatomical treatment indicated only in low-demand sedentary patients without any associated destabilizing injuries (rare to find). There is a possibility of development of distal radial ulnar joint (DRUJ) instability and proximal radius migration, if associated with Essex-Lopresti. Whenever done err on the side of delaying the surgery by at least 4 weeks or more (preferably 3 months).

Type IV Mason and terrible triad injuries—These need thorough evaluation of associated ligament and bony injuries. Restoration of ulnohumeral articulation is a priority along with elbow stability. So fix olecranon/coronoid, repair/reconstruct LCL/MCL and if osteosynthesis is possible then perform ORIF for radial head else replace the same.

The isolated radial neck fractures are not very common in adults and are managed conservatively if the angulation is less than 30°. Closed reduction with forearm in supination and under valgus stress may be attempted by direct pressure on the radial head fragment for improved alignment. The fragment commonly falls in place and immobilization is done in above elbow POP slab. For fractures angulated more than 30° closed reduction is performed and if angulation reduces to less than 30° then POP immobilization is done else ORIF is preferred. The implant of choice are small fragment (2.4 mm) T-plates placed in the "safe zone" of radial head. Anatomical radial head/neck plates have not been popular for these injuries anymore.

Management of radial head/neck fractures in children: Fat pad signs are a good aide to diagnose these injuries in children, as undisplaced fractures may be difficult to identify.

Fractures that are angulated <30° are better managed by immobilization alone in a long arm cast with quick restoration of ROM (passive followed by active mobilization, within 2 weeks).

For fractures angulated >30° closed reduction followed by immobilization is done (3 weeks for restoring ROM at elbow).

Operative: Closed reduction (Patterson/Israeli/Nehar and Torch technique) + percutaneous pinning (K-wire joystick or Metaizeau technique) is indicated for fractures angulated >30° or that is unstable after reduction.

Open reduction is needed for fractures that are displaced more and closed maneuvers cannot restore alignment to <40°. It has not been defined as to how much residual angulation constitutes a failed attempt at reduction. Commonly failed closed reduction has been variably defined as range from 15° to 45° of residual angulation.

The posterolateral (Kocher) approach to the radial head is used protecting the posterior interosseous nerve. After reduction of the proximal fragment, internal fixation is commonly used. The various described methods of internal fixation include:

Suture fixation of the fragment (not very popular).

Transcapitellar pin fixation (no longer recommended because these pins have a tendency to break in the joint).

The current recommendation is to place one or two K-wires obliquely from the lateral edge of the radial head, across the fracture site, into the distal fragment. The wires are left protruding from the wound for simple removal. Before closing the incision, the capsule and orbicular ligament should be repaired. The arm then is immobilized in 90° flexion and neutral rotation, because these fractures have a tendency to lose some supination and pronation. Remove wires at 3–4 weeks.

43. **What are the management principles in fresh fractures of proximal radius in children and malunited fractures of proximal radius?**

Ans: *The management principles for fresh fractures of proximal radius include*:

Nonoperative:
- <2 mm displacement of the radial head or neck
- <30–45° angulation of the radial neck (<30° age >10 years, <45° age <10 years)
- Full forearm pronation and supination

Operative: Operative treatment should be considered when displacement remains over 2 mm, angulation is >45° (age <10 years) or >30° (age >10 years), and for open injuries. Nerve palsy is generally not an indication for surgery because most will recover function over time.

Management principles in malunited fractures of proximal radius in children:
The malunions of proximal radius can be classified into:
- Malunions of the radial head
- Malunions of the radial neck and
- Malunions of the proximal radial shaft
- Malunions with radioulnar synostosis

Radial head and/or neck malunion is difficult to treat and even after corrective osteotomy methods of stabilization and fixation are not very satisfactory. Radial head excision should be avoided due to possibility of resulting ulna plus variance but this may have to be undertaken if functional limitation is severe.

The malunions of radial shaft of up to 10° are well accepted with minimal effect on forearm rotations (pronosupination). But malunions of >15° cause progressive limitation of pronosupination (25% and more). So, the possible upper tolerable limit of angular malunion of shaft of radius is possibly 15° beyond which it must be corrected. Osteotomy at the deformity site to correct angular deformity while preserving length is the most common practice.

Synostosis is managed on standard lines with excision and interposition of fat or synthetic membranes with aggressive physiotherapy and pharmacotherapy to gain function and prevent recurrence.

44. Classify elbow dislocation. Explain management of unreduced posterior elbow dislocation in a 10-year-old child.

Ans:

Classification:
- Simple versus complex (associated with fracture)
- *According to the direction of displacement of the ulna relative to the humerus*:
  - Posterior
  - Posterolateral
  - Posteromedial
  - Lateral
  - Medial
  - Anterior

Management: When dislocations of the elbow remained unreduced for 3 months or longer, a satisfactory functional result still could be obtained by an open reduction and the results were better than after extensive arthroplasty procedures in immature patients.

Open reduction of untreated (chronic) posterior dislocation of the elbow in children by Fowles et al.:
- Exposure—Campbell posterolateral approach
- Subperiosteal elevation of all muscle attachments from the distal humerus anteriorly and posteriorly. Release the attachments of the joint capsule around the humeral condyles. Expose the joint circumferentially, and detach the collateral ligaments from their proximal insertions.
- *A fibrous ankylosis forms in most patients with the elbow in 30–60° of flexion*:
  - Release the thick, fibrotic, contracted capsule, and resect portions as necessary.
  - Remove all the fibrous tissue from the joint, protecting the underlying cartilage.
  - Excise scar tissue carefully because it is often difficult to distinguish firm white scar from normal articular cartilage.
  - Clear subperiosteal new bone when it is an obstacle to reduction of the dislocation.
- If the triceps is tight, preventing reduction or limiting flexion to about 30° after reduction, lengthen the muscle using Speed's V-Y muscleplasty.
- Gently reduce the elbow if easy, else further release is necessary.

- Further, soft-tissues release for elbow reduction can be done proximally around the humerus and distally from the olecranon.
- Do not reattach the ligaments to bone to avoid making the repair too tight. If the ulnar nerve is tight, or was compressed preoperatively, transpose it anteriorly.
- If the stability at 90° of elbow flexion id precarious then insert one or two large Kirschner wires through the olecranon and into the humerus with the elbow flexed to 70°. Close the wound, and apply a long arm cast with the forearm in neutral rotation.

45. Briefly describe TRASH injuries of elbow in children.

Ans: A small subset of serious injuries to the pediatric elbow, deemed "TRASH" lesions, are easily missed on radiograph because of their benign appearance. These lesions, however, represent a group of osteochondral injuries, which if treated insufficiently result in chronic long-term consequences. Due to poor visualization on conventional radiographs (nonossification of the bone), these injuries are frequently missed. The following comprise group of TRASH injuries:

Elbow TRASH lesions:
- Unossified medial condylar humerus fractures
- Unossified transphyseal distal humerus fractures
- Entrapped medial epicondylar fractures
- Complex osteochondral elbow fracture-dislocations below the age of 10 years
- Osteochondral fractures with joint incongruity
- Radial head anterior compression fractures with progressive radiocapitellar subluxation
- Monteggia fracture dislocations
- Lateral condylar avulsion shear fractures

These injuries are usually seen in children less than 10 years of age who sustain high-energy trauma. The challenge is a prompt diagnosis requiring a high level of suspicion and early additional imaging. Many of these injuries are displaced and unstable requiring anatomic reduction, internal fixation with or without soft tissue repair for further stability. These injuries when diagnosed late, missed completely or treated improperly without aggressive surgical care can result in long-term complications. Surgical reconstruction of the late presenting malunion is difficult.

46. Describe the ligaments of elbow joint. Describe PLRI of elbow and briefly outline its management.

Ans: *(A question should never be asked in non-standard abbreviations like PLRI here—students may not know that PLRI is posterolateral rotatory instability)*

The ligaments of elbow:
- *Capsular ligament*: Superiorly, it is attached to the lower end of the humerus in such a way that the capitulum, the trochlea, the radial fossa, the coronoid fossa and the olecranon fossa are intracapsular. Inferomedially, it is attached to the margin of the trochlear notch of the ulna except laterally; inferolaterally, it is attached to the annular ligament of the superior radioulnar joint. The anterior and posterior ligaments are thickening of the capsule.
- The ulnar collateral ligament is triangular in shape comprises of various sub-parts that can be identified in anatomical specimens. These are primarily composed of the anterior oblique, posterior oblique and transverse ligaments. The anterior oblique bundle has separate anterior (primary restraint to valgus stresses at 30°, 60°, and 90° of flexion) and posterior (secondary restraint to valgus stress with the elbow held at 120° of flexion) bands that tighten in reciprocal fashion as flexion (posterior band) and extension (anterior band) of the elbow occurs. This is the primary stabilizer of the elbow to valgus stress. Ulnar collateral ligament originates from the anteroinferior surface of the medial epicondyle not from axis of rotation except the "Guiding bundle". The ligament is crossed by the ulnar nerve and it gives origin to the flexor digitorum superficialis. It is closely related to the flexor carpi ulnaris and the triceps brachii.
- *The radial collateral or lateral ligament* has lateral collateral (LCL), lateral ulnar collateral (LUCL) and annular ligaments components, but parts are not easily separable during dissection. The lateral collateral ligament origin is from the entire inferior surface of the lateral epicondyle as a blend of poorly demarcated fan-shaped ligamentous fibers. It

provides external rotation and varus stability as the elbow flexes toward 110°. It remains taut throughout flexion and extension as lateral collateral ligament originates from axis of rotation on lateral epicondyle.
- *The annular ligament*: It forms four-fifths of the ring within which the head of the radius rotates. It is attached to the margins of the radial notch of the ulna, and is continuous with the capsule of the elbow joint above.
- *The quadrate ligament* extends from the neck of the radius to the lower margin of the radial notch of the ulna.

PLRI: PLRI stands for posterolateral rotatory instability. The rotatory instability develops due to injury to lateral UCL that happens with a combination of axial compression, valgus stress and supination (or external rotation). The peculiar mechanism imparts a rotational force to the elbow resulting in a spectrum of soft tissue injury. Contemplating the *Hori circle* concept, the initial injury is to the ulnar portion of the LCL that progresses to capsular disruption (anterior and posterior capsule) and eventually may involve the UCL complex, if the injury is severe.

Pathomechanics:
- PLRI of the elbow results from a rotatory subluxation of the radius and ulna.
- Although the LUCL was considered to be the primary stabilizer to PLRI recent literature suggests that the injury pattern is not limited to LUCL alone. The secondary restraints such as the radial collateral ligament and capsule need to get injured for manifestations of PLRI.
- The only condition in which LUCL injury alone can produce PLRI is a proximal injury to the "Y" configuration of LUCL near the epicondyle.

Diagnosis and Clinical Features: Most patients have a vague elbow discomfort. Others often report nonspecific symptoms such as painful clicking, snapping, clunking, locking or giving way.

Provocative test of instability described by O'Driscoll et al. (the lateral pivot-shift test of the elbow). The pivot-shift test is performed with the patient supine and the examiner standing above the patient's head. The upper extremity is brought into full forward elevation over the head and the shoulder is placed in full external rotation to stabilize the humerus for the test. The forearm is held in maximal supination. A valgus force is applied to the elbow holding the wrist. Loading the elbow by valgus in full supination produces an axial joint compression forcing the combined radius and ulna into a posterolateral rotatory subluxation relative to the humerus. Sensation of instability and apprehension or guarding is reported a positive test. The subluxation is maximal with elbow in 40° flexion and further flexion results in a sudden clunk.

Radiology
Lateral stress radiographic studies or fluoroscopy during the pivot maneuver demonstrates posterolateral radial head dislocation and widening of the ulnohumeral joint (due to the subluxation of the ulna out of the trochlear groove). The ulna is rotated off the distal humerus (slight gapping of the ulnohumeral joint with otherwise maintained relationship), while the radial head is rotated with the ulna (differentiating from radial head subluxation) so that the radial head rests posterior to the capitellum.

MRI allows good visualization of the LCL and can be helpful in confirming the diagnosis in some cases.

Management: Posterolateral rotatory instability that markedly interferes with the patient's daily function only needs to be treated. For early cases, one can consider activity modification and a hinged brace support that puts forearm in pronation and gives an extension block.

Surgical treatment of PLRI is the treatment of choice. The primary aim is to restore the lateral ligamentous structures by reattaching the avulsed LCL or reconstructing the LUCL with a free tendon graft to the lateral epicondyle. If the condition is diagnosed acutely, primary repair of the LUCL may be performed back to the bone. Various methods of surgical reconstruction are described in addition to the technique originally described by O'Driscoll and include making the distal connecting tunnels perpendicular to the isometric point to the lateral epicondyle, using interference screw, etc.

47. How will you manage sideswipe injuries of elbow?
Ans: Sideswipe injuries (**Flowchart 3.3.3**) are complex elbow trauma that have also been colloquially called baby car injuries and commonly result from road-traffic elbow injuries, typically, when a patient travelling in a vehicle with elbow resting on the window is hit by oncoming object or a vehicle. These injuries have a high complication rate that includes stiffness, contractures, nonunion, deformity, and poor functional outcome due to functiolaesia.

Management:
Evaluation of these injuries involve (in addition to local bony injuries) thorough note of associated injuries:
- Nerve injuries—all three radial, median, and ulnar nerves
- Skin loss—if open injuries
- Forearm bone injuries—also note shoulder tenderness or dislocation (uncommon)
- Soft tissue injuries in closed ones that may predispose to compartment syndrome if missed.

Primary management: The most frequent combination fracture pattern is a supracondylar fracture of the humerus associated with intra-articular extension (intercondylar fracture pattern—usually comminuted) and/or fracture of radius and/or ulna. The injury may be closed or open and the management protocol is modified based on this most important independent factor along with associated injuries (*see* **Flowchart 3.3.3**).

Internal fixation is the preferred stabilization modality of choice in closed fractures, and in clean open grade one and grade two injuries. Dual plate fixation—perpendicular construct is favored—one plate over medial column and another plate placed posterolaterally, 90° from the medial plate. Parallel LCP can also be applied as described by O'Driscoll.

External fixation (articulated external fixator) should be limited to open fractures, or nonreconstructible markedly comminuted fractures, fractures with bone loss where articular reconstruction is not possible, extensive soft tissue damage and polytrauma patient [follow DCO (damage control orthopedics)].

Transfixation of the elbow joint (Morrey procedure) may be done as an alternate to external fixation in cases of severe comminution, instability and/or extensive soft tissue injuries but is not very popular.

Olecranon pin traction is a redundant method in modern orthopedics as it limits patient mobility.

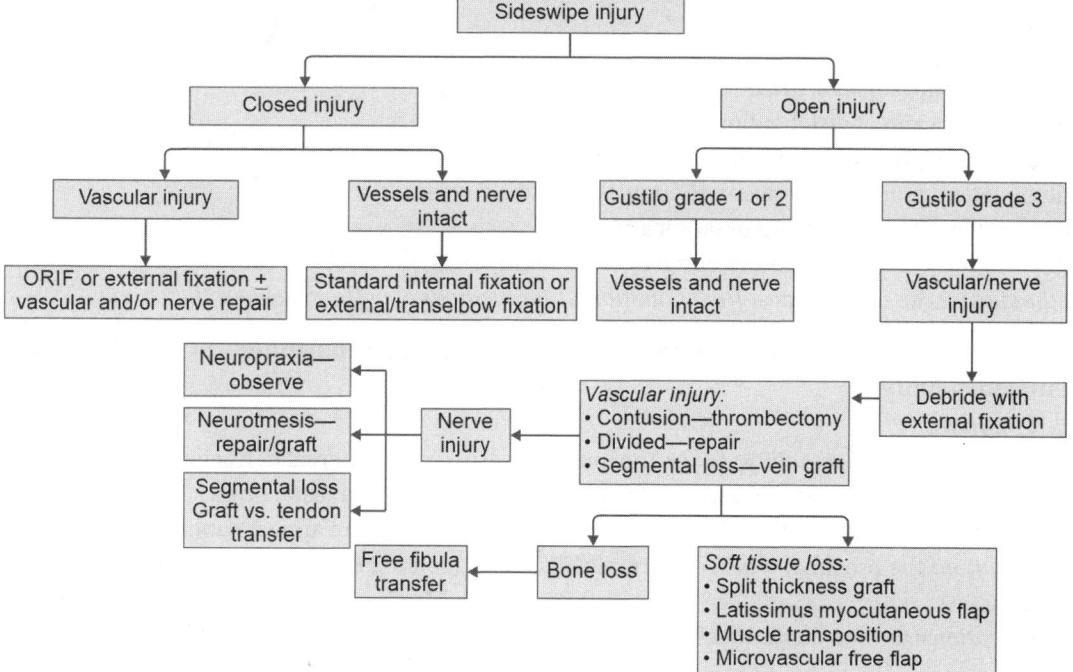

Flowchart 3.3.3: Classificaton of sideswipe injury.

Total elbow arthroplasty (semiconstrained) is preferred in osteopenic bone with markedly comminuted closed fractures.

Vessel injuries are best managed in association with vascular surgeon as for primary repair or vascular grafting.

Nerve injuries may be primarily repaired or tagged for repair later or nerve grafting may be done in index procedure depending on availability of resources or expertise.

Local rotational flaps are commonly preferred for management of skin loss rather than microvascular flaps.

Bone loss at index surgery may be managed by free fibula transfer if feasible.

Secondary (longer-term) management:
- Management of nonunion—due to high-velocity trauma and stripping of soft tissues ± open injury, there is often failure of bone to unite in one or both columns. This needs to be addressed later by bone grafting and/or revision fixation.
- Management of skin loss—this often needs local flaps at primary fixation stage or skin grafting later. Microvascular flaps are rarely used.
- Management of nerve injuries—nerve repair is a part of primary management but in case of axonotmesis or mixed nerve injuries neural reconstruction or delayed repair may be needed. Later tendon transfers may be required to regain function.
- Management of stiffness—this is quite common and aim should be to obtain at least the functional ROM of 100° (30–130°). Soft tissue or capsular releases may be performed, where feasible.

48. Describe the radiological indices of wrist. Discuss treatment principles of extra-articular distal radius fractures.

Ans: Radiological indices of wrist are tabulated in **Table 3.3.3**.

TABLE 3.3.3: Radiological indices.

Criterion	Normal	Acceptable
Ulnar variance (radial length)	±2 mm comparing level of lunate facet	No > 2 mm of shortening relative to ulnar
Radial height	12 mm	>9 mm
Palmar (lateral) tilt	11° volar tilt	Neutral
Radial inclination	20° as measured from lunate facet to radial styloid	No < 10°
Intra-articular step or gap	None	< 2 mm

Principles (goals) of management of extra-articular distal radius fracture:
- Radial shortening <5 mm at distal radioulnar joint
- Radial inclination on posteroanterior radiographs >15°
- Sagittal tilt on lateral projection between 15° dorsal tilt and 20° volar tilt
- Intra-articular step-off or gap <2 mm of radiocarpal joint
- Articular incongruity <2 mm of sigmoid notch of distal radius.

(*In addition the student can write Answer from Question 51 for methods of ORIF to achieve these goals*)

49. Describe instability patterns after wrist trauma. Discuss the management of VISI (volar intercalated segmental instability).

Ans: *Instability patterns*:
- *Dorsal intercalated segment instability (DISI)*: The lunate, regarded as an intercalated segment between the distal row and the forearm bones, is abnormally extended relative to its proximal and distal links.
- *Volar intercalated segment instability (VISI)*: In the sagittal plane, the lunate appears abnormally flexed.
- *Ulnar translocation*: The proximal row is abnormally displaced (rotated or translocated) relative to the radius in an ulnar direction.
- *Dorsal translocation*: Due to a malunited fracture of the radius, the carpus is subluxed in a dorsal direction.

Management of VISI: Disruption of the lunotriquetral ligaments results in a dissociative VISI pattern of carpal instability. For acute disruptions, anatomical reduction (usually open) and repair of both the intrinsic and extrinsic ligaments are done. Closed reduction and percutaneous pinning is acceptable for select cases. For delayed cases, when there is cartilage degeneration and/or triangular fibrocartilage deterioration, a lunotriquetral arthrodesis is preferred. In cases with ulnar positive variance, the long ulna may be impacting the triquetrum (ulna impaction syndrome) where arthroscopic debridement of lunotriquetral ligament can be combined to ulna shortening with acceptable results. (*For detailed discussion on instability patterns and management, kindly see Chapter 103 of the book Essential Orthopedics: Principles and Practice, 2nd edition.)*

50. Classify fracture of distal end of radius.

Ans: There are numerous classification systems for fracture distal end radius (*may be one can concentrate on any two of them like Melone and Frykman classifications and write answer with figures*).

Gartland and Werley (1951):
- *Group 1*: Simple Colles' fracture
- *Group 2*: Comminuted Colles' fracture and undisplaced intra-articular fragment
- *Group 3*: Comminuted Colles' fracture and displaced intra-articular fragment.

Frykman (1967):
- *Group 1*: Extra-articular without fracture of the distal ulna
- *Group 2*: Extra-articular with fracture of the distal ulna
- *Group 3*: Intra-articular involving the radiocarpal joint without fracture of the distal ulna
- *Group 4*: Intra-articular involving the radiocarpal joint with fracture of the distal ulna
- *Group 5*: Intra-articular involving the distal radioulnar joint without fracture of the distal ulna
- *Group 6*: Intra-articular involving the distal radioulnar joint with fracture of the distal ulna
- *Group 7*: Intra-articular involving both radiocarpal and distal radioulnar joints without fracture of the distal ulna
- *Group 8*: Intra-articular involving both radiocarpal and distal radioulnar joints with fracture of the distal ulna

Melone (1986):
- *Type 1*: Undisplaced, minimal comminution, and stable
- *Type 2*: Unstable, displacement of medial complex, and moderate-to-severe comminution
- *Type 3*: Displacement of medial complex as a unit plus an anterior spike
- *Type 4*: Wide separation or rotation of the dorsal fragment and palmar fragment rotation

Fernandez (1987):
- *Type 1 Bending*: One cortex of the metaphysis fails due to tensile stress; opposite cortex with some comminution
- *Type 2 Shearing*: Fracture of the joint surface
- *Type 3 Compression*: Fracture of the joint surface with impaction of subchondral and metaphyseal bone, and intraarticular comminution
- *Type 4 Avulsion*: Fracture of the ligament attachments of the ulnar and radial styloid process, and radiocarpal fracture-dislocation
- *Type 5 Combination*: High-velocity injuries.

Cooney (1990) Universal Classification:
- *Type 1*: Extra-articular and undisplaced
- *Type 2*: Extra-articular and displaced
- *Type 3*: Intra-articular and undisplaced
- *Type 4*: Intra-articular and displaced.

Modified AO:
- *Type A*: Extra-articular
- *Type B*: Partial articular
  - B1–radial styloid fracture
  - B2–dorsal rim fracture
  - B3–volar rim fracture
  - B4–die-punch fracture
- *Type C*: Complete articular.

51. Discuss modalities of surgical treatment of fracture of lower end of radius.

Ans:

Distal radius fracture can be treated by various modalities as follows:
- POP cast immobilization ± manipulation
- External fixator application ± pinning
- Pinning alone—intrafocal versus transfracture
- *Plate and screw stabilization:*
  - Volar buttress plate
  - Volar anatomical locked screw construct
  - Volar + dorsal plating
  - Dorsal only plating
  - Column plate fixation
- Nail-plate construct.

Details of all the techniques can be read from the book Essential Orthopedics: Principles and Practice, 2nd edition–Annexure 1.
Fracture pattern is first classified and then treated accordingly.

As per Fernandez classification, most type I distal radial fractures can be successfully treated nonoperatively. In younger patients, near-normal function, and clinical and radiographic appearance are expected. If maintenance of reduction of Colles' or Smith's fractures requires prolonged immobilization in extreme positions, or reduction is lost early in treatment, closed reduction followed by percutaneous pinning of the distal radius through the radial styloid can be performed.

Type II distal radial shear fractures usually require open reduction and internal fixation, especially if the fracture is a Barton type. These fractures are almost impossible to treat by closed means. Buttress plate fixation of volar Barton's fractures usually is necessary.

Type III compression injuries require operative treatment, if intra-articular damage is significant or radial shortening is severe. Careful restoration of the articular surface and radial angulation and length is crucial. Fixation with multiple Kirschner wires or plates often is necessary, and cancellous bone grafting is frequently required to fill impacted areas.

Type IV avulsion fractures usually are associated with radiocarpal fracture-dislocations and are unstable. Often the avulsed fracture fragments are so small that they can be repaired only with suture. Secure reduction of the carpus to the distal radius frequently can be achieved only with Kirschner wires. External fixation using the principle of ligamentotaxis is inappropriate in the treatment of radiocarpal fracture-dislocation because of the extensive ligament disruption.

Type V high-velocity fractures are always unstable, frequently open, and difficult to treat. A combination of percutaneous pinning and external fixation often is necessary. Many of these fractures are so severely comminuted that open reduction is impossible.

52. Describe management of volar Barton's fracture.

Ans: Fractures of the volar articular margin of the radius with volar dislocation or subluxation of the carpus are referred to as volar Barton's fractures. These fractures require special attention because the method of reduction and maintenance of reduction are the opposite of those used for Colles' or Smith's fractures. When the marginal fracture is small closed reduction and cast immobilization may be satisfactory. Volar Barton's fractures usually are most stable with volar flexion of the wrist and supination of the forearm. Stability is afforded by the intact carpal ligament opposite the fracture.

Open reduction and internal fixation is mostly needed in large fragments with subluxation as maintaining reduction is challenging and redisplacement is common. Because loss of reduction with subluxation of the carpus is so common, frequently used is a small buttress plate, as described by Ellis, as fixation for volar marginal fractures. Buttress plate fixation of volar Barton's fractures is commonly done, both locked fixation and buttress modes are available. Buttress plating is done primarily for shear fracture of the volar lip without dorsal comminution. Volar locked plating is the mainstay of modern fixation as it stabilizes even a dorsally comminuted fracture. The problem is irritation of both volar and extensor tendons (avoided by limiting the size of screws, using all locked screws, low-profile anatomical plates and avoiding placement beyond watershed line).

- Make a longitudinal incision about 7.5 cm long on the radiovolar aspect of the distal forearm. Develop the plane between the flexor carpi radialis and the palmaris longus.

- Retract the flexor pollicis longus tendon radialward, and the median nerve and the other tendons ulnarward.
- Sever the fibers of the pronator quadratus from their origin on the radius, and expose the fracture.
- Reduce the fracture and contour a T-plate so that, when it is applied and fixed to the proximal fragment, the distal transverse part acts as a buttress and holds the fracture reduced.
- Two screws are usually all that is required in the proximal fragment, and usually no screw is inserted through the distal part of the plate into the fracture fragments.
- The reduction of the fracture and restoration of the articular surface are confirmed by direct observation and by anteroposterior and lateral radiographs.
- Replace the pronator quadratus over the plate to its origin on the radius and close the wound.

53. Describe perilunate fracture dislocation and its management in acute case. Discuss potential complications of chronic perilunate dislocation.

Ans: Perilunate fracture dislocation—perilunate fracture dislocations (greater-arc injury) combine ligament ruptures, osseous avulsions and various types of fractures. The most common pattern of perilunate instability is the trans-scaphoid perilunate fracture-dislocation. Fractures of the capitate, hamate, lunate, triquetrum, and radial styloid can also occur. Displaced transverse fractures of the neck of the capitate and sagittal fractures of the triquetrum are also quite frequent.

Clinical assessment: Patients are often young males who present following a high-energy hyperextension injury (e.g., fall from height, motor vehicle accident, and sports), with persistent wrist pain, swelling, and deformity. Approximately a quarter of presentations will be associated with a polytrauma, with one in ten sustaining an associated upper limb injury. In around 16% of cases, clinical presentation includes median nerve symptoms and signs, but an ulnar neuropathy, arterial injury, or tendon disruption may also be seen.

Radiographic evaluation: PA, lateral, and oblique views should be obtained to confirm the diagnosis and rule out associated injuries. A CT scan may be useful in further defining the injury pattern.
- *Posterior-anterior (PA) view*:
  - The dislocated lunate appears to be wedge-shaped and more triangular, with an elongated volar lip.
  - Loss of normal carpal colinear "Gilula lines" and abnormal widening of the scapholunate interval >3 mm are noted.
  - Look for associated fractures, such as "trans-scaphoid" injuries.
  - A clenched-fist PA view obtained after closed reduction of the midcarpal joint is useful for checking residual scapholunate or lunotriquetral dissociation as well as fractures.
- *Lateral view (most important view)*: Carefully look at the outline of the capitate and lunate carefully. The "spilled tea cup sign" occurs with volar dislocation of the lunate.

Management: Management is with closed reduction followed by ORIF, as it is the best method of achieving anatomic reduction of the fracture. This also allows repair of associated ligament injuries, as well as primary bone grafting when there is comminution of the scaphoid. Cannulated screw fixation of the scaphoid is routinely recommended. Overall patient satisfaction is good with return to employment, although restoration of function is rarely complete with residual wrist stiffness and weakness of grip strength documented.

Complications of chronic perilunate dislocation include chronic pain, instability, and wrist deformity, often associated with tendon rupture or increasing nerve symptoms.

54. A. Describe trans-scaphoid perilunate fracture dislocation.
   B. Discuss potential complications and outcomes of a chronic neglected trans-scaphoid perilunate dislocation.

Ans:
A. In trans-scaphoperilunate dislocation, the distal row (including the fractures scaphoid and triquetrum) dislocates in dorsal or dorsoradial direction commonly (the greater arc injury). So, a trans-scaphoid perilunate dislocation will mean dorsally displaced distal fragment of scaphoid with other carpal bones and lunate rotated 90° volarly. Trans-scaphoid perilunate dislocation is the most common reported variety. The dislocations are most commonly seen in young individuals, as in children the radial physis undergoes separation while in older people the forces are dissipated by the distal radius fractures.

B. Perilunate dislocations produce injury to both the intrinsic and extrinsic ligaments of the wrist joint so a combined CID and CIND pattern of instability results in untreated cases (the CIC pattern). Failure to obtain stability of the joints of the proximal row may result in a chronic CID type of carpal collapse. The damaged extrinsic radiocarpal ligaments if do not heal or remain inefficient may lead to development of CIND (with ulnar translocation of the ulnar side of the carpus). On plain radiographs in CIC, the scaphoid is seen palmar flexed with widening of the scapholunate joint space. The ulnar translocation of carpus is prominent with dorsiflexed lunate. When neglected for long duration it results in SNAC wrist joint arthritis which is consequent upon chondromalacia and degeneration of radio-scapholunate articulation.

55. Describe in brief mechanism of injury and classification of perilunate injuries.
Ans:
Mechanism of injury:
Perilunate dislocations and fracture dislocation predominantly follow a high-energy mechanism of hyperextension, ulnar deviation, and intercarpal supination injury to the wrist.

Classification:
Mayfield suggested that carpal instability predominantly occurs in relation to the lunate, which is the carpal keystone. He put forward a pathoanatomic classification associated with progressive perilunate instability from a radial to ulnar direction.

- *Stage I*: Scaphoid fracture, SLD, or both—
  - As the distal carpal row is violently extended, supinated, and ulnarly deviated, the scaphotrapezium-trapezoid and scaphocapitate ligaments are tightened causing the scaphoid to extend. As the scaphoid extends, the scapholunate ligament transmits the force to the lunate, which cannot rotate as much as the scaphoid because it is constrained by the palmarly located radiolunate and ulnolunate ligaments. As a consequence, a scaphoid fracture or a progressive elongation and tearing of the scapholunate and palmar RSC ligaments may occur, potentially leading to complete SLD.
- *Stage II*: Lunocapitate disruption—
  - If the extension–supination force on the wrist persists once the proximal carpal row has been dislocated, transmission of the force distally to the capitate may lead to displacement and eventual dislocation dorsally through the space of Poirier. It is followed by the rest of the distal carpal row and the radial—most portion of the dislocated proximal carpal row. This may be the complete scaphoid or just its distal fragment.
- *Stage III*: Lunotriquetral disruption—
  - If the extension–supination force to the wrist persists, once the capitate is displaced dorsally lunotriquetral (most common), ulnotriquetral, and/or triquetrum-hamate-capitate ligament disruptions may occur. Stage III is complete when the palmar lunotriquetral ligament, including the medial expansions of the long radiolunate ligament, is completely disrupted and the joint has displaced.
- *Stage IV*: Perilunate dislocation—
  - If the extension–supination force to the wrist persists and the dorsally displaced capitate is pulled proximally, pressure is applied onto the dorsal aspect of the lunate, forcing it to dislocate in a palmar direction due to injury to the dorsal radiocarpal (DRC) ligament. As the palmar ligaments are much stronger than the dorsal capsule, such a dislocation seldom involves a pure palmar displacement of the lunate, but rather a variable degree of palmar rotation of the bone into the carpal tunnel using the intact palmar ligaments as a hinge.

56. A. What is the blood supply of scaphoid bone?
   B. Classify scaphoid fracture.
   C. Discuss management of displaced and undisplaced scaphoid fractures.

Ans: *Blood supply of scaphoid* **(Fig. 3.3.6)**: Typically, the scaphoid is supplied by two groups of small vessels. Majority of its blood supply comes from dorsal vessels at or just distal to waist area perfusing the proximal pole in a retrograde fashion.

These are branches of radial artery that enter scaphoid through foramina along its dorsal ridge. It supplies 70–80% of bone, including the entire proximal pole. The second group of vessels arises from palmar and superficial palmar branches of radial artery and enters carpal scaphoid in region of its distal tubercle. This perfuses distal 20–30% of bone, including tuberosity. The vascular supply of clinically distinct proximal and distal scaphoid can be summarized as follows:

- The proximal two-thirds to three-fourths of scaphoid are supplied by vessels entering dorsal surface through dorsal ridge in 79%. Alternatively, the vessels may enter distal to waist in 14% and proximal to waist in 7%.
- *Distal scaphoid*: The tubercle and distal 20–30% of scaphoid are supplied by palmar vessels predominantly. In a few persons, supplying vessels may enter tip of tubercle reaching the waist. There is no anastomosis between the dorsal and palmar vessels.

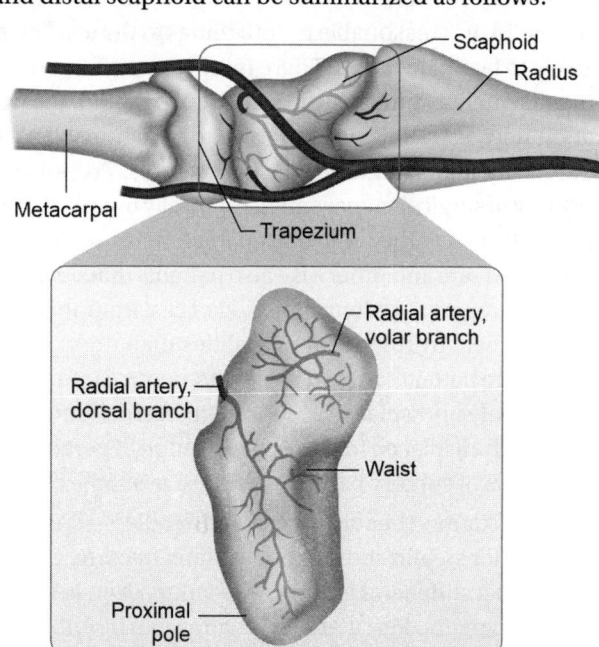

Fig. 3.3.6: Blood supply of scaphoid bone.

Classification:
- *Russe classification*: The Russe classification predicts instability according to the inclination of the fracture line; out of the three types—horizontal oblique, vertical oblique, and transverse, the vertical oblique fractures are most unstable.
- *AO classification*: The AO classification breaks the fracture down into comminution and then further into simple anatomic location (distal pole, waist, and proximal pole).
- *Herbert and Fisher classification*:
  - *Type A*: Stable acute fractures—
    - A1 (tuberosity)
    - A2 (non-displaced transverse waist).
  - *Type B*: Unstable acute fractures—
    - B1 (distal oblique/pole)
    - B2 (complete waist)
    - B3 (proximal pole)
    - B4 (trans-scaphoid perilunate fracture dislocation)
    - B5 (comminuted)
  - *Type C*: Delayed union
  - *Type D*: Nonunion further classified into four types (stable, unstable, nonunion with DISI and nonunion with AVN).
- *Mayo classification*: The criteria for instability they set out are as follows—
  - 1 mm of fracture displacement
  - A lateral intrascaphoid angle of >35°
  - Bone loss or comminution
  - Fracture malalignment
  - Proximal pole fractures
  - DISI deformity
  - Perilunate fracture-dislocation.

Management

Undisplaced fractures: Standard below-elbow cast with the thumb free is preferred for nondisplaced stable scaphoid fractures. If there is any doubt about the presence of displacement, particularly if there is fragmentation at the fracture line, we would progress to a CT scan. Based more on tradition than data, the duration of immobilization is 8–10 weeks. Tuberosity fractures are mostly managed in short-arm plaster of Paris (POP) cast for 4–6 weeks. There is no role for long-arm POP cast, as they do not offer any advantage in preventing interfragmentary motion. Radiographs and clinical examination should not be used to determine duration of immobilization because they are unreliable for diagnosis of union. Return to sport and use of the hand with force are delayed until there is clear radiographic evidence of union or 4–6 months have passed. At this point, it is reasonable to "put things to the test" no matter what the radiographs show since additional protection is unlikely to facilitate union. There is little controversy, if any to fix a displaced fracture scaphoid, however, when it comes to management of undisplaced fractured scaphoid, the world seems divided with the balance tilting toward percutaneous fixation now, especially when return to work is used as a criterion to assess endpoint. Union percentage is also higher in surgically managed undisplaced fractures. Proponents of POP cast management site-increased complications and morbidity of surgical management especially open reduction, percutaneous fixation limits these, although to a large extent. Around 90–95% of the undisplaced fractures of scaphoid heal in POP cast but on the other hand studies report 1.5–37% of nonunion rate and otherwise also patients that develop nonunion and scaphoid nonunion advanced collapse (SNAC) wrist often report a prolonged period of cast immobilization in their history. Nonunion after POP cast treatment is more difficult to heal by treatment modalities than those after surgical fixation. This then entails that undisplaced fractured scaphoid are better managed by percutaneous fixation when compared to nonoperative management or open reduction. Proximal pole undisplaced scaphoid fractures should be possibly fixed without controversy. Patients with nondisplaced or minimally displaced fractures have option of percutaneous screw fixation, including a balanced discussion on the risks and benefits of surgery based on the best available evidence.

Screw fixation (headless central threadless screw, 3D printed screw or conical fully threaded screw) is the main workhorse for stabilization of the scaphoid fracture. Conical screw provides better compression at the fracture site making the construct stiffer and less prone to failure even in eccentric screw placement; headless central threadless screws need central placement. Percutaneous fixation can be either by a dorsal or a volar approach. Advantages of the volar approach are that the scaphoid tubercle is very superficial, the wrist can be maintained in neutral which makes imaging easier and decreases the chance of bending the guidewire, and there is no need to open the radiocarpal joint. Care must be taken to ensure that an overhanging trapezium does not cause the surgeon to insert the screw too superficially (too volar) or too vertical. There may also be a risk of later scaphotrapezial arthrosis. Using this approach, the surgeon must be prepared to place the screw through the overhang of the trapezium which is usually extra-articular. If the screw is placed too vertically in the sagittal plane, the screw tip may penetrate the dorsal radial scaphoid cortex, which both endangers the radioscaphoid cartilage and usually provides inadequate fixation of the proximal fragment. Advantages of a dorsal approach include easier central placement in the proximal pole and body of the scaphoid. Disadvantages include the need to keep the wrist in a flexed position, greater risk of bending the guidewire, risk to digital extensor tendons, and creation of a hole in the scaphoid articular surface. The starting point of the wire can be identified arthroscopically and a large bore needle used as a guidewire or this can be done entirely with the image intensifier. The hand is placed on top of a stack of towels on the image intensifier to maintain the wrist in flexion to provide access to the starting point and limit the potential for bending the wire. The wrist is kept flexed and the images are perpendicular to the carpus. After determining the length of the screw, the wire is placed into the trapezium to prevent unintended extraction if predrilling is used.

Postoperatively, a bandage is applied and usually a cast is not required. Non-contact sports are allowed immediately. Contact sports, heavy lifting, or axial loading of the wrist can commence progressively 6 weeks after surgery.

Displaced fractures:
- If reduction can be achieved and monitored arthroscopically, percutaneous fixation is possible, but the standard treatment is open reduction and internal fixation. Arthroscopic-assisted fixation or ORIF of the scaphoid is recommended if there is any gapping or angulation in the scaphoid, even if the fracture appears stable and impacted, because displaced fractures are unstable and should be managed operatively. Reduction is facilitated by the use of K-wires used as joysticks in each fragment as well as other instruments used to push and guide the fragments into position.
- Bone grafting is considered in the face of comminution.
- Plate fixation and staples are for experienced surgeons who frequently deal with this injury.

A splint is applied for comfort after operative fixation. In most cases, the splint is maintained until suture removal, which takes place about 2 weeks later. In unreliable patients or some very unstable or very proximal fractures, a cast may be used for 4–8 weeks. Return to sports is risky until the fracture is healed (at least 2–3 months). Patients who wish to return sooner must agree to assume the associated risks.

(For details, refer to Chapter 15 of the book Essential Orthopedics: Principles and Practice, 2nd edition.)

57. Explain mallet finger.

Ans: Mallet finger deformity is the disruption of extensor mechanism (extensor zone I) to distal phalanx resulting commonly from trauma as in baseball (baseball finger) resulting in an extensor lag of the distal interphalangeal joint (DIP) (drop finger).

Mechanism: The common mechanism of mallet finger in sports injury is by a direct blow to the tip of the extended finger. This acutely flexes the distal phalanx resulting in strained tendon at the insertion due to existing tenodesis effect. The other mechanism is a direct blow to the dorsum of the DIP joint. The mallet finger may lastly be also produced by hyperextension injuries that fracture the dorsal base of distal phalanx. Although closed injuries are more common, open injuries caused by lacerations and crush abrasions also occur. Approximately 40% of mallet fingers result from minor injuries. Full passive extension of the distal interphalangeal joint usually remains, and over long period of time hyperextension of the proximal interphalangeal joint may develop because of secondary proximal migration of the extensor apparatus causing volar subluxation of extensor slips resulting in a swan neck deformity.

Presentation: The patient or athlete presents with pain and swelling on the dorsum of the DIP joint with lack of active extension at this joint.

Types: The mallet deformity may be purely soft tissue caused by tear of the terminal extensor mechanism through its substance or bony, associated with an avulsed bony fragment. Mallet fingers are classified into four types according to associated soft tissue injuries and the fracture pattern:

- *Type 1*: Closed or blunt trauma with loss of tendon continuity with or without a small avulsion fracture
- *Type 2*: Laceration at or proximal to the distal interphalangeal joint with loss of tendon continuity
- *Type 3*: Deep abrasion with loss of skin, subcutaneous cover, and tendon substance
- *Type 4*: *4A*—transphyseal fracture in children; *4B*—hyperflexion injury with fracture of articular surface of 20–50%; *4C*—hyperextension injury with fracture of the articular surface usually >50% with early or late volar subluxation of the distal phalanx.

Type 1 mallet fingers are the most common. Differentiating small avulsion type 1 fractures from the larger type 4 fractures is important because the subluxation or dislocation present in type 4 fractures determines treatment.

Treatment for type 1 mallet fingers, usually consists of continuous distal interphalangeal joint extension splinting with a molded polythene (stack) or aluminum splint for 6–8 weeks. Night splinting usually is recommended for an additional 2–6 weeks. Volar splints are mostly recommended. Hyperextension of the distal interphalangeal joint should be avoided because it causes skin blanching, which possibly contributes to skin breakdown over the fracture. Although open type 2 injuries can be treated with closed reduction after appropriate wound care, splint management can be difficult. Direct repair of the extensor tendon can be done using a roll stitch with Kirschner wire fixation of the distal interphalangeal joint in full extension.

Type 3 mallet fingers require soft tissue coverage and pinning of the distal interphalangeal joint and possible primary arthrodesis. Pediatric mallet fingers or Seymore fractures should be treated with closed reduction and splinting of the distal interphalangeal joint in neutral or slight extension for 4 weeks. These fractures frequently are open fractures. These injuries usually require soft tissue coverage and primary grafting or other soft tissue reconstruction along with correction of mallet deformity. The tendon avulsion can be repaired using suture anchors or tying them through button anchor on volar aspect using a pull through suture.

Type IVa injury, usually is a Salter-Harris type II injury and should be managed with closed reduction and splinting.

Type IVb injuries heal well with closed treatment for articular surface remodeling. Late presenting injuries with displaced bony fragment (>2 mm) can be treated with extension block wiring.

Type IVc injuries with palmar subluxation of the distal phalanx are usually treated with open reduction internal fixation (ORIF) with a K-wire and possibly using a pullout suture with a button.

(For further reading, kindly refer to Chapter 38 in the book Essential Orthopedics: Principles and Practice, 2nd edition.)

58. Describe pathoanatomy and brief management of most common ligamentous injury of thumb in adults.

Ans: The injury is gamekeeper's thumb.

Pathoanatomy: The ulnar collateral ligament (UCL) of the thumb has two components:
1. The accessory
2. The UCL proper

UCL proper gets taut in flexion and loose in extension and vice versa for the accessory UCL.

Both have to be completely injured for prominent instability but volar plate resists abduction even with complete UCL injury. For complete instability, the volar plate also has to be injured. UCL inherently provides lateral support and prevents volar subluxation of the MCP joint also. This stability is vital for key pinch, tip pinch, and thumb opposition. In Skier's thumb and most of the gamekeeper's thumb the distal attachment of the UCL is usually avulsed from the proximal phalanx of the thumb. Severed distal end gets caught under the adductor aponeurosis and gets separated from bone precluding healing (the classical Stener lesion). The severed ligament then folds on itself and loses its anatomical relationship, and hence function (stability). Adductor aponeurosis serves as an active restraint to thumb abduction but has no passive role in MCP stability, so the MCP becomes unstable and symptomatic.

Stener lesion is only produced if there is significant radial deviation of phalanx (60° and more) along with tears of both proper and accessory collateral ligaments and volar plate.

Management: In the presence of Stener lesion only operative intervention will allow apposition and healing of the traumatically displaced ligament in an anatomic position. In the absence of Stener lesion, splinting of the thumb such that the torn ligament ends are reduced may produce healing and restoration of joint stability in selected patients—one should be fully sure that there is no Stener lesion and it is only a type 1 or type 3 injury.

The indications of surgical intervention (one should be a bit more biased to it):
- Gross radiographic instability
- Presence of palpable torn ligament ends (Stener lesion)
- Type 4 injury
- Type 2 injury (relative) as better and secure fixation would help early mobilization.

59. A. Describe and draw Stener lesion of thumb.
B. Explain indications and functioning of Suzuki frame for fingers.
C. Discuss etiology, classification, and management of Profundus tendon avulsion.

Ans: For (A) Please see answer above. The asked figure is provided here (**Fig. 3.3.7**).

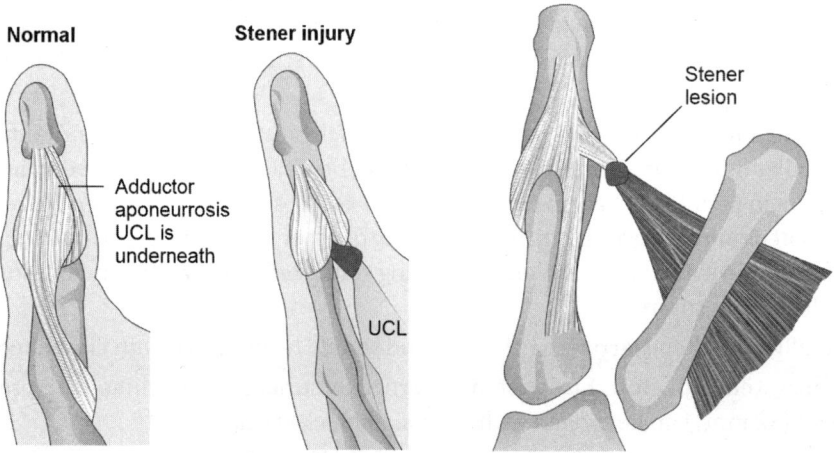

Fig. 3.3.7: The illustration of Stener lesion.

B. Indications and Functioning of Suzuki Frame for Fingers

Indications:

The Suzuki frame is indicated for:
- *Complex intra-articular fractures*: Comminuted or unstable fractures of the proximal interphalangeal joint (PIPJ) or distal interphalangeal joint (DIPJ) in the proximal or middle phalanges.
- *Fracture-dislocations*: PIPJ or DIPJ injuries with joint instability or subluxation.
- Severe phalangeal fractures: Cases where open reduction and internal fixation (ORIF) may lead to stiffness or poor outcomes.
- *High-risk cases*: Fractures with significant soft-tissue damage or where early mobilization is critical to prevent stiffness.

Functioning:

The Suzuki frame, developed by Yasushi Suzuki in 1994, is a dynamic external fixation device using Kirschner wires (K-wires) and rubber bands to treat finger fractures.
- Mechanism:
  - *K-Wire placement*: Two 1.2 mm K-wires are inserted—one in the proximal phalanx (center of rotation) and one distal to the fracture in the middle phalanx, parallel to the first. An optional third 1.0 mm K-wire in the middle phalanx prevents dorsal dislocation.
  - *Dynamic traction*: Rubber bands (or Foley catheter pieces) connect U-shaped hooks bent on the K-wires, applying longitudinal traction via capsuloligamentotaxis to align fracture fragments and maintain joint reduction.
  - *Early mobilization*: The frame allows controlled active range of motion (ROM) at PIPJ/DIPJ from day 1, preventing stiffness and promoting bone/joint remodeling.
- Advantages:
  - Minimally invasive, soft-tissue sparing, and cost-effective.
  - Enables early ROM (mean PIPJ ROM ~86° post-treatment), reducing adhesions and stiffness.
  - High union rate (~91%) with minimal complications (e.g., extensor lag and residual stiffness).
- Procedure:
  - Performed percutaneously under image intensification as a day procedure.
  - Postoperatively, a custom splint protects the frame; active flexion/extension exercises are encouraged.
  - Frame removal at ~6 weeks under local anesthesia, followed by hand therapy.

C. Profundus Tendon Avulsion *(Jersey Finger)*

Etiology:
- *Mechanism*: Sudden forced extension of a flexed DIP joint—Common in sports (e.g., tackling in rugby/football when opponent grabs jersey).
- *Most common digit*: Ring finger (due to its relatively weak FDP insertion and hand position in grip).
- *Pathophysiology*: Avulsion of flexor digitorum profundus (FDP) tendon from its insertion at the base of the distal phalanx ± fracture fragment.

Classification of Jersey finger **(Table 3.3.4)**

TABLE 3.3.4: Classification of Jersey finger.

Classification—Leddy and Packer (1977)

Type	Description	Retracted tendon level	Blood supply	Prognosis
Type I	Tendon retracts to palm	Palm	Both vincula ruptured → no blood supply	Poor—needs urgent repair
Type II	Tendon retracts to level of PIP joint	PIP joint	Long vinculum intact → some blood supply	Better prognosis
Type III	Large bony fragment avulsed and caught at A4 pulley	DIP joint level	Intact blood supply via bone	Best prognosis
Type IV	Bony fragment avulsed + FDP tendon avulsed from fragment	Variable	Variable	Requires fixation + tendon repair
Type V	Comminuted fracture of distal phalanx	Variable	Variable	Complex management

Management

General Principles
- Early diagnosis and surgical repair are essential to avoid permanent loss of DIP flexion.
- *Nonoperative treatment*: Rare; for chronic injuries, elderly, low-demand patients.

Surgical Options
- Type I: Urgent primary tendon repair (within 7–10 days) to prevent muscle retraction/fibrosis
- Type II: Primary tendon repair; less urgent but ideally within 3 weeks
- Type III: Open reduction and internal fixation (screw, K-wire, and pull-out suture) of bony fragment
- Type IV: Fix bone fragment + reattach FDP tendon
- Type V: ORIF or fragment excision + tendon repair, depending on comminution

Postoperative Care:
- Dorsal blocking splint (DIP and PIP joints flexed)
- Early passive motion protocol (Kleinert or Duran) under supervision
- Gradual strengthening after 6–8 weeks
- Return to sports usually after 3 months

60. Briefly discuss categories of dog bite, their first aid and postexposure prophylaxis.

Ans: The various categories of dog bites as described are as follows **(Table 3.3.5)**:

TABLE 3.3.5: Categorization of dog bite and indicative prophylaxis.

Categories	Characteristics	Postexposure prophylaxis
1	Touching or feeding animals, licks on intact skin	None
2	Nibbling of uncovered skin, minor scratches or abrasions without bleeding	Immediate vaccination and local treatment of the wound
3	Single or multiple transdermal bites or scratches, licks on broken skin, contamination of mucous membrane with saliva from licks, contacts with bats	Immediate vaccination and administration of rabies immunoglobulin, local treatment of the wound

First aid management: Local treatment of the wound is done as early as possible. Purpose is to remove as much virus as possible from the site of inoculation before it can be absorbed on nerve endings. Immediate flushing and washing of wound, scratches and the adjoining areas with plenty of soap and water, preferably under a running tap for at least 15 minutes is of paramount importance in the prevention. If soap is not available, simple flushing of the wound with plenty of water should be done as first aid.

Postexposure prophylaxis: All categories 2 and 3 exposures assessed as carrying a risk of developing rabies require PEP. PEP may be discontinued, if the suspected animal is proved by appropriate lab examination to be free of rabies or in case of domestic dogs, cats or ferrets, the animal remains healthy throughout a 10-day observation period starting from date of the bite.
- *Intramuscular administration of vaccine*: The schedule is based on injecting 1 mL or 0.5 mL (volume depends on type of vaccine) into the deltoid (or anterolateral thigh in children aged <2 years) of patients with category 2 and 3 exposures. The recommended regimen consists of either a 5-dose or 4-dose schedule.
  The 5-dose regimen prescribes 1 dose on each of days 0, 3, 7, 14, and 28 days.
  The 4-dose abbreviated multisite regimen (2-1-1) prescribes two doses on day 0 (1 in each of the deltoid or thigh sites) followed by one dose on each of days 7 and 21.
- *Intradermal administration of vaccine*: The two-site regimen prescribes injection of 0.1 mL at two sites (deltoid or thigh) on days 0, 3, 7 and 28.

61. First aid management of a firecracker hand injury in an adult.

Ans: The following are the first-aid management do's and don'ts for a firecracker hand injury:
- Pour ample water over the burns till the burning sensation stops or under cold running water for 10 minutes.

- Remove any constricting materials such as rings, bangles immediately as after setting-up of swelling they are difficult to remove later causing constriction of blood supply to the region.
- After cooling the burn for at least 15 minutes insert it into a sterile plastic bag
- *Do not*:
  - Apply agents such as ink, toothpaste, ointments and creams over the burn wound.
  - Touch the burn
  - Use adhesive dressings
  - Pop or puncture blisters

62. A. Describe and draw anatomy of nail bed, complete spectrum of nail bed injuries and its treatment.

B. Describe principles of treatment of "Fingertip injuries with tissue loss".

Ans:

1. Anatomy of the Nail Bed

A nail unit consists of several specialized components **(Table 3.3.6 and Fig. 3.3.8)**:
- *Nail plate*: Hard keratin structure.
- *Proximal nail fold*: Protects germinal matrix.
- *Germinal matrix*: Produces ~90% of the nail; damage can cause permanent deformity.
- *Sterile matrix*: Adds keratin to the underside of the nail; helps adhesion.
- *Hyponychium*: Skin under the free edge; barrier to infection.
- *Distal phalanx*: Bone support.

TABLE 3.3.6: Nail-bed anatomy.

Component	Description	Function
Nail plate	Hard keratinized structure	Protection
Nail folds	Proximal and lateral skin folds overlapping nail plate	Anchor and protect germinal matrix
Cuticle (Eponychium)	Distal projection of proximal nail fold	Barrier to infection
Germinal matrix	Proximal 3–4 mm of nail bed beneath nail root	Produces 90% of nail plate
Sterile matrix	Distal nail bed to hyponychium	Produces remaining 10% of nail plate, secures nail
Hyponychium	Skin under free nail edge	Seal to prevent infection
Perionychium	Soft tissue surrounding the nail unit	Support
Blood supply	Terminal branches of volar digital arteries form dorsal and ventral arcades	Nourishment
Innervation	Dorsal branches from volar digital nerves	Sensation

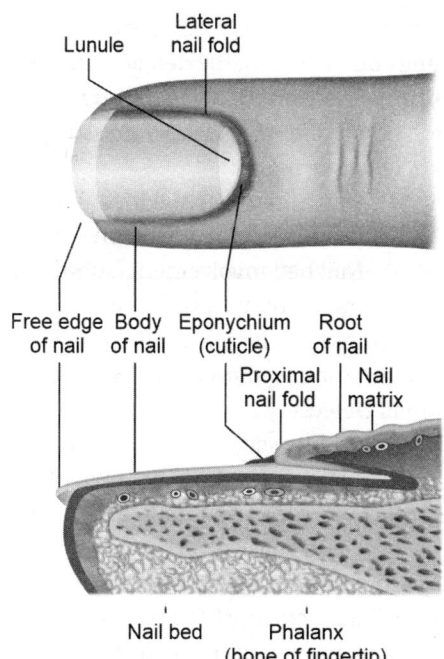

Fig. 3.3.8: Illustration of nail bad anatomy.

2. Spectrum of Nail Bed Injuries

A. Closed Injuries
1. *Subungual hematoma*: Blood under nail plate (often from crush injury)
2. *Sterile matrix contusion*: No visible nail deformity immediately

B. Open/Laceration Injuries
1. *Simple nail bed laceration*: From sharp objects.
2. *Complex laceration*: Irregular wound edges, often with nail plate disruption

3. *Crush injury*: Comminuted distal phalanx fracture + nail bed disruption
4. *Avulsion injury*: Nail plate and bed partially or completely torn off

C. Associated Injuries
1. Distal phalanx fracture (Tuft fracture)
2. Germinal matrix loss (risk of permanent nail deformity)

3. **Management Principles (Table 3.3.7)**

TABLE 3.3.7: Management of nail bed injuries.

Injury type	Treatment
Subungual hematoma (<50% nail, no fracture)	Nail plate left intact, trephination with heated needle or cautery for drainage
Subungual hematoma (>50% nail or with fracture)	Remove nail plate, inspect and repair nail bed
Simple laceration	Nail plate removal, microsurgical repair with 6-0/7-0 absorbable sutures, replace nail plate or use sterile foil/silicone sheet
Complex laceration/Crush injury	Debridement, meticulous repair, fracture stabilization (K-wire if unstable), replace nail plate
Avulsion with germinal matrix loss	Nail bed graft (split-thickness sterile matrix graft from great toe)
Distal phalanx fracture with nail bed injury	Repair nail bed + splinting; K-wire for unstable fractures
Complete amputation of fingertip	Consider replantation or composite graft in children

Principles of Treatment for Fingertip Injuries with Tissue Loss

Fingertip injuries with tissue loss are common in trauma (e.g., crush injuries, lacerations, amputations). Management depends on the size of the defect, bone exposure, and viability of remaining tissue.

1. **Initial Assessment and Emergency Care**
   - *Control bleeding*: Direct pressure, elevation, and hemostatic agents if needed.
   - *Evaluate injury*:
     - Skin and soft-tissue loss (partial vs. complete amputation)
     - Bone exposure (distal phalanx fracture or tuft fracture)
     - Nail bed involvement (subungual hematoma, avulsion)
   - Tetanus prophylaxis if contaminated
   - Antibiotics (if high-risk for infection, e.g., crush injury and contamination)

2. **Treatment based on Defect Size and Tissue Loss**

A. Small Defects (<1 cm) Without Bone Exposure
   - Healing by secondary intention:
     - Clean wound, apply nonadherent dressing (e.g., petrolatum gauze).
     - Allowed to granulate over 2–4 weeks.
     - Good sensory recovery in most cases.

B. Moderate Defects (1–2 cm) or Bone Exposure
   - Primary closure (if minimal tension)
   - Skin grafting (full thickness preferred for better durability and sensation)
   - Local flaps (if bone is exposed but minimal soft tissue loss):
     - V-Y advancement flap (Atasoy/Kleinert flap)—for volar defects.
     - Cross-finger flap—for larger dorsal defects.

C. Large Defects (>2 cm) or Complete Amputation
   - Replantation (if clean-cut injury and proximal amputation, especially in children)
   - Revision amputation + closure (if replantation not feasible):
     - Shorten bone slightly to allow tension-free closure.
     - Preserve nail matrix if possible.
     - Thenar flap or homodigital island flap for volar defects.

3.4 UPPER LIMB TRAUMA FROM HIP TO FOOT (Q63–113)

63. Mention the complications of fractured head and neck femur in children.

Ans:

Complications:
- Avascular necrosis
- Malunion (coxa vara)
- Physeal arrest
- Nonunion.

Nonunion: Prevention—
- Anatomic reduction, and open the fracture site, if necessary
- Stable internal fixation, and cross the physis, if necessary
- Spica cast supplemental immobilization for children, if there is a concern for stabilization.

Avascular necrosis: Prevention—
- Urgent reduction <24 hours
- Open reduction or capsulotomy, if reduction is closed
- Anatomic reduction.

Physeal arrest: Prevention—
- Stop the fixation distal to the physis but do not compromise stability. The majority of type II and IV fractures can achieve stable fixation without crossing the physis.
- Consider removal of implants once the fracture has bony union.

Other complications in hip fractures: Infection is uncommon after hip fractures in children. The reported incidence of 1% is consistent with the expected infection rate in any closed fracture treated surgically with ORIF. Care must be taken to avoid persistent penetration of hardware into the joint, which can cause chondrolysis in conditions such as slipped capital femoral epiphysis (SCFE). Finally, SCFE has been reported after fixation of an ipsilateral femoral neck fracture.

64. What is posterior dislocation of hip? Discuss clinical features and different methods of reduction. Write short notes on Stimson and Bigelow methods to reduce posterior dislocation of hip. Enumerate complications.

Ans: The hip joint is inherently stable, and hip dislocations generally are produced by high-energy trauma. Often they are associated with multiple injuries to different organ systems. Motor vehicle accidents remain the most common mechanism of hip dislocation, followed by falls from a height, industrial accidents, and, more rarely, sports such as football or wrestling. Posterior dislocations occur much more frequently than anterior dislocations and result from a posteriorly directed force to the flexed knee with the hip also in a flexed position. Lesser degrees of hip flexion and increasing amounts of hip abduction with similarly applied force often result in an acetabular fracture.

Clinical features: Severe pain, deformity [flexion, adduction, internal rotation (FADIR) in posterior, extension/external rotation (superior anterior dislocation) or FADER (obturator type anterior dislocation)], and inability to bear weight. Patients with an isolated posterior hip dislocation present with hip flexion, adduction, internal rotation, and a shortened extremity. Careful physical examination is crucial, with particular attention paid to associated pelvic, sciatic nerve or ipsilateral knee injuries.

Methods of reduction are many (vide below):
- Allis method
- Stimson method
- East Baltimore lift
- Bigelow method
- Lefkowitz maneuver.

Stimson method: For reducing posterior dislocation, the patient is placed prone on the stretcher with the affected leg hanging off the side of the stretcher/couch. This brings the extremity into a position of hip flexion and knee flexion of 90° each. In this position, the assistant immobilizes the pelvis, and the surgeon applies an anteriorly directed force on the proximal calf. Gentle rotation of the limb may assist in reduction. This technique is difficult to perform in the emergency department.

Bigelow method: This have been associated with iatrogenic femoral neck fractures and are not as frequently used as reduction techniques. In the Bigelow maneuver, the patient is supine, and the surgeon applies longitudinal traction on the limb. The adducted and internally rotated thigh is then flexed at least 90°. The femoral head is then levered into the acetabulum by abduction, external rotation, and extension of the hip.

Complications:
- *Osteonecrosis (AVN)*: Seen in 5–40% of injuries with risk proportional to delay until reduction (>6–24 hours). This is not always true as osteonecrosis may also result from the initial injury itself. Diagnosis of osteonecrosis may be delayed from several months to even years after injury. Repeated reduction attempts and harsh technique may also increase its incidence.
- *Post-traumatic osteoarthritis*: This is the most common long-term complication of hip dislocations and is particularly common in joints with residual incongruity such as dislocations with acetabular fractures or transchondral fractures of the femoral head.
- *Recurrent dislocation*: Although rare (<2%), patients with decreased femoral anteversion or those mobilized before substantial healing of soft tissues may sustain a recurrent posterior dislocation.
- *Neurovascular injury*: Sciatic nerve injury occurs in 10–20% of hip dislocations. It is usually caused by stretching of the nerve or from displaced acetabular fracture fragment or direct compression of the nerve from the dislocated femoral head. Recovery is seen in 40–50% cases. Electromyographic studies can be done at 3–4 weeks for prognostic guidance. No clinical or electrical improvement by 1 year, and sciatic nerve injury after closed reduction (entrapped nerve) are indications for surgical intervention. Injury to the femoral nerve and femoral vascular structures are even rarer as seen with anterior dislocations.
- *Femoral head fractures*: These occur in 10% of posterior dislocations (shear fractures) and in 25–75% of anterior dislocations (indentation fractures).
- *Heterotopic ossification*: This occurs in 2% of patients and is related to the initial muscular damage and hematoma formation. Surgery increases its incidence. Prophylaxis choices include indomethacin for 6 weeks or use of radiation.
- *Thromboembolism*: This may occur due to traction-induced endothelial injury of crossing vasculature. Prophylaxis is imperative in high-risk patients including chemoprophylaxis.

(For further reading of DVT prophylaxis, kindly refer to Chapter 18 of the book Essential Orthopedics: Principles and Practice, 2nd edition.)

65. Describe in details fracture of head of femur. Also, discuss the treatment for the same.
Ans:
Introduction: Femoral head fractures are almost always associated with hip dislocation. They occur in 5–15% of all hip dislocations and are seen in nearly 10% of posterior hip dislocations. There are two types of femoral head fracture with shear or cleavage type occurring in majority of the patients, and indention or crush type occurring in remainder.

Mechanism of injury: These fractures are secondary to motor vehicle accidents with axial load transmitted proximally through the femur. If the thigh is in the neutral or adducted position, posterior dislocation with or without femoral head fractures may result. These fractures may result from counter force from ligamentum teres resulting in avulsion of fragment or cleavage by the posterior acetabular edge (shear fracture).

Anatomy: Femoral head varies in size from 40 mm to 60 mm in diameter in proportion to body mass. Most of the femoral head articular surface is involved in the load transfer and thus damage to this surface may lead to the development of post-traumatic arthritis. So, maintaining the anatomy is crucial.

Clinical evaluation: Ninety-five percent of patients have injuries that require inpatient management independent of femoral head fracture. In addition to hip dislocation, femoral head fractures are also associated with acetabular fractures, knee ligament injuries, patella fractures, and femoral shaft fractures. A careful neurovascular examination is essential because posterior hip dislocations may result in neurovascular compromise.

Associated injuries: Hip dislocations, acetabular fractures, femoral shaft fractures, patella fractures, and knee ligamentous injuries.

Radiographic evaluation: Anteroposterior (AP) and Judet views of the pelvis—demonstrate the femoral head fractures and hip dislocations in majority of the cases.

Computed tomography: It is usually performed after the reduction of hip dislocation to assess the size, location, and reduction of femoral head fracture. CT is necessary to evaluate the reduction of the femoral head fracture and to rule out the presence of intra-articular fragments that may prevent hip joint congruity.

Classification

Pipkin Classification (Fig. 3.4.1):
- *Type I*: Hip dislocation with fracture of the femoral head inferior to the fovea capitis femoris.
- *Type II*: Hip dislocation with fracture of the femoral head superior to the fovea capitis femoris.
- *Type III*: Type I or II injury associated with fracture of the femoral neck.
- *Type IV*: Type I or II injury associated with fracture of the acetabular rim.

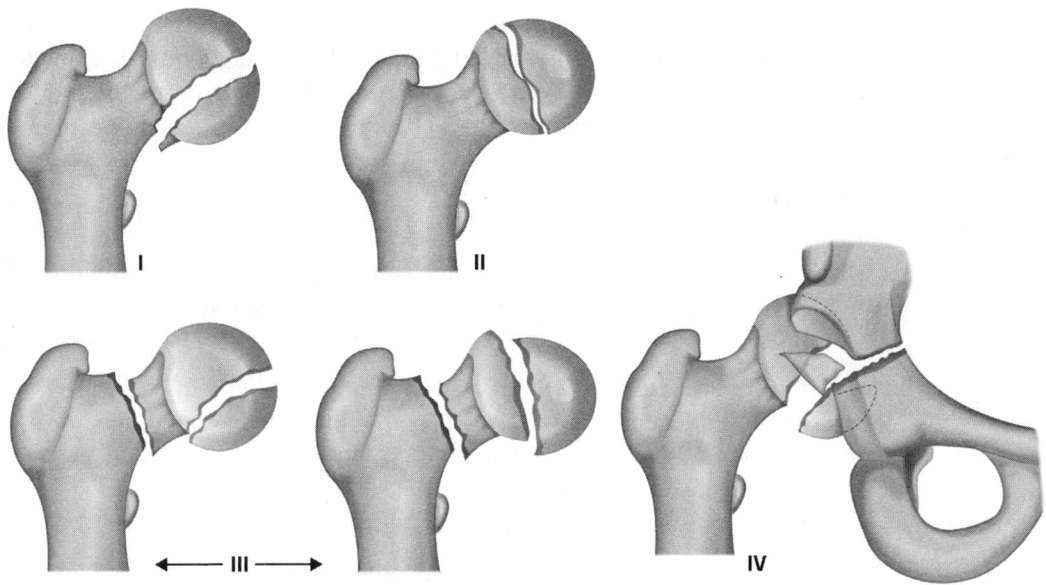

Fig. 3.4.1: Pipkin classification.

Brumback classification of femoral head fractures:
- *Type 1*: Posterior hip dislocation with fracture of the femoral head involving the inferomedial portion of the femoral head
- *Type 1A*: With minimum or no fracture of the acetabular rim and staple hip joint after reduction
- *Type 1B*: With significant acetabular rim and stable joint after reconstruction
- *Type 2*: Posterior hip dislocation with fracture of the femoral head involving the supermedial portion of the femoral head
- *Type 2A*: With minimum or no fracture of the acetabular rim and stable joint after reduction
- *Type 2B*: With significant acetabular fracture and hip joint instability
- *Type 3*: Dislocation of the hip (unspecified direction) with femoral neck fracture
- *Type 3A*: Without fracture of the femoral head
- *Type 3B*: With fracture of the femoral head
- *Type 4*: Anterior dislocation of the femoral head

- *Type 4A*: Indentation type—depression of the superolateral surface of the femoral head
- *Type 4B*: Transchondral type, osteocartilaginous shear fracture of the weight-bearing surface of the femoral head
- *Type 5*: Central fracture–dislocation of the hip with femoral head fracture.

Treatment

Pipkin Type I: The femoral head fracture is inferior to the fovea. These fractures occur in the nonweight-bearing surface. If reduction is adequate (<1 mm step-off) and the hip is stable, closed treatment is recommended. If the reduction is not adequate, open reduction and internal fixation with small subarticular screws using an anterior approach are recommended. Small fragments may be excised, if they do not sacrifice stability.

Pipkin Type II: The femoral head fracture is superior to the fovea. These fractures involve the weight-bearing surface. The same recommendations apply for the nonoperative treatment of type II fractures as for type I fractures, except that only an anatomic reduction as seen on CT and repeat radiographs can be accepted for nonoperative care. In general, the treatment of choice is open reduction and internal fixation through an anterior approach (Smith-Peterson). Mini fragment implants must be countersunk and/or headless screws utilized. Care must be taken to bury the implants below the articular cartilage.

Pipkin Type III: A femoral head fracture occurs with an associated fracture of the femoral neck. The prognosis for this fracture is poor and depends on the degree of displacement of the femoral neck fracture. In younger individuals, emergency open reduction and internal fixation of the femoral neck are performed, followed by internal fixation of the femoral head. This can be done using an anterolateral (Watson–Jones) approach. In older individuals with a displaced femoral neck fracture, prosthetic replacement is indicated.

Pipkin Type IV: A femoral head fracture occurs with an associated fracture of the acetabulum. This fracture must be treated in tandem with the associated acetabular fracture. The acetabular fracture should dictate the surgical approach (although this may not be possible), and the femoral head fracture, even if nondisplaced, should be internally fixed to allow early motion of the hip joint.

Femoral head fractures associated with anterior dislocations: These fractures are difficult to manage. Impaction fractures, typically located on the superior aspect of the femoral head, require no specific treatment, but the fracture size and location have prognostic implications. Displaced transchondral fractures that result in a nonconcentric reduction require open reduction and either excision or internal fixation, depending on fragment size and location.

Complications

Osteonecrosis: Patients with posterior hip dislocations with an associated femoral head fracture are at high risk for developing osteonecrosis and post-traumatic degenerative arthritis. The prognosis for these injuries varies. Pipkin types I and II are reported to have the same prognosis as a simple dislocation (1–10% if dislocated <6 hours). Pipkin type IV injuries seem to have roughly the same prognosis as acetabular fractures without a femoral head fracture. Pipkin type III injuries have a poor prognosis, with a 50% rate of post-traumatic osteonecrosis.

Post-traumatic osteoarthritis: Risk factors include transchondral fracture, indentation fracture greater than 4 mm in depth, and osteonecrosis.

66. **Classify fracture neck of femur in children. Discuss the treatment principles and prognosis.**

Ans: *Classification proposed by Delbet and popularized by Colonna* **(Fig. 3.4.2)**:
- *Type I*: Transepiphyseal separations with or without dislocation of the femoral head from the acetabulum
- *Type II*: Transcervical fractures, displaced and nondisplaced
- *Type III*: Cervicotrochanteric fractures, displaced and nondisplaced
- *Type IV*: Intertrochanteric fractures.

Treatment principles:
- Fix/treat on priority
- Gentle reduction

- Minimum number of attempts (senior personnel, especially a pediatric orthopedician preferred if available) if closed reduction attempted
- The physis should be crossed only by smooth pins when internal fixation is necessary
- Preserve vascularity to head, if open reduction is done.

Type I: Attempt gentle closed reduction and internal fixation (CRIF). If dislocation is present then gentle CRIF is performed but if unsuccessful, then immediate open reduction and fixation with pins or cannulated hip screws is done.

Type II: CRIF regardless of the amount of displacement

Type III: Gentle CRIF; if not displaced—abduction spica cast

Type IV: Skin or skeletal traction, abduction spica cast; internal fixation may be necessary if the fracture cannot be reduced/maintained in reduction and held in a spica cast or if traction followed by casting is not an option.

Prognosis: Osteonecrosis as per type is—
- Type I: 100%
- Type II: 52%
- Type III: 27%
- Type IV: 14%

Premature physeal closure: The incidence is ≤60%, increases with pins penetrating the physis. It causes femoral shortening, coxa vara, and short femoral neck.

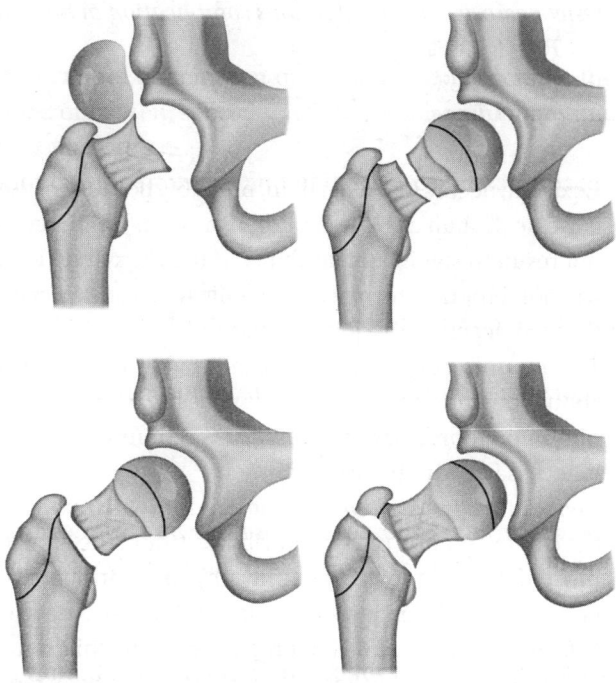

Fig. 3.4.2: Delbet and Colonna classification.

Coxa vara: The incidence is 20%, often follows inadequate closed reduction.

Nonunion: The incidence is 10% resulting from multiple factors (inadequate reduction or inadequate internal fixation, biological, etc.).

67. **Describe pediatric hip fractures along with its classification and management.**

Ans: Pediatric hip fractures:

Classification proposed by Delbet and popularized by Colonna:
- *Type I*: Transepiphyseal separations with or without dislocation of the femoral head from the acetabulum
- *Type II*: Transcervical fractures, displaced and nondisplaced
- *Type III*: Cervicotrochanteric fractures, displaced and nondisplaced
- *Type IV*: Intertrochanteric fractures.

Management:
- *Type I*: Transepiphyseal separations without dislocations—gentle closed reduction and internal fixation; with dislocation—gentle closed reduction, then, if unsuccessful, immediate open reduction and fixation with pins or cannulated hip screws
- *Type II*: Transcervical—closed reduction and internal fixation regardless of the amount of displacement
- *Type III*: Cervicotrochanteric fractures, if displaced—gentle closed reduction and internal fixation; if not displaced—abduction spica cast
- *Type IV*: Intertrochanteric fractures—skin or skeletal traction, abduction spica cast; internal fixation may be necessary if the fracture cannot be reduced and held in a spica cast or if traction followed by casting is not an option.

68. What are the complications of neck femur fractures in children?

Ans: The following are the complications of fracture femoral neck in children:
- *Osteonecrosis is the most serious complication of hip fractures in children*:
  - Type I: 100%
  - Type II: 52%
  - Type III: 27%
  - Type IV: 14%
- Coxavara occurs less often than, probably because of the routine use of internal fixation. In the children with coxa vara, if the neck-shaft angle was >120° in a young child, remodeling can occur to some degree, and even if it did not, it will not result in significant disability. If the neck-shaft angle is between 100 and 110°, however, the coxa vara deformity will not remodel and persists. Significant coxa vara causes a shortened extremity and an abductor or gluteal lurch and delayed degenerative joint changes.
- The nonunion rate is low. Use of internal fixation decreases chances for nonunion. Operative treatment for nonunion should be undertaken as soon as possible. Valgus subtrochanteric osteotomy as recommended by Ratliff; makes the nonunion more horizontal and allows compressive vertical forces to aid in union. This osteotomy can be augmented, if necessary, with bone grafts.
- *Premature physeal closure*: Of the children with pins crossing the physis, 87% have premature physeal closure. Because the capital femoral physis contributes 15% of the growth of the entire lower extremity and normally closes earlier than most of the other lower extremity physes, shortening is <2 cm in most of the children involved. The discrepancy is >2 cm only in children in whom osteonecrosis also develops.
- Infection is uncommon after hip fractures in children.
- Chondrolysis after hip fractures in children has been reported. They can also have osteonecrosis along with chondrolysis which have ever poorer results.

69. A. Describe the various techniques of osteosynthesis of adult fracture neck of femur including concept of "Femoral neck system (FNS)".
B. What are the pros and cons of FNS?

Ans:

A. Fracture neck of femur in adults has high risk of non-union and avascular necrosis. Choice of Fixation techniques **(Table 3.4.1)** depends on:
- Age (<60 years: preserve head)
- Displacement (Garden's classification)
- Pauwels angle (biomechanical stability)

TABLE 3.4.1: Various techniques for fixation of femoral neck fracture.

Technique	Indications	Principle/Biomechanics	Advantages	Disadvantages/Limitations
Multiple cannulated cancellous screws (CCS)	Nondisplaced/minimally displaced fractures (Garden I–II) in young adults	Parallel or slightly divergent screws across fracture	Minimally invasive, preserves bone	Poor rotational stability, weaker in vertical fractures (Pauwels III)
Dynamic hip screw (DHS) with derotation screw	Basicervical/Pauwels II–III fractures in young	Side plate with lag screw allows controlled collapse + derotation screw for rotational stability	Better control in vertical fractures	Larger exposure, more bone removal
Sliding hip screw (SHS)	Similar to DHS but more compact	Controlled collapse	Strong fixation in vertical fractures	Bulky implant for intracapsular fractures

Contd...

Contd...

Technique	Indications	Principle/Biomechanics	Advantages	Disadvantages/Limitations
Pauwels osteotomy (Valgus intertrochanteric osteotomy)	Vertical fractures with high shear	Converts shear → compression forces	Promotes union	Technically demanding; limb length discrepancy possible
Femoral neck system (FNS)	Garden I–III fractures, especially Pauwels II–III	Angular stable plate with central bolt + antirotation screw; minimal invasiveness	High rotational and angular stability, less soft-tissue disruption, early mobilization	Newer system → limited long-term data
Fixed angle devices (Blade plate/Angle nail)	Unstable patterns with comminution	Fixed angular stability	Strong fixation	Technically demanding; not commonly used today

Concept of Femoral Neck System (FNS)
The FNS is a minimally invasive implant for femoral neck fracture fixation, combining a central bolt, antirotation screw, and small side plate. It provides angular stability, dynamic compression (up to 20 mm), and preserves the native hip, ideal for subcapital, transcervical, or basicervical fractures.

B.

Pros:
- Superior stability versus cannulated screws (lower reoperation rate, $p < 0.001$)
- Minimally invasive (6 cm incision, shorter surgery)
- Faster healing, better function (e.g., Harris Hip Score)
- Preserves hip in younger patients.
- Compact design suits narrow necks

Cons:
- Slightly higher blood loss (~16 mL vs. CCS).
- Less effective for vertical fractures (Pauwels III).
- Technical complexity and learning curve
- Higher cost than traditional screws
- *Risks*: Nonunion (5–10%), avascular necrosis.

70. Describe stress fracture of neck of femur.

Ans: *Stress fracture*: Stress fractures of the femoral neck can occur in young and vigorous individuals with unaccustomed strenuous activity, such as athletics, running, or marching long distances. In elderly individuals, they can occur because of one of the metabolic disorders of bone. Frequently, routine anteroposterior and lateral radiographs initially are normal, with the diagnosis confirmed by bone scan or MRI.

Classification and treatment: Femoral neck stress fractures have been classified by Fullerton and Snowdy according to the location of the fracture in the femoral neck.
- Type A (lateral) fractures, often referred to as *tension fractures,* are more unstable and prone to displacement. We recommend internal fixation with multiple screws for this fracture.
- Type B (medial) compression fractures can be treated nonoperatively with rest followed by a period of protected weight bearing. Radiographs should be made at multiple intervals to confirm progression toward union without displacement. If a patient cannot comply with activity restriction, internal fixation is recommended.
- Type C fractures are displaced and require closed or open reduction with screw fixation or hemiarthroplasty, depending on the patient's age and medical circumstances.

(Detailed discussion on stress fractures of femoral neck is provided in Chapter 36 of the book Essential Orthopedics: Principles and Practice, 2nd edition.)

71. Discuss management of fractured proximal third of femur in an adolescent. Compare the advantages and disadvantages of each method.

Ans: Management of proximal third shaft femur fractures in an adolescent can be done by one of the following methods. The advantages and disadvantages of each are noted along:

- *Cephalomedullary nail*:
  - *Advantages*:
    - Rotationally stable
    - Small operative wound
    - Preserves fracture hematoma
    - Less chances of infection
    - Early and abundant callus formation.
  - *Disadvantages*:
    - Greater trochanteric physeal injury leading to deformity
    - Osteonescrosis of femoral head
    - Resurgery for implant removal.
- *TENS nailing*:
  - *Advantages*:
    - Early abundant callus
    - Small operative wound
    - Less chances of infection
    - Preserves fracture hematoma.
  - *Disadvantages*:
    - Use only in transverse or short oblique fractures
    - Mild varus or valgus angulation and mild anterior or posterior malalignment
    - Physeal injury
    - Limb length discrepancy
    - Poor rotation control
    - Reoperation for implant removal
    - Infection (superficial and deep)
    - Nail impingement/painful bursa at entry site.
- *Plating*:
  - *Advantages*:
    - Absolute fixation
    - Interdigitation of edges
    - Needed where TENS cannot be done, i.e. length unstable fractures.
  - *Disadvantages*:
    - Bigger operative wound and scar formation
    - Fracture hematoma is lost
    - High chances of infection
    - Reoperation for implant removal with same size incision needed.

72. Classify trochanteric fractures of hip. Mention the pros and cons of their management with DHS/PFN.

Ans: *Boyd and Griffin* classified fractures in the peritrochanteric area of the femur into four types **(Fig. 3.4.3)**.

- *Type 1*: Undisplaced fracture that extend along the intertrochanteric line (two part)
- *Type 2*: Posteromedial comminuted fractures with main fracture along the intertrochanteric line
- *Type 3*: Fractures that extend distal to lesser trochanter or fracture lines runs obliquely down from lateral to medial (reverse obliquity type)
- *Type 4*: Fracture of trochanteric region or proximal shaft with fracture line in at least two planes.

Evans classification: It classifies the fracture on the basis of stability **(Fig. 3.4.4)**.
- *Type 1*: The fracture line that extends up from lesser trochanter to the greater trochanter.
  - Undisplaced
  - Displaced two-part fracture and reducible
  - Three-fragment fracture with posterolateral support
  - Three-part fracture with lost medial support
  - Comminuted (four parts or more) with separate posterolateral and medial fragments.
- *Type 2*: Reverse obliquity type.

Russell-Taylor classification:
- *Type 1*: Fractures that do not extend to piriformis
  - Lesser trochanter is intact
  - Lesser trochanter is disrupted.
- *Type 2*: Fractures that involve the piriformis fossa
  - Lesser trochanter is intact
  - Lesser trochanter is disrupted

DHS (Dynamic Hip Screw) Plate Construct
Pros:
- Relatively easy reduction and manipulation of fracture site possible due to direct accessibility (open reduction)
- Relatively easy to perform due to wide experience and practice

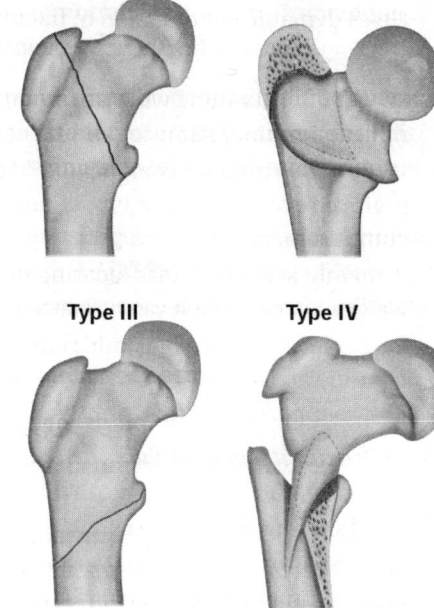

Fig. 3.4.3: Boyd and Griffin classification.

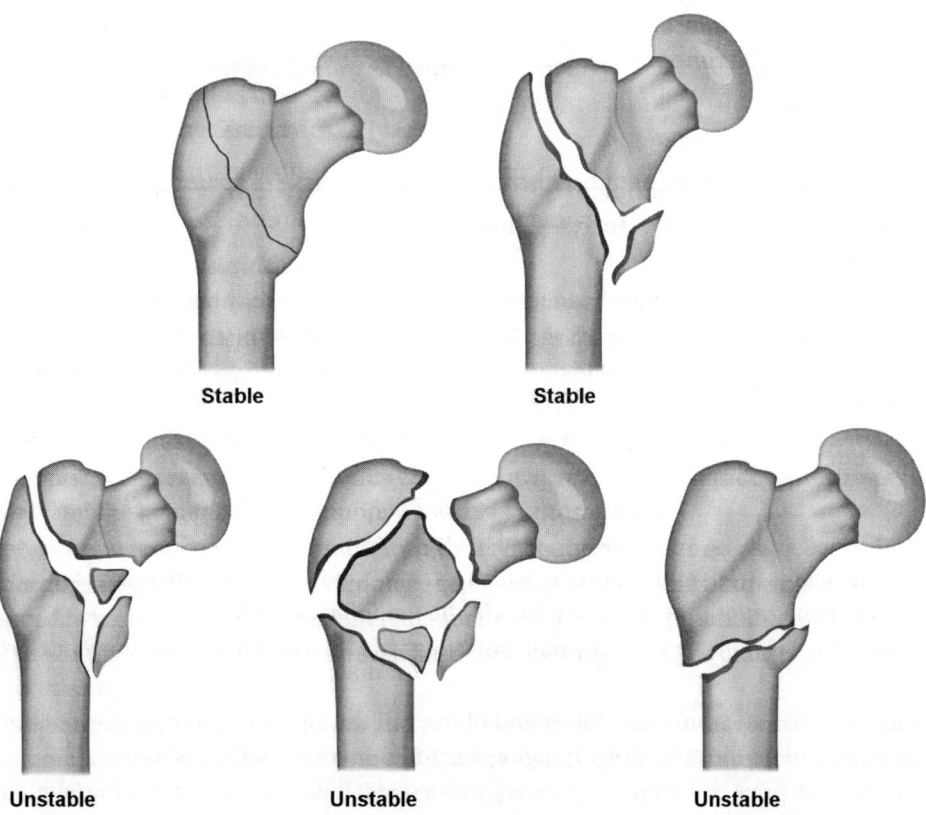

Fig. 3.4.4: Evans classification.

- Additional trochanteric stabilization possible, if needed (using TSP)
- Anterotation stabilization of head possible (if needed) with placement of additional screw
- Gives dynamic compression to fracture site when patient walks.

Cons:
- Large surgical wound with associated morbidity and increased infection rates. Also, it increases bleeding and surgical time as additional time for closure of wound needed.
- It cannot be used for complicated fractures like those with subtrochanteric extension or fractures of subtrochanteric region, reverse oblique types, unstable trochanteric fractures—posteromedial comminution/circumferential comminution.
- It mainly acts like a load-bearing device hence fracture union is a necessity for complete weight-bearing (partial weight-bearing albeit can be started very early).
- Larger lever arm for dynamic screw (plate fixation point to screw length) results in higher resulting forces, it has to bear in case patient bears weight—leading to higher chances of device failure, if reduction is less than perfect or if bony support is less than optimal (as in medial comminution).

PFN (Proximal Femoral Nail)
Pros:
- Load sharing device—so allows early rehabilitation and weight-bearing
- Smaller lever arm—due to intramedullary location of the fixation device results in lesser forces on the fixation bolt/anterotation screw producing lesser varus moment for failure (provided screw length is appropriate else smaller screw still results in varus failure)
- Small incision is needed for fixation of the fracture
- Implant of choice in subtrochanteric fractures and unstable fracture types of intertrochanteric fractures (comminuted/reverse obliquity)
- Less operative time.

Cons:
- Difficult reduction and many times open reduction is needed as indirect reduction may not be possible. Reduction of the fracture before implant placement is a must.
- Has a steeper learning curve if untrained.

73. A. Principle and mechanism of action of a PFN in the treatment of proximal femur fractures.
B. Write its complications and how to avoid them.

Ans:
A. *Principle*: The proximal fragment is reduced and locked in appropriate neck-shaft angle in line of compression forces. The fragment is forced into controlled compression at fracture line-enhancing union and maintaining reduction while weight bearing and force transmission. The controlled collapse is offered by sliding mechanism of the proximal bolt sliding into the tunnel in nail.
  - The increased proximal nail diameter and wall thickness, in combination with screw, design, provide greater fixation and stability.
  - The distal end of the nail is fixed to the cortex with two fully threaded screws. The screws statically lock the nail and help in control of rotation and telescoping of the fracture fragments.
  - The lag screw withstands the bending moment which is transferred to the intramedullary nail and counterbalanced by its locking mechanism with the femoral cortex in the medullary canal.
  - Almost the entire load is transferred to the nail and a negligible portion to the medial femoral cortex.

B. *Complications*:
  - Fracture of the femur shaft around the lower end of the nail during insertion due to excessive bow of the femur vis-à-vis straighter nail perforating and impinging the anterior cortex while insertion.
  - Tendency of nail to fix proximal fragment in varus due to shaft deformities and bowing/angulations.
  - Fat embolism during reaming.

74. What is unstable trochanteric fracture? What are the various methods of managing unstable intertrochanteric fracture?

Ans: Evans devised a widely used classification system based on the division of fractures into stable and unstable groups. He divided unstable fractures further into those in which stability could be restored by anatomical or near-anatomical reduction and those in which anatomical reduction would not create stability. In an Evans type I fracture, the fracture line extends upward and outward from the lesser trochanter. In type II, reverse obliquity fracture, the major fracture line extends outward and downward from the lesser trochanter. Type II fractures have a tendency toward medial displacement of the femoral shaft because of the pull of the adductor muscles.

Radiologically, the fractures with loss of lateral wall, posteromedial comminution, reverse obliquity type and four part or more are unstable types needing extra care while planning fixation.

Unstable fractures usually can be treated by anatomical reduction with the use of a collapsible fixation device, such as:
- Hip dynamic compression screw (DCS not DHS)
- Medoff plate (now obsolete)
- Cephalomedullary nail (commonly used).

Such collapsible internal fixation devices permit the proximal fragment to collapse or settle onto the fixation device, seeking its own position of stability, with the shaft usually displacing medially. Intramedullary nails seem to have some advantage in unstable fractures, especially fractures with reverse obliquity and subtrochanteric extension that cannot be treated easily with standard hip compression screws.

Studies have reported the results of unstable intertrochanteric fracture treated with 95° fixed-angle devices, compression hip screws, or intramedullary nails. These studies show worse results with extramedullary implants than intramedullary nails. So unstable intertrochanteric fractures, reverse obliquity, and fractures with a significant subtrochanteric extension (AO A2.2 through A3.3) usually are treated with an intramedullary device. Stable fractures (AO A1.1 through A2.1) may be treated by either device, but the literature does not support the routine use of intramedullary nails in stable fractures because of concerns over the added complexity of the procedure and added expense of the intramedullary implants.

Some authors have suggested that unstable trochanteric fractures in patients with severely osteoporotic bone are best thought of as pathological fractures, and that the use of polymethyl methacrylate (PMMA) to augment the fixation (Delta bolt® Depuy-synthes) can improve stability in these patients. PMMA augmentation provided early stability and allowed early mobilization of elderly patients, but when improperly used could cause late problems. PMMA augmentation for unstable trochanteric fractures in elderly patients with severe osteoporosis for whom no better form of fixation is available, and the bone is too porotic to hold a screw. Some orthopedic manufacturers have introduced "super lag" screws that have screw threads of an enlarged width to improve purchase in "soft" bone.

(For various classification systems and understanding of unstable fracture types, refer to Annexure 2 of the book Essential Orthopedics: Principles and Practice, 2nd edition.)

75. What are peritrochanteric fractures? Discuss its classification and management.

Ans: Boyd and Griffin classified fractures in the peritrochanteric area of the femur into four types.

- *Type 1*: Undisplaced fracture that extend along the intertrochanteric line (two part). Reduction usually is simple and is maintained with little difficulty.
- *Type 2*: Posteromedial comminuted fractures with main fracture along the intertrochanteric line. Reduction of these fractures is more difficult because the comminution can vary from slight to extreme. A particularly deceptive form is the fracture in which an anteroposterior linear intertrochanteric fracture occurs, as in type 1, but with an additional fracture in the coronal plane, which can be seen on the lateral radiograph.
- *Type 3*: Fractures that extend distal to lesser trochanter or fracture lines runs obliquely down from lateral to medial (reverse obliquity type). These fractures usually are more difficult to reduce and result in more complications at operation and during convalescence.
- *Type 4*: Fracture of trochanteric region or proximal shaft with fracture line in at least two planes. If open reduction and internal fixation are used, two-plane fixation is required because of the spiral, oblique, or butterfly fracture of the shaft.

Management: Two broad categories of internal fixation devices are commonly used for intertrochanteric femoral fractures—sliding compression hip screws with side plate assemblies and intramedullary fixation devices. Sliding hip screws include traditional compression hip screws that provide compression in the intertrochanteric plane and compression plates that provide additional compression axially. Intramedullary devices include cephalomedullary nails with two screws (Recon-type nails, Smith and Nephew, Memphis, Tenn) or compression-type screws [e.g., the gamma (Stryker Orthopaedics, Kalamazoo, Mich) or intramedullary hip screw]. The intramedullary compression-type screw may be short and end in the diaphyseal femur or long and end in the supracondylar region.

The preferred type of device is controversial. Intramedullary nails have a biomechanical and biological advantage over standard compression hip screws. Intramedullary nails can be inserted with less exposure of the fracture and less blood loss, although they require more fluoroscopic exposure and have been associated with fracture comminution. Biomechanically, nails allow for stable anatomical fixation of more comminuted fractures without shortening the abductor moment arm or changing the proximal femoral anatomy. These devices provide fracture stability by virtue of allowing the lateral aspect of the head and neck to come to rest against the nail in the medullary canal. In addition, intramedullary nailing is a more technically demanding procedure.

For management of unstable fracture types, kindly refer to Question 74.

(For details on various fixation devices and indications, kindly refer to Annexure 2 of the book Essential Orthopedics: Principles and Practice, 2nd edition.)

76. **Describe the various types of femoral intramedullary nails? What are the methods to remove a broken and/or struck nail in a nonunited fracture shaft of femur in an adult?**

Ans: Types of femoral intramedullary nails
- Intramedullary nails, akin to plates, are categorized by both anatomical and functional nomenclature. Centromedullary nails are inserted in alignment with the medullary canal, establishing contact with the bone through multiple longitudinal interference points. These nails rely on the restoration of bony contact and stability to prevent axial and rotational deformation of the fracture. Notable examples of centromedullary nails include the classic Küntscher cloverleaf and Sampson nails.
- Condylocephalic nails are introduced into the bone at the condyles of the metaphysis and typically extend into the opposite metaphyseal-epiphyseal region. They are often inserted in groups to enhance rotational stability, with Ender and Hackenthall pins serving as examples.
- Cephalomedullary nails possess a centromedullary component but also facilitate fixation into the femoral head. The Küntscher Y-nail and Zickel subtrochanteric nail exemplify this category.
- Interlocking techniques have further evolved these traditional designs by incorporating interlocking centromedullary and cephalomedullary nails. Interlocking nails extend the working length of the nail by incorporating interlocking screws to counteract axial and rotational deformation of the fracture. Modney is credited with the design of the first interlocking nail, while Küntscher developed the detensor nail, which was subsequently modified by Klemm and Schellman, and later by Kempf et al. and others. These innovators laid the groundwork for numerous contemporary designs and techniques.
- Cephalomedullary interlocking nails were specifically engineered to address complex fractures extending into the proximal femur that exhibit axial and rotational instability, such as complex subtrochanteric fractures, pathological fractures, and ipsilateral hip and shaft fractures. These nails enable fixation using bolts, nails, and specialized lag screws, as demonstrated by the Russell–Taylor reconstruction nail, the Williams Y-nail, and the Uniflex nail.

Current intramedullary nails designed for femoral fixation are characterized by their insertion site. Antegrade femoral nailing can be performed through either a piriformis or a trochanteric entry portal, while retrograde femoral nailing is conducted through an entry portal located between the femoral condyles.

Methods to remove: Removing a broken or struck intramedullary nail from a nonunited fracture of the femur can be a complex surgical procedure. Here are some of the methods commonly utilized for the removal of broken or struck nails in such cases:

1. Surgical exploration:
   A. *Open surgical approach*: An open surgical approach to directly expose the nail is often required when the nail cannot be removed through closed methods.
   B. Nail extraction techniques:
      i. *Using proximal locking screws*: If the nail is intact but cannot be removed due to interlocking screws, these may need to be removed first. If the screws are stripped or broken, special screw extraction techniques might be employed, such as using reverse threading or extraction devices.
      ii. *Reaming*: In some cases, the use of a reamer to ream out the proximal end of the nail can create space for removal, particularly if the nail is broken.
2. Closed methods:
   A. *Manual manipulation*:
      - *Liston type extraction tools*: Special tools that can grasp the nail and allow it to be pulled out may be used when there is sufficient good fixation around the fracture site.
   B. *Fluoroscopy*: Real-time imaging can help to guide the process and ensure that the correct sections of the nail are targeted for extraction.
3. Advanced techniques for broken nails:
   A. Extraction reamers and nail removal devices:
      - For broken nails, specialized instruments designed to grasp and extract the internal portion of the nail can offer a solution. These may include flexible or rigid reamers that can help in "screwing out" the broken segment of the nail.
   B. Drilling out the nail:
      - In extreme cases, the nail can be drilled out using a cannulated drill bit if options for extraction are limited. Care must be taken to avoid damaging surrounding bone or soft tissue.

77. Discuss classification and management of distal femoral fractures.
Ans: Classification

AO **(Fig. 3.4.5)** classify the distal femur fractures into group 33 which is further classified as extra-articular, partial articular, and intra-articular.

a. *Extra-articular*:
   - *33-A1*: Simple
   - *33-A2*: Metaphyseal wedge
   - *33-A3*: Metaphyseal complex.
b. *Partial articular*:
   - *33-B1*: Sagittal fracture of lateral condyle
   - *33-B2*: Sagittal fracture of medial condyle
   - *33-B3*: Coronal split fracture (Hoffa fracture).
c. *Intra-articular*:
   - *33-C1*: Articular simple and metaphyseal simple
   - *33-C2*: Articular simple and metaphyseal multifragmentary
   - *33-C3*: Articular multifragmentary.

   Seinsheimer (1980) classified the fractures of the distal 3.5 inches of the femur into 4 types:
- *Type I*: Nondisplaced fractures (less than 2 mm displacement)
- *Type II*: Distal metaphyseal fractures (extra-articular)
   - *II-A*: Two-part fractures
   - *II-B*: Comminuted fractures.
- *Type III*: Fractures involving the intercondylar notch in which one or both condyles are separate fragments.
- *Type IV*: Intra-articular fractures

- *IV-A*: Medial condyle fracture
- *IV-B*: Lateral condyle fracture
- *IV-C*: Comminuted fractures.

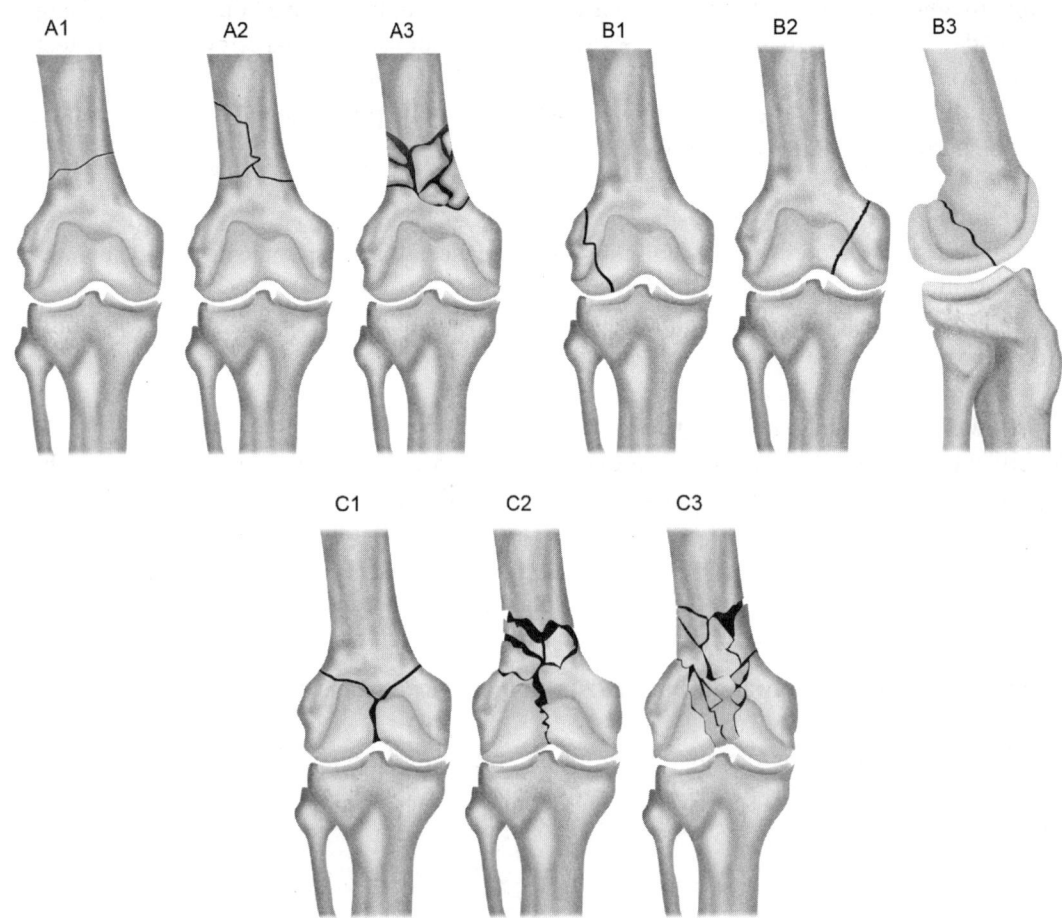

Fig. 3.4.5: AO classification.

Management

Nonoperative: It is indicated in stable, undisplaced or incomplete fracture. The patient with underlying medical conditions precluding surgery or patients unwilling to undergo surgery or nonambulatory patients are treated with hinged brace with early nonweight bearing mobilization out of the bed. The displaced fractures are treated with above knee cast for 6–12 weeks with acceptance of the residual deformity.

Operative: Operative treatment is recommended for all fractures of the distal femur, with the exception of simple, nondisplaced fractures. Early mobilization of the knee is important in obtaining a good result. The goal of the treatment is anatomical restoration of the articular surface, maintenance of the femoral length, and rotation.

Screws only: This may be used for reconstruction of type B3 fractures after anatomical reduction. Else screws are a common adjunctive fixation for stabilizing the condylar fragments.

Plate and screw fixation: The condylar blade plate was one of the first devices to gain wide acceptability in treatment. The blade plate provides stable fixation but it requires accurate insertion in three planes simultaneously. A minimum of 4 cm of uncomminuted bone in femoral condyles above intercondylar notch is necessary for successful fixation and is unsuitable for fractures with articular comminution, especially medial deficiency. As experience increased, more biological techniques of plating have been advocated using indirect reduction techniques, minimal soft tissue stripping, and gentle retraction. Femoral distractors or external fixators are used to regain length and alignment of the fracture, and metaphyseal comminution is left *in situ* with no attempt made to reduce comminuted fragments anatomically. Because the soft tissues are left relatively undisturbed, bone grafting is less often necessary.

Dynamic condylar screw: This is technically easier to insert than blade plate. It allows freedom in flexion extension plane and it also allows interfragmentary compression at the fracture site. Disadvantages are minimum 4 cm of noncomminuted bone required above intercondylar notch, insertion of lag screw requires removal of large amount of bone which makes revision surgery difficult, poor rotational control than blade plate and device is bulky. The interfragmentary movement on the bones fixed with blade plate is greater than on the bones fixed by DCS when medial defect is present.

Anatomical condylar locking plate: It is indicated in AO type A and C fractures requiring plate osteosynthesis, becoming the modality of choice for fixation of these fractures nowadays. Extra-articular and intra-articular condylar fractures, buttressing of comminuted distal femoral fractures, periprosthetic fractures and treatment of distal femoral malunion can all be achieved with it. Fracture reduction before plate application is a pre-requisite, reduction should not be attempted through plate. Anterolateral approach is commonly used to expose the fracture while parapatellar approaches may be needed for intra-articular comminution. These plates are fixed angle locking plates which allows the screws lock to the plate and provide angular stability to the construct. Variable angle locking option is also available to position screw in dense safe bone and for management of periprosthetic fractures. Long elastic construction is recommended for comminuted fractures.

Condylar buttress plate: These plates are used for the fractures with articular comminution and in fractures with less than 4 cm of uncomminuted bone above intercondylar notch. The advantage is that the multiple holes in distal end of plate allows multiple screws into the comminuted fragments.

Less invasive stabilization system (LISS): This system uses locked screws and percutaneous fixation. This system is made of titanium, so it has higher elastic deformation than other system, placing it between rigid fixation and intramedullary nail. LISS relies on the reduction being achieved before implant fixation. It is also called internal-external fixator where placing the locking screw near and far from fracture site provides greatest stability. The screw fixation is entirely unicortical in this system.

Intramedullary nailing: These devices obtain more "biological" fixation than plates because they are load sharing, rather than load-sparing, implants and there has been improvement in design of condylar blade for osteoporotic bone. They offer greater soft tissue preservation, and bone grafting is required less often. It is preferred for type A fractures with intact distal femur to fix with screws. The major disadvantage of nail fixation is that it provides less rigid stabilization of distal femoral fractures than plate fixation in biomechanical testing. Hardware failure in 15% of distal-third femoral fractures treated with antegrade interlocking nailing is seen with slotted designs. The incidence of hardware failure increases if the fracture is within 5 cm of the most proximal screw hole. It has been suggested that hardware failure can be prevented by driving the nail to subchondral bone, delaying full weight-bearing, and increasing the wall thickness of the nail. By using these principles, intramedullary nailing has been used successfully to treat fractures of the distal femur.

Retrograde femoral nails inserted through the intercondylar notch and, in addition to treating AO type A and type B supracondylar fractures, they can also be used for type C1 and C2 fracture fixation. Similar to antegrade nails, these "supracondylar" and "knee" nails have the theoretical advantages of being load-sharing devices, requiring little soft tissue dissection and infrequently needing bone grafting. Retrograde nailing of distal femoral fractures is preferable to antegrade nailing in obese patients. Distal femoral fractures below hip implants or above total knee implants with an open notch design also can be treated effectively with retrograde nailing. Other indications include fixation of distal femoral fractures associated with ipsilateral hip fractures, allowing the hip fracture to be stabilized with a separate device.

External fixation: It can be used as temporary or definitive fixation in severe open distal femoral fractures for later definitive fixation. The fracture with severe intercondylar comminution should be spanned by external fixator. Fractures associated with vascular injury are also treated with external fixator.

78. What is LISS? Discuss its role in stabilizing fracture of distal femur.

Ans: LISS stands for "Less Invasive Stabilization System".

Distal femoral fractures today are treated operatively almost without exception, whereby a broad spectrum of different operative techniques and implants is available. Regardless of these differences, the aim of treatment remains the same.

Treatment should lead to an optimal restoration of the joint surfaces and correct axial alignment of the distal fragment in relation to the shaft permitting early functional, cast-free rehabilitation.

For a long time, the aim of treatment was the anatomical reconstruction of all fragments, including the metaphyseal region, and high primary stability. This was achieved by extensive exposure of the fracture site and by insertion of numerous independent lag and plate screws. A potential complication of such excessive procedures, namely disturbed fracture healing, was handled by use of extensive primary bone graft, a procedure that was performed in up to 86% of the published cases.

Today, "biological" osteosynthesis and indirect reduction techniques without anatomical reduction of every individual fragment permit better conservation of the bone-to-soft tissue connections in nonarticulating regions and ensure higher fragment vascularization. The "rediscovered" relevance of iatrogenic soft tissue trauma and the influence of blood supply to the fragments led to new concepts in terms of surgical techniques: minimally invasive percutaneous plate osteosynthesis (MIPPO). It was proven experimentally that minimally invasive approaches caused less iatrogenic damage to the blood supply and led to increased restitution. Very good results were also obtained under clinical conditions. Extra-articular distal femoral fractures can be treated by extra- or intramedullary techniques. In general, it is preferable to perform indirect reduction and minimally invasive stabilization. Therefore, extramedullary treatment makes use of angular-stable implants (condylar plate, DCS, or internal fixator). For intramedullary procedures, antegrade and retrograde nailing techniques are available. Partially intra-articular fractures (type B fractures) are stabilized by screw fixation. In cases of exceptionally poor bone quality, a protective plate osteosynthesis or an internal fixator may become necessary.

Even completely intra-articular fractures can be stabilized by using extra- or intramedullary techniques. Sufficient anchorage in the distal fragment is a decisive factor for the choice of the implant. Today, the locked internal fixator is the standard implant in cases of severe comminution, open fracture with excessive bone loss or in a very small distal fragment.

79. Discuss Hoffa fracture in details.

Ans: The fracture is named after a German surgeon Albert Hoffa. Hoffa fracture is a specific type of intra-articular fracture of inter-/intracondylar distal femoral fractures where the fracture line(s) runs in coronal plane. It may be unicondylar (more common, mostly originating from lateral condyle) or bicondylar. It is classified as partial articular type B3 fracture pattern in Muller-AO classification and is intrinsically unstable. Isolated fracture is a rarity but the fracture fragment typified by definition may be a component of intercondylar fractures in 40% of cases.

Mechanism of injury: Specific mechanism is not there, though a shearing force to the posterior femoral condyle is postulated, both direct impact and vertical shear with twisting mechanism have been proposed. This particular situation is seen with knee flexed to 90° or more and an axial force is applied to the joint.

Clinical features: Clinical examination invariably reveals tenderness, fracture crepitance with thigh swelling, knee effusion, and subtle varus/valgus instability (that may be absent in minimally displaced isolated fractures).

- Limb deformity is absent in isolated condylar fractures but is a part of larger intercondylar fractures or bicondylar Hoffa.
- The skin should be examined for bruising, contusion, or open fracture.
- Other injuries to the same extremity should be suspected when there is pain or swelling in the limb above or below the fracture site.
- A careful neurovascular examination must be performed and documented including the presence or absence of distal pulses and sensorimotor assessment.

Imaging: An anteroposterior (AP) and lateral radiograph of the knee and femur should be obtained and is needed for diagnosis although it can be easily missed in undisplaced fractures. CT scan of the involved joint with 3D reconstruction (includes fine cuts) in axial, coronal, and sagittal planes of the distal femur is an important evaluation armamentarium for diagnosis, planning and prognostication purpose. Classification is usually done as per AO/OTA system.

Treatment: The fracture pattern is inherently unstable and it separates patellofemoral from tibiofemoral joint, so operative treatment is commonly recommended. Conservative management is unpredictable as adequate stabilization is challenging due to line of force transmission. Operative reduction is aimed for atraumatic anatomical reduction, secure fixation, and early functional rehabilitation.

Although transtibial osteotomy, posterior and medial approaches have all been described but swashbuckler approach or medial para patellar approach is most commonly used. Screw fixation is done in AP OR PA direction (4.5 or 6.5 mm partially threaded cancellous) with use of countersink for simple fractures. Plate fixation is necessary for more complicated/comminuted fracture types.

Complications—include loss of reduction, malunion, neurovascular damage, and osteonecrosis.

80. Which is the commonly preferred approach to bicondylar Hoffa fracture?

Ans: *Swashbuckler approach* is commonly preferred as a specialized exposure for bicondylar Hoffa fracture:
- Place the patient in supine position, preferably on a radiolucent table.
- Use a sterile tourniquet only if necessary to avoid medial retraction of the quadriceps.
- Place a roll or triangle under the knee. Make a midline incision from above the fracture laterally to across the patella.
- Extend the incision directly down to the fascia of the quadriceps. Incise the quadriceps fascia in line with the skin incision. Sharply dissect the quadriceps fascia off the vastus lateralis muscle laterally to its inclusion with the iliotibial band.
- Retract the iliotibial band and fascia laterally, continuing the dissection down to the linea aspera.
- Incise the lateral parapatellar retinaculum, separating it from the vastus lateralis.
- Make a lateral parapatellar arthrotomy to expose the femoral condyles.
- Place a retractor under the vastus lateralis and medialis, exposing the distal femur and displacing the patella medially.
- Ligate the perforating vessels, and elevate the vastus lateralis, exposing the entire distal femur.
- Proceed with the internal fixation as needed.
- Close the wound by suturing the fascia back in place.

81. What is tibial plateau fracture? Discuss its classification and management of each type.

Ans: Kindly see Question 82 for *classification* of tibial plateau fractures.

Management based on Schatzker classification:
- *Type I*: If displaced, it can be fixed with two transverse cancellous screws, with or without single hole plate (washer).
- *Type II*: Get CT scan done for quantification of depression. Less than 5 mm depression of articular surface can be managed conservatively. If the depression is > 5–8 mm, or instability is present, most should be treated by open reduction, elevation of the depressed plateau "en mass," bone grafting of the metaphysis, fixation of the fracture with cancellous screws, and buttress plating of the lateral cortex.
- *Type III*: If the depression is severe, or if instability can be shown on stress, the articular fragments should be elevated and bone grafted, and the lateral cortex is supported with a buttress plate.
- *Type IV*: Treated by open reduction and fixation with a medial buttress plate and cancellous screws.
- *Type V*: The more displaced and comminuted condyle can be stabilized with a buttress plate, whereas the less involved condyle is reduced by ligamentotaxis or with percutaneous techniques and stabilized with large cancellous screws. Alternatively, the less involved condyle can be stabilized with a small antiglide plate placed at the apex of the fracture with minimal soft-tissue dissection.
- *Type VI*: It should be treated with buttress plates and cancellous screws, usually a bicondylar fixation is recommended for optimal outcome. The usual mistake is trying to fix the medial condylar fracture from screws through lateral plate that often fails.

82. Classify tibial plateau fractures. What is the ideal time and technique for fixation of a type IV tibial plateau fracture?

Ans:

Classification

Schatzker classification (Fig. 3.4.6):
- *Type I*: Pure cleavage
- *Type II*: Cleavage combined with depression
- *Type III*: Pure central depression
- *Type IV*: Fractures of medial condyle
- *Type V*: Bicondylar fractures
- *Type VI*: Plateau fracture with dissociation of metaphysis and diaphysis.

Column concept for fracture classification for tibial plateau:

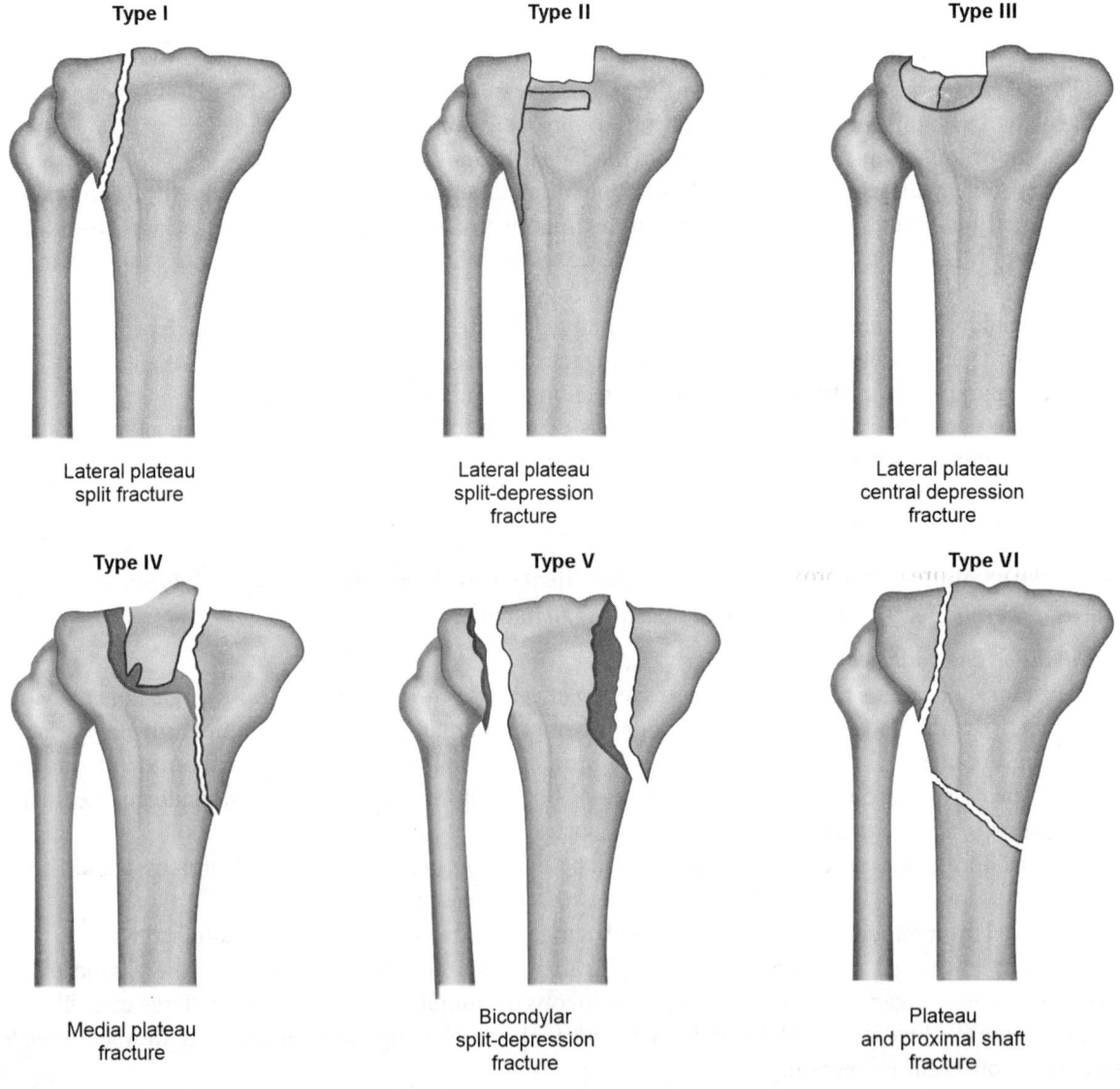

Fig. 3.4.6: Schatzker classification.

"Zero-column" fracture: Pure articular depression

"One-column" fracture: Split and split depression types. Newly described posterior shear fractures.

"Two-column" fractures: Anterolateral fractures with posterolateral articular depression and cortical breach. Anteromedial fragment + separate posteromedial fragment (type IV Schatzker).

"Three-column" fractures: At least one independent articular fragment in each column—the type V and VI Schatzker fractures.

Ideal time: The factors influencing type and timing of treatment are degree of displacement and joint depression along with extent of soft tissue injury. Two stage management is recommended for complex fractures and those with associated significant soft tissue injury. Joint spanning fixator maintains the fragments and alignment by ligamentotaxis. Take good pin-site care as there is evidence for increased incidence of infection on conversion to definitive fixation.

Type IV fractures should be treated by open direct reduction and fixation with medial buttress plate and cancellous screw. There is no described ideal time but surgery undertaken within 7 days from trauma is better for achieving good reduction. One should take care of soft tissues and if there is excessive swelling due to extensive soft tissue trauma or blood extravasation or reactive then one should wait with limb elevation, ice packs locally and conservative management till soft tissues stabilize. If prolonged time (>2–3 weeks) is deemed for stabilization of soft tissues or other co-morbidities, then indirect reduction and fixation with hybrid fixator or percutaneous screws and external stabilization may be undertaken.

Technique of open direct reduction and fixation:
- Incision is placed medially usually in the shape of inverted hockey-stick fashion with vertical limb along the medial border of gastrocnemius and horizontal limb just proximal to posterior joint line in popliteal fossa.
- Expose the main fracture line by a deep vertical incision between the tibial (medial) collateral ligament and posterior oblique ligament.
- Reflect the ligamentous borders to allow open reduction of the fragment. Use K-wires to provisionally fix the fracture. Definitive fixation is usually done with a small antiglide plate without compromising the thin soft-tissue envelope.
- Usually avoided and not recommended but if more access to the medial wall of the proximal tibia is necessary, make a transverse cut through the medial collateral ligament and strip the medial collateral ligament with periosteum off the bone down to its insertion as a single layer, exposing fracture lines of the medial wall.
- Suture the medial collateral ligament back at the end of the procedure.
- In complex fractures of the medial wall, take the anteromedial incision down to the bone, and detach the entire fascial-periosteal layer from anterior to posterior, including the insertions of the pes tendons of the medial collateral ligament. Leave the medial meniscus in continuity with this layer, and retract it out of the joint for entire medial and posteromedial exposure of the proximal tibia.
- Fix the fascial-periosteal layer back to the bone with a one-layer running suture.

83. Outline the principles of managing tibial plafond fractures.

Ans: Rüedi and Allgöwer four sequential principles for the management of fractures of the tibial plafond (1979).
1. Restoration of fibular length—provides lateral buttress and restores length.
2. Anatomic reduction of the articular surface—decreases the risk of post-traumatic arthritis.
3. Filling the residual bone defect with cancellous autograft using autologous bone graft, cancellous and structural allograft, calcium-based cements, and demineralized bone matrix products.
4. Stabilization of the medial column—buttress and correct any varus deformity.

84. A. Four-column classification in proximal tibia fractures.
B. Raft screw in proximal tibia fracture fixation.

Ans:

A. A four-column classification described by Chang **(Fig. 3.4.7)** includes the whole articular surface of the proximal tibia. Every column is designated with an alphabet:
1. Anteromedial column (A)
2. Anterolateral column (B)
3. Posteromedial column (C)
4. Posterolateral column (D).

Each fracture can be assigned a minimum of one letter and a maximum of four letters according to the degree of compromise in one or multiple columns. For example, a fracture in the anterolateral column would be represented as B; a fracture of the four columns as ABCD; a fracture of the anteromedial, posteromedial and posterolateral columns as BCD, and so on.

The main limitations of this classification are that it only gives information regarding the articular fragments but the status of distal part of tibia (meta-diaphysis) is unknown (Schatzker classification) also soft tissue injury is not accounted for (Tscherne classification).

B. Raft screws are small diameter parallel locking screws (commonly 4 in number) placed through low-profile proximal tibia lateral plating system. These screws are placed through the proximal portion of the plate from lateral to medial capturing the intact medial cortex. They form a supporting raft to bone in subchondral region preventing collapse of the articular surface. They are placed after elevation of the plateau and may obviate need for bone grafting.

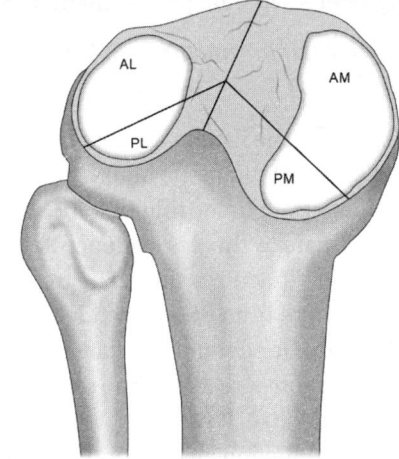

Fig. 3.4.7: The four columns of proximal tibia as used in classification of Chang.

85. What are potential complications of tibial condylar fractures and their management?

Ans: The following are the potential complications of tibial condylar fractures along with proposed methods to prevent/treat them:

- *Loss of reduction*: This can be managed by improved methods of fixing low-energy fractures such as—
  - Smaller precontoured plates allowing subchondral screws to raft under the reduced articular surface (reduces tendency for postoperative displacement).
  - Calcium phosphate cement used as void filler after reducing the articular fragments (synthetic substitutes have higher compressive strength)
- *Wound infection and breakdown*:
  - Irrigation and debridement in the operating room
  - Organism-specific antibiotics
  - In early postoperative infections, well-fixed hardware may be maintained and the wound packed open. If the infection can be suppressed until fracture healing, hardware removal will then give a chance for a cure.
  - If the infection is aggressive or the bone is involved, hardware removal followed by external fixation may be prudent.
  - Associated soft-tissue defects may require flap coverage. Definitive stabilization can be with external fixation or repeat internal fixation after infection control and soft-tissue coverage are accomplished.
  - Proximal tibial infections after internal fixation of tibial plateau fractures that involve the joint and the bone may be very difficult to control and cure. Proximal tibial resection with a cement spacer and subsequent arthroplasty, knee arthrodesis, or even above knee amputation may be necessary to eradicate infection.
- *Septic arthritis after external fixation*: This complication is now rarely seen.
  - Manage as standard for joint septic arthritis and remove all intra-articular hardware.
- *Knee stiffness*: Stiffness after a tibial plateau fracture is challenging to treat.
  - Knee manipulation may improve motion in some knees that are not progressing. It is preferable to wait until healing has likely occurred, usually around 3 months.
  - After 4 months, a surgical lysis of intra-articular adhesions, either open or arthroscopic, may be necessary.
- *Painful prominent hardware*: It is advised to wait till healing occurs and then removal of hardware. Titanium-locked plates may be difficult to remove because of cold welding of screws.
  - Because plates used to treat comminuted metaphyseal fractures are frequently long and are beneath a long length of the anterior compartment removal can require substantial dissection.
- *Tibial nonunion*: The presence or absence of infection is the first issue in deciding on treatment techniques. Infection is suspected based on the history, clinical examination, imaging, and laboratory studies. In periarticular nonunions

of the proximal tibia, the mobility of the joint and the presence or absence of post-traumatic arthritis both must be considered.
- If the joint is salvageable, the nonunion is repaired with internal or external fixation and usually some osteoinductive material such as autologous bone graft or bone morphogenic protein is added. Accurate alignment must be restored.
- If the joint cannot be salvaged, the nonunion should be treated along with the knee by arthrodesis or arthroplasty.
- *Malunion*: If correction is necessary, the surgical approach and technique will depend on the direction and amount of the deformity, the presence of pre-existing implants, and the condition of the soft-tissue envelope.
  - For metaphyseal malunions, either opening or closing wedge osteotomies may be chosen and can be fixed internally or with an external fixator.
  - Intra-articular malunions can contribute to limb malalignment. If the alignment is unacceptable, it can be corrected through an intra-articular osteotomy to restore the lateral articular surface and support the lateral femoral condyle. An alternative approach accepts the intra-articular deformity and aligns the limb with an extra-articular osteotomy. In certain challenging deformities, combined intra- and extra-articular osteotomies may be the best approach.
- Post-traumatic arthritis, depending on loss of function and demands of profession, the following options may be chosen:
  - *Knee arthroplasty*: This is most favorable because it maintains movements and removes pain.
  - Knee arthrodesis is not preferred nowadays but in a very heavy manual young laborer, arthroplasty may fail early so arthrodesis may be preferred.
  - A tibial osteotomy to change alignment was a frequently associated procedure and there was a trend to better results with concomitant meniscal transplantation.
  - Mosaicplasty has been reported as another possibility to reconstruct defects in the lateral tibial plateau after fracture.

86. What is floating knee? Discuss its management in a 25-year-old.

Ans: Floating knee is fracture of ipsilateral femur and tibia (or both bones leg commonly) so that the knee that is in between 2 fractures has no contact with any bony part of body hence remains "floating".

Management:

ATLS protocol is applied first. Shock is treated with aggressive IV fluid therapy and blood transfusion is indicated. Patient is evaluated for other injuries. Other body systems are simultaneously addressed if involved according to triage.

X-ray imaging of femur and tibia is done after secondary survey and planned for surgery.

Based on the assessment of performance status and other injuries DCO versus ETC is planned. In ETC, if fractures are closed, the indicated treatment is nailing of femur and tibia. In floating knee, femur is nailed in retrograde manner as floating knee is an indication for retrograde nailing. A DFN is used to fix femur fracture.

From that similar incision used to nail femur by a DFN, tibia is nailed by routine antegrade technique.

If fractures are compound and there is a suspicion of impending infection or DCO is planned, then a knee spanning external fixator is applied.

87. Discuss management principles in a young adult male presenting with floating knee.

Ans: Floating knee refers to ipsilateral fractures of the femur and tibia, often due to high-energy trauma (e.g., motor vehicle accidents and falls). This injury is associated with significant morbidity, including knee instability, nonunion, and long-term disability.

Initial Management (ATLS Protocol)
1. Primary survey (ABCs):
   - Airway, breathing, and circulation: Assess for life-threatening injuries (e.g., chest/abdominal trauma and hemorrhage).
   - Control bleeding (tourniquet if needed).
2. Secondary survey:
   - Neurovascular exam: Check for popliteal artery injury (absent pulses, ischemia) or peroneal nerve palsy (foot drop).
   - Compartment syndrome assessment (pain, pallor, paralysis, paresthesia, pulselessness).

3. Imaging:
   - X-rays (AP/lateral femur + tibia and knee views)
   - CT angiogram if vascular injury suspected
   - CT scan (if intra-articular extension)

Definitive Management
1. Surgical stabilization (Goal: Early mobility)
   A. Femur fracture fixation:
      - Intramedullary nailing (IMN): Gold standard for diaphyseal fractures.
      - Plate fixation: If IMN contraindicated (e.g., narrow medullary canal)
      - External fixation: Temporary if severe soft-tissue damage.
   B. Tibia fracture fixation:
      - IMN: For diaphyseal fractures.
      - Plate fixation: For metaphyseal/intra-articular fractures.
      - External fixator → Conversion to IMN/plate (in staged approach for open fractures).
   C. Knee ligament assessment:
      - MRI if instability post-fixation (common due to associated ligament tears)
      - Delayed ligament reconstruction after fracture healing
2. Open fracture management (Gustilo–Anderson Classification)
   - Early debridement + antibiotics (within 6 hours)
   - Temporary external fixation → Later conversion to internal fixation
   - Soft-tissue coverage (flap if needed)
3. Postoperative care
   - Early knee mobilization (CPM machine if stable fixation)
   - Weight-bearing progression (non-weight-bearing → partial → full over 8–12 weeks)
   - DVT prophylaxis (LMWH + mechanical compression)

88. What are the clinical features and assessment of floating knee injury?
Ans:

Clinical features:
- Floating knee should be suspected in polytrauma cases with injury to the lower limbs. There is deformity of the lower limb seen on either side of knee (in thigh and leg), associated with swelling, bruises, and variable shortening. Characteristics of fracture-like abnormal mobility and crepitus are present with local tenderness but too much elicitation of abnormal mobility should be avoided. Damage to the vessels (mainly popliteal and posterior tibial arteries) and lesions of nerves (peroneal nerve) are common. Vascular injury is common and may be life threatening if not recognized and addressed. Often, the vascular injury is to anterior tibial artery, resulting in ischemia only rarely and is not treated with vascular repair or reconstruction. However, vascular status should be thoroughly assessed.
- Incidence of open fractures is high with these injuries (either femoral or tibial or both). Most commonly the pattern is closed femoral fracture with an open tibial fracture.
- Injuries to knee ligaments commonly occur in association with these fractures. Anterolateral rotatory instability is the most common type present.

Assessment:
After thorough clinical examination keeping in mind the above-mentioned injuries, the imaging is done.
- *X-rays*: Anteroposterior (AP) and lateral views of femur and tibia with one joint above and below included
- Doppler sonography of the lower limb for assessing vascular injury
- Magnetic resonance imaging (MRI) of the knee joint in patients with suspected ligament injuries
- Computed tomography (CT) scan of metaphyseal and/or intra-articular fractures with 3D reconstruction
- Generalized radiological screening of suspected skeletal injuries

- Arterial blood gas (ABG) is done to see lactate levels. For levels >2.5, then apply fixators. If <2.5, then proceed with nailing both sites with single incision. After nailing of 1 bone, send intraoperative ABG to see for lactate levels. If still <2.5, then only proceed for second nailing.

89. What is the mechanism of injury of Unhappy Triad of O'Donoghue?

Ans: The most common mechanism is abduction, flexion, and internal rotation of the femur on the tibia when the weight-bearing leg of an athlete is struck from the lateral aspect by an opponent. This mechanism results in an abduction and flexion force on the knee, and the femur is rotated internally by the shift of the body weight on the fixed tibia. This mechanism produces injury on the medial side of the knee, the severity of which depends on the magnitude and dissipation of the applied force. When abduction, flexion, and internal rotation of the femur on the tibia occur, the medial supporting structures—the medial collateral ligament and the medial capsular ligament—are the initial structures injured. If the force is of sufficient magnitude, the anterior cruciate ligament (ACL) also can be torn. The medial meniscus may be trapped between the condyles of the femur and the tibia, and it may be torn at its periphery as the medial structures tear, thus producing "the unhappy triad" of O'Donoghue.

(For further reading and understanding, kindly read Chapter 34 of the book Essential Orthopedics: Principles and Practice, 2nd edition.)

90. Explain management of hemarthrosis of knee developed after a trauma.

Ans: Presence of blood in joint is called hemarthrosis. It commonly results from bony or ligamentous injury of intra-articular structures or structures that may become intra-articular postinjury (PCL for ex). Peripheral meniscal tear in red zone may also cause hemarthrosis.

Swelling developing immediately after injury usually indicates blood in the joint. The knee is very painful and it feels warm, tense and tender. Later there may be a "doughy" feel. Movements are restricted due to pain. X-rays are essential to see if there is a fracture, if there is not, then suspect a tear of the anterior cruciate ligament or meniscal injury. MRI demonstrates well the soft tissue injuries and blood in joint provides contrast effect.

The joint should be aspirated under aseptic conditions and PRICE should be followed. If a ligament injury is suspected, examination under anesthesia is helpful and may indicate the need for operation; otherwise a crepe bandage is applied and the leg cradled in a back-splint. Jones bandaging of three layers of alternating wet and dry bandage also provides good compression and support to joint. Quadriceps exercises are practiced from the start. The patient may get up when comfortable, retaining the back-splint until muscle control returns.

91. Discuss management of acute knee dislocation with absent pulsation.

Ans: The incidence of vascular injuries in knee dislocations ranges to 40%. Some centers use ankle-brachial indices to assess for vascular injury, but recommended is an arteriogram, if the dislocation required reduction. When there is doubt concerning an injury to the popliteal artery, a thorough evaluation, including arteriography and early surgical exploration, is mandatory. Continued observation in anticipation of improvement often leads to disaster.

A patient's foot usually can be warm while a thrombus was forming. The absence of pulses in the pedal vessels, tenderness, swelling, and ecchymosis in the popliteal fossa, and a cold, cyanotic foot are well-known danger signals and when present indicate the need for prompt arterial exploration. Results are best when arterial repair and knee reconstruction are done within 6–8 hours after injury. The amputation rate is approximately 11%, if vascular repair is made within 6 hours, and this increases to 86%, if repair is delayed beyond 8 hours.

The neurocirculatory status should be checked frequently for 5–7 days. A large transarticular pin can be placed through the intercondylar notch of the femur into the intercondylar eminence of the tibia to provide immediate stability for knees that redislocate in a splint or after vascular repair.

A knee-spanning external fixator can be used in open knee dislocations with extensive soft tissue injury or in unstable knees after vascular repair.

92. Describe acute management of traumatic knee dislocation. Classify multiligament knee injury and principle of managing such cases.

Ans: *Investigations:* AP and lateral view of the knee is needed. Knee dislocations are designated as anterior, posterior, medial, lateral, or rotary, according to the displacement of the tibia in relation to the femur. Rotary dislocations are designated further as anteromedial, anterolateral, posteromedial, or posterolateral. The dislocations often reduce spontaneously, so are commonly missed by the time they are seen in an emergency room on a casual examination.

Vascular and neurological injuries are common, should be looked for and comprehensively dealt with. Popliteal artery injury (30–50% cases) due to intimal injury and stretch (anterior dislocations or hyperextension injuries) should be suspected in most cases to mandate vascular evaluation for 6–8 hours even after injury. Neural injury is seen in 20–30% cases and although stretch neuropraxia is most common mechanism, no recovery has been reported in more than 50% cases suggesting that most are complete injuries (grade 3 and more Sunderland).

Schenck classification:
- *Knee dislocation 1*: Intact PCL with variable injury to collateral ligaments
- *Knee dislocation 2*: Injury to both cruciates with intact collaterals
- *Knee dislocation 3*: Complete injury to both cruciates with one collateral ligament disrupted
- *Knee dislocation 4*: Both cruciates and collateral ligament disrupted
- *Knee dislocation 5*: Dislocation with periarticular fracture.

Acute management comprises RICE, analgesics, medications to reduce swelling, evacuation of hematoma if it is tense, and management of vascular injury (emergent vascular reconstruction with reverse saphenous vein graft). If on exploration nerve injury is seen as a transaction then acute repair may be attempted immediately. Aspiration of the hemarthrosis using sterile technique and immobilizing the knee in full extension are satisfactory temporary treatments. The neurocirculatory status should be checked frequently for 5–7 days. A large transarticular pin can be placed through the intercondylar notch of the femur into the intercondylar eminence of the tibia to provide immediate stability for knees that redislocate in a splint or after vascular repair.

After acute management, obtain MRI to confirm and aid in planning reconstruction of the ligamentous structures. Maintain the patient in long leg brace for 3–4 weeks, if there is associated TCL and or LCL injury. For critically ill patients or those with sedentary lifestyle or patients with grossly contaminated wounds, immobilization in long leg cast may suffice. External fixators may also be used as a definitive management in such cases especially open injuries. For active individuals, the management is often a staged or single sitting reconstruction. Arthroscopic reconstruction for intra-articular ligaments is preferred.

93. Explain management of chronic ACL deficiency in an adult.

Ans: Isolated ACL insufficiency is uncommon and can usually be managed by physiotherapy. Splints or braces may be used to speed the return to weight-bearing.

Patients seeking to resume competitive sport may need something more; reconstructive surgery involves replacing the torn ACL with an autologous graft, usually a strip of patellar tendon with bone attachments at either end or with hamstring tendons. Combined injuries such as anterolateral or anteromedial rotatory instability are the commonest reasons for reconstructive surgery. When the ACL is damaged together with either the medial or lateral collateral ligament, reconstruction of the ACL alone often suffices. The torn ACL is replaced by an autograft (usually from the patellar tendon or from hamstring tendons) or by an allograft. Some surgeons advocate replicating the dual bundle arrangement of the original ligament. The ideal synthetic graft has yet to be developed. Postoperative care will depend on the fixation of the new ligament; in many cases a short period of splintage can be followed by regular physiotherapy to avoid joint stiffness and improve muscle control. Many patients return to sports within 6 months.

(For details of reconstruction options, kindly refer to Chapter 34 of the book Essential Orthopedics: Principles and Practice, 2nd edition.)

94. Classify ankle fractures. How will you manage supination external rotation injury?

Ans: *Classification of ankle fractures*: Various systems of classification are used as follows—

Lauge-Hansen classification:
- *Supination-Adduction (SA)* **(Fig. 3.4.8)**
  - Transverse avulsion-type fracture of the fibula below the level of the joint or tear of the lateral collateral ligaments
  - Vertical fracture of the medial malleolus.

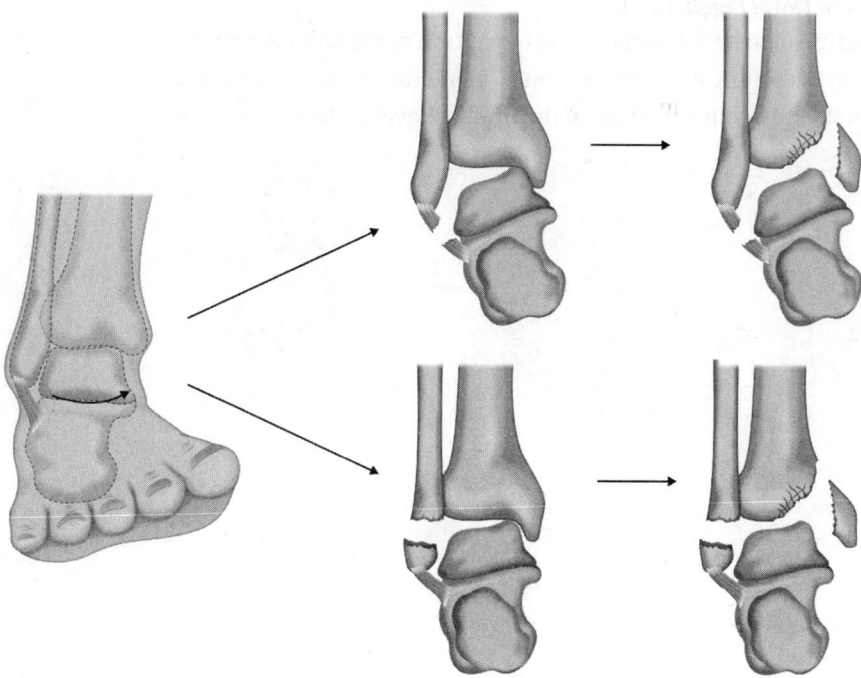

Fig. 3.4.8: Supination adduction injury.

- *Supination-Eversion (External rotation) (SER)* **(Fig. 3.4.9)**:
  - Disruption of the anterior tibiofibular ligament
  - Spiral oblique fracture of the distal fibula
  - Disruption of the posterior tibiofibular ligament or fracture of the posterior malleolus
  - Fracture of the medial malleolus or rupture of the deltoid ligament.

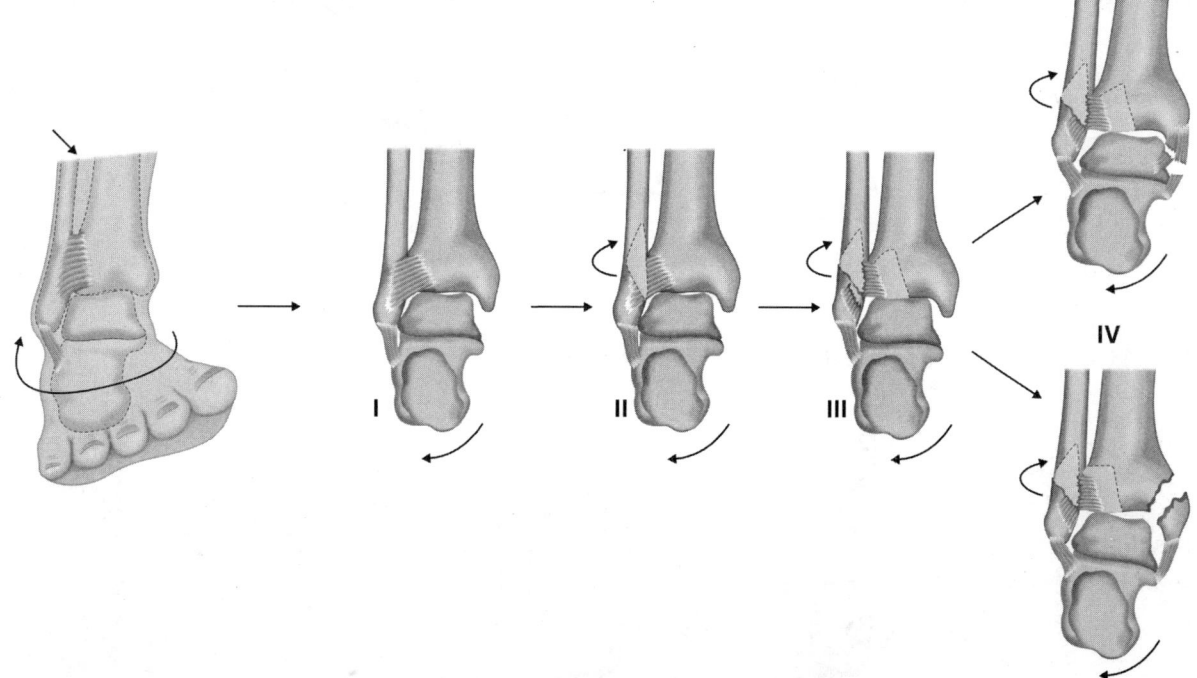

Fig. 3.4.9: Supination—external rotation injury.

- *Pronation-Abduction (PA) (Fig. 3.4.10)*:
  - Transverse fracture of the medial malleolus or rupture of the deltoid ligament
  - Rupture of the syndesmotic ligaments or avulsion fracture of their insertions
  - Short, horizontal, and oblique fracture of the fibula above the level of the joint.

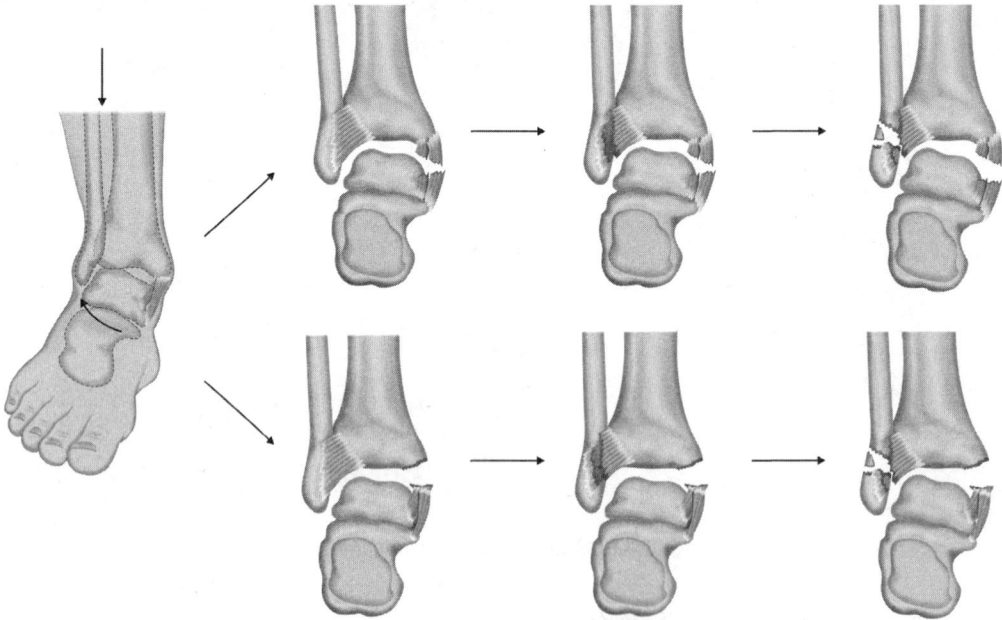

Fig. 3.4.10: Pronation abduction injury.

- *Pronation-Eversion (External rotation) (PER) (Fig. 3.4.11)*:
  - Transverse fracture of the medial malleolus or disruption of the deltoid ligament
  - Disruption of the anterior tibiofibular ligament
  - Short oblique fracture of the fibula above the level of the joint
  - Rupture of posterior tibiofibular ligament or avulsion fracture of the posterolateral tibia.

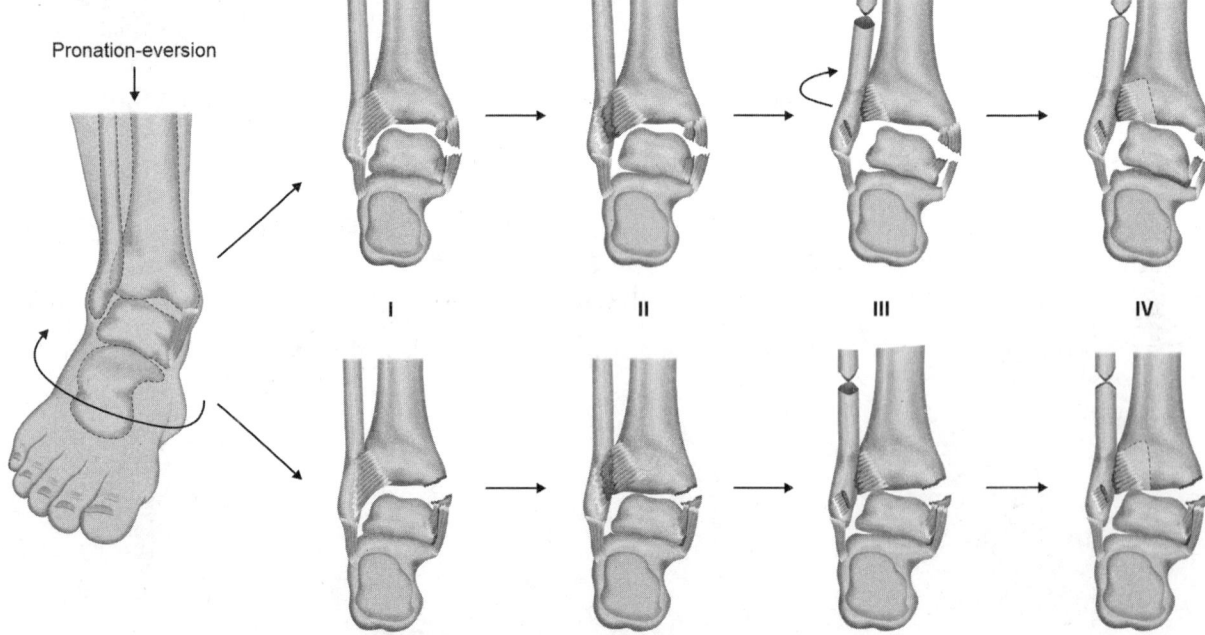

Fig. 3.4.11: Pronation—external rotation injury.

- *Pronation-Dorsiflexion (PD)*:
  - Fracture of the medial malleolus
  - Fracture of the anterior margin of the tibia
  - Supramalleolar fracture of the fibula
  - Transverse fracture of the posterior tibial surface.

AO classification:
- Type A: Fibula fracture below syndesmosis (infrasyndesmotic)
  - A1—Isolated
  - A2—With fracture of medial malleolus
  - A3—With a posteromedial fracture
- Type B: Fibula fracture at level of syndesmosis (trans-syndesmotic)
  - B1—Isolated
  - B2—With medial lesion (malleolus or ligament)
  - B3—With a medial lesion and fracture of posterolateral tibia
- Type C: Fibula fracture above syndesmosis (suprasyndesmotic)
  - C1—Diaphyseal fracture of the fibula, simple
  - C2—Diaphyseal fracture of the fibula, complex
  - C3—Proximal fracture of the fibula

Danis–Weber classification (**Fig. 3.4.12**):

- Type A fracture is caused by internal rotation and adduction that produce a transverse fracture of the lateral malleolus at or below the plafond, with or without an oblique fracture of the medial malleolus.
- Type B fracture is caused by external rotation that results in an oblique fracture of the lateral malleolus, beginning on the anteromedial surface and extending proximally to the posterolateral aspect. The injury may include rupture or avulsion of the anterior anteroinferior tibiofibular ligament, fracture of the medial malleolus, or rupture of the deltoid ligament.
- Type C fractures are divided into abduction injuries with oblique fracture of the fibula proximal to the disrupted tibiofibular ligaments (C-1) and abduction–external rotation injuries with a more proximal fracture of the fibula and more extensive disruption of the interosseous membrane (C-2).
  - Type C injuries may involve a medial malleolar fracture or a deltoid ligament rupture.
  - Fracture of the posterior malleolus may accompany any of the three types.

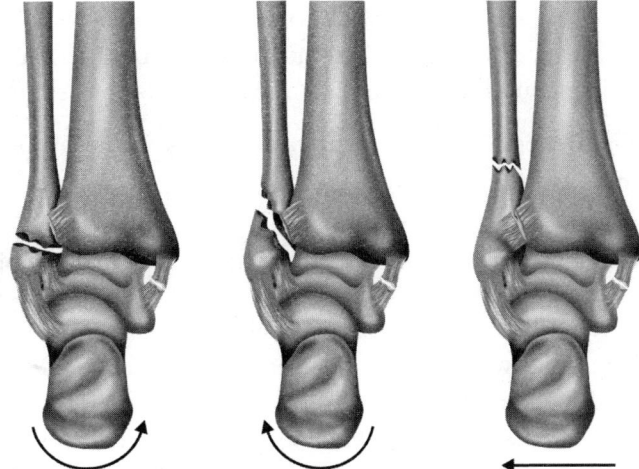

Fig. 3.4.12: Danis–Weber system of classification.

Management of Supination External Rotation (SER) Injury

The injury complex includes:
- Disruption of the anterior tibiofibular ligament
- Spiral oblique fracture of the distal fibula
- Disruption of the posterior tibiofibular ligament or fracture of the posterior malleolus
- Fracture of the medial malleolus or rupture of the deltoid ligament

Fix fibular fracture first with ORIF by plating or TBW through a lateral approach. The integrity of the syndesmosis is then evaluated intraoperatively by performing an external rotation stress test and Cotton test. *(Cotton described this test to determine incompetence of the ankle syndesmosis intraoperatively. Distraction is applied to the fibula with a bone hook* to try to separate it from the tibia to which an opposing force has been applied to prevent tibial motion. *If no significant motion is noted between the distal tibia and fibula, the syndesmotic ligaments are intact).* If more than 3 to 4 mm of lateral displacement occurs, syndesmotic fixation is necessary. Intraoperative radiographs should show a clear space of less than 5 mm between the medial wall of the fibula and the lateral wall of the posterior tibial malleolus. This injury occurs mostly in pronation types and less in supination types.

Next fixation of posterior malleolus fractures is needed if it involves >25% of the articular surface. Fixation may be achieved by indirect reduction and placement of an anterior to posterior lag screw, or a posteriorly placed plate and/or screws through a separate incision.

Management of medial malleolar fracture or deltoid rupture needs operative fixation. Medial malleolar fractures can usually be stabilized with cancellous screws or a figure-of-eight tension band. Deltoid ligament is repaired with suture anchor.

95. Briefly outline management of pronation abduction (PAB) injuries of ankle joint according to Lauge-Hansen classification.

Ans: The following are the progressive stages of pronation abduction (PAB) injuries:
- In the first stage (PAB 1), the abducting talus avulses the medial malleolus (resulting in a transverse fracture line) or causes a deltoid ligament rupture—screw fixation of the medial malleolus or tension band wiring would suffice.
- In the second stage (PAB 2), the fibula is pushed laterally resulting in rupture of the anterior inferior tibiofibular ligament (AITFL) or an avulsion fracture of the tubercle of Chaput—along with above the Chaput fragment needs fixation for syndesmotic stability and improved function. Prolonged immobilization would be needed for optimal ligament healing.
- In the third stage (PAB 3), the fibula fractures under compression and bending, resulting in a comminuted fracture at or above the level of the syndesmosis. Bridge plating of fibula with a small fragment DCP or equivalent is needed. The medial fracture can be addressed with orthogonal cancellous lag screws or with a tension band construct if the fragment is small. The integrity of the syndesmosis should be assessed.

96. Describe in brief the investigations and treatment of each type of ankle fractures.
Ans:

Investigations:

X-rays: The standard radiographs are an AP and a lateral projection of the ankle. Tenderness of the proximal fibula should be investigated with a full-length radiograph of the leg.

A mortise view of the ankle taken in 15° of internal rotation is also extremely helpful in assessing the lateral aspect of the ankle which is often poorly seen on the AP view because of the shape of the talus and consequent overlap of the tibia, fibula, and talus.
- In supination–external rotation injury, the identifying feature is a spiral oblique fracture of the distal fibula and a rupture of the deltoid ligament or fracture of the medial malleolus.
- The supination–adduction type of injury is characterized by a transverse fracture of the distal fibula and a relatively vertical fracture of the medial malleolus. Only type associated with medial displacement of talus.
- The pronation–abduction injury produces a transverse fracture of the medial malleolus and a short oblique fracture of the fibula that appears relatively horizontal on the lateral radiograph.
- The pronation–external rotation injury is characterized by a deltoid ligament tear or a fracture of the medial malleolus and a spiral oblique fracture of the fibula relatively high above the level of the ankle joint.

Neither CT nor MRI is used frequently in the investigation of ankle fractures. CT scanning is helpful in characterizing joint displacement in pilon fractures, assessing the size of a posterior malleolar fragment, and in assessing the accuracy of the reduction of the syndesmosis postoperatively. MRI has been used in the experimental setting to assess the integrity of the deep deltoid ligament where this is uncertain, but this is not common practice. Osteochondral lesions are frequently identified on MRI scans, but the importance of these remains uncertain.

Treatment:
Medial malleolus: Fractures of the medial malleolus should be treated surgically because persistent displacement allows the talus to tilt into varus. Avulsion fractures involving only the tip of the medial malleolus are not as unstable as fractures involving the axilla of the mortise and do not require internal fixation, unless displacement is significant. Fixation of the medial malleolus usually consists of two 4-mm cancellous lag screws-oriented perpendicular to the fracture. Vertical fractures of the medial malleolus require horizontally directed screws.

Smaller fragments can be fixed with one lag screw and one Kirschner wire to prevent rotation. Fragments that are too small or comminuted for screw fixation can be stabilized with two Kirschner wires and a tension band. Fixation with a small semitubular buttress plate may be necessary to stabilize adequately vertical fractures that extend high into the metaphysis.

Lateral malleolus: Recommended is open reduction and internal fixation of lateral malleoli.
If the stability of a lateral malleolar fracture is uncertain, stress radiographs can be obtained with the ankle in supination and external rotation to detect displacement of the talus indicative of medial injury.

Various methods are: Standard fixation of fibular fracture with one-third semitubular 3.5-mm plate and screws, multiple 3.5-mm lag screws, two lag screws for long oblique fracture, single 4.5-mm malleolar screw for low transverse fracture, tension band wiring for very small transverse chip fracture. Metaphyseal transverse fractures may also be fixed by percutaneous intramedullary 6.5 mm or 7.0 mm partially threaded cancellous screw but needs experience.

Syndesmotic injuries: Syndesmotic injuries are most commonly caused by pronation–external rotation, pronation-abduction and, infrequently, supination–external rotation mechanisms (Danis–Weber type C and type B injuries). These forces cause the talus to abduct or rotate externally in the mortise, leading to disruption of the syndesmotic ligaments. Anatomical restoration of the distal tibiofibular syndesmosis is essential. If the fibular fracture is above the level of the distal tibiofibular joint, this joint is assumed to be disrupted and must be anatomically reduced.

The integrity of the syndesmosis can be evaluated intraoperatively by grasping the stabilized fibula with a hook or clamp and pulling it laterally. If more than 3–4 mm of lateral displacement occurs, syndesmotic fixation is necessary.

Intraoperative radiographs should show a clear space of <5 mm between the medial wall of the fibula and the lateral wall of the posterior tibial malleolus.

There is general agreement that syndesmotic fixation is indicated for (1) syndesmotic injuries associated with proximal fibular fractures for which fixation is not planned and that involve a medial injury that cannot be stabilized, and (2) syndesmotic injuries extending >5 cm proximal to the plafond. Whether syndesmotic fixation should be used in lateral malleolar fractures located 3-5 cm from the ankle joint in which the medial injury (deltoid ligament) is not repaired remains controversial.

Various methods have been used to fix the syndesmosis, most commonly screws or oblique pins inserted through the lateral malleolus and into the distal tibia. These pins or screws not only hold the joint anatomically reduced, but also stabilize and fix the lateral buttress of the ankle mortise. Bioabsorbable screws also have been used for fixation of the syndesmosis. Tightrope method also is used nowadays.

Posterior malleolus: Ankle fracture involving >25% of the posterior malleolus should be managed operatively. The majority of cases are stabilized with percutaneous anterior to posterior screws. Large or irreducible fragments are treated with posterior buttress plating.

97. Discuss clinical features and imaging in chronic inferior tibiofibular diastasis. Briefly discuss its management in a young and active adult male.

Ans: *Clinical features*: The patient has recurrent episodes of pain and swelling along with history of repeated episodes of ankle giving way followed by inadequate treatment and improper physiotherapy. He may complain of ankle instability. On examination, areas of point tenderness should be identified and correlated with the underlying ligamentous structures. In neglected cases, ecchymosis is usually absent unless a fresh recurrent sprain occurs over the chronic injury. In patients with syndesmotic injuries pain can be elicited at the syndesmosis by squeezing the fibula at the midcalf. External rotation of the foot while stabilizing the leg reproduces the pain at the syndesmosis.

Imaging: X-rays include standard anteroposterior, lateral and mortise views of the ankle. Stress views are easier to perform and reveal dynamic instability.

MRI is the gold standard for determining the extent of ligament injury. The ligaments may be thickened due to a previous healed tear or more likely they may be attenuated or even absent. In patients with recurrent sprains, joint effusion and bone marrow edema may be observed. Osteochondral lesions may also be picked up on MRI.

Management: For neglected syndesmotic sprains, surgical treatment depends on whether any arthritic change is present. If the articular surface is destroyed, tibiotalar arthrodesis or arthroplasty is necessary. In patients with diastasis without significant tibiotalar arthritis, late reduction of the syndesmosis and reconstruction of the ligaments are recommended.

In the Indian context, salvage procedures such as ankle arthrodesis may be more beneficial to poor manual laborers who have no access to expensive rehabilitation programs, especially if the ankle instability has led to degenerative changes.

98. What is Dupuytren's fracture dislocation? Discuss its management.

Ans: Dupuytren's fracture is a vague term applied to bimalleolar fractures and fracture-dislocation. It is also known as Pott's syndrome I. Kindly refer to answer above for all details.

99. A. Describe the mechanism of Trimalleolar fracture.
B. Enumerate its classifications.
C. Explain the treatment guidelines and surgical approach.

Ans:

A. Mechanism of Trimalleolar Fracture
- Most commonly due to *rotational forces* on the ankle with foot fixed on the ground.
- Supination–external rotation or pronation–abduction injuries (per Lauge-Hansen classification).
- Posterior malleolus fracture usually results from:
  - Posterior displacement of talus pushing posterior tibial lip
  - Shearing by posterior talofibular ligament
- High-energy trauma can produce additional ligamentous injuries.

B. Classifications
1. **Lauge-Hansen Classification (Mechanism based)**
   - Supination–External Rotation (SER) stage IV
     - Stage I: Anterior tibiofibular ligament rupture
     - Stage II: Spiral fracture of fibula (distal 1/3)
     - Stage III: Posterior tibiofibular ligament rupture or posterior malleolus fracture
     - Stage IV: Medial malleolus fracture or deltoid ligament rupture *(Trimalleolar fracture appears at stage IV)*
   - Pronation–Abduction (PAB) stage III can also produce similar fracture pattern.
2. **AO/OTA Classification**
   - Type 44 (Ankle fractures)
     - 44-B3 or 44-C3 depending on fibular fracture height and syndesmotic involvement.

C. Treatment Guidelines and Surgical Approach

Principles:
- Restore articular congruity of ankle joint
- Restore fibular length, rotation, and alignment
- Stabilize medial and posterior malleolus
- Assess and repair syndesmotic instability

Indications for surgery:
- Displaced fractures
- Posterior malleolus fragment involving >25–30% of articular surface or >2 mm displacement
- Syndesmotic instability
- Open fractures

Surgical steps:
1. Fix fibula first (usually lateral approach):
   - Restores length and rotation, helps indirect reduction of posterior malleolus.
   - Fix with lag screw + plate (neutralization or antiglide).
2. Fix posterior malleolus
   - Approach:
     – Posterolateral approach (with patient in prone or lateral position) if direct fixation required.
     – Anteroposterior screws if indirect reduction is possible.
   - Fixation helps to restore incisura fibularis and syndesmotic stability.
3. Fix medial malleolus
   - Medial approach
   - Fix with cannulated screws or tension band wiring.
4. Check syndesmosis
   - Cotton test or external rotation stress test after fixation
   - If unstable → syndesmotic screw fixation.

100. Discuss mechanism of injury and classification of tibial pilon fracture along with its management.
Ans:

Mechanism: Most articular fractures of the distal tibial weight-bearing surface are the result of high-energy mechanisms that occur during motor vehicle accidents, falls from heights, motorcycle accidents, and industrial mishaps.

The ultimate fracture pattern depends on the direction and rate of application of the injurious force, and the position of the foot at the time of loading. Because of this, wide variations in fracture patterns occur. A vertical impact while the foot is in dorsiflexion results in cephalad and anterior force, resulting in significant anterior plafond comminution, although impact with the foot in the neutral position results in significant central comminution. These injury patterns are much more common than those of the posterior plafond, which are thought to occur during plantar flexion. The precise direction and position of the foot at the time of impact, however, leads to wide variations in fracture patterns.

Classification:

Rüedi and Allgöwer classification:
- Type I fractures are nondisplaced cleavage fractures that involve the joint surface.
- Type II fractures have cleavage-type fracture lines with displacement of the articular surface, but minimal comminution.
- Type III fractures are associated with metaphyseal and articular comminution.

AO/OTA classification:
- *43-A*: Extra-articular fracture
- *43-A1*: Simple
- *43-A2*: Wedge
- *43-A3*: Complex
- *43-B*: Partial articular fracture
- *43-B1*: Pure split
- *43-B2*: Split-depression
- *43-B3*: Multifragmentary depression
- *43-C*: Complete articular fracture
- *43-C1*: Articular simple and metaphyseal simple
- *43-C2*: Articular simple, metaphyseal multifragmentary
- *43-C3*: Articular multifragmentary

Management: Factors to consider in the formulation of a treatment plan include the fracture pattern, soft tissue injury, patient comorbidities, fixation resources, and surgical experience. The degree of articular comminution, talar damage, and soft tissue injury is dictated by the injury, however, the surgeon does have some influence over other prognostic factors. The goal should be to obtain the best possible articular reduction and axial alignment, while respecting the soft tissues. If the articular surface does not reduce by ligamentotaxis, some form of open reduction usually is indicated after the soft tissues have recovered.

Nondisplaced fractures, such as AO types A1, B1, and C1, have been treated successfully with operative and nonoperative methods. These are the only fracture types in which cast immobilization alone may be suitable. If casting is chosen, the patient should be followed closely for displacement, and weight-bearing should be restricted for at least 8 weeks if nonarthritic. Calcaneal traction alone often is helpful in temporarily stabilizing severe fractures associated with soft tissue swelling, but it seldom is used for definitive treatment. External fixation accomplishes the same goal of fracture reduction through ligamentotaxis and allows the patient to be mobilized. Limited fixation with 3.5-mm or 4-mm screws, inserted after either percutaneous or limited open reduction, combined with plaster immobilization may be adequate treatment for AO types B1, B2, and stable C1 fractures. If the stability of the fracture is uncertain, however, an external fixator should be used instead of a cast.

101. Enumerate surgical approaches to reduce and fix pilon fractures. Enumerate steps of posterolateral approach. Enumerate its advantages and disadvantages.

Ans: The *various surgical approaches* used to reduce and fix pilon fractures are as follows:
- Posterolateral approach (Konrath and Hopkins)
- Anterolateral Böhler approach
- Anteromedial approach

Steps of posterolateral approach:
- With the patient under general anesthesia, remove the temporary external fixator that was previously placed. Administer antibiotics preoperatively.
- Place the patient prone, and exsanguinate the extremity and inflate the tourniquet to 300 mm Hg.
- Make a posterolateral incision into the distal tibia between the peroneal tendons and flexor hallucis longus. The approach can be carried proximally if needed.
- Identify and protect the sural nerve.
- Apply a femoral distractor if necessary to gain length or view the joint. Apply the distractor through new pins in the tibia to the calcaneus.
- If necessary, plate the fibula through the same incision, and fix with a one-third tubular plate.
- Obtain articular reduction by direct manipulation of the fracture fragments through the fracture sites under direct exposure. Confirm reduction with fluoroscopy.
- Fix the articular fragments with 3.5-mm lag screws.
- Fix the metaphyseal section to the diaphysis with a plate.
- For large bone defects caused by comminution, use iliac crest bone grafting.
- Close the wounds primarily.

Advantages and disadvantages of posterolateral approach:

Advantages:
- Pilon fractures in which the articular displacement and comminution are predominantly located posteriorly
- When an anterior approach is not recommended because of the condition of the soft tissues.

Disadvantages:
- Wound problems (superficial infections, three deep infections).
- Poor exposure of the ankle joint, which limits its utility in fractures with anterior comminution leading to increased malunion/nonunion rates.

102. What is Tillaux fracture? Discuss Malgaigne fracture and clinical signs of fractured pelvis.

Ans: *Tillaux fracture (Tillaux-Chaput avulsion fracture)* **(Fig. 3.4.13)**: An avulsion fracture of distal tibia epiphysis occurring in older adolescents as originally described by Tillaux. The mechanism of injury is an external rotational force with stress placed on the anterior inferior tibiofibular ligament, causing avulsion of the distal tibial physis anterolaterally. This occurs after the medial part of the physis has closed, but before the lateral part fuses completely (typically within the one-year window period whence the distal tibial physis closure is completing at the end of growth). The resultant fracture through the physis runs across the epiphysis and distally into the joint, creating a Salter–Harris type III (commonly) or IV (uncommon) fracture. Typically, there is no fracture in the posterior part of physis.

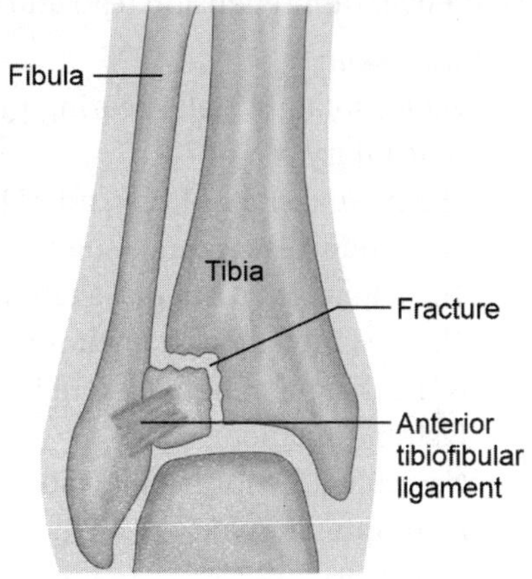

Note: Area-wise the distal tibial physis closes in the following pattern usually— central → posterior → medial → anterolateral.

Malgaigne fracture: The Malgaigne fracture named after Joseph–François Malgaigne is a hemipelvic unstable injury. There is a double vertical (two ipsilateral fractures) fracture in the pelvic ring or a fracture with a dislocation that renders the hemipelvis unstable. Usually one fracture line is anterior to acetabulum (involving the rami) and the other one posterior to it (involving the SI joint). The fragment containing acetabulum is rendered unstable (? floating acetabulum). It is less common in children than in adults. It results due to vertical shear energy vectors. A CT scan may be helpful in determining the amount of joint displacement.

Clinical signs of fracture pelvis:
- Pelvic, flank, or perineal contusions, ecchymoses, or abrasions. Open wounds of the groin, buttock, or perineum
- Leg length inequality
- External or internal rotation deformity of the hemipelvis
- Scrotal/labial edema, hematoma or ecchymosis
- Flank hematoma/ecchymosis
- Abnormal pelvic motion on anteroposterior or lateral compression of the anterior iliac spines and iliac crests
- Pain on palpation of posterior pelvis
- External or internal degloving (Morel-Lavallee lesion)
- Blood at the urethral meatus
- Blood in or around the rectum
- Blood out of the vagina (rule out laceration vs. menses)
- Neurologic deficit involving the lumbosacral plexus—reduced rectal sphincter tone and perirectal sensation
- High-riding prostate (urethral injury).

Fig. 3.4.13: Tillaux fracture.

103. Discuss classification, clinical features, and management of Lisfranc injuries.

Ans:

Classification: Myerson's modification of the original classifications of Quénu and Küss, **(Fig. 3.4.14)** and Hardcastle et al.
- *Type A injuries*: Displacement of all five metatarsals (MTs) with or without fracture of the base of the 2nd metatarsal. The usual displacement is lateral or dorsolateral, and the MTs move as a unit (homolateral injury).
- *Type B injuries*: One or more articulations remain intact.
  - Type B1 injuries are medially displaced, sometimes involving the intercuneiform or naviculocuneiform joint.
  - Type B2 injuries are laterally displaced and may involve the first MT–cuneiform joint.
- *Type C injuries*: These are divergent injuries that can be partial (C1) or complete (C2). These result from high-energy trauma, associated with significant swelling, and there is significant risk of complications, especially compartment syndrome.

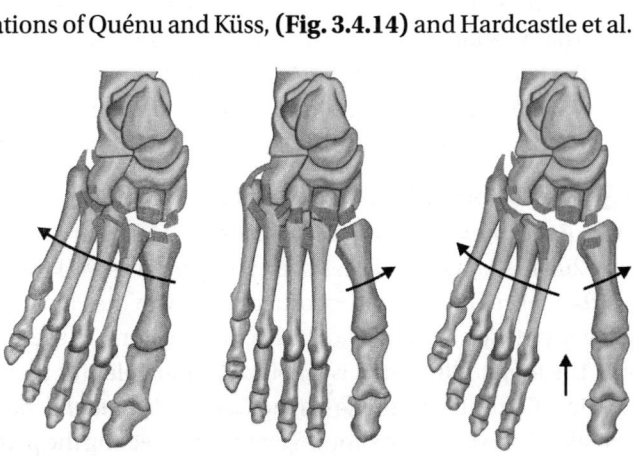

Fig. 3.4.14: Quénu and Küss classification.

Clinical features: Painful swelling, and functional disability (e.g., inability to perform pain-free weight-bearing or the inability to stand on tip-toe) are common. Presence of plantar ecchymosis should raise suspicion of a tarsometatarsal injury. The tarsometatarsal transition zone will be widened in comparison to the opposite foot. The abduction–pronation maneuver (apprehension test) and the transverse tarsometatarsal-1/2 squeeze test would elicit pain.

Management:

Imaging: Obtain weight-bearing radiographs of the patient preferably. Evaluate the following signs for documenting Lisfranc injury:
- The medial shaft of the 2nd MT is aligned with the medial aspect of the middle cuneiform on the anteroposterior view—any discordance suggests Lisfranc injury.
- The alignment of medial shaft of the 4th MT with the medial aspect of the cuboid on the oblique view is disturbed.
- The first metatarsal–cuneiform articulation is incongruent.
- A "fleck sign" should be sought in the medial cuneiform–second metatarsal space. This represents an avulsion of the Lisfranc ligament.
- Naviculocuneiform subluxation
- A compression fracture of the cuboid suggests TMT injury.

Treatment: The key to successful outcome in Lisfranc injuries is anatomical alignment of the involved joints. Closed, nondisplaced (<2 mm) injuries or patients with surgical contraindication (poor medical status, dysvascular foot, and Charcot foot) can be treated with a non–weight bearing cast for 6 weeks followed by a weight-bearing cast for an additional 4–6 weeks. Repeat radiographs should be obtained to ensure that no displacement is occurring in the cast.

Operative treatment: This is indicated in unstable and or displaced fracture dislocation injuries. Surgery is commonly performed within 24 hours before the foot swelling becomes unmanageable or after the foot swelling subsides and wrinkles appear (10–14 days). Till then the foot may be elevated in splint and swelling reduced by controlled crepe bandage application. If anatomical reduction is obtained by closed reduction, then the injury may be fixed with thick K-wires under C-arm guidance. Else if stable reduction is not obtained by closed method then open reduction is the preferred method (some prefer this to open straightaway). The tendons of tibialis anterior or peronei may interpose precluding reduction and after accurate reduction and confirmation under C-arm fixation can be done with K-wires or screw osteosynthesis or mini fragment plate fixation. In general K-wires are sufficient for lateral column fixation (as they have some mobility so rigid fixation compromises arch resilience) while multiple cannulated screws (preferable) provide best multidirectional stability for injury stabilization, especially 1st and 2nd metatarsals and tarsometatarsal stabilization. The 4th and 5th metatarsals (lateral column) can be reduced and pinned to the cuboid using K-wires. Due to concern of articular damage with screws, extra-articular fixation with plates is preferred by many (but it needs an open fixation). The foot is supported in a splint for 6 weeks after surgery and K-wires removed at 6 weeks followed by support to foot in a rocker style shoe. External fixation may be done for fractures where tissue condition does not permit screw/plate placement. Primary medial two rays TMT arthrodesis is indicated in comminuted fractures that cannot be reconstructed or in neuropathic foot. Some tend to fix the comminuted injuries using a "Lisfranc screw" and dorsal plate. Midfoot arthrodesis may be done in progressive arch collapse or chronic Lisfranc injuries that produced midfoot arthrosis.

104. **Describe pathoanatomy of Lisfranc injury. Describe management in a chronic Lisfranc injury.**

Ans: *Pathoanatomy*: The tarsometatarsal (TMT) joint complex forms the distal limit between the tarsal and metatarsal units. The 2nd metatarsal (MT) has been recognized as the keystone for substantial bony stability. The cuboid is the keystone in the lateral column of the foot articulating with the calcaneus and the bases of the fourth and fifth metatarsals in the axial plane, and the navicular and the lateral cuneiform in the coronal plane. The navicular forms the key in the medial column.

The longitudinal arch is stabilized by the plantar aponeurosis, the long plantar ligament, and the peroneus longus tendon. Out of these, the so-called *Lisfranc ligament bundle*, spanning from the first cuneiform to the second metatarsal (weaker), as well as the strong ligament connecting the plantar aspect of the medial cuneiform to the bases of the 2nd and 3rd metatarsals, provide substantial stability to the TMT joint line. Both ligamentous structures are important stabilizers of the medial TMT column, however, the more commonly found dorsal displacement is related to the easier failure of the dorsal Lisfranc ligament.

Management: The treatment of chronic Lisfranc's injury essentially involves restoration of joint anatomy.
- If there is no significant residual arthritis or fixed deformity → delayed open reduction and internal fixation with or without reconstruction of the Lisfranc ligament may be performed. Rigid fixation of the displaced TMT joints with screws/k-wires is recommended. Associated metatarsal fractures are treated with intramedullary K-wire fixation. In patients with intra-articular injury and joint destruction, the joints should be fused.
- Once arthritic changes develop then joint preservation and realignment will be painful mostly. Arthrodesis, including correction of deformity, is the treatment of choice for the 1st, 2nd and 3rd TMT joints. Resection arthroplasty of the 4th and 5th TMT joints may be preferable to arthrodesis in order to maintain physiologic motion. Arthrodesis is also beneficial in patients with advanced arthritic changes and Charcot's joints.

105. What are the complications of Lisfranc fracture dislocation?

Ans: The following are the complications of Lisfranc fracture dislocation:
- *Post-traumatic arthritis*:
  - Present in most, but may not be symptomatic
  - Related to initial injury and adequacy of reduction
  - Treated with orthotics initially and arthrodesis late for the medial column
  - Possibly treated with interpositional arthroplasty for the lateral column
- Compartment syndrome
- Infection
- Complex regional pain syndrome (CRPS, RSD)
- Neurovascular injury
- Hardware failure

106. Discuss potential complications and outcomes of a chronic neglected Lisfranc injury.

Ans: A chronically neglected Lisfranc injury presents a series of significant complications that can profoundly impact both the structural integrity of the foot and the overall functionality of the lower extremity. The Lisfranc joint complex, which encompasses the tarsometatarsal joints, is critical for maintaining mechanical stability and optimizing weight-bearing efficiency. Neglecting such injuries can precipitate a cascade of deleterious outcomes that warrant authoritative examination.

1. *Immediate complications*: The immediate repercussions of a neglected Lisfranc injury predominantly include chronic pain, joint instability, and the onset of osteoarthritis. Delayed intervention often results in malalignment of the tarsometatarsal joints, which produces abnormal wear patterns on the articular cartilage. Over time, this degeneration manifests as osteoarthritis, characterized by persistent joint pain, swelling, and substantially reduced range of motion, all of which significantly impair the patient's mobility and overall quality of life.
2. *Chronic instability*: Insufficient ligamentous support resulting from the neglect of the injury can lead to chronic instability. This instability predisposes the foot to recurrent sprains and dislocations, complicating the healing process of the initial injury. Furthermore, the resultant instability encourages compensatory gait alterations, subjecting adjacent joints—such as the ankle and knee—to undue stress, thereby increasing the risk of secondary pathologies.
3. *Forefoot deformities*: Another critical complication associated with chronic Lisfranc injuries is the development of forefoot deformities, including flatfoot and claw foot. These deformities arise from imbalances in muscle function and tendon dynamics that emerge as consequences of altered foot biomechanics. The structural changes associated with such deformities often necessitate surgical intervention aimed at restoring normal anatomical architecture and function.
4. *Psychological impacts*: The chronic pain and functional limitations stemming from a neglected Lisfranc injury may also invoke significant psychological ramifications, including anxiety and depression. These mental health issues frequently result from diminished physical activity and reduced social engagement. The compelling interplay between physical health and mental well-being underscores the necessity for a comprehensive and integrated management approach for individuals affected by these injuries.

5. *Surgical outcomes*: Regarding treatment, the prognosis for chronic Lisfranc injuries necessitates prompt and aggressive intervention. Therapeutic approaches typically include realignment of the bones, stabilization of the joint complex, and, when warranted, reconstruction of ligamentous structures. It is imperative to note that patients with chronic conditions generally exhibit poorer outcomes compared to those with acute injuries, primarily due to the presence of established arthritic changes and the potential development of chronic pain syndromes.

In conclusion, the multifaceted consequences of a chronically neglected Lisfranc injury extend far beyond mere physical impairment. The complications arising from such neglect mandate a multidisciplinary approach that incorporates both surgical and nonsurgical interventions. The overarching goal of treatment should be to restore not only the mechanical functionality of the foot but also to enhance the overall well-being of the patient. Recognizing and addressing these complexities is essential for achieving optimal outcomes in individuals affected by chronic Lisfranc injuries.

107. Classify calcaneal fractures. Management principles and complications of calcaneal fractures.

Ans: *Classification:*

Extra-articular fractures: These do not involve the posterior facet.
- Anterior process fractures
- Tuberosity fractures
- Medial process fractures
- Sustentacular fractures
- Body fractures not involving the subtalar articulation.

Intra-Articular Fractures

Essex–Lopresti Classification:

Primary fracture line: Runs obliquely through the posterior facet and divides the calcaneus into anteromedial or sustentacular fragment and posterolateral or tuberosity fragment. The fracture line exits anterolaterally at the crucial angle or as far distally as the calcaneocuboid joint.
- The anteromedial fragment is rarely comminuted and remains attached to the talus by the deltoid and interosseous talocalcaneal ligaments.
- The posterolateral fragment is usually comminuted and displaces superolaterally resulting in incongruity of the posterior facet along with heel shortening and widening.

Secondary fracture line: With continued compressive forces, there is additional comminution, creating a free lateral piece of posterior facet separate from the tuberosity fragment. This creates two commonly seen fracture patterns:
- *Tongue-type fracture*: A secondary fracture line appears beneath the facet and exits posteriorly through the tuberosity.
- *Joint depression fracture*: A secondary fracture line exits just behind the posterior facet. As this occurs, the tuberosity fragment will rotate into varus. The posterolateral aspect of the talus will force the free lateral piece of the posterior facet down into the tuberosity fragment, rotating it as much as 90°.

Sanders classification: This is based on the number of intra-articular fracture lines and their location on semicoronal CT images for intra-articular calcaneal fractures involving the posterior facet. The posterior facet is divided into three fracture lines (A, B, and C corresponding to lateral, central, and medial fracture lines on coronal image).
- *Type 1*: All fractures with less than 2 mm of displacement regardless of the number of fracture lines.
- *Type 2*: Two-part fracture of posterior facet, further divided into—
  - *2A*: One primary fracture line that courses through the lateral aspect of posterior facet
  - *2B*: One primary fracture line that courses through the middle of posterior facet
  - *2C*: One primary fracture line that courses through the medial aspect of posterior facet.
- *Type 3*: Three-part fracture with centrally depressed fragment, further divided into—
  - *3AB*: Two primary fracture lines, one coursing through the lateral aspect and another through the central aspect of posterior facet
  - *3AC*: Two primary fracture lines, one coursing through the lateral aspect and another through the medial aspect of posterior facet
  - *3BC*: Two primary fracture lines, one coursing through the central aspect and another through the medial aspect of posterior facet.

- *Type 4*: Four-part intra-articular fracture with greater than 2 mm displacement and is severely comminuted.

Management principles: Indications for nonoperative treatment:
- Nondisplaced or minimally displaced intra- and extra-articular fractures
- Sanders type 1 and type 4 intra-articular fractures
- Patient older than 50–55 years with severe osteopenia, limited ambulatory abilities, and significant medical comorbidities
- Patients with diabetes or insensate limb due to any cause.

Operative management is prescribed commonly for displaced tongue-type fractures, Sanders type II and III posterior facet displacement >2 to 3 mm, flattening of Bohler angle, large extra-articular fractures (>1 cm) with detachment of Achilles tendon and/or >2 mm displacement urgent if skin is compromised. The usual goals are:
- Restoration of congruency of the posterior facet of the subtalar joint
- Restoration of the height of the calcaneus (Böhler angle)
- Reduction of the width of the calcaneus
- Decompression of the subfibular space available for the peroneal tendons
- Realignment of the tuberosity into a valgus position
- Reduction of the calcaneocuboid joint, if fractured.

Complications:
- *Subtalar arthritis*: It may occur even in the presence of an anatomic reduction; it may be treated with injections or orthoses, or it may ultimately require subtalar or triple arthrodesis.
- *Wound complications*: It is most common at the angle of incision. It may need treatment with wet to dry dressing changes, skin grafting, or muscle flap if necessary.
- *Increased heel width*: Some degree of heel widening is always seen. It may result in lateral impingement on the peroneal tendons. It is aggravated by increased residual lateral width and may be treated by wall resection or hardware removal.
- *Peroneal tendon irritation and impingement*: This is generally seen following nonoperative treatment and results from lateral impingement.
- Compartment syndrome
- Complex regional pain syndrome
- *Sural nerve injury*: This may occur in up to 15% of operative cases using a lateral approach.
- Damage to FHL
- *Calcaneal osteomyelitis*: The risk may be minimized by allowing soft tissue edema to resolve preoperatively.
- *Malunion*: Calcaneal malunion has been classified on CT scan into three types—
  - *Type 1*: Lateral exostosis with no subtalar arthritis. This is treated with lateral wall resection
  - *Type 2*: Lateral exostosis with subtalar arthritis. This needs lateral wall excision and subtalar fusion
  - *Type 3*: Lateral exostosis with subtalar arthritis and varus malunion. Treat with lateral wall resection, subtalar fusion ± valgus osteotomy.

(For a detailed reading, kindly refer to Annexure 2 of the book Essential Orthopedics: Principles and Practice, 2nd edition.)

108. **Describe in brief mechanism of injury and treatment of calcaneal fractures.**

Ans: Mechanism of injury: Intra-articular fractures are uniformly caused by an axial load mechanism, such as a fall or a motor vehicle accident, and may be associated with other axial load injuries, such as lumbar, pelvic, and tibial plateau fractures.

Treatment:

Nonoperative:
- Nondisplaced to minimally displaced extra-articular fractures
- Nondisplaced intra-articular fractures (type 1) and in type 4 Sander's type
- Anterior process fractures with <25% involvement of calcaneocuboid articulation
- Fractures in patients with severe peripheral vascular disease
- Insulin-dependent diabetes mellitus, medical comorbidities prohibiting surgery
- Minimally ambulatory elderly patients

Operative: Operative treatment is primarily indicated for:
- Displaced intra-articular fractures involving the posterior facet
- Anterior process of the calcaneus fractures with > 25% involvement of the calcaneocuboid articulation
- Displaced fractures of the calcaneal tuberosity
- Fracture–dislocations of the calcaneus
- Selected open fractures of the calcaneus

Operative fixation methods:

Percutaneous or minimally invasive fixation: Indications—
- Sanders 2C tongue-type fractures in which the entire posterior facet is attached to the tongue fragment
- Displaced calcaneal tuberosity or beak fractures
- Emergent reduction and temporary stabilization of fractures with severe or impending soft-tissue compromise from displaced fracture fragments
- Fractures in patients with relative contraindications to open surgery, such as heavy smokers or patients requiring chronic anticoagulation. The initial closed or percutaneous reduction and temporary stabilization with K-wires may be converted to a formal open procedure or may be used as definitive treatment.

ORIF with plate and screws:
- Displaced intra-articular fractures involving the posterior facet (for type 2 and type 3 Sander's types)
- Anterior process fractures with >25% involvement of calcaneocuboid articulation
- Displaced fractures of calcaneal tuberosity
- Fracture-dislocations of calcaneus
- Open fractures of calcaneus

109. Compare extensile lateral approach and sinus tarsi approach for calcaneal fractures.

Ans: Comparison of lateral extensile approach and sinus tarsi approach is presented in Table 3.4.2.

TABLE 3.4.2: Comparison of extensile lateral and sinus tarsi approaches for calcaneum fractures.

Serial number	Variables	Extensile lateral approach	Sinus tarsi approach
1	Size of incision	Longer	Smaller
2	Accuracy of reduction	Slightly more or equal	Equal or a bit less
3	Time of surgery	More	Less
4	Infection rate	Higher	Lower
5	Implant related issues	More	Less
6	Post operative stay	More	Less

110. Classify fracture of neck of talus. Discuss principles of management. What is Hawkins sign?

Ans:

Classification

Hawkins classification **(Fig. 3.4.15)**:
- *Type 1*: Nondisplaced vertical fractures of the neck
- *Type 2*: Displaced fractures with subluxation or dislocation of the subtalar joint
- *Type 3*: Fractures with dislocation of the subtalar and the ankle joints
- *Type 4*: Fractured neck with body of the talus extruded from the ankle mortise, head of the talus subluxed or dislocated from the navicular articulation.

Principles of Management

Talar neck fractures: All cases with subluxed or dislocated talus should be immediately reduced to prevent further vascular compromise.

The goal of treatment is anatomical reduction.

- For nondisplaced (Hawkins I) fractures below knee, POP cast for 8–10 weeks with weight-bearing is delayed until trabeculation across the fracture usually suffice while all other fractures need ORIF. A talar neck fracture must be thoroughly evaluated before labelling it as a type I. Many fractures, if examined closely by CT scans display subtle displacement, or one can evaluate subtalar stability under fluoroscope. Regular follow-up is needed to identify early displacements.
- *Type II fractures*: Closed reduction is needed and after that unacceptable plantar flexion is needed to maintain reduction of head so surgery is indicated. Commonly a medial (anteromedial) approach is used or alternatively anterolateral approach also allows reduction. Screws are placed just off the articular surface fixing the fracture. If lag screws are used, then one needs to ensure that there is no comminution else impaction shortening may result. Often the medial neck is the location of the comminution of the fracture, however, and fracture alignment and reduction can be difficult to assess. This area also may offer only limited access for fixation. Adding an anterolateral approach,

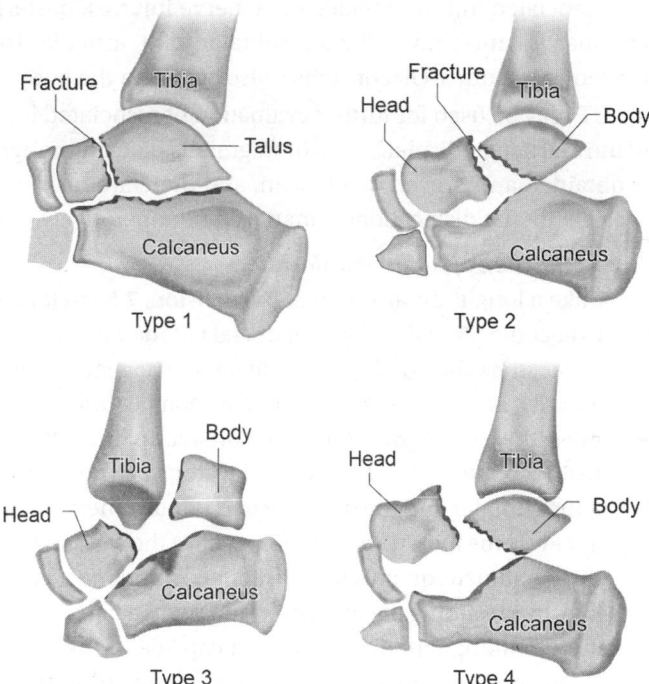

Fig. 3.4.15: Hawkins classification.

which may help to assess reduction and to offer a region for screw fixation. The screws can also be placed through posterolateral approach of Trillat. The best bone for fixation is located in the lateral talar head, using posterior-to-anterior screw placement. It is usual to combine the anteromedial with posterolateral approach, passing the screw (at least two screws, cannulated or solid core) from posterior to anterior. In case of comminuted fractures, it is better to place plate at the comminuted column while using a screw in neutralization mode. Plates offer a solid buttress as a bridging strut against collapse, supination or pronation of the fragments.
- *Type III fractures*: After emergent reduction, it is imperative to reposition the body that may be done by medial malleolus osteotomy (preserving the deltoid blood supply). In open fractures, it is better to debride, wash the site, and place a distractor while toggling the talar body in place with a pin. Fixation can be done as for type II fractures. If the body is totally extruded and wound is contaminated—it is better to discard the body fragment and plan a reconstruction by arthrodesis—usually in two stages.
- *Type IV injuries*: These are managed like type III while considering the fact that there are high chances of additional osteonecrosis of head fragment as the only remaining blood supply to the talus, the deltoid branch, may be rotated, and occluded, correctable only through emergency reduction of the body.

Hawkins sign: Subchondral lucency on X-ray present 12 weeks after injury (Hawkins line) is an indication that osteonecrosis will not occur, but this is not a foolproof measure. However, lack of a subchondral lucency at 3 months indicates that osteonecrosis has occurred, and appears to be more reliable prognosticator for osteonecrosis.

III. What is peritalar dislocation?

Ans: Peritalar dislocation is also known as subtalar dislocation.

In dislocation of the subtalar joint, the calcaneus, cuboid, navicular, and all of the forefoot become displaced from the talus. Most often, the foot is dislocated medial to the talus, although lateral, anterior, and posterior dislocations occur.

Medial subtalar dislocations, without marginal fractures of the calcaneus or talus, almost always are reducible by closed means. Lateral subtalar dislocations frequently are irreducible by closed manipulation, and the most common offending structures blocking reduction are the posterior tibial tendon and osteochondral fracture of the talus.

Associated injuries include tibial nerve injuries, posterior tibial tendon ruptures, posterior tibial nerve lacerations, articular fractures involving the subtalar joint, articular fractures of the talonavicular joint, talar dome fractures, and malleolar fractures. Osteonecrosis also occurs in the body of the talus in the patients.

CT may be used for further evaluation of associated injuries and often find fractures that require treatment because of intra-articular displacement or fragments blocking congruent reduction of the subtalar joint. If a congruent reduction is obtained and proved on CT scan, and there are no intra-articular fragments or displaced bone fragments requiring repair, subtalar dislocations is managed nonoperatively.

Open reduction of subtalar dislocation:
- Make a longitudinal anterolateral incision, 7.5 cm long from just proximal to the ankle joint to the cuboid. Carefully protect the medial and lateral dorsal cutaneous branches of the superficial peroneal nerve.
- Retract the extensor digitorum longus and extensor hallucis longus tendons medially and the peroneus tertius tendon laterally, and expose the talus and midtarsal joints.
- Incise the capsule over the head and neck of the talus, and extend the incision into the midtarsus.
- Insert a bone skid or periosteal elevator into the subtalar joint, and by leverage and traction reduce the dislocation of the subtalar and the talonavicular joints. When the dislocation is medial, have an assistant simultaneously abduct and evert the foot; when it is lateral, have the assistant adduct and invert the foot. In a lateral dislocation, the posterior tibial tendon frequently blocks reduction and must be lifted out of the talonavicular joint before reduction is possible. Also, by extending the medial wound seen in lateral subtalar dislocations and lifting the dorsal neurovascular bundle and offending tendons, the dorsal capsule of the talonavicular joint can be incised. With this structure loosened, the navicular may be levered around the head of the talus with a periosteal elevator. This may require a separate anterolateral incision.
- If necessary, hold the reduction with longitudinally placed Steinmann pins across the calcaneocuboid and talonavicular joints for 4 weeks.

112. What are unreconstructable fractures in elderly and discuss the management options?
Ans:
(This is a conceptual question and would entail very expandable answer, the students can expand the answer as needed).
Unreconstructable fractures in elderly would fall in either of the following categories:
1. Fracture that is too complex for anatomical/acceptable osteosynthesis by current available methods due to poor condition of bone:
   - Complex pelviacetabular fractures
   - Complex fractures of the spine
   - Complex and comminuted fractures of the distal humerus
   - Comminuted fractures of the proximal femur
   - Complex comminuted fractures of distal or proximal tibia
   - Comminuted fractures of distal femur
   - Proximal humerus comminuted fracture/fracture dislocations
   - Any periarticular fracture with bone loss
   - Late presentation of complex intra-articular comminuted fractures (>1 month)
   - Open fractures of long bones with significant bone loss
   - Old neglected fractures/fracture dislocations
2. Fracture not amenable to osteosynthesis due to comorbid conditions though they can be mended by the current technology
   - Poor soft tissue condition at fracture site due to skin diseases or skin loss or Morel-Lavallée lesion renders current osteosynthesis impossible: In these cases, the surgery has to be deferred till the skin cover could be satisfactorily achieved or the skin condition is improved to acceptable level. Then later osteosynthesis/replacement or corrective osteotomies may be done as needed.
   - Here any fracture would be rendered literally unreconstructible by operative osteosynthesis as fracture cannot be operated.

- Patients having cognitive problems—mental incapacity to understand the consequences of either approach. In this case, the institutional guidelines have to be followed rather than the state policy and legal implications have to be obtained keeping the family in confidence. Surrogate consent may not be valid in these cases depending on state laws.

For both categories of patients, principles of conservative management of fractures need to be applied if the fracture can neither be reconstructed (osteosynthesis) nor replaced (*reconstruction means osteosynthesis repair of bone and does not include replacement*). While using the conservative management principles pay attention to adequate analgesia, fluid and electrolyte balance, cognitive and psychological problems of the patient and nutrition requirements. The following are the common practices of management of different fractures:

- *Proximal femoral fractures*: The neglected fractures of proximal femur in osteoporotic patients may not be fixable and have to be alternatively managed:
  - *Neglected fracture neck of femur*: Replacement hemiarthroplasty with quick in and out procedure. If the patient is unfit for surgery, then "derotation boot and bar" ± traction (I do not prefer traction) application to the limb and bed rest. Take precautions for bed sore and chest complications.
  - Neglected femoral head fracture, replacement hemiarthroplasty or total hip replacement if possible. For nonoperable patients, the treatment usually includes mobilization as early as possible gradually from toe—touch walk to full-weight bearing as permissible by pain.
  - *Old intertrochanteric fracture*: Replacement with calcar replacing prosthesis in neglected cases. If patient is not fit for regional or general anesthesia; some have attempted applying external fixator in local anesthesia and sedation (I have never done this!). In nonoperable patients, classical "derotation boot and bar" ± traction (I do not prefer traction) application to the limb and bed rest. Take precautions for bed sore and chest complications. Traction may be essential for comatose patients or those with increased muscle tone.
- *Distal femoral and proximal tibial fractures (similar approaches remain so grouped together)*: Highly comminuted osteoporotic intra-articular fractures that cannot be stabilized with osteosynthesis need to be replaced with custom knee replacement prosthesis. External fixation is another nonanatomical method for stabilizing the injuries in shortening provided the intra-articular could be acceptably maintained with minimally invasive screws or otherwise. Another approach is maintaining the fracture in above knee cast as best as possible till union and then performing standard total knee arthroplasty later. This approach, however, is risky as knee stiffness may render later arthroplasty untenable. For nonoperable patients, the standard management is applying above-knee cast till union or for first 6 weeks followed by long knee brace to maintain hygiene and allow ankle movements.
- *Distal tibial fractures*: The option of replacement is also not very successful for ankle fractures. In such cases, it is best to use an external fixator to maintain alignment if primary osteosynthesis is not possible. Use of Ilizarov and hybrid frames improves chances of acceptable alignment. This can be followed by gradual mobilization once union occurs. Later arthrodesis of ankle may be performed if patient has persistent pain. For nonoperable patients, long knee cast for 3 weeks followed by below-knee cast for further 3–4 weeks is applied. Gradual motion is begun later as permissible.
- *Distal humerus fractures*: Osteoporotic comminuted distal humeral fractures are a challenge for reconstruction as fragments are small and hidden behind olecranon. The articular surface is also not a smooth curve so fitting the jigsaw puzzle and stabilizing with implant is sometimes impossible in anatomical position, despite having best of the implants. In such cases, "bag of bones" treatment may be followed or a hanging type above-elbow cast that will maintain alignment for 4–6 weeks for fracture to start uniting. Then hinge brace can be applied for gradual mobilization. Later stable elbow joint arthroplasty can be done for painful arthritic joint if persists. The other alternative is primary elbow replacement but then it would be a fully constrained prosthesis that has higher failure rates in future. In patients inoperable due to skin condition or otherwise external fixator is acceptable option that may be combined with K-wire fixation for temporary stabilization of fractures. In patients unfit for surgery, applying long elbow cast would suffice.
- *Proximal humerus fractures*: Replacement arthroplasty is quite rewarding for nonreconstructible fractures of proximal humerus. Hemi or total shoulder replacement provides improved result over suboptimal osteosynthesis in osteoporotic proximal humerus fractures. Most fractures would involve tuberosities and if they cannot be utilized then

reverse shoulder prosthesis would be needed. Shoulder arthrodesis is an option in patients unfit for arthroplasty or unaffording patients or in patients who present late with arthritis painful shoulder and stiffness where replacing the joint would not yield good results. Conservative management with arm-pouch immobilization or POP slab for 4–6 weeks is done in inoperable patients. Early graduated mobilization should be the aim in these patients to improve function and prevent stiffness.

- *Acetabular and pelvis fractures*: Due to poor fixation in osteoporotic bones and loss of maintenance of reduction over time, the results of osteosynthesis are unpredictable. In comminuted and complex fractures, osteosynthesis may not be possible at all. It is better in such cases to let the fragments maintain their position in situ by traction and after bone formation, total hip arthroplasty can be performed with augmented implants if needed. Malunions of pelvis unless compromising internal organs are well accepted so conservative management with bed-rest and supportive care for pain, bedsores, bowel, and bladder care is instituted. Gross opening of pelvis due to massive instability would be life-threatening in the beginning so these fractures may be maintained by pelvic C-clamp or external fixation to bind the pelvis and provide fixed volume.

113. Describe Morel–Lavallée lesion and briefly mention the management.

Ans: Morel-Lavallée lesion is considered equivalent of internal degloving in a shear trauma to body. It occurs when the skin is separated from the fascia. This separation creates a pocket in which considerable bleeding can occur. Usually this is a subcutaneous hematoma, but the hematoma can become so large that it seriously threatens the viability of the skin above. The microvasculature connecting the two layers and lymphatics are damaged so that resorption of the collected fluid is delayed and thus healing does not occur. The layers remain separated and are vulnerable to necrosis and infection lest another trauma (like surgery) occurs. This syndrome occurs frequently in patients with pelvic fractures, especially in obese individuals in whom there was a shear component to the injury.

Management: Multiple treatment options have been suggested for Morel-Lavallée syndrome ranging from radical incision/ excision (leaves behind a massive wound) to wound drainage to inactivity. The primary recommendation is to treat the soft-tissue problem at the same time the fracture is stabilized. Due to high complication rate of necrosis and open wound conservative policy of wait and watch initially rather than to proceed was practiced. Immediate decompression was frequently met with the risk of devascularizing additional skin by opening the wound. Percutaneous aspiration may cause recurrence of the swelling. As a change in practice draining the hematoma with a small incision and applying a compression bandage within 3 days has met with improved results.

3.5 AXIAL SKELETON INJURY, SPINE AND PELVIS (Q114–140)

114. What is Hangman's fracture? Discuss classification and management of Hangman's fracture.

Ans: Hangman fracture is traumatic spondylolisthesis of the axis (C2 cervical vertebra) resulting from hyperextension injury to the neck as may occur in people who try to hang themselves, contact sports or high-velocity motor vehicle accidents. Though uncommon it is mostly a lethal injury that results in respiratory center failure causing respiratory muscle paralysis. The hyperextension results in break of the pedicles of axis vertebra symmetrically while the dens process is mostly intact. There may be associated injury to anterior longitudinal ligament (ALL) and underlying intervertebral disk.

Classification with management:
Hangman's fracture classification with management is shown in **Table 3.5.1**.

TABLE 3.5.1: Classification (Levine and Edwards modification of Effendi system).

Type	Management
Type I fractures are minimally displaced and are believed to be caused by hyperextension and axial loading with failure of the neural arch in tension. ALL and posterior longitudinal ligament (PLL) are intact	These fractures are stable and usually heal with 12 weeks of immobilization in a rigid cervical orthosis

Contd...

Contd...

Type	Management
Type II fractures have more than 3 mm of anterior translation and/or 11° or greater angulation (unstable fracture) ALL damage → ± PLL and C2-3 disk injury → +	Treatment consists of application of skull traction through tongs or a halo ring with slight extension of the neck over a rolled-up towel. Immobilization in a halo vest does not achieve or maintain reduction, and halo traction with slight extension may be necessary for 3–6 weeks to maintain anatomical reduction
Type IIA fractures are a variant of type II fractures that show severe angulation between C2 and C3 with minimal translation. They usually have a more horizontal than vertical fracture line through the C2 arch	Treatment is application of a halo vest with slight compression applied under image intensification to achieve and maintain anatomical reduction. When reduction has been obtained, halo vest immobilization is continued for 12 weeks until union occurs
Type III injuries combine a bipedicular fracture with posterior facet injuries. They result from initial flexion and rebound extension with axial compression ALL and PLL damage → ++ C2-3 disk injury → ++ Unilateral or bilateral facet dislocation → +	Type III injuries are the only type of Hangman's fracture that commonly require surgical stabilization. Open reduction and internal fixation are usually required because of inability to obtain or maintain reduction of the C2–3 facet dislocation. Because the lamina and spinous process of C2 are a free-floating fragment, bilateral oblique wiring of C2–3 is necessary for stable reduction. After posterior cervical fusion at the C2-3 level, halo vest immobilization for 3 months is necessary for the bipedicular fracture and for consolidation of the fusion mass

115. A. Discuss unifacetal fracture dislocation of C5–C6 and its management.
   B. What are the types of cord injuries?
   C. Also, discuss the role of methylprednisolone succinate in spinal cord injuries.

Ans:
A. Unilateral facet dislocation
Unilateral facet dislocations usually result from flexion and rotation of the cervical spine. They are considered stage 2 distractive flexion injuries. The most common site of dislocation is at C5-6. Patients may present with an isolated nerve root injury or an incomplete neurological deficit. The injury may be purely ligamentous or may involve a facet fracture in addition to the dislocation.

Management: Unilateral facet dislocations may be difficult to reduce in skeletal traction. Closed reduction may be attempted to unlock the dislocated facet joint, however, this is successful in less than 50% of patients, and we do not routinely use manipulation of the cervical spine. The patients who undergo open reduction and fusion usually have better results than the patients whose fractures were left unreduced. Open reduction and internal fixation of unilateral facet dislocations have provided consistently good results. If a unilateral facet dislocation can be reduced in skull traction, halo vest immobilization can be used for 3 months, with the possibility that stability would be obtained by spontaneous fusion. If skull traction does not reduce the dislocation, however, proceed with open reduction and posterior cervical fusion with either triple wiring or oblique facet wiring for additional rotational control. Postoperative treatment consists of immobilization in a rigid cervical orthosis for 6-8 weeks.

Often patients present with chronic pain, limitation of rotation, and radiculopathy caused by a unilateral jump facet that was either missed initially or was allowed to heal unreduced. For these patients with nerve root impingement and chronic pain, foraminotomy with decompression of the involved nerve root and posterior cervical fusion over the involved segment is recommended. Reduction with traction may be attempted, but this usually is impossible.

B. Types of cord injuries
Complete and incomplete cord injuries: The importance of determining whether a patient has a complete or incomplete cord injury is needed. By definition, an incomplete spinal cord injury (SCI) is one in which some motor or sensory function is spared distal to the cord injury. A complete SCI is manifested by total motor and sensory loss distal to the injury. When the bulbocavernosus reflex is positive, and no sacral sensation or motor function has returned, the paralysis is permanent

and complete in most patients. An incomplete spinal cord syndrome may be a Brown–Séquard syndrome, central cord syndrome, anterior cord syndrome, posterior cord syndrome, or rarely monoparesis of the upper extremity 90% of incomplete lesions produce a central cord syndrome, a Brown–Séquard syndrome, or an anterior cervical cord syndrome.

Central cord syndrome is the most common. This syndrome usually results from a hyperextension injury in an older individual with pre-existing osteoarthritis of the spine. There is compression of the cord anteriorly by osteophytes and posteriorly by ligamentum flavum. The syndrome is also associated with fracture dislocation and compression fractures.

- More centrally situated cervical tracts tend to be more involved—possible explanation is relatively loose texture and rich vascularization of the central cord region which allows the extension of edema and hemorrhage along the central canal in a longitudinal direction. The other possibility is relative vascular insufficiency in the terminal area of the anterior spinal artery.
- Disproportionally greater motor impairment of the upper than of the lower extremities.
- Perianal sensation and some lower extremity movement and sensation may be preserved; hands are more severely involved than legs.
- In milder lesions, only the pain and temperature sensation are lost that are carried by the spinothalamic tracts and cross midline.
- High percentage of patients will attain ambulatory function, bladder and bowel control, and hand function.

Brown–Séquard syndrome: Result of hemisection of spinal cord caused by gunshot or stab wound. It is usually associated with fractures of lateral mass of vertebrae. The nontraumatic causes include neoplasms, multiple sclerosis, disk herniation, cervical spondylosis, direct herniation of the spinal cord through a defect in the dura, pressure due to an epidural hematoma, dissection in the vertebral artery, transverse myelitis, radiation, intravenously drug abuse, TB, decompression sickness, etc. A slowly progressive Brown–Séquard syndrome suggests spinal cord compression on one side, such as by a prolapsed intervertebral disk.

- Ipsilateral upper motor neuron (UMN) paralysis (corticospinal) one-two spinal segments below, Babinski sign ipsilateral to the lesion.
- Ipsilateral lower motor neuron (LMN) paralysis or weakness at and/or just below the level of injury.
- There is same sided derangement of fine touch, proprioception and vibration (dorsal column).
- There is same sided derangement of pain and temperature sense but only at the level of lesion.
- There is derangement of crude touch, pain and temperature sense (spinothalamic) on the opposite side at one-two levels below the lesion.
- Horner syndrome could be present on same side due to deranged autonomic function.
- *Brown–Séquard-plus syndrome*: Pure syndrome is extremely rare in clinical practice whereas often there are partial signs of the syndrome along with that of the hemisection syndrome plus additional symptoms and signs referred to as Brown–Séquard plus syndrome.
- If there is no traumatic hemisection, the motor recovery in this syndrome is good. The sequence of recovery is as follows:
  - The ipsilateral proximal extensor muscles recover before the ipsilateral distal flexors
  - The extremity with sensory loss recovers first as compared to the opposite extremity
  - It takes about 1-6 months for voluntary motor strength and a functional gait to recover.

Anterior cord syndrome: It is usually caused by cervical flexion ± rotation, which compresses and damages the anterior part of the spinal cord or anterior spinal artery. It usually occurs in an elderly patient with stenotic cervical spine due to osteophytes and ligament hypertrophy. It may also be produced by anterior dislocation/compression fracture of a vertebral body encroaching the ventral canal. Uncommonly, it may be seen in vascular lesions with thrombosis of the anterior spinal artery and resultant spinal infarction.

- Corticospinal and spinothalamic tracts are damaged either by direct trauma or ischemia of blood supply (anterior spinal arteries).
- Motor function below the lesion is lost bilaterally.
- Pain and temperature sensation are lost bilaterally below the lesion.
- Dorsal columns (vibration and proprioception) remain intact.

Posterior cord syndrome: It is a very rare syndrome caused by compression by tumor or infarction of the posterior spinal artery.
- Proprioception, stereognosis, two-point discrimination and graphesthesia are lost below the lesion—ataxia and faltering gait.
- Motor function is preserved.

A *mixed syndrome* usually is an unclassifiable combination of several syndromes. It describes the small percentage of incomplete spinal cord injuries that do not fit one of the previously described syndromes.

Conus medullaris syndrome, or injury of the sacral cord (conus) and lumbar nerve roots within the spinal canal, usually results in areflexic bladder, bowel, and lower extremities. Most of these injuries occur between T11 and L2 and result in flaccid paralysis in the perineum and loss of all bladder and perianal muscle control. The irreversible nature of this injury to the sacral segments is evidenced by the absence of the bulbocavernosus reflex and the perianal wink. Motor function in the lower extremities between L1 and L4 may be present if nerve root sparing occurs.

Cauda equina syndrome, or injury between the conus and the lumbosacral nerve roots within the spinal canal, also results in areflexic bladder, bowel, and lower limbs. With a complete cauda equina injury, all peripheral nerves to the bowel, bladder, perianal area, and lower extremities are lost, and the bulbocavernosus reflex, anal wink, and all reflex activities in the lower extremities are absent, indicating absence of any function in the cauda equina. The cauda equina functions as the peripheral nervous system, and there is a possibility of return of function of the nerve rootlets if they have not been completely transected or destroyed. Most often, cauda equina syndrome manifests as a neurologically incomplete lesion.

(Details on dissociated sensory loss, Foix-Alajouanine syndrome and contusion cervicalis posterior can be read from Chapter 95 of the book Essential Orthopedics: Principles and Practice, 2nd edition.)

C. Role of methylprednisolone (MP)

MP has been evaluated in various studies over past few decades and has found favors, but more importantly criticisms to its use. The applicability of MP was derived from animal studies and its theoretical ability to suppress or ameliorate many of the pathophysiological processes causing secondary SCI. The neuroprotective effects of MP have been proposed to be due to various mechanisms like:
- Inhibition of lipid peroxidation
- Attenuation of anti-inflammatory cytokines
- Suppression of proinflammatory cytokine expression
- Prevention of calcium influx into cells
- Improved microvascular perfusion
- Inhibition of nitric oxide production
- Inhibition of apoptosis.

The reason why MP was chosen was its higher efficiency to inhibit lipid peroxidation (compared to other peers). The use of MP has undergone three multicenter clinical trials collectively referred to as National Acute Spinal Cord Injury Study (NASCIS). These trials evoked the clinical practice of higher doses of MP to patients acute SCI and became popular world-wide. The impact of trials was so high and lasting that the practice still continues despite criticism and lack of definite evidence. The following is a summary of the three NASCIS trials:
1. *First trial*: Two relatively low doses of MP after traumatic SCI (Bracken et al., 1984) given within 48 hours of SCI.
2. *Second trial* much higher dose of MP (still currently practiced dose of 30 mg/kg bolus with 5.4 mg/kg/h infusion) compared to naloxone (opioid antagonist) and a placebo (Bracken et al. 1990).
3. *Third trial* evaluated the timing of initiation and duration of MP treatment (Bracken et al., 1997). NASCIS 3 compared the 24- and 48-hour infusions of NASCIS 2 doses of MP against trilazad mesylate (antioxidant that inhibits lipid peroxidation in steroid independent pathway). The treatments were given within 8 hours of SCI.

Criticisms of NASCIS trials: There are detailed publications outlining the criticisms on the conduct of the NASCIS trials (especially, NASCIS 2), statistical analysis interpretations and conclusion drawn from them. A few are outlined below:
- Actually, in none of the trials any definitive benefit of the therapeutic interventions was ever revealed. NASCIS 3 also revealed indifferent result with respect to the treatment duration and only post hoc analysis showed some benefit for earliest interventions. The trial failed to show improvement in primary outcome measures like motor scores, pinprick scores and light touch scores which could mean that improved recovery with methylprednisolone may be random

events, thus weakening the overall study findings. The significant difference was only revealed after subgrouping the patients.
- None of the studies addressed the confounding variables. NASCIS 2 trial did not include information about other interventions such as radiology, surgical manipulations, or the extent of rehabilitative therapies, which could contribute to improvements.
- One should clearly understand that the trials did not include pediatric spinal cord injuries, penetrating spinal cord injuries and cauda equine injuries so there is no rationale to use of MP in these patients (as is still blindly followed at some centers).

Conclusions that can be drawn from the above discussion are that:
- Methylprednisolone therapy should be avoided 8 hours after the SCI.
- In pediatric spinal cord injuries, penetrating injuries, and possibly cauda equina injuries also, MP should not be used until specifically studied.
- Expecting benefit in neurological recovery in patients after SCI from MP administrations is more theoretically guided than experimentally substantiated so false hope to self or relatives of patient should not be given over the use of this drug.
- If used, one should adequately cover the patients with appropriate management for complications of MP, which can even be fatal in due course.

116. Draw the cross-section of spinal cord.
Ans: The cross-section of spinal cord is depicted in **Figure 3.5.1**.

117. Discuss the pathophysiology and pharmacological treatment of acute spinal cord injury.
Ans: *Pathophysiology*: There are both primary and secondary mechanisms of injury that may affect the final outcome of SCI. The best prognostic indicator is the patient's neurologic grade at presentation, there are a further majority of patients that deteriorate or fail to respond to optimal treatment given due to secondary injury mechanisms. Both will, hence, be discussed below.

Primary injury: The central gray matter sustains most damage by the initial trauma and the white matter is relatively spared possibly due to the softness of former. These primary mechanisms cause blood flow disruption and hemorrhages within the cord. This leads to hypoxia and ischemia. A central hemorrhagic area of necrosis marks the "epicenter" injury. This is surrounded by surviving axons in a centrifugal distribution. This centrifugal pattern of loss occurs due to longitudinal displacement of the cord's central content. The toothpaste theory explains these events that are similar to those occurring in a compressed toothpaste tube.

The main five features of the primary injury are:
1. *Pinching or contact pressure*: The former is due to pressure on the cord from opposite side (hematoma, neoplasia, etc.) while latter is pressure transmitted from same side (prolapsed disk, infolded ligaments, osteophytes). In cervical spinal injuries, there may be persistent pinching, such as from bilateral facet interlocking or temporary pinching such as from hyperextension sprains.
2. Impact plus persistent compression (e.g., burst fractures with retropulsed bone fragment).
3. Impact alone with transient compression (hyperextension injury in patients with degenerative spine).
4. *Distraction*: The shearing and forcible stretching of spinal cord is a component of various SCI mechanisms. Possibly this is the common mode of injury in SCI without radiographic abnormalities (SCIWORA) in adults with degenerative spine and in children with cartilaginous vertebrae.
5. *Laceration/transection*: This results often from missile injury, sharp bone fragment dislocation, or severe distraction. The injury may be complete or incomplete as described above.

Axonal tear is caused in the cord when tissue velocity exceeds 0.5–1 ms^{-1}. As the central part of the cord is the place where stretch velocities are maximum, it becomes the most common site for tears due to stretch and shearing forces. Most of the neural stretch injuries are seen at nodes of Ranvier.

Secondary mechanisms of injury: These build upon the primary mechanisms at the primary injury sites as a focus of injury. The secondary mechanisms are either the continuations of primary injury (continued compression) or more or less the reactions of body to primary injury and in time though meant for recovery, prove to be deleterious. The disturbances ultimately lead to neuronal necrosis, apoptosis, scarring and cyst formation, demyelination and disruption of the morphofunctional nerve pathways (see below in rehabilitation). The most common secondary mechanism is persistence of compression from primary injury. The other causes of secondary injury are neurogenic shock, reperfusion injury after hemorrhage and ischemia, secondary injury mediated by intracellular calcium release, fluid electrolyte imbalance, immunologic injury, injury due to apoptosis and disturbed mitochondrial function and excitotoxicity.

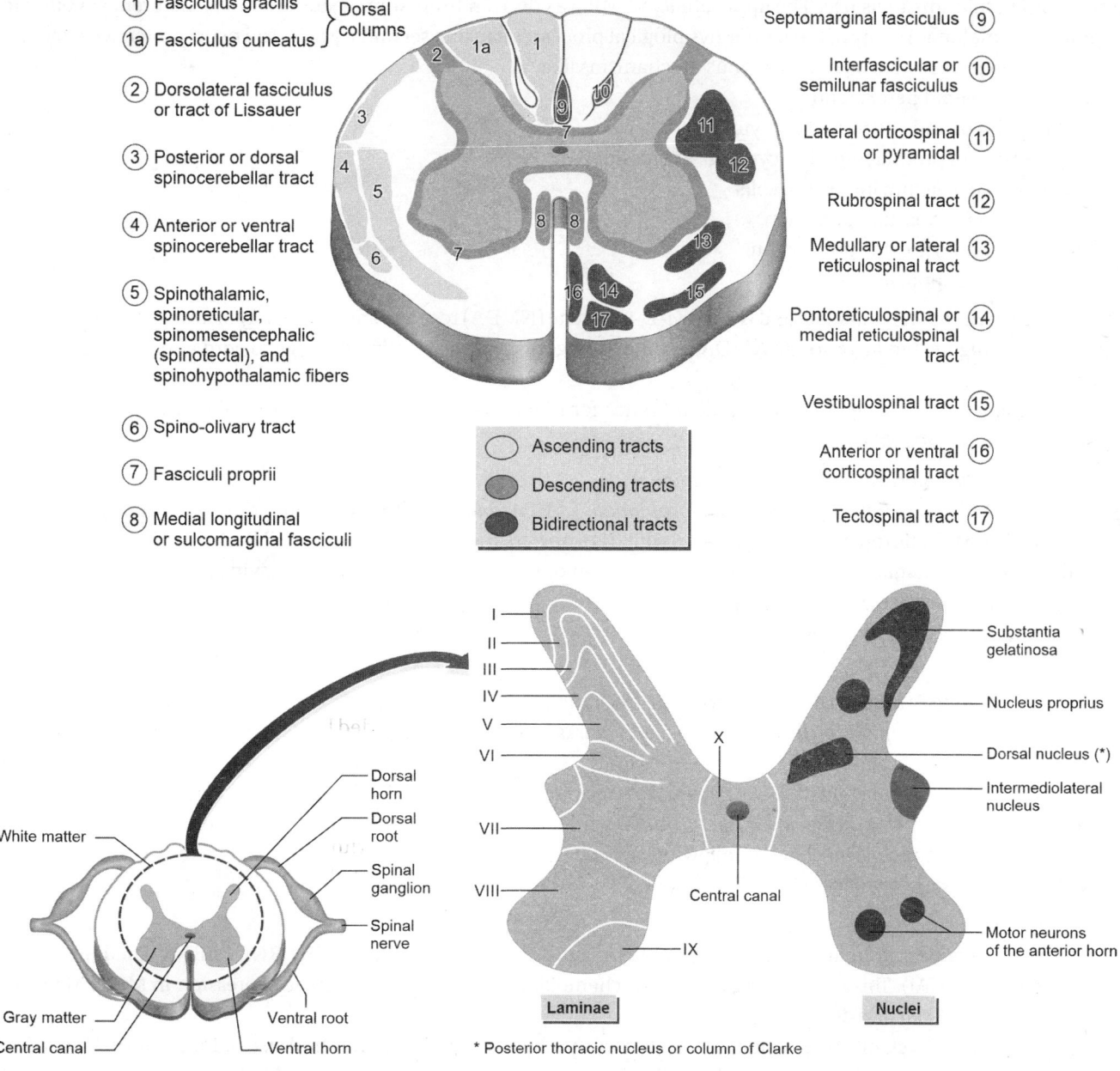

Fig. 3.5.1: The cross-section of spinal cord depicting various tracts and nuclei.

Pharmacological treatment: No standard or definitive recommendation for use of any neuroprotective agent exists, this includes steroids.

Methylprednisolone therapy if initiated is stopped as early as possible in neurologically normal patients and where prior neurologic symptoms have resolved.

Role of pharmacotherapy in immediate management: Based on the pathophysiology discussed above, there are a lot of experimental and evolutive strategies under development, some do have potential to become the future standard of care (none currently definitively recommended):

Anti-inflammatory Strategies
Corticosteroids: Typically, MP has been evaluated in various studies over past few decades and has found favors, but more importantly criticisms to its use. The applicability of MP was derived from animal studies and its theoretical ability to suppress or ameliorate many of the pathophysiological processes causing secondary SCI. The neuroprotective effects of MP have been proposed to be due to various mechanisms like:
- Inhibition of lipid peroxidation
- Attenuation of anti-inflammatory cytokines
- Suppression of proinflammatory cytokine expression
- Prevention of calcium influx into cells
- Improved microvascular perfusion
- Inhibition of nitric oxide production
- Inhibition of apoptosis.

Antiexcitotoxic agents: As glutamate and N-methyl-D-aspartate (NMDA) receptors are intimately involved in excitotoxicity, it is an intriguing idea to incorporate NMDA receptor antagonists for preventing damage to cord after SCI (secondary injury).
- Gacyclidine was evaluated in a large trial in France for human SCI based upon its observed neuroprotective effect seen in animal models.

Other strategies for antiexcitotoxic agents include:
- α-amino-3-hydroxyl-5-methyl-4-isoxazole propionate (AMPA) blockers: The KDI tripeptide domain of γ1-chain of laminin is a synthetic tripeptide (Lys–Asp–Ile) which is a universal and potent inhibitor of NMDA, AMPA, and of kainite subclasses of glutamate receptors. It facilitates axon guidance, modulated electrical activity, and has been found to promote the survival of rat hippocampal neurons.
- Metabotropic receptor-kainate-blockers

Antiapoptotic strategies:
- *Block the apoptotic trigger*: Drugs that scavenge free radicals, approaches target early premitochondrial alterations.
- *Activation of antiapoptotic pathways*: This strategy works by inhibiting caspase-3 activity and protects neurons from ischemic injury.
- An NMDA receptor antagonist MK-801 could reduce apoptosis and reverse impairment following SCI.
- *Protease inhibitors or caspase and calpain inhibitors*: Direct caspase inhibitors (caspase-9 inhibitor z-LEHD-fmk) decrease the morphological changes following SCI and improve outcome.
- Poly (ADP-ribose) polymerase (PARP) inhibitors.

Stem cell and gene therapy:
- Silencing of gene can be achieved by Micro RNA (miRNA) and small interfering RNA (siRNA) mediated RNA interference (RNAi). This can be used to stop CC chemokine receptor 1 (CCR1) gene expression in MCCLM3 cells, and thus inhibit cell invasion.
- Increasing local levels of cAMP enhances the efficacy of Schwann cell transplants and also reduces the production of inflammatory cytokine TNF-α. Stem cell therapy is being tried to increase the local cAMP levels.

118. Discuss whiplash injury of cervical spine, clinical features, diagnosis, and treatment.
Ans: (Also known as: acceleration injury, cervical sprain syndrome, soft tissue neck injury)

Definition: It is an unconventional and inconsequential ligamentous injury of the cervical spine due to an extension injury that follows sudden rapid acceleration-deceleration force following a rear-end collision in a road traffic accident (RTA). In original description in 1928 whiplash was considered to occur due to hyperflexion following a hyperextension of the cervical spine but it is now clear that such extreme movements are not mandatory rather the rapidity of occurrence of alternative movements is needed.

Incidence:
- It is seen in about one-fifth of rear-end collision of RTAs.
- Seventy percent of those affected are women.
- It is common in the 3rd or 4th decades.

Phases of whiplash: There are four phases of whiplash injury as follows:

Phase 1: Vehicle seat moves forward while the head is stationary → torso flattens against the seat resulting in upward acceleration on cervical spine (joints and disk compressed) → head strikes head restraint.

Phase 2: Torso accelerating forward (enhanced more by the forward recoil of seatback) but head still moving back (relative). This causes shear injury to the muscles of neck and soft tissues (ligaments, etc.).

Phase 3: Head and neck start forward movement while torso is rewinding into flexion.

Phase 4: Head and neck in peak forward flexion while torso moving back or stationary due to seat belt. Unrestrained forward movement of head causes stretching of the neck muscles and ligaments tearing the fibers in spinal disk. Concussion may occur if head strikes steering or windshield.

Clinical Features

Symptoms:
- Upper neck pain that becomes worse with movement—radiates to occiput and shoulder blades
- Occipital headache
- Temporomandibular joint dysfunction
- Neck stiffness
- Rarely vertigo, auditory or visual disturbances, etc.—related to concussion
- Low back pain—usually delayed onset.

Signs:
- Decreased range of neck movements
- Neck muscle spasm is seen.

Symptoms appear within 48 hours of injury and recovery is seen in most within three months. Some one-fifth of patients continue to suffer from pain, weakness, and restricted movements where final state is reached by 1 year.

Investigations: X-rays are usually normal. MRI helps to make a diagnosis.

Treatment

It is mainly conservative and consists of the following:
- *Drugs*: Nonsteroidal anti-inflammatory drugs, muscle relaxants, etc. are given.
- *Orthosis (SOMI brace)*: Recommended for the first 3 days.
- Short arc active movements are slowly begun.
- Active ROM exercises are slowly commenced. Trigger point injections and epidural/spinal injections may be given for pain control.
- After the pain subsides, isometric strengthening exercises are slowly commenced.
- Other modalities take ultrasound, traction, manipulation, massage, etc. also help.
- Surgery may be needed for prolapsed disk causing neural compression symptoms.

119. A. What is concept of spinal stability? Describe checklist for diagnosis of clinical instability in the lower cervical spine.

   B. Discuss Canadian C-spine rule.

Ans: A. According to White and Panjabi, spinal stability is its ability to maintain patterns of displacement and movement under normal physiological loads without incapacitating pain, progressive deformity, or increasing neurologic deficit.

- Clinical instability may be caused by trauma, neoplastic or infectious disorders, or iatrogenic causes. Instability may be acute or chronic.
    a. Acute instability is caused by bone or ligament disruption that places the neural elements in danger of injury with any subsequent loading or deformity.
    b. Chronic instability is the result of progressive deformity that may cause neurological deterioration, prevent recovery of injured neural tissue, or cause increasing pain or decreasing function.
- *Radiological stability is described as per Denis concept*: Denis developed a three-column concept of spinal injury using a series of more than 400 CT scans of thoracolumbar injuries. The anterior column contains the anterior longitudinal ligament, the anterior half of the vertebral body, and the anterior portion of the annulus fibrosus. The middle column consists of the posterior longitudinal ligament, the posterior half of the vertebral body, and the posterior aspect of the annulus fibrosus. The posterior column includes the neural arch, the ligamentum flavum, the facet capsules, and the interspinous ligaments. Denis noted that one or more of the three columns predictably failed in axial compression, axial distraction, or translation from combinations of forces in different planes.

The instability in cervical spine may be assessed clinically by stretch test as follows:

The stretch test (never do this in an obviously unstable injury): The cervical spine is stretched (using Crutchfield tongs traction or head halter traction + gradually increasing weights) and the changes are recorded on X-rays. Neural status is measured with each addition of weight until one third body weight traction has been applied (or the test becomes positive in between). The test is positive if there is a neurological deficit or some abnormal separation (>1.7 mm difference in interspace or angle between prestretch condition and maximal weights is 7.5°) of anterior or posterior elements occur (or both happens). This test measures the displacement patterns of the spine under carefully controlled conditions and identifies anterior or posterior disrupted ligaments.

Checklist for diagnosis of clinical instability in the lower cervical spine

White and Panjabi systematically cut the various supporting structures in cadavers and noted the resulting instabilities of the spine. Distinct anterior and posterior supporting structures were found for cervical spine. If a motion segment has all the anterior elements and one posterior element intact, or all the posterior elements and one anterior element intact, it can remain stable under physiological loads. White, Southwick, and Panjabi suggested that a motion segment should be considered unstable if all the anterior or posterior elements are not functional. They developed a checklist for the diagnosis of clinical instability of the lower cervical spine **(Table 3.5.2)**, in which a score of 5 or more indicates instability.

TABLE 3.5.2: Point system for evaluation of cervical spine instability.

Element	Point Value
Anterior elements destroyed or unable to function	2
Posterior elements destroyed or unable to function	2
Relative sagittal plane translation >3.5 mm	2
Relative sagittal plane rotation >11°	2
Positive stretch test	2
Medullary (cord) damage	2
Root damage	1
Abnormal disc narrowing	1
Dangerous loading anticipated	1

B. **Canadian C-spine rule (Flowchart 3.5.1)**

Flowchart 3.5.1: The Canadian Spine Rule flowchart to determine when imaging is needed in alert patient.

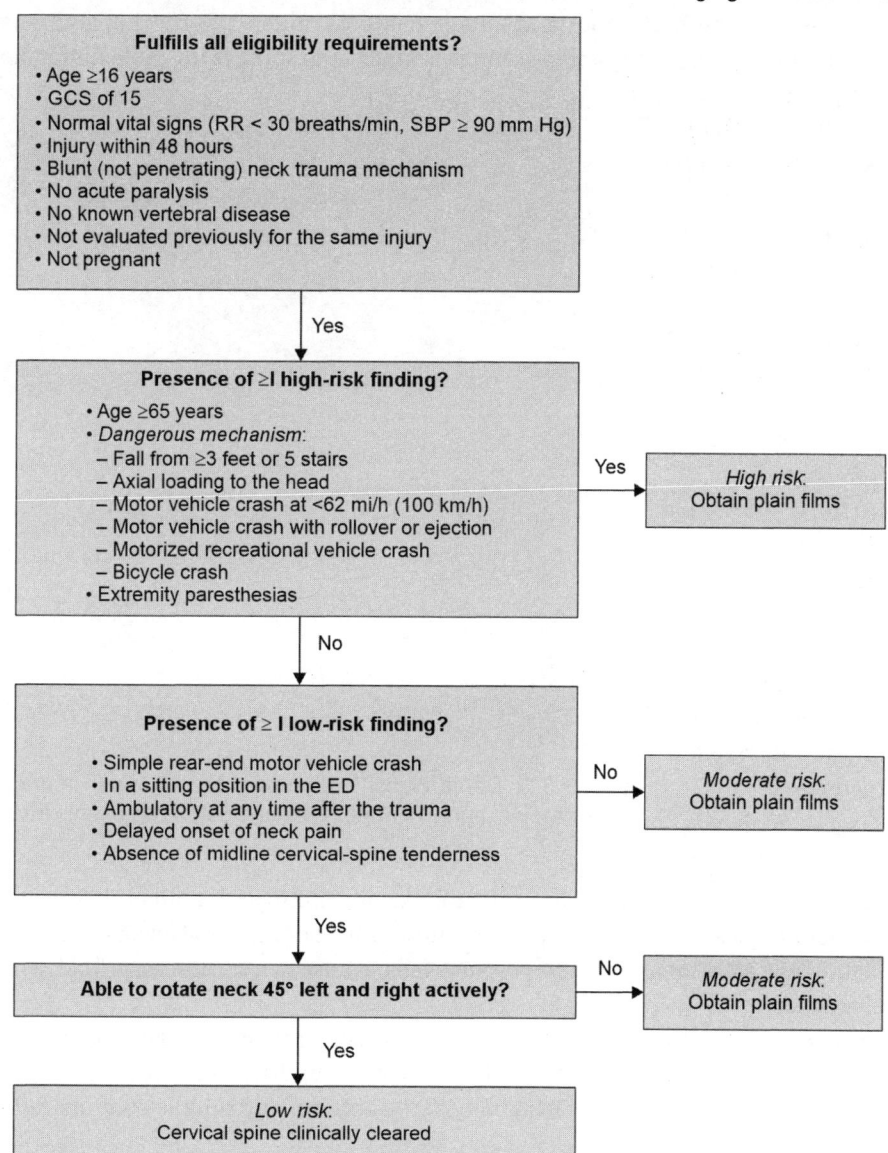

120. Classify injuries of thoracolumbar spine. Also, outline the management.

Ans: *Classification*: Holdsworth classified thoracolumbar fractures based on two columns concept that was improved by Denis three columns concept **(Fig. 3.5.2)**. Denis classification includes minor and major injuries. The major injuries include:

- *Compression fractures*: Anterior column fracture with middle acting as a hinge. Posterior column may fail under tension. Intact middle column prevents subluxation of retropulsion. This is further subclassified into four subtypes.
- *Burst fracture*: Both anterior and middle columns fail under axial load. Subtypes are:
  - *Type A*: Both endplates involved. Bone retropulsed into the canal.
  - *Type B*: Superior end-plate fracture under combined axial load and flexion.
  - *Type C*: Inferior end-plate fracture.
  - *Type D*: Burst rotation due to axial load and rotation moment.

- *Type E*: Burst lateral flexion, similar to lateral flexion but interpedicular distance increased.
- *Seatbelt type injury*: Failure of both posterior and middle columns under hyperflexion and tension forces. Though there is damage to anterior cortex but the anterior hinge is intact. The spine is unstable under flexion but there is no subluxation. Subtypes are:
  - *One-level injury*: This is a chance fracture going through bone or a ligamentous disruption passing through posterior ligamentous complex and the intervertebral disk.
  - *Two-level injury*: The middle column is ruptured either through the bone or the disk. This injury pattern is comparable to Hangman's fracture.
- *Flexion-dislocations*: They are failure of all three columns under compression, tension, rotation, or shear. It is similar to seat-belt-type injury with disrupted anterior hinge and some degree of dislocation is present. These are subclassified into flexion-rotation, flexion-distraction, and shear type fractures.

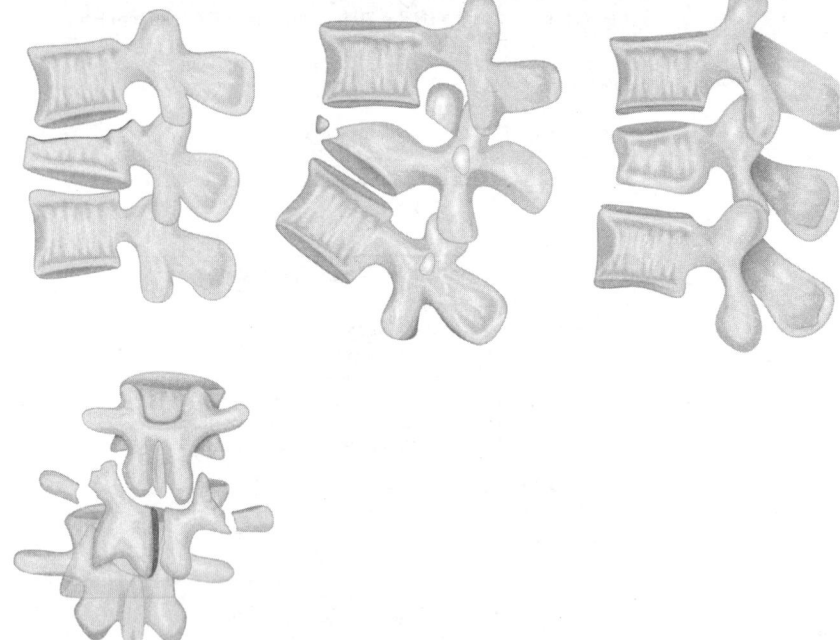

Fig. 3.5.2: Denis classification of thoracolumbar injuries (from left to right: compression, burst, seat-belt type and below represents fracture dislocation type).

Classification by McAfee et al.: This is a simplified version of Denis system **(Table 3.5.3)**.

- *Wedge compression fractures* cause isolated failure of the anterior column and result from forward flexion. They rarely are associated with neurological deficit except when multiple adjacent vertebral levels are affected.
- In *stable burst fractures,* the anterior and middle columns fail because of a compressive load, with no loss of integrity of the posterior elements.
- In *unstable burst fractures,* the anterior and middle columns fail in compression, and the posterior column is disrupted. The posterior column can fail in compression, lateral flexion, or rotation. There is a tendency for post-traumatic kyphosis and progressive neural symptoms because of instability. If the anterior and middle columns fail in compression, the posterior column cannot fail in distraction.
- *Chance fractures* are horizontal avulsion injuries of the vertebral bodies caused by flexion around an axis anterior to the anterior longitudinal ligament. The entire vertebra is pulled apart by a strong tensile force.
- In *flexion distraction injuries,* the flexion axis is posterior to the anterior longitudinal ligament. The anterior column fails in compression, whereas the middle and posterior columns fail in tension. This injury is unstable because the ligamentum flavum, interspinous ligaments, and supraspinous ligaments usually are disrupted.
- *Translational injuries* are characterized by malalignment of the neural canal, which has been totally disrupted. Usually, all three columns have failed in shear. At the affected level, one part of the spinal canal has been displaced in the transverse plane.

Management: Medical management and stabilization of patient with initiation of measures for SCI takes precedence over surgical stabilization. SCI management is done on standard lines like protection of cord from further injury, pharmacotherapy and decompression as needed. The management of thoracolumbar fractures can take nonoperative or operative path depending on various parameters.

Nonoperative management: All stable thoracolumbar injuries without involvement of neurology are managed with thoracolumbar orthoses. There may be an increase in kyphosis during the course of management but up to 30° worsening has not been found to clinically deteriorate the results.

TABLE 3.5.3: Thoracolumbar injury classification and severity score.	
	Points
Fracture mechanism	
Compression fracture	1
Burst fracture	1
Translation/rotation	3
Distraction	4
Neurological involvement	
Intact	0
Nerve root	2
Cord, conus medullaris, incomplete	3
Cord, conus medullaris, complete	2
Cauda equina	3
Posterior ligamentous complex integrity	
Intact	0
Injury suspected/indeterminate	2
Injured	3
Score of ≤3—nonoperative treatment	
Score of ≥5—operative treatment	
Score of 4—either nonoperative or operative treatment, depending on qualifiers such as comorbid medical conditions and other injuries	

Operative management: Operative management is indicated for all unstable thoracolumbar injuries (flexion distraction injuries, unstable burst fractures and fracture dislocations, AO type A4, B1, B2, B3 and C injuries, kyphosis >30°) that cannot be reliably stabilized by nonoperative measures and those injuries where involvement of neurology needs decompression (incomplete neurological deficit, progressive neurological deficit, and spinal cord compression) for deemed improvement in function. Surgical management also avoids the morbidity associated with conservative management in patients with polytrauma, obesity, and skin complications where early mobilization is needed. Ultimately an individual decision is needed weighing the benefits of surgical treatment against potential surgical morbidity. Also, progressive neurological deficit needs urgent decompression and stabilization. Compression of the neural elements by retropulsed bone fragments can be relieved indirectly by the insertion of posterior instrumentation or directly by exploration of the spinal canal through a posterolateral or anterior approach. The indirect approach to decompression of the spinal canal generally involves insertion of posterior instrumentation. These techniques use the distraction instrumentation and the intact posterior longitudinal ligament to reduce the retropulsed bone from the spinal canal. Severely comminuted fractures with multiple pieces of bone pushed into the spinal canal may not be completely reduced by distraction instrumentation. The posterolateral technique for decompression of the spinal canal is effective at the thoracolumbar junction and in the lumbar spine. In the thoracic spine, where less room is available for the cord, this technique involves increased risk to the neural elements. Posterior short segment fixation (pedicle screw and rods) is the commonly performed surgery that intends to decompress and stabilize the involved segment. The disadvantages include instrumentation failure, pseudarthrosis, infection, risks of SCI, inadequate neurological decompression, insufficient correction of kyphosis and the need for late instrumentation removal. For comminuted body fractures additional anterior reconstruction may be needed to prevent implant failure.

The anterior approach allows direct decompression of the thecal sac and should be combined with anterior instrumentation to achieve stability. To avoid anterior additional surgery various measures have been proposed like intracorporeal bone grafting, vertebroplasty and kyphoplasty, intracorporeal filling with hydroxyapatite or calcium phosphate, use of cross-links, supplemental hook fixation at the levels of the screws and the addition of "intermediate" screw into the fractured vertebra. Acutely painful vertebral compression fractures can be treated with a percutaneous procedure like vertebroplasty where large spinal needles are placed into the fractured vertebral body through a channel made in the pedicle and injecting bone cement into the fractured bone. Balloon kyphoplasty evolved as the next step in the treatment of vertebral compression fractures. This is a minimally invasive procedure involves reduction and fixation. The procedure is performed through small instruments that are inserted into the vertebral body through the pedicle. A small balloon is inflated to restore the height of a collapsed vertebral body and create a cavity inside. The balloon is deflated and withdrawn, and the remaining cavity is filled under low pressure with cement.

Fracture dislocations are severe injuries needing more sturdy stabilization in the form of multilevel spinal fixation (two to three segments above and below the injury).

121. Discuss the clinical presentation of burst fracture L1.

Ans: A burst fracture of the L1 vertebra is a severe spinal injury caused by axial compression (e.g., falls, car accidents). It involves vertebral body collapse with retropulsion of bone fragments into the spinal canal, potentially causing neurological deficits.

1. Symptoms and Signs
A. *Acute symptoms*:
- Severe back pain (localized to L1 region)
- Inability to stand/walk (if unstable or neurological injury)
- Decreased height (if significant vertebral collapse)

B. *Neurological deficits (if spinal cord/cauda equina involved)*:
- Paraplegia (if spinal cord compression at T12-L1)
- Bowel/bladder dysfunction (retention or incontinence)
- Sensory loss (numbness, tingling below injury level)
- Motor weakness (hip flexion/knee extension affected)

C. *Associated injuries*:
- Abdominal trauma (due to proximity to diaphragm/organs)
- Other spinal fractures (e.g., T12 and L2)

2. Physical Examination Findings
- Tenderness on palpation over L1 spinous process
- Kyphotic deformity (visible or palpable step-off)
- Neurological assessment:
  - *Motor*: Hip flexion (L2) and knee extension (L3–L4)
  - *Sensory*: Groin (L1) and anterior thigh (L2)
  - *Reflexes*: Patellar (L4) and Achilles (S1)
- Perianal sensation and anal tone (assess cauda equina syndrome)

122. A. Discuss Denis three columns concept in spinal injuries. B. Describe pathoanatomy of flexion rotation injuries in lumbar spine.

Ans: A. Denis developed a three-column concept **(Fig. 3.5.3)** of spinal injury using a series of more than 400 CT scans of thoracolumbar injuries. The anterior column contains the anterior longitudinal ligament, the anterior half of the vertebral body, and the anterior portion of the annulus fibrosus. The middle column consists of the posterior longitudinal ligament, the posterior half of the vertebral body, and the posterior aspect of the annulus fibrosus. The posterior column includes the neural arch, the ligamentum flavum, the facet capsules, and the interspinous ligaments. Denis noted that one or more of the three columns predictably failed in axial compression, axial distraction, or translation from combinations of forces in different planes.

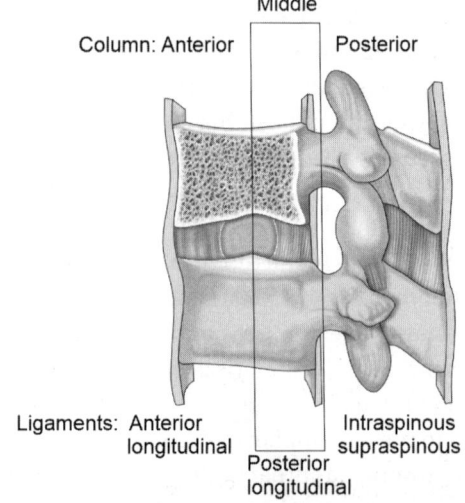

Fig. 3.5.3: The Denis three column concept of spinal injury.

B. (*See diagram in Answer to Question above*). It produces an unstable fracture-dislocation with rupture of the posterior ligament complex, separation of the spinous processes, a slice fracture near the upper border of the lower vertebra, and dislocation of the lower articular processes of the upper vertebra.

123. How will you classify spine injuries based on mechanism? Discuss in brief the clinical diagnosis and treatment of a patient with anterior wedge compression fracture of L1 vertebra.

Ans:
[*The classification of spine injuries will demand mentioning cervical and thoracolumbar injury classification, so the same have been included. Sacral classification is not based on mechanism of injury so excluded, else if you want to write then include Denis classification (kindly look up in Annexure 3 of the book Essential Orthopedics: Principles and Practice, 2nd edition)*].

Classification:
Cervical spine: **Allen–Ferguson classification** (see answer below also on cervical spine injury for detail)
This is based on major injury vector **(Fig. 3.5.4)** producing cervical injuries. The following common types are recognized and widely followed:
- Compression–flexion
- Compression–extension
- Vertical–compression
- Distraction–flexion
- Distraction–extension
- Lateral flexion

Thoracolumbar spine:
Holdsworth classified thoracolumbar fractures has been described above

Clinical diagnosis of anterior wedge compression fracture of L1 vertebra:
- Trauma
- Osteoporotic fracture
- Pathological fracture
- Central type of TB

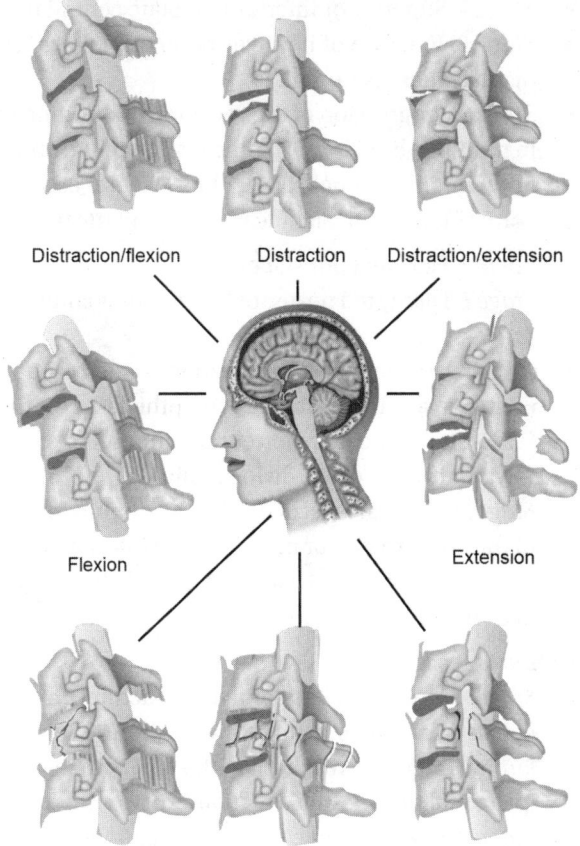

Fig. 3.5.4: The Allen-Ferguson classification of cervical spine injury.

Treatment of vertebral fracture injury management has been described above.

124. What are the current concepts of classification and management of thoracolumbar spine fractures?
Ans: Kindly see Answer to Question no. 120 above.

125. A. Classify cervical spine injuries.
B. Describe diagnosis and treatment of a patient with C5-C6 dislocation in brief.

Ans:
A. Classification by Allen et al.:
Compressive–Flexion—Five Stages:
- *Stage 1*: Blunting of the anterosuperior vertebral margin to a rounded contour + intact posterior longitudinal ligament (PLL)
- *Stage 2*: Stage 1 + anterior wedge compression. Anteroinferior vertebral body "beak" + increased concavity of the inferior end plate + possible vertebral body vertical fracture.
- *Stage 3*: Stage 2 + oblique fracture line from the anterior surface of the vertebra across the body and extending through the inferior subchondral plate + fracture of the beak.

- *Stage 4*: Deformation of the body and fracture of the beak with mild (<3 mm) displacement of the inferoposterior vertebral margin into the spinal canal
- *Stage 5*: Stage 3 + >3 mm of displacement of the posterior portion of the vertebral body into the spinal canal. Intact vertebral arch, the articular facets are separated, and the interspinous process space is increased at the level of injury (tensile posterior ligamentous disruption).

Vertical Compression: Three stages—
- *Stage 1*: Superior or inferior end plate central fracture with a "cupping" deformity.
- *Stage 2*: Fracture of both vertebral end plates with cupping deformities + possible fracture lines through the body, displacement is minimal.
- *Stage 3*: Progression of the vertebral body damage described in stage 2 + fragmented body + peripheral displacement in multiple directions. Significant impaction and fragmentation of body + possible posterior displacement of fractured body into the spinal canal. The vertebral arch may be intact with no evidence of ligamentous failure, or it may be comminuted with significant failure of the posterior ligamentous complex.

Distractive Flexion: Four stages—
- *Stage 1*: Disrupted posterior ligamentous complex (facet subluxation in flexion) + abnormal divergence of the spinous process
- *Stage 2*: Unilateral facet dislocation (Posterior ligamentous failure may be partial to complete [ALL + (Posterior ligament complex failure)]. Subluxation of the facet on the side opposite the dislocation suggests severe ligamentous injury. Widening of the uncovertebral joint on the side of the dislocation + displacement of the tip of the spinous process toward the side of the dislocation.
- *Stage 3*: Bilateral facet dislocations + approximately 50% anterior subluxation of the vertebral body + possible blunting of the anterosuperior margin of the inferior vertebra
- *Stage 4*: Full vertebral body width displacement anteriorly or a grossly unstable motion segment, giving the appearance of a "floating" vertebra

Compressive Extension: Five stages—
- *Stage 1*: Unilateral vertebral arch fracture ± anterior rotatory vertebral displacement. Posterior element failure may consist of a linear fracture through the articular process, impaction of the articular process, and ipsilateral pedicle and lamina fractures, resulting in the "transverse facet" appearance on anteroposterior radiographs, or a combination of ipsilateral pedicle and articular process fractures.
- *Stage 2*: Bilaminar fractures (laminar fractures occur at multiple contiguous levels)
- *Stage 3*: Bilateral vertebral arch fractures + fracture of the articular processes, pedicles, lamina, or some bilateral combination, without vertebral body displacement
- *Stage 4*: Bilateral vertebral arch fractures with partial vertebral body width displacement anteriorly
- *Stage 5*: Bilateral vertebral arch fracture + full vertebral body width displacement anteriorly. The posterior portion of the vertebral arch of the fractured vertebra does not displace, and the anterior portion of the arch remains with the body. Bifocal ligament failure (posteriorly between the fractured vertebra and the one above it and anteriorly between the fractured vertebra and the one below it).

Distractive Extension: Two stages—
- *Stage 1*: Either failure of the anterior ligamentous complex or a transverse fracture of the centrum. There is abnormal widening of the disk space.
- *Stage 2*: Stage 1 + failure of the posterior ligamentous complex, with displacement of the upper vertebral body posteriorly into the spinal canal. Radiographs may be normal because displacement of this type tends to reduce spontaneously when the head is placed in a neutral position.

Lateral Flexion: Two stages—
- *Stage 1*: Asymmetrical compression fracture of the centrum + ipsilateral vertebral arch fracture, without displacement of the arch on the AP view.

- *Stage 2*: Lateral asymmetrical compression of the centrum and either ipsilateral displaced vertebral arch fracture or ligamentous failure on the contralateral side with separation of the articular processes.

B. Diagnosis:
- Plain AP and lateral X-rays show listhesis of vertebrae. If the slip is <50% of the vertebral body, then it is a unilateral facet dislocation and if it is >50%, then it is bifacetal dislocation.
- *CT scan*: To see for locked facets, perched facets and fractures in addition to the degree of slip.
- Reverse hamburger on bun sign is seen at site of dislocated facet.
- *MRI*: To see for degree of cord compression and edema

Treatment:

Unilateral facet dislocation is already described in Q115A.

Bilateral facet dislocation: These injuries are more frequently associated with neurological deficits than are unilateral facet dislocations. These dislocations are more easily reduced with closed traction methods than are unilateral dislocations, but because they are so unstable, redislocation is frequent when they are treated with prolonged skeletal traction or even in a halo vest. Some bilateral facet dislocations heal with spontaneous anterior interbody fusions, but this is unpredictable, and preferred is open reduction and internal fixation with an interspinous process wiring technique, such as the Bohlman triple-wire technique, or oblique wiring from the inferior facet of the upper level to the spinous process of the lower level. Posterior cervical plating also provides stable fixation and is advantageous when laminar and spinous processes are deficient.

126. **A. Classify odontoid fractures. Describe B. Mechanism of injury of odontoid fractures, C. Clinical features, and D. Management.**

Ans:

A. Classification of odontoid fractures:

Anderson D'Alonzo classification of odontoid fractures:
- *Type I*: Fracture of odontoid tip
- *Type II*: Fracture at junction of base and body of odontoid
- *Type III*: Fractures that extend into body of axis

B. Mechanism of injury:

Odontoid fractures represent 20% of cervical spine injury that may result from high energy injury in younger patients or low-energy injury in elderly. Neurological damage is uncommon but may occur as incomplete involvement to quadriparesis.
- Type II odontoid fractures are likely caused by lateral or oblique forces.
- Type III fractures result from extension mechanisms.

C. Clinical features of acute odontiod fractures:

Symptoms: Neck pain worsened with motion, dysphagia may be present when associated with a large retropharyngeal hematoma.

Signs: Usually, mimics myelopathy findings if neurological damage is present. This is, however, very rare due to large cross section area of spinal canal at this level.

D. Management of acute odontoid fractures:

Conservative management: For undisplaced and/or reducible types II and III fractures, Halo vest immobilization is a good option of immobilization if patient can comply with the bulky orthosis. Traction via a halo ring may be initially used to reduce the fracture and then subsequently convert to a halo-thoracic vest.

Operative treatment: General indications for surgical treatment of an odontoid fracture in a younger patient include:
- Fracture displacement >5 mm
- Fracture angulation >10°
- Presence of neurologic deficit or substantial comminution
- Multisystem trauma where external immobilization may not be well tolerated.

Anterior odontoid screw: With respect to fracture morphology, transverse fractures or oblique fractures in which the fracture line runs from anterosuperior to posteroinferior, an odontoid screw is implant of choice for type II fractures. They should not be considered for type I and most type III fractures (barring some rare types).

Posterior C1-C2 fixation: This is the standard surgical procedure of choice. The methods to achieve this are:

Sublaminar wiring techniques, such as the Brooks or Gallie methods, carry the lowest risk of complications but necessitate adjunctive halothoracic immobilization and can accentuate posteriorly displaced fractures.

Transarticular screw fixation requires reasonable reduction of the fracture so that there is sufficient overlap of the C1–C2 lateral masses through which to pass the screws. C1 lateral mass C2 instrumentation is the most versatile fixation method, as it does not require anatomical reduction and, in fact, can be used to help reduce fractures. However, it has a higher risk of complications and is a technically demanding procedure.

Anterior C1-C2 fusion: Although not widely used. Indications include:
- Failure of posterior fusion
- Soft-tissue injury over the proposed posterior surgical incision site
- Contraindication to prone positioning.

127. Discuss the classification of thoracolumbar spine injuries and management of L1 burst fractures.

Ans: Please vide Answer to Question 120.

128. Classify pelvic fractures. Discuss various radiological views and management of rotationally unstable pelvic injuries.

Ans:

Classification

Tile classification had been most popular and describes nearly all important patterns of pelvic injury as shown in **Table 3.5.4 and Figure 3.5.5**.

TABLE 3.5.4: Tile classification of pelvic fracture.	
Type A: Stable (posterior arch intact)	
A1	Avulsion injury
A2	Iliac wing or anterior arch fracture caused by a direct blow
A3	Transverse sacrococcygeal fracture
Type B: Partially stable (incomplete disruption of posterior arch)	
B1	Open book injury (external rotation)
B2	Lateral compression injury (internal rotation)
B2-1	Ipsilateral anterior and posterior injuries
B2-2	Contralateral (bucket-handle) injuries
B3	Bilateral
Type C: Unstable (complete disruption of posterior arch)	
C1	Unilateral
C1-1	Iliac fracture
C1-2	Sacroiliac fracture-dislocation
C1-3	Sacral fracture
C2	Bilateral, with one side type B, one side type C
C3	Bilateral

Young–Burgess classification is now the recommended classification that describes associated instability (**Table 3.5.5 and Fig. 3.5.6**).

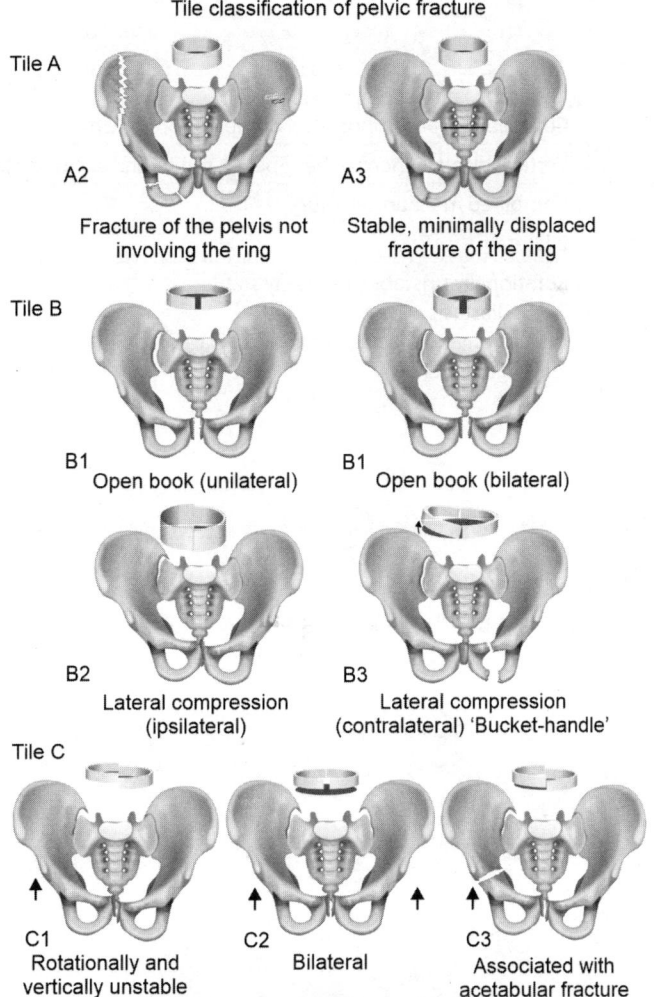

Fig. 3.5.5: Tile classification of pelvic injury.

TABLE 3.5.5: Young–Burgess classification.	
Stable pelvic ring	
Anterior-posterior compression I (APC I)	Pubic diastasis <2.5 cm
Lateral compression I (LC I)	Oblique fracture of pubic rami Ipsilateral anterior compression fracture of sacral ala
Combined mechanical injury	
Partial instability	
Anterior-posterior compression II	Rotationally unstable, vertically stable Pubic diastasis >2.5 cm Disruption and diastasis of anterior part of sacroiliac joint, with intact posterior sacroiliac joint ligaments
Lateral compression II	Rotationally unstable, vertically stable Fracture of pubic rami Posterior fracture with dislocation of ipsilateral iliac wing (crescent fracture)
Combined mechanical injury	

Contd...

Contd...

Complete instability	
Lateral compression III	Ipsilateral lateral compression (LC) Contralateral anteroposterior compression (APC)
Vertical shear	Vertical displacement of hemipelvis, pubic, and sacroiliac joint fractures
	Combined mechanical injury
	Bilateral
APC III	Rotationally unstable, vertically stable Pubic diastasis >2.5 cm Disruption and diastasis of anterior part of sacroiliac joint, with intact posterior sacroiliac joint ligaments

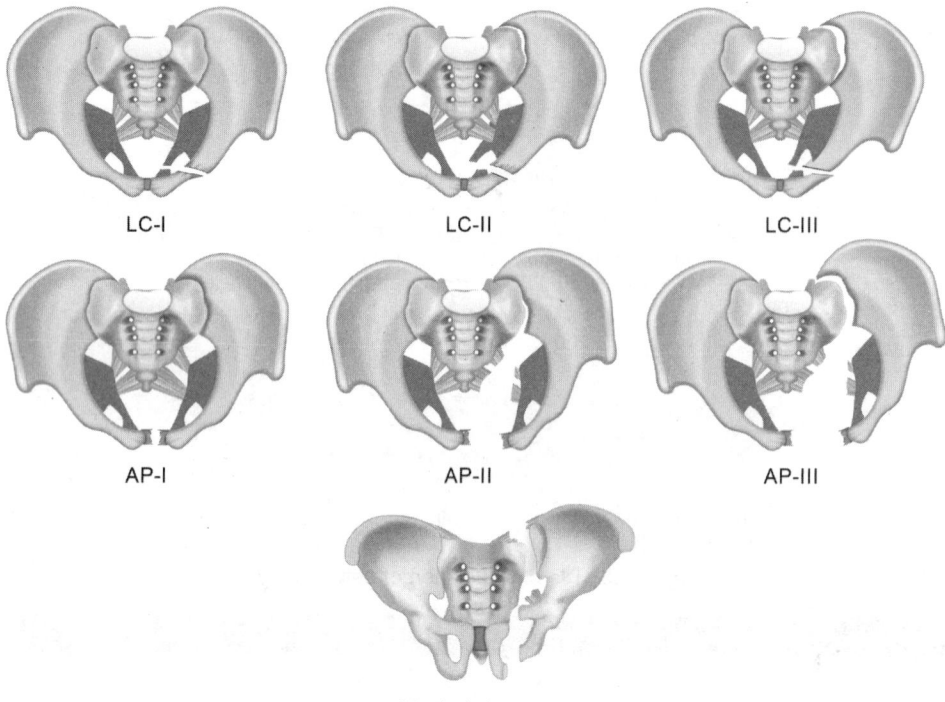

Fig. 3.5.6: Young–Burgess classification.

Radiological views: The standard radiographic projections required for evaluation of pelvic fractures are:
- Anteroposterior view of the pelvis
- *40° caudad inlet*: The inlet view shows rotational deformity or anteroposterior displacement of the hemipelvis.
- *40° cephalad outlet views*: The outlet view shows vertical displacement of the hemipelvis, sacral fractures, and widening or fracture of the anterior pelvis.
- *Stress views*: Push–pull radiographs are performed while the patient is under general anesthesia to assess vertical stability.

Radiographic signs of instability include:
- Sacroiliac displacement of 5 mm in any plane
- Posterior fracture gap (rather than impaction)
- Avulsion of the 5th lumbar transverse process, the lateral border of the sacrum (sacrotuberous ligament), or the ischial spine (sacrospinous ligament).

Management of rotationally unstable fractures: These fractures conform to type B according to Tile's classification. Operative treatment of rotationally unstable pelvic fractures can be accomplished by an anterior external fixator used for definitive treatment or open reduction and internal fixation with anterior plating. Retrograde pubic ramus screws placed percutaneously or with an open technique also have been described. External fixation has been widely described for the definitive treatment of Tile type B (Young and Burgess type AP II) injuries. In the type B injuries, if an adequate reduction (<1 cm displacement) was maintained, 100% of patients were functionally normal; but if the reduction was not maintained, 80% required analgesics for posterior pain. This method may be especially useful in patients with associated genitourinary or gastrointestinal injuries with significant contamination or other soft tissue problems that might preclude anterior open reduction and internal fixation.

129. Describe pelvic ring disruptions: Complications and management.

Ans: Complications—

- *Infection*: The incidence is variable, ranging from 0 to 25%, although the presence of wound infection does not preclude a successful result. The presence of contusion or shear injuries to soft tissues (Morel lesion) is a risk factor for infection if a posterior approach is used. This risk is minimized by a percutaneous posterior ring fixation.
- *Thromboembolism*: Disruption of the pelvic venous vasculature and immobilization constitute major risk factors for the development of deep venous thromboses.
- *Malunion*: Significant disability may result, but it is rare. It is associated with chronic pain, limb length inequalities, gait disturbances, sitting difficulties, low back pain, and pelvic outlet obstruction.
- *Nonunion*: This is rare, although it tends to occur more in younger patients (average age 35 years) with possible sequelae of pain, gait abnormalities, and nerve root compression or irritation. Stable fixation and bone grafting are usually necessary for union.
- Mortality:
  - Hemodynamically stable patients: 3%
  - Hemodynamically unstable patients: 38%
  - *LC*: Head injury major cause of death
  - *APC*: Pelvic and visceral injury major cause of death
  - *AP3 (comprehensive posterior instability)*: 37% death
  - *VS*: 25% death

Management: The recommended management of pelvic fractures varies from institution to institution. A general perspective is presented in **Flowchart 3.5.2**.

Nonoperative

Fractures amenable to nonoperative treatment include:
- Most LC-1 and APC-1 fractures
- Gapping of pubic symphysis <2.5 cm

Rehabilitation

- Protect weight bearing typically with a walker or crutches initially.
- Serial radiographs are required after mobilization has begun to monitor for subsequent displacement.
- If secondary displacement of the posterior ring >1 cm is noted, weight bearing should be stopped.

Operative treatment should be considered for gross displacement.

Absolute Indications for Operative Treatment
- Open pelvic fractures or those in which there is an associated visceral perforation requiring operative intervention
- Open-book fractures or vertically unstable fractures with associated patient hemodynamic instability

Relative Indications for Operative Treatment
- Symphyseal diastasis >2.5 cm (loss of mechanical stability)
- Leg-length discrepancy >1.5 cm
- Rotational deformity
- Sacral displacement

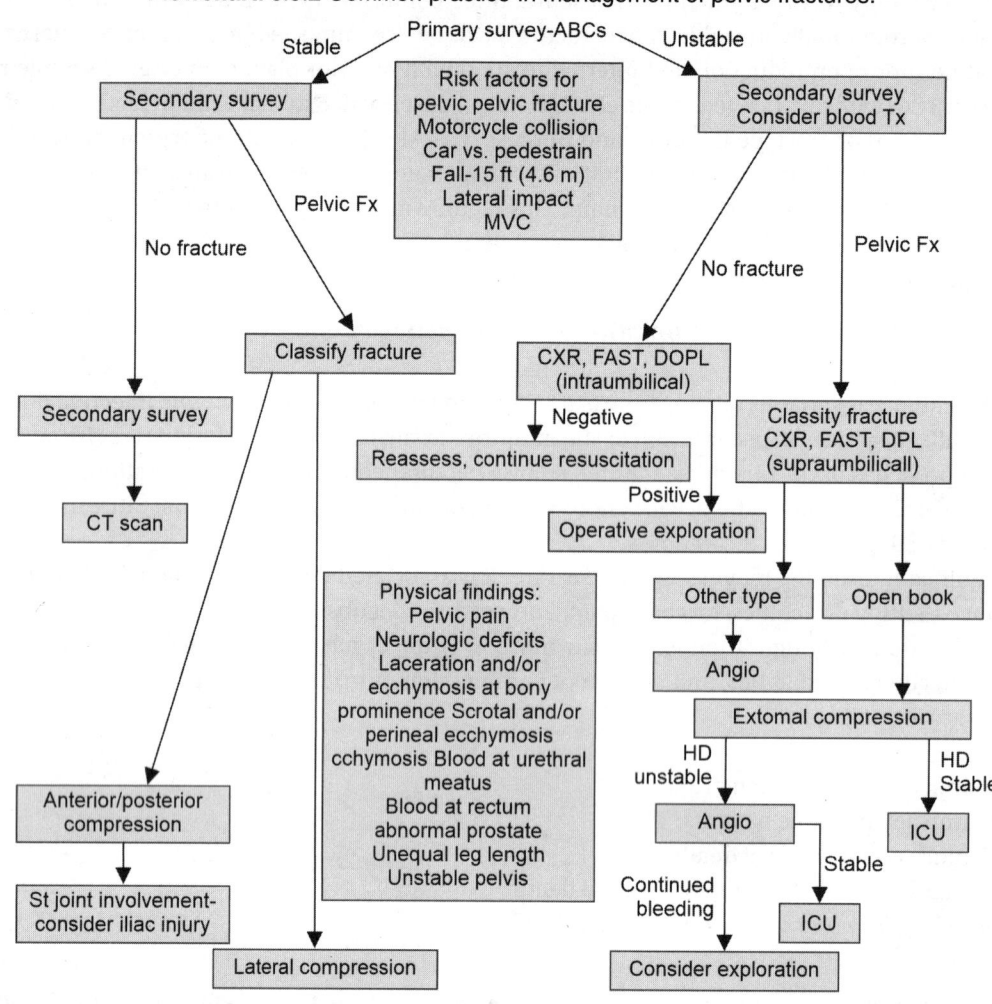

Flowchart: 3.5.2 Common practice in management of pelvic fractures.

130. Describe pathoanatomy, diagnosis, early and late management of urethral and bladder injuries in pelvic fractures.

Ans: Urethral and Bladder Injuries in Pelvic Fractures

I. Pathoanatomy

A. *Mechanism of injury*:
- High-energy trauma (road traffic accidents, crush injuries, and falls).
- Pelvic ring fracture transmits force to urogenital diaphragm and adjacent structures.
- Shearing force → disruption of membranous urethra at bulbomembranous junction (most common).
- Bladder injury from:
  – Blunt trauma with full bladder → rupture at weakest point (dome)
  – Associated pubic rami fractures → direct bladder wall injury

B. *Anatomical considerations*:
- *Male urethra*: Divided into *anterior* (penile and bulbar) and *posterior* (membranous and prostatic) urethra.
- *Posterior urethral injury*: Commonly associated with pelvic fractures.
- *Anterior urethral injury*: Usually from straddle injury (less commonly pelvic fracture).

- *Bladder injuries*:
  - *Intraperitoneal*: Rupture at bladder dome → urine leaks into peritoneum.
  - *Extraperitoneal*: Rupture adjacent to pelvic fracture → urine extravasates into pelvis/retropubic space.
  - Combined: Both patterns.

II. Diagnosis

A. *Clinical clues*:
- Pelvic fracture + any of:
  - Blood at urethral meatus
  - Inability to void
  - High-riding or non-palpable prostate on DRE
  - Perineal/scrotal hematoma
- Suprapubic tenderness/fullness → possible bladder injury.

B. *Investigations*:
- Do not attempt urethral catheterization if urethral injury suspected.
- Retrograde urethrogram (RUG):
  - Gold standard for urethral injury.
  - Contrast outlines urethra and shows extravasation.
- Retrograde cystography (X-ray or CT cystogram):
  - Gold standard for bladder injury.
  - Instill contrast via catheter → check for intraperitoneal/extraperitoneal leak.
- CT pelvis/abdomen with contrast for associated injuries.

III. Management

A. *Early management*:
- *Resuscitation (ATLS principles)*: Treat shock and control bleeding.
- *Bladder drainage*:
  - If urethral injury suspected → perform suprapubic cystostomy (SPC) for urine diversion.
  - If RUG excludes urethral injury → gentle catheterization allowed.
- *Posterior urethral injury*:
  - *Initial*: SPC + delayed repair after 3–6 months (once pelvic hematoma resolves and fibrosis stabilizes).
  - *Rarely*: Immediate endoscopic realignment in stable patients with minimal distraction defect.
- *Anterior urethral injury*:
  - Partial tear → catheterization.
  - Complete tear → SPC + delayed repair.
- *Bladder injuries*:
  - *Intraperitoneal*: Requires immediate surgical repair (2-layer closure + bladder drainage).
  - *Extraperitoneal*: Usually managed conservatively with catheter drainage for 10–14 days unless:
    - Bone fragment intravesical
    - Concomitant bladder neck/rectal/vaginal injury
    - Failure of healing

IV. Late Management (Complications and Treatment)
- Urethral stricture → definitive urethroplasty after 3–6 months.
- *Incontinence*: May require sphincter repair/artificial urinary sphincter.
- Erectile dysfunction: Neurovascular injury; may require counseling, PDE5 inhibitors, or surgery.
- *Chronic urinary tract infection*: Treat with antibiotics, address cause.
- Bladder diverticulum/fistula: Surgical correction.

131. A. Open book injury of pelvis. B. Give a flowchart of management of urethral injury following fracture pelvis.

Ans: A. The open book injury of pelvis is classified variously as follows:

Tile classification: Type B fractures of pelvis are rotationally unstable. Type B1 fractures include "open book" fractures or anterior compression injuries in which the anterior pelvis opens through a diastasis of the symphysis or through a fracture of the anterior pelvic ring. The posterior sacroiliac and interosseous ligaments remain intact. Tile described stages of this injury.
  i. In the first stage, the symphysis separation is less than 2.5 cm, and the sacrospinous ligament remains intact.
  ii. In the second stage, the diastasis is more than 2.5 cm with rupture of the sacrospinous ligament and the anterior sacroiliac ligament.
  iii. In the third stage, the lesions are bilateral, creating a B3 injury.

According to *Young and Burgess classification*, the "open-book" pelvis or APC injury was described as anterior–posterior in nature, but can be from posterior to anterior, and in most cases is caused by severe external rotation of one hemipelvis. With increase in force from anterior to posterior, an external rotation of one or both hemipelvises occurs that gets hinged open anteriorly. The hinge is formed posteriorly across the SI joints. Depending on the strength of forces following stages of incremental ligament damage are seen:

a. *APC type 1*: Intact posterior ligaments with <2.5 cm of symphyseal diastasis anteriorly.
b. *APC type 2*: >2.5 cm (newer studies find 4.5 cm to be more reliable cut-off) of symphyseal diastasis with disrupted anterior sacroiliac ligaments.
c. *APC type 3*: Complete disruption of anterior and posterior sacroiliac ligaments. This is the most unstable pattern resulting in vascular injuries.

Imaging: AP radiograph of pelvis shows widened symphysis. CT scan (Axial and Coronal) cuts showing measurement of > or <2.5 cm at symphysis. 3D reconstructions of AP, inlet, and outlet views.

Treatment: Resuscitate the patient for hemodynamic stability. Closing the pelvic diastasis in open-book–type injuries reduces the pelvic volume available for hemorrhage, thereby improving the chance of tamponade and clot formation. This is now performed using circumferential folded bed sheet or pelvic binders placed at the level of the greater trochanters or external fixators. Adduction and internal rotation of the extremities, if uninjured, can also assist in reducing the pelvic ring fracture. Pneumatic antishock garment (PASG) and MAST are not used now due to high complications and no added advantage. External compression provides the following:

- Closes the open-book pelvic injury, which reduces the pelvic volume thereby allowing for a tamponade effect. Reducing pelvic volume is debatable because pelvis is a hemielliptical and changed radius or diameter does not drastically increase or decrease the volume.
- Stabilizes the pelvic ring injury → compressing and stabilizing associated fractures appears to be the more significant factor controlling bleeding.
- Allows for autotransfusion by returning the blood from the lower extremities to the vascular system.

Pelvic binders are more commonly used than emergent external fixation. However external fixation has additional advantage for the definitive management of some pelvic ring injuries when combined with posterior internal fixation. This is especially useful when anterior stabilization is required and precluded by soft tissue problems or genitourinary injuries. C-clamp are the easiest and fastest to deploy as external fixators for pelvic injury. The fixator internally rotates each hemipelvis, thereby closing an "open-book" injury re-establishing some pelvic ring geometry, but when the posterior ligamentous structures are disrupted, perfect reduction is difficult to obtain and certainly cannot be treated definitively with the anterior frame. C-clamp are superior in this regard because they translate the hemipelvis medially instead of internally rotating it controlling the posterior lesions also better.

B. The **Flowchart 3.5.3** shows management of ureteric injury is as follows:

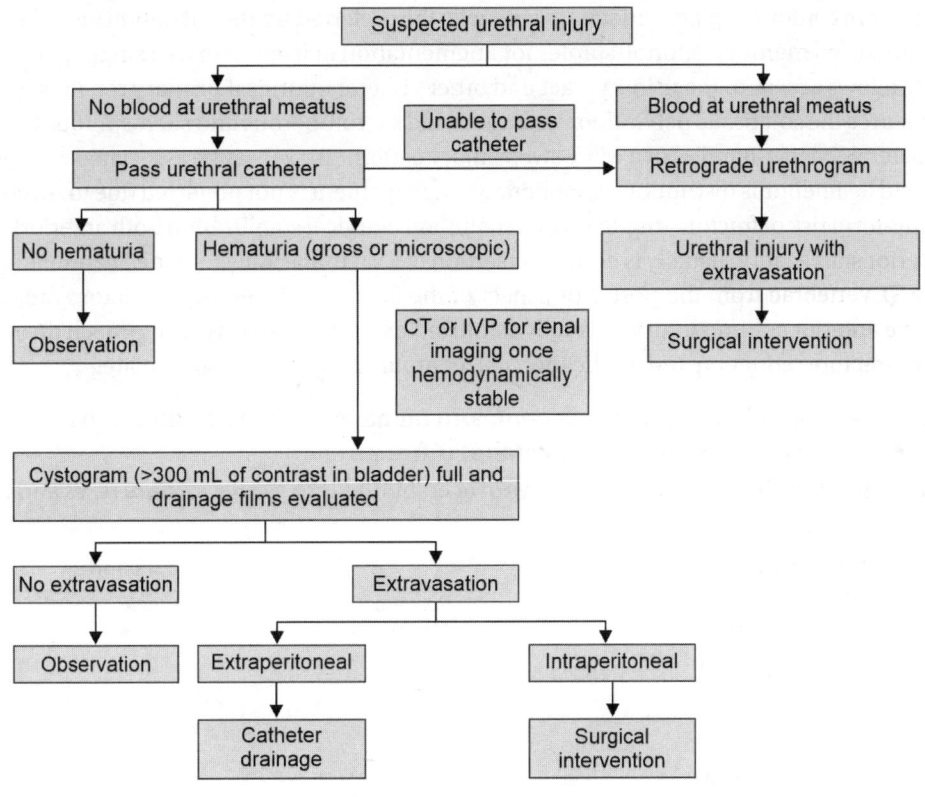

Flowchart 3.5.3: Management of suspected urethral injury in pelvic injury.

132. Principles of treating Tile's type B injury.

Ans: The Tile type B fracture of pelvis includes partially stable (incomplete disruption of the posterior arch), i.e., rotationally unstable, vertically stable fractures of pelvic ring:
- *B1*: Open-book injury (external rotation)
- *B2*: Lateral-compression injury (internal rotation)
  - B2-1: Ipsilateral anterior and posterior injuries
  - B2-2: Contralateral (bucket-handle) injuries
- *B3*: Bilateral

Management principles: The goals are to restore the shape of the pelvic ring and provide stability immediately while in long-term the aim is to avoid fracture non- and malunion that may result in chronic pelvic pain and disability. Immediate attention is to resuscitate the patient and evaluate on the lines of advanced trauma life support.

Definitive management: Type B fractures are vertically stable with intact posterior pelvic structures but are rotationally unstable.
- *B1*: Open-book injuries can be uni- or bilateral and can be minimally (<2.5 cm) or severely (>2.5 cm) displaced on plain radiographs or CT best assessed without pelvic bonder. Minimally displaced (<2.5 cm) pubic symphyseal injuries have an intact pelvic floor and can be managed nonoperatively. Weight-bearing allows compression at the injured site.
- Displaced (>2.5 cm) B1 injuries usually mean injury to pelvic floor structures, sacrospinous and sacrotuberous and anterior sacroiliac ligaments. Bleeding control and stabilization takes priority. Operative management options for displaced B1 fractures are external or internal fixation. External fixation restores volume and limits clot disruption maintaining the tamponade effect. Instead of conventional external fixator pelvic C-clamp may also be used. This is a

quick and relatively straightforward way of obtaining anterior pelvic stability. However, open reduction and internal fixation with a 3.5 mm contoured plate and screws is usually the preferred treatment option for definitive management. Surgeons have also used memory 'Nitinol' staples for augmentation of fixation or as a singular method. Additionally, open procedure allows access to the urinary tract and other visceral injuries if primary repair is needed.

- In type B2-1 fractures the soft tissue pelvic floor structures and sacrotuberous and sacrospinous ligaments are usually intact. A contralateral (bucket-handle) or a wind-swept injury pattern (B2-2) may be associated with vertically instability and soft tissue and ligamentous disruption. Nonoperative management is not preferred due to severe pain; immobility and a higher long-term risk of fracture migration and malunion. Surgical stabilization both anteriorly and posteriorly is preferred. Posterior stabilization usually is done by insertion of a sacroiliac fully threaded cannulated screw (6.5, 7.3 or 8 mm) into the S1 vertebrae from the posterior aspect of the iliac wing inserted well across the sacral ala avoiding compression. The anterior column injury is usually stabilized using a STOPPA-type approach through a Pfannenstiel incision to allow fracture reduction and application of a contoured rim type 3.5 mm plate.

133. **Discuss classification, radiological assessment, and management of acetabular fractures with a note on minimal access surgical management of acetabular fractures.**

Ans: Letournel and Judet classification divides fractures of acetabulum into *simple fracture types* and the more complex *associated fracture types* **(Fig. 3.5.7)**.

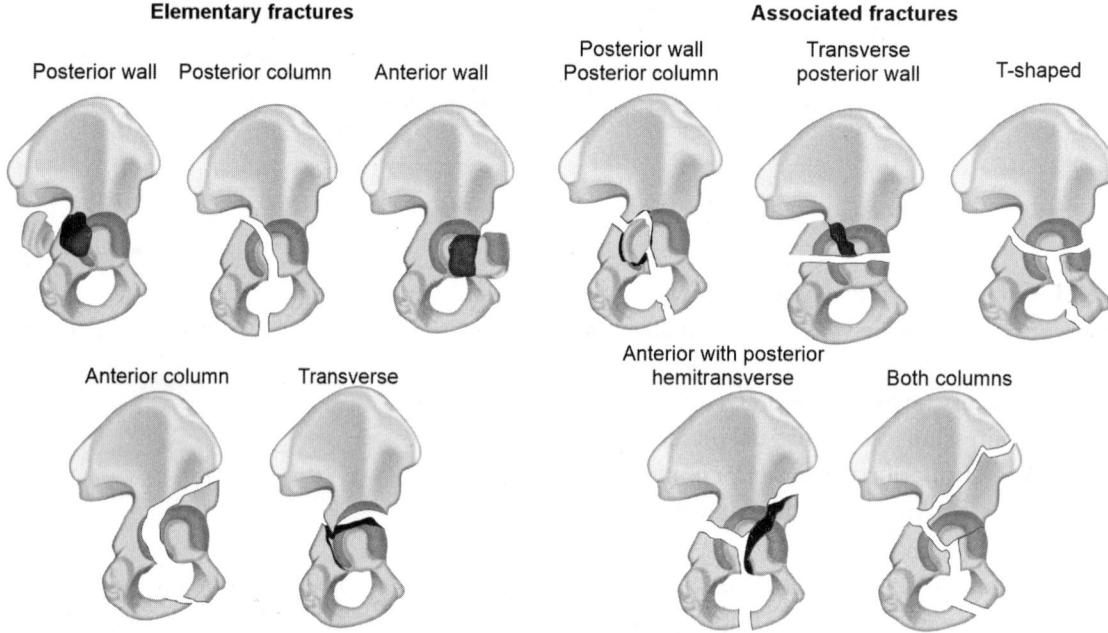

Fig. 3.5.7: Letournel and Judet classification.

Simple fracture types are fractures of:
- The posterior wall
- Posterior column
- Anterior wall
- Anterior column
- Transverse fractures.

Associated fractures include:
- T-type fractures
- Combined fractures of the posterior column and wall

- Combined transverse and posterior wall fractures
- Anterior column fractures with a hemitransverse posterior fracture
- Both-column fractures.

Radiological Assessment

The acetabulum is evaluated radiographically with:
- Anteroposterior pelvic view
- Inlet and outlet views
- 45° oblique views of the pelvis described by Judet and Letournel, commonly called Judet views.
  - In the iliac oblique view, the radiographic beam is roughly perpendicular to the iliac wing.
  - In the obturator oblique view, the radiographic beam is roughly perpendicular to the obturator foramen.

Inclusion of the opposite hip in the radiographic field on the anteroposterior and Judet views is essential for evaluation of symmetrical contours that may have slight individual variations and to determine the width of the normal articular cartilage in each view. The medial clear space between the femoral head and the radiographic teardrop in the injured and uninjured hips should be compared on the anteroposterior view as an indication of femoral head subluxation.

Fractures that traverse the anterior column disrupt the iliopectineal line, whereas fractures that traverse the posterior column disrupt the ilioischial line. Each fracture pattern in the classification of Letournel and Judet has typical radiographic characteristics with respect to the disruption or intactness of the radiographic landmarks.

Landmarks of standard anteroposterior radiograph of hip:
- Iliopectineal line beginning at greater sciatic notch of ilium and extending down to pubic tubercle
- Ilioischial line formed by posterior four fifths of quadrilateral surface of ilium
- Radiographic teardrop composed laterally of most inferior and anterior portion of acetabulum and medially of anterior flat part of quadrilateral surface of iliac bone
- Roof of acetabulum
- Edge of anterior lip of acetabulum
- Edge of posterior lip of acetabulum.

Management: Fractures that traverse the weight-bearing dome but are displaced less than 2 mm can be treated with nonweight-bearing for 6–12 weeks, depending on the fracture characteristics.

Displaced fractures through the weight-bearing dome should be treated with operative reduction and internal fixation, regardless of how they may "line up" in traction. These fractures have a tendency to displace, leading to inferior results. One exception to this rule is an extremely comminuted both-column fracture that attains secondary congruence. In reality, very few fractures are treated definitively by traction to maintain a reduction of the acetabular dome.

Posterior wall fractures associated with posterior fracture-dislocations of the hip require separate consideration and are evaluated after closed reduction. Larger posterior wall fragments lead to posterior hip instability and require fixation.

Minimal access surgical management: The ilioinguinal approach, modified Stoppa approach, and Kocher-Lagenback approaches have been used as a standard to reduce and fix the acetabular fractures but these may not be possible in some cases where skin has suffered significant damages. Some surgeons use two-incision minimally invasive (TIMI) method for the treatment of anterior acetabular fractures where the first incision is performed by a pararectal approach at the level of the proximal third of the arcuate line of the ilium. The iliac vessels are mobilized medially while the neuromuscular bundle is retracted laterally. The second approach lies above the medial pubic bone. Soft tissues are retracted and fractures fixed with reconstruction/pelvic plates and screws.

Other minimally invasive method involves percutaneous fixation of the fractures:

Anterior column fixation: Anterior column can be fixed using a long screw. The screw entry point is located at the junction of a line drawn along the lateral border of the femur through the greater trochanter and a line from the pubic symphysis through the anterior inferior iliac spine. The screw is placed over a guide wire under image intensifier.

Posterior column fixation: This is done through entry made through ischial tuberosity just 1 cm posterior to the most distal aspect of tuberosity located with hip in flexion and knee extended. Screw is placed over a guide wire.

134. Explain different approaches to manage acetabular injuries.

Ans: Surgical Approaches for Acetabular Fractures

1. *Posterior approach*: Kocher–Langenbeck
   - *Indications*:
     – Transverse + posterior wall fractures
     – T-shaped fractures with posterior displacement
     – Posterior column fractures
   - *Key techniques*:
     – Prone positioning aids reduction by counteracting medial displacement.
     – Trochanteric flip osteotomy (Siebenrock) improves exposure for transverse fractures or femoral head involvement (e.g., Pipkin fractures).
     – Preserves femoral head vascularity (high union rate).
   - *Advantages*: Direct access to posterior pathology.
   - *Risks*: Sciatic nerve injury (protect with knee flexion).

2. *Anterior approaches*:
   A. *Anterior intrapelvic (AIP/Modified Stoppa)*
      - *Indications*:
        – Anterior wall/column fractures
        – Anterior-column posterior-hemitransverse
        – Both-column fractures (alternative to ilioinguinal)
      - *Key steps*:
        – Pfannenstiel incision + linea alba split
        – Ligation of corona mortis (obturator-external iliac anastomosis)
        – Exposure of quadrilateral surface/internal pelvis
      - *Advantages*:
        – Avoids middle-window dissection (↓ neurovascular risk).
        – Better visualization in obese patients.
   B. *Ilioinguinal (Letournel's 3-Window)*:
      - *Windows*:
        1. *Lateral*: Iliac crest to iliopsoas (iliopectineal fascia).
        2. *Middle*: Between iliopsoas and external iliac vessels.
        3. *Medial*: Medial to vessels (rarely used; modern AIP replaces this).
      - *Modern hybrid*: Combine AIP + lateral window to minimize dissection.
   C. *Adjuncts for anterior approaches*:
      - Skeletal traction on radiolucent table
      - Triangular hip support relaxes iliopsoas for lateral window
      - ASIS osteotomy enhances anterior wall/psoas gutter access.

3. *Extensile approaches (Rare and high morbidity)*:
   - *Indications*:
     – Complex both-column fractures with posterior wall displacement
     – Young patients with severe displacement (transtectal T-shaped)
   - *Options*:
     – Extended iliofemoral (Letournel/Judet)
     – Triradiate (Mears/Rubash)
     – T-approach (Reinert)
   - *Critical Consideration*:
     – Preoperative superior gluteal artery angiogram (avoids abductor necrosis).

4. *Evolving strategies*:
   - Sequential anterior-posterior approaches preferred over "floppy lateral" (better visibility, avoids implant conflict).
   - Indirect reduction techniques minimize soft-tissue disruption.

Decision-Making Summary **(Table 3.5.6)**

TABLE 3.5.6: Preferred exposure for different types/combination of acetabular fracture.

Fracture pattern	Preferred approach	Key modifications
Posterior wall/column	Kocher–Langenbeck	Trochanteric flip if needed
Anterior wall/column	AIP or Ilioinguinal (lateral)	ASIS osteotomy for obese patients
Both-column	AIP + lateral window	Sequential anterior-posterior
Complex displacement	Extensile (caution!)	Confirm gluteal artery patency

Complication mitigation:
- *Posterior*: Protect sciatic nerve.
- *Anterior*: Ligate *corona mortis*, avoid femoral vessel traction.
- *Extensile*: Limit use; prioritize staged approaches.

135. **Describe the design of pelvic C-clamp. What are the indications of its application and method to fix an unstable fracture?**

Ans: In vertically unstable fractures an anterior-only fixation will not control motion in the posterior sacroiliac complex, the pelvic clamps were hence developed to control the posterior pelvis in the resuscitation phase.

The Ganz C-clamp: This device uses large, percutaneously placed pins over the region of the sacroiliac joint posteriorly. Compression is produced at SI joints by pushing through the iliac blades posteriorly. An iliac wing fracture close to the sacroiliac joint (transiliac fracture dislocation/transiliac instability) is a contraindication to the use of this device. The device is only a temporary stabilizing method that should be removed within 5 days if possible.

Indications:
- Vertically unstable pelvic fractures
- Grossly unstable pelvic fracture (type C) waiting for definitive stabilization due to need of resuscitation or other injuries
- Sacroiliac disruptions
- Fracture of sacrum (relative).

Contraindications:
- Major life-threatening hemorrhage that needs primary attention rather than obtaining pelvic instability
- Transiliac instability
- Type A pelvic injury with hemodynamic stability
- Type B pelvic injury that can be stabilized by external fixation and are hemodynamically stable
- Comminuted sacral fractures that would get compressed and cause injury to sacral plexus.

Steps of Application:
- Place the patient supine so that intraoperative fluoroscopy in AP, lateral, oblique (inlet/outlet) planes is available. Drape legs free for reduction.
- Part preparation and asepsis.
- Palpate the posterior superior iliac spine and draw an imaginary line between it and the anterior inferior iliac spine. Insert the nail on this line, approximately 3–4 fingerbreadths anterolateral to the posterior superior iliac spine. (*note*: avoid distal entry to protect gluteal vessels or the sciatic nerve).
- Insert the Steinmann pin until bone is contacted, and then use a hammer to drive the pins approximately 1 cm into the bone **(Fig. 3.5.8)**.

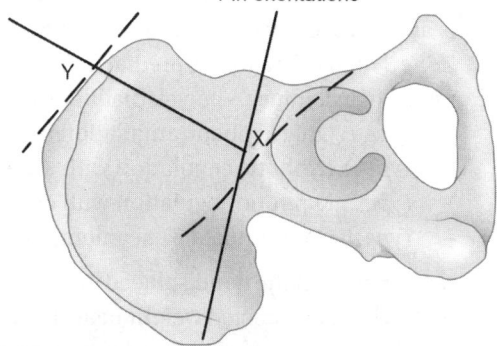

Fig. 3.5.8: Pin orientation.

- Slide the two side arms medially toward one another until the ends of the threaded bolts, sliding over the pins, come into contact with the bone.
- Correct cranial displacement of the hemipelvis by placing traction on the ipsilateral leg.
- Drive the threaded bolts inward with a wrench to apply compression to the unstable hemipelvis. This closes the diastasis and stabilizes the posterior pelvic ring (**Fig. 3.5.9**).
- Correct dorsal displacement by manual traction using the T-handle applied to a Schanz pin placed in the anterior superior iliac spine. Carry out other necessary manipulations in a similar manner.
- Check the reduction maneuvers radiographically, or if other procedures are necessary immediately, obtain a radiograph as soon as possible.
- The device can be applied in an oblique configuration by placing the Steinmann pin on the side of the stable hemipelvis in the anterior superior iliac spine. When the bolt is tightened, one component of the force vector on the unstable side is directed anteriorly, which helps reduce a posteriorly displaced hemipelvis (**Fig. 3.5.10**).

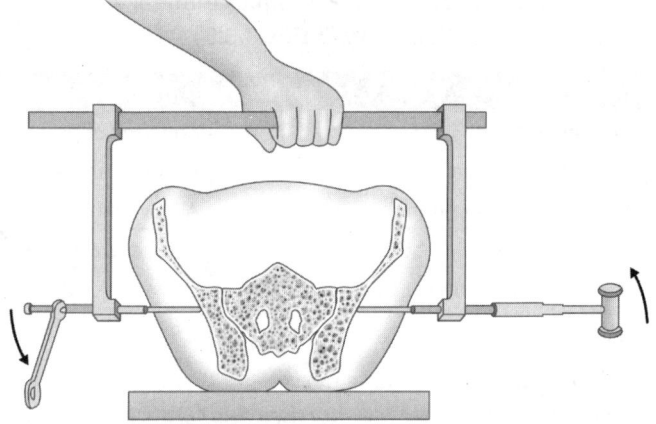

Fig. 3.5.9: Compression applied to the unstable hemipelvis.

136. What is sacral fractures? Discuss classification and management.

Ans: Fractures of the sacrum are commonly associated with pelvic ring injuries in up to 30–45% cases. Around 1/4th of these are associated with neurological injury. Currently, the classification used most often is that proposed by Denis, Davis, and Comfort.

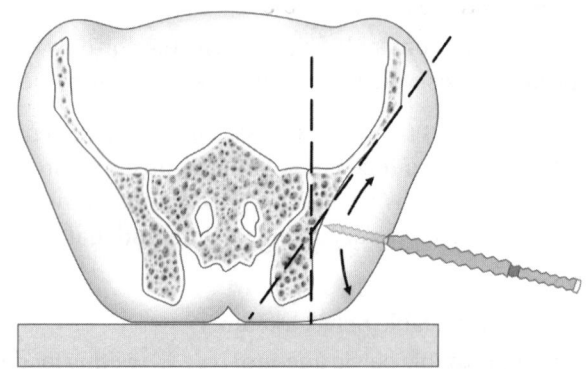

Fig. 3.5.10: Steinmann pin on the side of the stable hemipelvis.

Denis classifies the sagittal fractures into 3 types and subtypes along sagittal plane.
- *Zone 1 injuries*: Fracture lateral to foramina. This is most common injury and is associated with <5% incidence of neurological injury (mostly to L5)
- *Zone 2*: Fracture through foramina. Shear fractures are unstable and often associated with neurological injury. There is an increased risk of nonunion and poor functional outcome.
- *Zone 3 injury*: Fracture is medial to foramina extending to spinal canal. They are associated with highest incidence of neurological injury—bowel, bladder dysfunction. These are subclassified into 4 types as follows:
  - *Type 1*: Only kyphotic angulation at the fracture site (no translation)
  - *Type 2*: Kyphotic angulation with anterior translation of the distal sacrum
  - *Type 3*: Kyphotic angulation with complete offset of the fracture fragments
  - *Type 4*: Comminuted S1 segment, usually due to axial compression.

Treatment: Most of the nondisplaced fractures (<1 cm) and fractures without neurological deficit are treated conservatively by rest and then protected weight bearing beginning 6–8 weeks. Operative treatment is indicated in displaced fractures >1 cm displacement or those associated with neurological deficit. Other indications include soft tissue compromise, persistent pain after nonoperative management and fractures that displace with nonoperative management. In patients with neurological deficit additional decompression is a must usually.

Operative fixation techniques include:
- Percutaneous screw fixation—sacroiliac, transsacral or transiliac transsacral screws are commonly placed for reducible sagittal plane fractures. Loss of reduction and malreduction may result if not perfect. L5 nerve root may be damaged. One should avoid the temptation to over-compress the fracture and failure is high in osteoporotic bones.

- Posterior tension band plating is a viable option in patients not suitable for percutaneous screw especially those with osteoporotic bones.
- Iliosacral and lumbopelvic fixation using pedicle screw in lumbar spine and iliac screws joined by longitudinal and transverse rods have highest stiffness and stability but needs experience.

137. Discuss Ganz antishock pelvic fixator.

Ans: Please vide Answer to Question 135.

138. Discuss approach to pelvic trauma with abdominal injury.

Ans: The acute management of a patient with a pelvic fracture and unrelenting hemorrhage remains a challenge to the orthopedic surgeon. A multidisciplinary approach with orthopedic surgeons, general surgeons, and anesthesiologists is critical to optimizing outcomes. The initial trauma workup, including CT scan of the chest and abdomen, supraumbilical peritoneal lavage, and abdominal ultrasound, must rule out other sources of bleeding.

The patient with a pelvic ring injury who remains hemodynamically unstable even after circumferential pelvic binding should be considered for arteriography as corona mortis injury is common cause of internal bleed in them and may be managed by interventional radiologist with embolization. Hemorrhage otherwise results from fractured cancellous surfaces and small vessels in the retroperitoneum. Some 5–10% of patients with pelvic fractures bleed from arterial sources that can be embolized.

Open pelvic fractures are extremely difficult injuries to manage, with reported mortality rates of up to 50%. If the retroperitoneal space is open, no tamponade effect occurs to prevent excessive bleeding. Sepsis caused by fecal contamination is a major cause of mortality with this injury, and immediate diverting colostomy is indicated in patients with perineal wounds.

Routine vaginal and rectal examinations should be performed in patients with open pelvic fractures because fracture fragments can penetrate these structures, with devastating consequences if timely and appropriate debridement is not performed. External fixation can minimize fracture motion and further soft tissue injury.

Flowchart 3.5.4 Dictates the plausible emergency management of such injuries.

Flowchart 3.5.4: Emergency management algorithm for pelvic fractures.

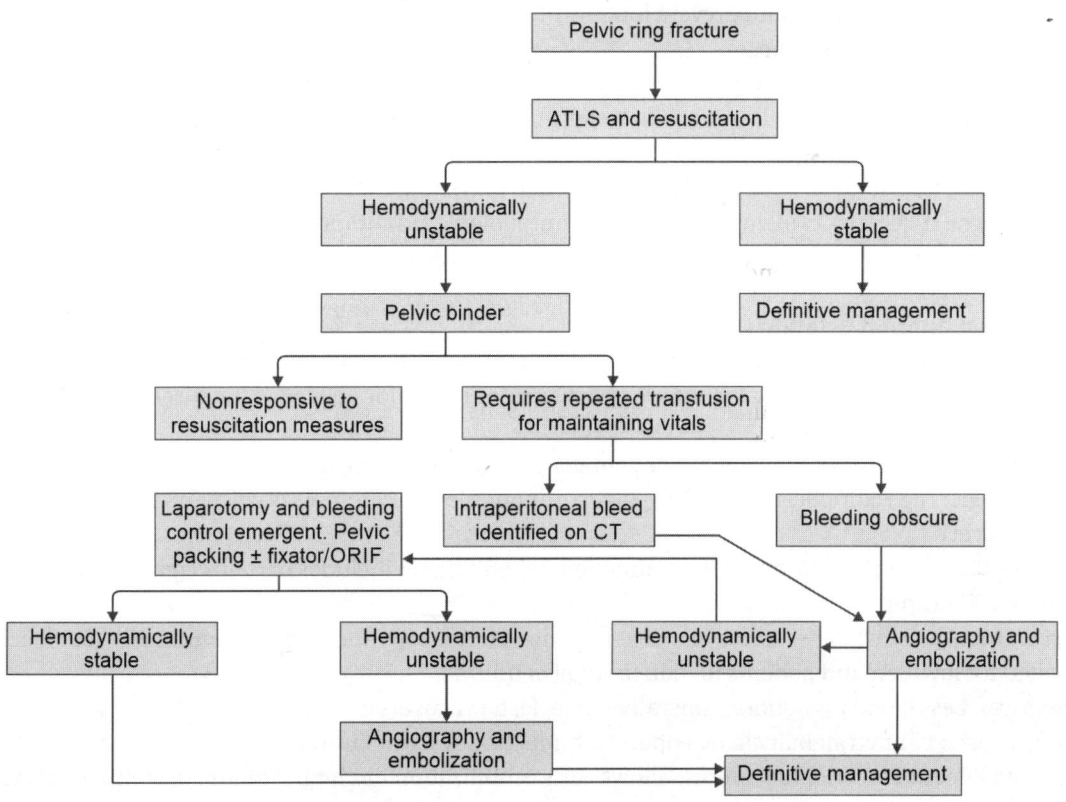

139. Discuss surgical management of posterior column acetabular fractures.

Ans: Fractures of the posterior column involve detachment of the entire ischioacetabular segment from the innominate bone and represent 3–5% of acetabular fractures. The fracture begins at the posterior border of the innominate bone near the apex of the greater sciatic notch. It descends across the articular surface, quadrilateral surface, ischiopubic notch (roof of the obturator canal), and finally across the inferior ramus. On the AP radiograph, the ilioischial line, the posterior rim, and the inferior ramus are disrupted. The disruption of the posterior rim will be seen in only one location where the fracture line crosses the rim. The iliac oblique radiograph demonstrates the fracture crossing the posterior border of the bone. The fracture of the ischiopubic ramus and posterior rim are confirmed on the obturator oblique. The iliopectineal line is preserved on all views. The femoral head follows the displacement of the posterior column posteriorly and medially. The ilioischial line is typically displaced.

Fractures of the posterior column are notoriously unstable and skeletal traction is frequently required to keep the femoral head reduced beneath the intact portion of the roof. The posterior column fracture frequently involves the greater sciatic notch at or above the location of the superior gluteal neurovascular bundle. In widely displaced fractures, it is common to find the neurovascular bundle in the posterior column fracture site and it must be carefully extracted before reduction of the fracture to prevent iatrogenic injury.

Posterior column fractures are relatively uncommon and, if significantly displaced, require ORIF. The Kocher-Langenbeck approach is used routinely. Rotational deformity in addition to displacement must be corrected by placement of a Schanz screw in the ischium to control rotation while the fracture is reduced with a small Jungbluth reduction clamp. Typical fixation is with a lag screw combined with a contoured reconstruction plate along the posterior column.

140. A. Describe the various methods of treating Geriatric Acetabular Fractures.
   B. Describe the indications, timing and approach for open reduction and internal fixation/acute total hip arthroplasty in geriatric acetabular fractures.

Ans: Treatment Methods for Geriatric Acetabular Fractures

Geriatric acetabular fractures [common in patients >60 years due to osteoporosis and low-energy falls) are managed based on fracture pattern (e.g., anterior column-posterior hemitransverse (ACPHT), associated both columns (ABC)], patient comorbidities, bone quality, and functional demand. Treatment aims to restore mobility, minimize complications (e.g., avascular necrosis, nonunion), and prevent long-term disability. No universal guideline exists, but options include nonoperative and operative approaches.

1. **Nonoperative (Conservative) Management**
   - *Concept*: Bed rest or early mobilization with weight-bearing restrictions, pain control, physical therapy, and DVT prophylaxis. Indicated for stable, minimally displaced fractures in low-demand or frail patients.
   - *Advantages*: Avoids surgical risks (e.g., infection, blood loss); rapid mobilization possible.
   - *Disadvantages*: Higher risk of malunion, prolonged immobility, and complications like pressure sores or pneumonia.
   - *Outcomes*: Suitable for non-displaced fractures; functional recovery in 70–80% but higher mortality in unstable cases.

2. **Open Reduction Internal Fixation (ORIF)**
   - *Concept*: Surgical realignment and fixation using plates/screws via approaches like ilioinguinal, Kocher-Langenbeck, or modified Stoppa for anterior fractures. Indicated for displaced fractures with joint incongruity in healthier geriatrics.
   - *Advantages*: Preserves native hip; good for younger geriatrics or stable patterns.
   - *Disadvantages*: High complication rate (20–30%, e.g., nonunion, heterotopic ossification) due to poor bone quality; longer recovery.
   - *Outcomes*: 80–90% union rate but variable function; rehabilitation includes partial weight-bearing for 6–12 weeks.

3. **Percutaneous Fixation**
   - *Concept*: Minimally invasive screw placement under fluoroscopy for stable or minimally displaced fractures. Indicated for low-demand patients to reduce surgical trauma.
   - *Advantages*: Less blood loss, shorter operative time, faster recovery.
   - *Disadvantages*: Limited stability in osteoporotic bone; risk of screw cut-out.
   - *Outcomes*: Effective for simple patterns; allows early mobilization but higher failure in complex fractures.

4. **Acute Total Hip Arthroplasty (THA)**
   - *Concept*: Immediate hip replacement, often with acetabular reconstruction (e.g., cages and augments) for unstable fractures. Indicated for displaced fractures in active geriatrics or those with pre-existing arthritis.
   - *Advantages*: Immediate weight-bearing, better pain relief and function; lower reoperation rate versus ORIF in RCTs.
   - *Disadvantages*: Higher infection/dislocation risk; not suitable for all (e.g., frail patients).
   - *Outcomes*: Superior Harris Hip Scores; rehabilitation focuses on early ambulation.
5. **Combined ORIF + THA ("Fix and Replace")**
   - *Concept*: ORIF of the fracture followed by acute THA in one stage. Indicated for complex, comminuted fractures in geriatrics.
   - *Advantages*: Stabilizes fracture while addressing joint damage; good for osteoporotic bone.
   - *Disadvantages*: Longer surgery, increased blood loss/complications.
   - *Outcomes*: High union rate (90%); allows early mobilization but variable long-term function.
B. Open Reduction and Internal Fixation (ORIF)

Indications: Displaced fractures with joint incongruity, in healthier geriatrics with good bone quality and stable patterns [e.g., anterior column-posterior hemitransverse (ACPHT)]. Suitable for low-demand patients or those without pre-existing arthritis.

Timing: Perform timely (within 3–7 days of injury) in stable patients to minimize blood loss and physiological stress; delay if comorbidities require optimization.

Approach: Ilioinguinal or modified Stoppa for anterior fractures; Kocher–Langenbeck for posterior. Use fluoroscopy for percutaneous screws in minimally displaced cases.

Acute Total Hip Arthroplasty (THA)

Indications: Unreconstructable displaced fractures (e.g., comminuted, both-column), subchondral impaction, pre-existing arthritis, or in active geriatrics with high functional demand.

Timing: Immediate (acute, within 24–72 hours) postinjury in stable patients, often combined with fixation for early mobilization.

Approach: Direct anterior for THA combined with anterior intrapelvic for fracture fixation; use cages/augments for reconstruction in osteoporotic bone.

3.6 OPEN INJURIES (Q141–149)

141. Classify open fractures.

Ans: Gustilo and Anderson classification is the most popular for classifying open injuries of bone:
The modified classification is based on the size of the wound, periosteal soft-tissue damage, periosteal stripping, and vascular injury.
- *Grade I*: Clean wound smaller than 1 cm in diameter or puncture wound that appears clean with a simple fracture pattern, no skin crushing or internal degloving.
- *Grade II*: A laceration larger than 1 cm but <10 cm, without significant soft-tissue crushing, including no flaps, degloving, or contusion. Fracture pattern may be more complex. High velocity trauma
- *Grade III*: An open segmental fracture or a single fracture with extensive soft-tissue injury (>10 cm). Injuries older than 8 hours, farm injuries, gunshot injuries, segmental fractures, and fractures with diaphyseal bone loss are also included in this type. Type III injuries are subdivided into three subtypes:
  1. Type IIIA open fractures have extensive soft-tissue lacerations or flaps, but maintain adequate soft-tissue coverage of bone, or they result from high-energy trauma regardless of the size of the wound. This group includes segmental or severely comminuted fractures, even those with 1-cm lacerations.
  2. Type IIIB open fractures have extensive soft-tissue loss with periosteal stripping and bony exposure. They usually are massively contaminated.
  3. Type IIIC open fractures include open fractures with an arterial injury that requires repair regardless of the size of the soft-tissue wound.

142. Explain reconstructive ladder for open fractures. What is fix and close protocol in open fractures?

Ans: *Reconstructive ladder*: The traditional reconstructive ladder proposes a plan for reconstruction where each step of the ladder denotes a reconstruction of increasing complexity starting from primary closure. It was originally suggested that the surgeon must choose the lowest possible step that will suit the defect. However, this concept is not strictly followed now **(Fig. 3.6.1)**.

In patients with established skin loss there are many options for providing skin cover over the fracture site from releasing incisions to microvascular free tissue transfer. Traditionally, it is viewed as a reconstructive ladder starting from simple split skin grafts and progressing to fasciocutaneous flaps, rotational muscle flaps, and free muscle flaps. Each step of the ladder provides a wound cover option of increasing complexity and the traditional advice was to choose the simplest option as the first choice for soft tissue cover. However, this approach has been questioned recently because of extensive advances in microsurgery. Free flaps are now undertaken with a high success rate and they have the advantage of providing versatile skin cover with vascular tissue. Hence, it has been suggested that the reconstructive ladder concept should be replaced by the "reconstructive elevator" concept as the ladder's top step option is often the one that provides the best wound healing.

Rather than adopting a stepwise algorithm for wound cover, surgeons now choose the appropriate method.

Recently, a "revised reconstructive ladder" has been advocated where newer developments such as vacuum-assisted closure (VAC) therapy, acute bone shortening, and bone transport are incorporated **(Flowchart 3.6.1)**.

Type III injuries are associated with wounds of varying size and complexity. Reconstruction should be tailored to the wound and also the surgeon's expertise. Every surgeon has certain preferences in reconstruction techniques but the following guidelines generally hold true:
- Lacerated wounds without skin loss, which can be opposed without tension, can be primarily sutured.
- In small linear vertical wounds, lying over bone, with minimal soft tissue loss cover can be achieved using a parallel releasing skin incision which will allow direct closure of the laceration. The releasing skin incision should be over a good muscle bed or fascia so that it will allow skin grafting of the defect.
- Wounds which are not directly over the bone and which have a healthy muscle bed can usually be treated by split skin grafting with good results. Small defects in the skin which are directly over bone and are exposing implants can be successfully covered with rotational fasciocutaneous flaps which may have either a proximal or a distal base.
- The commonly seen defect over the subcutaneous surface of the tibia can be treated by a rotational flap, provided there is no degloving and the zone of injury is not extensive. A distally based flap is commonly performed for a defect in the anterior part of the leg as it creates a donor area over healthy calf muscles that take skin grafts well. Larger defects

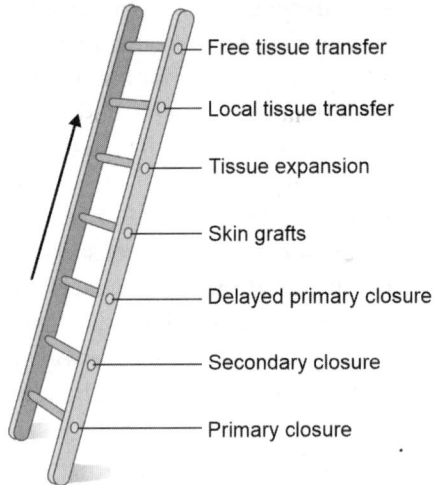

Fig. 3.6.1: The reconstructive ladder.

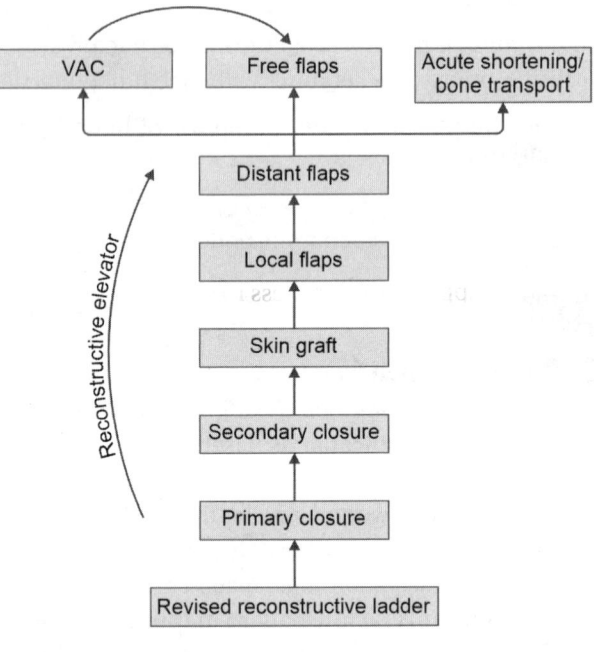

Flowchart 3.6.1: Revised reconstructive ladder.

and injuries exposing the bone and tendons require to be covered with vascularized tissue and the best option is a muscle flap covered with split skin graft.

Fix and close protocol: This is the emerging method for management of open fractures that are not grossly contaminated. Here the fracture is fixed using appropriate method and all attempts are made to achieve primary closure of the wound irrespective of "grade" of injury in the initial management itself. Primary closure has not been correlated with increased risk of deep infection, nor has it been associated with development of delayed or nonunion in an altered manner. There is also no correlation of time to closure to development of deep infection but instead early closure is recommended (against the older recommendation of delayed closure). This early "fix and close" protocol for open fractures has been found to be safe and potentially cost-effective treatment with improved healing rates and minimize complications. The current contraindications for this particular method is in patients with hand and foot injuries, hemodynamic compromise, sewage or farmyard contamination, and several pre-existing conditions, such as peripheral vascular disease, drug-dependent diabetes mellitus, and connective tissue disorders.

143. **How will you manage Gustilo Anderson type IIIB fracture of distal femur? Compare pros and cons of angular stable device and dynamic compression screw for distal femur fractures.**

Ans:

Management of type IIIB: Wound debridement (along prescribed guidelines by experienced surgeon) and external fixation are primary measures in open IIIB distal femoral fractures. If the fracture has a significant intercondylar component, the knee should be spanned by the external fixator (reserve this for the most severe open fractures for chances of pin-track infection and knee stiffness). It provides local traction, while allowing mobility for patients with multiple traumas. This technique also allows better CT evaluation of the distal femoral fracture. DICTUM IS SPAN, SCAN AND PLAN.

Conversion to internal fixation [nailing/dynamic condylar screw (DCS)/distal femoral locking plate (DFLP)] can be done up to 14 days but strict care should be taken for preventing pin-track infection. Chose a small wire fixator or Ilizarov frame or hybrid fixator if definitive fixation (nailing/plating) cannot be done by 2–3 weeks for soft tissue condition. The articular portions of the fracture can be treated with limited internal fixation.

Angular Stable Device

Pros:
- Allows higher elastic deformation of a level between rigid fixation and intramedullary nailing (so a favorable construct).
- Locking screws give angular stability
- Can be applied as LISS (Less Invasive Stabilization Technique)
- No need of minimum 4 cm of uncomminuted bone, i.e. can be used in comminuted intra-articular fractures with screws holding these fragments.

Cons: Technically demanding.

Dynamic Condylar Screw

Pros:
- Less technically demanding
- Allows freedom in flexion-extension plane.

Cons:
- Minimum of 4 cm of uncomminuted bone in the femoral condyles above the intercondylar notch is necessary for successful fixation.
- Insertion of the condylar lag screw requires removal of a large amount of bone, which makes revision surgery, should it be necessary, more difficult.
    - Nonunion in 3–5%
    - Malunion in 5–10%
    - Infection in 2–5%.

144. Explain Ganga trauma score and VAC closure of wounds.

Ans:

Ganga trauma score (**Table 3.6.1**):

TABLE 3.6.1: The Ganga Trauma score.

Covering Structures: Skin and Fascia	
• Wound with no skin loss and not over the fracture site	1
• Wound with no skin loss and over the fracture site	2
• Wound with skin loss and not over the fracture site	3
• Wound with skin loss and over the fracture site	4
• Wound with circumferential skin loss	5
Functional Tissues: Musculotendinous and Nerve Units	
• Partial injury to musculotendinous unit	1
• Complete but repairable injury to musculotendinous units	2
• Irreparable injury to musculotendinous units, partial loss of a compartment, or complete injury to posterior tibial nerve	3
• Loss of one compartment of musculotendinous units	4
• Loss of two or more compartments or subtotal amputation	5
Skeletal Structures: Bone and Joints	
• Transverse or oblique fracture or butterfly fragment <50% circumference	1
• Large butterfly fragment >50% circumference	2
• Comminution or segmental fractures without bone loss	3
• Bone loss <4 cm	4
• Bone loss >4 cm	5
Comorbid Conditions: Add Two Points for Each of the following Condition Present	
• Injury leading to debridement interval >12 hours • Sewage or organic contamination or farmyard injuries • Age >65 years • Drug-dependent diabetes mellitus or cardiorespiratory diseases leading to increased anesthetic risk • Polytrauma involving chest or abdomen with injury severity score >25 or fat embolism • Hypotension with systolic blood pressure <90 mm Hg at presentation • Another major injury to the same limb or compartment syndrome • Injuries with a score equal to 14 or below are advised salvage	
Scores:	
• Injuries with score 17 and above usually end up in amputation • Injuries with score 15 and 16 fall into gray zone where decision is made on patient-to-patient basis	

(VAC closure of wounds is discussed in detail in Chapter 2)

145. Explain the management of open fractures of tibia in a tertiary care setting.

Ans: The results of treatment of open high-energy tibial fractures have improved significantly. The following are the risks of open fractures that need to be addressed by stepwise, integrated approach:
- Increased risk of infection
- Higher chances of nonunion
- Management of associated skin and soft tissue injury that contribute to future comorbidities.

Limb salvage is the primary goal unless the following are present:
- Mangled extremity beyond reconstruction/repair
- Cold ischemia time of ≥6 hours
- Poor facilities for salvage
- Poor performance status that precludes prolonged and multiple treatment sittings.

The following are the commonly recommended steps to achieve goals based on understanding of above challenges:
- Timely irrigation of the wound and debridement (wound toileting). Ideal time and amount of irrigant is unknown still but should be done as early and with ample fluid. Aggressive and repeated debridement of all devitalized tissue, including large fragments of bone, is essential. The protocol is repeat drainage and debridement at 48 hours if there is evidence of inflammation. All Gustilo type III fractures routinely have repeat debridement.
- Because vascular soft tissue and bone are essential for resisting infection and providing a bed for reconstruction, the tibia should be stabilized with as little additional devascularization as possible.
- Antibiotics should be used routinely with open fractures and should be commenced as early as possible (within emergency care). Aminoglycosides are added to cephalosporins for type III open fractures, and penicillin is included for fractures with severe contamination.
- Primary wound closure if possible should be the priority but for wounds that need delayed closure/coverage, soft tissue coverage by 5–7 days should be obtained (delayed closure, skin grafting, or flap coverage) even if vacuum-assisted wound therapy is in place. There is no dispute that soft tissue management is the most important factor in determining the outcome of open tibial fractures.
- Currently, most traumatologists prefer intramedullary nailing for Gustilo type I, type II, and type IIIA open fractures. They are contraindicated if there is untreated compartment syndrome and in Gustilo type IIIC and possibly IIIB injuries.
- External fixation usually is indicated for severe open fractures (type IIIB and type C), especially fractures with gross contamination of the tibial canal, or if the adequacy of the initial debridement (shotgun wound, crush injuries) is a concern. Three distinct types of fixators are commonly used: half-pin fixators, wire and ring fixators, and hybrid fixators that combine half-pins and tensioned wires. External fixation provides stable fixation, preserves soft tissues and bone vascularity, leaves wounds accessible, and causes little blood loss. It should be converted into definitive fixation unless contraindicated. The conversion should be done within 28 days else chances of nonunion and infection increase.

146. Describe classification of open fracture of tibia.

Ans: Tscherne classification for open tibial fractures is given in **Table 3.6.2**.

TABLE 3.6.2: Tscherne classification for open tibial fractures.	
Grade 1	Skin lacerations caused by a bone fragment from inside, little or no contusion of skin
Grade 2	Any type of skin laceration with circumscribed skin or soft-tissue contusion and moderate contamination; can occur with any type of fracture.
Grade 3	Fracture must have severe soft-tissue damage, often with major vessel or nerve injury or both: all fractures accompanied by ischemia and severe bone comminution belong in this group and those associated with compartment syndrome
Grade 4	Subtotal and total amputation, defined as separation of all important anatomical structures, especially major vessels with total ischemia; remaining soft tissue may not exceed one fourth of circumference of extremity (any revascularization is grade 3)

147. Discuss management of grade-3 open tibial fractures.

Ans: Kindly see Answers to the Questions above.

148. A. Classify gunshot wounds.

B. Brief management outline for a high-velocity gunshot wound in thigh in an adult male with fracture shaft of femur.

Ans: A. The current system realizes transfer of energy to tissues from projectile so classification systems based on energy transferred should be used.
- *Low velocity/energy*:
  – Muzzle velocity less than 350 meters per second or less than 2,000 feet per second—meant for injuring person and not killing.
    - Most handguns (pistols and revolvers)
    - Wounds produced are comparable to Gustilo-Anderson type I or type II due to low energy transfer.

- *Intermediate velocity/energy*:
  - These weapons impart muzzle velocity of 350–500 meters per second to the bullet.
  - Shotgun blasts are typical example, magnums also reach this velocity.
    - The wound profile varies according to the firing distance from target.
    - If fired from close range (<21 feet) severe tissue trauma results that reproduce wounding potential of high velocity firearms. Same pattern may result from multiple intermediate-velocity shots fired.
    - Wound contamination is common due to shotgun wadding and causes infection when close ranges are used to fire.
    - Wounding potential of projectile depends on three major factors:
      1. Shot pattern
      2. Load (size of individual pellet)
      3. Distance from target
- *High muzzle velocity (high kinetic energy)*:
  - These are usually military grade weapons having muzzle velocity more than 600 meters per second or more than 2,000 feet per second.
  - Military rifles/assault rifles.
  - Due to high energy transfers from the projectile the wounds produced are comparable to Gustillo-Anderson type III even if the size on superficial inspection is small.
  - They have high risk of infection due primarily to contaminants sucked in during impact and traversal through tissue. Also responsible is the wide zone of injury and tissue necrosis that results from blast effect.

B. Already written in Answer to Question 145

149. Pathophysiology of gunshot wounds.

Ans: When a projectile passes through the tissue it causes tissue to move away from the front and sides of the projectile due to pressure wave created by the impact. This causes tissue laceration and injury by crush. The depth to which the projectile penetrates the tissue causing laceration and the amount of crush produced is governed primarily by the kinetic energy available in the projectile to do this work. The amount of kinetic energy is denoted by the well-known equation:

$$E \text{ (joules)} = 1/2 \, mv^2 \text{ (where, m = mass in kg; v = velocity in m/s)}.$$

Other theories realize the transfer of energy in the form of momentum (= mv) or power (based again on mv). Now, as the amount of energy is dependent heavily on velocity of the projectile so, injuries have been classically classified on the basis of velocity. The velocity of the M-16 bullet is thrice that of the 0.22 bullet. This explains: why although M-16 has almost the same caliber and mass as the 0.22 its kinetic energy is almost 10 times than the 0.22. The energy transfer is also affected by the tissue involved in the projectile tract (related to the density and rigidity of the tissue), direction of projectile (defined by rotation axis and yaw) and projectile characteristics (regular shape or hollow-point, copper or lead cover, metal or rubber projectile). The higher the rigidity of the tissue greater and faster is the energy transfer to cause tissue damage. For direction of projectile if a bullet wobbles and then tumbles to 90° to its initial direction, maximal energy transfer is achieved and tissue damage is three times than with bullet entering at 0 degrees. The movements of bullet and energy transfer are also governed by the additional motions imparted to it by the rifle. For example, projectiles often to rotate in a rosette pattern of motion due to combined action of spin on a yawing bullet (precession), and nutation (motion of higher frequency but lower amplitude). Rifling the barrel (creating helical grooves in the barrel) and increasing its length will cause a long narrow pointed bullet to achieve gyroscopic stability by imparting rotational speed of 1,500 and 6,000 rotations per second to the bullet in flight and reducing the tumble. Prescoring bullet so that it fragments at impact (dumdum bullet, declared inhumane now and banned), hollow-tip bullet, etc. have been used to increase energy transfer. Hollow-point or soft point bullets mushroom upon impact imparting higher energy to the tissues. Bullet injuries that have exit wound also transfer much less energy than retained bullets.

3.7 PERIPROSTHETIC FRACTURES (Q150–151)

150. Classify periprosthetic fractures around the knee. Outline the treatment strategy.

Ans: *Classification:*

Supracondylar femur fractures (Lewis and Rorabeck): This classification takes into account both fracture displacement and prosthesis stability **(Fig. 3.7.1)**.

- *Type I*: The fracture is nondisplaced, and the bone–prosthesis interface remains intact.
- *Type II*: The interface remains intact, but the fracture is displaced.
- *Type III*: The patient has a loose or failing prosthesis in the presence of either a displaced or a nondisplaced fracture.

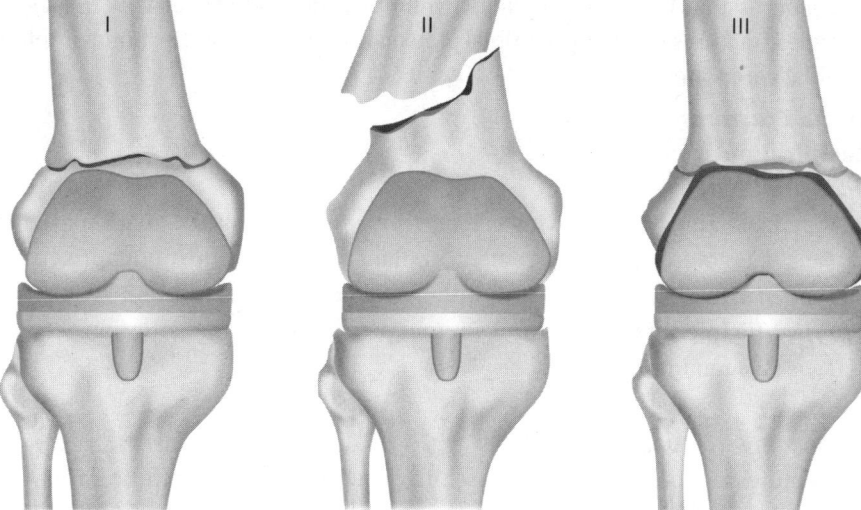

Fig. 3.7.1: Lewis and Rorabeck classification.

Treatment:

Principles:
- Anatomic and mechanical alignments are critical.
- Nondisplaced fractures may be treated nonoperatively.
- Open reduction internal fixation (ORIF) is indicated if the alignment is unacceptable by closed means and if bone stock is adequate for fixation devices.
- Immediate prosthetic revision is indicated in selected cases.

Nonoperative treatment: Long leg casting or cast bracing for 4–8 weeks may be used to treat minimally displaced fractures.

Operative treatment
- Displaced periprosthetic fractures around a total knee replacement are almost always managed with ORIF because of the difficulties in maintaining acceptable alignment after displacement.
- A fixed-angle plate, locked plate, or retrograde intramedullary (IM) nailing may be used for operative stabilization. (*NB*: Nonunion rates are reported higher with use of IM nail.)
- Primary revision with a stemmed component may be considered if there is involvement of the bone–implant interface and if the prosthesis is loose.
- Bone loss may be addressed with autologous grafting.
- Cases of severe bone loss, especially in the metaphyseal region, may be addressed with distal femoral replacement with a specialized prosthesis designed for oncologic management.

Tibial Fractures

Classification

Periprosthetic tibial fractures (Felix et al.): Classification is based on three factors, viz. location of the fracture, stability of the implant, and whether the fracture occurred intraoperatively or postoperatively.
- *Type I*: Occur in the tibial plateau
- *Type II*: Adjacent to the stem
- *Type III*: Distal to the prosthesis
- *Type IV*: Involve the tubercle.

Treatment

Nonoperative treatment:
- Closed reduction and cast immobilization may be performed for most tibial shaft fractures after alignment is restored.
- Early conversion to a cast brace to preserve knee range of motion is advised.

Operative treatment:
- Periprosthetic tibial fractures not involving the plateau require ORIF if closed reduction and cast immobilization are unsuccessful. Use of locked plating with unicortical screws to avoid the keel has made management easier.
- Type I fractures involving the tibial plateau typically involve the bone–implant interface, necessitating revision of the tibial component.

Patella Fractures

Classification

Goldberg:
- *Type I:* Fractures not involving cement/implant composite or quadriceps mechanism
- *Type II:* Fractures involving cement/implant composite and/or quadriceps mechanism
- *Type IIIA:* Inferior pole fractures with patellar ligament disruption
- *Type IIIB:* Inferior pole fractures without patellar ligament disruption
- *Type IV:* Fracture-dislocations.

Treatment

Nonoperative treatment:
- Fractures without component loosening, extensor mechanism rupture, or malalignment of the implant (type I or IIIB) may be treated nonoperatively (these situations compose the majority of clinical cases).
- The patient may be placed in a knee immobilizer for 4–6 weeks, with partial weight bearing on crutches.

Operative treatment: Indicated for patients with disruption of the extensor mechanism, patellar dislocation, or prosthetic loosening.

Treatment options include:
- *Open reduction internal fixation with revision of the prosthetic patella:* This is indicated for types II, IIIA, and IV fractures.
- *Fragment excision:* This may be undertaken for small fragments that do not compromise implant stability or patellar tracking.
- *Patellectomy:* This may be necessary in cases of extensive comminution or devascularization with osteonecrosis.
- Surgical considerations include adequate medial arthrotomy, adequate lateral release, preservation of the superior lateral geniculate artery, and preservation of the patellar fat pad.

151. **Classify periprosthetic fractures of femoral shaft after total hip arthroplasty and their treatment options.**

Ans: *Classification:* The Vancouver classification proposed by Duncan and Masri is more appropriate and is most commonly used **(Table 3.7.1)**.

TABLE 3.7.1: The Vancouver classification.			
Intraoperative fracture	Subtypes	*Postoperative fracture*	Subtypes
A. Proximal metaphyseal fractures not extending into the diaphysis	1. Simple cortical perforation 2. Undisplaced linear crack 3. Displaced or unstable fracture	A. Fractures around the trochanteric region	G. Around the greater trochanter LT. Around the lesser trochanter
B. Diaphyseal fratures not extending into the distal diaphysis	1. Simple cortical perforation 2. Undisplaced linear crack 3. Displaced or unstable fracture	B. Fractures around or just distal to the femoral stem	1. Femoral implant well-fixed 2. Femoral implant loose but good bone stock 3. Femoral implant loose and poor-bone stock
C. Distal fractures extending into the distal metaphysis	1. Simple cortical perforation 2. Undisplaced linear crack 3. Displaced or unstable fracture	C. Fractures distal to the femoral stem	

Treatment Principles
- *Treatment depends on*:
  - Location of the fracture
  - Stability of the prosthesis
  - A loose stem should be revised
  - Bone stock
  - Age and medical condition of the patient
  - Accurate reduction and secure fixation.
- *Options include*:
  - Open reduction internal fixation (ORIF) (with plate and screws or cable and/or strut allograft)
  - Revision plus ORIF.

Treatment
Vancouver Type B1 Fractures: These are usually treated with internal fixation. One may choose wires or cables or plate and screws and/or cables.

Technique:
- Open versus percutaneous plate placement
- Cortical onlay allograft—may or may not be added to fixation
- Combination.

Long-term results depend on:
- Implant alignment
- Preservation of the periosteal blood supply
- Adequacy of stress riser augmentation.

Vancouver Type B2 Fractures: Best treated by revision arthroplasty and ORIF. Most commonly one of the following options is used:
- Uncemented prosthesis
- Extensive-coated long-stem curved prosthesis
- Fluted long-stem prosthesis
- Modular implants
- Cemented prosthesis (very uncommon).

Vancouver Type B3 Fractures: The bone stock is insufficient to hold any type of prosthesis so this problem needs elaborate planning and treatment depending on the age and functional status of the patient and severity of bone defect. The options include:
- Proximal femoral reconstruction
- Composite allograft
- Scaffold technique
- Proximal femoral replacement.

Vancouver Type C Fractures: Treat as shaft femur fracture using plate/screw or cable construct but avoid any new stress riser by bypassing the implant.
(For a detailed reading and long answer for the question, kindly refer to Chapter 66 of the book *Essential Orthopedics: Principles and Practice*, 2nd edition.)

CHAPTER 4

Regional Orthopedics

4A. UPPER LIMB

4A.1 CONGENITAL SHOULDER GIRDLE AFFLICTIONS (Q1–3)

1. A. Classify torticollis.
B. Explain management of torticollis and
C. Sprengel shoulder deformity.

Ans: **A. Classification of torticollis:**
- *Adult onset variety:*
  - Cervical dystonia
  - Acute spasm of sternocleidomastoid (SCM) muscle
  - Acute cervical disk calcification
  - Bone tumors.
- *Pediatric variety:*
  - Congenital
  - Congenital muscular torticollis (CMT)
  - Congenital absence of SCM of one side
  - Pterygium colli
  - Klippel-Feil syndrome
  - Unilateral atlanto-occipital fusion
  - Vertebral anomalies
  - Positional torticollis (CPT).
- *Acquired:*
  - Infectious or inflammatory
  - Traumatic
  - Neurological
  - Ocular torticollis
  - Medications
  - Psychogenic
  - Postural
  - Sandifer syndrome
  - Benign paroxysmal torticollis.

B. Management: Radiographs of cervical spine should be obtained to identify bony abnormalities especially unilateral fusions (not very helpful in infancy) and identification of atlantoaxial subluxations in juvenile rheumatoid arthritis (JRA). Radiographs are especially ordered if there is cervical spine tenderness that persists following short course of analgesics, severe pain, JRA, ligamentous laxity or persistently restricted range of motion (ROM). Ultrasonographic imaging has high sensitivity and specificity of 96% and 83%, respectively and has good diagnostic and prognostic value. It is considered investigation of choice though findings vary in accordance with different CMT stages. MRI has limited role in CMT diagnosis with evident clinical features though the radiological findings have high concordance with histopathological findings.

Treatment: Initial management of CMT is always conservative manipulation to stretch the SCM muscle. This can be done by parents or dedicated physiotherapists. Some other modalities may be combined but exquisite details to their use have not been described.

Physical therapy: Manual passive stretching of the SCM muscle is recommended to be done for 2–4 times a day till the age of 12 months. Stretching is done by one hand lying between child's head and the ipsilateral shoulder to reduce lateral flexion (side-to-side stretch), while the other is applied on the face and chin to derotate the neck (ear-to-shoulder stretch). Ten to fifteen stretches of 30 seconds each are performed in one sitting. This is considered the most effective form of therapy with more than 90% patients showing positive response when performed correctly. Recurrence rate is estimated to be nearly 2% with physical therapy mainly due to carelessness. Higher recurrence rate and incomplete response is seen when the initial rotation of the head from the neutral position is greater than 15°, there is well palpable sternomastoid tumor, and initiation of the treatment done after first year of life. In between revaluation of the stretching program is done at the age of 4 months where if head tilt of the infant is found to be more than or equal to 6° then a cervical collar or brace [tubular orthosis for torticollis (TOT)] is added to the program during waking hours. With the increasing use of botulinum toxin it has been proposed that earlier injection of the toxin in less than optimally progressing or refractory cases of CMT at 3 months of age may improve the outcome significantly. This has also been found to be effective in cases of adult onset torticollis (cervical dystonia). Other forms of physical therapy have also been tried but their use is not prevalent as briefly mentioned here.

- Heat application using paraphino-therapy and thermotherapy.
- Iontophoresis from 2 weeks to 3 weeks of life (possibly for resorption, organization, and resolution the endomysial mass).
- Microcurrent therapy (may improve head tilt at supine and neck rotation ROM to the affected side).
- Massage of tight neck muscles and subcutaneous tissues to improve pain-free ROM.
- Kinesiology taping to improve muscular imbalance. Patients with suspected rotatory subluxation of atlantoaxial joint due to Grisel syndrome, postsurgery or trauma need to be evaluated by dynamic rotational computed tomography with neck in right and left lateral rotations. For symptoms last few days, treatment with anti-inflammatory and cervical spine immobilization would suffice. Symptoms lasting more than a week would need admission for injectable analgesics, traction and muscle relaxants, failing which 6 weeks halo vest traction would be needed. Patients presenting late or with fixed deformity would need posterior atlantoaxial fusion.

Surgical treatment: Failure of conservative and physical therapy would necessitate surgical release of the tight SCM muscle or neurotomy. Surgery is highly recommended when a restriction of movement up to 30° is present, as well in cases complicated with deformities of facial bones.

Timing of surgical intervention is contested for by authors. In general, surgical release may be considered in children with CMT between 1 year and 4 years of age (Chandler and Altenberg) resistant to conservative treatment. Manual stretching is not as effective after 1 year of age. For children aged more than 6 years of age, Chen and Ko recommended bipolar release. With the reporting of safe surgical release by Coventry and Harris the age for providing surgical treatment has been extended to 12 years. Cranial base and cranium deformities occur early in uncorrected torticollis while facial deformity develops in childhood. After puberty the remodeling potential of bones decreases tremendously, so surgery may not be very effective when the disease with deformity has fully settled. In these cases the crooked appearance may be improved along with improved ROM of cervical spine and elimination of head tilt to better their quality of life. All considerations and recommendations taken into account it has been believed that age at the time of release is an important determinant of outcome and that most favorable results are seen in children aged between 1 year and 4 years. This does not mean that surgery done within first few weeks of birth would be more successful. Rationale is that as most cases (>90%) resolve with stretching program with or without bracing and that there is a high tendency for surgical hematoma formation in infants, it is better to restrict use of knife in them. Also this does not mean that patients be deprived of surgery if they cross 4 years of age as then proper release will help prevent development of (or progression of) complications of torticollis like facial asymmetry, plagiocephaly, strabismus, blinding, cervical scoliosis, etc. Surgical lengthening of the contracted SCM is needed in only 3% of the cases. Two types of surgical procedures may be performed.

1. *Classical surgical division of the SCM muscle:* Here various options include endoscopic release, unipolar release at the sternoclavicular origin, bipolar open tenotomy (bipolar release), transection of the middle of the muscle, Z-plasties on the attachments of the sternal portion of SCM, and complete excision of the muscle. A section/release of the clavicular insertion of the SCM along with elongation in a Z-shape of its sterna insertion is commonly recommended and practiced. This provides adequate release and maintains normal outline of the SCM muscle. Bipolar release intends release of the mastoid insertion as may be needed in neglected cases (generally it is considered in children over age of 6 years as reported by excellent results of Arslan et al.). Once developed, facial asymmetry is difficult to correct and should be explained to the family and child that surgical release may not have any significant role in improving the facial discrepancies that have already set-in. An important practical guide to perform bipolar release is when unipolar release is unable to give satisfactory correction irrespective of age. Transaxillary endoscopic release of the fibrotic bands has been described by few author to provide neck scar free method. The advantages include quick and direct access with prevention of injury to neurovascular structures and cosmesis.
2. Surgical resection of the spinal accessory nerve and/or the anterior and posterior divisions of the first three cervical motor roots.

C. Sprengel shoulder: The superior border of scapula is situated normally at the seventh cervical vertebra and its inferior angle is at the level of the sixth rib. During embryonic development scapular enlarge is situated opposite the fifth cervical vertebra. Sprengel's deformity results from failure of scapular descent during embryologic development. The scapula remains hypoplastic, high-riding with varying degrees of reduced scapulothoracic movement.

Diagnosis: Primarily, the condition is identified on physical examination where the affected scapula appears small and high riding into the cervical spine. There is increased width to height ratio. The inferior pole is rotated medially with the glenoid pointing inferiorly. Due to weakening of parascapular muscles there could be scapular winging. Other findings include presence of webbed neck and a variable loss of ROM. Usually, the deformity is painless.

Investigations: Anteroposterior radiographs of shoulder confirm the diagnosis and a bony omovertebral bar may also be visualized. The condition can also be diagnosed prenatally by ultrasonography.

Treatment: The treatment is primarily surgical for conspicuous deformities with disability. Treatment is guided primarily based on Cavendish classification. The age of surgical intervention is of primary concern and often debated. Early intervention has chances of maximal correction during further growth before adaptive movements and restrictions develop. But the child may not bear the extensive nature of intervention and may succumb. So, the age of at least 3 years is considered by most as the optimal time for intervention. Surgical treatment involves primarily releasing the scapular tethers by resection of the superior angle of the scapula and the tethering omovertebral bar. Additionally, the scapula is derotated and relocated to a more caudal position. The greatest challenge put with caudal repositioning of the scapula, is the risk of compressive injury to the brachial plexus and it increases with age. This risk is greatest in children older than 8 years. Concomitant clavicular osteotomy may reduce the risk. Surgical techniques described for scapular relocation include:

- The Woodward procedure relocates the scapula by detachment and caudal relocation of the midline origin of the parascapular muscle (shifting the trapezius and rhomboids caudally along the spine). In addition, the superomedial scapular prominence may also be resected (Borges modification to Woodward's procedure). Clavicular osteotomy allows additional scapular descent. It is the most common surgical technique used for correction of a moderate or severe Sprengel's deformity with good cosmetic and functional improvement. The outcome of procedure is independent of the age of the patient or the presence of an omovertebral bone. Cervical spine anomalies, however, affect the outcome negatively.
- *The Green procedure:* Here scapula is derotated by extraperiosteal detachment of scapular muscles at their scapular insertion and scapula is laid free. After caudal relocation of the scapula and fixation using scapular traction cables, the parascapular detached muscles are reattached.

- *Vertical scapular osteotomy:* The lateral half of scapula is brought down caudally with concomitant clavicular osteotomy or morcellization. The clavicular osteotomy is recommended to reduce the risk of neurovascular injury and to provide anterior release. The correction achieved is limited, however, compared to other procedures.

2. A. Enumerate signs and symptoms of congenital torticollis in a 9-year-old child.
B. How will you manage spasmodic torticollis in a child?

Ans: A. Signs and symptoms of congenital torticollis is a 9-year-old (apparently untreated case):

Appearance of CMT is characteristic with tilt of the head toward the same side while chin points to the contralateral side due to torsional deformity of neck consequent upon shortened SCM muscle.

The other characteristic signs of torticollis include:
- Orbital dystopia (the eye on the unaffected side is higher up)
- Restricted rotation of the neck
- Dental malocclusion (the lower midline is deviated to the affected side, causing a unilateral crossbite, postnormal Class II molar relation on the affected side, and prenormal Class III molar occlusion on the unaffected side)
- Anteriorly shifted ear contralateral to the shortened SCM
- Secondary plagiocephaly (flattened parieto-occipital surface on the same side), frontal flattening (ipsilateral), and facial asymmetry
- Compensatory postures include shoulder elevation and side bending of the trunk on the ipsilateral side
- In late and neglected cases of CMT craniofacial asymmetry is seen that include:
  - Posterior displacement of ipsilateral ear (94%)
  - Posterior regression of ipsilateral zygoma (87%)
  - Posterior regression of ipsilateral forehead (81%)
  - Inferior positioning of the affected eye (31%)
  - Mandibular deviation toward affected side (44%)
  - Deviation of nasal tip toward affected side (31%)
  - Rhomboidal shape skull.

B. The management is described in Answer of Question 1.

3. Explain cleidocranial dysostosis.

Ans: Cleidocranial dysplasia is a condition that primarily affects the development of the bones and teeth. It is caused by a mutation of the core-binding factor α-1 (*CBFA1*) gene (also called *RUNX2*), a transcription factor that activates osteoblast differentiation. *RUNX2* gene (*CBFA1*) provides instructions for making a protein that is involved in bone and cartilage development and maintenance. *RUNX2* protein acts as a "master switch", regulating a number of other genes involved in the development of cells that build bones (osteoblasts). Due to mutational shortage of functional *RUNX2* protein the normal bone and cartilage development is interfered, resulting in the signs and symptoms of cleidocranial dysplasia. Although it should be remembered that one-third of the patients does not have a mutation of the gene and the cause of disease in these patients is unknown. The inheritance pattern is autosomal dominant. Incidence is nearly 1 per million individuals.

Clinical features: The affected individuals characteristically have the following features:
- *Clavicle hypoplasia or aplasia:* Their shoulders are narrow and sloping with an increased ability to appose the shoulders.
- Widening of the symphysis pubis.
- Delayed closing of fontanels (may persist up to adulthood)
- Coxa vara
- Short stature (3–6 inches shorter than family members)
- They may also have short, tapered fingers and broad thumbs; shortened middle phalanges of the third, fourth, and fifth fingers; short forearms; flat feet; knock knees; and an abnormal curvature of the spine (scoliosis)
- Characteristic facies may include a wide, short skull (brachycephaly); a prominent forehead; wide-set eyes (hypertelorism); a flat nose; and a small upper jaw.
- In females, due to abnormal shape of pelvis the rate of cesarean section is quite high.

- Dental abnormalities in these individuals are characterized by:
  - Delayed loss of the primary (baby) teeth.
  - Delayed appearance of the secondary (adult) teeth, often they are supernumerary and unless get absorbed, crowding of teeth occurs in adults requiring removal.
  - Unusually shaped, peg-like teeth
  - Misalignment of the teeth and jaws (malocclusion)
  - Extra teeth are sometimes accompanied by cysts in the gums.
- The individuals are also predisposed to ear and sinus infections, have hearing loss. Some children have delayed motor functions and development. Intelligence is but normal.

Treatment
- Clavicle hypoplasia does not require treatment unless there is irritation of brachial plexus in which case the clavicular fragments need excision.
- Valgus osteotomy is indicated for coxa vara with a neck shaft angle less than 100° and an associated Trendelenburg gait usually by 5 years of age to also prevent the worsening of deformity.
- Oral check-ups should be done regularly and otologist referral should be done for hearing problems.
- Craniofacial surgery may be needed in uncommon cases to correct skull defects.

4A.2 ROTATOR CUFF PATHOLOGY (Q4–20)

4. A. What is scapular dyskinesia?
B. Explain its role in rotator cuff impingement syndrome.

Ans: A. In brief, scapular dyskinesia is alteration in the normal static or dynamic position or motion of the scapula during coupled scapulohumeral movements. The scapula normally follows very rhythmic movement with the shoulder girdle. Movements of scapula however can become dyskinetic making the bone unstable for a number of reasons. A dysfunctional (as in arthritic joint) or nonfunctioning (as in distal clavicular resection) acromioclavicular joint or sternoclavicular joint (viz., post-traumatic) can also produce shoulder girdle abnormality causing an unstable scapula due to altered biomechanics. Seventeen muscles attach to the scapula; imbalance of muscular activity that primarily stabilizes the scapula can also hence cause an unstable scapula. Specifically, the muscles that stabilize scapula are the trapezius, the serratus anterior, the rhomboids, the levator scapulae, and the subscapularis. Abnormality in the stabilization of scapula produce broadly two groups of dysfunction—scapular dyskinesia which primarily involves nonrhythmic scapular rotations seen associated with the glenohumeral movements (primarily originating from muscular or neurological abnormalities of periscapular muscles) and altered scapulohumeral rhythm that is associated with impingement syndrome and later with rotator cuff tears.

B. Altered scapulohumeral rhythm that occurs with external impingement or rotator cuff tears, occurs due to alteration in the force-couple mechanism and hence noncoordinated position of scapula at rest and with dynamic motion. Typically, this is characterized by lost upward motion of acromion, excessive internal rotation of scapula, and excessive anterior tilt. There is poor patterning due to late activation of weak serratus anterior or early deactivation of it associated with early activation of trapezius and altered force couples. These produce scapular protraction which actually reduces subacromial space and decreases rotator cuff strength. Reduced space causes cuff impingement that may rupture into a full blown tear on repeated movements.

5. Explain painful arc syndrome.

Ans: It is also known as impingement syndrome of shoulder.

Subacromial impingement syndrome (SIS) or simply impingement syndrome is closely related to rotator cuff tear and often precedes nontraumatic cuff tears. With normal rotator cuff function, the humeral head translates less than 3 mm superiorly during the midranges of active elevation, whereas at extreme movements, anteroposterior (AP) and superoinferior translations of 4–10 mm do occur. An increase in superior translation with active abduction may result in encroachment of the coracoacromial arch. This encroachment produces a compression of the suprahumeral structures against the anteroinferior aspect of the acromion and coracoacromial ligament. Repeated compression of these structures, when coupled with other predisposing factors, results in SIS. It was first recognized by Jarjavay in 1867, and the term *impingement syndrome* was popularized by Neer in the 1970s. Now with detailed study various intrinsic and extrinsic factors have been implicated into the impingement process including the shape of acromion, cuff vascularization, functioning of dynamic stabilizers, acromioclavicular (AC) joint degeneration, position of arm during activities, capsular tightness, and repetitive activities. A number of impingement types and subtypes have thus evolved. Two of those broad types include the outlet (intrinsic) impingement, and the nonoutlet (extrinsic) impingement.

Outlet impingement: "Outlet impingement", classically described by Neer, is called so because it occurs at the supraspinatus outlet formed by the coracoid process, the anterior acromion, the AC joint, and the coracoacromial ligament. The term impingement syndrome refers to this outlet impingement per se. This type of impingement classically presents as a painful arc. Painful arc test is commonly used to diagnose SIS **(Fig. 4A.2.1)**. The patient is made to abduct the extremity to maximum possible overhead abduction. Reporting of pain in an arc between 45–60° and 120° is generally considered positive with a sensitivity of 33%, specificity of 81%, and positive likelihood ration of 1.7. One should further evaluate with positive Hawkins-Kennedy sign, Neer's test, Jobe's test and empty can sign and test to substantiate the diagnosis and identify the pathology.

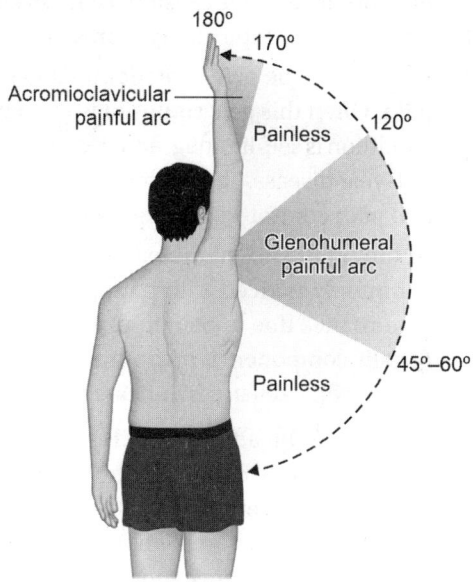

Fig. 4A.2.1: Painful arc test.

Outlet impingement *per se* is thought to be the cause of symptoms in 90–95% cases; however, with better understanding and evaluation of elderly, the role of degenerative changes is gathering importance. Neer divided the outlet impingement process into three stages, although the condition is a continuum of symptoms. These stages have specific findings and the intrinsic or extrinsic factors contributing to the problem.

- *Stage I:* This stage consists of localized inflammation, and edema of the rotator cuff typically observed in younger (<25 years of age) patients, although it can also be seen in older patients as a result of overuse. The patient has painful shoulder and a history of associated trauma or microtrauma. There is tenderness at the supraspinatus insertion and anterior acromion, the range of motion (ROM) is painful, and weakness arises due to pain. Scapular stabilization is jeopardized due to painful inhibition of the serratus anterior and trapezius.
- *Stage II:* This represents a progressive deterioration in the tissues of the rotator cuff typically seen in the 26- to 40-year-old age group. With continued irritation of the subacromial structures, secondary changes develop in the tissue. The subacromial bursa loses its ability to lubricate and tendonitis of the cuff develops. Especially the overhead activities are painful with pain commonly located on the top of the shoulder radiating to arm in the deltoid insertion region.
- *Stage III:* This is the end stage with destruction of the soft tissue and tear of the rotator cuff. It is commonly seen in patients above 40-year age. The wear of the anterior aspect of the acromion on the greater tuberosity and the supraspinatus tendon eventually results in a full-thickness tear of the rotator cuff. Degeneration of nearby AC joint is seen with osteophyte formation. Muscle atrophy is quite prominent especially of the infraspinatus and supraspinatus. There is progressive limitation in active and passive ROM. Rotator cuff tears hence develop.

Treatment: Nonsteroidal anti-inflammatory drugs (NSAIDs), physical therapy which includes the ultrasound massage and cryotherapy should be liberally used, especially in the stage 1 of SIS. Scapular and rotator cuff exercises, neuromuscular training exercises, and plyometric exercises will build the muscles around the shoulder girdle and are appropriate in stage 2 of SIS. This is usually effectively combined with passive joint mobilization and ROM. Conservative management should always include training for proper use and strengthening of core body and shoulder girdle musculature, and avoidance of aggravating activities that helps in preventing tear progression. Operative management is prescribed for patients whose symptoms are not relieved by above conservative measures for a minimum of 2–3 months, or for those who have a full-thickness symptomatic rotator cuff tear. For patients of impingement syndrome that failed with conservative management subacromial decompression gives good results. Subacromial decompression can be done by open or arthroscopic methods. The principles of surgery include removal of the subacromial bursa and removal of any bony spurs and, at times, the coracoacromial ligament.

6. Explain frozen shoulder. Also explain its clinical features and management.

Ans: The use of term frozen shoulder is more colloquial than scientific and usually describes end-stage adhesive capsulitis with rampant capsular and soft tissue contractures. The clinical features are as follows:

Patients of adhesive capsulitis have in general pain as the primary complaint with restriction of movements (so called frozen shoulder). Typically, two presentations can be seen:

1. In a subset, the pain is predominant complaint while the movement restriction does not corroborate to quantity of pain. Often this gets confused with rotator cuff disorder or impingement syndrome with incarcerated tendon. This condition is self-limiting, and the patient spontaneously recovers within 6 months to a year—the so-called connotation of 1-year disease. The treatment here is majorly supportive with stretching exercise program aimed to restore function and pain control with analgesics.
2. In the other subset, the pain is as prominent as restricted movements at shoulder and a radiation component is commonly noticed with pain going laterally from arm to elbow. The patient complains of pain at rest and sleep disturbance due to pain noticeable in specific postures. Typical restriction of external rotation is noticed. Because fibrotic component is predominant fibrolysis with manipulation, repetitive steroid injections, distension therapy, and arthroscopic release is indicated individually or in combinations.

Management: The advances in histopathological characterization or clinical judgment over time with recognition of various patterns have not contributed much to guide the treatment, which has been classically symptom based. Various modalities have been prescribed to basically improve movements and control pain without any logical reasoning as to how fast and how complete the relief of symptoms should be. Treatment options for adhesive capsulitis range from nonoperative to operative modalities. The various proposed methods by different authors for the treatment of frozen shoulder are education/watchful waiting; physical therapy (including physiotherapy, cryotherapy, and acupuncture), oral corticosteroids, NSAIDs, injections (corticosteroid, local anesthetic, and sodium hyaluronate), articular or arthrographic distension, manipulation under anesthesia, arthroscopic and open surgery, or a combination of these.

Conservative management is aimed at symptomatic relief and gradual return of shoulder function by stretching exercises. Patients need to be informed and counseled for protracted course of physiotherapy so that compliance is better. Interventions like local ultrasonics and guided program for intensive stretching in movement restricted patients. The steroids should be used to control pain and ongoing fibrosis keeping also in mind the prohibiting effects on collagen. Periarticular trigger point injection of subscapular tendon and pericapsular muscles provide at best temporary relief and are not effective in long term. Suprascapular nerve blocks improve patient's tolerance to deep pressure and may have possible role in patients associated with reflex sympathetic dystrophy. Despite aggressive maneuvers significant percentage of patients (30–50%) have long-term restriction of movements.

Various *interventional measures* have been reported to dilate capsule. Capsular distension or brisement relies on rupturing the capsule by fluid injection. Closed manipulation under anesthesia is recommended as a measure to stretch capsule but may be associated with recurrence of disease due to subsequent pain, neurological damage, uncontrolled damage due to stretching of tissue, and fractures in osteopenic patients. Sequential stretching of inferior, anteroinferior, anterior, posterior, and posteroinferior capsule should be done using force from only two fingers else arthroscopic release is recommended. Long-term diabetics are usually resistant to manipulation techniques.

Surgical management: Good return of function is achieved by arthroscopic anterior release and synovectomy combined with steroid injection. Prior to arthroscopic release the shoulder is manipulated to improve external rotation and abduction. This facilitates the arthroscopic visualization in an otherwise stiff, tight shoulder. Intra-articular steroid suppresses synovitis well compared to any oral therapy and controls the recurrence of fibrosis. Early intervention is the rule that should be followed and the technique is effective even in long-term diabetics. In general, the more the patient is delayed for treatment, the more protracted course he undergoes and takes longer time to recovery. Open release is rarely needed but may be used for recalcitrant shoulder stiffness following arthroscopic release.

7. Define adhesive capsulitis of shoulder.

Ans: It is aptly defined as "a condition of uncertain etiology characterized by significant restriction of both active and passive shoulder motion that occurs in the absence of a known intrinsic shoulder disorder" by the American Academy of Orthopedic Surgeons in 1993.

8. Describe boundaries of quadrilateral space (shoulder). Describe clinical features and treatment of quadrilateral syndrome briefly.

Ans: *Boundaries:*

Superior:
- Subscapularis in front.
- Capsule of the shoulder joint.
- Inferior border of teres minor behind.

Inferior: Superior border of teres major.

Medial: Lateral border of long head of the triceps brachii.

Lateral: Surgical neck of the humerus.

Contents:
- Axillary nerve
- Posterior circumflex humeral vessels.

Clinical features: Quadrilateral space syndrome results from compression of the axillary nerve that runs through this space. Compression of the nerve may occur from:
- Fibrous bands
- Trauma (scapular fracture)
- Paralabral cysts (inferior labral tear)
- Muscle hypertrophy
- Benign or malignant mass

Pain and paresthesias involving the lateral aspect of the shoulder and the posterosuperior region of the arm characterize the syndrome. Pain can be worse at night, and patients almost always point tender at the quadrilateral space itself. Weakness is most easily elicited in abduction and external rotation while overhead activities are painful. Eventually weakness and atrophy of the teres minor muscle may develop. It invariably spares the deltoid.

Radiology:

MRI: Sagittal oblique images best show the fatty atrophy of these muscles, seen as high signal intensity on T1W images.

Treatment: Medical management is initially conservative to control pain with NSAIDs and avoiding the movements causing aggravation of symptoms. Diagnostic lidocaine injections may be used while steroid injections may provide relief for 4–6 weeks. If conservative treatment has failed after 6 months, then surgical decompression is generally recommended.

9. A. Explain anatomy of rotator cuff and
B. Discuss clinical tests to diagnose rotator cuff tears, pathology, and outline its management.

Ans: A. *Anatomy:* The rotator cuff is a conjoint tendon made up of the lateral tendinous portions of the infraspinatus, supraspinatus, and subscapularis muscles that insert at greater and lesser tuberosity (supra- and infraspinatus, teres minor attaching to greater tuberosity and subscapularis to lesser tuberosity). The musculotendinous cuff passes beneath the coracoacromial arch, from which it is separated by the subacromial bursa; during abduction of the arm the cuff slides outward under the arch. Rotator interval is a triangular structure that lies between superior aspect of subscapularis tendon and anterior aspect of supraspinatus tendon. The base of triangle is located at coracoid. The deep surface of the cuff is intimately related to the joint capsule though microstructure of rotator cuff has been detailed into five layers near the insertion of supraspinatus and infraspinatus. The main function of the conjoint structure is to keep the humeral head firmly centered against the glenoid and stabilize it, when the deltoid muscle contracts and abducts the arm. Consequently, patients with rotator cuff tendinitis experience pain and weakness on active abduction and those with a severe tear of the cuff are unable to abduct the arm at all; while still they have the capability to hold arm into abduction over-head if done passively **(Fig. 4A.2.2)**.

B. *Clinical Tests (Table 4A.2.1):* Clinical examination reveals generally preserved motion of shoulder especially external rotation (it is usually restricted in adhesive capsulitis).
- Neer-Hawkins test and Jobe's test are positive in cuff impingement.
- Empty can and full can test for supraspinatus impingement/bursitis.
- Horn blower's sign will test the integrity of infraspinatus and teres minor tendons.
- External rotation stress test and drop sign for infraspinatus and teres minor.
- The "lift-off test" assesses the integrity of the lower subscapularis muscle.
- Belly press and Napoleon test estimate the integrity of upper subscapularis.
- Drop arm test if positive indicates complete rotator cuff tear.

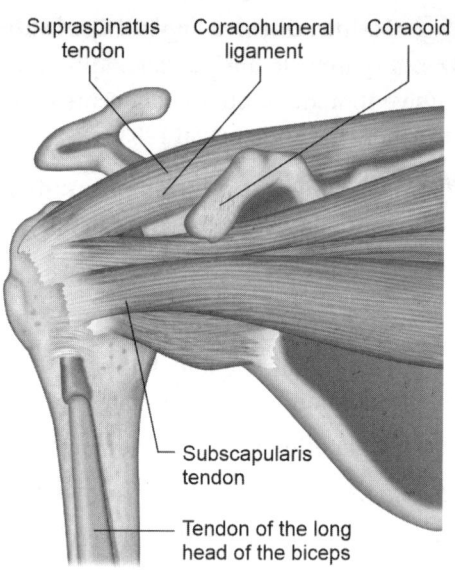

Fig. 4A.2.2: Anatomy of rotator cuff.

TABLE 4A.2.1: Clinical tests for rotator cuff tears.

Test	Finding	Muscle
Drop arm test	Patient unable to maintain arm in 90° elevation	Supraspinatus
External rotation lag test	Patient unable to maintain arm in maximum external rotation in adduction	Infraspinatus
Hornblower sign	Patient unable to maintain arm in external rotation 90° abduction, 90° external rotation	Teres minor
Belly press test	Paint while pressing on abdomen with hand and elbows anterior to midsagittal plane of body	Upper subscapularis
Lift-off test	Patient unable to maintain hand off lumbosacral spine in full internal rotation	Lower subscapularis

Pathology: The current understanding of rotator cuff pathology can be summarized into four mechanisms—
1. *Tensile overload:* The rotator cuff is subject to stretching forces when it attempts to resist horizontal adduction, internal rotation, anterior translation, and distraction forces eventually damaging the collagen fibers.
2. *Compression:* Compression of the cuff can either be primarily due to a reduction in the size of the subacromial space, or secondary (dynamic) due to joint instability.
3. *Internal impingement:* Stretching and impingement of the rotator cuff tendons in internal impingement leads to articular side tear of supraspinatus and infraspinatus [partial articular surface tendon avulsion (PASTA)]. The PASTA lesion term was coined by Snyder et al. to describe the articular side lesions at junction of supra- and infraspinatus tendons. Rotator cuff tears in throwers can extend into middle layers of infraspinatus tendon delineated by Conway et al. and termed partial articular-sided intrasubstance tears (PAINT) lesion.
4. *Acute trauma:* Tearing of the tendon results when forces generated by the trauma exceed the tensile strength of the tendon.

Diagnosis: Radiographs (AP in internal and external rotation, scapular Y-view) are usually unremarkable but may show subtle or prominent (depending on duration) greater tuberosity sclerosis, subacromial spurs or sclerosis (sourcil sign), and narrowing of the acromiohumeral distance. Glenohumeral arthritis should also be noted. Few patients may show a type 2 or type 3 acromion which has no bearing on the intensity of the symptoms. Cuff tear arthropathy obviously tells long-standing disorder.

Computed tomography (CT) scan is useful particularly for its ability to grade tears based on the Goutallier grading system which describes grades consequent to muscle fatty infiltration. A higher preoperative degree (≥ grade 3) is associated with recurrent tears and lower constant scores.

Magnetic resonance imaging (MRI) is an excellent method to confirm the diagnosis and the extent of involvement for a rotator cuff tear images show hyperintense signals of the supraspinatus tendon in T2-weighted images. MR arthrogram is beneficial for detecting small, full-thickness tears and depicting the extent of partial articular-sided tears. Ultrasound is an accurate, highly user-dependent, noninvasive, less expensive method of detecting rotator cuff tears. It can be as useful as MRI but requires a highly experienced person.

Treatment: Conservative therapy is best suited for patients having cuff symptoms with incomplete (partial thickness) tears. This includes rest, activity modification, gentle passive and active motion exercises, anti-inflammatory medication, and subacromial corticosteroid injections.

Surgical treatment options for rotator cuff tear: Surgical repair of rotator cuff tears can be performed through open, arthroscopically assisted mini-open, or all-arthroscopic techniques. Various anatomic types and configuration patterns of tears have been described but they are not helpful in defining the treatment. Acromioplasty and subacromial decompression are usual accompaniments to relieve pressure on the cuff preserving deltoid function.

Open rotator cuff repair: A diagnostic arthroscopy is recommended to be performed before open repair as restaging and visual examination often differs from the clinical and imaging picture. Also concomitant pathologies can be simultaneously identified. In large and massive tears, the degree of glenohumeral arthritis may be more severe than suggested by preoperative evaluation precluding repair. Typically, the biceps tendon pathology (subluxation, fraying, tenosynovitis, insertional detachment or hypertrophy) is not appreciated well on imaging and needs proper addressal in the form of tenodesis or tenotomy as the case may be. Skin incisions are planned with respect to addressing all current pathologies (including massive tears) and keeping in mind the future requirements of revision surgery including arthroplasty. An oblique incision from the posterior edge of the AC joint to the anterolateral corner of the acromion that extends 2–3 cm distally between the anterior and middle deltoid provides excellent visualization for cuff repair (simultaneously also it allows for anterosuperior access for revision surgery including reverse shoulder arthroplasty). With open repair, the arthroscopic portals should be closed and the shoulder draped again to prevent infection. Often a distal clavicle resection and acromioplasty and subacromial bursectomy are added to improve access to the subacromial space without compromising deltoid anatomy. The coracohumeral ligament is palpated in external rotation, adduction, and released if it is tight. This gives excellent exposure to the rotator cuff pathology for evaluation, mobilization, and repair. The repair techniques (single-row, double-row, transosseous, and transosseous equivalent) are similar in arthroscopic and open surgery and depend on surgeon preference and training. The deltoid should be meticulously repaired.

Arthroscopic repair: Arthroscopic rotator cuff surgery as stated above has become increasingly popular and more standardized. Often a beach-chair position with arm holder is preferred that also allows conversion to open repair if required. Some critical aspects are addressed as follows. For partial thickness tears, the typical treatment includes debridement, transtendinous in situ repair, or tear completion and repair. Tears that are at least 50% tend to progress to full-thickness tears and should be repaired. Repair with tear completion and transtendinous repair have both produced good and excellent results. Tear completion facilitates debridement of the degenerative tendon while the later has been boasted of avoiding the creation of a full-thickness tear.

The controversy of single-row versus double-row repair is unsettled by and large. Double-row fixation is costly, time-consuming, and technically more difficult when performed arthroscopically but biomechanically have higher initial fixation strength and stiffness, improved footprint restoration, and decreased gap formation. It is suggested that for larger tears (>3 cm), double-row fixation may be better as recent studies have reported higher American Shoulder and Elbow Surgeon and constant scores with double-row fixation in tears larger than 3 cm. Also better healing has been demonstrated with CT arthrography following double-row fixation but clinical superiority for smaller tears is unsubstantiated for smaller tears between the two methods. Further, it is notable that the transosseous and transosseous equivalent rotator cuff repair techniques produce low bone-tendon interface motion, excellent footprint restoration, a high number of cycles to failure in biomechanical and clinical evaluations and could improve the current repair technique scenario for large and massive tears but are technically demanding. They are preferred for cuff tears that can be adequately mobilized reattached to bone (through anchors) or tears juxtaposed to tuberosity.

10. Briefly describe 3 clinical tests to diagnose rotator cuff tendinosis of shoulder.

Ans: The tests are written in answer above. When there's pain but no weakness during the test, it implies tendinosis but when weakness plus pain is there then it is tear.

11. How will you investigate and manage a case of chronic full thickness rotator cuff tear in a 65-year-old osteoporotic female?

Ans: *Investigations:* Radiographs (AP in internal and external rotation, scapular Y-view) are usually unremarkable but may show subtle or prominent (depending on duration) greater tuberosity sclerosis, subacromial spurs or sclerosis (sourcil sign), and narrowing of the acromiohumeral distance. Glenohumeral arthritis should also be noted. Few patients may show a type 2 or type 3 acromion which has no bearing on the intensity of the symptoms. Cuff tear arthropathy obviously tells long-standing disorder.

MRI is useful particular for its ability to grade tears based on the Goutallier grading system which describes grades consequent to muscle fatty infiltration. A higher preoperative degree ($\geq$ grade 3) is associated with recurrent tears and lower constant scores. Also, it confirms the diagnosis and the extent of involvement for a rotator cuff tear. Images show hyperintense signals of the supraspinatus tendon in T2-weighted images. MR arthrogram is beneficial for detecting small, full-thickness tears and depicting the extent of partial articular-sided tears. Ultrasound is an accurate, highly user-dependent, noninvasive, less expensive method of detecting rotator cuff tears. It can be as useful as MRI but requires a highly experienced person. Also, MRI tells about the glenohumeral joint arthritis.

Management:
- Repairable tear without joint arthritis—Arthroscopic rotator cuff repair
- Irrepairable tear without joint arthritis—Superior capsular reconstruction
- Irrepairable tear with joint arthritis—Reverse shoulder arthroplasty

Arthroscopic repair: Arthroscopic rotator cuff surgery has become increasingly popular and more standardized. Often a beach-chair position with arm holder is preferred that also allows conversion to open repair if required. Tears that are at least 50% tend to progress to full-thickness tears and should be repaired. Repair with tear completion and transtendinous repair have both produced good and excellent results. Tear completion facilitates debridement of the degenerative tendon while the later has been boasted of avoiding the creation of a full-thickness tear.

Augmentation techniques for repair: It is logical that large and massive tears have high failure rates (up to 94% at 1 year) so augmentation techniques are yet another tool to strengthen the repair techniques. The recurrent tears are currently managed with augmentation; however, it is recommended to augment large and massive tear primary repair with allograft or xenograft tissues to improve repair strength and provide a bioreplaceable collagen network in an effort to decrease failure rates. Human dermal allograft is possibly the best method (not available in India currently) as porcine dermis, and porcine smooth intestine submucosa have been found to induce adverse immunological graft reactions.

Massive unrepairable tears: There are yet instances where tears are so large and massive that repair is not possible with current methods. For such cases, especially in young patients or active individuals with higher functional demands, tendon transfers are a viable option to reduce pain and restore function. Latissimus dorsi tendon transfer is recommended for patients with an intact subscapularis, an irreparable, painful posterosuperior rotator cuff tear with external rotation deficit. Though grade 2 or less fatty infiltration of the teres minor on preoperative imaging is ideal condition but satisfactory results are reported even with teres minor dysfunction. The tendon transfer improves external rotation and forward flexion. The pectoralis major tendon transfer is designed for treating symptomatic anterosuperior tears with an irreparable subscapularis tendon. The tendon transfer is commonly done over the conjoint tendon whereas underneath repairs have also been described. Interestingly like the confounding influence of teres minor on latissimus dorsi tendon transfer, an irreparable supraspinatous tear produces worse outcome with pectoralis major transfer so it should be concomitantly addressed. Reconstruction of superior shoulder capsule to provide stability to chronic massive irreparable cuff tears is also being explored.

12. Mention clinical and surgical significance of rotator interval.

Ans: *Clinical significance:* The rotator interval is composed of the coracohumeral ligament (CHL) and superior and middle glenohumeral ligaments deeper, even if the middle glenohumeral ligament contribution is relatively variable (different studies has reported its absence, from 10 to 40% of cases). Usually, it is larger in males than in females and becomes smaller with internal rotation. It is an important inferior stabilizer, and its insufficiency could be clinically appreciated with sulcus sign examination. A rotator interval defect could be a little foramen or could reach larger size, influencing significantly inferior stability.

Sulcus test: With the patient sitting and the arm in internal rotation, traction is applied to the arm. Sunken skin between the acromion and humeral head is a positive sign. In a nonpathological shoulder, with the arm in external rotation, the sulcus sign disappears. A positive sulcus sign means that there is laxity of rotator interval: 1+ means subluxation <1 cm; 2+ means subluxation of 1–2 cm; and 3+ means subluxation >2 cm.

Surgical significance: The rotator interval is characteristically involved in adhesive capsulitis. Scar tissue forms around the SGHL and the coracohumeral ligament in the rotator interval. Arthroscopic rotator interval release is thereby done in patients suffering from adhesive capsulitis. Also, in general, arthroscopists enter the shoulder joint through rotator interval to avoid damaging tendons. Rotator cuff interval tears may occur secondary to anterior glenohumeral dislocations or instability or due to surgical defect from arthroscopy. When torn, rotator interval becomes patulous.

13. Describe anatomy of subacromial space. What is morphology of acromion process in the pathogenesis of rotator cuff tear? How will you manage full thickness tear?

Ans: *Subacromial space:* The *subacromial space*, as the name suggests, is the space under the surface of the acromion and the coracoid process of the scapula with the coracoacromial ligament (aka "roof of shoulder") stretched between them **(Fig. 4A.2.3)**.

- The roof of space is formed by the coracoacromial arch and the acromioclavicular joint.
- The floor of the space is formed by the greater tuberosity and upper portions of the humeral head.
- The space is occupied by the rotator cuff tendons, the tendon of the long head of biceps brachii, and the subacromial and subdeltoid bursae.

Morphology of acromion: The pathology of impingement is more related to acromion anatomy and biomechanical strain. Three types of acromion were originally recognized by Bigliani et al. in 1986 based on the outlet view radiographs based on morphology of anterior edge, to which a fourth type has been added by Vanarthos (identified on sagittal oblique MRI) in 1995.

1. Flat inferiorly
2. Curved with undersurface parallel to humeral head—most common type
3. Hooked—where the most anterior part is bent downward forming a hook. Anteriorly hooked acromion (type 3 Bigliani) is associated with friction and degenerative tear due to extrinsic impingement on the tendon.
4. Convex—here the undersurface of the acromion is convex near the distal end.

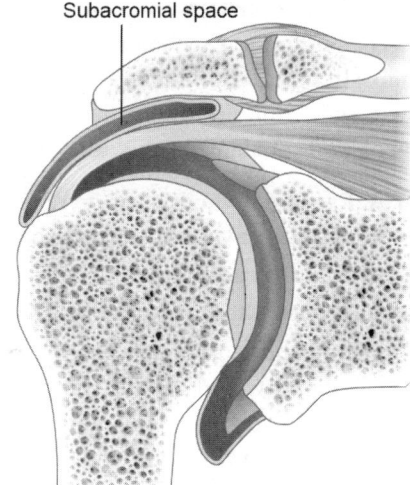

Fig. 4A.2.3: Anatomy of subacromial space.

Type 1 (straight) and type 2 (curved) do not cause supraspinatus impingement. The different shapes of acromion are not congenital but develop in response to traction forces applied by the coracoacromial ligament on it.

Management of full thickness rotator cuff tear

Investigations: Radiographs (AP in internal and external rotation, scapular Y-view) are usually unremarkable but may show subtle or prominent (depending on duration) greater tuberosity sclerosis, subacromial spurs or sclerosis, and narrowing of the acromiohumeral distance. Cuff tear arthropathy obviously tells long-standing disorder. CT scan is useful particularly for its ability to grade tears based on the Goutallier grading system. A higher preoperative degree (≥ grade 3) is associated with recurrent tears and lower constant scores. MRI is an excellent method to confirm the diagnosis and the extent of involvement for a rotator cuff tear images show hyperintense signals of the supraspinatus tendon in T2-weighted images. MR arthrogram is beneficial for detecting small, full-thickness tears and depicting the extent of partial articular-sided tears.

Conservative management of rotator cuff tears: Consider a combination of modalities individually in the conservative management of rotator cuff pathology. Avoid pain aggravating/producing movements, NSAIDs, physical modalities, subacromial steroid injection for documented subacromial bursitis. Some patients also benefit from suprascapular nerve block.

Surgical treatment options for rotator cuff tear
Surgical repair of rotator cuff tears can be performed through open, arthroscopically assisted mini-open, or all-arthroscopic techniques. Acromioplasty and subacromial decompression are usual accompaniments to relieve pressure on the cuff preserving deltoid function.

Open repair: Perform a diagnostic arthroscopy to identify associated lesions that might also need treatment. Skin incisions are planned with respect to addressing all current pathologies (including massive tears) and keeping in mind the future requirements of revision surgery including arthroplasty. An oblique incision from the posterior edge of the AC joint to the anterolateral corner of the acromion that extends 2–3 cm distally between the anterior and middle deltoid provides excellent visualization for cuff repair. The repair techniques (single-row, double-row, transosseous, and transosseous equivalent) are similar in arthroscopic and open surgery and depend on surgeon preference and training. Often a distal clavicle resection and acromioplasty and subacromial bursectomy are added to improve access to the subacromial space without compromising deltoid anatomy. The coracohumeral ligament is palpated in external rotation, adduction, and released if it is tight. This gives excellent exposure to the rotator cuff pathology for evaluation, mobilization, and repair.

Arthroscopic repair: Arthroscopic rotator cuff surgery as stated above has become increasingly popular and more standardized. Often a beach-chair position with arm holder is preferred that also allows conversion to open repair if required. The controversy of single-row versus double-row repair is unsettled by and large. Double-row fixation is costly, time-consuming, and technically more difficult when performed arthroscopically but biomechanically have higher initial fixation strength and stiffness, improved footprint restoration, and decreased gap formation. It is suggested that for larger tears (>3 cm), double-row fixation may be better as recent studies have reported higher American Shoulder and Elbow Surgeon and constant scores with double-row fixation in tears larger than 3 cm.

14. **A. Explain principles of reverse shoulder replacement. Enumerate its indications. How is it different from conventional shoulder arthroplasty?**
   B. Explain radial head prosthesis, its design, and technique of implantation.

Ans: A. Reverse shoulder arthroplasty (RSA) principles:
- Reversing the component design so that the weight-bearing part is convex and located at glenoid while the supporting moving part would acquire a concave shape attached to the humeral shaft. Initially, the glenoid component was two-thirds of a sphere centered at the center of rotation of native glenoid, this was then changed to a hemisphere positioning the glenohumeral center of rotation at the interface of the glenoid component and scapula (neck). Also the stemmed humeral component was introduced.
- Restricting glenoid translation by making the weight-bearing part at glenoid convex along with two essential modifications:
  1. Center of the sphere (glenosphere) should lie within the glenoid neck. This eliminated the neck totally and its associated complications. Neckless hemisphere was found to induce compressive forces at the implant bone interface rather than creating shear forces that were responsible for failure of initial designs.
  2. The center of rotation must be medialized and shifted a bit distally. Medialization of glenosphere by 10 mm increases deltoid moment by 20% at an abduction angle of 60°. Medializing the center of rotation in an almost horizontal humeral concave component however produces the so called "inferior scapular notching" by impingement of humeral poly component and inferior glenoid bony rim. This necessitates distalizing the component so that ROM is impingement free. Also with distalization of the glenosphere by 10 mm the abductor moment is further increased by 30% (increased deltoid efficiency). Some authors prefer to lateralize the glenoid component by

using a convex baseplate however increasing the tilting forces at the baseplate-bone interface. Medialization and distalization also impact the excursion of humerus tuberosities by increasing it, so for a given diameter of total shoulder arthroplasty (TSA) humeral sphere the tuberosities have to travel a greater distance when instead reverse total shoulder arthroplasty (RTSA) is used, the implications are unclear but some authors did find tuberosity impingement at the spine of scapula levering out the humeral socket and the risk in fact increases the more the humerus is lateralized.

- Providing intrinsic stability (albeit with some loss of movements)—this biomechanically implies zero mismatch in the radii of curvature of convex and concave surfaces as is provided in RTSA components. In the conventional TSA the spherical humeral component has shorter radius of curvature to that of the glenoid by a proportion of at least 5.5 mm to basically prevent rim loading, but in effect this is responsible for pseudoparesis of abduction (despite full ROM passively and absence of any neurological disease) in patients with inadequate rotator cuff. In a conventional TSA, the joint reaction force should be within 30° of the glenoid center line so that effective abduction can happen. In the absence of rotator cuff the unopposed action of deltoid results in superior translation of the spherical head and the joint reaction force vector lies beyond the required less than 30° of glenoid center line. So most of the effort goes waste in translation of the head instead of producing rotation at the joint—causing pseudoparesis. In RTSA, the deeper concave component and smaller convex component with shorter radius of curvature is responsible for increasing the joint force vector to 45° and even more without the risk of dislocating, hence increasing the inherent stability. Also rotation is quite subtly induced in a concave stem component oriented at 155° (neck-shaft angle) that is pulled up by deltoid against a spherical component, rather than translating superiorly.
- Compensating for deltoid dysfunction partially—RTSA offers methods to increase tension in the deltoid by distally translating the humerus (increasing the size of poly insert) and also distalizing the glenosphere. The other benefit is that even if the anterior deltoid is damaged by previous surgeries the elevation in RTSA is affected by lateral deltoid which is commonly preserved.

Difference from conventional prosthesis: The reverse prosthesis converts the conventional geometry of the shoulder joint of medial cup-lateral ball to lateral cup-medial ball design thereby changing the direction of pull of the deltoid muscle. With standard prostheses (that reconfigures original shoulder geometry), absence of rotator cuff allows the humeral head to subluxate superiorly (because of minimal restraint from the medial cup) during deltoid muscle contraction. The reverse prosthesis corrects the abnormal vector by moving the center of rotation of the arm laterally and by redirecting the pull of deltoid muscle more horizontally reducing the vertical vector. Moving the center of rotation with the prosthesis allows the deltoid to elevate the arm despite the shoulder joint having few or no rotator cuff tendons present.

Indications of RSA:
- Primarily the prosthesis is considered when shoulder pain due to arthritis and functional loss say rotator cuff tear or deltoid dysfunction cannot be managed by conventional surgical reconstruction methods. Such patients usually have paresis of anterior and/or lateral elevation of the arm. Fixed upper displacement of humeral head (anterosuperior escape) relative to glenoid and massive rotator cuff tears managed with hemiarthroplasty had inconsistent results due to recurrent instability and glenoid arthrosis but results have been superior with reverse prosthesis. One should notice that patients with both advanced arthritis and massive rotator cuff tears are ideal candidates for RTSA and not patients with any one of them.
- Other indications for RTSA include a failed prosthetic reconstruction with superior, anterior, or posterior instability (i.e., revision surgery); or a failed reconstruction for a traumatic injury with pseudoparalysis and instability.
- Possible indications—three or four part fractures in elderly older than 70 years of age; rheumatoid arthritis with adequate glenoid bone stock and revision of failed fracture fixation, revision of failed RTSA itself!

B. Radial head prosthesis:
Design: The many types of radial head implants now available have evolved from a monoblock design to modular prostheses, some of which incorporate bipolar features and different materials that may lessen the likelihood of capitellar wear from the prosthesis. Radial head replacement should be close to an anatomical substitute. Generally, the proximal edge of the radial head is 0.9 mm distal to the lateral coronoid edge, but patient variability might make imaging of the contralateral elbow useful for sizing purposes. To prevent capitellar wear from overstuffing the radiocapitellar joint, the

proximal edge of the prosthesis should be level with the lateral coronoid edge. Correct sizing and appropriate reattachment of the lateral ligamentous complex are necessary to prevent edge binding of the radial head prosthesis.

Technique:
- Position the patient *supine* or in the *lateral position* with the affected elbow up. Prepare and drape the extremity to expose the elbow with the arm across the chest (*supine position*).
- Use tourniquet for ease of surgery.
- *Using conventional Kocher posterolateral approach:* Begin the incision superior to the lateral epicondyle, and extend it distally approximately 6 cm across the joint in the interval between the extensor carpi ulnaris and the anconeus.
- Proceeding between the two muscles, expose the lateral capsule of the elbow. Else in traumatic cases the stripped lateral capsular structures from the lateral epicondyle, themselves allow removal of bone fragments and exposure of the radial neck.
- Dislocate the radial head or radial shaft as the case may be through the interval and cut the radial neck just proximal to the fracture site.
- Prepare the proximal radial medullary canal with burrs or rasps to accept the implant stem to achieve snug fit of the stem in the medullary canal.
- Prepare proximal radius in an even horizontal plane so that contact between it and the collar of the prosthesis is complete.
- Choose a prosthesis that allows good contact with the capitellum and does not overfill the joint.
- Check the radiocapitellar contact and reconstructed joint by moving the forearm through a range of flexion, extension, and rotation to observe in AP and lateral projections and rotations for stability.
- Insert the final prosthesis—cemented or uncemented depends on the type being used.
- Make drill holes or use a suture anchor at the capitellar rotation center to reattach lateral capsular structures, including the lateral ulnar collateral ligament to its isometric point with the ulnohumeral joint held reduced.
- Leave a suction drain in the wound, close the wound in layers, and protect the elbow with a compression dressing in 90° of flexion.

15. Radial head prosthesis:
   A. Discuss indications of surgery.
   B. Discuss complications.

Ans:
A. *Indications:* Radial head fractures associated with elbow dislocations frequently are comminuted and cannot be reconstructed. In this situation, the lateral ulnar collateral ligament is injured with concomitant elbow instability, and a radial head replacement is recommended to help stabilize the joint and facilitate early mobilization. These complex injury patterns may include either a coronoid fracture and/or a medial collateral ligament rupture. If the radial head is fractured and the distal radioulnar joint is dislocated (the Essex-Lopresti lesion), proximal migration of the radius after simple radial head excision may be mitigated by a radial head implant. Attempts to prevent recurrent elbow dislocation, proximal migration of the radius, and excessive instability after certain elbow and forearm axis injuries have led to an evolution of radial head prosthetic designs.
B. *Complications:* Nerve paresthesias, nerve entrapment/injury, ankylosis, loosening, instability, infection, and fracture.

16. What are the contraindications of reverse shoulder arthroplasty?
Ans: Contraindications of reverse shoulder arthroplasty include:
- Loss or inactivity of the anterior deltoid
- Excessive glenoid bone loss that would not allow secure implantation of the glenoid component. Some authors have suggested that the procedure is unsuitable for patients younger than 70 years old.
- Rheumatoid arthritis is a relative contraindication because of concerns about glenoid loosening.

17. Explain pathophysiology of cuff tear arthroplasty.
Ans: This is not an appropriate question, possibly it should be rotator cuff arthropathy that has been described above or it may be arthroplasty for rotator cuff arthropathy—that may be referred to in answer above.

18. Discuss briefly the biological treatment options for rotator cuff tears.

Ans: Please read Chapter no. 2 for detailed biological methods used for enhancing rotator cuff healing (like platelet-rich plasma, growth factors, stem cells, and exosomes).

19. Explain:
  A. Management of marrow edema syndrome and
  B. SLAP (superior labral tear from anterior to posterior) lesions.

Ans: A. *Marrow edema syndrome* is a transient clinical condition of unknown etiology.
It includes conditions like:
- Regional migratory osteoporosis
- Transient osteoporosis of hip
- Reflex sympathetic dystrophy.

Diagnosis

Conventional radiography: Radiographs may be normal in the early stages of transient osteoporosis. Usually at 3–6 weeks from the onset of symptoms there is periarticular osseous demineralization manifest as osteopenia. These findings may persist even weeks after the symptoms have resolved (sometimes up to 2 years). The joint space remains intact with preserved bony margins and there are no subchondral erosions. In advanced stages of transient osteoporosis, the femoral head may seem to completely disappear in osseous architecture—the "phantom appearance" of the femoral head. The trochanter, acetabulum, and iliac wings are rarely affected.

Bone scintigraphy: Though nonspecific, the findings of technetium Tc-99m methylene diphosphonate scintigraphy is useful in the early diagnosis of transient osteoporosis. Increased uptake (seen in all three phases) in the affected joint usually precedes radiologic features and can appear within a few days after the onset of symptoms. Bone scanning is sensitive, but not specific for detection of transient osteoporosis and can be used in symptomatic period when radiographs are normal. Scintigraphy however, appears to be very useful both for monitoring the progression of the disease and therapeutic response. It is also helpful in differentiating transient osteoporosis from other conditions that are characterized by regional osteopenia. With subsidence of symptoms reduced activity on the perfusion and blood pool phases are noted that indicate resolution of disease. Increased activity in the delayed bone phase may still persist for many months due to repair activity.

MRI: It is the modality of choice. On MRI, bone marrow edema (BME) is characterized by increased signal intensity on fat-suppressed T2-weighted and short tau inversion recovery images. These are complemented by low-signal intensity on T1-weighted images. BME is, however, a nonspecific finding and enhancement of the BME area after intravenous administration of contrast agents is indicative of hypervascularity and increased permeability of the capillary bed. Vasodilation and increased permeability may constitute a result rather than a cause of the BME disclosed on MRI. Differentiation from osteonecrosis is important as early stages may mimic transient osteoporosis lesion. The lack of subchondral changes other than BME on both T2-weighted and contrast-enhanced T1-weighted highly suggests transient lesions. Subchondral area of low-signal intensity at least 4 mm thickness on either T2-weighted or contrast-enhanced T1-weighted images suggests osteonecrosis. Presence of contour deformity and areas of subchondral low-signal intensity further support osteonecrosis.

Treatment

Transient osteoporosis is a self-limiting disease and treatment is mainly supportive primarily aimed to reduce pain and protect the bone due to reduced mechanical strength. Protected weight-bearing, mild analgesics, and administration of NSAIDs are main therapeutic approaches. Glucocorticoids are not found to be effective for remineralization though they improve pain symptoms in anti-inflammatory doses. Sympathetic blockade provides no definitive improvement of results in the treatment of transient osteoporosis. Bisphosphonates (especially intravenous) may help in reducing pain and improving bone strength. Oral calcium and corrective doses of vitamin D should be started. Iloprost, a prostacyclin analog, has shown pain relief in patients with transient osteoporosis of hip and BME syndrome by possibly dilating the vessels and reducing permeability.

B. *SLAP lesions:*

Diagnosis: A combination of positive O'Brien test, speed's test and apprehension with arm in 90° of abduction and maximal external rotation has been found to be 75% sensitive and 90% specific for diagnosis, though Crank and Yergason's tests are also positive. MRI will identify the lesion in doubtful cases though MR arthrogram is a more specific investigation.

Treatment: Conservative treatment is the preferred modality in low-demand patients and even in high-grade athletes. High-demand athletes also are first managed conservatively as they need to have enough intrinsic laxity while also stability to prevent subluxation (thrower's paradox). Even minimal decreases in ROM are potentially dangerous to career. There should be stress on dynamic stabilization exercises and stabilizing the shoulder thus usually suffices. Focused core-strengthening, trunk stability, and pelvic stabilization exercises should be stressed. Labral and rotator cuff pathologies are addressed by rotator cuff stretching and strengthening and correcting the internal rotation deficits (GIRD).

Repair of the lesion is indicated in high-level athletes for restoring function if the conservative management fails after 6 months of faithful perusal. The order of repair is usually as follows:
- Rotator cuff debridement
- Labrum debridement
- Posterior and superior labrum repair
- Articular-sided rotator cuff repair (PASTA lesions)
- Anterior labrum repair
- Intratendinous rotator cuff repair (PAINT lesions).

20. **What is the rocking horse effect after a total shoulder arthroplasty (TSA)? What are the methods to manage it after a total shoulder arthroplasty?**

Ans: The "rocking horse effect" in the context of TSA denotes a specific type of instability characterized by excessive movement of the humeral component relative to the glenoid component. This phenomenon may occur postoperatively, particularly when the humeral head retains a degree of mobility that allows it to oscillate, akin to the motion of a rocking horse. This instability can result from:
- *Improper component positioning:* Malalignment during the surgical procedure can lead to abnormal movement patterns.
- *Soft tissue imbalance:* Insufficient balance and tension in the surrounding soft tissues (capsule, ligaments, and muscles) can compromise stability.
- *Inadequate glenoid bone support*: Deterioration of glenoid bone or inadequate fixation can lead to loss of stability of the implant.

This effect often results in pain, decreased range of motion, and may significantly impact the functional outcome of the joint replacement.

Management of the Rocking Horse Effect

Management of the rocking horse effect following total shoulder arthroplasty involves multiple strategies:
- *Rehabilitation and physical therapy:*
  - Emphasize strengthening the rotator cuff and scapular stabilizers to enhance overall shoulder function and stability.
  - Implement specific exercises targeting the range of motion and stability without imposing excessive stress on the joint.
- *Activity modification:*
  - Advise patients to avoid high-risk activities that could exacerbate instability, particularly overhead and heavy lifting.
- *Surgical intervention:*
  - *Revision surgery:* If instability persists despite conservative measures, surgical revision may be necessary. This could involve:
    - Repositioning or revising the humeral component to enhance stability.
    - Addressing any bone loss with grafting techniques or using specialized implants designed for deficient bone.
    - Soft tissue procedures, such as capsular tightening or repairing any torn ligaments that may contribute to instability.

- *Orthotic support:* In some cases, a shoulder brace may be recommended initially to provide stability while rehabilitative efforts are ongoing.
- *Pain management:* Utilize analgesics, anti-inflammatory medications, and corticosteroid injections as necessary to manage discomfort and inflammation.
- *Monitoring:* Regular follow-up assessments are essential to evaluate progression and effectiveness of treatments and to make any adjustments to the rehabilitation plan as needed.

4A.3 SHOULDER INSTABILITY AND ARTHRODESIS (Q21–32)

21. A. Explain various clinical tests to assess glenohumeral instability.
B. How will you manage anterior dislocation of shoulder with Bankart lesion and Hill-Sachs lesion associated with dislocation?

Ans: A. **Clinical tests:**

The apprehension–relocation test is performed to diagnose suspected anterior instability cases. Apprehension test as described by Rowe consists of maximally externally rotating the shoulder with patient supine and shoulder in 90° of abduction and elbow flexed to 90°. Patients are asked for (and observed for apprehension) feeling of impending dislocation, mere pain is insignificant. Then either elbow is taken backward or a posterior to anterior force is applied to the posterior aspect of the humeral head. Increase in apprehension and retraction by patient are positive signs.

Relocation test of Jobe is performed in conjunction to above and consists of applying a posteriorly directed force on anterior humerus (attempting to reduce anterior subluxation); a decrease in apprehension with a posterior-directed force implies anterior instability.

Load-shift test: The humeral head is compressed into glenoid and then noting the amount of force needed to displace the humeral head "out" in anterior and posterior direction.

Drawer test: The examiner holds the humeral head while standing behind the patient and pushes forward (for anterior laxity) and pulls backward (for posterior laxity) in the glenoid to access translational stability. A clunk or snap on anterior subluxation can suggest Bankart lesion.

The push-pull test: Done in supine position with shoulder off the edge of bed and arm in 90° abduction and 30° flexion. Examiner pulls on the wrist while pushing the proximal humerus down. Normally, 50% posterior translation is allowed. The sulcus sign signifies anteroinferior labral tear/inferior shoulder laxity/instability. The patient is seated or standing with the arm relaxed by the side. The patient's arm is grasped by the examiner and pulled inferiorly. Dimpling of the skin below the acromion suggests widening of the subacromial space between the acromion and the humeral head with inferior subluxation of humeral head.

Fulcrum test: This tests the anterior shoulder laxity. The patient is made to lie supine on examination couch and arm is abducted to 90°. The examiner places his fist on the table under the proximal humerus. The arm is then extended with the fist as fulcrum in external rotation to elicit apprehension. Apprehension of the patient may cause subscapularis contraction to mask instability which can be fatigued by maintaining external rotation for a minute and hence revealing the instability.

Jerk test: The patient's arm is internally rotated and flexed forward to 90°. Axial load is applied by examiner toward a plane tangent to glenoid while moving the arm across the body. Sliding of humeral head off the posterior border of glenoid in a jerk indicates positive test. Jerk of return can be felt when the arm is returned to original position.

B. **Management:**

Hill-Sachs lesion: There are various approaches to manage the Hill-Sachs lesion, choice of a procedure can be decided based on individual needs:
- First is by way of tightening the shoulder to restrict external rotation as by double breasting subscapularis (Putti-Platt operation).
- Second approach is by filling the humeral head defect by matched or unmatched osteoarticular allograft.

- Partial articular resurfacing is available in select centers that avoid the issue of disease transmission or the need of dedicated bone bank.
- Failed primary surgery with shoulder remaining unstable at less than 90° of abduction and less than 90° of external rotation with large Hill-Sachs lesion can be successfully managed by *tendon transfers*. The *Saha procedure* involves transfer of latissimus dorsi muscle at the infraspinatus insertion, thus pulling the humeral head backward during abduction. Infraspinatus tendon transfer acts as an anterior block to humeral defect engaging the glenoid. Reverse Hill-Sachs lesions can be managed with subscapularis transfer.
- Older patients with large defects greater than 45% of articular surface can be very well managed with arthroplasty (hemi or total). Arthroplasty can also be used for chronic unreduced dislocations. Total arthroplasty is preferred for associated glenoid side degenerative changes.

Bankart lesion: Bankart lesion repair falls into anatomical reconstruction of shoulder instability by classical standards and can be done by open or arthroscopic technique. Though arthroscopic Bankart repair has gained immense popularity with the progress toward minimally access surgeries, open repairs are regaining lost grounds due to demonstrable better outcomes that are being reported lately.
- Arthroscopic Bankart repair involves repair of the avulsed capsulolabral structures from glenoid rim using suture anchors. This may be combined with other identified pathologies.
- Open repair usually adds capsulorrhaphy in addition to the labral repair.
- Staple capsulorrhaphy is largely not practiced due to better and widely successful alternatives.

22. Describe stabilizers of shoulder joint.
Ans: The *stability of shoulder* is outcome of complementary and in tandem working of various stabilizing structures. These structures have been typically classified into static and dynamic types.
- *The static ones* include the labrum, ligaments (discrete thickenings of capsule), capsule and to a certain extent the bones. The shoulder capsule has twice the surface area of humeral head and accepts 25–30 mL of fluid normally. The capsule fibers blend with ligamentous structures to provide static support.
- *The dynamic stabilizers* include the rotator cuff muscles, scapular muscles, scapulothoracic rhythm and even the axial core muscles of the body. Proprioception connects the dynamic stabilizers to each other and to the static ones. The most active primary stabilizers are the glenohumeral ligaments.
    - *There are four ligaments:* The superior glenohumeral ligament (SGHL), middle (MGHL), inferior (IGHL, its split anterior and posterior part) and the posterior glenohumeral ligament (it is the posterior split part of IGHL).
  The secondary stabilizers include the rotator cuff and the core muscles of the body.

23. What are the clinical features and management of posterior dislocation of shoulder joint?
Ans: Clinical features:
- Clinically, a posterior glenohumeral dislocation does not present with striking deformity; the injured upper extremity is typically held in the traditional sling position of shoulder internal rotation and adduction. These injuries may be missed if a complete radiographic series is not obtained.
- A careful neurovascular examination is important to rule out axillary nerve injury, although it is much less common than with anterior glenohumeral dislocation.
- On examination, limited external rotation (often <0°) and limited anterior forward elevation (often <90°) may be appreciated.
- A palpable mass posterior to the shoulder, flattening of the anterior shoulder, and coracoid prominence may be observed.

Management:
Radiographic evaluation:
- *Trauma series of the affected shoulder:* Anteroposterior (AP), Scapular-Y, and axillary views. A Velpeau axillary view may be obtained if the patient is unable to position the shoulder for a standard axillary view.

- On a standard AP view of the shoulder, signs suggestive of a posterior glenohumeral dislocation include:
  - Absence of the normal elliptic overlap of the humeral head on the glenoid.
  - *Vacant glenoid sign:* The glenoid appears partially vacant (space between anterior rim and humeral head is >6 mm).
  - *Trough sign:* Impaction fracture of the anterior humeral head caused by the posterior rim of glenoid (reverse Hill–Sachs lesion). This is reported to be present in 75% of cases.
  - *Loss of profile of humeral neck:* The humerus is in full internal rotation.
  - Void in the superior/inferior glenoid fossa, owing to inferosuperior displacement of the dislocated humeral head.
- Glenohumeral dislocations are most readily recognized on the axillary view; this view may also demonstrate the reverse Hill–Sachs defect.
- Computed tomography scans are valuable in assessing the percentage of the humeral head involved with an impaction fracture.

Treatment:
Nonoperative:
- Closed reduction requires full muscle relaxation, sedation, and analgesia.
  - The pain from an acute, traumatic posterior glenohumeral dislocation is usually greater than with an anterior dislocation and may require general anesthesia for reduction.
  - With the patient supine, traction should be applied to the adducted arm in the line of deformity with gentle lifting of the humeral head into the glenoid fossa.
  - The shoulder should not be forced into external rotation, because this may result in a humeral head fracture if an impaction fracture is locked on the posterior glenoid rim.
  - If prereduction radiographs demonstrate an impaction fracture locked on the glenoid rim, axial traction should be accompanied by lateral traction on the upper arm to unlock the humeral head.

Operative:
Indications for surgery include:
- Major displacement of an associated lesser tuberosity fracture
- A large posterior glenoid fragment
- Irreducible dislocation or an impaction fracture on the posterior glenoid preventing reduction
- Open dislocation
- An anteromedial humeral impaction fracture (reverse Hill–Sachs lesion)
- *20–40% humeral head involvement:* Transfer the lesser tuberosity with attached subscapularis into the defect (modified McLaughlin procedure)
- *Greater than 40% humeral head involvement:* Hemiarthroplasty with neutral version of the prosthesis
- Recurrent instability
- Surgical options include open reduction, infraspinatus muscle/tendon plication (reverse Putti-Platt procedure), long head of the biceps tendon transfer to the posterior glenoid margin (Boyd-Sisk procedure), humeral and glenoid osteotomies, and capsulorrhaphy.

24. A. Classify traumatic shoulder dislocation.

B. Explain diagnosis and management of neglected posterior dislocation of shoulder in a young adult.

Ans: A. *Classification:*
- Anterior—subcoracoid, subglenoid, intrathoracic
- Posterior—subacromial, subglenoid, subspinous
- Inferior
- Superior.

B. Obtain anteroposterior and axillary views of the shoulder. Computed tomography (CT) and three-dimensional CT techniques are helpful in evaluating the bony injuries. CT also demonstrates the extent of damage to the articular surface of the humeral head and glenoid that determines selection of treatment procedure.

Management: The various treatment options for an old unreduced dislocation of the shoulder are no treatment, closed reduction (arthroscopic-assisted), open reduction, hemiarthroplasty, and total shoulder replacement. Despite dislocated joint some patients need no treatment due to morbid physiology or they may be minimally crippled by the condition though motion is limited as the upper extremity remains functional because the arm rests at the side in internal rotation, allowing the patient to reach the face, head, and rear of the body.

For manipulative reduction consider the patient's age, the degree of osteoporosis of the humerus, the vascular status, and the duration of the dislocation, and the size of the humeral depression. After 4 weeks the soft-tissue contractures, the fibrous tissue within the glenoid cavity, and the retracted rotator cuff muscles usually make closed reduction impossible. In such cases arthroscopic-assisted closed reduction may be performed after adhesions are freed, and labroligamentous repair of the glenoid may also be simultaneously performed. In general, closed reduction is not possible for a shoulder with an impression defect involving more than 20% of the articular surface of the humeral head or for a shoulder that has been dislocated for more than 4 weeks. If a closed reduction is attempted, it should be done with minimal traction, no leverage, and complete muscle relaxation under general anesthesia.

Open reduction: Generally, it also needs some fixation method for stabilizing the joint postreduction. Because of fibrosis, shortening of the muscle, contracture, bowstringing of the capsule across the glenoid cavity, defect of the articular surface in the humeral head at the point of impingement at the glenoid, and scar tissue in the glenoid fossa extensive clearing of the joint is needed and primary instability makes maintaining closed reduction difficult so transfixation (k-wires/screw) is usually combined.

Impression defects in humerus and eburnation of glenoid need bony/soft-tissue stabilizing procedures to prevent recurrent instability. This may be done by filling the defect in the anterior part of the humeral head with the subscapularis tendon or transplanting the subscapularis tendon with the lesser tuberosity attached. Humeral derotational osteotomy may be performed for improving function in incarcerated joint.

Approach to joint is more or less surgeon's discretion but posterior or anteromedial approaches are commonly preferred.

25. Explain etiology and pathoanatomy of old unreduced dislocation of shoulder joint.

Ans: Etiology: These old dislocations most often are traumatic but frequently have been produced by a trivial injury as a result of the patient's increasing age and weakness and degeneration of the soft tissue around the glenohumeral joint, such as the rotator cuff and subscapularis tendon. In younger patients, unreduced dislocations often occur in those with alcoholism, seizures, or multiple trauma.

Pathoanatomy: These injuries produce pathological conditions in both the soft tissue and the bone. After a few weeks, fibrous and capsular contractures occur across the base of the glenoid. The rotator cuff muscles also are contracted. The fibrosis can include other structures, such as the axillary artery and nerve. The natural anatomy is therefore often markedly distorted. Literature has described a capsular "bowstringing" phenomenon. The capsule itself becomes adherent in the glenoid fossa, preventing closed reduction.

Bony pathological change is also apparent. In chronic anterior dislocations, a compression fracture occurs in the posterolateral aspect of the humeral head, where it impinges against the anterior glenoid rim. Because of the repeated efforts of the patient to achieve normal motion in the glenohumeral joint, this lesion is larger than the usual Hill–Sachs lesion seen in recurring anterior dislocations of the shoulder. There are also compression fractures of the apposing glenoid rim or sometimes a pseudoarticulation with the scapula. In chronic posterior dislocations, a bony lesion similar to the Hill–Sachs lesion of recurring anterior dislocations is found. This is a compression fracture caused by impingement of the posterior rim of the glenoid on the anteromedial aspect of the humeral head. These lesions also are usually large because of the patient's continual attempts to increase the range of motion of the affected joint.

26. Define recurrent anterior dislocation of shoulder.

Ans: Recurrent shoulder instability of shoulder simply means repeated dislocations (complete separation of glenohumeral articular surfaces) of the shoulder joint that need to be replaced either by a physician or self to maintain function. Only in FEDS (frequency, etiology, direction, severity) classification, the frequency of dislocation has been mentioned to

categorize it as recurrent. These entail >5 episodes of repeated complete glenohumeral separations including the first acute episode. *[Some texts and classical teaching of >3 episodes of shoulder dislocations are only arbitrary and not supported in literature anywhere.]* Instead of focusing on the frequency of dislocations (which is only more indicative or recurrence), one must focus on etiology and other systems such as classifying shoulder dislocations as traumatic anterior shoulder instability (TUBS) or atraumatic multidirectional bilateral instability (AMBRI) type would help better. There are various factors that lead to recurrent shoulder instability like:
- Young age at first dislocation (<20 years)
- Ease of dislocation with applied force (the less the force required to initially dislocate is associated with higher incidence of dislocation)
- Possibly shorter time of immobilization (not proven)
- Presence of associated lesions as described above (bipolar lesions are especially important.)

27. Explain etiology and pathoanatomy of recurrent dislocation shoulder. Outline the principles of management.

Ans: Recurrent shoulder dislocation is a symptom of shoulder instability and not a disease in itself. Although anterior shoulder instability is the most common, it can present in various forms/directions depending on the complex pathogenesis and etiological factors common of which are:
- Trauma—the most common
- Overuse injury to shoulder
- Constitutional—generalized joint laxity.

There are various associated risk factors that predispose a person for developing the recurrent instability, viz.
- Age
- Early return to contact or collision sports
- Presence of a significant anatomical abnormality like bony defect in the glenoid or humeral head
- Time from the first dislocation until surgery
- Ipsilateral rotator cuff or deltoid muscle insufficiency
- Ligamentous laxity.

Pathoanatomy: The pathogenesis of recurrent instability is complex and cannot be described in a generalized description. Nearly all known anatomical structures have been implicated in the development of recurrent shoulder instability one time or other by different researchers but a combination of them in variable quantity usually is responsible for individual cases. The following are the commonly described lesions for development of shoulder instability:
- *Bankart lesion:* Rowe et al. found Bankart lesions in 85% of traumatic recurrent dislocations, 64% of recurrent transient subluxations, and 84% of previous failed surgical procedures. Most authors agree that the Bankart lesion is the most commonly observed pathological lesion in recurrent subluxation or dislocation of the shoulder, but it is not the "essential" lesion as many shoulder with lesion are clinically silent. Perthes in 1906 described it as detachment of the labrum from the anterior rim of the glenoid cavity and also described surgical reattachment. In 1938, Bankart detailed the pathoanatomy of the lesion where he detailed the tear of not only the fibrocartilaginous labrum from almost the entire anterior half of the rim of the glenoid cavity, but also the capsule and periosteum from the anterior surface of the neck of the scapula as a cause of acute and possibly recurrent instability (later called Bankart lesion). He also described another mechanism of acute anterior shoulder instability in which humeral head is forced through the capsule where it is the weakest, generally anteriorly and inferiorly in the interval between the lower border of the subscapularis and the long head of the triceps muscle.
- *Excessive laxity of the shoulder capsule:* Rowe et al. found this excessive laxity in 28% of traumatic recurrent dislocations, 26% of transient subluxations, and 86% of previous failed surgical procedures. In arthroscopic studies it was identified that the generalized capsular laxity in most cases was either prominent intrasubstance ligamentous failures, or disruptions of the capsuloligamentous insertion into the glenoid neck. The terms like anterior labral periosteal sleeve avulsion (ALPSA), posterior labrocapsular periosteal sleeve avulsion (POLPSA), humeral avulsion of glenohumeral ligament (HAGL), etc. thus came into recognition for describing the recurrent shoulder instability. However, in a

smaller subset the capsular laxity could be a component of congenital collagen deficiency, shown by hyperlaxity of other joints, or by plastic deformation of the capsuloligamentous complex from a single macrotraumatic event or repetitive microtraumatic events. Warren et al. emphasized the importance of the "circle concept" of structural damage to the capsular structures. In cadaver studies, they showed that humeral dislocation does not occur unless the posterior capsular structures are disrupted in addition to the anterior capsular structures. Posterior capsulolabral changes associated with recurrent anterior instability often are identified by arthroscopy.

- *Bony defect:* Humeral head impaction fracture in the posterolateral aspect of the humeral head (Hill-Sachs lesion) can be produced as the shoulder is dislocated anteriorly, and the humeral head is impacted against the rim of the glenoid at the time of dislocation. Although the finding if Hill-Sachs lesion is quite common but for recurrent instability to occur the lesion should be large enough to engage the defect in glenoid rim in the functional arc of motion at 90° abduction and external rotation.
  - Glenoid rim fractures also can occur with an anterior or posterior dislocation. If these lesions involve more than 20% of the glenoid, they can result in recurrent instability despite having an excellent soft-tissue repair. Three-dimensional CT is indicated for their identification and quantization.

Treatment: As we have seen from above that the pathoanatomy is quite complex and various factors may remain unseen at the time of presentation for recurrent shoulder instability, the treatment is bound to be discrete for individuals. For all recurrent dislocations of the shoulder a variable combination of various possible primary deficiencies like erosion of the anterior glenoid rim, stretching of the anterior capsule and subscapularis tendon, and fraying and degeneration of the glenoid labrum, Bankart lesion, Hill-Sachs lesion all contribute. The surgeon must search carefully for and identify the deficiencies present to choose the proper procedure.

- *Conservative management:* The patient may choose to accommodate the inconvenience and simply try to avoid vulnerable positions of the shoulder. Although some studies suggest higher incidence of development of osteoarthritis but the jury is still open if it is due to the initial dislocation or due to recurrent instability as underlying cause. A subset of patients will be able to avoid surgery by doing rotator cuff and scapular rehabilitation exercise under the guidance of a physiotherapist and this is specifically true of AMBRI shoulders.
- *Operative treatment:* The indications for operation include—
  - Frequent painful dislocations
  - Recurrent subluxations or a fear of dislocation sufficient to prevent participation in everyday activities.

Two types of operation are commonly employed:
1. *Anatomical repairs:* These are essential methods for surgical repair of the anatomical defects and most commonly involve reconstruction of anteroinferior restrains of torn glenoid labrum and capsule, e.g., the Bankart procedure.
2. *Nonanatomical repairs:* These procedures are designed to counteract the pathological tendency to joint displacement and may be more effective than the anatomical repairs as the underlying pathology is mostly a combination of the deficiencies and not just involve Bankart lesion:
   - Glenoid augmentation because it indirectly increases the arc of contact preventing humeral head engagement
   - Restraining the external rotation of shoulder—these shorten the anterior capsule and subscapularis by an overlapping repair (e.g., the Putti–Platt operation)
   - Operations that reinforce the anteroinferior capsule by redirecting other muscles across the front of the joint (e.g., the Bristow-Latarjet operation)—the Bristow-Latarjet operation, in which the coracoid process with its attached muscles is transposed to the front of the neck of the scapula, produces less restriction of external rotation. It is a popular procedure for restoring shoulder stability nowadays
   - Filling the humeral head defect by matched or unmatched osteoarticular allograft.
   - Tendon transfer—like the Saha procedure
   - Partial articular surface replacement of humeral head
   - A bone operation to correct a reduced retroversion angle of the humeral head by osteotomy.

In general, if the labrum and anterior capsule are detached, and there is no marked joint laxity, the Bankart operation combined with anterior capsulorrhaphy is the procedure of choice. Bankart initially described this as an open operation through the deltopectoral approach; however, arthroscopic techniques have been developed with advanced anchor materials and the development of specialized arthroscopic instruments. After either type of operation there is still a significant recurrence rate (about 20%), usually following another injury. If there is bone loss on either the glenoid aspect or the humeral head the outcome following arthroscopic surgery is considerably worse.

28. Describe indications, advantages, and disadvantages of Latarjet procedure in shoulder instability.

Ans: Latarjet procedure involves transfer of a portion of coracoid process with conjoint tendon to anteroinferior portion of glenoid. The following are the common indications of the procedure:

- Glenoid bone defect (20–30% loss) causing recurrent anterior shoulder instability
- High-risk contact athlete with recurrent anterior shoulder instability despite minimal bone loss.

Advantages:

- High chances of obtaining a stable shoulder than other techniques
- Reduced rehabilitation time
- Reconstruction of bony defect
- Providing anterior bony block and sling effect to combine static and dynamic stability to shoulder joint

Disadvantages:

- Graft osteolysis/fracture/nonunion
- Development of arthritis in long run
- Neurological injury—axillary nerve > suprascapular nerve > musculocutaneous nerve.

29. Remplissage procedure.

Ans: Remplissage procedure was first described by Wolf et al. (2007) in arthroscopic anterior shoulder stabilization as an additional procedure 'to fill in' the large engaging 'Hill-Sach defect'. The anatomical Bankart repair does not provide sufficient stabilization in these patients.

Indication: Anterior shoulder instability in which the Hill-Sachs lesion is engaged/engaging on glenoid (off-track lesion).

Technique: Using the standard Bankart repair portals, the Hill-Sachs remplissage technique consists of fixation of the infraspinatus tendon and posterior capsule to the abraded surface of the Hill-Sachs lesion. Usually, a large triple loaded anchor is placed through the posterior portal into the created Hill-Sachs bed and infraspinatus muscle with capsule is tied down using 'parachute technique'. This effectively makes the Hill-Sachs lesion extra-articular by filling in defect and limiting the excursion of humeral head over glenoid.

Advantages: The addition of a remplissage procedure significantly reduces recurrence rates in contact athletes with Hill-Sachs lesions by preventing its engagement.

30. Define multidirectional instability (MDI) of shoulder joint. Discuss its management.

Ans: In MDI, laxity exists in more than one direction usually a variable combination of anterior, posterior and inferior and sometimes all. Despite uncertainties in etiology and pathogenesis, anatomical abnormalities (capsular stretching and thinning) can be detected in patients with MDI.

Management: An abnormally voluminous glenohumeral (GH) joint is noted on arthroscopy. Other findings include a large axillary pouch and broad rotator interval. The capsule is lax in more than one direction. It has been observed that in a subset of patients with MDI there is reduced scapular upward rotation during abduction while internal rotation is increased.

Majority of the patients can be managed with scapular stabilizing exercises and rotator cuff exercises. Changes in daily living activities and physical activities are the primary goals of rehabilitation. If physical therapy fails then the treatment is arthroscopic or open capsular tightening. Arthroscopic tightening gives better visualization and control over the tissues. In involuntary dislocators the labral tears could be circumferential that can be helped by arthroscopic stabilization with or without capsular plication. These procedures improve glenoid concavity while removing pathologic capsular redundancy.

The most popular open procedure is the Neer's inferior capsular shift but in any case, the surgical procedures alone have limited ability to cure atraumatic instability. The patient should be carefully chosen with a major functional problem clearly related to atraumatic GH instability and clear understanding by the patient of the limitations of this static procedure and future requirement of strict discipline. In the Neer's inferior capsular shift, the capsule is incised deep down inferiorly and medial capsule is taken superiorly and laterally under the lateral capsule. The sutures are placed and tied with arm in 20–30° of external rotation. Tough named inferior capsular shift the procedure tightens the capsule inferiorly, anteriorly and posteriorly.

31. **A. What is hypermobility syndrome?**
B. Enumerate its pathognomonic diagnostic criteria.
C. What is its role in management of shoulder instability?

Ans:

A. Hypermobility syndrome or joint hypermobility syndrome is mostly an inherited disorder that was first described in 1967 by Kirk et al. The individuals are otherwise healthy in growth and development, but their joints move beyond average range of mobility. It is more common in females of Afro-Caribbean and Asian descent. In case of well-developed disease, the typical symptoms include:

- Unstable joints and frequent dislocations/subluxations
- Acute or chronic pain in multiple joints, fatigue
- Frequent injuries
- Gastrointestinal symptoms such as reflux, constipation
- Pelvic floor and bladder symptoms
- Fragile easily bruised skin

Hypermobility is not a specific disorder but may arise from one of the four grouped conditions as follows:

1. Connective tissue inheritable disorders such as osteogenesis imperfecta, Marfan syndrome, Ehlers–Danlos syndromes, Stickler syndrome, etc.
2. *Excluding group A:* Abnormal joint shape, looser ligaments, or poor muscle tone
3. Down's syndrome, cerebral palsy, etc.
4. Repeated injury or stretching/training

B. The Beighton score **(Table 4A.3.1)** is a set of tests providing a nine-point scoring system for assessing generalized joint hypermobility. This epidemiological score is incorporated in Brighton criteria **(Box 4A.3.1)** for diagnosing joint hypermobility syndrome. The new Brighton criteria provide good method to assess benign joint hypermobility syndrome with reliable sensitivity and specificity.

TABLE 4A.3.1: The Beighton scoring system based on clinical examination.		
Beighton Scale	**Left**	**Right**
1. Passive dorsiflexion and hyperextension of the fifth MCP joint beyond 90°	1	1
2. Passive apposition of the thumb to the flexor aspect of the forearm	1	1
3. Passive hyperextension of the elbow beyond 10°	1	1
4. Passive hyperextension of the knee beyond 10°	1	1
5. Active forward flexion of the trunk with the knees fully extended so that the palms of the hands rest flat on the floor	1	1
The first four elements can be given a maximum score of 2, because these are performed bilateral. The last element is scored with 0 or 1. The maximum score for ligament laxity is 9. A score of 9 means hyperlax. A score of zero is tight. Several researchers appoint a score of 0–3 as normal and a score of 4–9 as representing ligamentous laxity.		

> **Box 4A.3.1:** New Beighton criteria.
>
> *Major criteria:*
> - A Beighton score of 4/9 or greater (either currently or historically)
> - Arthralgia for longer than 3 months in 4 or more joints
>
> *Minor criteria:*
> - A Beighton score of 1, 2 or 3/9 (0, 1, 2 or 3 if aged 50+)
> - Arthralgia (>3 months) in one to three joints or back pain (>3 months), spondylosis, spondylolysis/spondylolisthesis
> - Dislocation/subluxation in more than one joint, or in one joint on more than one occasion
> - Soft tissue rheumatism >3 lesions (e.g., epicondylitis, tenosynovitis, bursitis)
> - Marfanoid habitus (tall, slim, span/height ratio >1.03, upper:lower segment ratio less than 0.89, arachnodactyly [positive Steinberg/wrist signs].
> - *Abnormal skin:* Striae, hyperextensibility, thin skin, papyraceous scarring.
> - *Eye signs:* Drooping eyelids or myopia or antimongoloid slant.
> - Varicose veins or hernia or uterine/rectal prolapse.
>
> For diagnosis → the presence two major criteria, or one major and two minor criteria, or four minor criteria are needed. Two minor criteria will suffice where there is an unequivocally affected first-degree relative.

C. Hypermobility syndrome produces multidirectional instability (MDI) and some of the patients may even become voluntary willful dislocators. In MDI, laxity exists in more than one direction usually a variable combination of anterior, posterior and inferior and sometimes all. Despite uncertainties in etiology and pathogenesis, anatomical abnormalities (capsular stretching and thinning) can be detected in patients with MDI. An abnormally voluminous GH joint is noted on arthroscopy. Other findings include a large axillary pouch and broad rotator interval. The capsule is lax in more than one direction. Majority of the patients can be managed with scapular stabilizing exercises and rotator cuff exercises. Changes in daily living activities and physical activities are the primary goals of rehabilitation. If physical therapy fails then the treatment is arthroscopic or open capsular tightening. Arthroscopic tightening gives better visualization and control over the tissues. In involuntary dislocators, the labral tears could be circumferential, that can be helped by arthroscopic stabilization with or without capsular plication. These procedures improve glenoid concavity while removing pathologic capsular redundancy. The most popular open procedure is the Neer's inferior capsular shift but in any case, the surgical procedures alone have limited ability to cure atraumatic instability. The patient should be carefully chosen with a major functional problem clearly related to atraumatic GH instability and clear understanding by the patient of the limitations of this static procedure and future requirement of strict discipline.

32. Give a functional classification of muscles around the shoulder. Enumerate indications and various techniques for shoulder arthrodesis. What are the prerequisites for a good result? Describe any one technique.

Ans: The muscles around shoulder joint have been functionally classified (modified from Saha) into:
- *Scapular elevators:* Levator scapulae, trapezius, rhomboideus major, and rhomboideus minor.
- *Scapular depressors:* Pectoralis minor and major, serratus anterior, and trapezius.
- *Protractors of scapula:* Serratus anterior and pectoralis minor.
- *Retractors of scapula:* Trapezius and rhomboideus.
- *Rotators of scapula:* Trapezius and serratus anterior (upward rotator), rhomboideus and levator scapulae (downward rotator).
- Compressors of shoulder joint: Subscapularis (anterior compressor), supraspinatous (superior compressor), infraspinatous (inferior compressor), deltoid (the posterior and middle portions are important than the anterior part in producing concavity compression). Kindly note that there are NO "depressors" of shoulder joint as was once thought.
- Internal rotators of humerus: Deltoid (anterior), pectoralis major, subscapularis, teres major, and latissimus dorsi.
- External rotators of humerus: Infraspinatous, teres minor, and deltoid (posterior).
- Abductors: Supra- and infraspinatous and deltoid
- Adductors of humerus: Coracobrachialis, pectoralis major, teres major, and latissimus dorsi.

Indications of shoulder arthrodesis include:
- Infection
- Paralytic disorders
- Unreconstructable rotator cuff tears
- Combined insufficiency of rotator cuff and deltoid
- Failed shoulder arthroplasty
- Arthritic diseases unsuitable for arthroplasty
- Recurrent dislocations
- Neoplastic lesions
- Recurrent shoulder dislocations that persist after multiple surgical procedures
- Refractory multidirectional instability
- Tumor resections.

Various techniques for shoulder arthrodesis are:
- External fixation
- Screw fixation
- Tension band fixation
- Plate fixation (single- or double-plate method)
- Pelvic reconstruction plate.

Prerequisites for a good result:
- Sufficient strength of the axial and scapular musculature to maintain stability of the scapula
- Understanding patient.

Description: Arthrodesis of shoulder using reconstruction plate—Arbeitsgemeinschaft für Osteosynthesefragen (AO) shoulder arthrodesis:
- Prefer beach chair position and using extensile deltopectoral approach from spine of scapula to deltoid insertion exposes the deep structures.
- Protect deltoid and incise the rotator cuff to repair later.
- Retract humerus and decorticate glenoid using reamer and humeral head using curettes.
- Place bone graft between humeral head and acromion to bridge the gap and fix humeral head to glenoid using screws in the position of arthrodesis as above. Use side of body as reference point. Richards advocated translating the humerus head upward to acromion and did not use bone graft. Additional screw can be placed from acromion to humeral head.
- Place a long reconstruction plate from spine of scapula to proximal humerus as in many patients there is osteopenia of the bones.

Postoperatively place the upper limb in abduction pillow or a shoulder spica for 8–12 weeks. The former is preferred for better hygiene. Once fusion is demonstrated radiologically focus is shifted to periscapular muscle strengthening. The elbow and hand should be mobilized as early after the surgery as possible.

4A.4   MILWAUKEE SHOULDER SYNDROME (Q33)

33. A. What is Milwaukee shoulder syndrome?
B. Explain its clinical signs and symptoms, and
C. Its differential diagnosis and management.

Ans: The hemorrhagic shoulder of the elderly was first described in 1968 in a subtle form with not much detail. It consists of recurrent, blood-streaked effusions of the shoulder along with severely destroyed glenohumeral joint evident radiologically. The process is associated with chronic massive tears of rotator cuff and was labeled "cuff tear arthropathy" by Neer et al. Now the disease is thought to be a destructive shoulder arthropathy due to deposition of hydroxyapatite crystals identification of which in synovial fluid is the mainstay of diagnosis. The destructive changes are attributed to unrelenting collagenase activity released in response to hydroxyapatite crystals released from pathologic cuff, capsule, synovium, and possibly cartilage as described by McCarthy in 1981. McCarthy hailed from Milwaukee so possibly somehow this disorder now comes to be known in the name of "Milwaukee" shoulder. He is credited with the use of term "Milwaukee shoulder syndrome" where he described four elderly women from Milwaukee (Wisconsin, USA), with characteristic finding of recurrent bilateral shoulder effusions and radiologic description of advanced destructive changes in glenohumeral joint. The patients also had massive tears of the rotator cuff. Now it is known that though shoulder is most commonly involved the disease can also be found in wrists, hands, elbows, neck, lumbar spine, hips, knees, and feet.

Clinical features: The patients are typically elderly with long-standing history of shoulder pain. The shoulder somehow starts hurting more and becomes swollen and unstable over a few months. There is marked crepitus in the joint and loss of active movements. A characteristic finding has been reported by some authors of multiple small dilated blood vessels around the shoulder that produce repeated subcutaneous hemorrhages and ecchymosis in untreated shoulder. The vascular ectasia seems to disappear after surgical intervention spontaneously.

Differential diagnosis:
- Septic arthritis
- Tuberculosis of the shoulder joint
- Rapidly destructive arthropathy of unknown cause
- Neuropathic arthropathy
- Osteonecrosis
- Other crystal-associated arthropathy
- Inflammatory arthritis like rheumatoid arthritis
- Vanishing bone disease
- Syphilitic arthropathy (late).

Investigations: Radiographs demonstrate joint space narrowing, advanced degenerative changes, and loss of architecture of humeral head with flattening, osteophyte formation, and mixed subchondral sclerotic and cystic changes at the articular surface. Additionally, there may be calcification of the capsule and presence of multiple intra-articular loose bodies. Ultrasonography demonstrates intra-articular synovial proliferation and large effusions associated with rotator cuff tears.

Diagnosis: The diagnosis is made by clinicoradiological correlation of the above findings. Demonstration of the hydroxyapatite crystals in aspirate is not easy as they do not appear with characteristic findings on light or polarized microscopy. Aggregates of the crystals however appear as clumps of "shiny coins". These can be made conspicuous by the use of alizarin red S stain that produce a characteristic "halo" of orange-red stain around the clumps of hydroxyapatite crystals. Synovial histopathology reveals noncharacteristic findings like synovial cell hyperplasia, giant cell formation, and deposition of fibrin along with calcium phosphate crystals.

Treatment: Mostly the treatment is supportive and for a less troublesome shoulder initially a conservative approach serves to improve functionality. Mild anti-inflammatory medication and gentle stretching exercises to maintain or regain a functional ROM usually help gain patient confidence and reassess the situation. Colchicine has been found useful in management of Milwaukee shoulder syndrome. Physiotherapy is, however, the mainstay and a strengthening program should follow to improve the active use of the arm for activities of daily living. If conservative management fails or is unacceptable then resurfacing procedure will help pain relief and provide functional improvement. The functional gain is however much better with a reverse shoulder arthroplasty that takes care of the poor superior coverage and stability of shoulder. It only depends on the deltoid function rather than conventional arthroplasty that require good cuff integrity for functionality. It should be emphasized that reverse shoulder has higher chances of failure and glenoid loosening in young patients due to inferior glenoid rim impingement (inferior notching).

4A.5 MISCELLANEOUS ELBOW DISORDERS (Q34–39)

34. A. Enumerate causes of stiff elbow.
B. Explain surgical management of post-traumatic ankylosis of elbow in extension.

Ans: A. *The following are causes of stiff elbow:*
- *Soft tissue contracture:*
  - Skin burns
  - Wound contractures (post-traumatic) due to retractile fibrosis of the capsule, ligaments, and muscular tissue. Retracted medial collateral ligament (MCL) posterior band can cause a flexion contracture beyond 60°, while a tauter anterior produces an extension contracture beyond 80°
  - Hypertrophic scars
  - Spastic paresis (head injury)—contractures
  - Prolonged immobilization. Period of immobilization is directly proportional to elbow stiffness.
- Heterotopic ossification (HO).
- *Osteoarticular incongruity:* Due to high congruity of the articular surfaces, any incongruity in the surfaces produces altered motion and stresses the ligaments in different positions; this causes reduced movements at the joint.
- Malunions of following fractures produce stiff elbow:
  - Intercondylar fractures
  - Capitellum fractures
  - Olecranon fractures
  - Radial head fractures (displaced fragments)
  - Malunited supracondylar fracture with overriding of the fragments.
- Triceps/biceps adhesions (post-traumatic/postsurgical).
- Arthritis
  - Coronoid/olecranon/radial osteophytes.

B. *Surgical management:* Surgical release of soft tissue contracture or bony block is the standard management of stiff elbow. This can be achieved in various ways.

The lateral approach: This is the general approach used for treatment in most cases.
- *Limited "lateral column procedure":* Here proximal half of Kocher's skin incision is utilized. The lateral collateral ligament (LCL) complex is identified and preserved especially while identifying the annular ligament. This is best done before elevating the extensor carpi ulnaris. The LCL-sparing technique is useful to perform anterior and posterior capsulectomy without disturbing the extensor tendon insertion and LCL insertion. The advantage of this approach is to avoid instability after release. The disadvantage is however possible damage to posterior interosseous nerve and that there is greater difficulty in excising the medial half of the anterior capsule without disturbing the anterior bundle of the ulnar collateral ligament (UCL). If full flexion is not achieved then the most common cause is scarred posterior oblique bundle of the UCL that should be excised through a separate posteromedial skin incision.

Posterolateral approach for release of contractures and bony correction—this is most useful for bony deformities/bony blocks and fixed elbow as this provides extensive exposure to the joint. Anterior and posterior soft tissue contractures can be released while correcting bony blocks and fenestration of the fossa can be also done in a single sitting.

Arthroscopic approach is done in stiff elbows with intact articular surfaces with preserved congruity. The procedure is well-suited for limited pathologies and needs proficiency for moderately severe joint involvement.

Postoperative physiotherapy and continuous passive motion is an essential component to maintain the intraoperative gain in movements as there is a high tendency of the joint to again become stiff. Active assisted and passive elbow range of motion (ROM) is needed for a prolonged period of 3 months or more to maintain the gains.

35. What are the indications of excision of radial head? Describe the posterolateral approach.

Ans: The common indications for radial head excision are:
- Isolated type 3 fractures of radial head that cannot be reconstructed without concomitant valgus instability due to MCL injury.
- Some designs of hinge total elbow arthroplasty
- First step in radial head replacement for say isolated radiocapitellar arthrosis.

Posterolateral approach:
- Develop the Kocher interval between the anconeus and extensor carpi ulnaris muscle to expose the elbow capsule and lateral epicondyle
- Reflect the anconeus and triceps medially—this exposes olecranon fossa and distal lateral humerus.
- Elevate the common extensor origin anteriorly from the underlying capsule, lateral ulnar collateral ligament, and lateral epicondyle exposing the annular ligament and radial neck.
- Develop the interval between the extensor digitorum communis and extensor carpi radialis longus and brevis to the level of the deep radial (posterior interosseous) nerve where it enters the supinator at the arcade of Frohse. This allows reflection of the common extensor origin, lateral ulnar collateral ligament, and attached lateral epicondyle in an anterior and distal direction.
- Pronate the forearm to translate the posterior interosseous nerve anteriorly, and divide the annular ligament 5 mm from the edge of the lesser sigmoid notch.
- Release the supinator muscle from the supinator crest of the ulna, and retract it along with the posterior interosseous nerve to expose the proximal radius.

36. How will you manage a case of recalcitrant tennis elbow?

Ans: Some patients fail even surgical management (rare though) but then failures are the rule and can arise from wrong diagnosis or those with associated other symptoms that have not been addressed or true refractory tennis elbow. The treatment failures have been divided into two types by Morrey:
- *Type 1:* Those whose symptoms are identical to their preoperative symptoms (improper patient selection and incomplete diagnosis or incorrect procedure).
- *Type 2:* Those patients who have different symptoms following surgery resulting from possibly overzealous surgery resulting in elbow instability, capsular pathology, synovial herniation, bursitis, or capsular fistula.

The treatment for refractory lateral epicondylitis is commonly ineffective. The best possibility to treat is in fact those patients that had a wrong diagnosis. The opportunity now lies in treating the identified pathology provided patients trust is still maintained. Posterior interosseous nerve (PIN) compression is the most commonly missed associated pathology or confused pathology to tennis elbow, so one should always keep this in consideration while diagnosing a tennis elbow purely (one can easily differentiate by injecting local anesthetic distally into supinator and if it is due to PIN syndrome the symptoms will subside). To identify overtreatment (type 2), one should perform arthrography to identify capsular pathology and ligamentous injuries. The treatment is then directed to the same. As a matter of fact, only 15–20% of the refractory tennis elbow can be diagnosed and rest are more or less managed conservatively and majority improve surprisingly.

37. Describe briefly etiology, clinical features, diagnosis, and management of painful elbow following injury around elbow.

Ans: This is a very nonspecific question and incorrectly framed, if there is pain due to injury then what else will be the etiology. One basically needs to describe elbow trauma that is too vast if one begins to write all possible elbow bony trauma and then describe ligamentous injury.

38. Explain:
   A. Cubitus valgus and
   B. Bankart lesion.

Ans: A. *Cubitus valgus:* This is elbow deformity where the carrying angle of elbow exceeds beyond acceptable range. The normal carrying angle of the elbow is 5–15° of valgus; anything more than this is regarded as a valgus deformity, which

is usually quite obvious when the patient stands with arms to the sides and palms facing forward. The following are the common causes of cubitus valgus:
- Nonunion fracture lateral condyle
- Malunited supracondylar fracture humerus
- Osteonecrosis of lateral trochlea
- Malunited intercondylar fracture
- Radial head fracture dislocation
- Medial epiphyseal injury and growth stimulation.

    The most common cause is longstanding nonunion of a fractured lateral condyle; other causes are interference of epiphyseal growth on lateral side due to injury or infection, Turner syndrome.
- In type I lateral condyle fracture with healing there may be development of bony bar or arrest of lateral growth due to injury to ossification center. This leads to cubitus valgus deformity.
- Type II fractures cannot be held securely in place with conservative methods being inherently unstable, so there is always a tendency toward lateral and proximal migration; hence, development of cubitus valgus with nonunion. Even in united fractures there could be formation of bony bar which tethers lateral growth.

    The deformity may be associated with marked prominence of the medial condylar outline. The importance of cubitus valgus is the liability to delayed ulnar palsy; years after the causal injury the patient notices weakness of the hand, with numbness and tingling of the ulnar fingers. In late stages, claw hand deformity develops along with significant motor weakness.

    Not all cubitus valgus deformities will concern us, but particularly the one from lateral condyle nonunion or sometimes with united fracture is "progressive". This may lead to changed elbow mechanics or neurological complications or both. Mild deformity itself needs no treatment but for regular monitoring for progression whence it needs treatment. Moderate-to-severe deformity can be treated by osteotomy but for delayed ulnar palsy the nerve should be transposed to the front of the elbow. Great care is needed in performing the operation. Excessive dissection of the nerve or rough handling can impair nerve function.

B. *Bankart lesion:* The detachment of labrum from anterior glenoid (Bankart lesion) is common to the most if not all dislocations. The Bankart's lesion is seen in 87–100% of initial dislocation. Most often the glenoid labrum is detached along with osteoperiosteal structures from the anterior glenoid over a variable arc region. There may be avulsion from posterior aspect also in long-standing cases or inferior dislocations. The injury in some cases is not limited to soft tissue only (classical Bankart) while bony avulsion may also occur (Bony Bankart). The lesion is well diagnosed and characterized on magnetic resonance imaging while it is best evaluated on arthroscopy. Arthroscopic classification of anterior labral Bankart lesions was proposed by Green and Christensen as follows:
- Type I is the normal intact labrum.
- Type II is a simple detachment of the labrum from the glenoid.
- Type III is an intrasubstance tear of the glenoid labrum.
- Type IV is a detachment of the labrum with significant fraying or degeneration.
- Type V is complete degeneration or absence of the glenoid labrum.

(Pathology, pathoanatomy of Bankart lesion is further discussed with treatment in Q27.)

39. What are the indications and contraindications of total elbow arthroplasty? What are the complications? Describe the design changes to reduce complications?

Ans: Indications:
- Primary indications for total elbow arthroplasty are pain, instability, and bilateral elbow ankylosis. Rheumatoid arthritis with radiographic evidence of joint destruction, which is too far advanced to benefit from radial head excision and synovectomy, especially in patients with painful instability and painful stiffness that limit activities, is generally considered to be an indication. Bony or fibrous ankylosis with the elbow in a poorly functioning position also is considered an indication for elbow arthroplasty. In patients with rheumatoid arthritis, arthroplasty should be considered only after medical treatment has failed, and the disease has advanced beyond the stage at which synovectomy would be beneficial.

- *Juvenile rheumatoid arthritis (JRA):* Failed elbow arthroplasty of any type may be an indication for implant arthroplasty as a revision. Intractable pain with radiographic evidence of destruction of the radiohumeral and humeroulnar joints, instability, and failed synovectomy with radial head excision are indications for arthroplasty.
- Loss of bone stock caused by tumor, trauma, or infection also may be an indication.
- Total elbow arthroplasty is a satisfactory treatment for severely comminuted distal humeral fractures in elderly patients.

Contraindications:
- History of previous elbow sepsis
- Relative contraindications to the use of an unconstrained resurfacing arthroplasty included excessive bone loss, as in giant rheumatoid cysts, deficiency of the trochlear notch of the ulna, and post-traumatic or degenerative arthritis
- Excessive bone loss on either side of the joint, and poorly functioning flexor and extensor mechanisms are contraindications.
- Need for other than sedentary use of the elbow, ankylosis of the ipsilateral shoulder, and the presence of neurotrophic joints

Complications of elbow arthroplasty:
- Nerve paresthesias
- Wound problems
- Fracture, humerus
- Fracture, ulna
- Nerve entrapment
- Triceps problems
- Ankylosis
- Loosening (semiconstrained)
- Instability (unconstrained)
- Infection
- Fracture and loosening

Changes in design to decrease complications:

A principal complication of unconstrained total elbow arthroplasty has been loosening, usually of the humeral component. For semiconstrained prostheses, loosening of the humeral component, previously the most common cause for revision, has been reduced to <5% overall with improvements in prosthesis design, changes in operative technique, and better understanding of the anatomy and function of the elbow. In particular, use of a shorter (4 inch) stem in semiconstrained total elbow arthroplasty resulted in earlier time to revision than longer (6 inch) stems. Nevertheless, humeral stem loosening remained uncommon at a rate of approximately 2% at an average of 7 years of follow-up. Ulnar component loosening and osteolysis increased with the addition of a polymethylmethacrylate precoat in the 1990s but has decreased since the surface finish was changed to a plasma spray preparation.

Multiple recent reports have found that a semiconstrained device demonstrated better longevity than unconstrained replacements.

Most semiconstrained hinged prostheses use a high molecular-weight polyethylene bushing and titanium humeral and ulnar components. They are designed with 7° of rotary and side-to-side laxity. Humeral and ulnar stems match the shapes of the medullary canals. The triangular humeral stem is flattened near the base at the inferior flatter and wider portion of the medullary canal of the humerus. The large medullary stem enhances rigid fixation. The stem contour and distal anterior flange increase resistance to torque. Careful bone removal in the intercondylar area of the humerus is necessary to allow a tight fit of the humeral prosthesis.

The humeral and ulnar components typically are joined with a linking mechanism that, if necessary, can be disarticulated. The axis of rotation of these prostheses are near the anatomic center when the device is properly implanted. Because the components are relatively large, a disadvantage in smaller patients is that they occasionally require manufacture of custom components.

Instability in the form of dislocation or subluxation is the most common complication requiring revision of unconstrained prostheses and has been reported to occur in between 9% and 10% of total elbow arthroplasties. True dislocation occurs in fewer than 5% of unlinked implants and is dependent on surgical technique. Appropriate tensioning of the medial and lateral ligament complexes and preservation of the anterior capsule and triceps can help avoid this complication.

A number of measures have been recommended to minimize the occurrence of other complications of elbow implant arthroplasty, especially infection and problems with the triceps, ulnar nerve, and wound healing. These include the use of a straight incision medial to the olecranon tip, detachment of the triceps in continuity from the olecranon without division of the tendon or the use of a triceps-on approach, anterior transposition of the ulnar nerve, drainage of the wound with at least one suction drain, and initial splinting of the elbow in full extension.

4A.6 VOLKMANN ISCHEMIC CONTRACTURE (Q40–41)

40. Explain etiopathogenesis, clinical features, prevention, and management of Volkmann ischemic contracture (VIC).

Ans: *Etiology:*
- Compartment syndrome is the basis of majority of the VIC that can develop from various causes. The common causes of forearm compartment syndrome are:
  - Prolonged external compression
  - Internal bleeding (hemophilia) or fluid extravasation
  - Burns
  - Snake bites
  - Regional anesthesia (especially the intravenous regional anesthesia—Bier's block).
- The second most common recognized cause especially in children for VIC is the ischemic contracture following supracondylar fracture of humerus. Though terminally, it produces compartment like state but has a special mention due to frequent cause and distinctive vascular injury that needs specialty vascular intervention.
- The other major cause is the crush injuries and severe contusions of the forearm.
- Uncommon causes:
  - Chronic infections
  - Congenital
  - Idiopathic.

Pathogenesis: Whatever be the cause, VIC is the end result of prolonged ischemia of the muscles and nerves in an extremity. Muscles are the primary targets of ischemia while nerves are secondarily involved. Muscle undergoes necrosis, fibrosis and contracture while nerve injury causes further muscle dysfunction, sensory deficits, or chronic pain. Muscles retain the electrical response up to 3 hours and tolerate ischemia up to 4 hours. Irreversible damage occurs nearly around 6–8 hours of ischemia. Nerves retain electrical activity up to 1 hour and undergo physiological dysfunction by 4 hours (neuropraxia). They also undergo irreversible damage by 6–8 hours of ischemia.
- Development of ischemia can be explained by the Rowland's arteriovenous gradient theory supported by Matsen as depicted by the following equation:

Local blood flow = $(P_a - P_v)/R$

Where, P_a is the local arterial pressure, P_v is the local venous pressure and R is the local vascular resistance. Blood flow will reduce if the arterial pressure decreases (reduced P_a, arterial occlusion/thrombosis/injury) or increased P_v (venous stasis) or increased R (compression bandage/increased interstitial pressure).

Following ischemic necrosis, if infection does not occur (aseptic), the process of contracture formation begins. The process is due to the action of the myofibroblast—a cell with fibroblast and smooth muscle characteristics distributed throughout granulation tissue. Contraction of myofibroblasts shrinks the necrosed tissue. This is followed by collagen deposition and cross-linking to maintain contraction. The flexor digitorum profundus (FDP) and flexor pollicis longus (FPL) muscles are most affected. In mild affections only a portion of the FDP undergoes necrosis (usually to the ring and long fingers). In severe contractures, all four digits are involved. With increasing severity, flexor digitorum superficialis (FDS) and pronator teres (PT) with wrist extensors are also involved. The characteristic

distribution of ischemia and fibrotic pathological tissue can be explained by "the Seddon's ellipsoid infarct concept":
- Seddon described ischemic zone of injury usually following brachial artery injury that acquires ellipsoid shape which is in general different from conical ischemic zones observed in lung and liver ischemia.
- He described the "axial" oxygenation around anterior interosseous artery with center just above mid-forearm.
- So the middle thirds of muscles get most involved evolving in an ellipse with long axis along this region. He also noted that the center of muscle was most ischemic and the region was closest to the interosseous membrane (deeper aspect of forearm) while the peripheral parts escaped moderate reductions in main-line blood flow due to collateral circulation. In the modern unified concept of Holden one can view the ischemia as a global phenomenon affecting the muscles of forearm. As in developing and expanding osteosarcoma where the central cells get necrosed early due to loss of nutrition and blood supply, similarly in the growing sphere of ischemia the centrally lying muscles (FDP and FPL) get involved earlier and to a larger extent than the peripherally lying muscles (FDS and PT).
- Finally, hence the structures closest to the interosseous membrane are affected centrally.
- The FDP and FPL lying on either side of vessel are the most severely affected muscles.
- Median nerve at the center is most affected in VIC whereas ulnar nerve being in periphery is variably involved.
- Necrotic muscle is colloquially termed "muscle sequestrum".
- Nerves are also affected latter by the continuing fibrosis and autoamputation from resulting contractions and hence most pathological specimens report their diameter being reduced to one-third of the original.

Clinical features:
- *Volkmann's sign:* Inability to actively extend fingers [at interphalangeal and/or metacarpophalangeal (MCP) joints] without flexing wrist and passive extension of fingers possible only with wrist flexion (or conversely the wrist flexes with passive finger extension) this is a classical sign for type I VIC
    - In VIC type II, the fingers actively tend to extend when the wrist is flexed and hyperextension of the proximal phalanx is prevented (Bouvier's maneuver), though these are also the findings in a normal hand! Interphalangeal joints may not extend in patients with complicated claw hand (stiff joints).
    - For Volkmann's type III (Zancolli), characteristically the proximal interphalangeal (PIP) joint flexion increases only after the MCP joints are passively flexed. This is true of all intrinsic contractures of the fingers. Passive extension of the MCP joint produces hyperextension of the PIP joint and flexion of the distal interphalangeal joint.
- Wrist flexion
- Pronated forearm, wasting
- Flexed elbow
- Cord-like induration on the flexor side, extensors affected/spared
- Paresthesia or anesthesia in the hand and fingers
- Flexed and adducted thumb
- Claw hand
- Deformity and trophic changes due to ulnar and median nerve involvement.

Diagnosis:
Detailed examination as above followed by:
Radiology: This is an essential test to be done for the following reasons:
- *Radiographs of forearm and elbow in two projections:* To evaluate and understand the primary pathology (fracture type, location, status of union and nonunion, malunion, and degree of malunion).
- To determine if anything is needed to be done to the fracture itself now.
- Radiographs of the hand to determine joint subluxations and severity of flexion contracture/secondary changes in joints in long neglected cases (need joint procedures like fusion or capsulotomies in management).
    Electromyography can produce information concerning nerve function and nerve regeneration.

Angiography is required for information regarding the vascular status—especially to know the caliber of vessels and the best place to do anastomosis in case of free muscle transfer. (It is important to note that angiogram should not be done as therapeutic measure in cases of suspected thrombosis as else the thrombus will get dislodged to cause blockade distally and one may lose their hand).

Computed tomography (CT) scan and magnetic resonance imaging (MRI): Determination of the severity and the extent of muscle damage in Volkmann's ischemic contracture by use of CT scan or MRI—MRI demonstrates fibrosis and the extent of loss of muscular tissue, but the operative technique, as yet, has not been altered by this information. I find specific use of MRI in determining the extent of damage in early cases presenting to us (2 days to few weeks) as if the involvement is severe, the trend is tilted to early intervention now. This "severe" involvement in late acute cases is difficult to judge clinically.

Treatment: Often a variety of treatment options are used in combination. The following are the different methods deployed in customized combinations for management and functional improvement:

- *Conservative treatment*—consisting of a combination of exercises and orthoses for wrist, hand, and fingers. Stiffness of joints should at all times be prevented. Turnbuckle splint comes in handy to mobilize the fingers here.
- *Excision of fibrous tissue:*
  – Capsulotomy—needed if the fingers cannot be stretched after muscle sequestrum excision.
  – Neurolysis.
  – Tenolysis.
- *Proximal "muscle slide" of Max Page:* There are few vehement opposes to this procedure due to the fact that a fibrotic tissue is in any case not going to provide contractile function in any position. This procedure is logically possible only when there is adequate muscle mass left that can provide contractile function else prefer reconstruction by tendon transfer.
- *Tendon lengthening.*
- *Tendon transfers.*
- *Nerve grafting.*
- *Free, vascularized, innervated musculocutaneous flaps:*
  – *Gracilis muscle transfer:* This has only 17% of the contractile force of forearm flexors and is bulkier, but the minimal donor site morbidity and consistent pedicle makes it the first choice.
  – *Latissimus dorsi* provides 33% of the contractile force and has longer pedicle and is the second choice (disadvantage due primarily to its bulk).
  – *Rectus femoris* is the third choice though it has good contractile force, and cross-sectional area fit according to the region but donor site morbidity is obvious.

Determining factors: All the above-mentioned options are not used in all patients and the choice of procedure(s) usually depends on the following determinants:

- Severity of the infarction and contracture.
- Affected muscle and nerve tissue damage.
- Delayed cases—3 months after injury. We prefer two-stage procedure:
  – *Stage 1:* Releases and excision of the fibrotic masses followed by intensive physiotherapy and mobilization.
  – *Stage 2:* Reconstruction of the lost function.
- Condition of potential soft tissue coverage.
- Function of remaining muscles and nerves.
  – Preserved extensors can be used for tendon transfer.

The various procedures described above are adequate for discrete problems that are uniquely applied to individuals, either individually or in various combinations, so generalizations are not possible. The following is a more scientific approach:

- Evaluate the extent of infarction clinically (range-of-motion, grip strength, sensation testing, classify—Tsuge)
  – If mild or moderate, assess the remaining hand function and put the patient on aggressive physiotherapy to stretch the contractures and promote functional rehabilitation simultaneously (no surgery initially). If the function does

not improve or there is less than satisfactory function grade 3 or less at 3 months then do surgical reconstruction for individual deficits (no generalization). (*Specifics can be read in detail from Chapter 106 – VIC in the book Essential Orthopedics: Principles and Practice, 2nd edition.*)
- If the function is poor to start with and there is severe contracture then there is nothing further to lose, and surgery should be considered for excision and reconstruction planning anyway (as a two-staged procedure). Also early surgery is done for:
  - Cases with severe involvement presenting early (acute or late acute cases) to preserve as much function we can by improving ischemia.
  - Cases with neuralgic pain.

41. Define and classify VIC. Describe its surgical and orthotic management in grade 2 VIC of forearm.

Ans: Volkmann ischemic contracture is a condition which is characterized by ischemic necrosis of the structures in forearm (extending to lower arm and hand) and subsequent crippling contractures associated with varying degrees of neurologic deficit.

Classification:
- Bunnell classified VIC as simple or severe considering the involvement at the forearm and hand.
- Pedemonte (1948) classified the VIC into classic (favorable type) or useless hand depending on the possibilities of recovery with reconstructive procedure.
- Merle d'Aubigné (1955) also classified VIC into two types, one with claw hand and the other without.
- Seddon proposed classification according to increasing grades of involvement in 1956 and 1964, that was modified by Tsuge (pronounced "suj") in 1975 as follows:
  - Mild or localized type (Seddon described this as having diffuse but moderate ischemia without infarct and spontaneous recovery):
    - The deep flexor muscles are partly degenerated.
    - The fingers involved are most often the ring finger and the long finger. When the degree of muscle degeneration is more extensive, the little and index fingers may also be affected.
    - Joints are spared.
    - Sometimes, there is a contracture of the thumb.
    - Cord-like induration on the volar forearm.
    - There is usually no sensory disturbance but, if present, it is slight.
    - A tenodesis effect can be demonstrated (Volkmann sign).
  - Moderate or classic type (Seddon described this as intense but localized muscle damage with typical muscular infarct with or without nerve lesion):
    - The degeneration involves nearly all of the deep flexor muscles to the fingers and the pollicis longus, with partial involvement of the FDS and wrist flexors leading to contracture.
    - Flexion contractures of all fingers and thumb and wrist.
    - Neurologic signs are invariably present, most commonly involving the median nerve.
  - The severe type (Seddon's widespread necrosis and fibrosis with severe paralysis and deformity):
    - Degeneration of all flexor muscles and partial involvement of the wrist extensor muscles.
    - Extensor involvement is seen in 13% of all the patients seen.
    - The neurologic signs are severe.
- *Zancolli (1975):* The Zancolli classification **(Table 4A.6.1)** is based on the condition of intrinsic muscles of hand as it gives a rough idea of neurological involvement and deficits. It has been found that use of this classification leads to grouping of clinically discrete patients into same group despite obvious differences in pathology and requirement of management. However, the described pathology is true only of delayed presentations:
  - Normal intrinsic muscle type (type I, simple digital claw)—the contracture is limited to the forearm muscles.
    - Joints spared—no stiffness.
  - Paralytic intrinsic muscle type (type II, intrinsic claw hand).

- Simple claw type—flexed position of wrist, contracture of the long flexor muscles of fingers.
- Complicated claw type—severe intrinsic paralysis along with digital joint stiffness.
- Totally rigid claw hand—flexed interphalangeal joints while MCP joints stiff in extension.
– Retracted intrinsic muscle type (type III, intrinsic contracture of the interosseous and/or thumb muscles)—fingers have typical posture due to intrinsic muscle contracture and retraction of the interossei. MCP joints are flexed while the interphalangeal joints are in extension. Distal interphalangeal flexed due to FDP contracture. Wrist is also flexed.
– Combined type (type IV) usually a combination of type I and II.

Functional classification:

TABLE 4A.6.1: Zancolli Functional classification.

Functional grade description	Possible values of total active range of movement that can serve as guide at		
	Wrist	Fingers	Thumb
Grade I: Symptomatic tightness but no limitation in range-of-motion or function	>90°	>160°	>40°
Grade II: Mild decrease in range-of-motion or mild impairment of function, but without significant impact on activities of daily living, no distortion of normal architecture	>70°	>140°	>30°
Grade III: Functional deficit noted with early changes in normal architecture of the site or part	>25°	>120°	>20°
Grade IV: Loss of function of the site or part	<25°	<120°	<20°

- *Holden's classification:* This classification marked a breakthrough from the somehow developed misleading concept of ischemia as the sole cause of VIC during World War I.
  – Level I—injury is proximal to the ischemia and later contracture, as in a brachial artery injury say by supracondylar fracture. These injuries if treated early result in Tsuge type 1 injuries but, if untreated, lead to moderate and then severe type depending on the evolution.
  – Level II—ischemia is directly under the injury (pressure) usually by tight bandages and casts (classically reported by Volkmann)—these are moderate-to-severe types of Tsuge. These are commonly observed with unfortunate treatment from traditional bone setters.
- *Classification of the nerve lesions in VIC:* Ercetin et al. (1994) reported a classification of nerve lesions in three grades:
  – Grade 1—a pearly white nerve without vasa vasorum.
  – Grade 2—a constricted nerve section (hour-glass deformity).
  – Grade 3—continuation of the nerve is not detectable.

Treatment of Grade 2 VIC (what is grade 2 needs to be first ascertained as grading is available only for functional classification and that serves as a guide for specific function reconstruction but not an overall treatment guide, I feel the examiner meant type 2 Tsuge for which the treatment is as follows):

Initial stretching and correction of wrist flexor contracture by active stretching and use of Volkmann/turnbuckle splint (padded dynamic soft tissue stretching splint), followed by:
- For preserved muscle mass—muscle sliding operation (of Max Page) with neurolysis of median and ulnar nerve as neurological damage is characteristic of moderate type. Carpal tunnel release is done through a second approach. Again muscle slide is preferable only if finger movements are there else consider the following option.
- When there is no useful finger flexion left, or there is proximal skin problem then brachioradialis and extensor carpi radialis longus (ECRL) transfer to flexors (FPL and FDP respectively) and complete release of contracture and neurolysis is the usual option. Extensor indicis proprius (EIP) is used for thumb opposition.
- Sensation may be restored by nerve grafting.
- Other options are proximal row carpectomy or forearm shortening by 2–3 cm (Garre's operation).

4A.7 RADIAL CLUB HAND (Q42)

42. Classify radial club hand (RCH). Describe pathoanatomy and management of a 1-year-old child.

Ans: Classification based on the amount of radius present **(Table 4A.7.1)**:

TABLE 4A.7.1: Classification of radial club hand based on radial anlage.	
Type I deficiency	*Mildest form*: There is mild shortening of the radius (distal) without considerable bowing. Minor radial deviation of the hand is apparent, although considerable thumb hypoplasia may be evident. Ulna straight.
Type II deficiency	*Small radius with shortening from both ends*: There are distal and proximal physeal abnormalities and moderate radial deviation of the wrist. Ulna bows.
Type III deficiency	*Partial radius absent*: Significant part of the radius is absent (most commonly the distal portion) and there is severe wrist radial deviation.
Type IV deficiency	*Complete absence of radius*: It is the most common variant characterized by a complete absence of the radius. The hand acquires a perpendicular relationship to the forearm.

Pathoanatomy: Radial dysplasia involves various skeletal malformations from the most proximal parts of limb to distally but all on the radial (preaxial) side. These are paralleled by soft tissue deficiencies of the hand, wrist, and forearm. The severity of the soft tissue loss also parallels the skeletal deficiency. Associated skeletal anomalies with radial longitudinal deficiency include:
- Small scapula
- Short clavicle with an increased curvature
- The humerus may be short with deficiencies of the capitellum and trochlea
- Elbow movements are usually diminished (more restriction of flexion than extension)
- The forearm is always reduced in length
- The ulna is approximately 60% of the normal length at the time of birth. This discrepancy persists throughout the growth period
- True forearm rotation is absent in patients with partial or complete aplasia of the radius
- The articulation between the carpus and ulna is usually fibrous and abnormal
- Wrist motion is primarily in the radial or ulnar plane with limited flexion or extension
- Ossification of the carpal bones is delayed
- The scaphoid and trapezium are often absent or hypoplastic
- The capitate, hamate, and triquetrum ossify late.

Muscular anomalies include:
- The preaxial muscles arising from the lateral epicondyle (radial wrist extensors and brachioradialis) are often absent or deficient (normally innervated by the radial nerve) along with pronator quadratus. These structures are replaced by a fibrous tissue (radial anlage) that maintains or worsens wrist deformity during growth.
- The deltoid or pectoralis major muscle can be hypoplastic or partially absent.
- The biceps may be absent or fused to the underlying brachialis muscle.
- The extrinsic flexors and extensors of the fingers are usually adherent.
- The abnormalities of the thumb muscles are related to the degree of thumb hypoplasia.

Neurovascular structures include:
- The radial nerve often terminates at the elbow and interosseous sensory nerve is absent.
- An enlarged median nerve substitutes for the absence of the radial nerve and supplies a dorsal branch for dorsoradial sensibility.
- The radial artery is often absent, and the interosseous arteries usually remain patent.
- The blood supply to the hand comes through the ulnar artery, and possibly the interosseous vessels or a persistent median artery.

Treatment: The basic goals of treatment are—
- To correct basic deformity (radial deviation of the wrist)
- Balance the wrist on the forearm
- Maintain wrist and hand position and function (particularly finger weakness)
- Improve opposition by recreating thumb function
- Improve social and emotional aspect of patients.

Nonsurgical intervention: Corrective casting, bracing, and physical therapy are used in infancy to achieve passive correction of the radial deviation. Simultaneously the elbow flexion contracture is also corrected to improve function. In mild cases, a home exercise program of wrist ulnar deviation and distraction stretching is taught whilst in more severe cases it involves serial corrective casting or splinting to gradually stretch the contracted soft tissues. For failed attempts to passively correct the radial deviation contracture by 6–12 weeks of vigorous conservative treatment, usually external fixation with gradual distraction of soft tissues and obtaining musculoskeletal alignment is considered. To maintain the correction a nighttime corrective splinting program is combined till surgical stable correction. In patients with grade 1 or sometimes grade 2, this conservative treatment itself may suffice. Children with higher grades are candidates for operative correction generally undertaken at 10–12 months of age.

Surgical treatment: Surgery is usually undertaken at around 1 year of age that allows for bit maturation and formation of structures to be identified distinctly, improvement in forearm length and distinctive fixed learned motor skills of the patient have not fully developed. Correcting deformity hence will give the child adequate time for better adaption to motor functions and avoid trick movements. Also, this allows additional reconstruction for thumb hypoplasia in a staged manner (or sometimes even simultaneously). Children with bilateral deficiencies that affect both the forearm and thumb require staged treatment. Surgical intervention of RCH (centralization or radialization) improves cosmesis, function, and ease of performance of activities in comparison to nonoperative management especially in type III or IV (Bayne types). The contraindications for surgery include:
- Medically unfit patient or limited life expectancy in a child
- Mild deformity with acceptable carpus support
- An elbow extension contracture that prevents the hand from reaching the mouth
- Development of adaptive movements for grip and pinch (older children)
- Severe index digital deformity and weakness that will result in failed pollicization.

The surgical intervention for RCH is commonly divided into two aspects:
1. One to correct the wrist deformity and other
2. To correct the functionally limiting thumb deficiency.

The various surgical options for the wrist deformity correction and stabilization include:
- Centralization of carpus over ulna
- Radialization
- Wrist fusion
- Lengthening of radius by distractors
- Bone graft procedures to the ulna.

Centralization or radialization is indicated in RCH types III and IV, in which there is severe deformity and insufficient support of the carpus while controlled lengthening of radius by a distractor can be performed after osteotomy in patients with radius shortening (type II) to rebalance the wrist.

Surgical options for thumb anomalies are more limited and include:
- Recreating first-web space, opponensplasty
- Pollicization
- Microvascular toe-to-thumb transfer.

A hypoplastic thumb may be surgically corrected with first-web space deepening, metacarpophalangeal (MCP) joint stabilization, and opponensplasty tendon transfer while pollicization is required for aplasia. Bone grafting of ulna was the earliest form of surgical correction for RCH. Vascularized bone grafting has been advocated recently but is tedious and requires expertise. This finds limited usage in the current management of RCH.

Centralization of the carpus over the third metacarpal: This has been a standard treatment for long period practiced by surgeons' world over. The typical steps of centralization include:
- Transverse ulnar incision and removal of ellipse of skin
- Preserving the enlarged median nerve after identification in the skinfold
- Ulnar capsulotomy
- Soft tissue release of the radial contracture
- Contouring of the ulna to match the carpus
- Capsular reefing
- Extensor carpi ulnaris (ECU) tendon advancement
- Aligning the third metacarpal on ulna and stabilization with pin fixation until healing.

Lots of modifications to this technique have been advocated by many.

Buck-Gramcko introduced *radialization* for anatomical redirection of distractive forces during the thalidomide crisis. The carpals are overcorrected and preserved (no notching) and wrist is balanced by tendon transfers of the radial wrist motors (extensor carpi radialis, flexor carpi radialis) to the dorsal ulnar wrist. Tendon transfer is required to balance the carpals over small ulna.

Wrist fusion is not performed in young patients. This leads to loss of wrist motion and potential loss of ulnar physeal growth. People have tried concomitant lengthening of ulna with wrist fusion but as mentioned before loss of wrist movements produces poor functional results.

Thumb reconstruction should be done before 18 months of age as a staged (higher grade RCH deformity) or a concomitant procedure (milder forms) to better develop the pinch grip. In the mild forms of radial dysplasia, the thumb hypoplasia can be corrected by deepening the first web space with Z-plasties or rotation flaps. Additional release of adductor and first dorsal interosseous fascia is often necessary. The MCP joint should be stabilized by one of the following methods:
- Using local fascia or extra flexor digitorum superficialis (FDS) tendon length for ligament reconstruction.
- Metacarpophalangeal joint chondrodesis (fusion of the proximal phalanx epiphysis to the metacarpal head) or arthrodesis.

Opponensplasty is performed simultaneously with the use of the abductor digiti quinti or ring-finger FDS, or accessory digital extensors with equal success. Thumb aplasia is best addressed with pollicization of index finger. Toe-to-thumb microvascular transfers have been reported, but the results of index finger pollicization are fantastic. For microvascular transfer, the quality of index finger donor determines reconstructed thumb function.

The commonly reported unacceptable complications are stiff and weak thumb due to camptodactyly; frequent development of compensatory lateral pinch between adjacent digits. The results of pollicization are better only if additional opponensplasty is done else there are high chances of developing a weak and just structural thumb.

4A.8 DRUG AND ITS DISORDERS (Q43–48)

43. Discuss anatomy of DRUJ.

Ans: The distal radioulnar Joint (DRUJ) per se comprises of the following structures (**Figs. 4A.8.1 and 4A.8.2**):
- Bony articulation of the joint (sigmoid notch of ulna and articulating ulna head "articular seat")—a synovial joint. Radial sigmoid notch is shallow and ulna head is asymmetric. Sigmoid notch is triangular with a dorsal, palmar and distal (carpal margin). Articular cartilage on ulna head covers 90–135° arc. The radius of curvature of ulnar head is 10 mm while for sigmoid notch is 15 mm so they are concentric. This nonconcentric location causes rotational and significant sliding movement at DRUJ (translation of 2 mm volar and 5 mm dorsal in pronosupination). This volar position of ulnar head during supination and dorsal position during pronation produces a "centrode of rotation" rather than a single center of rotation. One must remember that it is the radius that rotates around the ulna, and hence it is the radius that dislocates/subluxates and not the ulna! The bony articulation is unstable as the sigmoid notch has inclination of 7.7° from longitudinal axis while head of ulna has inclination of 21°. The articulation is primarily stabilized by the palmar and dorsal radioulnar ligaments.

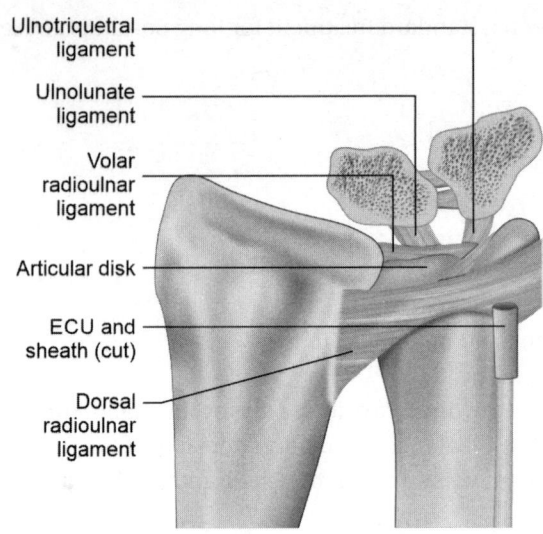

Fig. 4A.8.1: Anatomy of distal radioulnar joint (DRUJ).
(ECU: extensor carpi ulnaris)

Fig. 4A.8.2: The disposition of distal radioulnar ligament with respect to the articular disc.
(DRUL: dorsal radioulnar ligament)

- Interosseous membrane (IOM) of the forearm distally (syndesmosis).
- *Soft tissue support system of DRUJ:* These comprise of dynamic and static supports:
  - Static supports of DRUJ
    - *Triangular fibrocartilage complex (TFCC):* This is an extensive, complicated and recently studied in detail system comprising structures originating from dorsal lip of sigmoid notch and attach to the ulnar base of 5th metacarpal and ulnar styloid (complex 3D structure). It comprises of five predominant structures:
      - Triangular fibrocartilage (TFC)—the disk having three components.
      - Ulnocarpal ligaments (two)—these comprise of ulnolunate and ulnotriquetral ligaments. The ligaments form a "V" configuration originating from the base of ulnar styloid (apex of "V") and attaching to lunate or triquetrum distally.
  - IOM—transmits force between radius and ulna.

Dynamic stabilizers of DRUJ:
- Extensor carpi ulnaris (ECU)—tension in supination provides stability
- Infratendinous extensor retinaculum
- Pronator quadratus—acts in conjunction with the distal oblique fibers of IOM to provide stability in supination.

44. Describe anatomy of DRUJ. Describe indications and technique of performing Kapandji procedure.

Ans: Anatomy: The DRUJ per se comprises of following structures—
- Bony articulation of the joint (sigmoid notch of ulna and articulating ulna head "articular seat")—a synovial joint. Radial sigmoid notch is shallow and ulna head is asymmetric. Sigmoid notch is triangular with a dorsal, palmar and distal (carpal margin). Articular cartilage on ulna head covers 90–135° arc. The radius of curvature of ulnar head is 10 mm while for sigmoid notch is 15 mm so they are concentric. This nonconcentric location causes rotational and significant sliding movement at DRUJ (translation of 2 mm volar and 5 mm dorsal in pronosupination). This volar position of ulnar head during supination and dorsal position during pronation produces a "centrode of rotation" rather than a single center of rotation. One must remember that it is the radius that rotates around the ulna, and hence it is the radius that dislocates/subluxates and not the ulna! The bony articulation is unstable as the sigmoid notch has inclination of 7.7° from longitudinal axis while head of ulna has inclination of 21°. The articulation is primarily stabilized by the palmar and dorsal radioulnar ligaments.
- Interosseous membrane (IOM) of the forearm distally (syndesmosis).

- *Soft tissue support system of DRUJ:* These comprise of dynamic and static supports:
  - Static supports of DRUJ
    - *Triangular fibrocartilage complex (TFCC):* This is an extensive, complicated and recently studied in detail system comprising structures originating from dorsal lip of sigmoid notch and attach to the ulnar base of 5th metacarpal and ulnar styloid (complex 3D structure). It comprises of five predominant structures.
      - Triangular fibrocartilage (TFC)—the disk having three components.
      - Ulnocarpal ligaments (two)—these comprise of ulnolunate and ulnotriquetral ligaments. The ligaments form a "V" configuration originating from the base of ulnar styloid (apex of "V") and attaching to lunate or triquetrum distally.
    - IOM—transmits force between radius and ulna.
  - Dynamic stabilizers:
    - Extensor carpi ulnaris—tension in supination provides stability
    - Infratendinous extensor retinaculum
    - Pronator quadratus—acts in conjunction with the distal oblique fibers of IOM to provide stability in supination.

Indications of Kapandji procedure:
- Osteoarthritis/chondromalacia of DRUJ
- Posttraumatic ulnocarpal impingement
- Young rheumatoid arthritis (RA) patient with ulnar translocation with DRUJ disease
- Rheumatoid arthritis patient who may need a stable radioulnar surface for support of an arthroplasty.

Procedure:
- Position the patient supine on the operating table; apply a well-padded tourniquet; extend the arm on the hand table; prepare the skin; and apply drapes to expose the elbow, forearm, and hand. Exsanguinate the limb with an elastic wrap, and inflate a pneumatic tourniquet.
- The location of the incision may vary slightly if the patient has RA with extensor tenosynovitis. For rheumatoid patients, make a dorsal longitudinal incision to allow extensor tenosynovectomy and repair, grafting, or tendon transfers for ruptured tendons.
- For nonrheumatoid patients, make a dorsoulnar incision centered over the ulnar head. Avoid injury to the dorsal sensory branch of the ulnar nerve.
- Identify the interval between the ECU and the extensor digiti minimi.
- Open the extensor retinaculum, forming a proximal flap based laterally (radially) and a distal flap based medially (ulnarward). Use these flaps later to reinforce the extensor retinaculum and the capsule, or they can be discarded.
- Decorticate the radial and ulnar articular surfaces of the DRUJ with narrow osteotomes and a narrow rongeur.
- Temporarily stabilize the DRUJ with a 0.045-inch Kirschner wire.
- Just proximal to the ulnar neck and proximal to the DRUJ, make an ulnar osteotomy with an oscillating saw.
- For patients with neutral or negative ulnar variance, remove a 15-mm segment of ulna with its surrounding periosteum. For patients with positive ulnar variance, remove a larger segment of ulna to allow radioulnar arthrodesis at neutral variance and to allow removal of sufficient bone to allow pain-free rotation, a 15-mm gap, and stabilization by the pronator quadratus.
- Remove the temporary fixation from the DRUJ, and obtain permanent fixation with a 3.5-mm bone screw, using a "lag" technique. Use a washer if needed in poor-quality bone, or use Kirschner wires for permanent fixation.
- Use bone from the excised segment of ulna to graft the arthrodesis.
- Drill holes in the proximal ulnar stump to secure the pronator quadratus from the excised ulnar segment to the proximal segment for stabilization.
- Deflate the pneumatic tourniquet, ensure hemostasis, and close the skin.
- Apply a bulky compression dressing, supported by an above-elbow or below-elbow splint or cast. If a rheumatoid patient has had other procedures such as a tendon transfer, more immobilization may be required.

45. Discuss management of DRUJ disruption in 30-year-old software engineer.

Ans: Acute injuries that can be reduced congruously should be maintained in supination in an above elbow cast for 6 weeks. Many surgeons prefer arthroscopic TFCC repair intra-articularly when diagnosed early.

The typical operative indications are:
- Noncongruous reduction due to soft tissue interposition
- Locked DRUJ
- Persisting DRUJ instability due to fractured volar lip of sigmoid notch.

  Central tears (TFC tear) are debrided while peripheral tears are repaired often arthroscopically intra-articularly or by open technique. If successful, this anatomic intra-articular reconstruction may restore stability with minimal loss of motion. The intra-articular repair occasionally fails evidenced by continued instability and painful range-of-motion. These are managed by various extra-articular soft tissue reconstruction methods. In addition to this reconstruction, the bony abnormalities (malunions and length discrepancies) should be addressed as they may be one of the reasons of recurrent instability. In general the methods of reconstruction involve reconstructing some elements of TFCC by creating ulnocarpal or radioulnar tether (all these are non-anatomic reconstructions).

Following are the management options for acute injury:
- DRUJ instability following acute, isolated dorsal or volar dislocation—six weeks of forearm cast in forearm supination. Perform open reduction for irreducible joint and fix provisionally with K-wire that can be removed at 3 weeks.
- Acute distal radius fractures—assess for DRUJ instability using towel clip (perform lateral pull and dorsovolar translation to assess)—fix if unstable with K-wire.
- Ulnar styloid fractures—fix using K-wire—tension band technique.

46. Describe surgical anatomy of lower end radius.

Ans: The three-column concept is a helpful biomechanical model for understanding the pathomechanics of wrist fractures. The radial column includes the radial styloid and scaphoid fossa, the intermediate column consists of the lunate fossa and sigmoid notch of the radius, and the ulnar column comprises the distal ulna with the triangular fibrocartilaginous complex (TFCC).

The radial styloid is an important stabilizer of the wrist providing a bony buttress and attachment for the extrinsic carpal ligaments. Under normal physiological conditions, only a minor amount of load is transmitted along the radial column. A large proportion of load is transmitted across the lunate fossa to the intermediate column and so the lunate fossa is the key to the radiocarpal joint surface. The ulna is the stable partner in forearm rotation. The radius swings around the ulna and the two bones are firmly linked together by ligaments, at the level of the proximal and distal radioulnar joints, and by the interosseous membrane. The ulnar column represents the distal end of this stable pivot. The TFCC allows independent flexion/extension, radial/ulnar deviation, and pronation/supination of the wrist. It is therefore important in the stability of the carpus and forearm.

Significant forces are transmitted across the ulnar column, especially when making a tight fist.

The anatomy of distal radial fractures (DRFs) produces some unique surgical challenges. Dorsally placed implants have little soft-tissue cover and may irritate the overlying extensor tendons. Palmar implants are well covered by the pronator quadratus muscle. The thin cortex around the metaphysis of the distal radius means that the thread pitch of conventional screws gives insufficient purchase for fixation to be achieved with absolute stability, a problem that is increased in osteoporotic bone.

The pronator quadrates muscle is elevated from its radial origin proximally and the incision turned in an L-shaped fashion distally. The horizontal limb is placed at the fibrous transition zone between pronator quadratus and the watershed line. This fibrous zone lies a few millimeters proximal to the watershed line and is sharply elevated from the bone to expose the fracture lines and palmar fragments. The position of the joint line can be determined with a hypodermic needle placed inside the joint. The watershed line represents the margin between the structures which are elevated proximally and the palmar wrist extrinsic ligaments. They should not be detached from the radius (to expose the joint surface) as this may destabilize the wrist.

47. Describe the mechanism and pathoanatomy of dorsal intercalated segment instability (DISI). What are the radiological parameters to diagnose such an instability and outline management options in a chronic late presenting case?

Ans: *Mechanism and pathoanatomy of dorsal intercalated segment instability*

Mechanism:

DISI is a wrist condition characterized by abnormal mobility between the carpal bones, primarily affecting the scaphoid and lunate. Key mechanisms leading to DISI include:
- *Ligament injury:* The most common cause is the rupture of the scapholunate ligament, which destabilizes the joint.
- *Force imbalance:* Disruption between the flexor and extensor forces can lead to abnormal wrist movement.
- *Degenerative changes:* Conditions like arthritis weaken ligament support over time.

Pathoanatomy:

In DISI, the scaphoid flexes while the lunate extends, resulting in dorsal angulation of the lunate. This reduces joint congruency and increases the risk of further degeneration, potentially leading to osteoarthritis or scapholunate advanced collapse (SLAC) wrist.

Diagnosis: Diagnosis involves radiographic analysis, including:
- *Anteroposterior (AP) and lateral radiographs:*
  - *Scapholunate angle:* An angle greater than 60° may indicate instability.
  - *Lunate dorsiflexion:* A dorsal tilt of the lunate indicates DISI.
  - *Capitate position:* Displacement beneath the lunate suggests instability.
- *MRI or CT scans:* MRI can reveal soft tissue injuries, while CT provides detailed images of bone alignment.
  - *DISI angle:* Significant dorsal angulation between the scaphoid and lunate confirms DISI.

Management of chronic DISI may vary depending on the severity of the instability, symptoms, and the presence of degenerative changes. Options include:
- *Conservative management:*
  - *Activity modification:* Limiting activities that exacerbate symptoms.
  - *Wrist brace/orthosis:* Wrist immobilization may provide symptomatic relief and prevent further instability.
  - *Physical therapy:* Strengthening and stabilization exercises focusing on wrist mechanics may help.
- *Surgical management:*
  - *Ligament reconstruction:* If there is a significant scapholunate ligament tear, surgical repair or reconstruction may be necessary.
  - *Scaphoid osteotomy or fusion:* In cases where there is scaphoid nonunion or advanced degenerative changes, reconstructive procedures may be indicated; for instance, bridging the gap between the scaphoid and lunate.
  - *Wrist fusion:* In late-presenting chronic cases where severe degeneration has occurred (e.g., SLAC wrist), a midcarpal or dorsal wrist fusion may be considered to alleviate pain and restore function.
  - *Joint replacement:* In severe cases with significant arthritis where other options fail, consider partial or total wrist arthroplasty.

48. Describe causes of ulnar wrist pain after healing of distal radius fracture and discuss management.

Ans: The usual causes of ulnar wrist pain following a distal radius fracture arise from malunion producing shortening of radial length and loss of volar tilt. These produce some clinical conditions causing ulnar sided pain:
- Ulnocarpal impaction
- Ulnar impingement syndrome
- Ulnocarpal impaction secondary to ulnar styloid nonunion
- Unrecognized TFCC injury at the time of initial presentation.

Management

Ulnocarpal impaction

Imaging: Radiographic findings include—
- Subchondral sclerosis and cystic changes in the ulnar head, lunate bone, and proximal radial aspect of the triquetrum.
- Ulnocarpal osteoarthritis

- In subtle cases, the changes may not be present and in them recognition of the geographic nature of the abnormalities affecting the articular surfaces of the ulna, lunate and triquetrum is essential (MRI may be helpful).

The following etiological findings should be noted:
- Positive ulnar variance
- Neutral or negative variance
- Malunion of a distal radial fracture with residual radial shortening
- Abnormal dorsal tilt
- Premature physeal arrest of the distal radius
- Essex-Lopresti fracture or resection of the radial head may also be evident on conventional radiographs.

Magnetic resonance imaging is helpful in detecting occult disease that shows fibrillation of the joint cartilage of the ulnar head and ulnar carpus followed by bone hyperemia (low-signal intensity on T1-weighted images and high-signal intensity on T2-weighted images). In advanced stages sclerotic changes appear as areas of low-signal intensity on both T1- and T2-weighted images. Magnetic resonance arthrography may be done to demonstrate the integrity of the TFC and lunotriquetral ligament.

Treatment
The determining factors for the type of intervention are:
- The amount of ulnar variance
- The palmar lesion class
- The shape of the sigmoid fossa and ulnar seat
- The presence of concomitant lunotriquetral instability.

A simple algorithm to understand the basic treatment options are:
- Palmar class IIA and IIB lesions (no TFC perforation)—an open wafer procedure or formal ulnar shortening (preferred).
- Palmar class IIC and IID lesions (TFCC perforated)—arthroscopic wafer procedure (causes destruction of articular cartilage of ulna so may not be as prudent as considered by many).
- Class IIE lesions—Darrach's procedure or Sauvé-Kapandji procedure. They all however produce convergent instability (ulna impingement syndrome).

Ulnar impingement syndrome
Radiology:
- Ulnar impingement produces erosive cortical changes at the corresponding level of the radius (radial scalloping).
- There is subchondral sclerosis of ulna. Degenerative changes appear in the form of deformation, deshapening, and loss of ulnar profile.
- Magnetic resonance imaging may help in confirming the diagnosis before radiological changes are visible and may help diagnose it early.

Treatment:
- Aggressive ulnar shortening and stabilization by Breen and Jupiter or Bunnell-Boyes reconstruction.
- Ulna head replacement (see above).
- Distraction lengthening of the ulna—using external fixation, restores the length discrepancy, however, will not be suitable in cases of settled arthritis.
- Radial shortening in early cases—where the DRUJ can be specifically relocated and stabilized by soft tissue procedures additionally.

Ulnocarpal impaction secondary to ulnar styloid nonunion
Radiologically seen but MRI is the best modality for visualizing the integrity of the TFC complex and its ulnar attachments. It also reveals any associated chondromalacia of the ulnar carpus and degenerative changes.

Diagnostic arthroscopy is possibly the best investigation to guide treatment—loss of resilience of TFC (central disk) and loss of "trampoline effect" (bouncing back on hitting centrally) are the best indicator of the need to relocate the ulnar styloid at the anatomical location and reconstruction/repair of TFCC. Conversely if resilience is seen during arthroscopy and symptoms are significant then ulnar styloid can be removed (it indicates functional TFCC while styloid impingement as the cause of symptoms).

4A.9 MADELUNG DEFORMITY (Q49–50)

49. Describe the pathology, clinical features, diagnosis, and treatment of Madelung deformity.

Ans: Pathology: The characteristic anatomic abnormality is subnormal distal radial growth caused by disturbance of the volar and ulnar distal radial physis leading to asymmetric growth. The deformity is characterized by ulnar and palmar curvature of the distal radius, positive ulnar variance, and proximal subsidence of the lunate. The defect is filled by flame-shaped fibrotic ligament of Vickers that tethers lunate. It is a secondary pathologic structure rather than a primary abnormality.

Clinical features: Symptoms usually begin during adolescence only and most commonly in girls aged 10–14 years. Madelung deformity (MD) is observed very rarely in males. Patients experience increasing deformity and pain in the wrist with decreased range of motion (ROM). On physical examination, the deformity varies in degree from a slight protrusion of the lower end of the ulna abutting the carpus and becomes prominent dorsally relative to the carpus and hand. There is complete dislocation of the inferior radioulnar joint in advanced disease with marked radial deviation of the hand. The hand is translated volarly to the long axis of the forearm. ROM is decreased, with a limitation of supination, dorsiflexion and radial deviation. Pronation and flexion usually are normal. On the basis of etiology, MD is classified into four different groups (all of which should be evaluated accordingly) by Henry and Thorburn which are as follows:

1. Post-traumatic
2. Dysplastic
3. Chromosomal or genetic (Turner syndrome)
4. Idiopathic or primary.

Diagnosis:

Plain radiographs demonstrate:

- Lateral and dorsal curvature of the radius
- Widened interosseous space
- True shortening of the total length of the radius
- Premature fusion of the ulnar half of the distal radial physis
- Focal osteopenia in the area of the ulnar portion of the distal radius appearing as a "flame-like" lesion corresponding to the attachment of ligament of Vickers
- Exostosis at the distal ulnar border of the radius
- Triangularization of the distal radial epiphysis
- Ulnar and palmar facing distal radial articular surface
- Relative dorsal subluxation of the ulna
- Increased radiodensity of the ulnar head
- Carpal wedging with the lunate at the apex of the wedge
- An arched curvature of the carpal bones in direct continuation of the dorsal bowing of the radius on the lateral radiograph
- An increased radial tilt on the posteroanterior (PA) radiograph and the radial epiphysis becomes teardrop shaped, observation added by Carter and Ezaki. On the lateral view, the radius tilts volarward until the ulna appears dislocated from its normal articulation with the radius. The ulna lies dorsal to the proximal carpal row. The distal ulna does not actually sublux dorsally. Rather, the hand and radius are translated palmarward, resulting in incongruence of the distal radioulnar joint (DRUJ) injuries. The unaffected ulna continues to grow, ultimately becoming longer than the ulnar aspect of the radius.

Treatment:

Nonsurgical: Rest and nonsteroidal anti-inflammatory drugs are the treatments initially offered usually as interim measure till definite surgery is planned. If no improvement is made, a splint or brace can be used to keep the deviated arm straight.

If pain is predominantly DRUJ pain, then a sugar-tong-type splint is used to prevent joint irritation from overactivity. If pain is radiocarpal, then a volar splint should be used. Often the conservative measures fail as the malformation is progressive with a continuous conspicuous increase in deformity with growth and surgical intervention is designated. The acceptability to deformity and disability should be, however, always assessed individually before pushing surgery.

Surgical: In general, physiolysis with release of Vicker's ligament is proposed for treating younger skeletally immature patients. In older, skeletally mature patients, combinations of epiphysiodesis, lateral closing wedge osteotomy or dome osteotomy, and ulnar shortening osteotomy may be performed.

The surgical treatment is opted if the following criteria are fulfilled:
- Patient's age and the growth remaining in the distal radius
- Severity of the deformity
- Severity of the symptoms
- Clinical and radiographic findings.

Skeletally immature patient: These include—
- *Physiolysis (Vickers and Nielsen):* Here removal of the epiphyseal band is done that causes the abnormal growth of the wrist. A small incision is made at the volar-radial side. This approach is through flexor pollicis longus and palmaris longus leaving the median nerve and radial artery protected. The pronator quadratus muscle is identified and detached from the radius. The abnormal epiphysis is identified by a cut in the bone. After defining the epiphysis extra bone is removed to position the radius correctly and prevent formation of bone bar. This is always combined with a Vickers ligament release.
- *Correction of radius deformity by dome osteotomy:* This is done to straighten the abnormal radius by three-dimensional correction of the deformity with adequate bony contact. Here, an 8-cm incision is made from the wrist crease at the palmar radial side. The approach is made through flexor carpi radialis detaching the pronator quadratus muscle from the radius and releasing the Vickers ligament. The periosteum is elevated and a crescent-shaped osteotomy, concave at the end, is marked on the bone and bone cut and osteotomy fixed in desired corrected position. The distal end of the radius stays attached to the ulna.
- *Vickers ligament release:* The Vickers ligament originates on the radius in a fossa that is seen radiographically as a flame-shaped radiolucency distal to a bone spur on the ulnar aspect of the distal metaphysis. The purpose of its release is to release the tension and leave the wrist straight for further growth. Vickers and Nielsen described an ulnar-volar release for MD of the physis, called physiolysis. This allows normal and compensatory growth to correct the deformity. They were the first to describe a ligamentous lesion as part of the pathology and also were the first to use the volar approach to address it.

Skeletally mature patients: These include—
- *Ulna shortening:* Adults with Madelung's deformity may suffer from ulnar-sided wrist pain. Apart from the usual treatment by distal radial osteotomy if patients have a positive ulnar variance and focal wrist pathology, it is possible to treat with an isolated ulnar-shortening osteotomy. In these patients, the radial deformity may or may not be simultaneously treated.
- *Distal radioulnar joint injuries replacement:* An alternative treatment for patients with ulnar-sided wrist pain is a total replacement of the distal radioulnar joint. The prosthesis helps in managing the pain and may also improve the ROM of the wrist.
- *Correction of radius deformity:* As above corrective osteotomy can be performed.
- *Radioulnar length adjustment:* There is relative dorsal subluxation of normally growing ulna on the volar radius in MD. This disparity can be addressed by ulnar shortening, ulnar head resection, and a Sauve-Kapandji type (Lauenstein) DRUJ arthrodesis.

50. Describe the pathoanatomy of Madelung disease.

Ans: Kindly refer to Answer to Question 49 above.

4A.10 DISORDERS OF CARPAL BONES AND INSTABILITY (Q51–56)

51. **What is Kienböck's disease? Write in brief about etiology, diagnosis, and management of this condition.**

Ans: *Kienböck's disease:* Kienböck's disease is a painful disorder of the wrist of unknown cause in which radiographs eventually show osteonecrosis of the carpal lunate. If untreated, the disease usually results in fragmentation of the lunate, collapse with shortening of the carpus, and secondary arthritic changes throughout the proximal carpal area.

Etiology:
- *Aberrant blood supply to lunate:* Problems with arteries [single dominant nutrient arterial supply for lunate (20% patients)]—
  - Poorly organized intraosseous circulation—"I" pattern of anastomosis
  - Venous congestion leading to increased intraosseous pressure (Jensen)—this may also be partially responsible to finding Kienböck's in cerebral palsy (5–10% prevalence). The patients maintain a flexed posture of wrist and due to raised muscle tone the blood outflow is impeded, producing increased intraosseous pressure.
  - *Vasculopathies:*
    - Septic emboli
    - Raynaud's disease
    - Scleroderma
    - Systemic lupus erythematosus
    - Dermatomyositis
    - Rheumatoid arthritis
    - Juvenile idiopathic arthritis.
- *Coagulopathies and metabolic disorders:*
  - Sickle cell anemia
  - Gout
  - Antiphospholipid antibody syndrome
  - Crohn's enteritis.
- *Skeletal variations:*
  - Small lunate bone (Tsuge and Nakamura)
  - Negative ulnar variance (Hulten) putting extra pressure on the lunate due to large unsupported area of bone in certain wrist motions (extension and ulnar deviation). This extra stress causes microtrauma in the bone and can eventually lead to Kienböck's disease. Hulten advised radial shortening to reduce pressure on lunate while Persson advised ulnar lengthening procedure. The association is supported by finding higher incidence of lunatomalacia in cerebral palsy patients and patients with congenital shortening of the ulna in Langer-Giedion syndrome.
- Abnormal wrist biomechanics—pointed hammer effect of capitate along with higher force transmission through the bone (35% of forces across the wrist).
- Some diseases may be linked to a greater risk, including lupus, cerebral palsy, sickle cell anemia, and gout. One study found that 9.4% of cerebral palsy patients also had Kienböck's disease.
- Repetitive significant trauma as in power drillers (Jack Hammer), single major trauma as in motor vehicle accident—various methods of trauma have been proposed to cause avascular necrosis:
  - Trauma acting on vascular system directly (avulsion of pedicle)
  - Trauma acting on osseous system (fracture theory)
  - Trauma acting on vascular nervous system.

Diagnosis: Magnetic resonance imaging (MRI) helps in the diagnosis of early avascular changes in the lunate. Correlation of the patient's clinical and plain radiographic findings with MRI helps to diagnose Kienböck's disease.

Treatment:

Conservative: Spontaneous regression of the signs and symptoms has been observed in early Kienbock's disease. If the stress on the bone is taken away then revascularization can occur spontaneously. Immobilization and analgesics are commonly used. A combination approach utilizing bone marrow injection, ultrasonic therapy while simultaneously unloading the lunate using external fixator, has been found to be effective.

Operative management: The primary indication of surgery is a patient with persistent pain, not responsive to conservative treatment. The methods can be though grouped under following distinct categories:

- *Decompression of lunate:*
  - *Joint leveling procedure:* Joint "leveling" procedures include ulnar lengthening and radial shortening and usually are indicated for Lichtman stage I through IIIA Kienböck's disease, with an ulnar-minus variation and without degenerative changes in the radiolunate or capitolunate joints. Wedge osteotomy reduces the radioulnar inclination of the distal radius and can be alternately used to decrease the load on the lunate.
- *Revascularization procedures:* Lunate revascularization using a variety of pedicled bone grafts has been effective in preserving the lunate architecture. The reconstructed vascularity needs to be additionally protected by external fixator commonly.
- *Prosthetic replacement:* Excision of the lunate can give short-term relief. Prosthetic lunate replacement also may provide relief. While prosthetic replacement has been variably tried to reduce instances of carpal migration and instability.
- *Limited fusion and wrist fusion:* Limited intercarpal fusion can prevent proximal carpal migration after lunate excision and can help to decrease pressure on lunate prostheses. Development of intercarpal or radiocarpal arthritis needs wrist joint arthrodesis or else proximal row carpectomy.

52. Briefly mention principles of management of different stages of Kienböck's disease.

Ans: The following table **(Table 4A.10.1)** provides insight to the various treatment options depending on the different stages of Kienböck's disease:

TABLE 4A.10.1: Classification of Kienbock disease and proposed treatment.

Stahl-Lichtman	Bain and Begg	Magnetic resonance imaging	Treatment
0	0	A	Medical and preventive therapy
1	1	A	Medical and supportive therapy (temporary unloading of lunate), treat underlying disorder (autoimmune disorder, antiviral treatment) Surgical treatment (conservative failure)— Ulna minus → radial shortening ± revascularization Ulna neutral or plus → capitate shortening + capitohamate fusion ± revascularization
2	0 or 1	A	Joint leveling, revascularization as above
2	2	B	STT fusion ± revascularization procedure
2	4	C	Radiocarpal fusion
3A	1, 2	B	As for stage 2, bias toward doing revascularization
3A	3, 4	C	Wrist arthrodesis
3B	0	A	Salvage lunate—correct the scaphoid subluxation, rotation and perform scaphocapitate fusion to unload lunate ± revascularization procedure
3B	1	B	Proximal row carpectomy
3B	2	C	STT fusion, carbon implant ± wrist denervation
3B	3, 4	C	Wrist arthrodesis
3C (Proposed)	2b	C	Proximal row carpectomy ± wrist denervation
4	3, 4	C	Wrist arthrodesis

53. Describe the pathology, clinical features, diagnosis, and treatment principles of nonunion of fracture scaphoid. Describe the blood supply of scaphoid.

Ans: Pathology: The overall incidence of scaphoid fracture progressing to nonunion is around 10%, while it is 30% for proximal pole fragments due to precarious blood supply. Blood supply of scaphoid is precarious. The blood supply of the scaphoid is precarious. Only 67% of scaphoid bones have arterial foramina throughout their length, including the distal, middle, and proximal thirds. Of the remaining bones, 13% have blood supply predominantly in the distal third, and 20% have most of the arterial foramina in the waist area of the bone with no more than a single foramen near the proximal third. One-third of scaphoid fractures occurring in the proximal third may be without adequate blood supply. Apart from the precarious blood supply, nonunion of scaphoid fractures is also influenced by delayed diagnosis, gross displacement, associated injuries of the carpus. Of these fractures, an estimated 40% are undiagnosed at the time of the original injury. Displaced scaphoid fractures may have a nonunion rate of 92%. Nonunion is commonly associated with dorsal intercalated segment instability (DISI) carpal instability pattern because of dorsal displacement of proximal scaphoid (humpback deformity) as mentioned before. Proximal nonunions are associated with crescentic defects, while distal nonunions have large triangular defects with humpback deformity. Patients usually have variable amount of pain in the wrist, loss of grip strength, and on and off swelling at the site. Radiologically, there is discernible gap in the bone at the fracture site with rounded sclerotic fracture margins. The bone may be foreshortened or may have humpback deformity (commonly called flexed scaphoid). In advanced cases, there is radiocarpal arthritis and may develop into scaphoid nonunion advanced collapse (SNAC) wrist where advanced arthritis progresses from radial styloid to extend into midcarpal arthritis. If the arthritis extends into all carpal bones (pancarpal arthritis) then it is called SNAC plus.

Clinical features: Patients usually have variable amount of pain in the wrist, loss of grip strength, and on and off swelling at the site.

Diagnosis: Radiologically, there is discernible gap in the bone at the fracture site with rounded sclerotic fracture margins. The gap may be a linear defect or may have sclerotic margins with displacement. The defect may show bone absorption appearing as a cystic defect (Ikeda classification). Due to foreshortening, there may be humpback deformity. In advanced cases, there is radiocarpal arthritis → SNAC wrist that may progress to → pancarpal arthritis or SNAC *plus*.

Magnetic resonance imaging is the investigation of choice to identify osteonecrosis associated with nonunion scaphoid and to find associated ligament injury.

Scaphoid nonunion can be classified according to Herbert and Fisher system where fractures presenting after 6 weeks (nonunion, type D) or after 6 weeks of immobilization (type C, delayed union) are also classified. Type D fractures are further classified as:

- Type C—delayed union after 6 weeks of immobilization—manage like type D1/D2
- Type D1—stable (fibrotic)
- Type D2—unstable (sclerotic, pseudarthrosis)
- Type D3—nonunion with fixed DISI
- Type D4—nonunion with avascular necrosis (AVN).

Treatment principles

Blood supply of scaphoid: The prevalence of osteonecrosis can be 10–30% in scaphoid nonunion. Fractures in the proximal pole can be expected to take longer to heal and usually have higher rates of nonunion. Traditionally, bone grafting was suggested for all nonunions, but Type D1 and Ikeda's linear and cystic types have been successfully managed by solely compression screw fixation. Type D2/D3/D4 and Ikeda type sclerotic nonunions are usually due to delay in receiving treatment. The approach to nonunion can be distinctively chosen based on the location of nonunion and association of AVN **(Flowchart 4A.10.1)**.

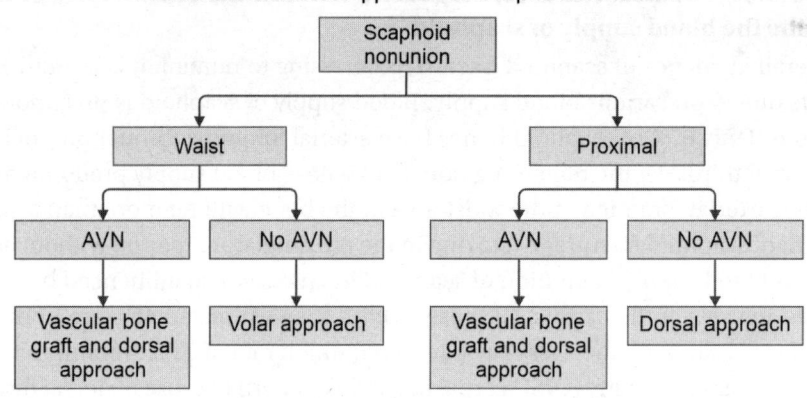

Flowchart 4A.10.1: Approach to scaphoid nonunion.

(AVN: avascular necrosis)

Depending on the delay in presentation, the operative management options are divided into two groups. In the first group, where no degenerative changes have set in one tries to achieve union by either of the following methods:
- *Nonvascularized bone grafting (NVBG):*
  - Cancellous inlay (Matti–Russe): Indicated in type D1 or cystic type Ikeda.
  - Wedge (Fisk–Fernandez): Indicated in nonunion with deformity as in some unstable D2 and D3 type nonunion.
  - Arthroscopic-assisted bone grafting.
- *Vascularized bone grafting (VBG):* This may be preferred for most type D2, D4 where there is high suspicion of osteonecrosis.
- Ilizarov fixation of scaphoid nonunion.
- Use of bone morphogenetic protein (BMP).

For patients who present late to the treating surgeon so that some form of degeneration has set in, only salvage procedures can be proposed as just achieving union will not treat the patient completely. These options include one of the following depending on the extent of degeneration that has set in:
- Distal scaphoid resection—indicated in cases with failed chronic nonunions with overgrown distal scaphoid pole ± arthritic changes at radioscaphoid joint
- Limited intercarpal fusion
- Proximal row carpectomy
- Scaphoid excision + four-corner fusion
- Scaphoid allograft and fixation for proximal pole nonunions and fragmentation.
- Proximal pole reconstruction using rib osteochondral autograft in unsalvageable proximal poles
- Proximal pole excision and filling by fascial/tendon spacer
- Wrist arthroplasty
- Wrist arthrodesis.

54. Clinical implication of blood supply of scaphoid on its fracture management.

Ans: The scaphoid bone has a retrograde blood supply, making it highly susceptible to avascular necrosis (AVN) and nonunion following fractures. Understanding its vascular anatomy is crucial in guiding diagnosis, treatment, and prognosis. The blood supply of the scaphoid is precarious.
- *Primary blood supply*: Dorsal branch of the radial artery (enters via the dorsal ridge).
  - Supplies 70–80% of the bone, including the proximal pole.
- *Secondary supply*: Volar branches (less significant).
- *Vulnerable zones*:
  - *Proximal pole* (relies on distal-to-proximal flow) → High AVN risk. *AVN risk:* 30–40% (due to disrupted retrograde flow).
  - *Waist fractures* (most common) → Moderate AVN risk. *Nonunion risk:* 10–15% if untreated.
  - *Distal fractures* → Good healing (direct blood supply).

Treatment Strategies Based on Vascular Risk
- Nondisplaced fractures
  - *Distal fractures:* Short-arm thumb spica cast (6 weeks).
  - *Waist fractures:* Long-arm cast (4–6 weeks) → Short-arm cast (until healing).
  - *Proximal fractures:* Prolonged immobilization (12+ weeks) or early surgical fixation due to AVN risk.
- Displaced fractures (> 1 mm) or high-risk cases
  - *ORIF (Open Reduction Internal Fixation) with a headless compression screw (e.g., Herbert screw).*
    - Preferred for proximal pole fractures (reduces AVN risk).
    - Early fixation improves healing in athletes/workers.
- Delayed presentation/nonunion
  - Bone grafting (vascularized vs. nonvascularized) + fixation.
    - Vascularized grafts (e.g., 1, 2 ICSRA graft) for AVN cases.

55. Explain carpal instability and its types, clinical features, and radiological assessment.

Ans: *Types:*
- *Dissociative carpal instability (CID):* It is a major dysfunction between bones of the same carpal row (fracture/ligament disruption). There is loss of linkage *between individual carpal bones*. It usually affects the *smaller ligaments* such as scapholunate and lunotriquetral that are difficult to repair. It can be subclassified into:
  - *Proximal (scapholunate and lunotriquetral dissociations):* It encompasses the terms DISI (scapholunate dissociation) and volar intercalated segmental instability (VISI) (lunotriquetral dissociation).
  - Distal (capitate-hamate axial disruptions).
- *Nondissociative carpal instability (CIND):* It is between carpal "rows", bones, and intercarpal relation and function is maintained. It usually affects the longer ligament such as triquetral capitate, radiolunate, and radiocapitate. It is also subclassified into:
  - Radiocarpal with rupture of several radiocarpal ligaments resulting in an ulnar translation of the carpus (often DISI).
  - Midcarpal with rupture of the triquetral-hamate capitate ligament complex (VISI).
  - Ulnar translocation.
- *Complex carpal instability (CIC):* It occurs when CID and CIND are found together. Perilunate dislocations are a good example that involves radiocarpal (radiolunate, radiocapitate ligaments) and intercarpal levels (scapholunate, lunotriquetral) that later evolve into chronic scapholunate and lunotriquetral dissociation (CID patterns) and also an ulnar translation of the lunate (CIND pattern). Progressive perilunate instability passes through the following stages:
  - *Stage I:* Scapholunate instability
  - *Stage II:* Capitate dislocation
  - *Stage III:* Triquetral dislocation
  - *Stage IV:* Lunate dislocation.
- *Adaptive carpal instability (CIA):* It occurs when carpal instability originates proximal or distal to the wrist and not located within the wrist (carpal bones individually or between rows). This instability arises secondary to adaptation of extrinsic pathology (like a malunited distal radius fracture).

Clinical features: The clinical features of different types of carpal instabilities are discrete and cannot be generalized. Most, however, present with pain in wrist in various parts of the joint and on specific activities that trigger the abnormal mechanics in particular pattern. The patient with scapholunate or lunotriquetral instability usually presents with pain and weakness of the wrist. This is commonly associated with clunking during movement or gripping actions but such clunks may be normal also. Most instabilities arise from trauma, so a deep enquiry is legible. There is swelling and tenderness over scapholunate joint. Chronic disruption of the S-L joint may progress to SLAC (scapholunate advanced collapse) wrist. The arthritis and degeneration arise due to abnormal distribution of the forces across the carpal bones while load bearing and movements. Arthritis progresses from the high-stress region of radioscaphoid joint to gradually involve the entire carpus, and finally a collapse of the carpal bones, radiologically, is characterized by proximal migration of capitate (reduced carpal height ratio). Patients with lunotriquetral dissociation have pain on ulnar aspect with pronation and ulnar deviation. The lunotriquetral ballottement test (Shuck test) is positive. Pain is also produced with shear forces across the lunotriquetral joint as in Kleinman's shear test.

On examination, there may be generalized tenderness over the carpus from synovitis or more localized tenderness, for example at the scapholunate junction or over the scaphoid itself. Grip strength is reduced.

Provocative tests *are useful.*

Watson's test for scapholunate incompetence: Thumb pressure is applied to the volar aspect of the wrist over the distal pole of the scaphoid (this restores the alignment of the volar-tilted scaphoid). Palpable clunk appears when the wrist is brought from ulnar deviation into radial deviation while pressure is applied to the palmar aspect of the scaphoid tubercle.

Lunotriquetral ballottement (Shuck test): It grasps the lunate between the thumb and index finger of one hand while applying alternative dorsal and palmar loads across the triquetrum with the thumb and index of the other hand-eliciting pain, crepitus, or laxity at lunotriquetral joint.

Kleinman's shear test: This test stabilizes the radiolunate joint with the forearm in neutral rotation, now with the contralateral hand load, the triquetrum in the anteroposterior plane—producing shear across the lunotriquetral joint.

Pivot shift test: The examiner grasps the patient's forearm with one hand and the patient's hand with the other; he then compresses the wrist axially while moving it from abduction to adduction. A painful "clunk" suggests midcarpal instability.

Radiological assessment:

- In scaphoid fractures, a fracture line or nonunion site is appreciable on anteroposterior X-ray. In an anteroposterior "clenched fist view", the scaphoid is seen to flex and a scapholunate gap becomes more apparent.
- In scapho-lunate (S-L) disruption, there may be widening of the scapholunate interval (*the Terry-Thomas sign*) **(Fig. 4A.10.1)**
- If the scaphoid is flexed, it will look foreshortened and the tubercle may appear as a dense "ring" in the bone—signet ring sign is more prominent with the wrist adducted and abducted.

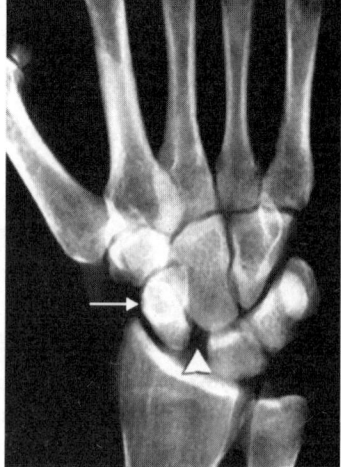

Fig. 4A.10.1: Appearance of signet ring (arrow) and Terry–Thomas sign (pointer).

- In SNAC wrist, there is radiocarpal arthrosis that advances to capitolunate joint and midcarpal joints in late stages with proximal migration of capitate–carpal collapse.
- A true lateral view is examined to assess the relative alignment of the distal radius, the lunate, capitate, and scaphoid. In the DISI deformity, the capitate axis is shifted dorsally but it flexes relative to the lunate, the lunate tilts backward and the scaphoid flexes; the scapholunate angle is greater than 70° **(Fig. 4A.10.2)**.
- In a VISI deformity, the lunate is flexed forwards and the scapholunate angle is less than 30°; the capitate tilts dorsally.
- Ulnar translocation of carpus is commonly seen in S-L instability.
- Destruction of Gilula's lines is seen in CIC.
- Malunion of distal radius fracture with loss of radial height and dorsal tilt is evident in CIND.

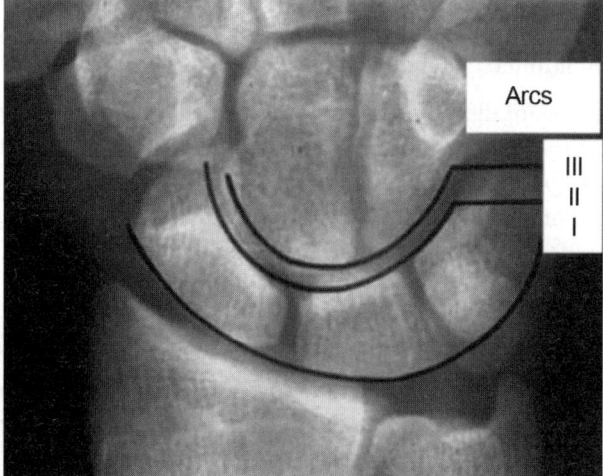

Fig. 4A.10.2: The appearance of Gilula's lines in normal carpus.

56. What is midcarpal instability?

Ans: We know from wrist biomechanics that under the loaded conditions of wrist:
- The triquetrum is pulled into extension by the palmar triquetrum-hamate ligaments.
- There is opposing movement of scaphoid to counter this, which goes into flexion.

This results in a twisted force transmitted across the lunate (scaphoid flexion and triquetrum extension) that remains neutral. With torn palmar triquetrum-hamate ligaments (or its laxity), the lunate is forced by the scaphoid into palmar flexion that drags triquetrum along, resulting in a nondissociative VISI deformity of the proximal carpal row. This VISI relationship is maintained throughout the movements of the wrist. In full ulnar deviation, the scaphoid extends and the triquetrum-hamate joint is also fully engaged that throws the proximal carpal row to suddenly extend, producing a quite typical snap (that can be tested clinically—positive ballottement test). This is most commonly referred to "VISI pattern" in loose terms when unspecified.

Treatment: Soft tissue reconstructions can correct this problem. Procedures described are palmar capsulorrhaphy or tenodesis but most have significant complications. So, commonly partial or total *fusion of the midcarpal joint* is done when causing symptoms are poorly controlled by conservative measures. For advanced cases with pancarpal arthritis, wrist fusion is best.

4A.11 DISORDERS OF HAND (Q57–66)

57. Discuss various functions of hand. How will you attain key pinch in quadriplegic with no useful power?

Ans: *Functions:*
- *Subjective sensory perception of the surrounding environment:* The tactile function is specialized for object identification, calibration, and distinction. Apart from the visual, auditory, taste, and smell such intricacy is not provided by any other part of body. Hand excels one step further that these functions can be done anywhere in space by virtue of mobility of upper limb and ability to place the hand anywhere (within limits) and does not require the object to be introduced to body.
- *Objective sensory contact.*
- *Communication with others by direction and demonstration:* Gestures are a very important part of communication and most of the sentences can be completed or emphasized by particular gestures that are common to community. It is amazing to see that dumb/mute persons are able to communicate almost as easily like others just by way of gestures.
- *Mechanical grips:* Gripping is a very important function of hand and used most often in day-to-day activities. The following are the common grips of hand. The grips may be used for power function or the advanced precision function. Thumb is an essential component for both types of grips.
    - *Power grip:* Most powerful grip (the fingers flex in one direction to hold the object while the thumb goes around in the opposite direction to provide the counterforce). This keeps the object supported in the palm and fingers. The strength of power grip is proportional to the range of flexion in the interphalangeal (IP) and metacarpophalangeal (MCP) joints, so that any cause of IP joint stiffness weakens the power grip. The final torque in grasping objects comes from hand intrinsics and the loss of this transverse arch movement is noted in ulnar nerve palsy. The little finger is mechanically very important in power grip, as it adds to the breadth of the palm and increases strength of power grip. Hence, amputation of little finger should not be lightly advised. The power grip is also aided by the typical distribution of fat and creases in the palm.

    The power grip is of three types:
    1. *Cylindrical grip:* All fingers are flexed around the object, which is usually at a right angle to forearm. The thumb overlaps the fingers wrapping the object around.
    2. *Spherical grip:* All of the fingers and the thumb are adducted around an object, and unlike the cylindrical grip, the fingers are more spread apart. The palm of the hand is often not involved. This is further classified into:
        - Spherical
        - Box
        - Lateral
        - Cylindrical
        - Flipped cylindrical types.

3. *Hook grip (briefcase grip):* It involves the second through fifth fingers flexed around an object in a hook-like manner. The MCP joints are extended, and the proximal interphalangeal (PIP) and distal interphalangeal (DIP) joints are in some degree of flexion. The thumb is usually not involved.

- *Precision grips:* These tend to hold the object between the tips of the fingers and thumb, especially when the objects are small or fragile where no palm support is needed or proximal joints are not moving. They involve actions of both extrinsics and intrinsics. Thumb remains abducted in all. The grip is responsible for most of the fine movements and accuracy of hand. These are of four types:
    1. *Pinch grip:* MCP and PIP of the fingers are flexed, thumb is abducted and the distal joints of both are extended bringing the pad of the finger and thumb together. If both the index and middle fingers are used then it is called "chuck pinch" (three jaw chuck). The pinch grip depends on the intrinsic muscles for posturing, stability, and strength. Weak or lost function of first dorsal interosseous weakens the radial abduction of the index against the thumb, while the loss of action of adductor pollicis breaks the longitudinal arch of the thumb that collapses under pinch grip stresses.
    2. *Lateral prehension:* Pad of the extended thumb presses an object against the radial side of the index finger as in holding the car key—"key grip" or in holding straps of objects. Most importantly, pen is held in this fashion!
    3. *Side-to-side grip:* It requires adduction of two fingers, usually the index and middle fingers. It is a weak grip and does not permit much precision.
    4. *Lumbrical grip:* MCP and PIP joints are flexed and the DIP joint extended the thumb and opposed the fingers holding and object horizontal. The lumbricals flex the MCPs while extending the IP joints.

Attain key pinch in a quadriplegic with no useful power: Personally, I feel there should be some utilizable motor to power pinch grip else I am unaware of any other method except futuristic approach of amputation and prosthetic fitting that can perform pinch on cerebral circuitry command! Otherwise, the motor restoration in quadriplegic is by one of the following methods:
- Brachioradialis (BR) to flexor pollicis longus transfer
- *Möberg key pinch procedure—tenodesis effect:* This can be possibly used as a very crude method to produce pinch, if proximal (elbow and wrist extension) restoration is possible. The BR is transferred to the extensor carpi radialis brevis (ECRB) to restore wrist extension, and a passive key pinch is obtained by tenodesis of the flexor pollicis longus (FPL), extensor pollicis longus (EPL), and abductor pollicis longus (APL) to the distal radius. Still, you need some motor!

58. Describe anatomy of palmar deep fascia.
Ans: The volar deep fascia of wrist and hand is specialized to form:
- The flexor retinaculum at the wrist
- The palmar aponeurosis in the palm
- The fibrous flexor sheaths in the fingers

All three form a continuous structure which holds the tendons in position and thus increase the efficiency of the grip

Flexor retinaculum at wrist:
Flexor (Latin to hold back) retinaculum is a strong fibrous band which bridges the anterior concavity of the carpus and converts it into a tunnel, the carpal tunnel.

Attachments
Medial:
- The pisiform bone
- To the hook of the hamate

Lateral:
- The tubercle of the scaphoid
- The crest of the trapezium

On either side, the retinaculum has a slip:
- The lateral deep slip is attached to the medial lip of the groove on the trapezium which is thus converted into a tunnel for the tendon of the flexor carpi radialis.

- The medial superficial slip (volar carpal ligament) is attached to the pisiform bone. The ulnar vessels and nerves pass deep to this slip.

Relations:
The structures passing superficial to the flexor retinaculum are:
- The palmar cutaneous branch of the median nerve
- The tendon of the palmaris longus
- The palmar cutaneous branch of the ulnar nerve
- The ulnar vessels
- The ulnar nerve
- The thenar and hypothenar muscles that arise from the retinaculum itself

The structures passing deep to the flexor retinaculum are:
- The median nerve
- Four tendons of the flexor digitorum superficialis
- Four tendons of the flexor digitorum profundus
- The tendon of the flexor pollicis longus
- The ulnar bursa
- The radial bursa
- The tendon of the flexor carpi radialis lies between the retinaculum and its deep slip, in the groove on the trapezium.

Palmar aponeurosis:
This term is often used for the entire deep fascia of the palm. However, it is better to restrict this term to the central part of the deep fascia of the palm which covers the superficial palmar arch, the long flexor tendons, the terminal part of the median nerve, and the superficial branch of the ulnar nerve.

Features:
Palmar aponeurosis is triangular in shape. The apex is proximal that blends with the flexor retinaculum and is continuous with the tendon of the palmaris longus. The base is directed distally. It divides into superficial and deep strata, superficial is attached to dermis. Deep strata divide into four slips opposite the heads of the metacarpals of the medial four digits. Each slip divides into two parts which are continuous with the fibrous flexor sheaths. Extensions pass to the deep transverse metacarpal ligament, the capsule of the metacarpophalangeal joints and the sides of the base of the proximal phalanx. The digital vessels and nerves, and the tendons of the lumbricals emerge through the intervals between the slips. From the lateral and medial margins of the palmar aponeurosis, the lateral and medial palmar septa pass backward and divide the palm into compartments.

Functions:
Palmar aponeurosis fixes the skin of the palm and thus improves the grip. It also protects the underlying tendons, vessels, and nerves.

Fibrous flexor sheaths of the fingers:
The fibrous flexor sheaths are made up of the deep fascia of the fingers. The fascia is thick and arched. It is attached to the sides of the phalanges and across the base of the distal phalanx. Proximally, it is continuous with a slip of the palmar aponeurosis. In this way, a blind osseofascial tunnel is formed which contains the long flexor tendons enclosed in the digital synovial sheath. The fibrous sheath is thick opposite the phalanges and thin opposite the joints to permit flexion. The sheath holds the tendons in position during flexion of the digits.

59. Define trigger finger. What are the causes? Describe the clinical features and surgical management of trigger thumb.

Ans: Trigger digits occur due to stenosing tenosynovitis primarily of A1 pulley resulting from various pathologies [including congenital causing hypertrophy of A1 pulley (commonly) or tendon thickening or both; however in congenital form, the tendon thickening is the primary pathology and not the pulley thickening]. The flexor tendon gets irritated as it slides through the hypertrophic tendon sheath constricting the tunnel causing progressive tenosynovitis and further thickening of the sheath resulting in a vicious cycle of tunnel narrowing. With continued irritation, the tendon may thicken and nodules form within it, making its passage through the tunnel more difficult (**Fig. 4A.11.1**). The patient develops painful hand grasp or the finger/thumb triggers during finger flexion or extension movements (opening of the finger with sudden jerk).

Causes:
- Diabetes
- Rheumatoid arthritis
- Amyloidosis
- Workers doing repetitive hand job.

Other causes:
- Tendon or tendon sheath tumor
- Tight Camper's chiasm that causes flexor digitorum profundus (FDP) entrapment and trigger
- Sesamoid bone abnormalities
- Floating bodies in the MCP area
- Intrinsic tendon involvement due to metacarpal head abnormalities
- Flexor digitorum profundus tendon thickening that causes trigger at the A3 pulley.

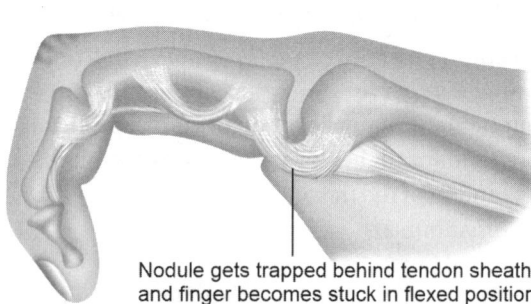

Fig. 4A.11.1: Trigger finger.

Clinical features: Trigger fingers are more common in women than men. They occur most frequently in people who are between the ages of 40 years and 60 years of age. Thumb is the most commonly involved digit followed by fourth (ring), third (middle), and fifth (pinky) finger, respectively. Symptoms of trigger finger are not associated with trauma although they may follow a period of heavy hand use. The symptoms commonly include:
- Pain on finger movements
- A tender nodule on volar aspect of the palm near the A1 pulley region often proximal to it
- Swelling
- Catching or popping sensation in finger or thumb, especially on extension stiffness and catching tend to be worse after inactivity, such as when the patient wakes up in the morning. Your fingers will often loosen up as you move them.
- *Pain in proximal interphalangeal (PIP) region:* The exact mechanism is unknown but may be related to excess stress put on the joint due to forceful pulling of the finger of snapping injury to the collateral ligaments. The other reason might be synovitis extending to the region and lastly may be related to referred pain.

Without treatment, the tendon meets one of the two fates:
1. *Incarceration of the tendon and adhesions in the region:* This prevents finger straightening and commonly the finger is fixed in mid-flexion.
2. The tendon breaks free and the finger fails to flex. There is a sensation of "dislocating" finger and complete weakness.

Surgical management: The definite indications of surgical treatment are—
- Incarcerated tendon
- Failed multiple injections.

Broken tendon is also a definitive indication for surgical treatment, but management is done on the lines of tendon reconstruction rather than typically for the trigger finger. Long-standing cases with active disease are a relative indication for surgical release, as conservative treatment often gives incomplete relief. The goal of surgery is to widen the opening of the tunnel, so that the tendon can slide through it more easily. A transverse skin incision is preferred for surgical release of the tendon and the A1 pulley is partially released in the distal half, else bowstringing of the tendon would occur. The procedure can be also done on out-patient basis under local anesthesia. I would prefer needle percutaneous release for most stage 1 and 2 cases except recurrent cases and cases failed with multiple injections. Various authors have described the percutaneous procedure using custom-designed tenotome, a scalpel and a hook, or an extra-thin scalpel and a hypodermic needle. We prefer using a blood transfusion set needle, as adequate force can be transmitted to cut the thickening in the pulley. Open release is also done for long-standing cases (>4–6 months of symptoms) and later stages.

No attempt is made to repair the released sheath, as the new sheath should be loose enough for tendon to glide easily. Local anesthesia is advantageous as adequacy of the release can be judged simultaneously by making the patient move finger through full flexion and extension. In children, the A2 pulley or one of the limbs of FDS tendon may need to be simultaneously released.

60. Infantile trigger thumb.

Ans: Trigger thumb is actually an acquired (as opposed to congenital) abnormality of the FPL tendon and its sheath at the A1 pulley. This is a relatively common condition having an estimated incidence of 3 infants per 1,000 live births that are acquired in first 2 years of life. There is a palpable mass, a nodule called Notta nodule that represents the FPL constriction at the A1 pulley.

The condition is caused by a size mismatch or a differential growth of the tendon and its pulley leading to progressive constriction. There is no inflammatory component involved (as opposed to adult form). The condition has been found to spontaneously resolve by 9 months of age in 30–50% of patients, but the chances of such favorable outcome diminish as the child grows older (< 10% after 1 year). It occurs sporadically and as many as 30% of patients have bilateral involvement.

Clinical Examination:
It reveals a palpable nodule of the FPL tendon at A1 pulley with either triggering (less common) or a fixed flexion contracture (more common) of the interphalangeal joint. Long-standing trigger presents as compensatory hyperextension at MCP joint in an effort to bring the thumb out of palm.

Treatment:
Surgical release of the A1 pulley is the treatment of choice and is almost always successful. It is recommended for patients who are older than 1 year and fail to resolve spontaneously or those presenting after 1 year of age with fixed PIP. Care should be taken to preserve neurovascular bundle and the oblique pulley (and hence avoid bowstringing). Transverse incision is much more cosmetic. Recurrence is extremely rare.

61. Discuss the clinical features, diagnosis, and treatment of de Quervain's tenovaginitis.

Ans:

Clinical features: Middle-aged patients between 40 and 60 years are commonly affected and the disease is much more common in females than males. Classic triad consists of tenderness over the radial styloid, swelling over the first extensor compartment, and a positive Finkelstein's test. Persistent pain 1–2 cm proximal to radial styloid process occurs during certain movements. The pain is present often for few weeks to months and at times there is loss of function. Crepitus or squeaking with movements of involved tendons (wet leather sign) may be palpable. Swelling is found in 85% of cases. Finkelstein's sign is pathognomonic. It consists of ulnar deviating the partially flexed wrist, with thumb in opposition eliciting severe pain. Locking or triggering is uncommon but when present is a definitive indication of surgical release.

Diagnosis:
- Most of the bony differentials should be ruled out by plain radiographs of the wrist and hand.
- *Ultrasonography:* It is important for diagnosis if clinically dubious. It can verify that there is a reduction in tendon gliding and an increase in the abductor pollicis longus (APL) or the EPB tendon sheath's thickness. Now this is considered a reliable test for diagnosis.

Treatment:
Medical treatment: Local ointments, plaster splint, physiotherapy, heat, and hydrotherapy are the mainstay of treatment along with the most useful drug—nonsteroidal anti-inflammatory drugs (NSAIDs). Injection of local steroids may give satisfactory results if the noninterventional management is not effective. It should be realized that most of the patients have anatomical variation with respect to first dorsal extensor compartment (see hand and wrist anatomy) so injecting all the stenotic canals is imperative else the relief will be partial or incomplete. Although commonly insoluble preparations of the steroid are used; however, local complications such as depigmentation, subcutaneous atrophy, and adipose necrosis are much more common. Preparations of dexamethasone are possibly soberer. Also only the tendon sheath should be infiltrated rather than injecting the steroid preparation intra-articularly.

Surgical treatment: This is indicated for recurrent disease or resistant one that does not respond to conservative management. Other definitive indication is extensor tendon triggering. Surgical release through a radial longitudinal or transverse incision aims at decompression of the twin tendons by the excision of the thickened sheath. Again the highly varying anatomy should be properly recognized and the multiple cutaneous branches of the radial nerve lying at the spot should be all protected.

62. What is felon? Discuss its preferred management and its difference from paronychia.

Ans: A deep space abscess of the distal pulp of finger or thumb is termed as felon. It usually is caused by bacterial infection, but herpes virus (called herpetic whitlow) and, more rarely, fungi also can cause felons **(Fig. 4A.11.2)**. The distal pulp space is walled off by fibrous septa at the level of the distal crease. These form small compartments separated by vertical 15–20 fibrous septa extending from skin to periosteum, filled with connective tissue and fat globules. If unchecked, the infection can progress to produce a sinus, skin sloughing, or osteomyelitis and further to septic arthritis of the DIP joint or pyogenic tenosynovitis.

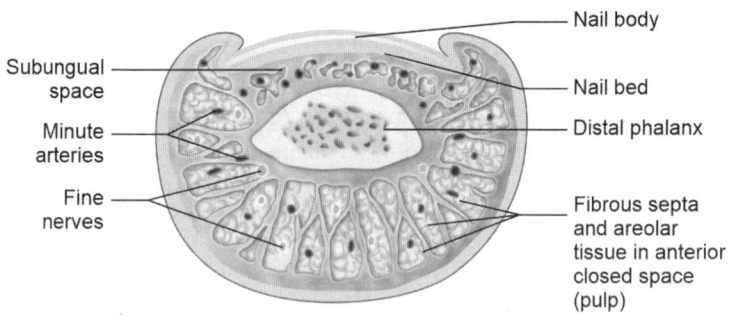

Fig. 4A.11.2: Felon.

Diagnosis: It is usually evident clinically. Patient has history of injury in the area. Initially, it presents with cellulitis and severe throbbing pain. Tenderness, redness, firmness, and enlargement of the fingertip are all signs of a felon containing tense abscess and are warning signs indicating the need of surgical evacuation. If there is small bubble-like cyst on the skin, called vesicles, and repeated episodes, it is a herpetic whitlow. Radiographs should be obtained for evaluating osteomyelitis (in order to prognosticate the patient).

Treatment: The initial treatment (<24 hours) is by antibiotics and rest. Give appropriate tetanus prophylaxis. If the symptoms are present for more than 48 hours, incision and evacuation of pus is the treatment of choice. Presence of throbbing pain is an indication of abscess formation. Pus is evacuated by "a unilateral longitudinal incision" (usually preferred but may have higher chances of ischemia and anesthesia by injuring one or both neurovascular bundles) over the most tender spot on the pulp or ideally performed on the noncontact surface of the involved digit. This includes the ulnar sides of the index and long fingers and the radial sides of the ring finger, small finger, and thumb. Fish-mouth incision should be avoided (causes unstable painful fingertip). "A longitudinal central midline incision" is advocated to avoid skin slough, digital nerve injury, or creation of an unstable fat pad. This incision is especially useful in the presence of a sinus track that can be incorporated within the incision. In any case, the following precautions are imperative:

- The incision should not cross the DIP joint to prevent formation of a flexion contracture at the DIP flexion crease.
- Probing is not carried out proximally to avoid extension of infection into the flexor tendon sheath.

Wick is then placed to prevent premature closure of the incision and recurrence of abscess. Obtain cultures from the evacuated pus. Empiric antibiotic coverage with a first generation cephalosporin or antistaphylococcal penicillin usually is adequate treatment for an uncomplicated felon. This should be later changed to culture and sensitivity patterns. Especially one should look for methicillin-resistant *Staphylococcus aureus* (MRSA) or gram-negative organisms.

Paronychia versus Felon
- A paronychia is an infection of eponychial fold (around the edge of nail plate), while a felon is an infection of the fingertip pulp.
- Felon usually results from penetrating injury or uncommonly through rupture of paronychia into pulp space, while paronychia results from violation of the seal between the nail plate and nail fold as in hangnails, manicure, or nail-biting habit.
- There is classical presentation of fluctuation and local purulence at the nail margin that rapidly progresses to subungual abscess and nail-bed destruction, if untreated in paronychia, while felon presents with tense swelling in finger pulp space over palmar aspect.

63. Describe the potential spaces of hand. Discuss clinical features and management of deep space infection of hand or describe the pathoanatomy of bursae of hand. Discuss etiology, clinical features, and management of acute infections of those bursae.

Ans: Potential spaces of hand:
- Dorsal subaponeurotic space is located deep to the extensor tendons and dorsal to the metacarpals.
- *Web space:* There are three interdigital web spaces containing loose fat and communicate proximally along the lumbrical canals with the middle palmar space.
- *Midpalmar space:* This space is bounded ventrally by flexor tendons and lumbricals and dorsally by volar fascia investing the second and third volar interossei and the third and fourth metacarpals.
- *Thenar space:* The thenar space is bound ventrally by the palmar fascia and dorsally by the transverse head of adductor pollicis.
- *Hypothenar space:* It contains the hypothenar muscles and is enclosed by their investing fascia.
- *Dorsal adductor space:* It is a potential space located dorsal to the adductor pollicis and palmar to the first dorsal interosseous.

Etiology of deep space infections: These are either primary infections from direct inoculation or secondary extending from the adjacent anatomical structures. The diagnosis is clinical and based on an abscess forming at the distal edge of the palm separating the adjacent fingers. The attachment of the palmar fascia to the skin results to the spread of the pus into the dorsal subcutaneous space with the typical picture of a collar-button abscess in web space infections.

Clinical features:
- In *a midpalmar space* infection, the concavity of the palm is usually lost. There is exquisite tenderness over the infected area, which is usually pallid and sometimes red. Fingers are held rigidly flexed, with decreasing rigidity from the little to the index finger. However, finger rigidity in case of midpalmar infections is less severe than the rigidity of septic tenosynovitis. There is usually a pitting edema in the remaining palm (over the thenar) and at the dorsum of the hand, while in the case of pus extension along the lumbrical channel, swelling of the web space is also observed. The midpalmar space is drained and debrided through a palmar incision (transverse, longitudinal, or along one of the lumbrical channels) taking care to avoid injury of the neurovascular bundle or contamination of the surrounding tissues (the ulnar bursa in particular).
- In *thenar compartment* and *thenar space* infections, a painful swelling of the thenar eminence is observed. The concavity of the palm is lost and often soft edema on the dorsum of the hand is present. The 1st metacarpal and the thumb are abducted and distal phalanx flexion becomes more marked. In extensive infections, a double incision over the volar and dorsal side is necessary for drainage of the infected spaces/compartments.
- In *hypothenar compartment* and *space* infections, the abscess is more localized. There is often limited swelling in the palm but always painful swelling of the hypothenar eminence. The incision is located over the hypothenar with care to avoid injury to the neurovascular bundle.
- In *subaponeurotic space* infections, the dorsal edema is more soft and the ischemia of the skin is less severe than in cases of subcutaneous pus accumulation. Attempts of finger extension may be limited by pain. The dorsal incisions for the drainage of the subaponeurotic space are longitudinal, over the 2nd and between 4th and 5th metacarpals.

Treatment of deep space infections: Surgical treatment includes drainage of the often multiloculated abscess, through a palmar and/or a dorsal incision. The incision should never cross the edge of the web to avoid the formation of dysfunctional scars.

Pathoanatomy of bursae:
- The little finger flexor sheath of FDP tendon (and on occasion, the ring, long, and index fingers) communicates with the ulnar bursa. The ulnar bursa extends proximal to the wrist level thus infections in these spaces may well spread to wrist proximally.

- The flexor sheath of the *flexor pollicis longus* (FPL) (to thumb) communicates with the radial bursa that also extends proximal to the wrist level.
- The flexor sheaths of ring and middle finger are usually isolated in most patients and do not communicate with other spaces.
- The radial and ulnar bursae communicate with each other at the level of the transverse carpal ligament through space of Parona (space between the pronator quadratus and the FDP tendons). Infection in any one of them may communicate to the other side when profuse and produce a "horseshoe abscess" (80% patients).

Etiology: Penetrating injury is the mode of injury leading to deposition of skin flora and subsequent disease.

Clinical features: Kanavel's four cardinal signs are quite characteristics to diagnose—
- Semiflexed posture of involved finger in rest.
- Symmetric enlargement of the whole finger (sausage digit).
- Excessive tenderness limited to the course of the sheath.
- Excruciating pain in extending the finger passively (the most dependable sign).

It causes a cylindrical swelling of the finger, which is kept semiflexed. Infection of the ulnar bursa causes edema of the whole hand with fullness above the flexor retinaculum. Infection of the radial bursa causes pain, swelling, and tenderness along the bursa. When the two bursae communicate through space of Parona, there forms horseshoe abscess. The gliding mechanism of the tendon can be damaged or ischemic necrosis of the tendon may take place. If not treated early, it may lead to protracted tendon sheath infection or osteomyelitis. This may eventually lead to loss of finger and hand function. Depending on the duration of infection and tissue changes, the pyogenic flexor tenosynovitis has been classified into three stages:
1. *Stage 1:* Increased fluid in sheath mainly serous exudate.
2. *Stage 2:* Cloudy/purulent fluid, synovium may be granulomatous.
3. *Stage 3:* Septic necrosis of the tendon, pulleys, or sheath.

Treatment: Treatment should be prompt and effective. The infection is treated conservatively with antibiotics, if detected within first 24 hours. If this causes relief of pain, conservative treatment is continued, else surgery is the treatment of choice.

Surgery: If signs and symptoms are not abating, decision to surgically drain the infection is taken. For stages 1 and 2, the incision is made classically through midlateral crease in case of index and little fingers, where the entire sheath can be laid open. Pus is expressed from terminal part to over the MCP joint. In case of middle or ring finger volar, a zigzag incision (Brunner's) or a combination of midlateral incision in finger and a transverse incision in palm over the proximal end of the flexor tendon sheath can be made. The fibrous flexor sheath should not be completely incised along its whole length, but important pulleys should be left intact particularly A2 and A4 pulleys. After a thorough decompression, drain is put for 24 hours; hand is splinted, elevated, and treated by systemic antibiotics.

A two-incision approach is preferred (for middle and ring fingers) in which the A1 pulley is approached proximally through a preferred transverse incision at the level of the metacarpal head. After entering the sheath, pus and debris are aspirated and a small infant feeding tube or 16-gauge suction catheter is passed up the sheath. Another palmar incision is made transversely distal to the A4 pulley in the finger and the sheath is irrigated using saline. We commonly use last wash with antibiotic before withdrawing the catheter back. Another catheter is then inserted and sutured to act as drain for next 24 hours. The radial and ulnar bursae are exposed through open technique. Horseshoe abscess is drained through both radial and ulnar bursae. For stage 3, the treatment is more extensive with extensive debridement and patient should be counseled in advance for possible need of amputation, the decision of which is taken by two consultants after independent evaluation.

64. Describe pathological anatomy of bursae of hand. Discuss the etiology, clinical features, and management of acute infection in those bursae.

Ans: Kindly see Answer to Question 63 above.

65. A. What is Kanavel's sign?
    B. Discuss management of suppurative flexor tenosynovitis of hand.

Ans: Kindly see Answer to Question 63 above.

66. Briefly describe management of human bites on hand.

Ans: Treatment is done through cleaning with a topical antiseptic agent in running water. Broad-spectrum antibiotic coverage should include a beta-lactam antibiotic (usually a cephalosporin) with beta-lactamase inhibitor along with fluoroquinolone. If infection of the wound has occurred surgical excision of the wound, thorough irrigation, appropriate antibiotics and the wound is left open. When the infection has subsided, the wound is then closed. The surgical debridement as a primary measure is used for pyogenic tenosynovitis and osteomyelitis.

Human bites are classified into four types:
1. Self-inflicted
2. Traumatic amputations
3. Full-thickness bite wounds to the hand or digits
4. Clenched-fist (e.g., blow to the mouth producing a knuckle-tooth wound) injuries.

The bacterial flora is same as described for animal bites while there is predominance of *Streptococcus* and *Staphylococcus* species and *Eikenella corrodens*. The latter is found commonly in the dental scrapings.

Clenched fist injuries (as may occur during street fights) are interesting as the penetrating tooth track is effectively sealed with digital extension, creating a closed-space environment. The potential spaces that may be entered are the dorsal subcutaneous space between the skin and extensor mechanism, the subtendinous space between the extensor mechanism and joint capsule and the joint space itself but importantly the site of entry of all changes with the position of hand during examination with fingers extended. Bites seen within 24 hours should be treated with cleansing and local therapy, especially if there is no evidence of joint or tenosynovium penetration. Oral antibiotics should be added commonly the combination of amoxicillin and clavulanic acid. Close follow-up with review at 12–24 hours should be done for spreading infection. Surgical debridement is done primarily for obvious infection (presenting late) or joint/tendon space penetration as the coverage with antibiotics is not sufficient at these places.

4A.12 NERVE INJURIES, TENDON TRANSFER, AND CARPAL TUNNEL SYNDROME (Q67–101)

67. Discuss Sunderland classification of nerve injuries.

Ans: Sunderland classification of nerve injuries is described in **Table 4A.12.1**.

TABLE 4A.12.1: Sunderland's classification of nerve injuries.

Cohen/Seddon types	Sunderland grades	Description
Neurapraxia	1	Local conduction block, variable myelin damage, no axonal discontinuity
Axonotmesis	2	Loss of axonal continuity, endoneurium intact, no conduction
	3	Loss of axonal and endoneurial continuity, perineurium intact, no conduction
	4	Loss of axonal, endoneurial and perineurial continuity, epineurium intact, no conduction
Neurotmesis	5	Epineurium also damaged—neural discontinuity with separation of ends, no conduction
	6	Mixed nerve damage along the nerve trunk, all types of nerve injuries seen 1–5, recovery is hence variable with nearly no recovery in combined types 4 and 5

68. Explain methods of nerve repair and methods of closing gaps between nerve ends.

Ans: The methods of nerve repair depending on time duration from injury are classified into:
1. *Primary repair:* Within hours it is not always possible and though considered ideal may actually be suboptimal in the absence of skilled repair done often by junior surgeons. Also, there is a phenomenon of "conditioning effect" that may improve the chances of a delayed primary repair.
2. *Delayed primary:* Within 5–7 days. This is the common scenario, where the repair is undertaken as an elective procedure with all available tools and possibilities so is the clinically preferred scenario. It also takes the advantage of conditioning effect on nerves following an injury. "Conditioning effect" is based on the premises that a "primed" neuron will regenerate faster at its peak metabolic activity due to "conditioning effect". Conditioning effect presupposes that axons regenerate quickly, if they have been damaged previously.
3. *Secondary:* Any repair more than 7 days. This may be done in grossly contaminated wounds, delayed referrals, or in polytrauma patients.

Methods of nerve repair, depending on type of tissue at which repair is being done, can be divided into:
- *Epineural:* This is the most common technique of nerve repair. A series of simple interrupted sutures are placed through the epineurium under low-power magnification. The epineurium is grasped and tensed with the Jeweler's forceps. Placement of sutures should be approximately 0.5–1.0 mm from edge. The suture material (3-0–5-0 prolene often) is placed from the surface of the nerve to emerge just subepineurially. It is then brought out to the free edge and the process continued in the opposing nerve stump to begin subepineurially and emerge on the surface. This completes one simple interrupted suture. The number of sutures required for adequate alignment of the stumps varies depending upon the diameter of the nerve. Optimal alignment is guided by epineural vessels. Smallest number of sutures possible is placed, so that the inflammatory reaction is minimized. However, adequate alignment is paramount for the success of the surgical procedure. Often four equidistant sutures as suggested by Swaim provide sufficient strength for healing.
- *Perineurorrhaphy:* This means the suturing is done through the perineurium. There is improved nerve alignment, but slightly increased risk of scarring.
    - *Epiperineurorrhaphy:* The needle is passed through both the epineurium and perineurium. Strong coaptation and better alignment (preferred).
    - *Interneural neurorrhaphy:* This is an alternative to epineural neurorrhaphy. It involves use of a double-armed suture material. Needle is centrally inserted into one of the two nerve stumps and directed down the longitudinal axis, so that it emerges 180° from its counterpart. The suture is hence placed centrally increasing the chances of proper alignment with minimal injury. Each end of the nerve is sutured to a button through which slip sutures are passed and tied together. Stump rotation may be prevented by single epineural stitch.
- *Group Fascicular:* Placement of one or two sutures of 10-0 suture material in the perineurium to anastomose individual funiculi has found favor in the past 10 years. This avoids lateral growth and allows best possible coaptation of the fascicles. Clinically, there have not been any demonstrable advantages of this technique over epineural neurorrhaphy. The technique can be improved with the use of simultaneous nerve stimulation.
    - *Anchor funicular suture technique of Tsuge:* It uses both epineurial and funicular repair. A horizontal mattress sutures is utilized to incorporate both the epineurium and perineurium, thereby aligning the major funiculi and also improves the holding strength by including the epineurium in the stitch. One of the major disadvantages of this technique is inability to achieve approximation in all the funiculi.
- *Fascicular (Funicular for small nerve):* Individual fascicles are identified and sutured. This is even more precise but cumbersome.

Methods of closing gaps between nerve ends:
- *Mobilization:* It is usually done proximally as in the distal region the nerves thin down and gives branches so tethering effect is more pronounced distally. In general, up to 4 cm of mobilization can be done. Mobilization more than 6–8 cm reduces perfusion. Distal nerve mobilization is also associated with increased collagen production and cross-linking. Eminent author (Zachary) have but mobilized nerves extensively with good results—the median and ulnar nerves mobilized 7–9 cm and with anterior transposition an ulnar nerve gap of 13 cm were also filled.
- *Transposition:* The nerves are placed in position where the change in length effect, resulting from joint motion, is minimal and the nerves are relaxed like anterior transposition of ulnar nerve. Median nerve can also be transported anterior beneath pronator teres.
- *Limb positioning:* For upper limb, placing the elbow in flexion (not more than 90°) and wrist in flexion (not more than 40°) for radial nerve repair helps. Limb can be then gradually extended.
- *Resection osteotomy:* If, for example, a nonunion is being addressed then the bone ends can be cut to provide better contact area and simultaneously this also relaxes the nerve by increasing the relative length. This also holds true for comminuted fractures.
- Nerve stretching and bulb suture (neuroma to glioma suture).
- Neuromatous neurotization (e.g., intercostal nerve for brachial plexus).
- *Nerve grafting:* Nerve grafting was first reported by Philipeaux and Vulpian in 1870. The first human allograft was reported in 1878 by Albert. This is a commonly employed technique to address nerve gaps. Fresh nerve grafts are the best choice. The nerve grafts can be harvested from various autogenous sites of body like:
    - Lateral cutaneous nerve of thigh
    - Medial brachial and antebrachial cutaneous nerve
    - Radial sensory nerve

- Sural nerve (up to 40 cm of graft)
- Lateral cutaneous nerve of forearm (up to 20 cm)
- Terminal branch of posterior interosseous neuropathy (PIN) (for digital nerves).

69. Enumerate expendable nerves. How donor-site morbidity is associated with nerve harvesting?

Ans: *The common nerves that can be used for nerve grafting and repair include the following:*
- Sural nerve
- Medial and lateral cutaneous nerves of the forearm
- Dorsal cutaneous branch of the ulnar nerve
- Superficial and deep peroneal nerves
- Intercostal nerves
- Posterior and lateral cutaneous nerves of the thigh

Donor site morbidity with nerve harvesting:
- Harvest site morbidity (scarring, surgical scar, neuroma formation, loss of donor function)
- Painful donor site, cold sensitivity, function alteration
- Harvest time/cost
- Limited size and length available
- Other postoperative complications such as wound infections and wound complications

70. Discuss course of radial nerve and its applied surgical significance.

Ans: The radial nerve is formed in front of subscapularis muscle from posterior cord receiving components from all roots of brachial plexus (C5-T1) and follows the course as below:

It passes anterior to latissimus dorsi muscle → to enter the triangular space accompanied with profunda brachii artery → spirals around the posterior aspect of humerus into radial groove (not spiral groove; radial groove is few millimeter above spiral groove) where it is separated from bone by medial head of triceps (it is not in direct contact with bone here) coursing obliquely laterally → pierces the lateral intermuscular septum around 122 mm above lateral epicondyle (gets tethered at this point limiting its translation) → the nerve then enters into anterior compartment emerging beneath brachioradialis → divides into two branches → the deep branch [posterior interosseous neuropathy (PIN)] pierces supinator muscle to emerge into extensor compartment of forearm → forms cauda equina of spinner 8 cm distal to elbow joint. So along the course, the nerve supplies triceps, anconeus, radial half of brachialis, brachioradialis, extensor carpi radialis longus (ECRL), ECRB, supinator, extensor digitorum communis (EDC), extensor carpi ulnaris (ECU), extensor digiti minimi (EDM), abductor pollicis longus (APL), extensor pollicis brevis (EPB), extensor pollicis longus (EPL), and extensor indicis propolis (EIP) in that order.

Depending on the site of injury the radial nerve palsy involves following muscles that help in clinically distinguishing the level of injury:
- *Complete radial nerve palsy (very high):* Triceps and all distal muscles supplied by the nerve are paralyzed (injury in axillary region).
- *High radial nerve palsy:* Triceps and often anconeus are spared, but rest all other distal muscles are paralyzed (injury around radial groove till it pierces septum, typified by Holstein–Lewis injury).
- *Low radial nerve palsy:* BR and ECRL are preserved [≡ posterior interosseous nerve (PIN) palsy as in high both bone forearm fractures, local penetrating injuries like bullet injury and iatrogenic injury during radial head/neck surgeries. ECRB in only 58% cases is supplied by PIN, so it may also be spared in some cases].

Functional deficit produced by nerve injury at various levels include (numbers indicate the five digits; one is thumb while five is little finger):
- Inability to extend fingers (1, 2, 3, 4, and 5) (low) and wrist (low + high).
- Inability to stabilize the wrist (wrist drop) and thumb (radial abduction of thumb) (low + high).
- Loss of grip strength (accessory forearm flexion) (high).
- Accessory forearm supination (very high).
- Accessory elbow flexion (high), there is mild weakness only as biceps is intact.

- Unstable CMC joint (low + high).
- Sensory loss (radial two-thirds dorsal sensation) (high and above).

71. Discuss algorithm for management of radial nerve palsy.

Ans: The **Flowchart 4A.12.1** is a comprehensive algorithm depicting the decision making and management of radial nerve palsy.

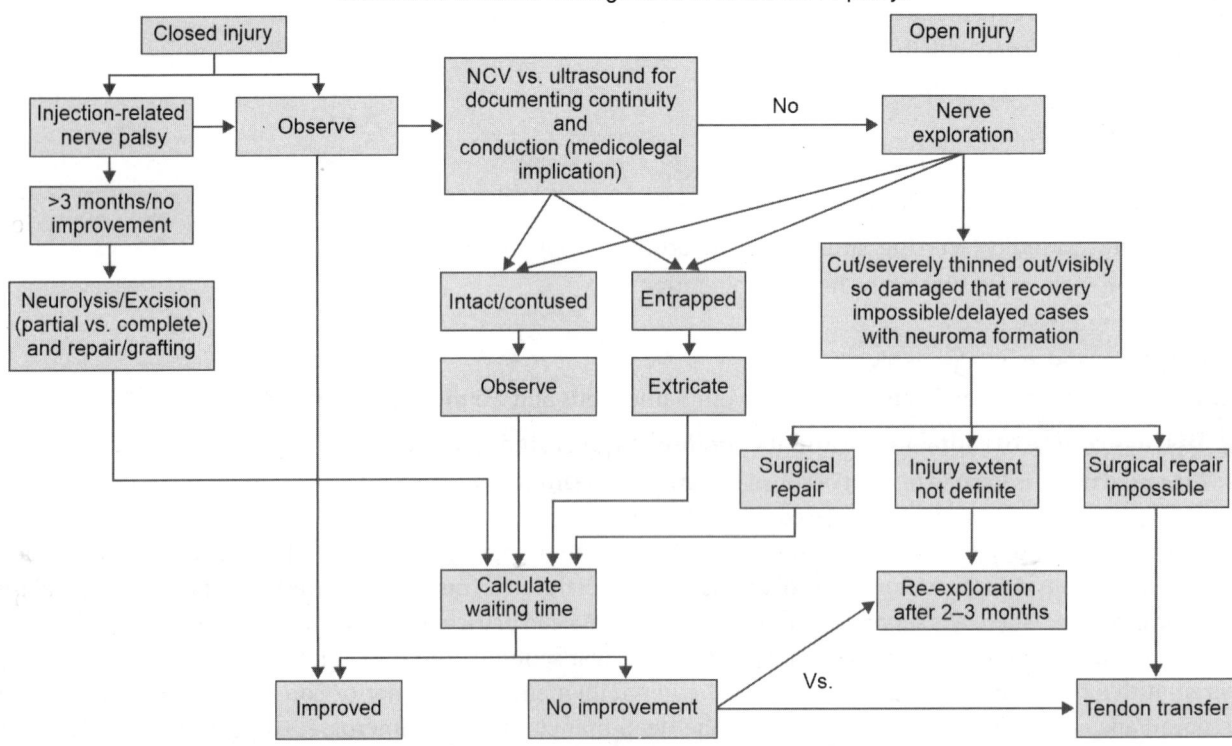

Flowchart 4A.12.1: Management of radial nerve palsy.

72. Discuss surgical anatomy of posterior interosseous nerve.

Ans: It is the chief nerve of the back of the forearm. It is a branch of the radial nerve given off in the cubital fossa, just below the level of the lateral epicondyle of the humerus.

Course:

It begins in cubital fossa and passes through supinator muscle to reach back of forearm, where it descends downward. It ends in a pseudoganglion in the 4th compartment of extensor retinaculum.

Relations:
- Posterior interosseous nerve leaves the cubital fossa and enters the back of the forearm by passing between the two planes of fibers of the supinator. Within the muscle, it winds backward round the lateral side of the radius.
- It emerges from the supinator on the back of the forearm. Here it lies between the superficial and deep muscles. At the lower border of the extensor pollicis brevis, it passes deep to the extensor pollicis longus. It then runs on the posterior surface of the interosseous membrane up to the wrist where it enlarges into a pseudoganglion and ends by supplying the wrist and intercarpal joints.

Branches:

Posterior interosseous nerve gives muscular and articular branches:
- *Muscular branches:*
  - Before piercing the supinator, branches are given to the extensor carpi radialis brevis and to the supinator.
  - While passing through the supinator, another branch is given to the supinator.
  - After emerging from the supinator, the nerve gives three short branches to:

- The extensor digitorum.
- The extensor digiti minimi
- The extensor carpi ulnaris

It also gives two long branches:
1. A lateral branch supplies the abductor pollicis longus and the extensor pollicis brevis
2. A medial branch supplies the extensor pollicis longus and the extensor indicis

- *Articular branches:*
Articular branches are given to:
  - The wrist joint
  - The distal radioulnar joint
  - Intercarpal and intermetacarpal joints
- *Sensory branches:* Sensory branches are given to the interosseous membrane, the radius, and the ulna.

Clinical anatomy: The deep branch of radial nerve may be damaged during an operation for exposure of the head/neck of the radius. Since the extensor carpi radialis longus and brevis are spared wrist drop does not occur while fingers loose dorsiflexion (finger drop).

73. Explain principles of tendon transfer. Describe the tendon transfers for high radial nerve palsy.

Ans: *Principles:*
- Correction of contractures (all joints must be supple)
- Adequate strength of the transferred tendon (4/5 power)
  - 85% of power is a must (Steindler)—graded as good power
  - "Omer" stated that a muscle loses at least one grade of strength after transfer.
- *Straight line of pull:* No pulley is ideal or minimum number of pulleys should be made.
- One tendon–one function, i.e., flex or extend:
  - *Synergism:* Synergistic transfer should be preferred as much as possible; however, there are a lot of violations of this rule.
- *Expendable donor:* There should be no functional morbidity following use of a tendon.
- Tissue should be in equilibrium (tissue equilibrium—termed by Steindler)
  - Soft tissue induration should subside
  - No reaction in wounds
  - Joints are supple
  - Scars should be as soft as possible.
- Pass tendon below fascial planes/sheaths and not below incision line/scar (best between subcutaneous fat and fascial sheath).
- Amplitude of transferred tendon should be as near to the original tendon for which the transfer is being done.
- Try preserving the nerve and vascular supply to muscle and vascular supply to tendon.
- Insertion of the tendon should be as close to the insertion of paralyzed tendon; at same angle, if split transfers then keep both slips in same tension.
- Try to restore sensibility of distal organ before treatment.
- Arthrodesis/joint procedure should be done before tendon transfer.
- The disorder should be a nonprogressive one.
- Keep dissection to a minimum around the muscle to be transferred and achieve meticulous hemostasis to prevent adhesion formation.

Tendon transfer in high radial nerve palsy:
- *Jones transfer:*
  Classical (1916):
  - PT → ECRL and ECRB;
  - FCU → EDC III-IV;
  - FCR → EPL; EDC II, EIP.

Classical (1921):
- PT → ECRL and ECRB
- FCU → EDC III-IV
- FCR → EDC II, EIP, EPL, EPB, APL.

Modified Jones: PT → ECRB and rest as above

- *FCR transfer (of Starr; Brand; Tsuge):*
  - PT → ECRB
  - FCR → EDC II-V
  - PL → rerouted APL.
- *Boyes transfer (superficialis transfer):*
  - PT → ECRB
  - FCR → APL and EPB
  - FDS III → EDC II-V via interosseous membrane
  - FDS IV → EIP; EPL via interosseous membrane.
- *FCU Transfer (standard transfer, this is not modified Jones transfer):*
  - PT → ECRB
  - FCU → EDC
  - PL → rerouted EPL.

74. Discuss early tendon transfer in radial nerve palsy.

Ans: When a precise neurorrhaphy has been performed early in a patient, selected tendon transfers may be performed early as internal splints to support partial function and prevent deformity, while awaiting the potential nerve recovery. These substitute also the function of external splints and immobilizers. The selected early tendon transfers (internal splints) enhance function while awaiting the return of nerve control and total muscle activity. The combined results of early tendon transfer plus the return from nerve repair often are better than those of either procedure separately by stimulating sensibility reeducation and improving the coordination of residual muscle-tendon units.

Principles of early tendon transfer:
- Should not ↓ function in remaining hand
- Should not create deformity
- Should be phasic or capable of phasic conversion, e.g., Pronator teres (PT) → extensor carpi radialis brevis (ECRB) transfer, described by Burkhalter, for radial nerve palsy or a wrist flexor in substitution for a finger extensor. A synergistic muscle-tendon unit will be able to use spinal reflex arcs and other autonomic feedback mechanisms to enhance re-education.

Indications:
- Substitutes function during nerve regrowth eliminating the need of splintage.
- Helper following reinnervation → aiding power of normally innervated muscle or helping a suboptimally innervated muscle.
- Substitute in cases where results of repair are poor or nerve irreparable.

75. Enumerate causes of claw hand deformity. Discuss its management in short with principles.

Ans: The common causes of claw hand deformity are:
- Low/high ulnar nerve paralysis (partial claw hand) or due to combined ulnar and median nerve paralysis (total or complete claw hand).
- Soft tissue contractures as in hand compartment syndrome and sequel, forearm compartment syndrome, and Volkmann ischemic contracture (VIC).

Management: The goals of correction of claw deformity are—
- Primary requirement in claw hand is to provide flexion at metacarpophalangeal (MCP) joint.
- Secondary is to achieve flexion at IP joint and coordination and power.
- Restoration of key pinch.

X-ray is done to look for condition of bones and joints—bony or joint pathology usually precludes attempts at correction by soft tissue reconstruction alone, hence, additional bony correction is needed.

Passive (static) treatment methods to provide flexion at MCP joint (achieve only first goal and also do not address adduction of fingers):
- Zancolli anterior capsulorrhaphy of MCP joint
- Extensor diversion graft (Srinivasan)
- Palande's technique (capsulorrhaphy and flexor pulley advancement)
- ECRL tenodesis.

Tendon transfer (dynamic): Even if ring finger (RF) and little finger (LF) are involved, transfer of tendon to all four tendons must be done to provide coordinated and powerful movements—
- *Sublimis transfer (modified Stiles-Bunnell FF4T phasic transfer):* Flexor digitorum superficialis (FDS) of RF (in low ulnar nerve palsy, else use MF or index finger flexor digitorum superficialis (IF FDS) is fashioned into tail/slips and attached to dorsal lateral extensor expansion. Specific attachment provides, in addition, adduction of fingers. Tendon should pass anterior to MCP joint (Bunnell originally used all 4 FDS slips that led to intrinsic plus deformity). Also, this transfer can cause IP joint hyperextension due to attachment done to extensor expansion and usually lax IP joints found in these patients. Modification, hence, is to attach the slips to proximal phalanx (Burkhalter) rather than into the extensor expansion.
- *Zancolli Lasso:* Transfer of FDS of RF/MF to all fingers. Here, a lasso is created around A2 pulley system (modified lasso) to provide dynamic MCP flexion (remember unassisted angle should be <30°).
- *Extensor to flexor 4 tailed (EF4T nonphasic, Brand):* ECRL tendon with fascia lata or palmaris or plantaris extension attached as mentioned. Brand originally described it with ECRB tendon and later modified with ECRB/ECRL.
- Palmaris longus many tailed graft, if fingers are hypermobile. (This weaker muscle will not cause swan neck deformity.)
- Extensor indices transfer.
- *Attaining key pinch:* For restoring key pinch, we need to restore the first dorsal interosseous and adductor pollicis function most importantly the latter (ADP function). Use of wrist and finger extensors, finger flexors, EDQ, the index EDC, and the EIP and the brachioradialis have been described in literature to power adductor pollicis function. The following are commonly employed methods for restoring key pinch:
    - *Smith ECRB transfer:* The tendon is lengthened by tendon graft that is passed between 2nd and 3rd MC into volar aspect of palm. The grafts are attached to adductor pollicis insertion routing over 2nd metacarpal that functions as a pulley here.
    - *Boyes brachioradialis transfer:* Tendon graft is used and passed similar to the detail given for Smith ECRB transfer.
    - *Littler FDS transfer:* The MF FDS if not used for correction of claw deformity then can be used to power adductor pollicis by passing beneath flexor tendons and attaching to adductor pollicis. This is less effective than ECRB transfer.

76. **Define ulnar claw hand. Enumerate causes of it. Discuss its management.**

Ans: *Ulnar claw hand:* It is the most characteristic deformity ascribed to ulnar nerve injury due to loss of intrinsic function of flexion at the MCP joint, while long flexor tendons flex the IP joints.

Causes:
- Trauma
- Compressive neuropathy
- Brachial plexus injury
- Infective (leprosy, polio)
- Peripheral neuropathy (systemic diseases, drugs and toxins, hereditary)
- VIC
- Primary nerve neoplasm.

Management:
- *Thumb adduction:* ECRB transferred and attached to abductor tubercle (Smith/Boyes). In other scenario, ECRB can be better attached to the APB insertion that additionally provides pronation for pinch. Tendon graft has to be used

to accomplish the transfer, which is done through third metacarpal space and passed volar to AP and deep to flexor tendons.
- *Metacarpophalangeal flexion with integrated IP flexion:* ECRL (Brown's 4 tailed; EF4) or FCR (if flexion contracture at wrist); tendon grafts passed volar to transverse carpal ligament attached to A2 pulley or radial band of dorsal apparatus.
- *Maintenance of palmar (transverse metacarpal) arch and adduction of little finger:* EDM tendon split and ulnar half transferred to radial collateral ligament of PP or radial band of dorsal apparatus of little finger. If the little finger is clawed and abducted then the tendon slip is inserted into A2 pulley of the flexor sheath.
- *Thumb–index finger "tip pinch":* Accessory slip of APL to first dorsal interosseous and MCP joint arthrodesis. If MCP joint already arthrodesed, EPB may be transferred.
- This procedure does not increase the power, but only stabilizes the index finger.
- *Volar sensations:* Vascular nerve grafts or proximal medial digital nerve translocated to distal ulnar digital nerve.
  To this, one can add Zancolli capsulodesis detailed in Answer to Question 76.

77. What is the pathogenesis of claw hand?
Ans: The clawing of fingers is due to loss of intrinsic muscles especially the lumbricals that produce extension at the interphalangeal joint (IP) joint so there is flexion at the IP joints. The clawing is more apparent in low ulnar nerve palsy as the maintained basal tone of long flexors make the clawing prominent while in a high palsy even the long flexors are paralyzed so flexion at interphalangeal joint is less pronounced and is only due to tenodesis effect. Complete claw hand (involving all four fingers) results from combined median and ulnar nerve palsy.

78. Explain tendon transfer in ulnar nerve palsy.
Ans: The ulnar nerve palsy may occur from injury to the nerve at wrist (low) or higher. The functional deficits resulting from isolated ulnar nerve palsy are as follows:
- Loss of grip strength (impairment of power grip is more than precise grasp) (High)
- Flexion of distal phalanx 4,5 (High)
- Digital balance 4,5 (High)
- Loss of finger function [flexion (partial), adduction, and abduction] (High + Low), there is loss of power flexion of the proximal phalanges and integration of metacarpophalangeal and interphalangeal joint motion. Normally, the fingers start flexion at distal interphalangeal (DIP) joint with simultaneous or just followed by (but in smaller amplitude) flexion at MCP joints. In ulnar nerve palsy, the flexion at DIP is associated with MCP extension instead and the fingers curl up in the palm instead of making a fist.
- Loss of thumb adduction and weakness of thumb flexion (High + Low)
- Sensory loss (medial 1 1/2 digits—Low; ulnar 1/3 volar—High).

Transfers for low ulnar nerve palsy (simplified version):
- *Thumb adduction:* ECRB to abductor tubercle (Smith/Boyes).
- *MCP flexion with integrated IP flexion:* ECRL (Brown's 4 tailed; EF4) or FCR (if flexion contracture at wrist); tendon grafts are passed volar to transverse carpal ligament attached to A2 pulley or radial band of dorsal apparatus).
- *Palmar arch and adduction of little finger:* EDM tendon split and ulnar half transferred to radial collateral ligament of PP or radial band of dorsal apparatus.
- *Thumb–index finger "tip pinch":* Accessory slip of APL to 1st dorsal interosseous and MP joint arthrodesis. If MP joint already arthrodesed, EPB may be transferred.
- *Volar sensations:* Proximal medial digital nerve translocated to distal ulnar digital nerve.

For high ulnar nerve palsy:
In addition to above points the following are required:
- Wrist flexion (ulnar side) (*not frequently done*): FCR transfer to FCU or Palmaris longus transfer to FCU
- *DIP flexion for RF and LF:* FDP (IF and MF) tenodesed to FDP (RF and LF).

(*For detailed description and additional transfers, kindly refer to the Chapter 108 on Peripheral Nerve Injuries in the book Essential Orthopedics: Principles and Practice, 2nd edition.*)

79. A. Describe anatomy of ulnar nerve.
B. Describe differences between low and high ulnar nerve palsy.
C. Algorithm for management of ulnar nerve palsy.

Ans: (A) The ulnar nerve is one of the major terminal branches of the brachial plexus; it takes origin from the medial cord of the brachial plexus with a root value of C8 and T1. In the axilla the nerve lies medial to axillary artery, from the axilla it enters the arm and stays between the axillary artery and vein. Near the insertion of coracobrachialis it pierces the medial intermuscular septum and enters the posterior compartment. The superior ulnar collateral artery joins ulnar nerve that then run together over the medial head of the triceps till cubital tunnel. The fibers of the nerve are arranged in layers with the sensory nerves for the hand lying superficially, followed by the intrinsic muscle nerves. The branches to the FDP and flexor carpi ulnaris (FCU) lie deep against the ulnar collateral ligament.

The ulnar nerve in forearm lies deep to the FCU. Distally, it becomes more superficial as it crosses the myotendinous junction of FCU. Radially, it is accompanied by the ulnar artery and FCU lies on the ulnar aspect as it progresses further and enters the ulnar canal/tunnel (Guyon's canal).

B. The differences between high and low ulnar palsy are summarized in the **Table 4A.12.2**.

S. No.	Features	Low ulnar nerve palsy	High ulnar nerve palsy
1	Inspection and palpation	Low ulnar nerve palsy mainly results in loss of intrinsic muscle function to hand due to injury in distal third forearm and/or wrist	• Atrophy of first web space and the interosseous muscles • Clawing of the ring and fifth finger • Benediction hand, this is less marked than in lower level ulnar nerve palsies (due to weakness of long flexors here) • MCP joint hyperextension • Subluxation of ulnar nerve on the medial epicondyle during flexion of elbow
2	Sensory examination		*Hypoesthesia in ulnar 1½ digits and dorsal ulnar half of hand:* The latter is a localizing sign of high ulnar nerve palsy
3	Treatment	• *Thumb adduction:* ECRB transferred and attached to abductor tubercle (Smith/Boyes). In other scenario, ECRB can be better attached to the APB insertion that additionally provides pronation for pinch. Tendon graft has to be used to accomplish the transfer which is done through third metacarpal space and passed volar to AP and deep to flexor tendons • *Metacarpophalangeal flexion with integrated IP flexion:* ECRL (Brown's 4 tailed; EF4) or FCR (if flexion contracture at wrist); tendon grafts passed volar to transverse carpal ligament attached to A2 pulley or radial band of dorsal apparatus • *Maintenance of Palmar (transverse metacarpal) arch and adduction of little finger:* EDM tendon split and ulnar half transferred to radial collateral ligament of PP or radial band of dorsal apparatus of little finger. If the little finger is clawed and abducted then the tendon slip is inserted into A2 pulley of the flexor sheath • *Thumb-index finger "tip pinch":* Accessory slip of APL to first dorsal interosseous and MCP joint arthrodesis. If MCP joint already arthrodesed EPB may be transferred. This procedure does not increase the power, but only stabilizes the index finger • *Volar sensations:* Vascular nerve grafts or proximal medial digital nerve translocated to distal ulnar digital nerve	For high ulnar nerve palsy in addition the following are done: • Wrist flexion (ulnar side) (*not frequently done*): FCR→FCU or PL→FCU • *DIP flexion for RF and LF:* FDP of MF is tenodesed to FDP (RF and LF) • *Ulnar deviation:* For persons requiring strong wrist flexion we need ulnar deviation so that FCR can be transferred to the FCU attachment

(APL: abductor pollicis longus; DIP: distal interphalangeal; ECRB: extensor carpi radialis brevis; EPB: extensor pollicis brevis; FDP: flexor digitorum profundus; FCR: flexor carpi ulnaris; FCU: flexor carpi radialis; MCP: metacarpophalangeal)

Algorithm: (The question is regarding "palsy" and not "injury" per se so acute cut and lacerated injuries have not been included in the below description, if one wants then the management is obviously surgical and in acute cases primary nerve repair vs. delayed primary repair is attempted while in old cases tendon transfers can be done as described above for high vs. low injuries). The management of ulnar nerve palsy involves a systematic approach for evaluation and treatment. Here is a simplified algorithm for the management of ulnar nerve palsy.

- Initial assessment
  - *History and symptoms:* Document symptoms such as weakness, sensory loss (tingling/numbness) along the ulnar nerve distribution (ring and little fingers), and any history of trauma, overuse, or existing medical conditions (e.g., diabetes, arthritis).
  - *Physical examination:* Assess muscle strength (intrinsic hand muscles), sensory function, and look for signs of muscle atrophy or deformities (e.g., claw hand).
- Investigations
  - *Electrodiagnostic studies:* Perform nerve conduction studies (NCS) and electromyography (EMG) to confirm the diagnosis and determine the extent of nerve damage.
  - *Imaging studies (if indicated):* Use ultrasound or MRI to evaluate for compressive lesions or structural abnormalities.
- Determine cause of palsy
  - Identify underlying causes (e.g., compression due to trauma, anatomical anomalies, tumors, systemic diseases).
- Initial management
  - Conservative treatment.
  - *Activity modification:* Avoid activities that exacerbate symptoms.
  - *Splinting:* Use a wrist splint to maintain the wrist in a neutral position and relieve pressure on the nerve, especially at night.
  - *Physical therapy:* Engage in therapeutic exercises to maintain strength and mobility.
- Monitor progress
  - Follow-up on symptoms and functional status. Monitor for improvement or worsening of symptoms over a specified period.
- Surgical intervention
  - If conservative management fails (typically after 3–6 months) or if there is severe weakness, atrophy, or significant functional impairment.
  - *Ulnar nerve decompression:* Surgical release of the nerve at the cubital tunnel or other sites of entrapment.
  - *Ulnar nerve transposition:* Moving the ulnar nerve to a different location if it is chronic or recurrent.
  - *Assess for other surgical options:* Such as neuroma resection or grafting if there is significant nerve injury.
- Rehabilitation postsurgery
  - Engage in physical and occupational therapy focused on strengthening and improving functionality.
  - Gradually return to normal activities; monitor recovery closely.
- Long-term management
  - Regular follow-up to assess symptoms and functional status. Adjust treatment plans as necessary based on progress and any emerging issues.

80. Discuss in detail about:
  A. Intrinsic plus hand
  B. Ulnar paradox.

Ans: A. *Intrinsic plus hand:* It is caused by muscle imbalance between spastic intrinsics (interossei and lumbricals) and weak extrinsics (FDS, FDP, and EDC), so that intrinsics have "plus" power compared to the extrinsics. This is opposite of the claw-hand deformity of hand. It may also be caused by contracture of the intrinsic muscles of the hand. Shortening of the intrinsic muscles in the hand produces a characteristic deformity:

- Flexion at the MCP joints with extension of the IP joints and adduction of the thumb (the so-called *"intrinsic-plus"* hand).

Slight degrees of deformity may not be obvious, but can be diagnosed by:
- *Bunnell "intrinsic-plus" test*—with the MCP joints pushed passively into hyperextension (thus putting the intrinsics on stretch), it is difficult or impossible to flex the IP joints passively; if the MCP joints are then placed in flexion, the IP joints can be passively flexed.

The causes of intrinsic plus deformity are:
- Neurological conditions (e.g., in cerebral palsy, stroke, Parkinson's)
- Volar subluxation of the MCP joints (e.g., in rheumatoid arthritis)
- Scarring after trauma or infection
- Shrinkage due to ischemia.

Symptoms: Difficulty in gripping large objects.

Imaging: No radiographs are required for diagnosis but for treatment they are obtained to look for presence of any secondary or primary structural bony changes or joint damage that needs to be addressed.

Treatment:
- Nonoperative—passive stretching in mild cases.
- Operative—by proximal muscle slide or distal intrinsic release. Moderate contracture can be treated by resecting a triangular segment of the intrinsic "aponeurosis" at the base of the proximal phalanx (Littler's operation).

B. *Ulnar paradox:* This is a clinical finding where it is commonly assumed that the higher the neurological injury the more severe/complete is the distal involvement producing characteristic deformities; however, this notion is altered in ulnar nerve injury. Ulnar nerve injury at wrist causes more clawing (severe interphalangeal flexion deformity due to unopposed and strong flexor digitorum profundus). In high ulnar nerve injury, say at elbow, the flexor digitorum profundus is also paralyzed/weak and leads to less evident clawing (less severe interphalangeal flexion deformity).

This is known as the ulnar paradox—one expects a more pronounced deformity due to high ulnar nerve injury at elbow as compared with wrist level but in fact the opposite occurs.

81. Describe indications and surgical method of Zancolli capsulodesis.

Ans: Zancolli capsulodesis is principally intended to prevent MCP hyperextension as is seen in claw hand deformities. In claw deformity, the primary hyperextension at the MCP joint spoils the rhythmic flexion at IP and MCP joints needed for grasping and making fist producing the claw deformity and finger flexion within the palm rather than into the palm. This precludes prehension. Zancolli capsulodesis shortens the volar capsule preventing preceding hyperextension at MCP joint to maintain normal fist and grip (*compare from*—Zancolli lasso). The most common indications are:
- Simple ulnar claw hand from ulnar nerve palsy from leprosy, trauma, or tardy ulnar nerve palsy
- Ancillary procedure with tendon transfers for ulnar nerve palsy
- Traumatic deformity of hand with dorsal contractures causing hyperextension at MCP joints.

Surgical method of Zancolli capsulodesis:
- Make a transverse incision in the palm at the level of the distal crease. Making thick flaps exposes the flexor tendon sheaths and protects neurovascular bundles.
- Over each metacarpophalangeal joint, make a longitudinal incision in the paratendinous fascia and tendon sheath and expose the flexor tendons.
- MCP joint is exposed by retracting the tendons.
- In classical method, an elliptical segment of the volar fibrocartilaginous plate with capsule is resected to produce a 10–30° flexion contracture when the tissue is reapproximated. Alternatively, the volar plate can be imbricated or its proximal attachment is advanced proximally to neck of metacarpal and secured with suture anchor.
- Close the volar plates with nonabsorbable sutures placed laterally. If needed, insert transarticular K-wires to maintain the MCP joint in position.
- Close the wound and apply a dorsal plaster splint, holding MCP joints in flexion and the wrist in extension.

82. Explain etiopathogenesis, clinical features, diagnosis, and management of carpal tunnel syndrome.

Ans: Carpal tunnel syndrome can develop acutely or have an insidious onset. Acute onset carpal tunnel syndrome (CTS) is characterized by rapid and sustained increment in pressure in the carpal tunnel and requires urgent decompression. These factors are few but not uncommon and include wrist trauma, infection, hematoma, and high-pressure injections. Most common presentation of CTS is chronic symptoms having varied pathology, and among these idiopathic one is the most common. In idiopathic variety, the exact cause is not identifiable; however, there is notable hypertrophy of fibrous tissue and chronic edema with minimal inflammation of the nerve. As compared to males, females are more commonly involved. In the carpal tunnel, the most common location of compression is 1 cm distal to proximal border of ligament, which corresponds to the thickest part of the ligament. Anatomic factors operate locally and have in common the characteristic of behaving as space-occupying lesions. Factors operating systemically either raise the interstitial pressure or may deposit pathological material that constricts the already tenuous space of the carpal tunnel. Pregnancy deserves special mention as the reported incidence is 20–45%. Symptoms typically develop during the third trimester, vary in severity, and abate postpartum with nonsurgical treatment. The etiology of gestational CTS is unknown, but is thought to be due to fluid retention. Keyboarding and occupational exposure to vibration have also been symptomatically associated to CTS. Repetitive movements of the wrist and fingers are associated with exertional CTS. It has been shown experimentally that extremes of wrist flexion and extension are associated with increased pressure in the carpal tunnel.

The following are etiological factors responsible for development of carpal tunnel syndrome:

Idiopathic

Local anatomic:
- *Acute* (fracture, crushing hand injury, hemorrhage, burn, median artery thrombosis, infection, and pregnancy)
- *Distal radius malunion*
- *Carpal canal stenosis* (deformity congenital or acquired)
- *Anomalous structures* (palmaris profundus, proximal origin of a lumbrical, reversed palmaris longus, and anomalous branch of radial artery)
- *Space-occupying lesions* (ganglion, lipoma, fibroma, synovial sarcoma, neuroma, neurofibroma, neurilemmomas, and hemangioma).

Occupational (use of vibrating tools)

Systemic:
- Disorders affecting fluid balance (pregnancy, congestive heart failure, renal failure, acromegaly, and myxedema)
- Endocrinopathy (diabetes mellitus, thyroid disease, and growth hormone)
- Collagen and autoimmune diseases
- Inflammatory conditions (scleroderma, dermatomyositis, tenovaginitis, rheumatoid arthritis, scleroderma, gout, etc.)
- Amyloidosis
- Polyneuropathy
- Alcoholism
- Myeloma
- Obesity
- Constitutional (advancing age and female gender)
- Hemorrhagic conditions (hemophilia and anticoagulation)
- Consequential forms (oral contraceptives, anticoagulants, and lack of vitamin B_6)
- Congenital diseases (mucopolysaccharidosis and mucolipidosis).

Clinical features and diagnosis
- The most common symptom is "nocturnal acroparesthesia", consisting of a painful tingling and numbness in the thumb and one of the radial digits, which may even disturb sleep; however, daytime paresthesias may also occur with activities, which involve extremes of wrist flexion. Certain activities or position of the hands that may trigger paresthesias

in daytime are pray position, the act of sewing, and holding the phone or a book while reading. In the initial stages of the disease, the patients find it difficult to exact distribution of paresthesia, whereas aggravating maneuvers can aptly localize the paresthesia to the radial three digits and the radial side of the fourth digit. A self-completed Katz and Stirrat hand symptom diagram may be used to make a correct clinical diagnosis.
- The most sensitive test for detecting early CTS is the Semmes–Weinstein monofilament test and probably vibrometry. These threshold tests reflect both sensory changes and decreases in sensory nerve function quite reliably and early. Innervation density tests (2-point discrimination and moving 2-point discrimination) correlate poorly due to subjective sensation and remain normal until all sensation has ceased.
- Carpal tunnel syndrome may involve both the limbs but usually the symptoms may be more in one hand. In chronic cases, grip strength and pinch may diminish.
- Bilateral CTS is common; however, the symptoms may be more marked in one hand.
- There may be symptoms of autonomic dysfunction like finger blanching, Raynaud's phenomenon, subjective swelling of fingers, etc.
- Thenar atrophy is a late sign often in neglected cases over a long duration of disease and patients often report less pain by this time!

Various "provocative tests" for CTS are:
- *Tinel's sign:* An electric shock-like or tingling sensation is felt in the distribution of median nerve after a firm, but gentle tap on the median nerve at the transverse carpal ligament (TCL) region. Truly speaking this has not been described for CTS, as it is mainly a sign of regenerating sensory nerves after injury and should not be present for an ongoing damaging process.
- *Phalen's wrist hyperflexion test:* Paresthesia in the median nerve distribution on flexion of the wrist for 60 seconds.
- Durkan's direct median nerve compression at TCL for 30 seconds (variously described as 15–120 seconds) also elicits similar response in a patient with CTS. Performing Durkan's after Phalen's might increase its sensitivity.
- Reverse Phalen's test has also been found positive and useful but in moderate to advanced compression predominantly.
- *Scratch collapse test or hierarchical scratch collapse test:* It is relatively a new provocative clinical test of nerve compression. The use of ethyl chloride allows for a hierarchical test, which can even reveal additional sites of compression. In various studies it shows a sensitivity of 64% and specificity of 69% for diagnosing CTS.

Diagnostic studies: Electrodiagnostic testing is described in next Q83.

Imaging: Radiographs in standard anteroposterior and lateral projections are commonly ordered, carpal tunnel view is also sometimes ordered but is helpful only to identify and study cause of CTS due to:
- Trauma
- Arthritis
- Degenerative cases may show calcification at the carpal region in carpal tunnel view.

Magnetic resonance imaging (MRI) and ultrasonography have been shown to be of useful to a variable extent defining the pathology and also provide measurements of the canal size. Flattening of the nerve at the level of hook of hamate is a usual finding. Cross-sectional diameter ratio of median nerve: In normal individuals it should be 1 cm or less, an increase in the diameter is diagnostic. It is checked at the level of pisiform to distal radius.

Additional findings on MRI may be inflammation of other structures, fatty infiltration of median nerve, bursitis, and demonstration of neuroma or other space-occupying lesions:
- Scarring
- Algodystrophy
- Inflammation
- Incomplete resection of ligament
- Real canal widening.

Treatment: Treatment options for CTS range from—
- Nonsurgical measures
- Steroid injections
- Surgical carpal tunnel release (CTR) including endoscopic methods.

The decision for specific modality relies on severity of nerve involvement judged by clinical examination and electrophysiological studies, chronicity of symptoms, and individual patient choices.

Nonsurgical measures

Splinting, activity modification and oral medications: Splinting may be appropriate in initial disease or mild chronic symptoms. Surgical release is typically prescribed in acute CTS due to infection, trauma, or hematoma formation. Findings of evident denervation in typical symptoms confirmed by electrodiagnostic studies are primary candidates for surgical release.

- About 80% patients respond to wrist immobilization in night and intermittently during day within days.
- Particularly helpful in patients with positive Phalen's test or a positive fist test. It keeps the lumbricals out of the tunnel.
- The position of splint is debatable, it has been demonstrated that the pressure is lowest $2° \pm 9°$ of extension and $2° \pm 6°$ of ulnar deviation. Ergonomic modifications may be of some help.

Anti-inflammatory medications like nonsteroidal anti-inflammatory drugs (NSAIDs) and supplementation with pyridoxine (B6) and methylcobalamin for its neurotropic action may have a beneficial role. Oral steroids and diuretics are prescribed to lower the interstitial fluid pressure with documented benefit in some studies.

Local corticosteroid injections: The benefits and effectiveness of local steroids are controversial, the use has been empirical and little information is available at present regarding the dosage, site of injection, and number of repetitions. The reported recurrence of symptoms after local corticosteroid injection has been demonstrated to range 8–100%. Some investigators have even found the benefit of injection to be similar to NSAIDs and splinting. Up to 3 months, local injection with a steroid is better than oral steroids.

Adjunctive measures: Laser therapy, local ultrasound therapy, and iontophoresis are variably being used but the benefits have been inconsistent.

Surgical Release: Various methods of CTR include—

- Open release
- Limited open method
- Endoscopic methods.

Choice of method of release is mainly surgeon dependent and as per comfort of the surgeon (while advanced methods like endoscopic release may also have a marketing motive). The different methods have their own pros and cons. A number of methods have been developed so as to reduce recurrence rates, limit the postoperative weakness, and to avoid complications.

Open release: It is the most common used method for carpal tunnel decompression. Various authors have described different incisions although the shape of incisions varies, they commonly involve similar deep dissection releasing palmar fascia and carpal ligament longitudinally. The proximal point for starting the incision is determined by flexing the fourth finger toward the distal wrist crease. The cutaneous incision line is ulnarly located with respect to the thenar crease and is located 2 mm ulnarly to the fourth ray. It is important to keep the superficial and the deep dissection lateral so as to prevent injury to motor branch and palmar cutaneous nerve of median nerve. Some principles for the nerve release are as follows:

- Care is taken to prevent laceration to recurrent motor branch and palmar cutaneous branch of median nerve.
- Internal neurolysis, epineurotomy, and tenosynovectomy often initially performed commonly lead to skin adhesions, neurodermodesis phenomenon, and algo-paresthesias. Hence, internal neurolysis has been definitively abandoned.
- Immediately after skin incision, one should be extremely cautious for anomalies that cross over the same incision line.
- The sectioning of the TCL is performed in layers and is kept along the 4th ray.
- While sectioning the midpalmar adipose tissue, one should also be extremely careful not to injure the superficial vascular arch.
- In majority of cases, there is hourglass constriction in the median nerve at the level of hook of hamate, while occasionally there is marked compression of the nerve with ecchymosis.

Limited open carpal tunnel release: Limited-incision CTR techniques similar to endoscopic surgery were developed to decrease palmar discomfort and hasten the return to activities. Modified instruments, light source, and availability of magnification have led to development of this technique. A "palm-only" less than 2 cm mini-incision is used to release the transverse carpal ligament. Some authors have recommended both proximal and distal release.

Endoscopic technique: In an attempt to reduce the complications of open release like scar tenderness and prolonged healing time, endoscopic procedures were developed. Both single and dual portals have been described. In single portal technique, a portal placed midway between flexor carpi ulnaris (FCU) and flexor carpi radialis (FCR). With wrist extended and endoscopic blade assembly aligned to ring finger, distal edge of ligament is identified and sectioned from distal to proximal in controlled fashion. Contraindications of endoscopic procedures include:
- Proliferative synovitis
- Stiffness of wrist joint
- Space-occupying lesions in the tunnel that obliterate the view of canal.

83. Describe electrodiagnosis in carpal tunnel syndrome.

Ans: The goals of an electrodiagnostic examination in CTS are basically to:
- Localization of lesion
- Determine evidence of reinnervation or of ongoing axonal loss
- Find the type of fibers involved motor, sensory fibers, or both
- Define the extent of injury to neural tissue (axon loss and demyelination)
- Define degree of axonal loss, the continuity of axon.

The primary objective of nerve conduction velocity (NCV) in a suspected case of CTS is to confirm the diagnosis of compression of the median nerve at the wrist. Also, it may help to rule out other causes of the symptoms like plexopathies, radiculopathies, and other causes not evident from clinical examination. Neurophysiologic examination in the preoperative workup of a CTS patient allows quantification of the severity and the type of nerve lesion; moreover, it can be of some value in litigation. It has been proposed that neurophysiological testing for CTS is more sensitive than routine clinical testing and may be positive in clinically silent patients. In the phenomenon of increased excitability and generation of ectopic impulses in the initial CTS (irritative stage), discharge cannot be demonstrated and the test will be normal.

Diagnostic criteria based on electrodiagnostic study:

Evidence of sensory nerve fiber compression:
- Delayed or absent motor nerve sensory action potential (SAP) >3.4 ms
- Increased median-to-ulnar latency difference of the fourth finger SAP (and 0.5 ms).

Evidence of motor nerve fiber compression:
- Prolonged distal motor latency (>4.2 ms)
- Denervation signs in the abductor pollicis brevis muscle.

84. Describe cross-section of peripheral nerve.

Ans: Cross-section of peripheral nerve has been shown in **Figure 4A.12.1**. A peripheral nerve (or parts like root, ramus, trunk, branch, etc.) is composed of orderly arrangements of the axonal and dendritic processes of many nerve cell bodies. Axons are arranged in bundles. A small bundle of such fibers enclosed in a tubular sheath (perineurium) is called a funiculus (termed by Sunderland, it is the smallest unit of nerve that can be manipulated surgically) and several such bundles form fascicles of variable sizes arranged together form a nerve. Depending on the number of fascicles present a nerve may be monofascicular (single fascicle), oligofascicular (few fascicles) or polyfascicular (many fascicles). These fasciculi are bound

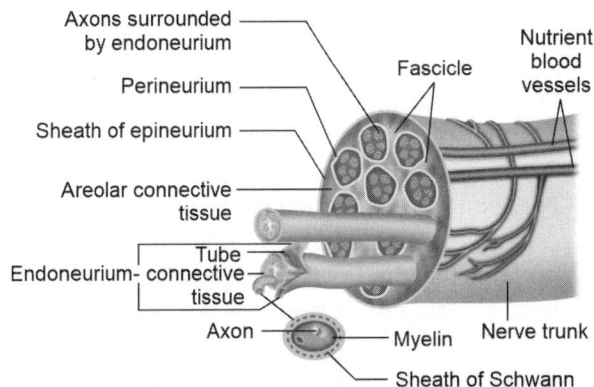

Fig. 4A.12.1: Cross-section of peripheral nerve.

together in a common membranous investment or sheath of the whole nerve called epineurium. These fascicles are hence united together by the epineurium. The coverings of peripheral nerve are:
- Epineurium typically is what we see from eyes when we see a naked nerve and has two parts. The dense connective tissue portion makes the fibrous coat of the whole nerve. The loose connective tissue portion of epineurium fills the spaces between the bundles of nerve fibers.

- Perineurium is an important structure physiologically and anatomically flattened epithelial cells (the perineural epithelium) with basal lamina on both sides. Perineurium provides mechanical support to the nerve and is dense (increased number of perineural cells), where the nerve crosses joint for greater need of mechanical strength.
- Endoneurium (analog of the pia mater) is the loose connective tissue between nerve fibers representing analog of the pia mater. It contains a basal layer of Schwann cells along with reticular tissue, blood capillaries, endoneural fluid, type I and type II collagen fibers (forming the so-called basement membrane), and endothelial cells sealed by zonula occludens (sort of maintains the "blood brain barrier" of nerve).

85. Classify peripheral nerve injuries. Describe management of a 1.5-year-old child with median nerve injury in the middle of the arm.

Ans: *Classification:* There are three main systems for classifying nerve injuries, Cohen's system (1941) popularized by Seddon in 1943, Sunderland in 1951 **(Table 4A.12.3)**, and Mackinnon in 1992. Cohen (Seddon) described three basic progressively increasing damage to nerves to which Sunderland added two degrees in between axonotmesis and neurotmesis. Mackinnon added the concept of mixed nerve injury.

TABLE 4A.12.3: Classification of nerve injuries.

Cohen/Seddon	Sunderland	Description
Neurapraxia	1	Local conduction block, variable myelin damage, and no axonal discontinuity
Axonotmesis	2	Loss of axonal continuity, endoneurium intact, and no conduction
	3	Loss of axonal and endoneurial continuity, perineurium intact, and no conduction
	4	Loss of axonal, endoneurial and perineurial continuity, epineurium intact, and no conduction
Neurotmesis	5	Epineurium also damaged—neural discontinuity with separation of ends and no conduction
	6	Mixed nerve damage along the nerve trunk, all types of nerve injuries seen in 1–5, recovery is hence variable with nearly no recovery in combined types 4 and 5

Neurapraxia (Sunderland first-degree):
- No disruption of internal structure only a localized conduction block exists (physiological disruption with anatomical preservation)
- Tinel's sign absent
- Loss of function is often complete initially but recovery can be expected to be complete within 3–6 weeks or maximum up to 3 months
- Nerve conduction velocity (NCV) shows increased latency.

Axonotmesis (Sunderland second-degree):
- Disruption of axons and Wallerian degeneration (WD)
- Maintenance of gross architecture of the nerve
- Tinel's sign positive as axonal regeneration occurs
- For Seddon's classification, there is no differentiation between partial or complete loss of axons but Sunderland classifies them further. For second-degree injury, there is limited loss of axons and minimal endoneurial scarring will occur, so that the Tinel's will proceed distally.
- Recovery should be complete.

Sunderland third- and fourth-grade neural disruption:
- *Third-degree:* Axonal injury is associated with endoneurial scarring. Nerve is in continuity. It yields the most variable ultimate, clinically, recovery. The Tinel's sign is characteristically positive both at the injury site (due to entangled regenerating axons in scar) and also proceeds distally due to retubulating axon regenerates. There is erroneous alignment of axons.
- *Fourth-degree:* Nerve still in continuity, but at the level of injury, there is complete scarring so that no conduction will ever across. Scar prevents axonal regeneration into distal tubes. Tinel's sign is present at site of injury, but does not progress or proceed distally. Excision repair is the best option for treatment. These often result from severe stretch, traction, crush or nerve injection.

Neurotmesis (Sunderland fifth-degree): There is complete transection of the nerve and anatomical interruption of continuity of all neural tissues. They may result from severe stretch resulting into avulsion, but often they are result of penetrating injury or iatrogenic nerve damage during dissection.
- No spontaneous recovery expected without surgical intervention.
- Electromyogram (EMG) shows fibrillation potentials (FPs), and positive sharp waves (PSWs) (2–3 weeks postinjury).

Mackinnon's mixed injury (1992, colloquially called Sunderland's sixth-degree):
- This is a combination injury where the pattern of injury varies from fascicle to fascicle (among fascicles) and even along the length of the same fascicle.
- There is often a "neuroma in continuity" (Mackinnon) that needs resection anastomosis.
- Surgically, the challenge is to protect good fascicles and correct the damaged ones.
- Tinel's sign and recovery patterns differ according to pattern and severity of injury.
- This nerve injury demonstrates variable recovery patterns.

Management: Management of a clinically identified nerve injury depends on the type of injury (classification, complete/incomplete), associated injuries (fracture/crush/open injury/head injury), level of injury (stronger repair needed at mobile regions), availability of facilities and expertise, and duration of presentation. Diagnosis of injury should be confirmed using clinical examination and electrodiagnostic studies (EDS). The indications for primary open exploration and repair of a nerve are as follows:
- Nerve injury secondary to manipulation of fracture (absolute indication) that was previously absent.
- *Open fractures:* Here, the surgeon has a good chance to evaluate the nerve injury, explore them and others, and possibly do a primary repair before edema or infection sets in.
- Fractures in which satisfactory alignment is not possible by closed methods—obviously these fractures are taken-up in operation theater to be fixed primarily and simultaneous nerve injury should be explored and repaired.
- Fractures with associated vascular injury—again vascular exploration and repair will be a must so that the associated nerve injuries should be addressed.
- *Patients with multiple trauma:* This is a relative indication. Proceed with nerve exploration only if it is easily assessable and good expertise is available that could make a remarkable difference between primary repair and secondary repair.

Mid-arm median nerve injury is very uncommon in a child though it is commonly observed around elbow following supracondylar fracture. If the child sustained only nerve injury (without any other injury) that can be repaired, then neurorrhaphy should be done utilizing primary/delayed primary repair as the case may be. This option can be explored possibly up to 1 year following injury with guarded prognosis for later presentations. If there is defect in the injury site, then mobilization, transposition, neuromatous neurotization or other methods like grafting can be used to affect repair.

If more than 1 year has passed following injury and there are no signs of progression of nerve regeneration, then possibly parents can be counseled for need of tendon transfers later as the child is intelligent enough for retraining of muscles.

(For details on individual techniques of nerve repair and tendon transfer, kindly refer to Chapter 108 of Essential Orthopedics: Principles and Practice, 2nd edition.)

86. Describe the pathophysiology of peripheral nerve regeneration following axonotmesis. Detail the anatomy and contents of carpal tunnel with suitable diagram.

Ans: Axonotmesis is also known as second-degree injury as per classification. In *second-degree injury,* disruption of the axon is evident with WD distal to the point of injury and degeneration proximal for one or more nodal segments. The process of degeneration and regeneration (WD)—WD is also called anterograde degeneration. The proximal stump degenerates till nearest node of Ranvier from where new sprouts grow (2–5 sprouts within 6 hours). Distally, by 72–96 hours, the myelin lamellae are disrupted into small fragments known as myelin ovoids (bead-like pattern formation along the degenerating axon) described by Lubinska in 1977. This is the basic criterion used by investigators to define WD in various studies. There is increased neuronal permeability by the breakdown of blood-neuron barrier. Neuronal permeability approaches four times the normal over a course of 4 days.

Myelin and axonal debris are removed by resident and newly recruited inflammatory cells (monocytes/macrophages), microglia [in the central nervous system (CNS)] and by Schwann cells [in peripheral nervous system (PNS)]. The neurolemma of axons (the outermost layer of the neuron made of Schwann cells) does not degenerate and remains as a hollow tube. Immediately after axonal degeneration and fragmentation, Schwann cells in the PNS enter continuous cell division, degrade their own membrane, and phagocytose myelin and axonal debris. In CNS, the oligodendrocytes undergo apoptosis (Schwann cells are absent from CNS) and are not involved in chemotaxis of inflammatory cells so the process is delayed there. If an axon sprout reaches the tube, it grows into it and advances about 1 mm/day (3 cm/month, Steindler). The tubes provide pathways for the sprouting (regenerating) axons to follow to muscles and skin (topographic sensitivity, discussed below in role of Schwann cells). The Schwann cells then remyelinate, the newly formed axons which eventually reach and innervate the target tissue. Motor reinnervation is accomplished in a progressive manner from proximal to distal in the order in which nerve branches leave the parent trunk. Commonly, an advancing Tinel's sign can be followed along the course of the nerve usually at the rate of 1 inch per month, tracing the progression of regeneration.

Contact guidance and neurotropism (The term "neurotropism" implies an ability to stimulate nerve maturation): Contact guidance refers to homing of the nerve sprouts to the empty tubes. It has been seen that the motor axonal sprouts migrate toward the motor Schwann cell tubes, while sensory to their specific tubes preferentially. There is a possible role of the cellular adhesion molecules (CAMs) upregulation after axonotomy.

Diagram of carpal tunnel has been shown in **Figure 4A.12.2**.

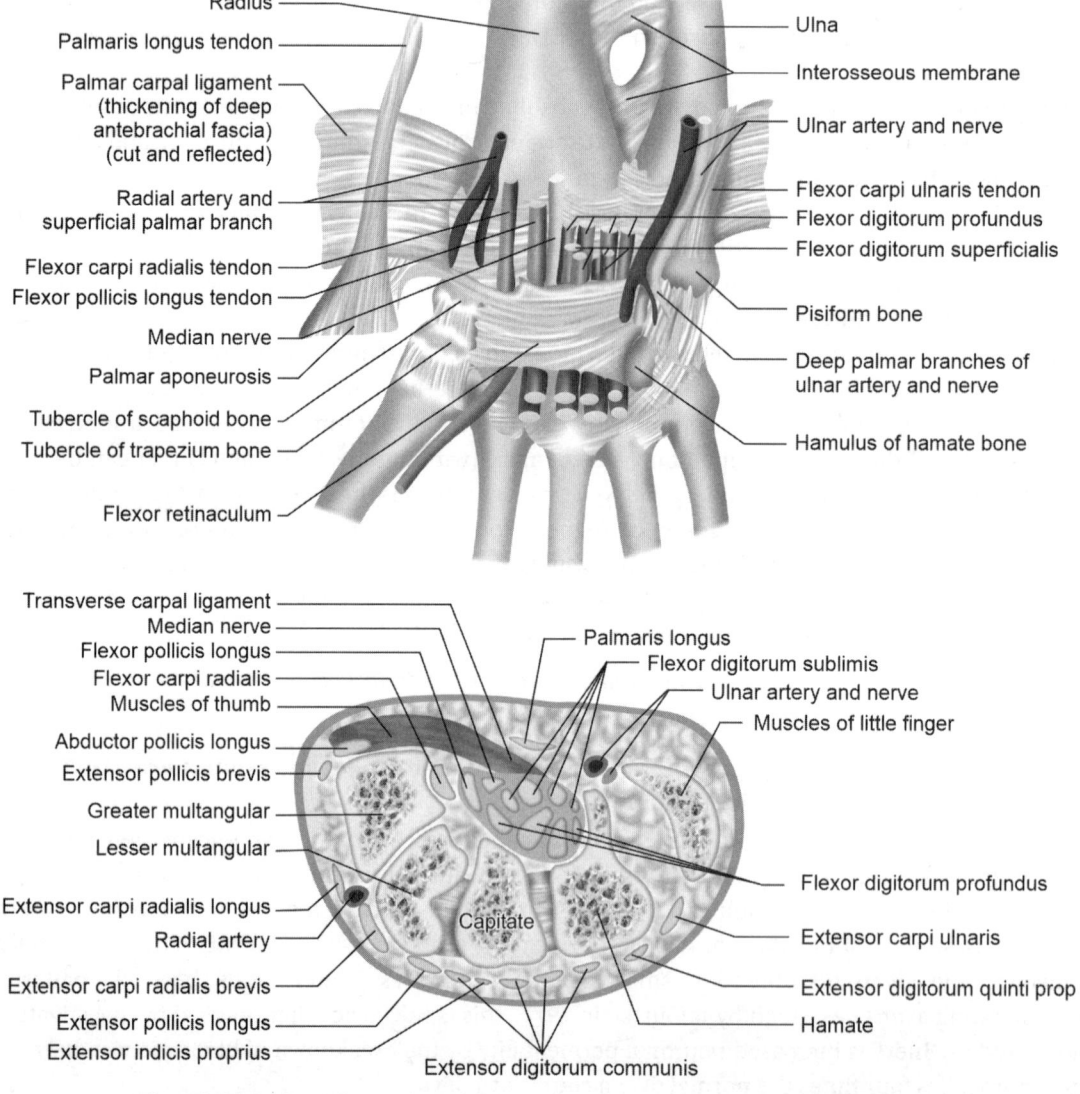

Fig. 4A.12.2: Carpal tunnel anatomy and various structures passing through it.

87. Explain the classification and EDS for nerve injuries.

Ans: For classification, kindly vide answer above.

Electrodiagnostic studies: EDS comprise of electromyography (EMG), nerve conduction studies (NCS), and strength-duration curve (SDC).

Electromyography is a technique of recording the electrical activity within a striated muscle belly by inserting needle in it. The electrical signal generated by the muscle tissue is detected by an electrode which is further amplified and monitored by oscilloscope or a speaker or recorded in system. Alterations in this signal are seen in various neuromuscular diseases. The signal detected by EMG reflects actions of motor unit (a motor neuron branch and the muscles fibers innervated by it). The EMG is used to:

- Demonstrate quantitative or qualitative changes in electrical activity of the muscle motor units in the resting state.
- Changes in electrical activity following direct or indirect electrical stimulation, or during voluntary or reflex motor unit activation.
- It can also be used to evaluate nerve conduction velocity and nerve terminal conduction time.

There are two common ways of performing EMG either using three small monopolar needle electrodes or by coaxial/concentric electrodes. The latter has the advantage of sampling a smaller volume of tissue than the monopolar design. Commonly, a record shows:

- A brief burst of electrical activity upon electrode insertion (normal in neutrally intact person). This activity is a result of sarcolemmal depolarization by electrode placement.
- After this, quiescence should return (straight line) except for voluntary muscle contraction or passive limb movement. Normal muscle is electrically silent at rest (embryonic muscle show fibrillation till ≈ 6 weeks of fetal life).
- In neural, neuromuscular or muscular disease aberrant patterns are seen. Changes in frequency, amplitude, and character of electrical signals occur and/or bursts of spontaneous electrical activity without stimulation may be noted. These changes are usually related to specific disease processes that can be recognized.
- In peripheral nerve injury, denervation to a group or region of muscles occurs. The muscle fibers develop spontaneous electrical activity due to the loss of innervation 5–7 days after injury represented as complex bizarre repetitive discharges. This baseline activity continues for a variable period until either reinnervation happens or muscle fibrosis ultimately occurs producing either reversal to near normal pattern of activity (reinnervation) or complete absence of electrical activity due to muscle fibrosis.
- Fibrillation and fasciculation waves are commonly seen in neuromuscular injury.
    - Fibrillation potentials could be in the form of PSW—monophasic waves with an initial positive deflection. These are frequently associated with denervation of tested muscles. They have characteristic appearance as above along with an irregular rate and rhythm. PSWs are produced by lack of inhibitory "feedback" (stabilization) that nerves normally exert on muscle fibers to maintain quiescence during the resting phase. PSW produces sound of "claps of distant thunder". They are initiated by insertion of a needle electrode into a muscle belly, but electrical activity continues in excess of that associated with electrode insertion "the bizarre repetitive discharges" heard as "rain on a tin roof". On an oscilloscope, they can be graded into increasing severity of four grades.
        - *Grade 1:* Rare occasional waves
        - *Grade 2:* Several
        - *Grade 3:* Abundant while
        - *Grade 4:* Innumerable filling the screen.
- *Endplate fibrillation potentials (EPFPs):* These are closely associated with the end-plate region. The end-plates become unstable following denervation and this causes aberrant membrane potentials that are picked up as fibrillations. This is different from PSW waves and has an initial negative deflection in the end-plate region, while in other areas of the muscle an initial positive deflection is noted. EPFP are mainly monophasic or biphasic in configuration. They appear usually within 8–14 days post injury, but may take 21 days in some cases. It is to be noted that as long as viable denervated muscle fibers are present, fibrillations will occur. With reinnervation, a marked decrease in fibrillation

occurs 2 weeks prior to reappearance of motor unit action potentials (MUAPs) of low magnitude. Polyphasic waves are also noted with reinnervation.
- Giant MUAPs are seen in a partially denervated muscle, which is additionally reinnervated by nearby nerve. There is decreased muscle recruitment with denervation.

Nerve conduction velocity (NCV): Normal conduction velocity in humans is approximately 50 m/sec (slightly more in sensory nerves). Motor nerve conduction velocity is more commonly measured although it is always better to measure both sensory and motor nerve velocities. Demyelization reduces conduction speed as is evident from the NCV in unmyelinated fibers that have nearly 10 m/sec of conduction velocity. Sunderland type I injury may show delay at the site of injury, but otherwise NCS and EMG is normal.
- Two sets of stimulating electrodes along the nerve trunk to be tested. A recording electrode is placed in a muscle belly known to be innervated by the nerve to be tested. After applying stimulus along the nerve, evoked muscle depolarization is noted. When the nerve is stimulated at two different points, the time difference between evoked potential can be determined. With a known distance between the two electrodes, the velocity of conduction along the nerve trunk can now be determined.
- Incomplete nerve injury only slightly alters the results of EMG and NCV testing that may not be discernible. Reduced amplitude in evoked potentials and/or prolongation of the potential evoked from a point distal to the injury site may be noted (due to delayed conduction in the injured fascicle). After complete transection, normal conduction in the distal stump is noted for 4–6 days post injury.

Strength-duration curve: A graph plotting the intensity of electrical stimulus to the length of time, it must flow to produce response. The SDC was first discovered by G Weiss in 1901. The curve is defined by rheobase and chronaxie (the strength-duration time constant). These curves are used to identify various neurological diseases and pathologies.
- *Rheobase (Rheos = current or flow; base = foundation):* It is the minimal amount of stimulus strength that will produce a response (action potential or muscle contraction) when applied indefinitely (practically a few milliseconds–300 milliseconds). It is used to measure membrane excitability. Louis Lapicque coined the term "rheobase" in 1909.
- *Chronaxie (chronos = time; axie = axis):* It is the stimulation duration that yields a response when stimulus strength is set to exactly 2X rheobase. For two nerves that have same rheobase, chronaxie gives an indication of relative excitability, this also holds true for sequential SDC plots done for neuropathic diseases. It is evident by right shift in the curve (showing poorer excitability).
- *F wave:* Stimulation of motor nerve and recording action potential from muscle supplied by it. The stimulus travels up the nerve to spinal cord then back to limb. It measures the conduction between nerve and spinal cord (others measure conduction within limb).
- *H-reflex:* In this case, afferent impulse travels up the sensory nerve and travels down motor nerve to produce discharge.
- Upward kink in SDC indicates partial denervation.

88. Draw a diagram of SDC and write about its clinical significance.

Ans: Strength-duration curve is a two dimensional (2D)-polygon graph plot between electrical stimuli of different intensities (y-axis) and the time needed (x-axis) by each stimulus to start the response in an excitable tissue (nerve/muscle) **(Fig. 4A.12.3)**. It indicates the strength of impulses of various durations required to produce a propagating electrical wave in the tissue. Not only the strength of stimulus but also its duration is important in generating an action potential (depolarization of the excitable tissue). Thus, it is the amount of charge delivered at the point (minus the leak or charge dissipation) that will determine if depolarization will happen or not. The amount of charge delivered is product of current and duration of application so a curve

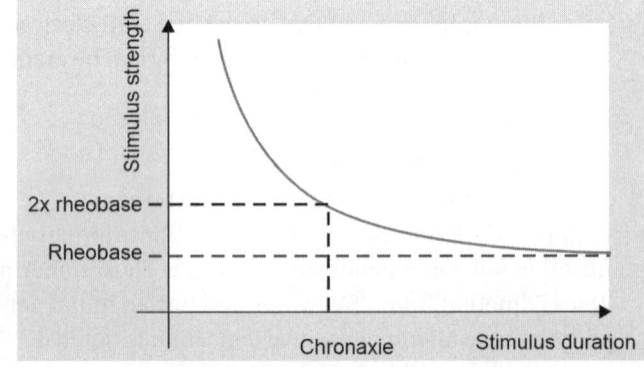

Fig. 4A.12.3: Strength-duration curve.

plotting the two is helpful. The normal curve shape is a reverse parabola. Two basic terms are commonly used to define various parameters in an excitable tissue:
- Rheobase is the minimal current amplitude of infinite duration (practically this duration is about 300 milliseconds) that results in the depolarization threshold of the cell membranes being reached—generating a muscle action potential or a depolarization wave in nerve
- Chronaxie (time constant of the cell membrane) is defined as the time on a SDC for twice the minimum (rheobase) current is needed for producing depolarization. Chronaxie is small at the nodes of Ranvier and axon initial segment and larger at the soma and dendrites.

  Shift in the curve to right or other curve abnormalities help one understand the anomalies of excitable tissue.
A. Right shift of SDC suggests reduced excitability of nerve (may occur with neuropathies) or demyelination or may be seen in slow excited nerve fibers when compared to fast nerve fibers.
B. At the same rheobase, two nerves with different excitabilities show different chronaxie.
C. Upward kink in SDC indicates partial denervation.
D. In case of neuropathies, sensory SDC representing properties of afferent nerve fibers are expected to be smooth also in case of partial denervation. Stimulus strength at sensory threshold is shown to be a reproducible measure of sensory deficit, increasing parallel to the degree of axonal failure **(Figs. 4A.12.4A and B)**.

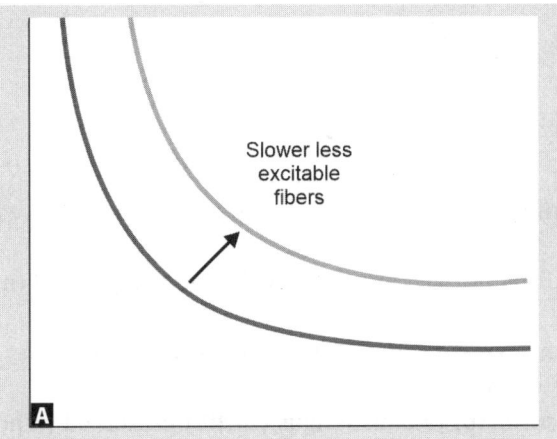
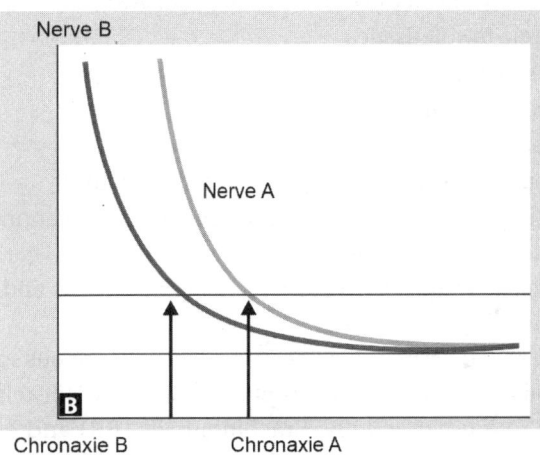

Figs. 4A.12.4A and B: Shift in strength-duration curve with respect to neural pathology (A) and type of nerve (B).

89. Describe changes in strength duration curve after nerve injury and following regeneration.
Ans:
- In peripheral nerve injury, denervation to a group or region of muscles occurs. The muscle fibers develop spontaneous electrical activity due to the loss of innervation 5-7 days after injury represented as complex bizarre repetitive discharges. This baseline activity continues for a variable period until either reinnervation happens or muscle fibrosis ultimately occurs producing either reversal to near normal pattern of activity (reinnervation) or complete absence of electrical activity due to muscle fibrosis.
- Fibrillation and fasciculation waves are commonly seen in neuromuscular injury.
    - Fibrillation potentials could be in the form of positive sharp wave (PSW)—monophasic waves with an initial positive deflection. These are frequently associated with denervation of tested muscles. They have characteristic appearance as above along with an irregular rate and rhythm. PSWs are produced by lack of inhibitory "feedback" (stabilization) that nerves normally exert on muscle fibers to maintain quiescence during the resting phase. PSW produces sound of "claps of distant thunder." They are initiated by insertion of a needle electrode into a muscle belly, but electrical activity continues in excess of that associated with electrode insertion "the bizarre repetitive discharges" heard as "rain on a tin roof." On an oscilloscope, they can be graded into increasing severity of four grades.
        - *Grade 1:* Rare occasional waves
        - *Grade 2:* Several

- *Grade 3:* Abundant while
- *Grade 4:* Innumerable filling the screen
- *Endplate fibrillation potentials (EPFP):* These are closely associated with the endplate region. The endplates become unstable following denervation and this causes aberrant membrane potentials that are picked up as fibrillations. This is different from PSW waves and has an initial negative deflection in the endplate region, while in other areas of the muscle an initial positive deflection is noted. EPFP are mainly monophasic or biphasic in configuration. They appear usually within 8–14 days post injury, but may take 21 days in some cases. It is to be noted that as long as viable denervated muscle fibers are present, fibrillations will occur. With reinnervation, a marked decrease in fibrillation occurs 2 weeks prior to reappearance of motor unit action potentials (MUAP) of low magnitude. Polyphasic waves are also noted with reinnervation.
- Giant MUAP are seen in a partially denervated muscle, which is additionally reinnervated by nearby nerve.
- There is decreased muscle recruitment with denervation.

90. Discuss radial nerve palsy.

Ans: The radial nerve may be damaged anywhere in its course from axilla to forearm. The nerve is formed in front of subscapularis muscle from posterior cord receiving components from all roots of brachial plexus (C5-T1). The nerve can be injured by one of the following mechanisms:
- Trauma to soft tissues
- Gunshot injury
- Fracture of humerus
- Intramuscular injection induced
- Iatrogenic (surgical fixation of humerus fracture).

For reconstruction purpose and clinical identification, terminology has been developed to classify the nerve injuries into various levels as follows:
- *Complete radial nerve palsy (very high):* Triceps and all distal muscles supplied by the nerve paralyzed (injury in axillary region).
- *High radial nerve palsy:* Triceps and often anconeus spared, but rest all other distal muscles paralyzed (injury around radial groove till it pierces septum, typified by Holstein–Lewis injury).
- *Low radial nerve palsy:* Brachioradialis (BR) and extensor carpi radialis longus (ECRL) preserved [≡ posterior interosseous nerve (PIN) palsy as in high both bone forearm fractures, local penetrating injuries like bullet injury, and iatrogenic injury during radial head/neck surgeries. Extensor carpi radialis brevis (ECRB) in only 58% cases is supplied by PIN so it may also be spared in some cases].

Functional deficit produced by nerve injury at various levels include (numbers indicate the five digits; one is thumb while five is little finger):
- Inability to extend fingers (1, 2, 3, 4, and 5) (low) and wrist (low + high).
- Inability to stabilize the wrist (wrist drop) and thumb (radial abduction of thumb) (low + high).
- Loss of grip strength (accessory forearm flexion) (high).
- Accessory forearm supination (very high).
- Accessory elbow flexion (high) there is mild weakness only as biceps is intact.
- Unstable carpometacarpal (CMC) joint (low + high).
- Sensory loss (radial two-thirds dorsal sensation) (high and above).
- The disabilities that need reconstruction for optimal functional gain are as not all listed above. The priority includes:
- Wrist extension
- Finger [metacarpophalangeal (MCP)] extension
- Combination of thumb extension and abduction.

After following the prerequisites of tendon transfer, surgeon can perform motor reconstruction using various options. Till the time patient awaits surgery, wrist can be managed in extension using static or dynamic cock-up splint. The motors supplied by median and ulnar nerves are all available. The various methods have their own merits and utility. Surgeon must always check for the presence of palmaris longus (PL) before proceeding for surgery as this will change the reconstruction plan completely. The procedures described in literature for motor reconstruction following the radial nerve palsy are:

- *Jones transfer:* Quite a lot of transfers done around the wrist for radial nerve palsy have been colloquially named Jones transfer, but in reality the tendon transfers described by Jones have met lot of criticism and are seldom if ever done. Jones transfer (and modified one also) uses both the primary wrist flexors causing unacceptable functional loss at the wrist.

Classical (1916):
1. Pronator teres (PT) → ECRL and ECRB
2. Flexor carpi ulnaris (FCU) → extensor digitorum communis (EDC) III–IV
3. Flexor carpi radialis (FCR) → extensor pollicis longus (EPL), EDC II, and extensor indicis proprius (EIP).

Classical (1921):
1. Pronator teres → ECRL and ECRB
2. Flexor carpi ulnaris → EDC III–IV
3. Flexor carpi radialis → EDC II, EIP, EPL, extensor pollicis brevis (EPB), and abductor pollicis longus (APL).

Modified Jones: PT → ECRB and rest as above.

- *Flexor carpi radialis transfer (of Starr; Brand; Tsuge):* This is the preferred transfer. Additionally, I usually tend to improve the thumb proximal stability by tenodesing the EPL to EPB.
1. Pronator teres → ECRB
2. Flexor carpi radialis → EDC II–V
3. Palmaris longus → rerouted APL.

- *Boyes transfer (superficialis transfer):* This is possibly the best alternative in cases with absent PL. However, surgeon should be meticulous enough to create large interosseous window to avoid tethering the tendons and developing adhesions and protect the interosseous nerve and artery. Complete FCU transfer is also an alternative but less preferred.
1. Pronator teres → ECRB
2. Flexor carpi radialis → APL and EPB
3. Flexor digitorum superficialis (FDS) III → EDC II–V via interosseous membrane
4. Flexor digitorum superficialis IV → EIP; EPL via interosseous membrane.

- *Flexor carpi ulnaris transfer (standard transfer, this is not modified Jones transfer):* This is the oldest described transfer for providing digital extension. The FCU is freed from fascial attachments to increase excursion, but mobilization is still limited by the innervation that enters muscle in its proximal 5 cm. Extensor digiti minimi (EDM) is included in transfer only if the EDC to little finger is absent. Classically, the FCU was itself used to motorize the EPL also, but over time the practice was discouraged (one muscle one function).
1. Pronator teres → ECRB
2. Flexor carpi ulnaris → EDC
3. Palmaris longus → rerouted EPL [the EPL is taken out of dorsal retinaculum (junction is made between PL and EPL in the region of snuff box). This gives a combination of abduction and extension force on thumb].

The disadvantage of FCU transfer is that there is slight radial deviation after the surgery and loss of the most powerful wrist flexor causes weakness of grip strength, this may be unacceptable to laborers.

Postoperatively, a plaster of Paris (POP) slab or splint is applied to immobilize the forearm in 30° pronation, wrist in 45° of extension, MCP joints in 0° of extension, and the thumb in maximum extension and abduction. Six weeks after surgery, the patient is explained the retraining and placed in a dynamic splint to obtain independent action for wrist and finger extension.

91. Clinical role of EMG in peripheral nerve injuries.
Ans: Answer already written in above questions.

92. Discuss the diagnosis of radial nerve palsy.
Ans:
- Clinically, first classify the nerve injuries into various levels as follows:
  - *Complete radial nerve palsy (very high):* Triceps and all distal muscles supplied by the nerve paralyzed (injury in axillary region)

- *High radial nerve palsy:* Triceps and often anconeus spared, but rest all other distal muscles paralyzed (injury around radial groove till it pierces septum, typified by Holstein–Lewis injury).
- *Low radial nerve palsy:* Brachioradialis (BR) and extensor carpi radialis longus (ECRL) preserved [posterior interosseous nerve (PIN) palsy as in high both bone forearm fractures, local penetrating injuries such as bullet injury and iatrogenic injury during radial head/neck surgeries. ECRB in only 58% cases is supplied by PIN so it may also be spared in some cases].

Functional deficit produced by nerve injury at various levels include (numbers indicate the five digits, one is thumb while five is little finger):
- Inability to extend fingers (1, 2, 3, 4, and 5) (low) and wrist (low + high).
- Inability to stabilize the wrist (Wrist drop) and thumb (radial abduction of thumb) (low + high)
- Loss of grip strength (Accessory forearm flexion) (high)
- Accessory forearm supination (very high)
- *Accessory elbow flexion (high):* There is mild weakness only as biceps is intact.
- Unstable CMC joint (low + high)
- Sensory loss (Radial two-thirds dorsal sensation) (high and above)

- *Electromyography (EMG) and nerve conduction velocity (NCV):* The goals of an electrodiagnostic examination are basically for:
  - Localization of lesion
  - Determine evidence of reinnervation or of ongoing axonal loss
  - Find the type of fibers involved motor, sensory fibers, or both
  - Define the extent of injury to neural tissue (axon loss, demyelination)
  - Define degree of axonal loss, the continuity of axon.

93. What is motor march?

Ans: This refers to the physiological recovery of progressively distal muscle groups in the neural supply of a nerve that gets sequentially recruited with advancement of neural recovery following injury. Nerves supply muscle in limbs in a "root-like" fashion. The branches keep coming off the peripheral nerve to supply the muscles along its path. When a nerve is damaged by trauma or otherwise, all neurological supply below the injury ceases causing paralysis due to loss of motor supply. During the physiological process of neurological recovery when nerve axons recover, they start migrating in the left over and cleaned neural tubes of the distal fragment of nerve. The axonal sprouts then grow up to the muscles that regain their innervation. This happens progressively along the course of nerve, thus supplying the muscles sequentially distally. Such motor recovery that happens over time is clinically assessed as motor march phenomenon.

Importance:
- Presence of motor march suggests neural recovery
- Motor march is absent in recovery from neurapraxia
- Motor march that stops suddenly from initial recovery suggests poor prognosis and formation of neuroma
- Grade 4 and above Sunderland injury to nerve usually have incomplete or absent motor march.

94. Discuss:
  A. Tardy ulnar nerve palsy
  B. Anterior interosseous nerve (AIN) syndrome.

Ans:

A. Tardy ulnar nerve palsy refers to traction injury or friction-induced slow fibrotic injury to nerve that develops over a period of time. Traction on nerve that ultimately decompensates causes damage to the axons and also induces intraneural fibrosis filling up the space created by thinning axons. Dislocation of unstable nerve (subluxating and dislocating nerve) and entrapment syndromes also have similar effect where friction causes neural fibrosis results in

loss of intraneural axons. The causes of tardy ulnar nerve palsy include etiologies resulting in traction, subluxation or entrapment of nerve at elbow that include:
- Malunited fractures of the lateral humeral condyle in children—late cubitus valgus causes ulnar nerve traction and injury. Cubitus varus deformity also produces tardy ulnar nerve palsy.
- Displaced fractures of the medial humeral epicondyle
- Dislocations of the elbow
- Contusions of the nerve
- *Subluxating ulnar nerve:*
  - Patients with shallow ulnar groove on the posterior aspect of the medial humeral epicondyle
  - Hypoplasia of the humeral trochlea
  - Inadequate fibrous arch.

Treatment for refractory tardy ulnar nerve palsy usually requires anterior transposition of the nerve less often combined with neurolysis. Conservative treatment is uncommonly prescribed (usually for 3 months), but includes avoiding prolonged elbow flexion in the workplace and elbow splinting in extension while sleeping.

(*Details of the treatment and procedures can be read from Chapter 107 of the book Essential Orthopedics: Principles and Practice, 2nd edition.*)

B. **Anterior interosseous nerve syndrome:** It is a compressive neuropathy involving the AIN manifesting as isolated motor deficit of muscles innervated by the nerve without any sensory symptoms. The compressive neuropathy is deemed as a syndrome now that has two specific presentations:
1. An acute self-resolving nontraumatic and inflammatory syndrome
2. A chronic often traumatic compression that needs release commonly.

Various causes can be attributed to the compression of AIN:
- Spontaneous compression
- Anatomic variations
- Trauma—supracondylar fractures (usually traction injury)
- Infections
- Iatrogenic cause—venipuncture, catheterization, etc. in cubital fossa
- Compartment syndrome and ensuing Volkmann ischemic contracture (VIC).

Clinical features: The palsy may be complete or incomplete. In a complete palsy, the following is usually observed.

Motor deficits only: Patient with complete AIN palsy loses motor function of all the four muscles supplied by AIN. The patient is unable to flex the interphalangeal (IP) joint of the thumb and the distal interphalangeal (DIP) joint of the index and long fingers. A typical pinch attitude occurs where patient is unable to make a ring by bringing together the tips of thumb and index finger and rather it transforms into a "peacock's eye".

Differential diagnosis:
- Partial median nerve lesion—so called pseudo-AIN syndrome.
- Attritional rupture of flexor pollicis longus (FPL) (seen in rheumatoids)
- Parsonage-Turner syndrome—brachial plexopathy
- Cervical spondylosis
- Bilateral AIN signs caused by viral brachial neuritis.

Nonoperative treatment is commonly effective for acute onset lesions while long-standing ones do not always improve with these measures. Empirically, observation, rest, and splinting in supination help if no organic lesion for compression is identified. Systemic disorders should be corrected (diabetes mellitus, alcoholism, and hypothyroidism). Additional vitamins like pyridoxine 100 mg for a few weeks (6–8 weeks) may be given.

Operative indication is needed for surgical decompression of AIN in case nonoperative measures fail or if the cause of nerve compression is evident (supracondylar spur and forearm mass). The cause of compression should be relieved and surgical decompression is done by a long incision beginning 5 cm proximal to elbow near the supracondylar spur to medially along the biceps tendon in forearm and further 5 cm into forearm. The nerve is decompressed all along.

95. Define entrapment syndrome. Enumerate various entrapment syndromes.

Ans: Definition: Entrapment syndrome or entrapment neuropathies are a group of disorders of the peripheral nerves that are characterized by pain and/or loss of function (motor and/or sensory) of the nerves as a result of chronic compression. Various entrapment syndromes are:
- Carpal tunnel syndrome
- Anterior interosseous nerve (AIN) entrapment
- Pronator syndrome
- Cubital tunnel syndrome
- Ulnar tunnel syndrome
- Radial tunnel syndrome/supinator syndrome
- Wartenberg syndrome
- PIN compression syndrome

96. Describe diagnostic tests for AIN syndrome.

Ans:

Clinical tests:
- *Motor deficits only:* Patient with complete AIN palsy loses motor function of all the four muscles supplied by AIN. The patient is unable to flex the interphalangeal (IP) joint of the thumb and the distal interphalangeal (DIP) joint of the index and long fingers. A typical pinch attitude occurs where patient is unable to make a ring by bringing together the tips of thumb and index finger and rather it transforms into a "Peacock's eye."
- *Electromyography (EMG):*
  - Helpful adjunct to clinical diagnosis and rule out differential diagnosis
  - Reveals abnormalities in the flexor pollicis longus (FPL), flexor digitorum profundus (FDP) index and middle finger, and pronator quadratus muscles (in 85% patients)
  - Can define the severity of involvement and can also rule out more proximal lesion

97. Draw diagrams of brachial plexus. How will you clinically differentiate pre- and postganglionic lesions?

Ans: For diagram of brachial plexus, see **Figure 4A.12.5**.

Preganglionic and postganglionic injuries should be differentiated for prognostication and management purpose. The preganglionic lesions (root avulsions) are irreparable and have worst prognosis while postganglionic lesions may either recover or can be surgically helped. The features that point to a preganglionic lesion (root avulsion) are:
- Presence of Horner's syndrome (see above)
- Burning pain or excessive pain out of proportion in an anesthetic hand
- Associated major vascular injury and/or fractures of the cervical spine
- Accompanying paralysis of scapular muscles or diaphragm
- Spinal cord dysfunction due to traction injury of the cord
- To diagnose root avulsions, the function of muscles innervated by the branches from the root level should also be assessed. Presence of function in this muscle group denotes an intact root with a good surgical prognosis.
  - *Serratus anterior:* The long thoracic nerve (C5–C7)
  - *The levator scapulae and the rhomboid muscles:* The dorsal scapular nerve (C5–C6)
  - Phrenic nerve (C4–C5)
  - Nerve to the subclavius muscle
  - Histamine test has been proposed to help diagnose a root or near root avulsion. Following the intradermal histamine injection if flare reaction (triple response) persists, then the lesion is a root avulsion as the ganglion is in continuity with the injured root. Ganglion is needed for flare response. If the flare was absent then ganglion is discontinuous with the injured root (a postganglionic lesion).

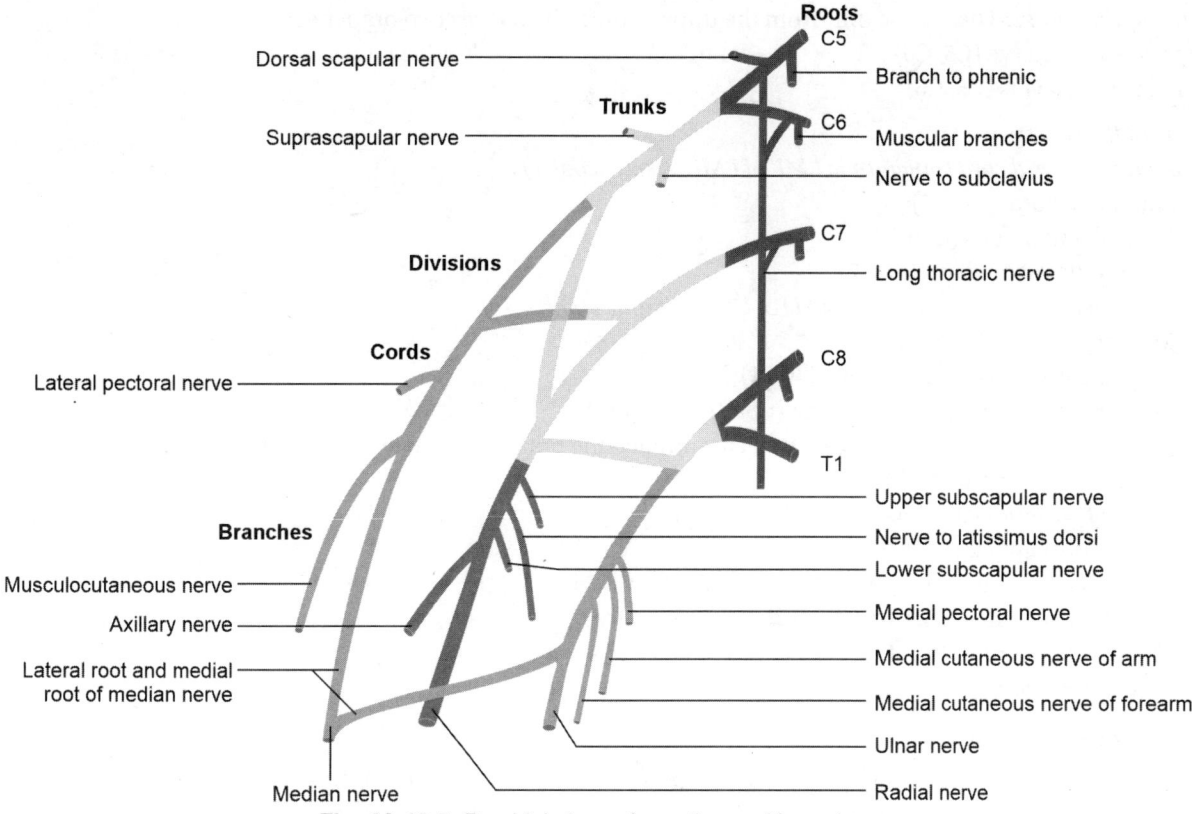

Fig. 4A.12.5: Brachial plexus formation and branches.

98. Discuss anatomy of brachial plexus.

Ans: The brachial plexus consists of roots, trunks, divisions, cords and branches *(See diagram in above question and use it in your answer)*.

Roots: These are constituted by the anterior primary rami of spinal nerves C5, C6, C7, C8 and T1, with contributions from the anterior primary rami of C4 and T2. The origin of the plexus may shift by one segment either upward or downward, resulting in a prefixed or postfixed plexus respectively. In a prefixed plexus, the contribution by C4 is large and that from T2 is often absent.

In a postfixed plexus, the contribution by T1 is large, T2 is always present, C4 is absent, and C5 is reduced in size. The roots join to form trunks as follows:

Trunks: Roots C5 and C6 join to form the upper trunk. Root C7 forms the middle trunk. Roots C8 and T1 join to form the lower trunk.

Divisions of the trunks: Each trunk (three in number) divides into ventral and dorsal divisions (which ultimately supply the anterior and posterior aspects of the limb). These divisions join to form cords.

Cords:
1. The lateral cord is formed by the union of ventral divisions of the upper and middle trunks (two divisions).
2. The medial cord is formed by the ventral division of the lower trunk (one division).
3. The posterior cord is formed by union of the dorsal divisions of all the three trunks (three divisions).

Branches: The roots value of each branch is given in brackets.

Branches of the roots:
1. Nerve to serratus anterior (long thoracic nerve) (C5, C6, C7)
2. Nerve to rhomboids (dorsal scapular nerve) (C5)
3. Branches to longus colli and scalene muscles (both C5-C8) and branch to phrenic nerve (C4)

Branches of the trunks: These arise only from the upper trunk which gives two branches:
1. Suprascapular nerve (C5, C6)
2. Nerve to subclavius (C5, C6)

Branches of the cords:
A. *Branches of lateral cord (mnemonic LML of LML Vespa Scooter):*
   a. Lateral pectoral (C5-C7)
   b. Musculocutaneous (C5-C7)
   c. Lateral root of median (C5-C7)
B. *Branches of medial cord (mnemonic M4U, i.e., 4M's and 1U):*
   a. Medial pectoral (C8, T1)
   b. Medial cutaneous nerve of arm (C8, T1)
   c. Medial cutaneous nerve of forearm (C8, T1)
   d. Ulnar (C7, C8, T1). C7 fibers reach by a communicating branch from lateral root of median nerve.
   e. Medial root of median (C8, T1)
C. *Branches of posterior cord (mnemonic ULNAR):*
   a. Upper subscapular (C5, C6)
   b. Nerve to latissimus dorsi (thoracodorsal) (C6, C7, C8)
   c. Lower subscapular (C5, C6)
   d. Axillary (circumflex) (C5, C6)
   e. Radial (C5-C8, T1)

99. Discuss Erb's palsy.

Ans: The **upper trunk** of the brachial plexus (C5 and C6) is most frequently injured, resulting in Erb palsy, which is characterized by the "waiter's tip" posture. Erb's palsy is the most common form of BRBPP. It has following components:
- Weak abductors and external rotators of the shoulder + weak flexors and supinators of the elbow + weak radial extensors
- Good power in internal rotators and adductors of shoulder + elbow extensors and wrist flexors (all supplied by the middle trunk and C7)
- Sensory loss occurs over the outer aspect of the arm and forearm.
- **Associated phrenic nerve damage** may cause diaphragmatic paralysis. Erb's palsy carries the best prognosis of recovery.

100. A. What are the types of brachial plexus injuries around birth? B. Describe the mechanism of causation. C. Discuss clinical features. D. What is the management of neglected undiagnosed Erb palsy in a 3-year-old child?

Ans:
A. Types of brachial plexus injuries around birth are given in **Table 4A.12.4**.

TABLE 4A.12.4: Types of birth-related brachial plexus injuries.

Primary involvement of brachial plexus	Roots involved	Narakas group	Description
Upper	C5, C6	I–Erb/Duchenne	Weakness of shoulder external rotation or abduction of arm and elbow flexion/supination
Middle	C5, C6, C7	II–Erb/Duchenne	Along with the findings for upper there is also elbow flexion/supination paralysis and loss of wrist extension
Lower	C8, T1	Klumpke's	Floppy hand with claw Deformity
Complete	C5, C6, C7, C8, T1	III–IV = III + Horner's	Flail arm

B. Mechanism of causation:

Birth-related brachial plexus palsy (BRBPP):
- *Excessive lateral traction on the brachial plexus at the time of delivery:* This mechanism is considered central to development of BRBPP as it also explains the concomitant presence of facial nerve palsy, fracture clavicle and humerus, and torticollis. The common cause is traction on the shoulder in shoulder dystocia when pressed against symphysis pubis.
- *The process of labor itself:* Maternal propulsive forces possibly are responsible for BRBPP otherwise unexplained. It appears that BRBPP in the absence of shoulder dystocia has a different mechanism and is a distinct entity.
- *In utero insult:* McFarland et al. suggested an in utero mechanism possibly resulting in BRBPP (compression, infiltration, ischemia, etc.). These may explain the bilateral occurrence of palsy in 10–20% cases.

Other less commonly accepted mechanisms for BRBPP include:
- Clavicular compression
- Fracture of the proximal humerus
- Neurotoxic effects of effusions escaping from the torn capsule of an injured glenohumeral joint

C. Clinical features in a newborn:
The clinical features depend on the part of plexus involved:
The upper trunk of the brachial plexus (C5 and C6) is most frequently injured, resulting in Erb palsy, which is characterized by the "waiter's tip" posture. Erb's palsy is the most common form of BRBPP. It has following components:
- Weak abductors and external rotators of the shoulder + weak flexors and supinators of the elbow + weak radial extensors
- Good power in internal rotators and adductors of shoulder + elbow extensors and wrist flexors (all supplied by the middle trunk and C7)
- Sensory loss occurs over the outer aspect of the arm and forearm.
- Associated phrenic nerve damage may cause diaphragmatic paralysis. Erb's palsy carries the best prognosis of recovery.

Total plexus palsy (C5–T1) presents with total paralysis of the arm and hand and is often associated with Horner's syndrome, and has a less favorable outcome. Horner's syndrome reflects injury to the preganglionic fibers serving the hand and neck region and is a valuable sign in severe traction injuries to the brachial plexus. The eye is examined for the presence of ptosis, loss of ciliospinal reflex, enophthalmos, miosis, and anhidrosis. If present, it indicates injury to the white rami of the T1 root to the stellate ganglion and signifies a partial or complete avulsion of the T1 root and other neighboring roots as well.

Pure lower plexus injuries: Klumpke's palsy (C8 to T1), involving only the lower trunk, is most uncommon, accounting for only 0.6% of all BRBPP. These injuries may cause claw hands, drop wrists and severe loss of hand function. Sensation is lost in the ulnar forearm and hand. There may be unilateral Horner's syndrome.

D. Management of neglected undiagnosed Erb palsy in a 3-year-old child: These unfortunate children need secondary reconstructive surgery. Unresolved upper trunk palsy is associated with internal rotation contracture of shoulder, glenohumeral dysplasia, subluxation, and dislocation. Various operative procedures including glenohumeral capsulorrhaphy, biceps tendon lengthening, tendon transfers, muscle releases, axillary nerve decompression, humeral osteotomy, anterior capsule release or a combination of these are variably applied.
- Posterior glenohumeral capsulorrhaphy tightens the posterior capsule surrounding the humeral head and repositions it anteriorly, addressing the posterior subluxation temporarily at least.
- For C5-C7 asymmetric nerve injury, biceps tendon lengthening or the Z-lengthening is an option to overpower triceps and add length to straighten elbow.
- Internal rotation contracture release involves sectioning internal rotators (the subscapularis and/or pectoralis major) and transferring functioning muscles [latissimus dorsi (LD) and/or teres major) to the posterior or posterosuperior rotator cuff
- *Modified Quad procedure:* Transfer of the LD muscle to give external rotation and abduction, transfer of the teres major muscle to stabilize the scapula, release of the subscapularis, pectoralis major and minor contractures and decompression and neurolysis of the axillary nerve.

- *Triangle tilt:* Osteotomy of the clavicle at the junction of the middle and distal thirds, osteotomy of the acromion process at its junction with the spine of the scapula, ostectomy of the superomedial angle of the scapula to reduce scapular winging and splinting of the extremity in adduction, external rotation, and forearm supination.

101. What is the clinical difference between pre- and postganglionic brachial plexus injury?

Ans: The preganglionic lesions (root avulsions) are irreparable and have worst prognosis while postganglionic lesions may either recover or can be surgically helped. The features that point to a preganglionic lesion (root avulsion) are:
- Presence of Horner's syndrome (see above)
- Burning pain or excessive pain out of proportion in an anesthetic hand
- Associated major vascular injury and/or fractures of the cervical spine
- Accompanying paralysis of scapular muscles or diaphragm
- Spinal cord dysfunction due to traction injury of the cord
- To diagnose root avulsions, the function of muscles innervated by the branches from the root level should also be assessed. Presence of function in this muscle group denotes an intact root with a good surgical prognosis.
    - *Serratus anterior:* The long thoracic nerve (C5–C7)
    - *The levator scapulae and the rhomboid muscles:* The dorsal scapular nerve (C5–C6)
    - Phrenic nerve (C4–C5)
    - Nerve to the subclavius muscle.

Histamine test has been proposed to help diagnose a root or near root avulsion. Following the intradermal histamine injection if flare reaction (triple response) persists, then the lesion is a root avulsion as the ganglion is in continuity with the injured root. Ganglion is needed for flare response. If the flare was absent then ganglion is discontinuous with the injured root (a postganglionic lesion).

4A.13 RHEUMATOID HAND (Q102–103)

102. Describe clinical features in rheumatoid hand and pathoanatomy of these lesions.

Ans: The rheumatoid hand deformities can be grouped as to those occurring at wrist, metacarpophalangeal (MCP) joint and fingers. The hand characteristically has a Z-deformity with ulnar deviation of fingers at MCP joint while radial deviation at the wrist. The proximal phalanges sublux or dislocate palmarly, lying beneath the metacarpal heads.

The palmar displacement of the proximal phalanges could occur from a combination of various causes like:
- Migration/displacement of the long flexor tendons
- Lax collateral ligaments of the MCP joint
- Attenuation of the dorsoradial support system
- Intrinsic muscles of hand undergo contracture or may be involved in spasm from joint inflammation.
- Destruction of the metacarpal heads.

Clinical features: The early stages of rheumatoid affection of small joints of hands are characterized by active inflammation and initial involvement of tendons and intrinsic muscles. The deformities are subtle at this stage but joint symptoms are prominent. Tendon involvement may cause pain, "triggering" and difficulty in active finger flexion. With poor remission permanent deformities may arise in the joints, the tendons, or the small muscles of the hands.
- Ulnar drift of the digits at MCP joints (combination of ulnar shift, ulnar deviation and volar dislocation, and also involves several deforming factors in combination). The pathoanatomic factors responsible are:
    - Synovitis of MCP and interphalangeal (IP) joints
    - Ulnar displacement of the extensor tendons, due to various factors:
        - Synovitis in the radial extensor triangle
        - Stretching of the radial-sided transverse extensor fibers (sagittal bands)
    - Increased ulnar pull tag due to lost extensor power (following tendon subluxation)
    - An increased ulnar pull of the junctura tendinae.
    - Intrinsic muscle tightness and a weakened dorsoradial support system

- *Radial deviation at wrist:* Produces vectorial forces favoring ulnar deviation at MCP joint. Rheumatoid involvement of the wrist leads to obligatory radial deviation of the metacarpals; the mechanism is not fully understood but may be due mainly to ulnar translocation and supination of the carpus. This produces abnormal vectorial force on the fingers pulling them into ulnar deviation.
- *Swan neck deformity (SND):* This is the most common finger deformity. The distal interphalangeal (DIP) joint is flexed and the proximal interphalangeal (PIP) joint is hyperextended (also termed as "recurvatum"). MCP flexion, although common in rheumatoid arthritis (RA) and other intrinsic-plus SND, need not be present. Hyperextension of the MCP joint and flexion at IP joint is termed as "Swan Neck Deformity of the thumb".
- *Boutonniere deformity:* The deformity is converse to SND with the PIP joint flexed and the DIP and MP joints hyperextended. The abnormal finger posture in RA starts with PIP joint flexion that leads to the changes in the other joints.

Pathoanatomy of SND: Zancolli has emphasized the fact that the two constituent deformities (PIP recurvatum and DIP flexion) are interrelated and are a logical consequence of the normal kinesiology of the digit. Any hyperextension of the PIP for any reason will secondarily produce flexion of the DIP. Conversely, a DIP flexion deformity produces hyperextension at PIP due to alteration of forces. The deformities also tend to vary equally in severity. The greater the recurvatum of the PIP, the greater is the flexion deformity of the DIP and vice-versa. Primary PIP hyperextension is more frequently a cause of SND as seen in RA. Mechanisms that contribute to the secondary DIP flexion from a primary PIP hyperextension.

- *Proximal interphalangeal* recurvatum relaxes the normal tension on the lateral extensor bands. These hence move centrally and dorsally. In such a lax position the bands lose ability to extend the DIP, which hence drops into flexion.
- The flexor digitorum profundus (FDP) is pulled by recurvatum of the PIP causing prominent flexion of DIP by the law of maintaining constant length.
- The mechanical advantage of FDP flexion at DIP produces equivalent mechanical disadvantage of the spiral oblique retinacular ligament (SORL) in extending the DIP.
- The last possible factor producing PIP recurvatum is the stretching of the capsule secondary to active synovitis or ruptured flexor digitorum superficialis (FDS) tendon, removing the restraint to PIP joint hyperextension (commonly seen in RA).

Pathoanatomy of Boutonniere deformity:
- Synovial proliferation due to RA in the PIP stretches and weakens the extensor mechanism: Full extension cannot be achieved.
- Also the effusion and distended joint due to the synovitis forces joint to go into partial flexion (position of maximum capsular volume).
- Over time the lateral bands are displaced volarly and the SORL are shortened. SORL shortening causes DIP hyperextension.
- The MP joint hyperextends to compensate increasing PIP joint flexion.

103. Discuss the management of various deformities of rheumatoid hand.

Ans:
- **Finger deformities:**
  - *Swan neck deformity (SND):*

The management is best discussed on the basis of Nalebuff classification as follows:
- *Nalebuff type I deformity:* Treatment focuses on correcting the proximal interphalangeal (PIP) hyperextension and hence the distal interphalangeal (DIP) secondarily corrects.
  - *Nonoperative:* Using silver rings (permits active PIP flexion and limits hyperextension of the PIP joint) or thermoplastic figure of 80 splints.
  - *Operative:*
    - Distal interphalangeal fusion along with PIP flexor tenodesis. Tenodesis is produced proximal to the A1 pulley by removing flexor digitorum superficialis (FDS) from the sheath creating a flexion deformity at the PIP.

- Spiral oblique retinacular ligament reconstruction ± dermodesis (removing elliptical skin wedge from volar aspect of the PIP and resuturing under tension).
- *Nalebuff type II deformity:* The treatment here is focused on relieving the intrinsic tightness that is produced due to malposition of the finger at metacarpophalangeal (MCP) joint.
  - Surgical resection of the lateral bands is done through which the lumbricals produce deformity. Ulnar extensor aponeurosis release is also done to prevent ulnar subluxation of the tendons and reduce extensor tightness. Silicone arthroplasty is done in cases of severe involvement of the MCP joint.
- *Nalebuff type III deformity:* The treatment focuses on restoration of passive motion to the PIP joint. The following measures help in achieving the goals:
  - *Proximal interphalangeal joint manipulation:* By doing a dorsal skin release distal to PIP joint and leaving the scar to heal over 2–3 weeks.
  - *Lateral band mobilization:* The lateral bands are freed from the central slip and PIP mobilized to full flexion completing the release passively.
  - *Ancillary procedure:* Flexor tenolysis may be needed in above additionally to provide adequate motor power.
- *Nalebuff type IV deformity:* Only salvage is possible for this type of deformity in the form of:
  - Arthrodesis of PIP joint is particularly useful for the index and middle fingers, because these digits need lateral stability when opposed to the thumb during pinch. Arthrodesis is also commonly done/preferred traditionally if concomitant MCP joint arthroplasty is being done (recently, however, arthroplasty has been favored concomitantly).
  - Arthroplasty is performed when the soft-tissue and ligamentous support is adequate especially for ring and small fingers, where mobility aids grasp.

Boutonniere deformity: There is specific classification of the Boutonniere deformity and its management can be better discussed by grade of deformity (mild, moderate, and severe).
- *Mild Boutonniere deformity:*
  - Minimal distortion of the joint positions and functional loss
  - Slight extensor lag (10–15°) at the PIP joint
  - Slight hyperextension at the DIP joint
  - No involvement of the MP joint

  Mild deformity is usually corrected by extensor tenotomy (usually limited) to increase DIP joint flexion.
- *Moderate Boutonniere deformity:*
  - Flexion deformity at the PIP joint increases to 30–40°
  - The MCP joint begins to hyperextend (compensatory mechanism).

  Moderate deformity is managed by reconstruction of the extensor mechanism to shorten the central slip and moving the lateral bands dorsally in their native position (repositioning). For success of soft-tissue reconstruction good dorsal skin, smooth joint surfaces, functional flexor tendons and flexible PIP joint should be present. Wrist deformity should be corrected before addressing the PIP extensor mechanism.
- In "severe Boutonniere deformity," the PIP joint can no longer be passively extended. This stage is treated by fusion of the joint or arthroplasty. Fusion of the PIP joint is performed in a functional (flexed) position. Functional position of PIP flexion increases from the index finger (25°) to small finger (40°). PIP joint arthroplasty is acceptable option if the extensor mechanism is healthy enough to be repaired. As mentioned for SND arthroplasty is useful for Boutonniere deformities of the small and ring fingers to improve grip strength.
- **MCP joint involvement:**

  The various methods for management of rheumatoid MCP joint affection are as follows:
  - Conservative management by medications [disease-modifying antirheumatic drugs (DMARDs) or biologics] hardly improves established deformities but is the most important aspect in prevention of deformities.
  - *Operative management:*
    - *Synovectomy:* Typically done for joint swellings not remitted by >6 months of medical therapy. Joint erosions should be absent.
    - *Extensor tendon relocation:* This is usually combined with synovectomy for patients who also demonstrate ulnar subluxation of the tendon and early ulnar drift. The extensor expansion is release from the ulnar aspect (tight

side) while radial imbrications or tightening is done. Overtightening should be avoided to avoid loss of MCP flexion. This should be performed early in young patients with a stable disease (remission or partial remission). In a progressive disease, the procedure may ultimately fail. Patient should be counseled that though he may not be actively able to extend fingers, the procedure will relieve him from extensor lag at least.
  - *Intrinsic balancing:* This is done by release of intrinsic muscles that relaxes the dorsal digital expansion. Crossed intrinsic transfer from ulnar side to radial side is another option taking not to excessively tension the dorsal expansion.
  - MCP joint replacement is by far the most popular method of restoring alignment and flexibility of MCP joint. The procedure is combined with ulnar extensor expansion release and tendon balancing. The metacarpal head and the base of proximal phalanx are cut perpendicular to the long axis. Shafts are reamed and the prosthesis is seated. The osteophytes and synovium should be debrided before prosthesis fitting using "no touch technique".
- *Wrist joint:* Ideally wrist should be managed before development of deformity at the joint but this is neglected most often. In most cases, wrist joint is addressed as a composite hand reconstruction plan where correction of finger deformities should follow wrist deformity correction.
  - *Synovectomy:* It helps to control pain and reduce disease load. It may also help in reducing joint destruction if managed well in accordance with medical management.
  - *Wrist fusion:* This is a salvage procedure but a preferred option to sturdily balance the wrist. Functional loss due to arthrodesis still produces better results for functional gained by the procedure and stability. This is hence a preferred option for composite hand and wrist reconstruction of late and neglected cases.
  - Interposition arthroplasty has not been well-accepted by orthopedic community.
  - *Wrist arthroplasty:* This is a growing field and not many replacements have been done world over compared to large joint replacements. The primary reason is the late introduction of the implants and patients already spend so much on other joint replacements that this comes in later stage of reconstructive ladder; cost is also a deterrent.
- *Thumb deformity:* The treatment of specific deformities depends on the severity of disease in each involved joint and the type of deformity (as follows). In general, fixed joint deformities with bony destruction are usually more amenable to fusion than arthroplasty.
  - *Type I deformity:* MCP joint synovectomy + extensor pollicis longus (EPL) rerouting in early cases. In late cases with 90–90 deformity, it is better to fuse the MP joint or do an arthroplasty.
  - *Type III (and type II):* Metacarpal adduction correction is the focus of treatment of type III deformity (and type II also but is uncommon to see). Block arthrodesis to restore abduction of metacarpal [± carpometacarpal (CMC) arthrodesis] is done that usually corrects the secondary deformities. If not, then MCP hyperextension is corrected by capsulodesis, sesamoidesis, or arthrodesis (if fixed deformity or minimal active flexion is present) in a slightly flexed position.
  - *Type IV deformity:* It is managed by stabilizing the MCP joint and correcting the adduction contracture by Z-plasty. Ulnar collateral ligament reconstruction is done to stabilize the MCP joint but if not possible then an arthrodesis usually helps (arthroplasty can be also considered). Thumb abduction can be efficiently done by the thenar muscles then.
  - *Type V deformity:* Best corrected by stabilization of the MP joint by a capsulodesis, sesamoidesis or fusion (if fixed deformity or minimal active flexion) in a slightly flexed position. Volar plate advancement is a good option or even arthroplasty is now being preferred.
  - *Type VI deformity:* Deformity is treated by fusion of the involved joints in functional position. Arthroplasty has no role at all. The IP joint should be fused at 0–20° of flexion.

4A.14 DUPUYTREN'S CONTRACTURE (Q104)

104. Discuss Dupuytren's contracture.

Ans: Dupuytren's contracture (DC) is a thickening and hypertrophic fibrosis (proliferative fibroplasia) of the palmar aponeurosis and its extensions into the digits (palmodigital extensions). It is the most common contracture of the palmar aponeurotic fascia, giving rise to flexion deformities of the distal palm and fingers. The fascia contains strands of fibers, like cords, that run from the palm upward into the fingers. In DC, these cords tighten, or contract, causing the fingers to curl forward. In severe cases, it can lead to crippling hand deformities.

Pathogenesis/Etiology: Dupuytren's contracture is the most common inherited connective tissue disease of humans and is hypothesized to be associated with aberrant wound healing of the palmar fascia. Both inherited and sporadic forms have been identified.
- Incidence among affected families has been reported to approach 70%. Autosomal dominant form of the disease has been mapped to the long arm of chromosome 16.
- Although, the genetic predisposition in Dupuytren's disease has been well established, the condition is seen more commonly in patients with epilepsy, patients who use alcohol and tobacco, and patients with diabetes, cirrhosis, and human immunodeficiency virus (HIV) infection. Diabetes could be a pathological cause as the combination of carpal tunnel syndrome (CTS), trigger finger, and DC has been increasingly found in the diabetic population.

The underlying etiology is poorly understood but the following are important contenders:
- Trauma may be a possible cause and explain a male gender bias.
- Dysregulation of multiple structural proteins like type I and type III collagens, the extracellular matrix (ECM) proteins fibronectin, tenascin C, and laminin.
- The various other putative pathogenic pathways and proteins possibly involved in the pathogenesis are listed below:
  - Oxidative stress molecules, including superoxide radical (O_2^-), hydrogen peroxide (H_2O_2), and the hydroxyl radical (OH^-).
  - Serum/glucocorticoid-regulated kinase (SGK) message is downregulated in DC.
  - Downregulation of Chitinase-3-like 2 (CHI3L2).

Pathology: The condition belongs to larger group of superficial fibromatosis (that may involve hand or foot) and begins as fibrous nodules in the palmar fascia. The earliest change is the thickening of Grapow's fibers (these connect the fascia to dermis). Initially, this tissue is hypercellular and vascular. Local proliferation continues to form a nodule or if skin retraction occurs then a pit. The palmar aponeurosis and the various ligamentous bands, when involved in the disease process, form the classical nodules and cords, giving rise to the characteristic flexion contractures of Dupuytren's disease. The pathoanatomy in fingers is much complex. The two fibrotic structures, which are clearly identifiable in Dupuytren's disease, are the nodule and the cord.
- Nodule is a relatively vascular tissue containing a dense population of fibroblasts, with a high proportion being myofibroblasts. As the nodule hardens, it gets adhered to subcutaneous tissue and skin, causing the cord formation leading to flexion contracture of the metacarpophalangeal joint (MCP) and proximal interphalangeal (PIP) joints.
  - In the palm, they are located adjacent to distal palmar crease; while in fingers, the nodules are commonly found at PIP joint or at the base of fingers.
- The cord is a collagen-rich structure that is relatively avascular and acellular and with a lesser (but still significant) abundance of myofibroblasts.
  - The cords involve the palmar, palmodigital, and digital regions.

Dupuytren's diathesis implies a more advanced form of the disease with multiple afflictions, presence of anyone should indicate a need to search for the other two:
1. "Knuckle pads" (Garrod nodes, thickening over the extensor surfaces of the PIP joints)
2. Plantar fibromatosis (Ledderhose disease)
3. Fasciitis of the penis (Peyronie's disease).

Clinical features: The condition is commonly seen in Caucasians and occurs more commonly in men between 50 years and 70 years of age. It has a familial tendency (autosomal dominant with variable penetrance).
- The most commonly affected digit is the ring finger followed by pinky finger (then middle and index, uncommonly thumb), but any finger can be affected.
- Pain is never a characteristic feature. It is the deformity that concerns patient. Patient generally presents with a nodule in the palm proximal to the base of the ring finger that has over the course of months or years become a thickened

fibrous cord running along the palm to the fingers. Nodules typically are painless, unless nerve compression or tenosynovitis is present.
- Over time, as the contracture develops, the fingers become clawed as they are pulled toward the palm. This leads to the flexion of the digit. The skin is adherent to this fibrous cord. Subsequently, other digits are involved and the patient has painful nodules in the pretendinous bands of palmar fascia of the ring and little fingers. Flexion contracture of the MCP joint occurs first, followed by finger contractures. The hand bows and the fingers are completely pulled against the palm gradually. This produces difficulty in maintaining hygiene due to inability to open up the hand.
- Often, the skin of the palm is dimpled and puckered.

Associated conditions are:
- Plantar nodules
- Peyronie's disease
- Diabetes
- Epilepsy
- Chronic alcoholism
- Smoking
- Pulmonary tuberculosis (TB)
- Vascular insufficiency.

Physical examination:
- Firm nodules (that may be tender to palpation) are closely adherent to the skin and their movement with finger motion suggests an association with the tendon and not DC.
- Thinning of subcutaneous fat
- Painless cords proximal to the nodules causing finger flexion contracture
- Active finger extension causes skin blanching
- Pits or grooves represent skin adherence to the underlying fascia by vertical bands through the fibrous tissue
- Garrod's nodes are tender knuckle pads over the back of (dorsal aspect) the PIPs in a more aggressive disease. These occur in 40-50% of patients.
- Ledderhose disease is concomitant involvement of plantar fascia seen in 5-30% patients and should be always examined, as this is associated with poorer prognosis.
- Presence of MCP and PIP joint contractures. True contracture is difficult to assess but objectively measure and record the degree of flexion deformity and also assess compensatory distal interphalangeal (DIP) joint hyperextension.
- *Hueston "table top test":* If the patient is unable to lay the palm flat on a table top, the findings are considered positive. We do not consider this to be additionally of any help. It used to be a good guideline to decide need of surgical release. Positive table top test indicates flexion contracture of 30-40° at MCP joint, but is also affected by finger joint contractures. It has been found that the surgical release of PIP contractures yields better functional outcome, while decisions based on MCP joint contracture either yield no improvement or worsening of contracture. So, now it seems that table top test that basically is an indirect indicator of MCP contracture may be useless.

Treatment: Spontaneous resolution does not occur, so nonoperative and operative regimes are followed depending on stage of disease, physician experience, and availability of resources.

Nonoperative treatment: A lot of attempts to improve nonoperative management have occurred due to dismal overall findings of operative management.

Physical therapy: Stretching with the application of heat and ultrasonographic waves may be helpful in the early stages of DC.
- A custom splint or brace to stretch the fingers passively, worn over the day may slow progression.
- Range of motion (ROM) exercises should be performed several times a day.
- Postsurgical physical therapy is very important and comprises of wound care, massage, passive stretching, active ROM exercises, and splinting.

Occupational therapy: These make the patient learn adaptive techniques and to use assistive devices that enhance functional abilities (like to open jars, wear clothes despite contractures).

Local injections:
- *Corticosteroid injection:* It may be effective for inflammatory tender nodules. The injection softens nodule and reduces inflammatory symptoms.
- γ-interferon injections
- Use of creams based on vitamin E and dimethyl sulfoxide
- *Clostridial collagenase injection:* Direct injection of clostridial collagenase into nodules and cords has been shown to cause lysis and rupture of digital cords, releasing MCP joint and PIP joint contractures.

Oral drugs like allopurinol.

Operative treatment: The best-known treatment is surgical. The surgical treatment is a partial or total excision of the palmar fascia depending on the extent of involvement. The contracture at the MCP joint is always correctable whereas the contracture at the PIP joint is more difficult to correct completely. The surgical procedures used in treatment of DC are:

- *Subcutaneous fasciotomy [also known as percutaneous needle fasciotomy (PNF)]:* This is the simplest of the procedures that has been popularized to relieve contracture in frail elderly who may be unable to bear anesthetic insult. It may also be done as a temporizing measure to improve skin hygiene before any definitive surgery or in those not willing for limited fasciectomy. It is usually performed as an outpatient procedure under local anesthesia. A large 16-gauge needle is used (as is available in some blood transfusion sets) to create multiple puncture sites and sectioning of the cord using the needle bevel. PNF is contraindicated in infiltrating disorders that would cause progressive and extensive contractures; rapid recurrence in a young patient, difficult to access multiple cords, and long-standing digital disease that would cause contractures additionally in other structures and postsurgical recurrence.
- *Regional fasciectomy (open fasciectomy):* It is used to manage severe cases of DC. It is an outpatient procedure performed under local anesthesia. An incision is made over the diseased cord and direct visualization of the cord and neurovascular structures is possible. The offending cord is divided at a point immediately underlying the skin incision. Fasciotomy is usually most successful for MCP flexion contracture. The recovery is rapid, but the recurrence rate is high. Open fasciotomy is usually reserved for patients who cannot tolerate a more extensive procedure.
- *Limited fasciectomy:* Popularized by Hueston (Hueston, 1961); in this procedure, only the involved fascia is removed, preserving the overlying skin. This is the most widely used technique. Skin incisions may be transverse, longitudinal, or diagonal/zigzag with Z-plasty, Y-V-plasty, and Bruner-type zigzag incision.
- *Extensive radical fasciectomy:* This involves extensive resection of the palmar and digital fascia. This technique though portended to be more successful due to extensive release of the pathological tissue but the recurrence rates have been similar to limited fasciectomy but with significantly higher complication rates. Patients are also prone to prolonged postoperative edema and stiffness.
- *Dermofasciectomy:* Now, it is known as the open palm technique (McCash, 1964). Here, excision of the fascia and overlying skin is done. The wounds may be closed using skin grafts or left open. Skin grafts may reduce disease recurrence. Because of the radical nature of this procedure, it is usually reserved for patients with recurrent or severe disease.
    - The technique involves making two incisions, one from the DIP joint of the affected digit to the distal palmar flexion crease joined to a transverse palmar incision forming an "L" shape.
    - A selective fasciectomy is done with partial closure of the incision site to maintain some flexibility. The open portion is then covered with a full-thickness skin graft harvested from the hypothenar eminence. Padded dressing is applied with support to the skin graft and an extension splint is maintained to prevent any recurrence of contracture.
    - In another technique, the harvested graft is applied after 4 days in another setting whence some vascularity and granulation tissue develops at the open raw surface. This also gives advantage of performing the first wound inspection simultaneously and then closing the wound for adequate time to allow graft to settle. The palm is re-splinted for next 1 week till wound inspection.
- Segmental aponeurectomy/fasciotomy of Moermans is a procedure that is intermediate between regional (open) fasciotomy and limited fasciectomy. Segments (1 cm in length) of fascia are excised to relieve contractures albeit partially.
- *Amputation:* Sometimes, the contracture is so severe as to form an unyielding stricture of rolled up finger into palm that precludes any other function from the hand including activities of daily living. In such severe and neglected cases

that often present late or else in multiple recurrences after surgery, amputation may be indicated. The threshold is particularly low for little finger. Amputation is by no means any benign surgery and acceptance may be low particularly due to complications like neuroma formation, neurogenic pain, increased stump sensitivity, development of reflex sympathetic dystrophy, reduced grip strength, and even proximal recurrence (1%) of disease. The cosmetic or psychological issues always exist with amputation.
- *Joint fusion:* This is considered a more cosmetic and ethical procedure to amputation. PIP fusion is a useful alternative to amputation. This is, however, achieved by shortening bone ends to account for the tight volar structures and then fused in a functional position.

4A.15 FLEXOR TENDON INJURY (Q105)

105. Flexor zones of hand. Describe the clinical features and management of a 2-month-old with zone 2 injury.

Ans: The synovial sheaths mark the various classically described zones for flexor tendons (**Fig. 4A.15.1**):
- Zone I represents the region distal to the synovial sheath occupied only by flexor digitorum profundus (FDP) tendon. It is represented by insertion of FDP tendon at distal phalange to insertion of flexor digitorum superficialis (FDS) at middle phalanx (MP).
- Zone II (no man's land) extends the length of the fibro-osseous sheath (insertion of FDS at MP to A1 pulley) of the digit occupied by both FDS and FDP. The tendons are nourished by synovial fluid within the sheath and through direct vascular inflow by way of the vincula dorsally. So repairs should avoid approaching the tendons dorsally.
- Zone III extends from the proximal aspect of the digital synovial sheath to the distal aspect of the transverse carpal ligament. For pinky finger, the zone III is considered to begin with A1 pulley as the sheath may be continuous in the palm.
- Zone IV (enemy territory) lies beneath the transverse carpal ligament—here it is easy to expose the tendons but repair often leads to cross adhesions. Also the presence of median nerve and closed space for tendon healing it is given the name of "enemy territory" as this will be the region where you would like your enemy to get injured.
- Zone V is the area proximal to transverse carpal ligament—injuries here involve multiple structures and neurovascular contiguity/repair takes a precedence. This region is often affected in crush injuries where extensive laceration of muscles has been colloquially called "Spaghetti wrist/full house injuries".

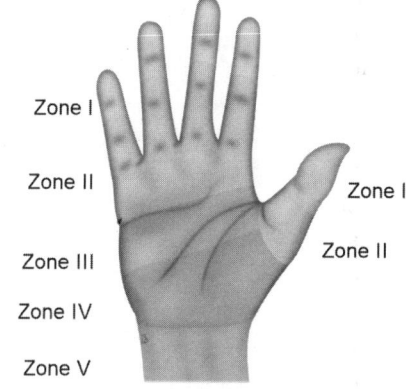

Fig. 4A.15.1: Flexor tendon zones of hand.

Management for neglected zone 2 injuries: There is a high chance that the repair is not possible as the cut ends would have retracted, contracted and hypertrophied. Tendon grafting is the best possible option in this scenario. This can be done as a single-stage or a double-stage technique. Mostly for cases with intact pulley system single-stage tendon graft using palmaris longus tendon or plantaris tendon if the former is absent suffices. There are a few prerequisites that must be fulfilled before tendon grafting procedure:
- There should be no extensive scarring and hand should be supple. Passive joint movements should be nearly normal.
- Circulation should be adequate.
- At least one digital nerve of the finger should be intact.
- Cooperative patient.

Tubiana recommended some principles for a successful tendon grafting that hold true for both primary procedure and two-staged one but especially true for the former.
- Only one tendon for one finger.
- Do not sacrifice intact superficialis tendon.
- Graft should be of smaller caliber.
- Ends of tendon graft should be fixed away from tendon sheath.
- Save as much pulleys as possible.

Two-stage tendon grafting—if the tendon bed and peritendinous tissue are badly disrupted so that the gliding sheath for tendon is not available and/or pulley system is damaged, place a silicone sheath in place (as spacer) so that pseudosheath develops around it which will act as tendon sheath for the future graft preserving or reconstructing A2 and A4 pulley. It is often difficult for the surgeon to know beforehand the condition of flexor sheath (which is deemed normal in fresh cases). But if one finds excessive fibrosis, poor tendon bed or incompetent pulley then it is better to do a two-staged procedure. One should preserve as much of the flexor sheath as possible in stage I. Stage II is performed at least 3 months after; requires extrasynovial grafts from palmaris longus (present in 85% population) or plantaris (present in 93% population) or toe extensor passed through the formed tunnel using railroad technique. The formed pseudosheath should never be opened proximal to distal interphalangeal joint. The tendon graft is attached to the distal end of silicone implant and pulled proximally into forearm wrist incision. The distal graft is secured to bone using suture anchors. The motor tendon graft is then sutured in the wrist wound using weaving technique.

4B. LOWER LIMB

4B.1 CONGENITAL, GENETIC, AND DEVELOPMENTAL DISORDERS OF LOWER LIMB (Q1–45)

1. Describe in brief development of proximal end of femur.

Ans: Ossification of the femur begins in the 7th fetal week. In early childhood, only a single proximal femoral chondroepiphysis exists. During the first year of life, the medial portion of this physis grows faster than the lateral, creating an elongated femoral neck by 1 year of age. The capital femoral epiphysis begins to ossify at approximately 4 months in girls and 5–6 months in boys. The ossification center of the trochanteric apophysis appears at 4 years in boys and girls. The proximal femoral physis is responsible for the metaphyseal growth in the femoral neck, whereas the trochanteric apophysis contributes to the appositional growth of the greater trochanter and less to the metaphyseal growth of the femur. Fusion of the proximal femoral and trochanteric physis occurs at about the age of 14 years in girls and 16 years in boys. The confluence of the greater trochanteric physis with the capital femoral physis along the superior femoral neck and the unique vascular supply to the capital femoral epiphysis makes the immature hip vulnerable to growth derangement and subsequent deformity after a fracture.

The neck represents the upper end of the shaft as it ossifies from primary center.

The epiphyseal line of the head coincides with the articular margins, except superiorly where a part of the monoarticular area is included in the epiphysis for passage of blood vessels to the head. The plane of this epiphysis changes from oblique to a more vertical one with age.

2. Classify congenital skeletal limb deficiencies.

Ans: Frantz and O'Rahilly classification of congenital long bone deficiencies (1961) is a widely used system that describes deficiencies as terminal or intercalary. In terminal deficiencies, there is an amputation with no body parts distal to the site. In intercalary deficits, a middle segment is missing, but the distal segments are present. Both may be transverse or longitudinal, for example, complete absence of a hand at the wrist is a terminal transverse deficiency while presence of hand without a radius or ulna is an intercalary transverse deficiency.

- *Terminal deficiencies*: No unaffected parts distal to and in line with deficient portion
  - *Transverse*: Defect extends transversely across entire width of limb
  - *Paraxial*: Only preaxial or postaxial portion of limb is absent
- *Intercalary deficiencies*: Middle portion of limb is deficient, but proximal and distal portions are present
  - *Transverse*: Entire central portion of limb absent with foreshortening
  - *Paraxial*: Segmental absence of preaxial or postaxial limb segments; intact proximal and distal.

3. What is the Pappas classification for congenital femoral deficiency? What is the management protocol according to the Pappas classification?

Ans: The nine Pappas classes along with management protocol are described in **Table 4B.1.1**.

TABLE 4B.1.1: Pappas classes along with management protocol.

	1	2	3	4	5	6	7	8	9
Femoral shortening (%)	–	70–90	45–80	40–67	48–85	30–60	10–50	10–41	6–20
Femoral-pelvic abnormalities	• Femur absent • Ischiopubic bone structures underdeveloped and deficient	• Femoral head absent • Ischiopubic bone structures delayed in ossification	• No osseous connection between femoral shaft and head • Femoral head ossification delayed	Femoral head and shaft joined by irregular calcification in fibrocartilaginous matrix	• Femur incompletely ossified, hypoplastic, and irregular	• Distal femur short, irregular, and hypoplastic	• Coxa vara • Hypoplastic femur • Proximal femoral diaphysis irregular with thickened cortex	• Coxa valga • Hypoplastic femur • Femoral head and neck smaller • Proximal femoral physis horizontal	• Hypoplastic femur

Contd...

Contd...

	1	2	3	4	5	6	7	8	9
Femoral shortening (%)	–	70–90	45–80	40–67	48–85	30–60	10–50	10–41	6–20
		• Lack of acetabular development		• Acetabulum may be absent • Femoral condyles maldeveloped • Irregular tuft on proximal end of femur (rare)		• Midshaft of femur abnormal	• Irregular distal femoral diaphysis	• Lateral femoral condyle deficiency common • Valgus distal femur	• Abnormality of femoral condyles common, with associated bowing of shaft and valgus of distal femur	
Associated abnormalities	Fibula absent	• Tibia shortened • Fibula, foot, knee joint, and ankle joint abnormal	• Tibia shortened 0–40% • Fibula shortened 5–100% • Patella absent or small and high riding • Knee joint instability common • Foot malformed	• Tibia shortened 0–20% • Fibula shortened 4–60% • Knee joint instability frequent • Foot small with infrequent malformations	• Tibia shortened 4–27% • Fibula shortened 10–100% • Knee joint instability frequent • Severe malformations of foot common	• Single-bone lower leg • Patella absent • Foot malformed	• Tibia shortened <10–24% • Fibula shortened <10–100% • Lateral and high-riding patella common	• Tibia shortens 0–36% • Fibula shortened 0–100% • Lateral and high-riding patella common • Foot malformed	• Tibia shortened 0–15% • Fibula shortened 3–30% • Additional ipsilateral and contralateral malformations common
Treatment protocol	Prosthetic management	Pelvic-femoral stability through prosthetic management	• Union between femoral shaft and hip for stability • Prosthetic management	• Union between femoral head, neck and shaft • Prosthetic management	Prosthetic management	Prosthetic management	• Extremity length equality • Improved alignment of (a) proximal and (b) distal femur	• Extremity length equality • Improved alignment of (a) proximal and (b) distal femur	Extremity length equality

4. Classify coxa vara. What is adolescent coxa vara.

Ans: Classification:

- *Congenital*: Due to embryonic limb bud abnormality. The deformity is present at birth itself and is seen associated with proximal femoral focal deficiency (PFFD), congenital short femur and congenital bowed femur, and fibular hemimelia.
- *Acquired*:
  - Metabolic (rickets)
  - Neoplastic (fibrous dysplasia)
  - Traumatic
  - Slipped upper femoral epiphysis (SUFE)
  - Inflammatory
  - Perthes
  - Infective (tuberculosis).
- *Developmental [infantile coxa vara (ICV)]*: This is a progressive coxa vara with associated neck lesion that makes it characteristic. Usually, there are no other associated musculoskeletal abnormalities.

Adolescent coxa vara: This is a totally different entity. This is now called *slipped upper (capital) femoral epiphysis*. Use of the term adolescent coxa vara has been dropped now altogether—it is given here only for creating confusion in student's mind. *For details of SUFE, kindly see Chapter 29 of the book Essential Orthopedics: Principles and Practice, 2nd edition.*

5. Describe the clinical features, radiological features, differential diagnosis, and management principles of unilateral coxa vara in a toddler.

Ans: *Clinical features*:
- *Progressive Trendelenburg gait*: This results from the reduced length—tension relationship of the hip abductors from tucked-up greater trochanter
- Decrease in hip abduction, internal rotation (progressive decrease in anteversion), and later global restriction (painless)
- Flexion contracture of hip
- Limb-length discrepancy (unilateral)
- Lumbar lordosis
- Prominent trochanters palpable on affected side
- Positive Trendelenburg sign.

Radiological features: There is decreased neck-shaft angle variable and progressive on sequential films. Vertically oriented proximal femoral physis with a triangular metaphyseal fragment in the form of inverted radiolucent "Y". This fragment is often called the "Fairbank fragment" and the triangle as "Fairbank triangle". There is reduced femoral anteversion that may actually become retroversion. There is usually associated coxa breva and mild acetabular dysplasia. The vertical position of the physis is the cause of progression of pathology due to nonphysiological transmission of forces. This position on a radiograph is quantifiable and also a guide for treatment.

- *Hilgenreiner physeal angle (HPA, used to quantify the verticality of proximal femoral capital physis)*: HPA is defined by the angle subtended by intersection planes of the physeal plate and the Hilgenreiner line. This angle is normally 25° or less, but in developmental coxa vara, it is usually in the range of 40–70°.
- *Neck-shaft angle*: This is another method to guide surgery and commonly used. Angles more than 110° have possibility for better resolution of the disease while those less than 90° should always be operated.
  Angles between 90° and 110° should be observed for progression or resolution of disease.

Differential diagnosis: Malunited femoral neck femur fracture and sequel of septic arthritis.

Management principles:
- Neck-shaft angle of less than 90° + limp should be operated.
- HPA greater than 60° should be operated, especially if associated with limp.
- Children with HPA between 45° and 60° (at risk cases) and progression of deformity should be considered for surgery after proper counseling.

6. A. Define coxa vara.
B. Etiology, clinical features, and management of congenital coxa vara.

Ans:
A. Coxa vara is defined as any decrease below the normal values of the neck-shaft angle of the proximal femur that can arise from various conditions.
B. *Etiology*: The exact etiology is unknown but there have been a lot of hypothesis projected to explain the disorder—
   - *Defective endochondral ossification*: Metabolic abnormality causing a deficient production of (or delayed) normal ossification process of the proximal end of the femur.
   - *Mechanical abnormality occurring during hip development*: Excessive intrauterine pressure on the developing hip results in a depression in the neck of the femur (Hoffa and Alsberg).
   - Partial vascular insult, causing an arrest in the early development of the femoral head and neck (Nilsson).
   - Secondary to a developmental error, resulting in faulty maturation of the cartilage and metaphyseal bone of the femoral neck (Duncan).
   - Variant of metaphyseal chondrodysplasia (Schmidt type) localized to hip joint (similar to Blount's disease at knee).

Clinical features: Kindly see Answer to Question 5.

Management: The treatment is guided primarily by HPA or neck-shaft angle as follows—
- Neck-shaft angle of less than 90° + limp should be operated.
- HPA greater than 60° should be operated, especially if associated with limp.
- Children with HPA between 45° and 60° (at risk cases) and progression of deformity should be considered for surgery after proper counseling.

Conservative treatment is done for patients with HPA less than 45° and patients under observation (at risk) of progression. These patients are taught range of motion (ROM) exercises and strengthening exercises to retain good muscle power and unload hip. Spica cast immobilization and skeletal traction with bed rest are not favored in modern orthopedics anymore due to lack of literature support.

Surgical treatment is commonly recommended for indicated patients older than 2 years of age to prevent further damage to the region (dysplasia at femoral head, neck and acetabulum). The bones are softer at this tender age but adequate fixation can be achieved with modern implants but some surgeons are concerned that physeal closure will produce shortening. Physeal growth at the capital physis does not significantly contribute to femoral length (at most providing 2-3 cm overall length to lower limb). Delaying surgery for better skeletal growth and fixation and gaining as much length before surgery may thus not be a wise recommendation. Goals of surgical treatment are to:
- Restore a more anatomic alignment—creation of neck-shaft angle that permits normalization of the femoral head and acetabulum.
- Repositioning of the femoral head in acetabulum so that the upper pole of femoral heads points up rather than medially.
- Gradual lengthening of the abductors. Often however, the length gain is done acutely with osteotomy. This can be done with ilizarov method.
- Creation of leverage to increase the efficiency of abductors eliminating the Trendelenburg sign.
- Eliminating the knee deformity and correcting shortening.
- Improve the hip ROM and mechanics.

Corrective intertrochanteric or subtrochanteric valgus osteotomy (Pauwel's "Y-shaped" or Langenskiold type) is the preferred method to restore the proximal alignment.

The osteotomy is done to overcorrect the neck-shaft angle to 150–160° (HPA < 30°). Because of reduced anteversion or actual retroversion in these cases, a rotational corrective option (*derotation*) needs to be added to the osteotomy. This is done by internally rotating the distal fragment during fixation. The physis must be protected from the fixation implant. Additional *adductor tenotomy* and/or *proximal femoral shortening* can be done to unload the femoral head and ease valgus correction.
- These convert the shear forces to compressive forces.
- Mechanical redirection of forces to improve acetabular dysplasia (dysplasia does not improve, if the angle is <140°).

Brackett procedure has high morbidity and is not done anymore considering the favorable outcome of valgus plus derotational osteotomy. In Brackett procedure, the pathological portion of neck is resected followed by insertion of the remaining shaft into femoral head and advancing the greater trochanter.

After surgery, it is seen that when the desired valgus correction has been obtained the triangular fragment heals spontaneously in 3–6 months. Unfortunately, in many of these patients (>90%), the physis also closes at 12–24 months postoperatively.

7. Management principles of developmental dysplasia of the hip (DDH) in a child of 2 years of age.

Ans: At 2 years of age, DDH is considered late-presentation, requiring aggressive management due to established bony changes and soft tissue adaptations. The goal is to achieve concentric reduction and prevent long-term complications like osteoarthritis.

Key Management Principles

Confirm diagnosis and assess severity:
- *Clinical exam*:
  - Limited hip abduction (< 60°)
  - Leg length discrepancy (Galeazzi sign)
  - Asymmetric thigh folds

- *Imaging*:
  - X-ray *[anteroposterior (AP) pelvis + frog-leg lateral]*: Assess acetabular index, migration percentage
  - Magnetic resonance imaging (MRI)/computed tomography (CT) (if needed for surgical planning)

Closed versus open reduction:
- *Closed reduction (Attempt first if possible)*:
  - *Indication*: If hip is reducible under anesthesia.
  - *Procedure*:
    - Gentle manipulation under general anesthesia + arthrogram.
    - Apply hip spica cast in human position (90° flexion, 40–50° abduction).
  - *Postreduction check*:
    - CT/MRI to confirm concentric reduction.
    - Cast for 3–6 months, changed periodically.
- *Open reduction (If closed fails or severe dysplasia)*:
  - *Indications*:
    - Failed closed reduction
    - Significant acetabular dysplasia [acetabular index (AI) > 30°]
    - Soft tissue interposition (labrum, ligamentum teres)
  - *Surgical approaches*:
    - *Medial approach (Ludloff/Ferguson)*: For younger infants (< 12 months).
    - *Anterior approach (Salter/Bikini)*: Preferred for older children (allows acetabular correction).
  - *Postoperative*: Hip spica cast for 6–12 weeks, followed by abduction bracing.

Acetabular osteotomy (If needed):
- *Indication*: Persistent dysplasia (AI > 25° after reduction).
- *Options*:
  - Salter osteotomy (for mild dysplasia)
  - Pemberton osteotomy (for moderate-severe dysplasia)
  - Dega osteotomy (posterior deficiency)

Posttreatment rehabilitation and monitoring:
- *Bracing*: Abduction orthosis (Pavlik harness no longer effective at this age)
- *Physical therapy*: Strengthening and range of motion (ROM) exercises
- *Follow-up*:
  - X-rays every 6–12 months until skeletal maturity.
  - Monitor for avascular necrosis (AVN) (risk: 5–15%).

8. **A. Describe clinical and radiological features of developmental dysplasia of the hip (DDH) and treatment of unilateral DDH in an 18-month-old child.**

B. Types of pelvic osteotomies for acetabular dysplasia.

Ans: A. *Clinical features*: The clinical presentation varies with the age. A small child less than 6 months with congenital dysplasia may go unnoticed by the parents. Such cases may be diagnosed by good and careful clinical examination. Hart mentioned that the classic signs for diagnosis of hip dysplasia include limited hip abduction with 90° knee flexion, positive Ortolani sign found up to 3 months and apparent shortening of thigh. The prominent findings are:
- Uprising trochanter riding above Nelaton's line, shortening of the limb
- Adduction contracture
- Absent femoral pulse (due to lack of support from underlying femoral head in a dislocation)—the Narath sign for femoral pulsations. Often the pulsations are less marked than totally absent to an experienced finger
- Asymmetric thigh folds—increased in number on the side of dislocation
- Higher buttock fold on side of dislocation
- Widened perineum in bilateral dislocation
- Galeazzi sign positive

- ROM—restricted abduction, increased internal rotation
- Positive Ortolani and Barlow's sign—once the infant is calm and pacified, the examiner places his/her hand around the infant's knee such that the thumb lies on the inner side and index and long finger at the greater trochanter (avoid Ilfeld phenomenon).
  - Now Ortolani (1937) test is performed by gently abducting the initially adducted and flexed hip through 90° arc while applying an anteromedial force to the greater trochanter (from fingers) to detect any reduction of the femoral head into acetabulum. If one of the hips is dislocated then a clunk or "scatto" of entry is produced in 90° arc somewhere along.
  - On the other hand, Barlow's test (modification of Ortolani test) is a provocative measure, which detects the potential of hip joint instability. The first part of the test is similar to Ortolani test while the second part is the provocative maneuver. For second part of the test (Barlow's test for dislocatable hips) outward pressure is exerted by the thumb onto inner aspect of thigh and pushing the shaft of femur along longitudinal axis posteriorly the clunk/jerk of exit is felt as the head slips out over the posterosuperior lip of acetabulum. This indicates a dislocatable hip and not a dislocated one.

As the child grows and reaches between 6 months and 18 months of age, it is usually not possible to abduct the hip and reduce it on clinical examination. The following are the findings in a walking child:

- Limitation of abduction and asymmetric thigh and gluteal folds are the most common clinical findings in such children.
- The Galeazzi sign may be positive when the femoral head is displaced laterally as well as proximally causing an apparent shortening of the femur.
- A child in walking age may walk with Trendelenburg gait (unilateral dislocation) described as waddling by parents with exaggerated lumbar lordosis. For bilateral cases the child has a duck-like or Sailor's gait.
- Increased lumbar lordosis.
- Positive Trendelenburg sign—amount of hip drop is proportional to the degree of displacement. The glutei are inefficient due to proximal migration of head and absent/unstable fulcrum.
- Ludloff sign—in a normal child with hips fully flexed and abducted, the knee cannot be fully extended due to hamstring tightness while in a dislocated hip due to proximal shortening knee can be fully extended.
- Galeazzi sign is positive.
- Klisic test—keep index finger on anterosuperior iliac spine (ASIS) and middle finger on greater trochanter. A line joining them meets at umbilicus while in bilateral dislocation the lines meet below it. In unilateral dislocation, a line drawn in a similar way would pass beneath the umbilicus.

Radiological features:
- Obliquity of the acetabulum depends on the ossification of the outer third.
- Uprising of trochanter and limb shortening.
- Proximal femoral epiphysis begin to ossify around 4–6 months of age, is delayed in DDH. In these cases, the line drawn-up the femoral long axis with radiograph taken in 45° of abduction (Andren-Von-Rosen line) should transect the triradiate cartilage and is true irrespective of the position of hip joint.
- *Hilgenreiner's line*: It is the horizontal line drawn joining the uppermost aspect of triradiate cartilage of both sides.
- *Perkin's line (Ombredanne's line)*: It is the line perpendicular to Hilgenreiner's line drawn at lateral margin of acetabulum. It divides the hip into four quadrants:
  - Normal hip—femoral epiphysis lies in the lower inner quadrant
  - Subluxated hip—femoral epiphysis lies in the upper medial quadrant
  - Dislocated hip—epiphysis in the lower outer quadrant
  - High dislocation—epiphysis in the upper outer quadrant.

Quite often a grading system is used for DDH to evaluate hips in research papers and studies based on this "quadrant position of the femoral head". The system gave rise to the classification of hip dysplasia by Tönnis (one should note that both systems are not exactly identical, and the authors feel that the Tönnis system is correct to follow) as follows:

- *Grade 1*: Capital femoral epiphysis medial to Perkins line.
- *Grade 2*: Capital femoral epiphysis lateral to Perkins line but below the level of the superior acetabular rim.
- *Grade 3*: Capital femoral epiphysis at the level of superior acetabular rim.
- *Grade 4*: Capital femoral epiphysis above the level of superior acetabular rim.

Acetabular index:
- Normal = 27.5° (mean in newborns)
- 6 months = 23.5°
- 2 years—decreases to less than 20°
- 30° is the upper limit of normal hence for any age
- Anteroinferior zone of weight-bearing or sourcil is less than 15° of the curve.

Medial gap: This is the distance between the ossified proximal portion of the femur and lateral wall of teardrop. Normal is less than 4 mm, 5 mm is suspicious and greater than or equal to 6 mm is dislocation.
- Dimension "H" is the distance from top of ossified proximal portion of femoral head to Hilgenreiner line.
- Dimension "D" is the distance from middle of the proximal ossified femur to the inner border of teardrop. These measures are useful in unossified or absent femoral head to grade the dislocation or displacement of femoral head.

Center-edge (CE) angle of Wiberg:
- 6–13 years; greater than 19° is normal
- 14 years and more; greater than 25° is normal
- Acetabular depth and femoral head extrusion index are other measures used to describe severity of DDH.

Treatment—Toddler (18–36 months)

Though manageable but extensive procedures in combination are often needed with less successful results than for previous group. Often an "open reduction and capsulorrhaphy" is accompanied by a "femoral or pelvic osteotomy or both".
- When the primary dysplasia exists in acetabulum, a pelvic redirectional osteotomy will be more appropriate. Generally, pelvic osteotomies are indicated only after the femoral head has been concentrically reduced, but the acetabulum is dysplastic, or the joint has failed to develop satisfactorily or the growth potential for acetabulum no longer exists. An upper age limit of 8 years is generally assumed after which acetabular dysplasia does not remodel even after open reduction.
- The femoral osteotomy for correcting rotation or anteversion is generally associated with shortening of femoral length to decrease pressure on the reduced femoral head, thereby diminishing the chances of avascular necrosis. After exposing the proximal femur through lateral incision, a transverse line is marked with an osteotome at the level of or just distal to the lesser trochanter. A longitudinal mark is also made on the anterior femoral cortex to determine correct rotation. After making an osteotomy at the transverse mark, the proximal femur is internally rotated by 15–30° to correct excessive anteversion. An appropriate wedge of bone is now removed from the medial cortex to achieve neck-shaft angles of 120–135°. The osteotomy is fixed with an appropriate device followed by spica cast application, which is worn for 8–12 weeks. The fixation device is removed after 12–24 months.

B. Types of acetabular osteotomies:
- Innominate osteotomy (Salter)
- Acetabuloplasty (Pemberton)
- Osteotomies that free the acetabulum (steel triple innominate or Ganz acetabular osteotomy)
- Shelf operation (Staheli)
- Innominate osteotomy with medial displacement of the acetabulum (Chiari).

9. Which orthoses are used in developmental dysplasia of the hip (DDH)?

Ans: The following are some of the orthoses used in DDH:
- *Von rosen splint*: It is a passive restraining or positioning device being adjustable in both abduction and flexion. It is made up of malleable plastic with frame for shoulders, waist, and thighs.
- *Pavlik harness* is a dynamic flexion abduction orthosis which has a chest strap, two shoulder straps and two stirrups. The harness is applied with the child in supine position. The harness works on the mechanism of dynamic flexion-abduction of hip
- *Denis Browne bar*: It has cuffs that go around thighs and are attached to a bar. This holds hips and knees up (flexed) with legs abducted.
- *Ilfeld orthosis* is a primarily abduction orthosis that promotes flexion to some degrees. It is a passive device and does not promote motion of hip joint.

10. Indications and principles of pelvic osteotomies and their merits and demerits.

Ans: The common osteotomies done in pediatric patients around pelvic region are given in **Table 4B.1.2**.

TABLE 4B.1.2: Common osteotomies done in pediatric patients around pelvic region.

Osteotomy	Age	Indications
Salter innominate osteotomy	18 months to 6 years	Congruous hip reduction; <10–15° correction of acetabular index required
Pemberton acetabuloplasty	18 months to 10 years	> 10–15° correction of acetabular index required; small femoral head, large acetabulum
Steel or Ganz osteotomy	Late adolescence to skeletal maturity	Residual acetabular dysplasia; symptoms; congruous joint
Shelf procedure or Chiari osteotomy	Adolescence to skeletal maturity	Incongruous joint; symptoms; other osteotomy not possible

Salter osteotomy: Kindly see Answer to Question below.

Pemberton osteotomy: Pemberton described a pericapsular approach which is made through full thickness (cf-Dega osteotomy done through outer cortex only) of ilium using the triradiate cartilage as hinge around which the acetabular roof is rotated anteriorly and laterally. The osteotomy is curvilinear beginning between anterior superior iliac spine (ASIS) and anterior inferior iliac spine (AIIS) ending at the posterior limb of triradiate cartilage near the inner-wall of acetabulum (cf-Dega). Stability is achieved by forward, lateral, and downward rotation of the anterosuperior acetabulum over femoral head improving coverage. The osteotomy is performed in several steps: The medial and lateral cortices are resected separately, and then the cancellous zone is resected using a curved osteotome. If lateral tipping is to be increased, the resection of the medial cortex must be more distal than the lateral cortical section. Posterior limb is deemed to remain intact at the inner wall of ilium but often fractures due to thin support. The deeper extent of osteotomy toward inner wall (posterior hinge/limb) is farther than in Dega osteotomy so that the hinge is thinner in Pemberton osteotomy.

The *advantages* over innominate osteotomy includes:
- Absence of internal fixation and thus need of a second operation to remove the implants
- Also a greater degree of correction can be achieved by acetabuloplasty as the fulcrum of rotation; the triradiate cartilage is near the site of desired correction.

The *disadvantages* include technical difficulty and alteration in the configuration and capacity of acetabulum which may result in incongruous relationship between femoral head and acetabulum and that it reduces the diameter of acetabulum (though overall volume is increased). The osteotomy fails to improve the coverage of posterior part of acetabulum as the posterior—most point remains untouched in the repositioning maneuver.

Dega osteotomy: It comprises a transiliac osteotomy designed for treatment of residual acetabular dysplasia secondary to congenital hip dysplasia and subluxation.
- It consists of an incomplete transiliac osteotomy involving the anterior and middle portions of ilium leaving a posterior hinge (inner-wall) intact.
- The osteotomy is placed just above acetabulum (closer than Pemberton) and ends at the triradiate cartilage.
- The osteotomy line is located 15 mm above the acetabular rim, following the contour of the acetabulum.
- It extends from the anteroinferior iliac spine to the greater ischiatic incisura (greater sciatic notch).
- The procedure begins at the two extremities (anterosuperior iliac spine and greater ischiatic incisura) with bicortical resection for a few millimeters.
- It passes toward the triradiate cartilage and stops just above it. The medial cortex is not resected.
- The osteotomy is levered open with a lamina spreader or and cortical graft is inserted anteriorly and posteriorly to open up the osteotomy.
- The graft insertion can change the direction of coverage. Larger graft placement posteriorly may lead to posterior coverage, vice versa resulting in an anterior coverage. The osteotomy can be done before or after closure of triradiate cartilage. The osteotomy reaches the triradiate cartilage closer to acetabulum than in Pemberton osteotomy.

Osteotomies that free the acetabulum: The osteotomies that free the acetabulum devised by Steel, Eppright, and Ganz can provide much more correction and improve femoral head coverage. These operations free the part of pelvis that contains acetabulum which can be placed in desirable position. These surgeries are indicated in adolescents and adults with residual dysplasia or subluxation where potential to remodel has been lost. The triple innominate osteotomy developed by Steel involves division of the ischium, the superior pubic ramus, and the ilium superior to the acetabulum. Now the acetabulum is repositioned over femoral head and stabilized by bone grafts and pins. The articular surfaces must be congruous or became congruous after acetabular redirection for the operation to yield successful results.

The complications include excessive external rotation of the acetabulum, posterior coverage, and nonunion of the ischial and pubic osteotomies.

The *pericapsular dial osteotomy* of the acetabulum described by Eppright consists of freeing the acetabulum superiorly, posteriorly, inferiorly and anteriorly as a single segment and redirecting it to cover the acetabulum.

The *Bernese periacetabular osteotomy (Ganz)* has been developed for adolescent and adults with dysplastic hips which achieving congruency and containment are desirable. The *advantages* include:
- Use of single approach to create all osteotomies
- Achieving larger amount of correction in all directions
- Preservation of blood supply to acetabulum
- No change in the shape of pelvis
- The intact posterior column of hemipelvis which allows immediate weight bearing (WB).

Shelf procedure: The shelf procedures have been used to enlarge the volume of acetabulum. The shelf procedure of Staheli involves extension of the acetabular roof laterally, anteriorly, or posteriorly by a graft or by turning part of the lateral cortex of ilium distally superior to the femoral head.

The primary indication for shelf is a deficient acetabulum that cannot be corrected by a redirectional pelvic osteotomy. This procedure is used when no other osteotomy can establish a congruous joint with apposition of acetabulum and femoral head.

Innominate osteotomy: The osteotomy of the innominate bone is performed at the superior margin of the acetabulum and the part inferior to the osteotomy along with femur is displaced medially (deepens acetabulum). Osteotomy proceeds in a direction medially—upward from just below AIIS to the greater sciatic notch. The starting point is important as higher starting point fails to provide support. The superior fragment of osteotomy then becomes a shelf and the capsule is interposed between it and femoral head.

Indications:
- Congenital subluxation in patients between 4 and 6 years or above
- For untreated congenital dislocation of hip in patients older than 4 years soon after open or closed reduction
- For dysplastic hip with osteoarthritis (OA)
- For paralytic dislocation caused by muscle weakness or spasticity
- For coxa magna following Perthes disease or osteonecrosis (ON) of head following treatment of congenital dysplasia.

11. Describe Salter's osteotomy.

Ans: Osteotomy of innominate bone (devised by Salter) can be done in a child from 18 months to 7 years of age for unilateral cases (not recommended above 5 years of age for bilateral cases) to provide coverage to femoral head anteriorly and laterally. The osteotomy is not done below 18 years of age as iliac wings cannot support the bone graft and fixation. The osteotomy is recommended in the prescribed age limit for:
- Primary treatment of congenital subluxation in early childhood.
- Secondary treatment of any residual or recurrent dislocation persisting after primary treatment.
- Persistent subluxation along with other methods of treatment (with inadequate coverage after closed/open reduction).
- Failure of acetabular angle to improve within 2 years following reduction or persistent dysplasia at 3–5 years (neglected cases).

The prerequisites include:
- Concentric and congruent reduction of femoral head inside the acetabulum.
- The femoral head must be seated into the depth of acetabulum completely.
- Ability to bring down the head to a position opposite acetabulum—the contractures of iliopsoas and adductor should be released.

- The ROM of the hip must be good, especially abduction, internal rotation, and flexion.
- Mild (preferable) to moderate (upper limit) dysplasia of acetabulum.

The level of osteotomy is just above the acetabulum at the anteroinferior iliac spine through the sciatic notch done is a transverse direction, completed using a Gigli saw. Entire acetabulum together with pubis and ischium is rotated forward, downward, and outward as a unit with symphysis pubic acting on a hinge. The osteotomy is then held open anterolaterally by a wedge of bone fixed by K-wire, which shifts the roof of acetabulum anteriorly and laterally. Patient is kept in a hip spica for 6 weeks after the procedure. Strict subperiosteal dissection is recommended to reduce bleeding and minimize nerve and vessel injury.

Complications:
- The sciatic nerve may be crushed or irritated by wrong placement of bone retractors in the sciatic notch.
- Prolonged retraction on iliopsoas may cause femoral nerve compression.
- Inadequate subperiosteal application of bone retractor medullary may compress the obturator nerve.
- The anterior approach may endanger the lateral cutaneous nerve of thigh.
- The approach also risks the nutrient vessels of the tensor fascia lata muscle, if retraction is prolonged.
- Posterior displacement of the distal fragment.

Disadvantages:
- Unstable osteotomy and requires internal fixation.
- Correction is limited by the size of graft and length of pubic ramus.
- "Defect" (pseudo) is created in the posterior acetabulum (due to repositioning) with narrowing of joint space.
- Limb lengthening approximately 1 cm is created.

12. Explain the role of USG in DDH.

Ans: Clinical assessment of the neonatal hip is performed routinely in the first day of life, and it has become diagnostic modality of choice for DDH due to its ability to evaluate cartilaginous structures. During first month of life, clinical examination is more relied upon as ultrasonography (USG) tends to overestimate the incidence of DDH. Graf (1980) described a static nonstress ultrasound measurement technique utilizing the nonossified head as a transmitting material. This is a morphological assessment relying on anatomic landmarks. The transducer is placed on the greater trochanter allowing visualization of the deeper structures (Fig. 4B.1.1).

The image include lateral surface of iliac bone above acetabulum, deepest portion of acetabulum roof, and proximal femoral metaphysis. Draw three lines, one baseline from lateral margin of ilium (intersecting the bony and cartilaginous portions), second line from bony acetabular roof (the acetabular roof-line), and third line from lateral aspect of acetabular labrum and cartilage (the inclination line). Measure the alpha (angle between the roof and baseline) and beta (angle between the inclination line and base-line) angles. The acetabular angles are carefully measured on a coronal view of the hip and subcategorized depending on labral echogenicity.

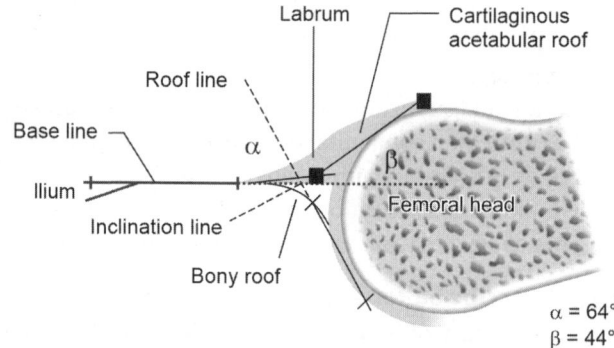

Fig. 4B.1.1: Clinical assessment of the neonatal hip.

Transverse scanning from the lateral aspect of the hip can also be used. Utilizing these techniques and assessing the hip stability by giving the head a push from posterior aspect Harcke and Grissom described dynamic stress sonography where the hip is scanned in transverse and coronal planes. While scanning the posterior lip of the acetabulum, a posterior push is performed to assess joint instability. As the child usually gives little time to examine, a dynamic standard minimum examination (DSME) is commonly done by the physicians succinctly looking for the pathology and diagnosis. Ultrasound examination thus not only establishes static relationship between femoral head and acetabulum but also allows dynamic examination. It is also now a preferred modality for evaluation of children on treatment with Pavlik harness. Role of USG as a screening test is still contested. While in Europe it is done for all newborn babies, in the United States it is recommended only for doubtful newborn cases that have been evaluated by standard clinical examination. A good use of USG could be to evaluate infants with risk factors for DDH like breech position, family history, torticollis, etc.

Observations for developmental dysplasia of hip:
Morphologic evaluation of the location of femoral head and degree of acetabulum development:
- Dynamic evaluation of the location of femoral head and degree of hip instability with stress
- The depth of acetabulum and displacement of femoral head are measured by alpha and beta angles
- Alpha angle is between body weight base line and acetabular base line
- Beta angle is measured between body weight base line and acetabular labrum line.

13. **A. Define Perthes disease.**
B. Etiological factors, classification systems, prognostic factors, and head-at-risk signs of Perthes disease.

Ans:
A. **Definition:** Legg-Calvé-Perthes (LCP) disease is a self-limiting disease of hip in children produced by varying degrees of idiopathic osteonecrosis of the capital femoral epiphysis and often the most proximal part of the metaphysis.
B. **Etiological factors:** Although the etiology remains unknown, the disease is associated with following factors—
- Deprived populations. It is much more common in deprived white population as compared to Asians and Africans.
- Global growth disorder is characterized by delayed and disproportionate growth. Some investigators found a "standstill phenomenon" where new carpal bones did not ossify while the existing ones kept growing; this relationship of delayed bone age was more prominent in patients with bilateral Perthes. Disproportionate growth pattern has been recognized in the form of subtle dysmorphic pattern called "rostral sparing".
- Hormones—it is difficult to establish relationship and even the levels of thyroid hormones have been found to be normal but the age of occurrence of Perthes is similar to hypothyroidism.
- Third born or later child of older than average parents.
- Exposure to smoke (particularly cigarette smoke but also *chulah* smoke).
- Role of intravascular mechanisms—any role of heritable thrombophilic factor is unproven but some reports suggest factor V Leiden deficiency.
- Local anatomical abnormalities—there is finding of increased anteversion at the affected hip.
- Developmental anomaly—this theory is promulgated based on finding of nongenetic associations of inguinal hernia, undescended testis, renal abnormalities (females with bilateral affection), pyloric stenosis, congenital heart disease, etc., in some cases.

Classification systems: "Salter-Thompson" is a two-category classification system—Group A denotes involvement of less than half of femoral head and Group B denotes involvement of more than half of the femoral head.

The "lateral pillar classification" introduced by Herring is a four-category system based on the height of lateral pillar (defined as the lateral 15–30% of epiphysis). The head is simply divided into three sectors or pillars. The lateral pillar occupies the lateral 15–30% of the width of head, 50% of width is occupied by the middle or central pillar, while medial pillar forms 20–35% of the width of head. Group A represents no loss of lateral pillar height; B represents less than 50% loss of height and group C more than 50% loss of height.

Table 4B.1.3 shows the Stulberg classification.

Stulberg class	Descriptive feature	Radiographic sign of OA at mean follow-up of 40 years	Radiographic evidence of joint space narrowing at mean follow-up of 40 years
I	Normal hip joint	0	0
II	Spherical enlarged head short neck or sleep acetabulum	16%	0
III	Nonspherical head (ovoid-, mushroom-, or Umbrella-shaped)	58%	47%
IV	Flat head	75%	53%
V	Flat head with incongruent hip joint	78%	61%

TABLE 4B.1.3: Stulberg classification.

Catterall classification

Group 1
- Affects the anterior aspect of femoral head
- No sequestrum
- No subchondral fracture
- No metaphyseal rarefaction
- Maintained epiphyseal height.

Group 2
- Affects anterolateral one-third to one-half of femoral head
- Sequestrum formation with clear junction
- Subchondral formation with clear junction
- Subchondral fracture does not extend into posterior half of femoral head
- Anterolateral metaphyseal rarefaction
- Lateral pillar is preserved.

Group 2½
These cases have intact lateral pillar, but a radiolucency is present in the lateral column.

Group 3
- Affects three-fourth of femoral head
- Sequestrum is large and junction is sclerotic
- Subchondral fracture extends into posterior half
- Diffuse metaphyseal rarefaction
- Lateral pillar is not preserved.

Reverse group 3
Affects three-fourths of femoral head but in anteromedial aspect of femoral head rather than anterolateral aspect.

Group 4
- Affects entire femoral head
- Dense well-marked sequestrum
- Subchondral fracture extends throughout the head
- Diffuse or central metaphyseal rarefaction
- Posterior remodeling seen.

Prognostic factors: The long-term outcome is affected by shape and size of the femoral head. The shape of femoral head can be assessed by Moses circles or separate circular discs of different sizes.

Head-at-risk signs

Clinical head-at-risk signs:
- Children aged 5 years or younger have the best prognosis. The outcome is especially dismal when the onset of disease is in adolescence (>8 years).
    - Younger patients have more time to remodel
    - Acetabulum in older patients loses remodeling potential
    - Older patients are heavier and more likely to damage the epiphysis
- Contrary to popular belief, there is no strong evidence to suggest a worst prognosis in girls. Most of the other important prognostic signs can be identified on plain radiographs. It was proposed that the girls achieve skeletal maturity early so get less time for bone remodeling. Age for age however the girls seem to be more severely affected for unknown reason(s).
- Extent of epiphyseal involvement (as classified by Catterall and Salter-Thompson) and extent of epiphyseal collapse (Herring's lateral pillar) do determine the prognosis. More involvement is expected with extrusion of the epiphysis. This can be measured by assessing the femoral head coverage by acetabulum. Center-edge angle of Wiberg is usually

not used because it is generally impossible to ascertain the center of the femoral head, which is deformed. Reimer's migration index and acetabular head index are much more commonly used.
- Obese patient has more stress at the epiphysis compromising the blood supply and rapid collapse of the head
- Patient with limited ROM—flexion less than 80° and abduction <30°.
- Increasing abduction contracture—increases the tendency of hip to subluxate laterally.
- Subluxating hips on clinical examination.

Radiological head-at-risk signs:
- The metaphyseal abnormalities like osteoporosis, metaphyseal cyst, and widening of the central femoral metaphysis have been identified as poor prognosticators
- Altered centers of acetabulum (bicompartmentalization) are also associated with poor outcome. In this, the central femoral head articulates with the lateral part of the acetabulum and the lateral part of femoral head extrudes out
- Catterall in addition mentioned some head-at-risk signs, the utility of which is debatable
    - Diffuse metaphyseal reaction
    - Calcification lateral to the epiphysis
    - Gage's sign—a V-shaped defect in lateral bony epiphysis indicating cartilage overgrowth without ossification
    - Horizontal alignment of the femoral epiphysis and lateral extrusion of the epiphysis. This lateral subluxation of femoral head is the most important prognosticator as mentioned earlier.

14. Discuss the management of Perthes disease.

Ans: The approach is to save the affected part of femoral head from bearing these transmitted forces by preventing or reversing the extrusion of head.

It is called "containment" which ensures that the anterolateral part of the epiphysis is positioned within the acetabulum, so that edge of acetabulum does not transmit any force on to this part of femoral epiphysis. This may be achieved by abduction and internal rotation or abduction and flexion through either casting or bracing but more reliably through surgery. All children older than 8 years at onset of disease must undergo containment procedure because there will be extrusion invariably. Those who are younger than 8 years need to be monitored regularly and the containment procedure offered as soon as extrusion is detected. For containment to work, it is imperative that it is carried out before the stage of fragmentation. If done at right time containment will prevent femoral head deformation and produce a spherical and congruent head on healing. *Good range of motion (ROM) is a prerequisite for achieving containment.* This can be effectively done by applying traction which relieves muscle spasm. Alternatively, abduction casts are applied serially, increasing range of abduction every 2 weeks. More recalcitrant hips may gain motion by applying abduction casts under general anesthesia for 6 weeks. *Status of the lateral pillar and the extent of extrusion are not used* widely for decision-making to perform containment because this procedure needs to be done before stage of fragmentation.

Cast or brace if used as method for containment should be continued for 12–13 months and should be worn for most of day. Ambulatory brace treatment has declined in use due to noncompliance especially in older children. Bracing is done as an attempt to prevent deformity of femoral head by prolonged mechanical unloading and immobilization of femoral head.

Also active joint motion and physiotherapy are encouraged. Strict mechanical unloading is not required and also patients can be allowed to participate in lighter sporting activities such as swimming and cycling strictly avoiding jumping and activities associated with extreme stress. Along with physiotherapy, the use of prostacyclins as vasoactive analogs is investigational. Pain control should be done with adequate use of analgesics.

Surgical containment procedures are most widely used to provide containment. Surgical procedures should be done with proper prerequisites and reasonable patient selection. Preoperative arthrogram is a must for containment procedures to understand the extent of cartilaginous femoral head and congruency and adequacy of reduction. Various modern authors prefer varus derotation osteotomy (VDRO) of proximal femur to contain the femoral head and do it as a standard procedure. Staheli, however, suggested the combination of VDRO and pelvic procedure to enhance the containment while limiting the complications of VDRO (abductor weakness, shortening, and coxa vara).

The acetabular remodeling capacity drastically reduces after 8 years of age, so containment procedure is less reliable in children > 9 years. The major disadvantage of this procedure is potential for residual shortening with coxa breva and trochanteric prominence. This may be associated early abductor lurch. Open-wedge varus reduces the limb length shortening. Derotation is generally not added because this leads to an externally rotated gait. Trochanteric apophysiodesis may be added in an older child to reduce trochanteric prominence.

The advantages of this proximal femoral varus osteotomy are:
- This method can be undertaken even when there is moderate restriction of motion.
- Relocates the femur in normal attitude of limb
- It shortens the femur so in turn reducing joint reaction forces and mediation the direction of such forces.
- Surgically simpler to perform

Pelvic osteotomies: Anterolateral coverage can also be improved by Salter's osteotomy. A 30° wedge of bone graft can improve anterior coverage by 25° and lateral coverage by 15°. The prerequisite but for this procedure is a completely round or almost round head.

Shelf procedures and Chiari's osteotomy may also be utilized for increasing the coverage of anterolateral hips, especially in coxa magna (large deformed heads). However, containment with *triple pelvic osteotomy* allows greater amount of coverage. The triple pelvic osteotomy basically combines the transverse osteotomy of Salter with complete osteotomies of superior pelvic ramus and ischium. This allows acetabulum to be redirected over femoral head without interfering with the growth of triradiate cartilage.

(Additionally one can write about the management of hinged abduction here)

15. Describe stage-wise management of Perthes' disease?

Ans: Stage-wise management of Perthes disease is presented in Flowchart 4B.1.1.

Flowchart 4B.1.1: Management of Perthes disease according to stage and age.

Age <6 years
- Mild disease
  - Conservative treatment
- Severe disease
  - Intertrochanteric osteotomy

Age 6–10 years
- Head contained
  - Conservative (mobilization, weight-relieving calipers, physiotherapy maintain ROM)
- Uncontained or at high risk for subluxation
  - Surgical containment—femoral (preferred) or pelvic

Age >10 years
- Contained head:
  - Trochanteric apophysiodesis (for coxa magna)
  - Valgus osteotomy (for coxa vara)
  - Lengthening of femoral neck (for coxa vara et magna)
- Uncontained head no hinge abduction:
  - Femoral varus osteotomy (should not reduce neck shaft angle below 105°)
  - + Pelvic osteotomy for additional coverage if unable to centralize by femoral osteotomy alone or if coxa vara present)
  - + Trochanter transposition (for coxa vara)
  - + Femoral neck lengthening (for coxa magna)
- Uncontained head with hinge abduction:
  - Selective and cautious soft tissue release + manipulative reduction and cast immobilization
  - Femoral valgus osteotomy and secondary coverage by triple pelvic osteotomy (preferred)
  - Garcie cheilectomy
  - Chiari osteotomy for large mushroom head

16. What is hinged abduction? What are the management principles/technique for hinged abduction, coxa magna in healed Perthes?

Ans: Some children with severe Perthes disease present later in the course, when the head has already collapsed and deformed. In such patients, abnormal hinge movement of the hip joint, so called "hinge-abduction" occurs due to extrusion of the femoral head. It is a phenomena of impingement of the outer part of the femoral head on the lateral lip of acetabulum, typically showing widening of medial joint space by levering of inferomedial part of femoral head against the lateral edge of acetabulum. *Hinge abduction is thought to be presented if there is lateralization of femoral head by >2 mm on an abduction radiograph.*

Management principles/technique for hinged abduction, coxa magna in healed Perthes:
The hinged abduction may be *reducible* when the soft extruded part can be gently reduced inside acetabulum as in transitional phase of disease; or it may be *irreducible* when the head cannot be reduced. Arthrography forms an important part of investigation to deduce the type of hinged abduction.
- The treatment in reducible hinge abduction includes closed reduction after adductor and psoas tenotomy. It may be augmented by medial capsular release through medial approach. This is followed by Petrie's cast for 3–6 weeks followed by ROM exercises. At the end of this period, appropriate containment procedure may be performed.
- The surgical treatment for irreducible hinged abduction aims to improve the joint congruity by reducing femoroacetabular impingement. Proximal femoral valgus osteotomy alleviates abnormal hinge movement. This may be later augmented by acetabular procedures to improve coverage of the femoral head, which may provide hyaline cartilage to hyaline cartilage of acetabular osteotomy (triple pelvic or periacetabular) or hyaline cartilage to fibrocartilage salvage procedure (Chiari or shelf procedure). Other procedures which may be done in irreducible hinge abduction include acetabular enlarging procedures, hip joint distraction, osteochondroplasty and femoral head reshaping (Garceau's cheilectomy). Soft-tissue releases should not be done with cheilectomy as it increases the tendency to hinged abduction by proximal migration.

17. **A. Describe clinical features and pathophysiology of slipped capital femoral epiphysis (SCFE).**
   B. Medical conditions associated with it.
   C. Difference in radiological picture of Delbet type 1 fracture nonossifying fibroma (NOF) and SCFE.

Ans:
A. **Clinical features:** Patients with SCFE present with limp and pain in the hip, groin, thigh, or knee. Knee or distal thigh pain is the initial presenting symptom in 46% of patients with the condition.

   The patient is overweight and has features of early puberty in general. He may be unable to bear weight with a severe slip or else walks with an abductor lurch or antalgic gait. The limb is in external rotation deformity with limitation in internal rotation, abduction, and flexion, which should immediately arouse suspicion of SCFE. The hip goes into obligatory external rotation with passive flexion to 90°. Unless the patient has bilateral SCFE, it is helpful to compare ROM with the uninvolved hip.

   Pathophysiology: The physis is already in strain due to external rotation of the femoral shaft with posterior counterforce on the femoral head. The head thus moves posteriorly while neck moves cephalad. Also the position of physis changes from horizontal to oblique in preadolescence and adolescence changing the direction of force from horizontal to oblique increasing vertical strain. The separation in SCFE results from the hypertrophic zone of physis that may occupy up to 80% of the width of the physis in affected patients. There is abnormal cartilage maturation, endochondral ossification, and perichondral ring instability. The physis is wide and undergoes disruption with reduced numbers of cartilage cells and disorganization.

B. **Medical conditions associated:** Endocrinopathy (hypothyroidism, panhypopituitarism, hyperparathyroidism, hypogonadism), craniopharyngioma, Down's syndrome, renal osteodystrophy, pituitary tumors, and adiposogenital syndrome.

C. **Radiological difference:** Chronic slips are easier to differentiate from acute fractures as they have—rounding of superior portion of femoral neck, reduced height of epiphysis, and presence of callus at epiphyseometaphyseal junction. For early slips following help differentiation on a standard radiograph:
   - Widening and irregularity of physeal plate
   - *Trethowan's sign*: Failure of Klein's line to intersect with the femoral head
   - *Blanch sign of steel*: Area of decreased bone density in the proximal femoral neck.

18. **Define slipped capital femoral epiphysis (SCFE). Describe its diagnosis and treatment in brief.**
Ans: Definition: The condition is defined as the posterior and inferior slippage of the proximal femoral epiphysis on the metaphysis (femoral neck) through the epiphyseal growth plate (physis).

Diagnosis:

History and physical examination: Patients with SCFE present with limp and pain in the hip, groin, thigh, or knee. Knee or distal thigh pain is the initial presenting symptom in 46% of patients with the condition. This pain is usually disregarded as muscle pull making prone to misdiagnosis and missing the condition. History of trauma is uncommon. The patient is overweight and has features of early puberty in general. He may be unable to bear weight with a severe slip or else walks with an abductor lurch/antalgic gait. The limb is in external rotation deformity with limitation in internal rotation, abduction, and flexion which should immediately arouse suspicion of SCFE. The hip goes into obligatory external rotation with passive flexion to 90°. Unless the patient has bilateral SCFE, it is helpful to compare ROM with the uninvolved hip.

Radiographs: Anteroposterior (AP) and true (cross-table) lateral radiographs are obtained for patients aged 8–15 years of age with new-onset limping and/or pain in the hip, groin, thigh, or knee.
- *Early mild SCFE*:
  - Widening and irregularity of physeal plate
  - *Trethowan's sign*: Failure of Klein's line to intersect with the femoral head
  - *Blanch sign of steel*: Area of decreased bone density in the proximal femoral neck.
- *Chronic SCFE*:
  - Rounding of superior portion of femoral neck
  - Reduced height of epiphysis
  - Callus at epiphyseometaphyseal junction

Radiography is used to grade the severity of the slip in SCFE.
- The Wilson method on a frog-leg lateral radiograph. Measure the relative displacement of the epiphysis on the metaphysis.
- *Mild slip*: Epiphysis displacement less than one-third of the width of the metaphysis
- *Moderate slip*: Displacement between one-third and one-half of the width
- *Severe slip*: Displacement greater than one-half of the width
- The Southwick method measures angular displacement between the epiphysis and shaft on lateral radiograph. The angular displacement is calculated by the difference between affected and unaffected sides.
- Mild slip is <30°
- Moderate slip is angular displacement between 30° and 50°
- Severe slip is >50°

Ultrasonography:
- Hip effusion—indicates acute event or infection.
- Metaphyseal remodeling—chronic slips

Computed tomography (CT) scan: Three-dimensional imaging may be done in cases of unclear cases and to confirm the status of growth plate.

Technetium-99 bone scintigraphy: Cold scan usually indicates loss of blood supply to the femoral epiphysis with 80–100% incident risk of ON.

Treatment: Patient should be immediately kept nonweight-bearing (prevents slip progression) and surgical treatment is also aimed to prevent slip progression and avoid complications.

There are three broad treatment methods available for management of SCFE based on the evolving notion that long-term outcome depends on reduction of original deformity during surgery:
1. Treatment to prevent further slippage (usually in situ fixation of fusion of growth plate)
2. *Treatment to reduce the degree of slippage*: Corrective osteotomies to correct the deformities and reduce the severity of slip from moderate and severe-to-mild or anatomical levels
3. Salvage procedure

Prophylactic treatment of the contralateral hip in patients with SCFE is controversial but it is not recommended in most patients. Prophylactic pinning may be indicated in patients at high risk of subsequent slips, such as patients with obesity or an endocrine disorder, or those who have a low likelihood of follow-up.

Unstable SCFE:
Unstable SCFE is a severe injury than stable SCFE with rate of ON is as high as 20–50%. The acceptable treatment recommendations include in situ percutaneous fixation or open epiphysiodesis with bone graft. In situ percutaneous screw fixation is the most common method of fixation; the screw must not penetrate joint (high chances of chondrolysis) but provide adequate stability and must not disturb the vascularity of head. The screw is so placed that the screw tip is central in femoral head in all views and the screw crossed the growth plate perpendicularly.

Stable SCFE:
The standard acceptable treatment of stable SCFE is in situ fixation with a single screw. Other methods include hip spica cast, open epiphysiodesis with bone grafting, open reduction internal fixation (ORIF) with cuneiform osteotomy, intertrochanteric osteotomy with internal fixation, and base of neck osteotomy with in situ stabilization.

For larger slips (grade 3), it is better to perform neck osteotomy and place in situ screw to reduce the deformity. Persistence of deformity will cause late-onset arthritis.

Correction by osteotomy: Correction of femoral neck deformity by performing osteotomy allows good anatomical realignment of epiphysis and improves the chances of future functioning hip. Osteotomies at various levels have been described, some close to physis and some away from it. The closer the osteotomy is to physis, the greater are chances of correction of deformity while it risks the vascularity more. The osteotomies done away from physis will result in lesser amount of correction but reduce the risk of complications.

- *Fish and Dunn osteotomy*: These are performed close to physis; the fish's cuneiform osteotomy differs from Dunn in the fact that it involves complete removal of physis so that there is good bone-to-bone apposition and revascularization. These are contraindicated if the physis is fused.
- Osteotomy at the base of neck
- *Intertrochanteric osteotomy*: This is preferably done for residual deformity. Though the complication rates are low, it may be associated with difficult future total limb arthroplasty (THA).

Salvage procedure: Arthrodesis of hip joint

19. Classify congenital dislocation of knee. Comment on differential diagnosis and management.

Ans: Clinically, based on the movements and possibility of passive corrections, the congenital dislocation of knee (CDK) has been classified into three grades. These grades are important to help elucidate the extent of knee deformity and guide the treatment initially.

- *Grade 1 (hyperextended knee)*: The knee has hyperextension deformity (>15°) but reduces with gentle stretching of the quadriceps and passive knee flexion goes past 45°. Radiologically, the tibia is seen reduced on femur but knee is hyperextended.
- *Grade 2 (subluxated knee)*: The knee does not flex beyond 45° and in most cases not beyond neutral. Tibial and femoral epiphysis are in contact and do not subluxate on attempted flexion. Anterior subluxation of the tibia onto the distal aspect of the femur can be seen on radiographs.
- *Grade 3 (dislocated irreducible knee)*: Knee flexion is not possible and anteriorly subluxated or translated tibia further translates laterally over femur on attempted flexion. There is significant anterior quadriceps contracture. The tibia is dislocated anterior to femur and proximally migrated with absent suprapatellar pouch (knee in reverse position appearance). Hamstring tendons can be palpated anterior to femur.

Differential diagnosis: Myelodysplasia, arthrogryposis, or Larsen syndrome.

Management: The treatment of congenital hyperextension of the knee depends on the severity of the subluxation or dislocation and the age of the patient. In a newborn with mild-to-moderate hyperextension or subluxation, conservative treatment methods, such as the use of the Pavlik harness for posturing of the knee in a continued position and serial casting to increase knee flexion, are most likely to succeed. Nonoperative treatment can be continued for 3 months. In children who do not respond to conservative measures, the use of skeletal traction for correction is an option, but the deformity is difficult to correct with this method. In older children with moderate or severe subluxation or dislocation, surgery is indicated. In a child with congenital dislocation of the knee and congenital dislocation of the hip, surgical correction of the knee first is advisable.

Surgical procedure for correction of congenital dislocation of the knee is recommended for fixed knee dislocation or failure of conservative management. Two surgical approaches have been described:
- For children younger than 3 months, a percutaneous section of the quadriceps tendon and suprapatellar retinaculum is performed, followed by early serial casting and motion. Performing extensive bilateral surgeries may not be a feasible option due to general health of the child.
- For older children, a VY quadricepsplasty (advancement) is performed, with release of the contracted structures of the suprapatellar pouch and the quadriceps tendon. For severe cases, the Z-plasty of whole extensor mechanism can be performed to obtain better length.

(Details should be read from Chapter 29 of the book Essential Orthopedics: Principles and Practice, 2nd edition.)

20. A. What is Gower sign?

B. Clinical features, investigations, pathology, and treatment with prognosis of Duchenne muscular dystrophy.

Ans: Clinical features:

A. *Gower sign*: A characteristic feature of muscle dystrophy is the child's method of rising from the floor by climbing up his own legs (Gowers' sign); this is due to weakness of the gluteus maximus and thigh muscles.

B. *Clinical features*: The condition is usually unsuspected until the child starts to walk. He has difficulty in standing and climbing stairs, he cannot run properly and he falls frequently. Weakness begins in the proximal muscles of the lower limbs and progresses distally, affecting particularly the glutei, the quadriceps and the tibialis anterior, giving rise to a wide-based stance and gait with the feet in equinus, the pelvis tilted forward, the back arched in lordosis, and the neck extended. The calf muscles look bulky, but much of this is due to fat and the pseudohypertrophy belies the obvious weakness. A characteristic feature is the child's method of rising from the floor by climbing up his own legs (Gowers' sign); this is due to weakness of the gluteus maximus and thigh muscles.

Shoulder girdle weakness follows around 5 years after the clinical onset of the disease, making it difficult for the patient to use crutches. Facial muscle involvement follows later. By the age of 10 years the child has usually lost the ability to walk and becomes dependent on a wheelchair; from then on there is rapid deterioration in spinal posture with the development of scoliosis and, subsequently, further deterioration in lung function. Cardiopulmonary failure is the usual cause of death, generally before the age of 30 years.

Investigations: The diagnosis is usually based on the clinical features and family history and by testing for serum creatinine phosphokinase levels which are 200–300 times the normal in the early stages of the disease (and also elevated, but less so, in female carriers). Confirmation is achieved by muscle biopsy and genetic testing with a DNA polymerase chain reaction.

Pathology: This is a progressive disease of sex-linked inheritance with recessive transmission. A defect at locus p21 on the X chromosome results in failure to code for the dystrophin gene, which is essential for maintaining the integrity of cardiac and skeletal muscle cells. Absence of functional dystrophin leads to cell membrane leakage and muscle fiber damage and replacement by fat and fibrous tissue.

Treatment: While the child can still walk, physiotherapy and splintage or tendon operations may help to prevent or correct joint deformities and so prolong the period of mobility. Corticosteroids are useful in preserving muscle strength but there are significant side effects such as osteoporosis, increased risk of fractures, and cataract formation. Research studies in which dystrophin in the form of myoblasts is introduced into diseased muscle have been successful in animal models. Gene therapy has also been tried but there have been difficulties with the viral vectors and associated immunological responses. If scoliosis is marked (more than 30°), instrumentation and spinal fusion helps to maintain pulmonary function and improves quality of life although not necessarily lifespan. Preoperative cardiac and pulmonary function evaluation should be performed.

Family counseling is important. Up to 20% of families already have a younger affected sibling by the time the proband is diagnosed.

21. **Describe biomechanics of patellofemoral joint.**

Ans: The primary function of the patella is to increase the lever arm of the extensor mechanism around the knee, improving the efficiency of quadriceps contraction.

Kinematics of patellofemoral joint:
- Motion of patella occurs in two planes—frontal and transverse (sliding articulation). In frontal plane, patella traverses nearly 7 cm of distance.
- Due to poor bony congruity the patellofemoral articulation is primarily supported by dynamic forces of muscles:
  - *Laterally*: Lateral retinaculum, vastus lateralis and iliotibial tract.
  - *Medially*: Medial retinaculum and vastus medialis.
  - *Superior*: Quadriceps via quadriceps tendon.
  - *Inferior*: Patellar tendon.
- The mean directional force vector across patella acts toward the knee joint pushing the bone into trochlear groove of femur. This patellofemoral compression force varies with the flexion of knee joint and primarily maintains the patella in the groove. Patellofemoral stability is maintained by a combination of the articular surface geometry and soft-tissue restraints. The Q angle is the angle between the extended anatomical axis of the femur and the line between the center of the patella and the tibial tubercle. The quadriceps acts primarily in line with the anatomical axis of the femur, with the exception of the vastus medialis obliquus, which acts to medialize the patella in terminal extension. Limbs with larger Q angles have a greater tendency for lateral patellar subluxation. The quadriceps and patellar tendons insert anteriorly on the patella lengthening the lever arm throughout the arc of knee motion. The length of the lever arm varies as a function of the geometry of the trochlea producing varying joint reaction forces in different activities.

Joint reaction forces across patellofemoral joint:
- The forces are generated by the quadriceps primarily, but manipulated by disposition and orientation of various structures, position of which changes constantly with knee movements.
- The forces increase with knee flexion. The magnitude of various forces at the joint are:
  - Walking—half body weight = 850 N
  - Riding bike—half body weight = 850 N
  - Open chain—half body weight (full extension)
  - Stair climbing—3.3 body weight = 1,500 N
  - Stair descending—5 body weight = 4,000 N
  - Jogging—7 body weight = 5,000 N
  - Squatting—7 body weight = 5,000 N
  - Full squatting (Indian toilet)—20 body weight = 20,000 N
  - Impact of abnormal tracking—results in higher forces/unit area. Minor lateral shift of the patella decreases the contact area by 60% and increase stress by 2.5 times.
- Impact of surgical procedures:
  - The joint reaction force can be reduced by up to 50% at 45° angle by elevating the tibial tuberosity by 2 cm. It also increases the quadriceps moment arm.
  - By reducing the Q angle, patellar stress can be reduced. For example, by reducing the angle from 15° to 5°, there is 50% decrease in patellar stress.

22. Define, clinical features, and management of recurrent dislocation of patella in a child.

Ans:

Definition: When patella dislocates more than once it is termed as "recurrent" (older definition of >3 episodes is a mere confirmation that dislocation is truly recurrent and patient is not just a chance dislocator).

Clinical features: Patients who have recurrent dislocation frequently report diffuse pain around the knee that is aggravated by going up and down stairs or hills. The pain usually is located anterior in the knee and often is described as an aching pain with intermittent episodes of sharp, severe pain. A feeling of insecurity in the knee and occasionally of "giving way" or "going out" of the knee may be present. Patient has symptoms of recurrent instability at knee, particularly during pitching activities and movements that require rotation at the knee, like turning. Also patient complains of instability while stair climbing and general activities that involve tracking of patella in compression. Patient often complains of knee hurting all of the time and often giving way; sometimes, it slips out and causes a lot of pain.

- The gait of patient changes due to adaptive changes to avoid the recurring episodes. There may be hyperpronation of feet and valgus thrust at knee while walking.
- Examine for patella baja, Q-angle, extensor lag, patellofemoral crepitus, and apprehension by Fulkerson's relocation test.
- Evaluate the quadriceps mass by thigh and leg girth measurements and signs of generalized laxity.
- Look for signs of damage in extensor apparatus particularly medially in retinaculum and for medial patellofemoral ligament (MPFL) tear. Palpate for articular cartilage damage and facet tenderness.
    - Medial-sided patellar tenderness over retinaculum (over MPFL).
    - Increase in passive patellar lateral translation (hypermobility of patella).
    - Fulkerson relocation test—apprehension test.
- Patellar grind test.
- J-sign indicates poor patellar tracking.
- In prone position, examine for rotational malalignment, Ely's test (for rectus tightness).
- Examine for tight ITB by Ober's test in side lying position. Iatrogenic medial patellar subluxation can also be examined.
- Thigh circumferences measured proximal to the patella often show quadriceps atrophy on the involved side.
- Look for malalignment (i.e., femoral anteversion, genu valgum, external tibial torsion, and pes planus).

Management

Investigations:
- X-rays of knee AP and lateral, skyline view
- Insall-Salvati ratio
- Computed tomography (CT) scan for TT: TG distance, trochlear dysplasia.

Treatment: Nonsurgical conservative management is to be done in only infrequent dislocators or isolated dislocations and if the surgeon feels that the patellar mechanics are able to accommodate the rehabilitation process. No single operation is universally successful in correcting recurrent patellar dislocation and subluxation. The operation must be chosen after assessing the skeletal maturity, the Q-angle, retinacular tightness, patellar tilt, TT-TG distance, trochlear dysplasia and patellar height specifically for each patient. The extent of the malalignment, the patient's age, the level of activity, and the condition of the joint also are important. Procedures that involve transplantation of the tibial tuberosity are contraindicated until the proximal tibial physis has closed. During all operative procedures for recurrent dislocation of the patella, a thorough arthroscopic inspection of the articular surfaces and intra-articular structures is important. The proximal realignment procedures (Madigan's quadricepsplasty, arthroscopic medial imbrication, MPFL reconstruction, etc.) have been classically advocated in skeletally immature patients or those skeletally mature patient in whom TT-TG distance, Q-angle, medial patellar facet and patellar height are normal with or without trochlear dysplasia. When surgery is indicated, the best approach is an MPFL reconstruction. Distal realignment procedures (Elmslie–Trillat, Fulkerson, Hauser, etc.) on the other hand are performed in patients who have an increased TT-TG distance or where Insall-Salvati ratio is >1.2 (patella alta). Guiding algorithm for treatment is presented in adjoining **Flowchart 4B.1.2**.

Flowchart 4B.1.2: Guiding algorithm for treatment of recurrent dislocation of patella.

```
Recurrent patellar dislocation
├── Skeletally mature patient
│   ├── Medial deficiency (Normal Q-angle) → MPFL reconstruction ± lateral lengthening or minimally invasive procedure
│   ├── Medial deficiency with Q-angle increased → Fulkerson's procedure ± MPFL reconstruction
│   ├── Patella alta → Distalization of tibial tuberosity
│   ├── Trochlear dysplasia → Trochleoplasty
│   └── Rotational or angular malalignment → Corrective osteotomies
└── Skeletally immature patient
    ├── Normal Q-angle → Minimally invasive soft tissue procedure (medial and lateral)
    └── Increased Q-angle → Medial imbrication + Roux procedure/ selected cases VMO advancement → Or wait for skeletal maturity if possible and treat as above
```

23. Discuss principles of management of recurrent dislocation of patella.

Ans: Guiding algorithm is written in answer above.

24. Describe recurrent dislocation of patella. Describe its etiology.

Ans: Kindly see Answer to Question above.

25. Describe:
  A. Metatarsus adductus.
  B. Congenital dislocation of patella.

Ans:

A. **Metatarsus adductus:** Metatarsus adductus is the most common foot deformity commonly seen in newborn infants with incidence approaching 1 in 1,000 to 1,500 live births. There is adduction of forefoot with normal hindfoot alignment or minimal valgus. Half of patients have bilateral involvement and there is no predilection. The exact cause of metatarsus adductus is not known, although intrauterine positioning (packaging defect) is commonly implicated. There is increased incidence in:
- First pregnancy
- Twin pregnancy
- Oligohydramnios.

Metatarsus adductus may be associated with few conditions like:
- Clubfoot
- Torticollis
- Developmental dysplasia of the hip (1–5%, recent studies have not confirmed this theory).

Clinical features: Metatarsus adductus is a common cause of intoeing gait. The forefoot is deviated medially with respect to the hindfoot that may show some valgus (higher valgus equates to skewfoot). Lateral border is convex with variable medial crease depending on severity (see below). The hindfoot and subtalar motion is usually normal. Metatarsus adductus may be seen as a residual deformity in patients previously treated surgically or nonsurgically for congenital clubfoot. This residual metatarsus adductus is often rigid (fixed positioning of the forefoot on the midfoot and hindfoot) but can be dynamic also, caused by imbalance of the anterior tibial tendon during gait. Late sequelae of metatarsus adductus may include an increased risk of stress fractures of the lateral metatarsal bones, due to altered biomechanics.

Classification: The deformity is classified by its magnitude and the stiffness of the metatarsus adductus—
- *The mild form*: The forefoot can be clinically abducted to the midline of the foot and beyond. This can be clinically tested by gently stroking the lateral border of foot that elicits spontaneous movements and active correction. The heel bisector line passes through 3rd toe (in a normal foot, it passes through 2nd web space).
- *The moderate form*: Heel bisector line passes through 3rd and 4th toe webspace. There is enough flexibility to allow abduction of the forefoot to the midline, but usually not beyond.
- *Rigid metatarsus adductus*: Heel bisector line passes through 4th and 5th toe webspace. The forefoot cannot be abducted at all. There is often a transverse crease on the medial border of the foot or an enlargement of the web space between the great and second toes.

The other classification (Berg) incorporates the metatarsus adductus and skewfoot together:
- Simple metatarsus adductus
- *Complex metatarsus adductus*: Metatarsus adductus with lateral shift of midfoot
- *Skewfoot*: Metatarsus adductus with valgus hindfoot
- *Complex skew foot*: Metatarsus adductus along with abducted midfoot and valgus hindfoot.

Radiology: Metatarsus adductus is best viewed on a dorsoplantar view and diagnosed with metatarsus adductus angle more than 21°. This angle is made by intersection of two lines, one bisecting the second metatarsal and the other perpendicular to the midfoot bisector (one can also use a perpendicular to second cuneiform bisector instead). When using the cuneiform bisector upper limit of angle is taken as 24°.

Berg considered metatarsus adductus to be present, if the bisector of first metatarsal was medial to the bisection line of talus.

Treatment: The primary treatment of mild flexible metatarsus adductus is observation. Most of the patients have a benign natural history (>90% cases) with good correction of the deformity by the age of 4–5 years. Mild residual deformity is rarely if ever a problem to patient or parents. Most of the deformity corrects in walking age group with corrective footwear. Patients with moderate or rigid, severe metatarsus adductus can be treated with manipulation and serial casting after the age of 6 months. Manipulation involves abduction of the forefoot against counterpressure placed over the calcaneal cuboid joint. To maintain the correction after manipulation, children are placed in a long leg plaster cast, and the cast is changed every 2 weeks for three or four sessions. Serial stretching and casting is done for 6–12 weeks or until the foot is clinically flexible. Medial release is described for resistant rigid foot that can then be manipulated. After the deformity is fully corrected, the child must wear a Denis Browne bar and shoes to prevent a recurrence. Surgical intervention can be used for the rare child with severe, stiff residual deformity.

Surgical indications include:
- Pain
- Objectionable appearance
- Difficulty in fitting shoes 2–4 years.

The common surgical technique involves medial column opening and lateral column shortening:
- Medial column opening consists of medial tarsometatarsal capsular release, abductor hallucis recession (recession only as a procedure is done in young patients with rigid resistant feet) and release of intermetatarsal ligaments. Soft tissue only procedures are helpful in younger patients. Medial cuneiform opening osteotomy is done in older patients to change its shape from trapezoid to rectangular. This also improves the 1st metatarsocuneiform relationship.
- Lateral column shortening involves cuboid closing wedge osteotomy, which can be combined with medial cuneiform osteotomy in severe deformities (double osteotomy).
- In children more than 5-year-old, multiple metatarsal osteotomies (Berman and Gartland), medial cuneiform, and lateral cuboid double osteotomy can be done to correct deformity. In Berman and Gartland osteotomy, all five

metatarsal bases are exposed dorsally. A small power drill is used to make a dome-shaped osteotomy in each with the apex of the dome proximally. Forefoot is rotated in corrected position and foot transfixed using small Steinmann pins through the shafts of the first and fifth metatarsals across the osteotomies.

B. **Congenital dislocation of patella:** Congenital dislocation of the patella often is familial and bilateral. It may be associated with arthrogryposis multiplex congenita or Down syndrome. The patella is permanently dislocated and irreducible and quadriceps contracture is essential feature with this anomaly. The vastus lateralis may be absent or severely contracted. When absent the patella is dislocated laterally and attached to the anterior aspect of the iliotibial band. Often the patella is small and misshapen and in an abnormal location in the quadriceps mechanism. Secondary deformities like genu valgum and external rotation of the tibia on the femur commonly develop, medial knee capsule is stretched, the lateral femoral condyle is flattened, and tibial tuberosity is commonly shifted more laterally than normal. In less severe condition, the patella may be seated in the misformed trochlea during knee extension but dislocated everytime the knee is flexed—habitual dislocation of patella. Eilert noted the difference between two clinical syndromes and called them: congenital dislocation of the patella and habitual dislocation of the patella, respectively. The differences between them are outlined in the **Table 4B.1.4**.

TABLE 4B.1.4: The differences between congenital and habitual dislocation of patella.

Congenital dislocation of patella	Habitual dislocation of patella
Patella is dislocated lateral and persistent in that location	Patella dislocates and reduces spontaneously with flexion and extension of knee joint
Often obvious in infancy	Usually present at 5–10 years old
Frequently associated with generalized syndrome	Usually isolated anomaly
Knee flexion contracture is present	Range of knee motion usually normal
Nearly always produces functional disability	May be well-tolerated with little functional disability
Early surgical correction	Surgical correction can be delayed until patient is symptomatic

The diagnosis of congenital dislocation of the patella is usually apparent after 3–4 years of age. Clinical suspicion and magnetic resonance imaging (MRI) can confirm the diagnosis early. The increasing use of ultrasound can also be exploited for early diagnosis.

Treatment is surgical correction as early as possible as the severity of the deformity is directly related to the length of time that the deformity is allowed to remain uncorrected. This effectively prevents valgus, flexion, or external rotation deformity of the knee developing later. The primary objective is release of the contracted structures on the lateral side of the patella (the lateral capsule, iliotibial band, and lateral portion of the quadriceps) to allow reduction of the patella. Medial plication of the lax capsule is necessary to stabilize the reduced patella. In older children, advancement of the vastus medialis often is necessary to tighten the muscle and improve muscle action.

Other surgical procedures include—extensive lateral release, medial plication, and transfer of the lateral half of the patellar tendon, lateral release and medial transfer of the patellar tendon, lateral release, and vastus medialis obliquus advancement and entire patellar transfer in skeletally immature patients and medial transfer of the tibial tubercle in skeletally mature patients.

26. Describe habitual dislocation of patella.

Ans: In habitual dislocation (or obligatory patellar dislocation), the patella dislocates every time knee flexes and is associated with quadriceps contracture. The vastus lateralis may be absent or is usually severely contracted, and the patella may remain dislocated laterally. In some cases, there may be dysplastic attachment of patella to anterior aspect of the iliotibial band. In any case the development of patella is hampered and it remains small and misshapen. Due to regular dislocation, the sesamoid bone develops in abnormal position in the quadriceps mechanism.

Lower limb alignment also suffers and there is commonly genu valgum and tibial external rotation laterally shifting the tibial tuberosity. The lateral femoral condyle is hypoplastic and the capsule on the medial side of the knee is stretched. The patellar tendon may be inserted more laterally than normal.

Clinical features:
- Patella dislocates and reduces spontaneously with flexion and extension of knee joint
- Patients usually consult at 5–10 years of age
- Usually isolated anomaly
- Range of motion of knee is normal.

Pathomechanics: Contracture of the quadriceps mechanism is present in all other bony findings are variable in presence and extent.

Treatment: The primary objective is release of the contracted structures on the lateral side of the patella (the lateral capsule, iliotibial band, and lateral portion of the quadriceps) to allow reduction of the patella. Medial plication of the lax capsule is added in nearly all patients to stabilize the reduced patella. In older children, additional advancement of the VMO (Madigan procedure) is often necessary to tighten the muscle and improve muscle action.

27. Describe extensor mechanism of knee and the factors that predispose to recurrent dislocation of patella.

Ans: *Extensor mechanism of knee*: The extensor mechanism of knee comprises of patella with quadriceps tendon, patellar tendon and whole extensor expansion. The details can be read from Chapter 2 and the reader is also encouraged to read it from *Chapter 34 of the book Essential Orthopedics: Principles and Practice, 2nd edition*.

Factors predisposing to recurrent dislocation of patella are:
- Incompetence of MPFL
- Increased Q angle
- Small or dysplastic patella
- Patella alta
- Dysplasia of femoral condyles.

28. Describe quadriceps contracture of infancy and childhood.

Ans: The quadriceps contracture can be congenital or acquired types and rarely may have features of both. Intramuscular injections have been long considered to cause these contractures due to compression of the muscle bundles and capillaries by the volume of medication injected and the toxicity of the drug. There is always some lag between injection and development of contracture. There are three pathological types:
1. Rectus femoris type—restricted knee flexion and hip flexes with knee flexion
2. Vastus type—restricted hip flexion but no effect with knee flexion
3. Mixed type—knee flexion restricted with hip flexion and hip flexes with knee flexion.

Components of quadriceps contracture:
- Fibrosis of the vastus intermedius muscle tying down the rectus femoris to the femur
- Adhesions between the patella and the femoral condyles
- Fibrosis and shortening of the lateral expansions of the vasti and their adherence to the femoral condyles,
- Shortening of the rectus femoris muscle.

Clinical features: There is progressive, painless limitation of knee flexion. Hyperextension and subluxation of the knee may occur with continued growth. Characteristic dimple may be present over the area of fibrosis, especially when the knee is flexed. Habitual dislocation of the patella and hypoplastic patellae are usually associated.

Radiographically hypoplasia of the patella, flattening of the femoral condyles, genu recurvatum, anterior dislocation of the tibia, and gross degenerative changes in the joint can be seen.

Treatment: Early recognition and prevention of quadriceps contracture through passive exercise in children for stretching is imperative. When the scar tissue is matured, however, surgical treatment is indicated to prevent late changes in the femoral condyles and the patella. Surgical treatment is indicated early in patients with habitual dislocation of the patella. Thompson's quadricepsplasty is the usual surgical approach while its extent depends on whether the rectus femoris muscle has escaped injury, and how well this muscle can be isolated from the scarred parts of the quadriceps mechanism. In early stage of contracture, limited proximal release to eliminate extensor lag and hemarthrosis of the knee is commonly done while in extensive contractures, Thompson type of quadricepsplasty is indicated. Supracondylar femoral osteotomy can be done to restore flexion in recurvatum knee.

29. Describe Osgood-Schlatter disease.

Ans: Repeated microtrauma at the insertion of the patellar tendon at tibial tuberosity causes traction apophysitis. In active adolescents, the disease presents as avulsion fracture of the tibial tubercle and occurs usually in patients who jump or kick, often boys as compared to girls. It is bilateral in 25–50% cases and is seen at 12–15 years of age in boys; the onset in girls may be slightly earlier (8–12 years). Paget originally described in 1891 the clinical symptoms, which later came to be known as Osgood-Schlatter disease. The condition was separately described (1903) by Robert B Osgood, a Boston orthopedic surgeon and Carl Schlatter, a Swiss professor of surgery.

Pathophysiology and natural history: The tibial tuberosity fragment is cartilaginous initially and with continued traction a bony callus forms and the tuberosity enlarges with growth. This condition usually resolves when the patient reaches approximately at the age of 18 years. The only remnant is an enlarged tibial tubercle. Repeated irritation causes swelling, hemorrhage, and gradual degeneration of the apophysis as a result of impaired circulation (osteochondrosis). Complete avulsion of the patellar tendon is a major complication seen in extremely rare and neglected circumstances else the condition spontaneously resolves once the physis closes by 16–18 years.

Clinical features: Patient complains of pain and swelling over the tibial tuberosity, exacerbated with exercise. The pain increases with kneeling, jumping, and running. There is point tenderness over the anterior proximal tibial tubercle which is enlarged. Pain aggravates with resisted knee extension. The knee has full ROM but may have hamstring tightness.

Investigations

Radiographs: Fragmentation of the tuberosity fragment, calcification within the patellar tendon, ossicle formation within, etc. may be seen on a lateral view of knee especially taken in 10–20° of internal rotation.

Ultrasound: This is the investigation of choice; the chief findings are:
- Swelling of the unossified tibial tuberosity cartilage and overlying soft tissues.
- Fragmentation and irregularity of the ossification center with reduced internal echogenicity.
- Thickening of the distal patellar tendon.
- Infrapatellar bursitis.

Magnetic resonance imaging: It is not indicated routinely but may demonstrate— thickening and edema of infrapatellar tendon, loss of sharp inferior angle of infrapatellar fat pad (IFP), soft tissue swelling anterior to the tibial tuberosity and sometimes infrapatellar bursitis.

Differential diagnosis: Sinding-Larsen-Johansson disease, quadriceps tendon avulsion, chondromalacia patella, Hoffa's syndrome, tibial tubercle fracture, tumor, plica syndrome, pes anserine bursitis, osteochondritis dissecans, etc.

Management: As the disease is self-limiting and the disorder stops progression with rest the management is usually conservative and includes the following:
- RICE in acute phase with strict immobilization for 2–4 weeks. Anti-inflammatory medications reduce pain and swelling. Counsel patients that rest is the best medicine.
- Also explain that reduction in stressful activities until the epiphyseal closure will prevent any aggravations. Use a cylindrical cast in severe and noncompliant cases.
- Perform isometric strengthening of the quadriceps and hamstring muscles once pain subsides.
- Steroid injections are totally discouraged as they may in fact cause tendon weakness and are also responsible for atrophy of the subcutaneous tissue over the tuberosity.
- Surgery is not commonly indicated. In skeletally immature patient, in fact surgery is contraindicated as it may cause premature fusion of tibial physis. The only indication of surgery in children could be avulsion of tibial tuberosity that

may be fixed in place by pins (preferably bioabsorbable ones). The other indication of surgery is in adults where ossicle formation or prominence causes undue irritation at the site locally. This is treated by removal of ossicle, bursa, and any prominence if any, but carefully protecting the patellar tendon.

30. Describe clinical signs of fat pad syndrome and briefly outline its management.

Ans: There are two most important fat pads of the knee one located beneath the patellar tendon—the infrapatellar pad (IFP) and the other one above it—the suprapatellar fat pad. The IFP separates the synovial membrane from the patellar tendon. Due to its large size and predilection for activity related injury, the IFP is more often injured and is also subjected to frictional wear chronically (Hoffa's disease). Fat pad irritation (Hoffa's syndrome or disease) is a common cause of anterior knee pain and is often mistaken for patellofemoral pain syndrome (PFPS) or knee osteoarthritis.

Clinical signs:
- Pain beneath the patellar ligament especially during knee extension.
- Pain getting worse with physical activity and sports.
- Frog eye deformity with pain may be seen in chronic cases with protrusion of the fat pad on either side of tendon anteriorly. Do not label females with hypertrophied fat pads as having Hoffa's disease.
- The knee may display weakness and stiffness during movement.
- Pressing on the inferior pole of patella increases symptoms.
- Tipping patella away from inferior pole relaxes the symptoms and pain.
- Hoffa's test—palpate the tenderness in IFP and ask the patient to contract quadriceps to tense the quadriceps tendon. This pulls patellar tendon and limits the access to IFP. The pain reduces with this maneuver in Hoffa's disease. If the pain increases, then pathology is more likely in the patellar tendon.

Management:
Conservative management consists of:
- *Management of swelling*: Ice application 2–3 times a day for 15–20 minutes. Local ultrasonic therapy. Rest from irritating activities until inflammation has subsided.
- Heel elevation of ½–1 inch (1.25–2.5 cm). Heel elevation prevents added irritation during full extension; taping to lift the inferior pole of patella and prevent impingement. Taping may also be done to prevent knee hyperextension.
- *Stretching exercises*: This is done to stretch the rectus femoris especially.
- *Strengthening exercises*: Quadriceps strengthening and improvement in muscle coordination.
- *Biomechanics*: Avoid heels.

Surgical option: If the above conservative measures fail, then release of tight fascial bands, inflamed synovium and ligamentum mucosae is required. The bands that tether the lower pole of patella need to be selectively released during arthroscopy. Fat pad may be debulked to avoid further impingement.

31. Describe classifications and principles of management of congenital pseudarthrosis of tibia.

Ans: Classification: The classification has been described in **Table 4B.1.5**.

TABLE 4B.1.5: Classification of congenital pseudarthrosis of tibia.		
Boyd	**Description**	**Anderson equivalent**
I	Patients born with anterior bowing and tibial defect	
II	Anterior bowing + hourglass contracture (Fracture by 2 years) associated with neurofibromatosis (worse prognosis)	Dysplastic type
III	Bone cyst	Cystic type
IV	Sclerotic segment of tibia (no narrowing), usually develops stress type fracture–nonunion	Late/sclerotic type
V	Also have dysplastic fibula	Fibular type
VI	Intraosseous neurofibroma/Schwannoma (rarest type) Foot deformity (CTEV/Streeter's band associated)	Clubfoot/congenital band type

Principles of Management

Conservative management: This is the initial preferred treatment for all cases, especially for patients without fracture or pseudarthrosis (prepseudarthrosis). Total contact plastic clamshell orthosis, AFO (prior to walking), and KAFO (after they start walking) are commonly employed methods as they are easier to manage than plaster casts. The bracing is discontinued, if:
- There is sufficient straightening of tibia
- Medullary canal is reformed
- Adequate cortical thickness is achieved.

Principles of surgical management:
Surgical treatment: Goals of surgical treatment include—
- Lasting union at fracture site
- Maintaining alignment to avoid undue stress at the pseudarthrosis site
- Obtaining acceptable limb length.

(Details of surgical methods can be read from Chapter 29 of the Essential Orthopedics: Principles and Practice, 2nd edition.)

32. Discuss various conventional and modern methods of management of congenital pseudarthrosis of tibia.

Ans: Conventional treatment options: The following are commonly described surgical treatment options mentioned here in decreasing order of popularity.

- *Intramedullary (IM) nailing with iliac crest bone graft and transfixation of ankle (Charnley)*: It involves extraperiosteal pseudarthrosis excision and IM stabilization of the tibia and fibula. An autogenous bone graft, with or without iliac crest periosteum, is used at the resection site. The success rate for IM nailing and bone grafting approaches 80–90%, although the pseudoarthrosis may recur and necessitate repeated bone grafting, with or without bone stimulation units. This technique is generally practiced with variously described modifications from different authors:
  - *IM bone graft with vascularized fibula and iliac crest cancellous graft*: Transfixes ankle and subtalar joint (retrograde insertion of rod)
  - *IM nailing with two parts of solid Peter Williams rod, pseudoarthrosis excision and iliac crest bone grafting*: The rod is advanced into the talus and calcaneus correcting the calcaneovalgus deformity of the foot simultaneously and then the rod is advanced retrograde into the proximal fragment. The gap at osteotomy site is filled with bone graft obtained from iliac crest. Another osteotomy may be required proximally in case of extensive deformity and tibial bow.
  - Bone morphogenic protein can be added to the procedure to stimulate bone formation at the site.
  - After surgery, children are placed in a cast for 3–4 months and then in an ankle-foot orthosis, with the ankle locked.
- *Microvascular fibular graft (contralateral), rib, iliac crest with excision of tibial pseudarthrosis*: The microvascular procedures are particularly useful and have shown better healing rates than other procedures, especially in cases with severe atrophied bones at the ends of fracture. For this procedure to be successful, the pathological region should be excised extraperiosteally. The graft bone is then fitted in a dowel-like manner and protected with plate osteosynthesis or external fixator. Subsequent additional surgical procedures are, however, required due to inadequate consolidation of the grafted bone in the form of secondary bone grafting commonly.
- *Ilizarov method*: The method is versatile in producing consolidation at the fracture site and simultaneous correction of the deformity. It can be applied in various forms including compression only, compression plus tibial lengthening, compression followed by distraction, distraction alone for hypertrophic nonunion. This method can also be used in children who were not successfully treated using the previous method or those who are older or in patients with atrophic bone ends at the fracture site. The pseudarthrosis is resected, and the two bone ends are impacted. A proximal corticotomy allows for bone transport to make up for the tibial shortening. The bone is compressed distally.
- As in other techniques, autogenous bone graft and bone morphogenetic protein are used to facilitate union at the distal site. The success rate of this method is 70–90%. Variations include implantation of an IM nail throughout the distraction–compression process [SCONE (slow compression over nail using external fixator)] or after union has been obtained. Compression using an external fixator often leads to deformation at the pseudoarthrosis site while placing an IM nail will prevent deformation in sagittal or coronal plane but allow axial compression to occur.

- Amputation (McCarthy), Boyd/Symes type to produce end-bearing stump: This is a mutilating surgery but may need to be employed judiciously in some cases:
  - Failed three surgical attempts
  - Shortening >5 cm
  - Deformed foot
  - Prolonged hospitalization
  - Pseudoarthrosis <2.5 cm from ankle joint.

Modern method(s):
Physeal (PDO) and subphyseal distraction (SPDO) osteogenesis in atrophic type of congenital pseudoarthrosis of tibia:
- *PDO*: A preconstructed Ilizarov frame with three rings is applied for lengthening through the physis causing epiphysiolysis or chondrodiastasis. Corticotomy is done at the proximal one-fourth to one-fifth of fibula protecting the nerve. Acute distraction is done from the first day until the occurrence of physeal separation of proximal tibia that could be recognized by sudden intense pain around knee. Immediately after confirming physeal separation by radiographs, the distracted physis is acutely shortened so that the separated physis was restored to its normal height.
- *SPDO*: Procedure same as PDO, except corticotomy is done below the physis and acute distraction is avoided.

33. Discuss Paley classification of congenital pseudoarthrosis of tibia. Describe principle of latest approach to its management.

Ans: The Paley classification is as follows:
- *Type 1*: No fractures
- *Type 2*: No fracture tibia, fracture fibula with fibula
  1. At station
  2. Proximal migration
- *Type 3*: Fracture tibia, no fracture fibula
- *Type 4*: Fracture tibia and fibula, with fibula
  1. At station
  2. Proximal migration
  3. Bone defect tibia with proximal migration fibula

Choi/Paley cross-union concept and method of treatment: This method is based on the premises of dismal (50%) union rates of contemporary methods while it was found that cross-union cases did not refracture. The idea was first reported as a method treatment for CPT by Johnston in 2002. Choi had been using this method since 1999 while Paley started using this after observation that cross-union had minimal refracture rates in 2007.
- *Choi et al. method*: Choi et al. (2011) recommended creation of a cross-union between the tibia and fibula for CPT cases where the fibula was broken but minimally proximally migrated. They converged the two fibula bone ends towards the two tibia bone ends in what they called a '4-in-1 Osteosynthesis'. They used a cortico-cancellous sheet of the inner table of the ilium with or without its periosteum and when necessary additional cortical bone from the contralateral tibia combined with cancellous bone chips to achieve the cross-union. The cortical graft was placed posterior to the two bones and then cancellous chips between the bones and another layer of cortical bone anterior to the bones. They did not recommend this method when the fibula was intact or when the fibula was significantly proximally migrated.
- *Paley method (pharmacological + surgical)*: The treatment protocol is presurgical infusion of zoledronic acid (ZA) + hamartoma resection around tibia and fibula with resection of the interosseous membrane + tibial rodding with a telescopic growing rod and fibular rodding with a wire + decancellousization of the ilium to harvest a large cancellous bone graft + harvest of periosteal graft from the underside of the iliacus muscle + application of a three-layer graft composed of: (1) periosteum around the CPT; (2) cancellous bone between and around the tibia and fibula; and (3) BMP2 posterior and anterior to the bone graft covered by soft tissues. The last step is application of the Ilizarov apparatus/internal fixator to compress the CPT site and to give rotational stability. The smooth nonlocking telescopic rod only gives angular support but does not prevent the bone ends pulling apart or rotating to each other. More recently in 2017, the author replaced the external fixator with an internal fixator (locking plate).

34. Bowing of tibia in children:
- Describe causes and types.
- Discuss management of congenital bowing of tibia.

Ans: Angular deformities of tibia are rare but do occasionally occur. The deformity can be:
- Anterior angulation or bow—seen commonly with fibular hemimelia. Fibular hemimelia is treated with amputation and prosthetic fitting or limb reconstruction and lengthening. Syme or Boyd amputation is considered for patients who have a nonfunctional foot with severe valgus positioning or fewer than three rays, as well as a projected limb-length discrepancy >30% compared with the contralateral side. Limb lengthening is considered for children who have a projected length discrepancy of <10%, compared with the contralateral side, as well as the potential for good foot function after ankle and foot reconstruction. Children with a discrepancy of between 10% and 30% can be managed with either amputation and prosthetic fitting or limb reconstruction and lengthening. The decision is based on the preference of the treating physician and the family.
- Posteromedial angulation or bow—seen commonly with calcaneovalgus foot deformity. It is a benign congenital anomaly without fracture or pseudoarthrosis. The foot deformity usually corrects itself within the first year of life but eventual limb-length discrepancy of 2–5 cm is commonly seen that is the main reason why an orthopedic surgeon is consulted. At birth, the foot is grossly dorsiflexed with limited plantar flexion. Tibial bow is evident only on palpation. There may be a small skin dimple at the site of bow. Stretching and casting are occasionally used to improve the deformity, and, rarely, an ankle-foot orthosis is used for weight-bearing. Gradual correction is expected to occur over several years until the tibia is straight or has a mild S shape. Treatment of the tibial deformity consists of observation versus correction of the limb-length discrepancy and residual bow. Lengthening of the extremity may be done with distraction osteosynthesis and bow corrected with guided growth. Contralateral physiodesis may be considered in individuals with a limb-length discrepancy but no residual tibial bow.
- Anterolateral angulation or bow—The anterolateral bowing of tibia is commonly seen in few congenital disorders apart from malunion resulting from trauma:
  - Congenital pseudoarthrosis of tibia
  - *Congenital anterolateral bowing of tibia with polydactyly*: Here, the bowing resolves spontaneously often. There may be associated duplication of great toe, clinodactyly, tibial shortening, and carpal or metacarpal anomaly.
  - *Neurofibromatosis type 1*: This is associated in 50% of anterolateral bowing cases with or with congenital pseudoarthrosis of tibia. It may be unilateral. Fibula may or may not be hypoplastic. The stigmata of neurofibromatosis including the skin and other osseous lesions are present.
  - Tibial hemimelia (congenital longitudinal deficiency of tibia)
  - Fibular hemimelia (congenital longitudinal deficiency of fibula)
  - Nonunion or malunion following osteomyelitis
  - *Fibrous dysplasia*: The bone is of poor quality due to geographic defect in bone quality. There may be associated skin lesions.
  - Amniotic band syndrome

The management of congenital pseudoarthrosis of tibia is written in detail in questions 30-32 above.

35. Describe tibial hemimelia.

Ans: Tibial hemimelia is also known as congenital longitudinal deficiency of the tibia, congenital dysplasia of the tibia, paraxial tibial hemimelia, tibial dysplasia, and congenital deficiency or absence of the tibia. These are extremely rare occurring in 1 in 1 million but tibial deficiency is associated with high likelihood for deformities in later generations. It is characterized by deficiency of the tibia with relatively intact fibula. The deficiency is bilateral in 30% of patients. Most of the affected children (60% and 70%) have concurrent musculoskeletal disorders that include:
- Equinovarus foot
- Congenital short femur
- Congenital dislocation of the hip
- Cleft hand.

The associated syndromes with tibial hemimelia include:
- Tibial hemimelia diplopodia
- Polydactyly triphalangeal thumb syndrome (Werner syndrome)
- Tibial hemimelia-split-hand or foot syndrome
- Tibial hemimelia-micromelia-trigonal brachycephaly syndrome.

Tibial deficiency is classified based on the presence of a proximal tibia (and hence a functional quadriceps mechanism). The jones classification divides tibial hemimelia into four groups:

1. *Type I deficiency*: No tibia is seen on radiographs. Cartilage tibia anlage may appear on ultrasonography or MRI which ossifies later.
    - In type 1 A, fibula is dislocated proximally, tibia is not radiographically evident and distal femoral epiphysis is smaller than on normal side.
    - In type 1 B, fibula is dislocated proximally and proximal tibial cartilaginous anlage may be visible at birth on ultrasound or MRI, but not on plain radiographs that may ossify later.
2. Type 2 deficiency has proximal dislocation of fibula and radiographically visible proximal tibia with normal appearing knee joint.
3. In type 3 deficiency, fibula is dislocated proximally, distal tibia is radiographically visible, but proximal tibia is not seen.
4. In rare type 4 deformity, fibula has migrated proximally, with congenital diastasis of the ankle joint (tibiofibular joint).

Clinical features: There is shortening of the involved leg. The fibular head is palpable and foot is held in severe equinovarus. The knee generally has flexion contracture and in more severe deformities quadriceps insufficiency causes lack of knee extension. The superficial peroneal nerve may extend up to ankle. The anterior tibial artery is absent, and the plantar arterial arch is incomplete. Tendons of leg muscles that insert on the plantar surface of the foot often fuse into single mass. The talus and calcaneus are often fused.

Treatment: The type of surgical treatment depends on the radiographic classification and clinical appearance. Type IA deficiency is usually treated with transarticular amputation (knee disarticulation) followed by prosthetic fitting. Fibular centralization is not considered unless an intact functional quadriceps mechanism is present that can be reconstructed to provide active knee extension. Type 1B deficiencies can be reconstructed to give a functional knee joint. The foot and sometimes distal leg are amputated to be fitted later with prosthesis. A type II or even the type 1B deficiency is treated with Syme amputation of the dysfunctional foot and a proximal tibial-fibular synostosis is created to produce a functioning below-knee amputation. Type III deficiencies are extremely rare to occur and are managed with foot amputation (Syme or Chopart) and prosthetic fitting. Patients with type IV deficiencies need individualized treatment after explaining the options. Easiest and quite reliable method is to do a Syme amputation and prosthetic fitting. Exquisite procedures like customized reconstruction of the ankle joint to retain the foot and ankle by combinations of distal tibiofibular synostosis and distal fibular epiphysiodesis have been described but require multiple surgeries followed by soft tissue releases for equinovarus deformities of the foot.

36. Describe tibial hemimelia.
Ans: Kindly see Answer to Question above.

37. Describe classification, clinical features and management of tibial hemimelia
Ans: Kindly see Answers to Questions above.

38. A. Describe the clinical signs and symptoms of a rigid pes planus deformity.
   B. Radiological features of congenital vertical talus, differential diagnosis, and management.

Ans: Pes Planus Deformity:
A. **Clinical features:**
   - Severe uncorrectable equinovalgus deformity of hindfoot.
   - Rocker bottom foot (loss of medial longitudinal arch with prominent rounded talar head as lowermost part of arch).

- Forefoot is abducted, pronated, and dorsiflexed with fixed dorsal subluxation of navicular over talar head.
- Lateral toes are outward looking and everted.
- Soft tissues (tendons of tibialis anterior, long toe extensors, and 3 peronei) on dorsolateral side of foot are contracted.
- Deep creases inferior and lateral to lateral malleolus.
- Tendo-Achilles contracture
- Callosities beneath anterior end of calcaneus and along medial border of foot superficial to talar head.
- Tendons of peroneus longus, brevis and tibialis posterior are tight and may come to lie anterior to malleoli (acting as dorsiflexors rather than plantar flexors).

B. **Congenital vertical talus (CVT)—Radiological features:** The films are obtained in AP and lateral projections in forced plantar flexion and dorsiflexion.
- The *forced plantar flexion lateral view* confirms rigid dorsal displacement of the first metatarsal axis to the longitudinal axis of the talus [Meary's angle >20° (*See* chapter of foot)], also called TAMBA—talar axis 1st metatarsal base axis. There is persistent dislocation of the talonavicular joint (reduced joint will come under the category of *oblique talus*). In patients with oblique talus, the forced plantar flexion lateral radiograph shows collinearity of the first metatarsal and the longitudinal axis of the talus, suggesting that the primary disorder is a posterior lateral contracture and not true congenital vertical talus (CVT).
- Forced dorsiflexion lateral radiograph is needed to confirm and demonstrate the equinus deformity of the ankle.
- Anteroposterior view shows the midfoot valgus and a talocalcaneal angle greater than 40° (normal range 20–40°).
- Mostly as the foot bones are not ossified in infants, an ultrasonographic evaluation is needed to demonstrate and document the vertical position of talus. Forced plantar flexion should be done while sonography also.

CVT—Differential diagnosis:
- Flexible flat foot
- Inflammatory and infective foot disorders
- Neurological like AMC and meningomyelocele
- *Compensatory*: Tight tendo-Achilles with/without equines deformity, external rotational deformity of lower limb
- Congenital oblique talus
- Tarsal coalition
- Pes valgus deformity either congenital, paralytic, or pes planovalgus.

CVT—Management

Manipulation of the deformity: Serial casting was thought to be an unsuccessful method of correction while lately described "reverse Ponseti" method of reducing navicular over talus has been found satisfactory. It is indicated in a child with mild or oblique CVT and is getting popular as initial treatment for CVT.

Dobb's method: Manipulation is done to stretch the foot in plantar flexion to elongate anterior structures and achieve inversion while applying counterpressure to the medial aspect of the talus. This prevents compression of the navicular. Dobbs used to fix the navicular to talus once satisfactory correction was obtained. To correct the equinus, an additional Achilles tendon tenotomy is always necessary.

Surgical treatment: This has been the standard method of correcting the deformity. Coleman and others described two-stage two incision procedure but this method had higher complication rate. In this procedure, lengthening of extensor digitorum longus (EDL), extensor hallucis longus (EHL), and tibialis anterior is done along with anterior capsular releases (talonavicular and calcaneocuboid joints). The second stage consists of tendo-Achilles release and posterior release (ankle and subtalar capsulotomies). Single-stage approach has become popular as described by Seimon and others. Here, the EHL and peroneus tendons are tenotomized and talonavicular joint reduced by open reduction and K-wire fixation. Achilles tenotomy is mandatory as usual. In children 2 years of age or younger, surgical reconstruction involves lengthening the Achilles, peroneus longus and peroneus brevis tendons, and performing a posterolateral subtalar release. Talonavicular joint is then reduced and pinned. The tibialis anterior, EHL, and EDL tendons are lengthened. The above procedure can be done in children up to 4 years of age with less severe deformities.

Older children with residual deformities may require a salvage procedure, such as a naviculectomy, talectomy, triple arthrodesis or subtalar fusion. Children 3 years or older often require navicular excision at the time of open reduction. Children 4–8 years of age often require open reduction and soft-tissue procedures along with extra-articular subtalar arthrodesis. Neglected cases presenting after 12 years of age often have developing arthrosis and deformities so rigid that cannot be corrected. They are best treated by triple arthrodesis for correction of the deformity.

39. Define congenital vertical talus. Describe clinical features.

Ans: Definition: Congenital vertical talus is a rare foot deformity consisting of an irreducible dorsal dislocation of the navicular on the talus, producing a rigid flatfoot deformity.

Clinical features: Congenital vertical talus usually can be detected at birth by the presence of a rounded prominence on the medial and plantar surface of the foot. The clinical features are secondary to the displaced position of talus:
- The talus is almost vertical and displaced plantarward and medially.
- The calcaneus is also in equinus position.
- The forefoot is dorsiflexed at the midtarsal joints.
- The navicular lies on the dorsal aspect of the head of the talus.
- The sole is convex, and there are deep creases on the dorsolateral aspect of the foot anterior and inferior to the lateral malleolus.

Late changes:
- Once WB begins, adaptive changes occur in the tarsal bones.
- The talus becomes shaped like an hourglass.
- The longitudinal axis of talus is almost the same as that of the tibia (only the posterior third of its superior articular surface articulates with the tibia).
- The calcaneus remains in an equinus position.
- The anterior part of calcaneus becomes rounded.
- Callosities develop beneath the anterior end of the calcaneus and along the medial border of the foot superficial to the head of the talus.
- The forefoot becomes severely abducted, and the heel does not touch the floor.
- All the capsules, ligaments, and tendons on the dorsum of the foot become contracted.
- The posterior tibial and peroneus longus and brevis tendons may come to lie anterior to the malleoli and act as dorsiflexors rather than plantar flexors.

40. A. Describe pathoanatomy and Pirani scoring in congenital talipes equinovarus (CTEV).
B. Steps of Ponseti manipulation and serial cast application.

Ans: Congenital talipes equinovarus (CTEV).

A. *Pathoanatomy*: There are two basic components of CTEV deformity:
1. Malposition of tarsal bones and joints, which are in extreme position of flexion, inversion, and adduction producing the primary deformity.
2. Ligaments and muscles on the posterior and medial aspect of ankle and tarsal joints are very thick and taut, thereby severely retaining and maintaining the foot in equinus, inversion and adduction.

Bean-shaped deformity of clubfoot is due to varus and adduction of heel, medial displacement of navicular on the medially angulated head and neck of the talus and forefoot adduction. Overall size of tarsals is reduced. Talus is the least displaced and shows most severe and consistent changes in form. Since, no muscle attachment occurs at talus, it is passively forced into equinus by calcaneus and navicular. Deformity in clubfoot hence is due to abnormal relationship of tarsal bones, that is, navicular and calcaneus is displaced medially around the talus. Severity of deformity depends upon degree of bony displacement. Resistance of deformity is determined by rigidity of soft tissue contractures.

- Adapted alteration in shape of tarsal bones is acquired in accordance with *Wolff's law,* which states that every change in the use of static functions of a bone causes changes in its internal form and architecture, external formation and function according to mathematical law.
- Soft tissue contractures are explained by *Davis law*, which states that ligaments and soft tissues in loose or lax state will gradually shorten.

The detailed bony and soft tissue changes are described below:

Talus: This bone is in severe plantar flexion with its head displaced medially and deflected plantarward.
- Normal angle between long axis of neck and head with body is 150°. But in clubfoot, the medial deviation is increased so that angle (angle of declination) is between 115° and 135° (i.e., more acute). Hence, neck is medially deviated and foreshortened.
- Normal constriction at neck which accommodates anterior lip of tibial plafond on dorsiflexion is absent, which decreases the dorsiflexion.
- Head and facet for navicular face medially instead of facing forward. It is broader, with varying degree of flattening. In severe cases, it may be wedge shaped.
- Posterior facet on the inferior surface of talus is underdeveloped and shallow. The three plantar facets on head appear as a single surface.
- Medial borders of talus and calcaneus are congruent and underdeveloped.

Calcaneum: The calcaneus is involved in all three components of the deformity, i.e., (1) equinus, (2) varus, and (3) adduction.
- Its posterior tuberosity is displaced upward and laterally
- The anterior end is displaced downward, medially and is inverted
- Sustentaculum tali is medially displaced, underdeveloped and fails to provide usual pulley for flexor hallucis longus tendon (FHL).

Navicular: The navicular is usually medially displaced. Its articular surface faces laterally to articulate with medially deviated head and neck of talus. In severe deformities, dorsomedial subluxation of navicular is present. Normal concavity of the proximal articular process is flattened. The navicular tuberosity is elongated and in close proximity to medial malleolus.

Cuboid bone: Cuboid bridges the midtarsal and tarsometatarsal joint and as it occupies a position in both rows of tarsal bones, hence significant medial displacement of cuboid is obstructed by navicular. Minimal changes occur in calcaneocuboid joint.

Metatarsals: Medial migration and inversion of all five metatarsals cause forefoot adduction, which contributes to the convexity of the lateral border of the foot and composite varus adduction deformity.

Soft tissue contractures: This involves muscles, tendons; tendon sheaths, ligaments, joint capsule, and skin. Posterior tibial neurovascular bundle may also be shortened. The prime contractures, which are common to all patients, are tendo-Achilles, tibialis posterior, deltoid ligament, spring ligament, and talonavicular capsule. Contractures may be divided into posterior, medial, plantar, and subtalar.
- Posterior contractures (tendo-Achilles, tibiotalar capsule, talocalcaneus capsule, post-talofibular ligament, calcaneofibular ligament) resist equines deformity and correction of calcaneus and ankle joint. Contracted tendo-Achilles, posterior talocalcaneal capsule, and the calcaneofibular ligament are the structures, which maximally resist correction by preventing downward excursions of the postcalcaneal tuberosity. Contracted tibiotalar capsule and posterior talofibular ligament resist dorsiflexion of talus by preventing the downward exit of posterior part of trochlea out of the mortise. Of the two capsules talocalcaneous joint capsule is more contracted. Tendo-Achilles tendon in clubfoot is broader and inserts distally on medial surface of calcaneus because tendon attaches itself to the deviated posterior end of calcaneus.
- Medial plantar contractures [tibialis posterior (TP) tendon and sheath, tendon of FHL and flexor digitorum longus (FDL), deltoid ligament, talonavicular capsule and spring ligament] form an indistinguishable scar, which maintain navicular tuberosity and sustentaculum in close proximity with medial malleolus causing atresia

of "acetabulum" of TCN joint. They prevent forward and lateral migration of navicular and prevent eversion and lateral movement of anterior end of calcaneus. The tendons of TP, FDL, and FHL do not contribute to the deformity but may increase resistance to correction. The contracted Henry's knot (annular ligament for 2 tendons) restricts mobility of navicular because of its attachment.

- Subtalar contractures comprise of talocalcanean interosseous ligament and bifurcate Y-ligament. These are usually seen in older children.
- Plantar contractures consist of abductor hallucis, intrinsic toe flexors, quadratus plantae, and plantar aponeurosis. Plantar aponeurosis is palpable as a tight band along medial plantar surface and is less prominent in children less than 4 years. Abductor hallucis has an abnormal attachment to TP tendon sheaths, the sheaths of FDL and FHL and to the navicular tuberosity. Intrinsic toe flexors are short and the first metatarsal is plantar flexed. The TA tendon may be attached till mid shaft of first metatarsal.

Pirani scoring: **Table 4B.1.6** shows Pirani scoring.

TABLE 4B.1.6: Pirani scoring.

Physical examination findings	Score of 0	Score of 0.5	Score of 1
Curvature of lateral border of foot	Straight	Mild distal curve	Curve at calcaneocuboid joint
Severity of medial crease (foot held in maximal correction)	Multiple fine creases	One or two deep creases	Deep creases change contour of arch
Severity of posterior crease (foot held in maximal correction)	Multiple fine creases	One or two deep creases	Deep creases change contour of arch
Medial malleolar–navicular interval (foot held in maximal correction)	Definite depression felt	Interval reduced	Interval not palpable
Palpation of lateral part of head of talus (forefoot fully abducted)	Navicular completely "reduces"; lateral talar head cannot be felt	Navicular partially "reduces"; lateral head less palpable	Navicular does not "reduce"; lateral talar head easily felt
Emptiness of heel (foot and ankle in maximal correction)	Tuberosity of calcaneus easily palpable	Tuberosity of calcaneus more difficult to palpate	Tuberosity of calcaneus not palpable
Fibula-Achilles interval (hip flexed, knee extended, foot and ankle maximally corrected)	Definite depression felt	Interval reduced	Interval not palpable
Rigidity of equinus (knee extended, ankle maximally corrected)	Normal ankle dorsiflexion	Ankle dorsiflexes beyond neutral, but not fully	Cannot dorsiflex ankle to neutral
Rigidity of adductus (forefoot is fully abducted)	Forefoot can be overcorrected into abduction	Forefoot can be corrected beyond neutral, but not fully	Forefoot cannot be corrected to neutral
Long flexor contracture (foot and ankle held in maximal correction)	MTP joints can be dorsiflexed to 90°	MTP joints can be dorsiflexed beyond neutral but not fully	MTP joints cannot be dorsiflexed to neutral

B. **Steps:** Stages to Ponseti method of correction—
The first stage is manipulative correction to stretch out the tendons and straightening of the foot. This is gradually achieved as follows:

- The first deformity to be corrected is cavus, which is because of excessive plantar flexion of the first ray. The fifth ray, in contrast is well-aligned with the cuboid. Consequently, although the entire foot is supinated, the forefoot is pronated as compared to the hindfoot resulting in the cavus deformity. Therefore, the cavus deformity is corrected by supinating the forefoot gently, thereby placing the first metatarsal in alignment with the rest of metatarsals. Although the foot now may seem to be more deformed, it actually corrects the cavus. An attempt to correct the supination of the foot by forcibly pronating will only increase the cavus deformity by producing further plantar flexion of the foot.

- The varus and adduction deformity are corrected next. The inverted and adducted calcaneus and medially displaced navicular and cuboid produce a severe heel varus and forefoot adduction deformity respectively. The correction of the cavus brings all the metatarsals, cuneiforms, navicular and the cuboid in the same plane of supination. This provides the necessary lever arm to displace the navicular and cuboid laterally and slightly downward. This manipulation includes stretching the tight medial structures by abducting the foot held in flexion and supination while counterpressure is applied by thumb to the lateral aspect of head of the talus.
- The abduction is gradually increased with each consecutive cast to achieve reduction of navicular on the head of talus. At least 60–70° of abduction is achieved at the end of treatment to reduce rate of relapse. *Under no circumstance, the foot is everted which locks the calcaneus under talus and prevents further correction.* On the other hand, gradual abduction of forefoot in flexion and supination unlocks the calcaneus from underneath the talus producing eversion of the heel.
- The equinus is corrected by stretching the tight posterior structures. The foot is extended by placing the flat of the hand under entire sole and pulling the heel down with the other hand. The above knee cast applied weekly from toe to groin produces correction in an average of five casts when the treatment is begun in the first month of life.

41. What is a relapsed clubfoot? Describe surgical options for a clubfoot not corrected with Ponseti method.

Ans: *Relapsed clubfoot*: Some (usually equinus) or a combination or all of deformities developing after the foot has been declared corrected. It should be noted that continuing treatment nowadays with Ponseti method is very short (older manipulation methods entailed treatment for 2–3 years and further maintenance for 7–8 years of age), so often the foot develops deformities after being fully corrected so the distinction between words recurrent and relapse is difficult as most will fall under the term "relapsed".

Surgical options: When proper treatment of clubfeet is started shortly after birth a good clinical correction is a rule. After advent of the Ponseti's treatment there has been a worldwide decline in the surgical intervention. The classical operations such as posteromedial release and complete subtalar release are no longer required where Ponseti's method is being practiced correctly. Still surgery might be mainstay in rigid, relapsed, and neglected clubfeet in developing countries where Ponseti method is not practiced. The kind of surgeries done for a clubfoot may be classified as:

- *Soft tissue surgery*: The soft tissue surgeries which are commonly required even after Ponseti's method include percutaneous tenotomy, tendo-Achilles lengthening and lateral transfer of the TA tendon, posteromedial soft tissue releases (PMSTR), *Modified McKay's procedure* (complete subtalar release of McKay and Simon).
- *Bony surgery*: Bony procedures are generally done in children above 5 years of age will almost always require a bony procedure in addition to soft tissue release. The following are the commonly described bony procedures as in literature [Osteotomy of calcaneus (Dwyer's osteotomy), resection and arthrodesis of calcaneocuboid (Dillwyn's-Evan's procedure), medial release and osteotomy of distal calcaneus (Lichtblau's), enucleation of the cuboid, anterior part of the calcaneus, and head of the talus may be used for more resistant and syndromic feet in older children. Talectomy has also been used for the same indications with variable results. Supramalleolar osteotomy (for persistent intoeing gait) and osteotomies of the bases of metatarsals are used to correct residual deformities. The triple arthrodesis is used for the correction of equines and varus in adolescents and adults (neglected clubfoot) and also for varus or valgus overcorrected feet.
- Combined soft tissue and bony surgery.
- Correction of deformities by external fixation application—three types of external fixators have been used in clubfoot:
  1. Wagner's device.
  2. Joshi's device.
  3. Ilizarov's apparatus.

42. What is treated, untreated, and neglected congenital talipes equinovarus (CTEV). Write differences between typical and atypical CTEV.
B. Discuss the severity classification of CTEV.
C. Briefly describe roles of Achilles tenotomy and tibialis anterior transfer.

Ans: A. *Treated*: All deformities corrected by manipulative or other method on defined parameters.

Untreated: A patient presenting for first time with CTEV < 2 years of age who has not received any treatment.

Neglected: A patient remaining untreated after 2 years.

Differences:

Atypical foot: This term applies to certain feet that are difficult to treat than others. The atypical features in a foot are any one or a combination of the following (though their presence is never a certainty that the feet will really be difficult to treat):

- Short, fat, and swollen foot
- Great toe pointing outward
- Sole crease deep and running from side to side
- Rigidly in turned heel
- Tugged-up heel with emptiness felt at the heel point
- Rigid and fixed equinus with downward flexion. The heel cord is small and very tight
- Deep crease in the skin above heel
- Calf muscle is small and bunched up high in the calf.

B. *Severity classification of CTEV*: Pirani scoring already written in answers above.

C. *Achilles tenotomy*: The correction of the equines can be hastened by percutaneous tenotomy of the tendo-Achilles.

Tibialis anterior transfer: Transfer of the tendon is usually indicated after relapse in a child older than 3 years of age where the tendon has significant supination pull or in patients with a relative "evertor insufficiency." In both the conditions the patients walk on lateral border of foot.

43. Briefly describe principles of Ponseti method of CTEV correction.

Ans: The "principle" of the method is based on relative and interdependent intertarsal motion. The movement of each tarsal bone involves simultaneous shifts in the adjacent bones. These are determined by the opposing joint surfaces, their curvature and ligamentous anatomy. Individual joints have its own specific motion pattern but that influences the adjacent joint by producing requisite shift. Therefore, it is logical that correction of the medial displacement and inversion of the tarsal bones will require a simultaneous gradual lateral shift of the navicular, cuboid, and calcaneus into proper apposition (by correcting cavus, before they can be everted into a neutral position). These displacements can be achieved by gradual correction utilizing the creep in ligaments.

[*Interesting details of technique and procedure can be learnt from chapter 43 of the book Essential Orthopedics Principles and Practice, 3rd edition, 2022 and answer above*]

44. Discuss management of neglected CTEV at 1 year.

Ans: Now-a-days all clubfeet deformities till 2 years of presentation are corrected with standard Ponseti method of manipulative correction as described above. Neglected clubfoot is defined as untreated deformity after 1 year of age because the child starts walking on deformity. These have been successfully managed with Ponseti manipulative correction (some even describe efficacy of correction up to 5 years of primary neglect!). Following soft tissue surgical procedures may be needed on *ale carte* basis as follows:

- Percutaneous tenotomy of the tendo-Achilles
- Tendon transfers
    - Tibialis anterior transfer
    - Peroneus transfer
    - Tibialis posterior transfer
- Limited posterior release
- Limited medial release

45. Discuss various bony procedures to correct hindfoot varus in a neglected clubfoot in a 5-year-old child.

Ans: The various bony procedures are as under:

- *Dwyer osteotomy in cases of isolated heel varus*: For isolated heel varus with mild supination of the forefoot, a Dwyer osteotomy with a lateral closing wedge osteotomy of the calcaneus can be performed. Opening wedge osteotomy of the calcaneus occasionally is followed by sloughing of tight skin along the incision over the calcaneus. Consequently, although some height of the calcaneus is lost after a lateral closing wedge osteotomy, most authors now prefer lateral closing wedge osteotomy with Kirschner wire fixation, if necessary. The ideal age for the operation is 3–4 years, but there is no upper age limit.
- *Dillwyn Evans procedure in cases of short medial column*: Resection and arthrodesis of calcaneocuboid (Dillwyn Evans procedure) joint may be carried alone or with soft tissue release, it often produces hindfoot stiffness. But this is preferred for so-called short medial column CTEV where soft tissue release is the essential surgery rather than correcting the lateral aspect of foot.
- *Lichtblau procedure in cases of long lateral column*: This is preferred for residual heel varus + internal rotation of the calcaneus with a long lateral column of the foot. This procedure corrects the long lateral column of the foot by a closing wedge osteotomy of the lateral aspect of the calcaneus. The best results with this procedure are obtained in children 3 years old or older. Potential complications include the development of a "Z"-foot, or "skew"-foot, deformity.

(Details can be read from Essential Orthopedics: Principles and Practice, 3rd edition Chapter on Clubfoot: Congenital Talipes Equinovarus)

4B.2 MECHANICAL AXIS OF LOWER LIMB AND FEMORAL ANTEVERSION (Q46–49)

46. Draw diagrams of anatomical and mechanical axis of lower limb. Describe the various axes of lower limb.

Ans: For diagrams of anatomical and mechanical axis of lower limb, see **Figure 4B.2.1**.

- *The coronal mechanical axis of the limb* on a full-length film. This is drawn by joining the center of head of femur to center of the ankle [mechanical axis—lower extremity (MALE)]. Center of ankle is defined as a point midway across the tibial metaphysis (this point coincides with the ankle center). The coronal mechanical axis line passes within 1 cm on either side of the tibial spines in both knees. Any deviation from this is the *mechanical axis deviation (MAD)*, which is measured as the perpendicular distance from the mechanical axis line. Normally, the line is 6–7 mm medial to the knee *center*. In varus deformity, the MAD would increase while in valgus deformity, the MAD would decrease or turn negative. Knee center has not been taken into account as tibial subluxation in coronal plane is common causing unwanted errors in measurement. For MAD however, the tibial spines are taken into consideration which is a source of error. In varus knees for example, the tibia often subluxates laterally so that the MAD is exaggerated. Given a choice femur center would represent a better landmark but has not been defined well in literature. Commonly center of femur is represented by the midpoint at superior aspect of intercondylar sulcus.

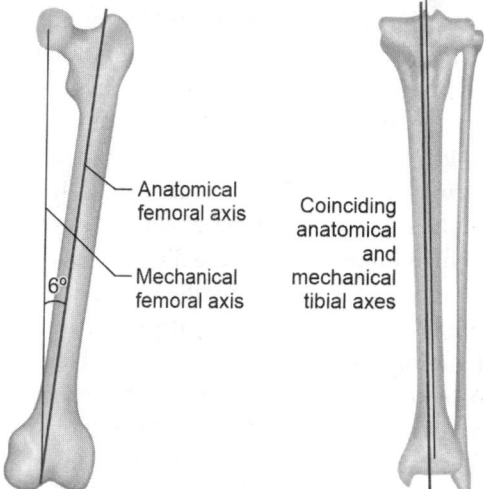

Fig. 4B.2.1: Anatomical and mechanical axis of lower limb.

- *The individual axis of femur and tibia* (truly speaking, these are not the "axis" per se but somehow the nomenclature is fixed in literature). *For femur*, determine the:
    - Mechanical axis of femur (line from the center of the femoral head to the center of the distal femur or center of the knee).
    - Femoral shaft axis: Line drawn from the center of the proximal femur to the center of the distal femur or center of the knee. The difference between femoral shaft axis and mechanical axis of femur is 6°. The femoral shaft axis exits from the piriformis fossa superiorly.
- *Mechanical axis of tibia and tibial shaft axis*: These two coincide in normal tibia, a line extending from the center of the proximal tibia to the center of the ankle.

47. Draw the diagram of normal parameters of lower extremity alignment and label the normal values of each parameter by drawing a scanogram.

Ans: The various parameters of normal lower extremity are depicted in **Figure 4B.2.2**.

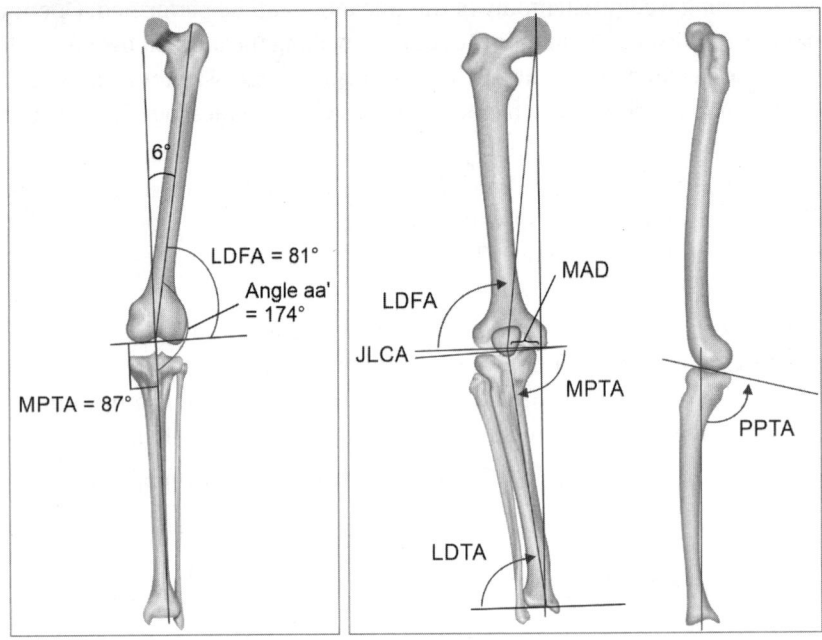

Fig. 4B.2.2: The various normal parameters of lower extremity.
(JLCA: joint line convergence angle; LDFA: lateral distal femoral angle; MAD: mechanical axis deviation; MPTA: medial proximal tibial angle; PDFA: posterior distal femoral angle; PPTA: posterior proximal tibial angle)

48. Describe the anatomical and physiological differences between neck shaft angle and version in a child and adult.

Ans: The neck shaft angle (NSA) is the angle formed by shaft axis and axis of the femoral neck (line drawn from the center of the femoral head to the center of the femoral neck at the narrowest part of the neck). The angle is also named as caput collum diaphysis (or) cervicodiaphyseal angle (CCD). In normal hips, the NSA should cause the longitudinal axes of the femoral necks to cross at the point of body weight. The NSA is very high in neonatal age (>140°), and then gradually it decreases during development and reaches adult values (120–130°). If the angle of inclination is greater than 125°, is termed as coxa valga or Alsberg angle. If the angle is decreased, is termed as coxa vara. The enlargement and maturation of the hip joint increases at 20th week of gestation, and the NSA ranges from 135° to 140° at birth. The femoral NSA is of high importance for the diagnostics and treatment of various conditions of the hip. It is essential in the diagnosis of various pathological conditions of the hip and femur including developmental dysplasia of the hip (DDH), osteogenesis imperfecta (OI), cerebral palsy (CP), and Perthes disease in children and in adults for femoroacetabular impingement, femoral head necrosis, and proximal femoral fractures. In particular, the planning of operative interventions including osteotomies, hip replacement surgery, and internal fixation of fractures requires adequate preoperative measurements and assessment of this angle. In children genu varum is a deformity of the knee concerned with coxa valga causing bow legs and genu valgum is related with coxa vara causing knock knees and pes planus (flat foot). Osteoporosis reduces NSA and predisposes to pathological and stress fractures.

Femoral neck anteversion (FNA) is represented by the angle between the longitudinal axis of the neck of—femur and the axis passing horizontally through femoral condyles and it depicts the degree of rotation of the femoral neck in reference to the coronal plane. The FNA is a result of fetal development, heredity, mechanical forces, and intrauterine position. The value of FNA angle at birth is commonly about 40° and decreases gradually to approximately 20° by the age of 10 years, to finally achieve value around 8–15° in adulthood. The physiological decline in FNA in children is influenced by dynamic forces produced during upright walking. Therefore, the magnitude of the angle is attributed to appropriate motor control, muscle balance and ligament-integrity. FNA of greater than 20° is considered excessive femoral anteversion, whereas a torsion angle of less than 10° is considered femoral retroversion. Excessive femoral torsion is seen in cerebral palsy and has also been associated with other neurologic and orthopedic conditions. Increased FNA produces in-toeing gait while reduced FNA produces out-toeing.

49. Define femoral anteversion. How do you detect it clinically? Discuss the role of anteversion in orthopedics.

Ans: *Definition*: Anteversion of the femur is the angle between the axis of femoral neck and the axis of knee joint in coronal plane.

Clinical tests to detect

Craig test or Ryder test: The patient lies prone with the knee flexed to 90°. The examiner palpates the lateral aspect of the greater trochanter of the femur. Hip is then passively rotated medially and laterally until the greater trochanter is parallel with the examining table or reaches its most lateral position as evident by being most prominent on palpation. The degree of anteversion can then be estimated, based on the angle of the lower leg with the couch and compared with other side.

Clinical significance:
- Increased femoral anteversion results in in-toeing gait while reduced anteversion causes grasshopper patellae with out-toeing gait and result in rotational malalignment of femur.
- During total hip arthroplasty (THA), orientation of the femoral neck osteotomy in the correct anteversion should always be assessed after hip dislocation by reference to the shaft of the femur with the knee flexed at 90°, because there is a wide variation in anteversion of the femoral neck. If the femoral neck osteotomy is made without reference to FNA, an inaccurate cut may result, and subsequent malpositioning of the prosthesis may occur.
- In cases of femoral dysplasia, there is frequently a marked increase in the femoral anteversion. This possibility should be assessed preoperatively with computed tomography (CT) scanning. If the anteversion is greater than 15°, then there are several different strategies available. A small femoral component may be used in association with a low neck cut to correct the anteversion. If using uncemented components of a tapered design, then cutting out a piece of the back of the femoral neck allows the component to be inserted in the correct degree of anteversion. The anterior neck may have to be trimmed to prevent impingement. If the anteversion is severe, then a modular prosthesis that allows the femoral component to be rotated within a proximal metaphyseal sleeve may be used. If a femoral shortening needs to be performed, then the proximal fragment can be rotated back to its correct position.
- All children with DDH have associated FNA. In general, children reduced before they are 2 years of age rarely require derotation osteotomies to correct the anteversion. Anteversion usually corrects once the reduction is obtained. Aseptic necrosis is the most devastating complication associated with the treatment of DDH.
- Excessive femoral anteversion can lead to significant knee valgus in stance phase as well as in-toeing with the feet hitting in swing phase.
- Excessive femoral anteversion is seen in patients of juvenile rheumatoid arthritis (JRA).

4B.3 ANGULAR DEFORMITY OF KNEE (Q50–58)

50. Discuss angular deformity of knee in children.

Ans: *Assessment and Principles of Correction of Angular Deformities*

Assessment should include a good medical history, physical examination, and, for some patients, detailed standard radiographs. These assessments are aimed to differentiate:
- Progressive versus stable
- Painful versus painless deformity
- Associated abnormalities like neurologic and circulatory disturbances that may require special modifications in the treatment
- Deformities of spine like scoliosis and foot abnormalities that may contribute to the angular deformity and may make them appear worse. These actually change the prognosis of treatment
- Leg-length discrepancy (LLD) that may need to be simultaneously corrected during the index surgery.

History should note the time when the deformity was noticed first, any change or improvement with walking or time, the time when child started walking (children with Blount's disease walk early). Take nutritional history, history of vitamin or other deficiency (PEM), treatment received, etc.

Examination for angular deformities:
- *Measure the intercondylar and intermalleolar distance* for genu varum and valgum, respectively expressed in centimeters for bilateral deformities.
- *Measure the femorotibial alignment*: Measure the angle formed between lines joining anterior superior iliac spine to center of patella and another line joining center of intermalleolar line to center of patella. Subtract normal valgus from the measured alignment (7° for males, 8° for females >7 years) for a valgus malalignment and add the same for varus to give the clinical magnitude of angular deformity (in degrees).
- *Measure the Q-angle.*
- *Look for features of ligament laxity and fibular overgrowth.*
- *Look for tight structures* [iliotibial band (ITB) in polio, etc.].
- *Look for features of neurological causes* [cerebral palsy (CP), polio, metabolic bone disease, toxicity, etc.].

Special examination that needs to be done includes:
- An observational gait analysis to:
  - Document foot progression angle
  - Lateral thrust (shifting of proximal tibia and fibula laterally due to capsular and ligament laxity—seen in pathological varum)
  - Antalgic gait
  - To rule out global pathologic conditions like limb scissoring, hyperlordotic gait (spastic conditions)
  - A Trendelenburg gait.

Radiology: A standing alignment radiograph (orthoradiogram) is obtained to document the direction and magnitude of the deformity. Mostly a computed tomography (CT) scanogram is ordered. CT also can be used to assess lengths, rotational deformity and is especially useful if the deformity is in the sagittal plane. Standing lateral radiographs of the femur and tibia are taken to confirm a sagittal plane deformity and tibial slope.

Commonly, the radiological assessment is done for the following two purposes:
1. Measure the femorotibial angle, mechanical and anatomical axis, and the metaphyseodiaphyseal angle.
2. Apart from measurement of deformity, it is also important to assess a patient's current *level of skeletal maturity* by radiology (see below in genu varum).

   Radiological analysis of deformity is very important and has been detailed by specialty authors. In simpler method, the analysis of a deformity can be done in following steps:
   - Assess the radiographs to document any obvious anatomic coronal or sagittal limb deformities (step 1, bowing or angulation of bones).
     - *Draw the coronal mechanical axis of the limb* on a full-length film. This is drawn by joining the center of head of femur to the center of ankle [mechanical axis—lower extremity (MALE)]. Center of ankle is defined as a point midway across the tibial metaphysis (this point coincides with the ankle center). The coronal mechanical axis line passes within 1 cm on either side of the tibial spines in both knees. Any deviation from this is the mechanical axis deviation (MAD), which is measured as the perpendicular distance from the mechanical axis line. Normally, the line is 6–7 mm medial to the knee center. In varus deformity, the MAD would increase while in valgus deformity, the MAD would decrease or turn negative. Knee center has not been taken into account as tibial subluxation in coronal plane is common causing unwanted errors in measurement. For MAD however, the tibial spines are taken into consideration which is a source of error.
     - *Draw the individual axis of femur and tibia. For femur*, determine the:
       - Mechanical axis of femur (line from the center of the femoral head to the center of the distal femur or center of the knee).
       - *Femoral shaft axis*: Line drawn from the center of the proximal femur to the center of the distal femur or center of the knee.
       - *Mechanical axis of tibia and tibial shaft axis*: These two coincide in normal tibia, a line extending from the center of the proximal tibia to the center of the ankle.

- *Anatomic tibiofemoral angle*: Angle formed between tibial and femoral shaft axis; this indicates the anatomic misalignment. This is usually an average of 6° of valgus in normal adult population.
- *Mechanical tibiofemoral angle*: The angle formed between the mechanical axis of femur and mechanical axis of tibia, indicates the mechanical misalignment (it averages to 180° in normal population). This is typically used to determine the amount of varus or the valgus deformity referred to commonly in literature. Now a measured mechanical tibiofemoral axis of 15° will be called 15° of valgus, but if anatomical axis were used then the same would indicate 21° of valgus.

However, if one refers to anatomical femorotibial alignment then it will be 173–174° measured on lateral side (LTFA).

- After first step where one identifies if there is any deformity (MAD) and the direction of the deformity (varus/valgus), next *determine the bone containing the deformity* (step 2)—it should be determined, if the deformity is in femur or tibia, or both bones. There are two ways to do this.
  1. If the deformity is in one limb then the other limb serves as reference for determination of magnitude of true deformity. The mechanical axes of the normal-side leg, affected-side leg, and individual mechanical axis of femur and tibia are constructed and compared.
  2. If the disease is bilateral, the comparison is made with established norms. The mechanical axis of the femur drawn from the center of the hip to the center of the knee normally intersects the articular surface of the distal femur to produce a lateral distal-femoral angle of 87°; this will be 81°, if angle is calculated from the anatomical femoral (femoral shaft) axis. Similarly, tibial mechanical axis is drawn as a line from the center of the knee to the center of the ankle that normally intersects the articular surface of the proximal tibia to produce a medial proximal tibia angle of 87°. The distal tibial articular surface normally is 90° with the mechanical axis of the tibia.
     - Extra-articular deformities are determined by drawing the anatomical axes from proximal and distal bone fragments. The point of intersection of these two lines is considered the site of deformities or technically the center of rotation of angulation (CORA). Percentage contribution of the extra-articular deformity to deformity at the knee is calculated by multiplying the proportion of length deformity is away from the joint.
     - Degenerative deformities are common in the joint itself due to asymmetric wear of the cartilage. To determine this, draw lines along the articular surface of femoral and tibial condyles. If these are not parallel then deformity at knee is confirmed. The femoral line is drawn by connecting the center points of two distal femoral condyles and the tibial articular line is similarly drawn by connecting two center points from medial and lateral plateau.
- After the existence of a bony deformity has been confirmed then its exact location within bone is determined by drawing the normal mechanical axes of the proximal and distal ends of the bone in coronal plane. Similar approach is applied on lateral radiographs and can be used for assessment of sagittal plane deformity—sagittal CORA.

Magnitude of deformity: For this in a typical case use mechanical axis alignments as reference to determine the magnitude of deformity. The steps in detail can be *read from Chapter 29 of the book Essential Orthopedics*: Principles and Practice, *2nd edition with Illustrations.*

Finding CORA by anatomical axis: Anatomical axes of femur and tibia can also be used to determine the deformity as follows—

- The normal proximal femoral angle is 84° (6° varus from mechanical axis) but as it is difficult to construct instead a neck-shaft angle of 130° is used.
- The lateral distal-femoral anatomic angle is 81°, the medial proximal tibial anatomic angle is 87°. The distal tibial articular surface is at 90° angle from the tibial shaft.
- In the lateral plane, the angle subtended by the femoral shaft and Blumensaat line is normally 83°.
- The tibial plateau is sloped posteriorly at 80° to the shaft of the tibia, and the tibial plafond is sloped anteriorly at 80°.
- If abnormal articular angles are found then it can be concluded that a deformity exists within that bone.
- Constructing the normal anatomic axis of the proximal and distal ends of the bone in both the coronal and sagittal planes reveals the location of the CORA.

Treatment: The bones in children keep growing till physeal fusion. This bony growth can be in fact utilized to guide the future growth of bone in order to produce a reverse "compensatory deformity" which would either reduce or fully correct the original deformity depending on the time available. This method of treatment is called *"guided growth method"* detailed as follows:

The continuous growth of physis can be modulated by principles laid down by Heuter-Volkman.

This is principally based on the fact that restricting the growth by "clamping" physis increases physeal pressure which inhibits the growth temporarily in that region but the other side of bone will continue to grow. If performed correctly, the deformity slowly corrects, and the inhibition can be removed (temporary methods) or if growth charts are properly utilized then permanent inhibition of the physis can be done to utilize the remaining growth potential by performing ablation at predetermined age.

Hemiepiphysiodesis is a well-accepted method of correcting long bone deformity, especially in children who have significant remaining bone growth. This method has been found to be associated with lesser morbidity than the osteotomy method.

It is a compensatory method for correcting LLD and not a corrective operation as the longer leg is treated in this manner to equalize limb length, thus making normal limb abnormal.

There are various *methods of performing hemiphysiodesis*:
- *Temporary*: Here in any method, care should be taken to remain outside periosteum and not damaging the same. One should avoid directly exposing the growth plate for the sake of preventing injury to physis.
    - Staples
    - *Two-hole plate and screws.*
- *Permanent*: These procedures should be done only after logical and thorough judgment of the deformity and remaining growth (Bowen's tables). As the growth on the side of hemiphysiodesis will be halted permanently, the patient will have residual deformity if the growth period was too short or deformity was too much. Else the patient will have overcorrection and even reverse deformity, if the deformity was too small compared to remaining growth.
    - Removal, rotation and reinsertion of bone piece (Phemister, White's, Blount's methods)
    - Bone grafting
    - Dowel grafts
    - Physeal curettage—done with a curette, should remove 50% of the central and peripheral region of the physis on that side
    - Percutaneous physeal curettage using burr.

51. Causes of genu varum?

Ans: *Causes*:
- Nutritional rickets (most common cause in India)
- Tibia vara (Blount's disease)
- Traumatic physeal injury
- Tumors
    - Direct affection of physis by tumors [aneurysmal bone cyst (ABC), chondroblastoma, etc.]
    - Mechanical effect of the neoplasm (exostosis)
    - Iatrogenic injury to physis
    - Alteration of bone anatomy (fibrous dysplasia)
- Infection (osteomyelitis—acute, chronic, tubercular, treatment-related injury)
- Renal osteodystrophy
- Osteogenesis imperfecta
- Hypophosphatemic rickets
- Skeletal dysplasia (achondroplasia, enchondromatosis, metaphyseal chondrodysplasia, and focal fibrocartilaginous dysplasia)
- Osteogenesis imperfecta

52. What is CORA? Draw a diagram to show how to calculate it.

Ans: CORA **(Figs. 4B.3.1 and 4B.3.2)** stands for center of rotation of angulation. Details can be read above in Answer to Question 47.

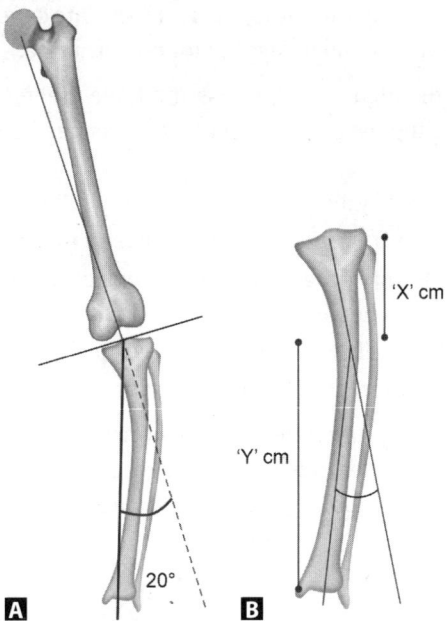

Figs. 4B.3.1A and B: Measuring extra-articular deformity. In compound deformities, where there is extra-articular deformity contribution to total angular deformity, one needs to calculate the percentage contribution of extra-articular deformity. In this example, the varus angle is 20° as calculated from mechanical axes (A). The extraarticular deformity contribution seems to be 15° as done from anatomical axes drawing (B), but this is an apparent measurement only. Suppose the deformity exists 'y' cm from the ankle, then the proportional distance is calculated as {y/(y+x) X 100} = Z%. Now calculate the Z% of 15° (say 'E') and this will give the real contribution of the extra-articular deformity for knee malalignment.

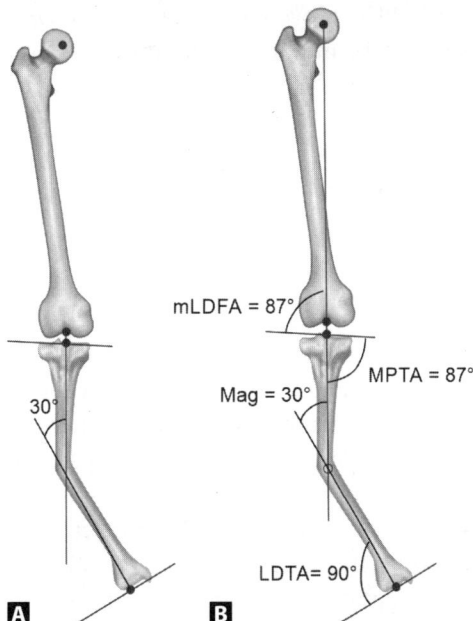

Figs. 4B.3.2A and B: Determining pure extra-articular deformity. If the deformity is purely extra-articular then the measurement is pretty simple. The deformity is determined by drawing the shaft axes of the parts proximal and distal to the deformity (A). The angle at the intersection gives the anatomical deformity (30° in this case). Draw also the LDFA and MPTA to find if there is deformity at the joint as that may coexist (B).

53. A 5-year-old child starts developing a progressive valgus deformity of tibia after an insignificant trauma to the knee. What is the possible cause and pathogenesis of such a deformity? How will you treat this condition?

Ans: This case represents the classic Cozen phenomenon—this refers to late development of valgus deformity in children between 3 years and 6 years of age following trivial or significant bony trauma.

Pathogenesis: Typically, low-energy with valgus force across the knee creates incomplete fracture of proximal tibia, which later develops into valgus on healing. NO specific pathogenesis has been explained but possible causes are as follows:
- Hyperemia of healing cause overgrowth of medial physis of proximal tibia
- Lateral periosteal tether due to initial injury while medial periosteal rupture uninhibiting medial growth
- Usually, this is the time when knee goes into progressive physiological valgus from physiological varus; this could get stimulated following injury added upon a healing response.
- Greenstick injury that tethered bone laterally while medial cortex healed by growing callus resulting in bowing.
- In a displaced fracture at the onset—underreduction of primary injury can be the cause.

Management: Serial and close follow-up is recommended and the parents should be counseled that the deformity corrects itself spontaneously in majority by 1–2 years. Remodeling quite successfully treats the deformity. In children where the deformity fails to improve with time one can utilize guided-growth method or temporary epiphysiodesis (2-hole plate) for correction of deformity.

54. Describe timed epiphysiodesis.

Ans: Epiphysiodesis is a guided-growth method that can be temporary or permanent. The temporary epiphysiodesis can be used to correct or overcorrect the deformity and repeated, if deformity recurs within growth period but for permanent epiphysiodesis, the procedure has to be performed at calculated time. "Calculated time" means surgeon has to calculate the duration of growth remaining (Bowen's tables), expected correction that can be achieved during that period and whether it can be matched to the present deformity. This is called timed epiphysiodesis. As the growth on the side of hemiphysiodesis will be halted permanently, the patient will have residual deformity, if the growth period was too short or deformity was too much. Else the patient will have overcorrection and even reverse deformity, if the deformity was too small compared to remaining growth. Some of the methods commonly used are:
- Removal, rotation, and reinsertion of bone piece (Phemister, White's, Blount's methods)
- Bone grafting
- Dowel grafts
- Physeal curettage—done with a curette, should remove 50% of the central and peripheral region of the physis on that side
- Percutaneous physeal curettage using burr.

55. Explain genu valgum.

Ans: This is outward deviation of legs so that there is medial angulation at the knee. The ankles are shifted outward while the knee is deviated toward each other. Though commonly the overshooting corrective valgus recorrects by 4 years of age but in normal variation, it is deemed that normal limb alignment is produced by 7 years of age only. Genu valgum is a physiological deformity so not considered so deforming by parents or even physicians. Also this does not readily result in knee degeneration or excess abnormal stress distribution as seen with genu varum, so the acceptability to this deformity is a bit higher. Genu valgum is definitely but pathological, if the deformity is greater than 2 standard deviations (SD) from normal for the age. Now, a normal limb alignment of 7° valgus at knee for males and 8° for females plus 2 SD of 5° comes to around 12–13° of acceptable upper limit of valgus at knee. It is deemed that valgus (anatomical femorotibial alignment not MAD) of more than (taking into consideration the measuring error) above 8 years of age is pathological (if we take mechanical axis then angle of more than 5° from normal mechanical axis would also qualify for genu valgum).

Excessive valgus deformity (say >20°) in a child older than 4 years of age may be associated with numerous conditions, including idiopathic genu valgus, skeletal dysplasia, metabolic bone disease, and renal abnormalities. Unilateral, progressive valgus deformity at the tibia, known as Cozen phenomenon, may follow a greenstick fracture of the proximal tibia metaphysis. Trauma in the metaphyseal region can lead to angular deformities, such as tibia valgus or overgrowth, and a longer limb.

Clinical features:
- Pain in the thigh and/or calf and easy fatigability
- Child walks with his knees rubbing together and one leg swinging around the other
- Unstable patellofemoral joint and recurrent lateral subluxation of patella. This is due to exaggerated Q-angle of quadriceps extensor mechanism
- Pronated feet and toeing-in to shift the alignment medially
- Laxity of medial collateral ligament (MCL)
- Genu recurvatum [genu varum, there is usually fixed flexion deformity (FFD) at knee]
- Lateral knee pain, patellar facet tenderness due to recurrent patellar subluxation, and increased patellofemoral pressure syndrome.

Assessment:
- Look for etiological cause of genu valgum:
    - Short stature [multiple epiphyseal dysplasia, multiple metaphyseal dysplasia, multiple enchondromatosis (Ollier's disease), multiple hereditary exostosis, Ellis-Van Creveld syndrome]
    - Swollen hot knees for rheumatoid arthritis
    - Fibular hemimelia
    - Iliotibial band contracture—Ober's test
    - Tibia valga is usually associated with tibial external torsion
    - Measure the anatomical femorotibial alignment (for magnitude of deformity) and Q-angle
    - Measure the predominant bone contributing to deformity—in genu valgum, it is the femur where the deformity predominates rather than tibia which is the common culprit bone in genu varum
    - Measure the sitting and standing height
    - Measure any limb-length discrepancy: Limb-length discrepancy is associated with conditions such as congenital short femur, infection, paralysis, tumor, mechanical factors, vascular inflammation, and skeletal dysplasia.

Imaging:
- Obtaining the patella views for assessment of patellar instability
- Full-length radiographs or scanogram for radiological assessment of deformity, MAD, CORA, and templating the osteotomy
- Assessment of skeletal maturity.

Treatment: Orthosis and special shoes are ineffective for preventing progression or correcting the deformity. However, University of California Biomechanics Laboratory (UCBL) orthotics helps the child during walk by supporting the foot. They relieve foot strain, easy fatigability, and foot-calf pain.

Orthotics may somehow help in preventing the developing ligament laxity in unrestricted cases that are not being operated. Children with a discrepancy greater than 2 cm can compensate by walking on their toes or, as they grow older, vaulting over the short leg. Deformities more than 15° need surgical management. The treatment of these deformities includes one of the two options used according to their merits and requirement:
- *Guided growth*: Hemiphysiodesis is done by stapling or fusing the medial part of the distal femoral and/or proximal tibial growth plates. Timing is crucial for permanent methods and should be judged from remaining skeletal growth

(assessed by radiological skeletal maturity) and the magnitude of deformity. Stapling is more forgiving and flexible to be used as a growth control method. After hemiphysiodesis, the physis is weak and protected in knee immobilizer for 2 weeks. This also allows for skin and soft tissue healing.

- *Osteotomy with deformity correction*: Principles of osteotomy correction remain the same. The gradual correction of deformity by a progressive gradual opening osteotomy of lateral aspect of tibia or femur is more feasible done laterally. As the deformity commonly lies in the femur, distal femur osteotomy is commonly done. This also corrects the lateral tilt to joint line usually associated with the deformity. Medially, the vascular structures are located so, commonly the osteotomy is done from lateral aspect; hence, lateral opening wedge osteotomy is preferred. Puddu plates, if available are often handy here else a synthetic bone graft block or autogenous iliac crest bone graft with locking plate can be used. Attention should be given to the fact that for moderate to severe deformities (>25°) the nerve may get stretched so gradual correcting methods or doing osteotomy in both distal femur and complementary osteotomy in proximal tibia may be better. By no way are medial femoral osteotomies contraindicated, if properly done. Dome osteotomies are better avoided in distal femur as they are difficult in this region. If present in proximal tibia then closing wedge option is very common and easier option. However, there is often external torsion of the bone associated with deformity which should be simultaneously corrected and given priority. Correcting the rotational deformity first often reduces the magnitude of deformity, which is then corrected. Partial fibular diaphyseal osteotomy has to be done if the method chosen for correction is acute else for gradual correction no surgery to fibular aspect is needed. Healing takes 4–6 weeks, till then the osteotomy should be protected. Knee bending and exercises are gradually begun thereafter with night brace for first two weeks and without protection later.

Additionally, correct the limb-length discrepancy: Here, it is important to predict the extent of limb-length discrepancy at skeletal maturity. Ilizarov method of correction is useful in cases where the deformity is associated with significant limb-length discrepancy (shortening >2.5 cm). Limb-lengthening may also be needed for patients where the deformity is corrected by closing wedge osteotomy with a wedge size of greater than 2.5 cm producing significant shortening.

56. What is malalignment test? Discuss the principles of focal dome osteotomy.

Ans: *Malalignment test*: It is used in patients in whom frontal MAD exists. This is done by drawing a z-line (zero line) on full leg anteroposterior (AP) radiograph taken with patella pointing forward joining the center of femoral head and center of ankle (distal tibia). It passes normally just medial to center of knee joint; if not then an MAD is present and measured in millimeter (normal range is 0–15 mm). It is used as a part of preoperative planning in high tibia osteotomy (HTO).

Principles of focal dome osteotomy:
- Cylindrical cut to correct the deformity
- Deformity should be in one or maximum two planes. Three-dimensional deformities and rotational deformities are very difficult to correct
- The locus of cylindrical cut should correspond to the CORA
- Arc of osteotomy should be neither two large (more translation and lesser bone contact) nor too small (limited correction possible)
- Correction achieved by rotation of bone and no bone is removed
- As far as possible avoid creating secondary translational deformities.

57. What is tibia vara? Classify tibia vara. Describe conventional management and recent advances in its management.

Ans: Definition: Growth retardation at the medial (specifically posteromedial) aspect of proximal tibial epiphysis, physis, and metaphysic resulting in persistent bow legs is called tibia vara.

Classification of tibia vara: Two types are commonly seen as initially described by Blount:
1. Infantile tibia vara (early onset) where the onset is before 3 years of age
2. Adolescent tibia vara (late onset) where the onset is at or after 10 years of age

Langenskiold classified infantile tibia vara into six stages according to the severity, which increases with the stage (**Table 4B.3.1**).

TABLE 4B.3.1: Classification of infantile tibia vara by Langenskiold according to severity.	
Stage 1	Mediodistal beaking of the upper proximal tibial metaphysis
Stage 2	Wedging of the medial part of the upper tibial epiphyseal secondary ossification center plus a saucer-shaped defect of the upper surface of the metaphyseal beak due to its dissolution, fragmentation, and collapse
Stage 3	Stepping of the inferomedial border of the secondary ossification center but without extending distal to the physeal plate level plus deepening of the metaphyseal saucer into a step in the medial metaphysis
Stage 4	The epiphyseal secondary ossification center passes more distally and cross distal to the physeal level to fill the metaphyseal step
Stage 5	Separation of the most medial part of the ossification center from the bulk of the secondary ossification center and resides now in the depth of the metaphyseal step below the physis. This is radiologically expressed as either a horizontal cleft (double epiphysis) or complete absence of the medial secondary ossification center as it will be overshadowed by the upper medial tibial metaphysis
Stage 6	Medial epiphyseal plate closure with a bony bridge

Conventional management and recent advances in its management:

Conventional:

Infantile type: Lot of treatment options have been described for the management of infantile tibia vara including observation, orthotic treatment, corrective osteotomy (acute or gradual correction), elevation of medial tibial condyle, resection of physeal bar, lateral hemiphysiodesis, and guided growth of proximal tibial physis (inhibiting lateral growth and promoting medial physeal growth).

A child younger than 3 years, especially in stage I and II can be effectively treated by orthoses. A knee ankle foot orthosis (KAFO) may be used to correct the mechanical axis using the principle of three-point fixation. To be effective, it should be applied during the day time for a period of at least 1 year. Night application is also recommended by some. The orthoses must be used till there are radiological signs for healing of the metaphyseal lesion.

Usually, children above 4 years of age do not respond to this treatment and therefore should be treated by osteotomy. Brace treatment is more effective for patients with initial low malondialdehyde (MDA) and those who are not obese. Patients with stage I and II deformity who do not respond to bracing should be taken up for corrective osteotomy (closing/opening wedge or dome) of the proximal tibia.

Surgical overcorrection of the mechanical axis to at least 5° with lateral translation of the distal fragment reduces the rate of recurrence. The level of osteotomy is just below the patellar tendon insertion. Some external rotation should be added to the distal fragment to compensate the internal rotation deformity. A fibular osteotomy in the proximal third is routinely added through a separate incision. Prophylactic fasciotomy is recommended for impending compartment syndrome. Postoperative weakness of flexor hallucis longus may denote partial peroneal nerve palsy. Stage III deformities should be treated aggressively because delay in surgery after 4 years of age increases the chances of recurrence. Osteotomy should also address the internal rotation deformity by appropriate external rotation correction otherwise the negative foot-progression angle would persist. Surgeon should also make additional compensation for out of plane correction as the center of rotation angle (CORA) lies at epiphysis but corrective osteotomy is often done distally. Lesions greater than stage III (stage IV and V) cannot be treated satisfactorily by simple corrective osteotomy alone due to the physiological physeal arrest that occurs on the medial side. There are very high chances of recurrence following simple osteotomies alone and therefore these should be accompanied by lateral epiphysiodesis or medial epiphysiolysis or both. The former, however, is not preferred due to unacceptable limb shortening that it is likely to produce. Thus, treatment of choice is realignment osteotomy with the excision of the medial bridge and lesion consisting of abnormal fibrocartilaginous structures and use of an interposition substance (usually methyl methacrylate) to prevent the rebridging.

Stage VI lesions are difficult to treat due to established bony bridge across the medial physis. If the child has <2 years of growth potential, realignment may be accompanied by lateral epiphysiodesis which reduces the chances of recurrence. This may be followed by limb lengthening procedures when indicated. External fixators can be planned for realignment osteotomy and lengthening together. The osteotomy can be carried through the physis itself in the older children. If significant incongruity and depression of the joint surface exist, an intra-articular osteotomy may be performed to elevate the medial tibial plateau which corrects the instability and restores alignment.

Adolescent type: Bracing is ineffective to treat such patients due to obesity and maturity of age. The treatment is, therefore, surgical with a goal to correct the mechanical axis. This can be achieved most successfully by a valgus producing high tibial osteotomy (HTO) with rigid internal fixation. *Overcorrection in adolescent tibia vara is contraindicated.* Even neutral correction in these patients may result in apparent excessive valgus with thighs rubbing against each other while walking. Some authors, therefore, recommend an undercorrection so as to produce a femorotibial angle of 0–5° varus. The common complications are nonunion, malunion, compartment syndrome, common peroneal nerve palsy, infection, and sometimes deep vein thrombosis due to obesity. Some authors have recently felt the need to correct the distal femoral varus simultaneously. External fixators give the advantage of postoperative adjustability but may be very difficult to apply and maintain in these obese patients and are therefore best avoided. Lateral epiphysiodesis is an attractive alternative procedure provided at least 2 years of growth potential is left. Proximal fibular epiphysiodesis is not necessary. The main disadvantage of lateral epiphysiodesis is that rotational deformity cannot be corrected. The advantages are significantly simpler technique, minimal morbidity, and subsequent correction can be carried out without added complications if the final correction is inadequate.

Recent advances: None reported but only modifications of existing techniques described!
- *Gradual correction*: Taylor spatial frame instead of Ilizarov
- *Guided growth method*: Using modified implants
- *Physeal bar resection*: CT-guided and using minimally invasive methods
- Hemiplateau elevation

58. **A. Clinical and radiological features of infantile tibia vara.**
   B. Indications of its treatment and brief treatment outline.

Ans:

A. *Clinical features*: The child has exaggerated genu varum with a clinically apparent lateral thrust of the knee during stance phase of the gait. This is because of varus instability due to ligamentous laxity that frequently develops on the lateral side of the knee. The typical child is obese and often exceeds 95th percentile for weight. Indeed, increased weight produces sufficient compressive forces to retard the physeal growth by Hueter-Volkmann principle.

Radiological features: Standard AP view of lower limbs in standing position from hip to knee is obtained. The characteristic findings include sharp varus angulation and prominent beaking of the medial metaphysis with radiolucent areas denoting cartilage islands; irregular and wide medial physeal line; and irregularly ossified and medially sloping epiphysis. The entire ossific zone of metaphysis shows irregularity. Little lateral islands of calcified tissue may appear that are separated from metaphysis by clear zones. These features are usually not seen before 18 months of age, but when appear are progressive. Beaking is due to sloping away from joint line distally. Attempts have been made to diagnose the condition before pathognomonic radiographic signs appear. Tibial MDA of Drennan greater than 11° and tibial epiphyseal-metaphyseal angle greater than 20° identify the toddlers at risk of developing Blount's disease. These values for distinction, however, have not been fully supported in newer studies (MDA of more than 15° is possibly more appropriate reference). MDA of less than 10° is associated with resolution of deformity in 95% cases. A child without the characteristic metaphyseal lesion also called the Blount's lesion cannot be labeled as infantile tibia vara.

B. *Indications*:
- *For brace management*: Age <3 years with Langenskiold stage upto 2
- *For operative management*:
    - Progressive deformity—despite brace treatment as above
    - Age ≥4 years (all stages)
    - Langenskiold stage I and II in children >3 years
    - Langenskiold stage III, IV, V, VI any age
    - Metaphyseo-diaphyseal angle >20°

Treatment outline: A child younger than 3 years especially in stage I and II can be effectively treated by orthoses. A KAFO may be used to correct the mechanical axis using the principle of three-point fixation. Patients with stage I and II deformity who do not respond to bracing should be taken up for corrective osteotomy (closing/opening wedge or dome) of the proximal tibia.

Stage III deformities should be treated aggressively because delay in surgery after 4 years of age increases the chances of recurrence. Osteotomy should also address the internal rotation deformity by appropriate external rotation correction otherwise the negative foot-progression angle would persist.

For lesions greater than stage III (stage IV and V), treatment of choice is realignment osteotomy with the excision of the medial bridge and lesion consisting of abnormal fibrocartilaginous structures and use of an interposition substance (usually methylmethacrylate) to prevent the rebridging.

Stage VI lesions are difficult to treat due to established bony bridge across the medial physis. If the child has less than 2 years of growth potential, realignment may be accompanied by lateral epiphysiodesis which reduces the chances of recurrence. This may be followed by limb-lengthening procedures when indicated.

4B.4 CEREBRAL PALSY AND LOWER LIMB AFFECTION (Q59-61)

59. A. Define cerebral palsy (CP) and its classification based on pattern of involvement.
B. Describe clinical features of crouch gait and its management.

Ans:
A. *Definition*: Cerebral palsy describes a group of permanent disorders of the development of movement and posture, causing activity limitation, that are attributed to nonprogressive disturbance that occurred in the developing fetal or infant brain.

Classification Based on Pattern of Involvement
Monoplegia: Monoplegia is very rare and usually occurs after meningitis. Most patients diagnosed with monoplegia actually have hemiplegia with one extremity only very mildly affected.

Hemiplegia: In hemiplegia, one side of the body is involved, with the upper extremity usually more affected than the lower extremity. Patients with hemiplegia, approximately 30% of patients with CP, typically have sensory changes in the affected extremities as well. Severe sensory changes, especially in the upper extremity, are a predictor of poor functional outcome after reconstructive surgery. Hemiplegic patients also may have a leg-length discrepancy, with shortening on the affected side.

Diplegia: Diplegia is the most common anatomical type of CP, constituting approximately 50% of all cases. Patients with diplegia have motor abnormalities in all four extremities, with the lower extremities more affected than the upper. The close proximity of the lower extremity tracts to the ventricles most likely explains the more frequent involvement of the lower extremities with periventricular lesions. This type of CP is most common in premature infants; intelligence usually is normal. Most children with diplegia walk eventually, although walking is delayed usually until around age 4 years.

Quadriplegia: In quadriplegia, all four extremities are equally involved, and many patients have significant cognitive deficiencies that make care more difficult. Head and neck control usually are present, which helps with communication, education, and seating. Treatment goals for patients with quadriplegia include a straight spine and level pelvis, located mobile hips with 90° of flexion for sitting and 30° of extension for pivoting, plantigrade feet that can fit in shoes, and an appropriate wheelchair.

Total body: Patients with total body involvement typically have profound cognitive deficits in addition to loss of head and neck control. These patients usually require full-time assistance for activities of daily living and specialized seating systems to assist with head positioning. Drooling, dysarthria, and dysphagia also are common and complicate care.

Other types: Some patients have a double hemiplegia pattern as a result of bleeding in both hemispheres of the brain. It often is difficult to differentiate this from diplegia or quadriplegia; however, in double hemiplegia, the upper extremities typically are more involved than the lower.

Paraplegia is very rare and is characterized by bilateral lower extremity involvement with—in contrast to diplegia—completely normal gross and fine motor skills in the upper extremity. Many patients diagnosed with paraplegia actually are diplegic with very mildly involved upper extremities. Although occasionally mentioned, triplegia, the involvement of three extremities, probably does not exist. With careful examination, most patients believed to have triplegia actually have subtle motor deficits of the least involved limb.

B. *Clinical features of crouch gait*: *Crouch gait* comprises increased hip and knee flexion with excessive ankle dorsiflexion. This gait pattern is generally seen in weaker patients with diplegia. The cause may be dynamic muscle contraction, spasticity, lever arm dysfunction, bony deformity and/or fixed joint contractures. Another significant cause is iatrogenic, where the calf muscle weakness is produced by lengthening of the calf muscles in the absence of a true equinus. The crouch pattern is usually seen in gross motor function classification system (GMFCS) levels II, III, and IV patients. In sagittal plane, the body's center of mass falls behind the already flexed knee, providing and increasingly larger deforming force as the child grows and increases his weight. Such body forces place quadriceps mechanism into disadvantage and increase all three components of the crouch gait. The excessive knee flexion gradually becomes fixed with overstretching and lengthening of the quadriceps resulting in patella alta, anterior knee pain, and sometimes avulsion fracture of the patella. The muscles responsible for the gait pattern include an overactive or spastic iliopsoas and rectus femoris at the hip and spastic hamstrings at the knee. Rectus femoris is especially responsible for the hip flexion deformity. Excessive ankle dorsiflexion results from uncontrolled tibial advancement in the second rocker during midstance due to weak or over-lengthened calf muscles.

Management of crouch gait: This is essentially aimed at correcting the flexion deformity at hip and knee, reducing the power of hamstrings, and also stabilizing the joints (by increasing extension power) so that they do not buckle under laxity. The various methods that are usually combined include:
- Shortening of the femur
- Plication of the patellar tendon
- Transfer of the semitendinosus to the back of the femur
- Fractional lengthening of the other hamstrings.
  Usually, the bony and soft tissue procedures are segregated into two different stages.

60. Define diplegia and double hemiplegia.
Ans: *Diplegia*: Diplegia is the most common anatomical type of CP, constituting approximately 50% of all cases. Patients with diplegia have motor abnormalities in all four extremities, with the lower extremities more affected than the upper. The close proximity of the lower extremity tracts to the ventricles most likely explains the more frequent involvement of the lower extremities with periventricular lesions. This type of CP is most common in premature infants; intelligence usually is normal. Most children with diplegia walk eventually, although walking is delayed usually until around age 4 years.

Double hemiplegia: Some patients have a double hemiplegia pattern as a result of bleeding in both hemispheres of the brain. It often is difficult to differentiate this from diplegia or quadriplegia; however, in double hemiplegia, the upper extremities typically are more involved than the lower.

61. Discuss the types of equines contracture and foot, ankle deformities in cerebral palsy and its management.
Ans: *Types of equines contracture with management*:
- Equinus
- Equinoplanovalgus
- Equinocavovarus.

Typically, in spastic CP, the ankle plantar flexor muscles are overactive and dorsiflexors are ineffective leading to equinus deformity.

Equinoplanovalgus deformities are characterized by equinus of the hindfoot coupled with pronation of midfoot and forefoot. The lateral column of the foot is structurally and functionally shorter than medial column. Ankle valgus and hallux valgus are frequently seen to be associated with equinoplanovalgus.

Equinocavovarus is characterized by equinus of hindfoot coupled with supination of the midfoot and forefoot. The lateral column is structurally and functionally longer than the medial column. Compensatory ankle valgus deformities may be seen in equinuocavovarus. These deformities are usually supple (Level I) but may exacerbate to level II or III with age and suboptimal treatment. The foot and ankle malalignment may disrupt the function in both stance and swing phase. The heel strike does not occur in any of the deformities.

Equinus and equinocavovarus pattern disrupt the ankle rocker by blocking ankle dorsiflexion resulting in compromised stability in midstance. Equinoplanovalgus deformity maintains the midfoot and forefoot in segments in unlocked alignment resulting in excessive loading of medial plantar aspect of the midfoot. Interventions to correct foot deformities are performed to improve cosmesis and function. It is presumed that improved foot shape can restore the stability and function by restoring the relative length of columns. However, increased stiffness of the foot by surgical procedures like arthrodesis may result in reduction of the shock absorption function of the foot.

- For level I (*equinus deformity*), the interventions are designed to reduce muscle tone and spasticity. This is accomplished by pharmaceutical methods (oral baclofen, botulinum toxin injection), neurosurgical methods (selective dorsal rhizotomy, intrathecal baclofen) or orthotic interventions. Split or complete muscle transfer may also be performed to produce balance. The level II deformities are best dealt with soft tissue surgical procedures like release, lengthening or transfer of muscle tendon unit. Level III deformities are dealt with a combination of soft tissue surgeries and skeletal intervention like osteotomy and arthrodesis. The true equinus deformity may be level I (due to overactivity) or level II (tightness of ankle plantar flexors). True equinus must be differentiated from the apparent equinus. Intervention done for ankle plantar flexors in apparent equinus may result in hindfoot calcaneus leading to severe crouch. Level I equinus deformity in young children (<5 years) is an ideal candidate for botulinum toxin injection in each head of gastrocnemius, where equinus deformities are due to isolated overactivity of gastrocnemius. Silfverskiold test helps in identifying the causative muscle. A short course of lasting, use of ankle foot orthosis, and physiotherapy may help to prolong the time limited effect of botulinum toxin.
- Level II deformities where the shortening of plantar flexors results in equinus need to be surgically treated. Isolated limitation of ankle dorsiflexion with knee extended suggests gastrocnemius muscle involvement; limitation of ankle dorsiflexion with knee flexed suggests soleus involvement while limitation in both positions suggests involvement of both muscles. A selective fractional lengthening of gastrocnemius (Baumann/Strayer) is required for the first instance; which is done in the muscle belly (called Zone I). This will achieve 5% or less of ankle dorsiflexion. When both muscles are involved; selective fractional lengthening at myotendinous junction (Zone II, Vulpius/Baker) or formal lengthening of tendo-achilles (Zone III, White/Hoke) may be required. Of course, tendo-achilles lengthening gives more dorsiflexion (Zone 3) at the cost of weakness of ankle plantar flexors.

Equinocavovarus deformity is a consequence of overactivity (Level I) or tightness (Level II) of ankle plantar flexors and invertors. Physical examination not only differentiates between dynamic (Level I) and static (Level II) deformities, but can also pinpoint the inverter muscle responsible for varus foot in majority of cases. Confusion test is done by asking the child to flex hip against resistance applied to knee in sitting position (hip and knee flexed to 90°). When the flexion is accompanied by dorsiflexion and inversion of ankle, tibialis anterior is the overactive muscle. This can be confirmed by dynamic electromyography (EMG) and pedobarography. The ankle dorsiflexion in midstance generally occurs due to tibialis anterior overactivity.

- Level I equinocavovarus deformities in young children (<5 years) may be treated with intramuscular injection in plantar flexors and inverters; requiring general anesthesia and ultrasonic or EMG guidance for the latter.
- Level II deformities may be managed by fractional lengthening of the ankle plantar flexors. Split transfer of tibialis anterior is considered when this muscle is found to be overactive in physical examination or EMG. In cases of doubt or when EMG assessments are not available, dynamic varus deformity may be treated by simultaneous split transfer of tibialis anterior and fractional lengthening of the tibialis posterior. Level II deformities may require further fractional lengthening of flexor hallucis longus and flexor digitorum longus muscles; abductor hallucis muscle on the medial border of foot and sequential release of plantar fascia and intrinsic muscles of the foot. Peroperative reassessment (clinical as well as radiological) of the foot after soft tissue release is necessary to plan any bony procedures. Gross

alignment and dynamic loading of the foot may improve by sequential osteotomies. Lateral closing wedge osteotomy of calcaneus is used to correct heel varus. Lateral column shortening through cuboid using a dorsolateral closing wedge osteotomy is used to correct midfoot supination deformity.
- Dorsally based closing wedge osteotomies of medial cuneiform or first metatarsal when the physis has closed may be used to treat residual forefoot inversion and varus.
- Triple arthrodesis is used in older patients with very stiff feet.
- Subtalar arthrodesis is used to correct hindfoot varus; calcaneocuboid arthrodesis corrects midfoot supination and talonavicular arthrodesis corrects forefoot inversion.

Equinoplanovalgus deformity is a consequence of overactivity (Level I) or tightness (Level II) of ankle plantar flexors and evertor group of muscles.
- Level I deformities in younger children (<5 years) may be treated with selective botulinum toxin injection in the muscle belly of gastrocnemius and, sometimes, peroneus brevis. Static deformities are usually seen in children between 6 years and 8 years of age and will require fractional lengthening of ankle plantar flexors with transfer of peroneus brevis to peroneus longer muscle distal to the lateral malleolus.
- Level II deformities where skeletal changes have started to appear require lengthening of the lateral column. The procedure may be performed at the neck of calcaneus; calcaneocuboid joint or in the body of cuboid, with the help of a tricortical iliac graft. A lengthening of 1–2 cm usually corrects deformities of all these segments of the foot.
- If there is residual forefoot varus deformity due to shortening of medial column (after surgical lengthening of lateral column), then a plantar-based closing osteotomy may be performed through the medial cuneiform or at the base of the great toe metatarsal.
- A triple arthrodesis is required, if lateral column lengthening fails to correct the deformity. It may be combined with lateral column lengthening through calcaneocuboid joint.

Ankle valgus may result due to tightness of the ankle plantar flexors. Overall hindfoot valgus alignment is a contribution from both subtalar and ankle joint. Ankle valgus is best seen on drawing tibiotalar angle on an anteroposterior view of ankle in standing position. Narrowing of lateral part of distal tibial epiphysis and shortening of distal fibula (called high fibular station) are frequently associated with it.
- Ankle valgus should be corrected when it contributes to overall hindfoot valgus alignment. It is not treated when ankle valgus is due to compensation for equinocavovarus deformity.
- Growth modulation is one of the best methods available to treat ankle valgus sufficient (>2 years) remaining growth. Reversible or temporarily hemiepiphysiodesis can be performed on the medial side of distal tibial epiphysis using a single fully threaded medial malleolar screw placed percutaneously under image guidance. The screw is removed after an overcorrection of approximately 5° has been achieved. The screw is preferred over a figure of eight plate on staples to minimize unintentional joint penetration by the distal screw.

4B.5 IN-TOEING GAIT (Q62–64)

62. How will you treat in-toeing gait due to hip disorders?

Ans: In-toeing gait or pigeon-toed gait may result from various pathologies; common of which are:
- Metatarsus adductus
- Tibial in-torsion
- Increased femoral anteversion
- *Neuromuscular disorders (usually unilateral, asymmetrical, and progressive)*:
  – Cerebral palsy (CP)
  – Myelomeningocele
  – Iliotibial band (ITB) contractures.
- *Protective in-toeing*:
  – Genu valgum
  – Flexible pes planus.

Management: Measure the clinical and radiological anteversion at hip and also assess the foot progression angle.

Most of the rotational deformities correct by 8–10 years of age and less than 1% needs surgical correction. Femoral anteversion is the most common cause of in-toeing after 3 years. These children often have habit of sitting in "W-posture". Their internal rotation at hip is more than 75° and external rotation often limited below 25°. Waiting for spontaneous correction is futile and primary corrective osteotomy should be done. Children should be encouraged to sit in Buddha position though waiting for prolonged periods may produce genu valgum or foot abduction. Derotation osteotomy of proximal femur is the preferred treatment that should be performed after 8 years of age. Typical indications include anteversion greater than 45°, internal rotation at hip greater than 80°, and external rotation less than 20° with gait disturbance. The proximal intertrochanteric osteotomy is judged intraoperatively for correction by equal resulting internal and external rotations. Osteotomy performed at other places (shaft or distal aspect) is neither cosmetic and may produce knee stiffness, respectively. Proximal osteotomies heal well due to wide opposing cancellous surfaces.

(For further details on radiological and clinical assessment kindly read Chapter 29 of the book Essential Orthopedics: Principles and Practice, 2nd edition.)

63. **A. Classification and clinical features of traumatic anterior hip dislocation.**
   B. Discuss the method of closed reduction and potential complications of traumatic anterior hip dislocation.

Ans: A. *Classification of traumatic anterior hip dislocation*:
Anterior dislocations also have been classified by Epstein as follows **(Box 4B.5.1)**:

Clinical features:
- *Pain*: Patients typically present with acute, severe pain in the hip region, which may radiate to the thigh or groin.
- *Position of the limb*: The affected hip is often held in a flexed, abducted, and externally rotated position. The leg may appear longer than the opposite leg due to the position of the femur.
- *Reduced range of motion*: Patients usually exhibit a significant reduction in the range of motion of the affected hip joint. Attempting to move the hip can elicit considerable pain.
- *Swelling and bruising*: There may be localized swelling and bruising around the hip joint, though this may develop over time.
- *Sensory and motor deficits*: Depending on associated neurovascular injuries, patients may exhibit altered sensation (paresthesia) or weakness in the lower limb, particularly if the obturator or femoral nerves are involved.
- *Crepitus*: Palpation of the hip may reveal crepitus due to associated soft tissue injury.
- *Deformity*: Visibly, the hip may appear deformed. The greater trochanter may be prominent, and the normal contour of the hip may be lost.
- *Inability to bear weight*: The patient usually cannot bear weight on the affected leg and may require assistance to move.

> **Box 4B.5.1:** Epstein classification of anterior hip dislocation.
>
> *Pubic (superior):*
> - With no fracture (simple)
> - With fracture of the head of the femur
> - With fracture of the acetabulum
>
> *Obturator (inferior):*
> - With no fracture (simple)
> - With fracture of the head of the femur
> - With fracture of the acetabulum

B. *Method*:
Regardless of the direction of the dislocation, an attempt to reduce it can be made by applying in-line traction while the patient is in a supine position. The ideal approach is to conduct a closed reduction under general anesthesia, but if this is not possible, conscious sedation can be used for the reduction. There are three well-known techniques for performing a closed reduction of the hip:
- *Allis method*: This involves applying traction aligned with the deformity. The patient lies supine while the surgeon stands above them on the stretcher or table. Initially, the surgeon applies in-line traction, and an assistant provides countertraction by stabilizing the patient's pelvis. As the traction force is increased, the surgeon should gradually increase the flexion to about 70°. Gentle rotational movements of the hip and slight adduction often aid the femoral head in clearing the acetabulum's edge. Applying lateral force to the proximal thigh may also facilitate reduction. A successful closed reduction is often indicated by an audible "clunk".

- *Reverse Bigelow Maneuver*: For anterior dislocations, the reverse Bigelow maneuver involves applying traction along the line of the deformity. The hip is then adducted, sharply internally rotated, and extended.
- The *Stimson method* for closed reduction of anterior hip dislocation involves positioning the patient supine with the affected leg hanging off the table to utilize gravity. Weights, typically 5-10 pounds, are attached to the ankle to create traction for about 15-20 minutes, allowing muscle relaxation. Afterward, the knee and hip are flexed to 90°, and the hip is gently rotated internally while stabilizing the pelvis. This technique aims to guide the dislocated femoral head back into the acetabulum, and successful reduction is confirmed through physical examination and imaging.

Complications:
- *Fractures*: Associated fractures of the acetabulum or femur can occur during the dislocation or during reduction maneuvers.
- *Avascular necrosis*: Injury to the blood supply of the femoral head can lead to avascular necrosis, a serious condition that may arise in the weeks or months following the injury.
- *Recurrent dislocation*: The hip may become unstable and prone to recurrent dislocations.
- *Nerve injuries*: Damage to nerves, particularly the femoral, obturator, or sciatic nerves, may occur and can lead to motor and sensory deficits.
- *Vascular complications*: Injury to the blood vessels supplying the femoral head can occur, which may result in complications such as thrombosis or necrosis.
- *Soft tissue injuries*: Ligamentous and muscular injuries may also occur, potentially leading to complications such as adhesions or chronic pain syndromes.
- *Infection*: Although rare, there is a risk of infection, especially if surgical intervention is required after the dislocation.
- *Posttraumatic osteoarthritis*: Damage to the articular surface may contribute to future osteoarthritis of the hip joint.

64. What are the causes of in-toeing gait? Discuss radiological investigations and their interpretation. What is the management protocol?

Ans: For causes of in-toeing gait kindly refer to answer to question 62.

Radiological investigations and interpretation:
- *Radiological measurement of tibial version*: On tomogram axial cuts the horizontal line is determined proximally by joining the most posterior aspect of tibial condyles. Distal axis is obtained by joining the two malleoli. These are superimposed to determine any torsion. Normal is around +20° (external tibial torsion) by and after 8 years of age.
- *Radiological measurement of femoral version*: Radiologically, the femoral version is determined by tomography. One image is taken to determine the axis of femoral neck–head proximally while other is drawn distally at the level of femoral condyles. The distal horizontal line is obtained by joining the most distal aspects of femoral condyles while the anteversion is measured by superimposed head-neck angle on this line. The normal value is <25° at the age of 8 years or older for both male and female.

Management protocol:
Most of the rotational deformities correct by 8–10 years of age and <1% need surgical correction. Orthotics are proven to be of no therapeutic or preventive value still very frequently prescribed (instead they confuse the young graduates to wrongly assume that rotational malalignment is pathological and should be quickly intervened!). Hallux adductus is often a dynamic deformity secondary to overstrain of abductor pollicis longus. This resolves with increasing age and nervous system maturity. Metatarsus adductus if flexible resolves spontaneously while rigid type needs treatment. Tibial intorsion if uncorrected by 8–10 years and if transmalleolar axis lying greater than 3 standard deviations from the mean (<-10° or >35°) causing significant gait abnormalities need correction by supramalleolar tibial derotation osteotomy. The osteotomy is fixed with K-wires and a cast.

Femoral anteversion is the most common cause of in-toeing after 3 years. These children often have habit of sitting in "W-posture." Their internal rotation at hip is >75° and external rotation often limited <25°. Waiting for spontaneous correction is futile and primary corrective osteotomy should be done. Children should be encouraged to sit in Buddha position though waiting for prolonged periods may produce genu valgum or foot abduction. Derotation osteotomy of proximal femur is the preferred treatment that should be performed after 8 years of age. Typical indications include anteversion >45°, internal rotation at hip >80° and external rotation <20° with gait disturbance. The proximal intertrochanteric osteotomy is judged intraoperatively for correction by equal resulting internal and external rotations. Osteotomies performed at other places (shaft or distal aspect) are not cosmetic and may produce knee stiffness. Proximal osteotomies heal well due to wide opposing cancellous surfaces. Angular deformity can increase the likelihood that degenerative arthritis eventually develops. So, angular deformities are to be corrected if they are beyond the acceptable physiological range. Treatment is basically done by realigning via osteotomy or by altering the forces within the growth plate to correct the deformity via asymmetric growth (guided growth method).

4B.6 SURGICAL EXPOSURES AND PROCEDURES AROUND HIP JOINT (Q65–72)

65. Discuss about trochanteric flip osteotomy in surgical exposures of the hip joint.

Ans: Trochanteric flip osteotomy is commonly added to lateral and anterolateral approaches to ease the hip exposure.

Indications:
Wider than normal exposure of the hip needed as in:
- Complex primary total hip arthroplasty (THA)
- Protrusio acetabuli (trochanteric slide is better suited)
- Complex acetabular reconstruction
- Total hip arthroplasty in a patient with unacceptable laxity of abductors that cannot be corrected otherwise as in developmental dysplasia of the hip (DDH)
- Cases where femur needs to be shortened as in high hip center making the hip lax.

Contraindication: Total hip arthroplasty or revision done using Hardinge approach.

Steps:
- Expose the hip joint.
- Protect capsule by placing Hohmann retractor between it and gluteus minimus.
- Release the origin of the vastus lateralis from the vastus tubercle.
- Make an osteotomy cut 1 cm distal to the vastus tubercle at the sulcus between the lateral portion of the origin of the vastus intermedius muscle and the insertions of the gluteus medius and minimus in a distal to proximal direction. When using a Gigli saw proximal to distal direction osteotomy progression is done.
- The trochanter is released from short external rotators and flipped proximally.
- Reattachment—after completion of procedure the attachment is made by a four-wire technique.
  In cases with poor bone quality (revision, osteoporotic, rheumatoid, etc.), it is recommended to use a wire mesh for reattachment.

Complications:
- Nonunion
- Migration
- Abductor insufficiency
- Instability
- Lateral hip pain, mainly due to hardware but removal does not guarantee alleviation
- Heterotopic ossification.

66. Explain surgical anatomy of hip joint. Enumerate various surgical approaches of hip. Mention advantages and disadvantages of each type.

Ans: Surgical anatomy of hip joint:
The hip joint is a diarthrodial joint of ball and socket type. Unlike shoulder joint, hip joint has well-developed bony constraints conferring static stability along with ligaments and capsules. The hip joints are located within pelvic girdle and provide attachment of lower limbs to it. Stability of hip joint is provided by the following:

Osseous structures:
- Head/neck offset
- Acetabular coverage of femoral head
- Acetabular anteversion
- Femoral anteversion

Ligamentous structures:
- Capsular ligaments
- Iliofemoral (limits extension)
- Pubofemoral (limits abduction)
- Ischiofemoral (limits internal rotation)
- Ligamentum orbicularis
- Internal ligaments
- Ligamentum teres (secondary constraint to external rotation)
- Transverse ligament
- Torn/stretched/lax ligaments → greater excursion, marginal contact

Neuromuscular factors:
- Strength of muscles bridging hip joint
- Balanced strength of opposing muscles
- *Muscle tone*: Complex neural feedback

Cartilaginous structures:
- Normal, intact labrum
- Concentric seal against femoral head.

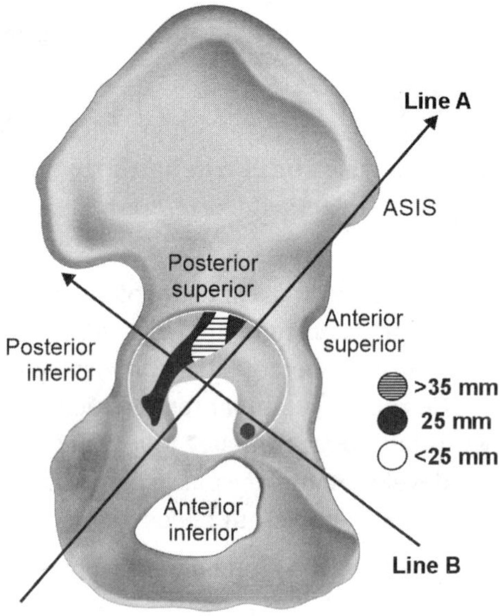

Bony anatomy:

Fig. 4B.6.1: Acetabular quadrant system.

Acetabulum: Formed at the trijunction of ilium, ischium, and pubis, it is in the shape of quasi-hemispherical shell covering the femoral head. It is outlined by labrum. The acetabular labrum is a rim of triangular fibrocartilage (in cross-section) that attaches to the perimeter of acetabulum. It serves the following purposes:
- Enhances joint stability—deepens the acetabulum for femoral head coverage by 21%
- Preserves joint congruity
- Distributes synovial fluid
- Pressure distribution—increases surface of acetabulum by 28% reducing point contact forces.
- Maintaining seal around the femoral head

The acetabular fossa is orientated inferiorly (45°) and anteriorly (15°) and laterally. The acetabular rim is circular but deficient in the lower one-fifth—completed by transverse acetabular ligament. Transverse acetabular ligament provides a landmark to identify the inferior most aspect of the acetabulum, especially in dysplastic hips. The landmark is quite often preserved in most pathologies and nearly always in dysplasia. Acetabular quadrant systems (**Fig. 4B.6.1**) demonstrate the nerves and vessels that course around the acetabulum and proximal femur. The quadrants are formed by two perpendicular lines:
- A line drawn from the ASIS through the center of the acetabulum defines anterior and posterior quadrant locations.
- Second line is perpendicular bisector of the first line at midpoint in acetabulum.

The quadrant helps surgeon to know the location of intrapelvic structures with respect to fixed points of reference within the acetabulum. Anterior quadrants should be avoided for the placement of screws or anchoring hole. Sharp-pointed retractors should not be used here (injury to external iliac artery and vein and the obturator nerve, artery, and vein). Posterior quadrant—sciatic nerve and the superior gluteal nerve and vessels course opposite the posterior superior quadrant and the inferior gluteal and internal pudendal structures are opposite the posteroinferior quadrant.

Femur:
The head of the femur forms approximately two-thirds of a sphere and is covered by articular hyaline cartilage in approximately 60–70% of a sphere. The neck of the femur is approximately 5 cm long. The proximal metaphysis and neck are anteverted by approximately 14°. The angle between the femoral shaft and the neck is approximately 125°. The proximal femoral metaphyseal orientation and shape have great variability that may create problems for a cementless stem with fixed proximal geometries. Cementless stems must fit the anterior, posterior, and medial–lateral dimensions of the canal that should be maintained down the canal for maximum contact. One should evaluate the preoperative radiographs for what is called "funnelization" of the canal. As the canal calcar isthmus ratio (the Dorr index) approaches 1, prosthesis fill proximally and distally is compromised.

The capsule is attached to the femur anteriorly along the intertrochanteric line, but posteriorly it attaches to middle of the neck so that the basicervical portion and intertrochanteric crest are extracapsular posteriorly. The iliofemoral (strongest ligament) and the pubofemoral ligaments reinforce anterior portion of the capsule while ischiofemoral ligament reinforces the posterior capsule.

The blood supply to femoral head is derived from three primary sources (as described by Crock), the metaphyseal system, retinacular system, and the foveolar system as follows:
- *Extracapsular arterial ring (ECA)*: This is the chief system giving rise to both IM and extramedullary arterial systems. The ECA gives less prominent metaphyseal branches to intertrochanteric region which also supply the head through neck (IM metaphyseal system). It is located at the base of femoral neck and is formed:
  - Posteriorly by branch of medial circumflex femoral artery
  - Anteriorly by branch of lateral circumflex femoral artery more often a branch of profunda femoris artery (main branch of femoral artery)
  - Ascending cervical branches of ECA (also known as epiphyseal arteries of Trueta or retinacular arteries) that arise from ECA (more prominent system) and ascend up the neck partly also supplying the neck in due course:
    - Divided into anterior, posterior, medial, and lateral groups
    - Anteriorly, these vessels penetrate the capsule at intertrochanteric line while, posteriorly they pass underneath the orbicularis fibers of the capsule
    - Lateral group (lateral ascending cervical vessels) is the most important group carrying major portion of blood supply to head and neck of femur.
- Subsynovial intra-articular arterial ring of Chung (Circulus articuli vasculosus of Hunter) is formed from lateral ascending cervical vessels:
  - Located at the margins of articular cartilage on surface of neck of femur
  - It is either a complete or incomplete ring.
  - Provides epiphyseal vessels (that penetrate the head just outside the articular cartilage to supply major portion of head).
- Artery of ligamentum teres:
  - Branch of obturator artery (more often) or medial circumflex femoral artery
  - Variable supply in adults
  - Supply head around the region of fovea

Movements at hip:
- Flexion of 120°
- Extension 30°
- Abduction 45–50°
- Adduction of 20–30°
- Internal rotation 35°
- External rotation 45°

Functional ROM of hip needed for walk on level surface is 30° of flexion, 10° of hyperextension, 5° of both abduction and adduction, and 5° of both internal and external rotation.

(*In addition, the muscular and neural anatomy of the hip joint may be read and written in detail from chapter 57 of the book, Essential Orthopedics Principles and Practice*)

Surgical approaches to hip joint:

Anterior approach: Smith-Petersen approach and modified mini-incision approach, Somerville "bikini" incision.

Advantages:
- Preservation of the vascularity—the medial circumflex femoral artery and its branches are preserved.
- Better stability following the procedure with less chance of dislocation—key muscle groups like the extensors and the abductors are intact.
- The approach involves muscle cutting.
- Easier to take intraoperative radiographs as the patient is supine.

Disadvantages
- Limited access makes it technically demanding to place components in arthroplasty as the femoral exposure is limited.
- Damage to lateral cutaneous nerve and the anterior cutaneous nerve

Anterolateral: Watson Jones, Cave, and Gonder

Advantages:
- Preferred for open reduction of fracture neck of femur
- Internervous approach

Disadvantages:
- Weakening of abductors during dissection or by denervation
- Injury to the superior gluteal nerve
- Injury to lateral circumflex femoral artery
- Rarely injury to the femoral nerve and vessels.

Lateral: Hardinge, Harris, McLauchlan approach, McFarland and Osborne

Advantages:
- Good access to the hip with preservation of vascularity
- Minimal risk of damage to sciatic nerve

Disadvantages:
- Damage to gluteal muscle mainly gluteus medius and loss of abductor function
- Heterotopic ossification may be a problem.

Posterior: Moore/Southern, Osborne

Advantages:
- Good exposure of both acetabulum and the femoral head and neck

Disadvantages and complications:
- The blood supply to femoral head is likely to get damaged resulting in ON restricting its use in conservative hip surgery such as open hip debridement, open surgery for hip impingement.
- Damage to sciatic nerve: Palpate the nerve through fat pad to identify its lateralized variation. The nerve is retracted by the reflected cut short external rotators (not piriformis—it lies superficial to nerve). The knee should be kept flexed minimum 45° throughout to prevent traction on the nerve.
- Injury to inferior gluteal vessels, branches of profunda femoris vessels and rarely femoral vessels
- Higher dislocation rate if soft-tissue reconstruction is inadequate.

Posterolateral: Kocher–Langenbeck, Gibson
- Advantages and disadvantages similar to posterior approach

Medial: Ludloff, Ferguson: Hoppenfeld and Deboer

Advantages:
- Minimal dissection and blood loss
- Allows direct approach to common obstacles to reduction, e.g., psoas tendon, capsular constriction, transverse acetabular ligament.

Disadvantages:
- Poor access to acetabulum
- Does not allow capsulorrhaphy
- Risk of avascular necrosis (AVN): 15%
- Approach cannot be used if head has migrated proximally.
- Approach cannot be used when child has started walking.

67. What are the steps of posterior approach to hip joint while performing total hip arthroplasty (THR)? What are the potential complications?

Ans: Posterior approach to hip joint: Moore approach—

Position: Lateral position.

Incision: 10–15 cm long curvilinear extending from 10 cm distal to posterior superior iliac spine (PSIS) to greater trochanter and extends down along the shaft of the femur as required. Small incisions ≈ 10 cm are also enough, however, can always be extended.

Soft-tissue dissection: The gluteus maximus fibers are split and upper part of fascia lata is split.
- The hip is internally rotated and short external rotators are identified and held with stay sutures.
- Obturator internus and externus, two gemelli, and piriformis are detached and reflected backward to protect the sciatic nerve. I personally preserve the piriformis in most hemiarthroplasty procedures and some of the total hips. Quadratus femoris is commonly separated from femur shaft in proximal thirds or half to improve exposure of the joint. For THR, the muscle may be detached at its attachment but for hip-preserving procedures, the muscle is cut at least 1 cm away from its femoral attachment to prevent injury to medial circumflex femoral artery.
- Superior extension and reflection of gluteus minimus may be done for acetabular reconstruction as needed.

Internervous plane: No internervous plane

Arthrotomy: Capsule is incised with a classical T/H-shaped incision or better an L-shaped incision to preserve the iliofemoral ligament.

Closure: This is the most important after arthroplasty as meticulous closure only has the greatest impact on reducing the dislocation rate seen with this approach:
- Capsular closure is imperative and possibly the most important factor in reducing dislocation rate.
- Reattach the external rotators and obturator internus and piriformis

Complications:
Kindly see Answer to Question above.

68. What are the indications and steps of safe surgical dislocation of hip?

Ans: *Indications*:
- Femoral head fractures (Pipkin fractures)
- Complex femoroacetabular impingement (FAI) deformities:
  - Repairing of acetabular labrum
  - Reshaping the bony acetabular rim (acetabuloplasty)
  - Removing bony bumps (cam lesions) on femoral head (femoral osteoplasty).
- Correction of major structural abnormalities of the hip joint:
  - Reduction osteotomy (intraosseous and head splitting) of femoral head in Perthes
  - A deformed femoral head as seen in Perthes disease (cheilectomy)
  - Slipped upper femoral epiphysis (SUFE)—intra-articular osteotomy of femoral neck.

- Articular cartilage defect reconstruction: Autologous cartilage implantation (ACI) and matrix autologous chondrocyte implantation (MACI)
- Loose body removal in fracture dislocation of hip
- Post-traumatic hip deformities
- Hip arthrodesis
- *Other conditions*: Includes—
  - Rheumatoid synovitis
  - Synovial chondromatosis
  - Pigmented villonodular synovitis.

Steps:

Position and approach: Patient is placed in lateral decubitus position and hip is exposed using posterior Kocher-Langenbeck approach. The incision is made and fascia lata splits. The leg is then internally rotated by assistant.

Superficial dissection:
- The posterior border of gluteus medius is only identified but neither mobilized nor retracted to view the piriformis.
- The trochanteric fine vascular plexus is cauterized superficially to minimize bleeding.
- Small length incision is made along the posterosuperior edge of greater trochanter that extends distally to the posterior border of the vastus ridge to expose the trochanter and identify landmarks for trochanteric osteotomy.

Deep tissue dissection:
- Mark the tip of greater trochanter, region of piriformis fossa, and vastus ridge.
- A trochanteric flip osteotomy is done. One should try to maintain thickness of 1.5 cm at least for the osteotomized fragment. One can also modify it into Z-osteotomy for improved stability.
- To make the cuts, one must ensure that the osteotomy does not incorporate anterior portion of the femoral neck or hip joint capsule. The osteotomy exits proximally just anterior to the most posterior insertion of gluteus medius muscle. This protects the profundus branch of the medial circumflex femoral artery (MCFA) at the soft spot where it becomes intracapsular to supply the ascending lateral retinacular vessels at the level of the superior gemellus muscle. To prevent the osteotomy becoming too oblique, it is useful to ask the assistant rotate flexed leg internally by 15–20°. This makes head parallel to the floor and avoids inadvertent injury when saw is used to make osteotomy.
- The greater trochanteric fragment is translated anteriorly after releasing at posterior border the tendon of gluteus maximus and inserting posterior fibers of gluteus medius. Usually a part of the tendon of piriformis is attached to the fragment that has to be freed to accomplish this.
- To ease external rotation at hip, the vastus lateralis and intermedius muscles are elevated from the lateral and anterior aspects of the proximal femur.
- Next, the inferior border of gluteus minimus is separated from the relaxed piriformis; usually there is a vascular anastomosis between underlying joint capsule and the muscle that needs to be preserved while freeing muscle. This anastomosis is formed by inferior gluteal artery and MCFA. The latter is seen running along the distal border of the piriformis.
- One should protect and retract the sciatic nerve from getting injured as the piriformis is mobilized and anomalous relationship of the nerve and muscle might cause nerve compression or traction damage.
- If the piriformis muscle is sandwiched between split branches of sciatic nerve, then muscle should be released from greater trochanter to avoid stretching the nerve during dislocation/anterior flip of entire flap.
- After anterior flip of the fragment with attached medius and vastus lateralis, the gluteus minimus is retracted anteriorly and superiorly to expose the superior capsule.
- To further enhance exposure to anterior, superior, and posterosuperior capsule, the leg can be further flexed and externally rotated.
- Hip joint capsule is then incised in a straight line along the long axis of the femoral neck anterolaterally as this zone is relatively watershed/avascular and avoids the deep branch of the MCFA. The incision is extended distally in the anteroinferior capsular along the base of femoral neck.

- It is important that this vertical limb of osteotomy remains anterior to the lesser trochanter to avoid damaging the main branch of the MCFA. The artery lies here just superior and posterior to lesser trochanter.
- The anterior and inferior half of the labrum can be well visualized once the anteroinferior flap of capsule is reflected.
- To expose rest of the labrum and hip joint, the first capsular incision (straight anterolateral) is extended along the superolateral acetabular rim using capsulotomy scissors or knife. The limb is extended till it sharply turns posteriorly. It may reach as far as the retracted tendon of piriformis protecting the labrum. This completes the capsulotomy.
- The hip joint is now dislocated by flexion, externally rotating the leg and bringing it over the front of the operating table. The leg can be placed in a sterile bag allowing inspection of most of the acetabulum.
- After completion of the procedure, greater trochanter is reattached using two or three cancellous screws or better cerclage wire.

69. Discuss Hardinge approach to hip.
Ans:
- *Position*: Patient supine with the greater trochanter at the edge of the table and the muscles of the buttocks freed from the edge.
- *Incision*: Make a posteriorly directed lazy-J incision centered over the greater trochanter.
- *Dissection*: Divide the fascia lata in line with the skin incision and centered over the greater trochanter.
    - Retract the tensor fasciae latae anteriorly and the gluteus maximus posteriorly, exposing the origin of the vastus lateralis and the insertion of the gluteus medius.
    - Incise the tendon of the gluteus medius obliquely across the greater trochanter, leaving the posterior half still attached to the trochanter.
    - Carry the incision proximally in line with the fibers of the gluteus medius at the junction of the middle and posterior thirds of the muscle.
    - Distally, carry the incision anteriorly in line with the fibers of the vastus lateralis down to bone along the anterolateral surface of the femur.
    - Elevate the tendinous insertions of the anterior portions of the gluteus minimus and vastus lateralis muscles. (Abduction of the thigh exposes the anterior capsule of the hip joint).
- Incise the capsule as desired.
- *Closure*: Repair the tendon of the gluteus medius with nonabsorbable braided sutures.

70. Discuss about the anterolateral exposure of hip.
Ans: Smith-Petersen described a modification of the anterior iliofemoral approach that he used for open reduction and internal fixation of fractures of the femoral neck. This approach retains the advantages of the anterior iliofemoral approach but exposes the trochanteric region laterally; this makes aligning a fracture or osteotomy of the femoral neck and inserting pins or nails under direct vision easier. This approach is also useful in reconstructive procedures such as osteotomy for slipping of the proximal femoral epiphysis and procedures for nonunions of the femoral neck. It gives a continuous exposure of the anterior aspect of the hip from the acetabular labrum to the base of the trochanter.
- Make the skin incision along the anterior third of the iliac crest and along the anterior border of the tensor fasciae latae muscle; curve it posteriorly across the insertion of this muscle into the iliotibial band in the subtrochanteric region (usually at a point 8–10 cm below the base of the greater trochanter) and end it there.
- Incise the fascia along the anterior border of the tensor fasciae latae muscle. Identify and protect the lateral femoral cutaneous nerve, which usually is medial to the medial border of the tensor fasciae latae and close to the lateral border of the sartorius.
- Cleanly incise the muscle attachments to the lateral aspect of the ilium along the iliac crest to make reflection of the periosteum easier. Reflect it as a continuous structure, without fraying, distally to the superior margin of the acetabulum.
- Divide the muscle attachments between the anterior superior iliac spine and the acetabular labrum. The flap thus reflected consists of the tensor fasciae latae, the gluteus minimus, and the anterior part of the gluteus medius.
- Inferiorly carry the fascial incision across the insertion of the tensor fasciae latae into the iliotibial band, and expose the lateral part of the rectus femoris and the anterior part of the vastus lateralis muscles.

- Begin the capsular incision on the inferior aspect of the capsule just lateral to the acetabular labrum; from this point, extend it proximally, parallel with the acetabular labrum, to the superior aspect of the capsule, and curve it laterally, continuing on beyond the capsule to the base of the greater trochanter. This incision divides that part of the reflected head of the rectus femoris that blends into the capsule inferior to its insertion into the superior margin of the acetabulum. By reflecting it with the capsule, the capsular flap is reinforced, and repair is made easier.

71. What is a rotationplasty?

Ans: Rotationplasties have been described as an alternative to amputation in cases of malignant tumors involving distal femur and proximal tibia to salvage the limb. These are based on the principle of rotating the distal part of the lower limb by 180° so that the ankle joint functions like a knee joint and a below knee prosthesis can be used. It is especially useful in children where the growth potential of distal end tibial is preserved. These rotationplasties basically evolved from the Van Nes rotationplasty which was originally described for congenital proximal femoral deficiencies. Winkelmann classified rotationplasty into five groups, which are as follows:

- *Group AI*: Here the lesion is in the distal femur and requires resection of the distal femur, knee joint, and proximal tibia. The lower leg is rotated 180° and the tibia is joined to the remaining femur.
- *Group AII*: Here the lesion is in the proximal tibia requiring the resection of distal femur, knee joint, and proximal tibia.
- *Group BI*: The lesion is in the proximal femur but spares the hip joint and gluteal muscles. The upper femur and hip joint require resection. The distal femur is joined to the pelvis to make the knee function as the hip and the ankle as the knee.
- *Group BII*: The lesion is also in the proximal femur but involves the hip joint soft tissue. The entire hemipelvis requires resection. The femur is joined to the remaining ilium and the knee functions as a hip joint and the ankle functions as the knee.
- *Group BIII*: The lesion is in the mid femur, requiring the entire femur to be resected. The tibia is attached to the pelvis with the help of an endoprosthesis.

The basic principles of rotationplasty are as follows:
- The ankle and foot must be disease free.
- Adequate nerve supply to the foot and ankle.
- Adequate blood supply to the foot and ankle must be restorable after resection.
- It must be possible to restore adequate muscle power to the ankle joint.
- Complete resection of the tumor must be possible while preserving the neurovascular structures.

The most commonly used rotationplasty is for lesion involving the distal femur. The skin incision is made in the shape of a rhombus with its long axis on the anterior surface and its two lateral points meeting on the posterior surface. If a biopsy scar is present, it must be included in the incision and the incision must be about 5–10 cm longer than the intended bone resection. The common peroneal, tibial, and sciatic nerves are identified and dissected away from the tumor. The femoral vessels are identified in the adductor canal and are similarly dissected distally. If the tumor involves the vessels, then part of the vessel is removed with the tumor and reconstructed later ensuring that the ischemia time does not exceed 2 hours. The femur is transected with a healthy margin of 5 cm. The tibia is transected just distal to the knee joint capsule in adults and distal to the proximal physis in children.

Frozen sections are taken to ensure adequate resection. The limb is then rotated to 180° so that the peroneal and tibial nerves lie on the medial side and the femur is joined to the tibia with a compression plate. In adults, the ankle joint should be at the same level as the contralateral knee joint. In children, an estimate of the growth potential of the contralateral leg should be made using a green Anderson table and the ankle should be lower than the knee to compensate for this growth. The muscles of the thigh are sutured to the leg fascia and skin is closed. After adequate bone union, a modified below knee prosthesis can be worn.

72. Define hip arthrography.

Ans: It is used in a variety of conditions:

Developmental dysplasia of the hip: It is a wonderful tool to assess the reduction (closed reduction), depth of acetabulum, and stability of reduction. The width of medial dye pool indicates the likely stability of reduction. Fair reduction is indicated by 5–6 mm of medial dye pool. Medial space greater than 6 mm indicates poor reduction, which is difficult to hold.

An arthrogram may help in determining the acetabular dysplasia, degree of femoral head dislocation, extent of soft tissue obstruction to closed reduction, condition of the limbus, and the quality of reduction.

- To perform an arthrogram, the child is laid supine under general anesthesia
- A 22-gauge spinal needle is inserted into the hip joint under image intensifier.
- Alternatively, the needle may be inserted medially, anterior to the adductor musculature.
- Resistance is met as needle passes through the hip joint capsule followed by sudden give way.
- Now saline solution is injected into capsule.
- If the joint has been successfully entered, the saline solution under pressure will reverse the plunger of the syringe.
- The saline is now aspirated and 1–3 mL of 25% hypaque solution is injected into the capsule.
- The needle is quickly removed and an arthrogram is made in unreduced position in adduction and extension.
- Further arthrograms are made after reducing the hip in flexion and abduction.
- Best position for concentric reduction and safe zone is noted carefully.

Perthes disease: Arthrography offers an opportunity to evaluate coverage and mobility under direct vision. It should be performed prior to surgery to help in determining the best position for femoral head containment and demonstrate absence of hinged abduction before containment procedures are performed. Laredo classified hips into five types depending upon arthrographic findings.

- Type 1 hips are normal.
- Type 2 hips have spherical femoral head which is larger than normal.
- Type 3 hips have ovoid femoral head.
- Type 4 has large and flattened femoral head, with straight and elevated labrum, hinged abduction may be present.
- Type 5 hips show a femoral head larger than normal and saddle-shaped, and the labrum is straight and elevated.

All hips from Type 2 to Type 5 show femoral head extrusion in neutral position and normal coverage at about 30° of abduction with some internal rotation.

Labral tears: Contrast-enhanced magnetic resonance *(MR) arthrography* is more sensitive than standard magnetic resonance imaging (MRI) at detecting intra-articular lesions of the hip with 95% and 88% sensitivity and specificity. Posterior tears are less effectively identified; the diagnostic accuracy increases after joint distension that causes the contrast to fill and outline tears more definitely. The procedure is performed in two stages: First, fluoroscopically guided hip arthrography performed through anterior approach. The joint is distended using diluted (2.5 nM) gadopentetate dimeglumine (by mixing 0.1 mL of contrast to 20 mL saline). The hip joint space is around 8–20 mL and is completely distended. In the second stage, MRI is performed using recommended protocols. The diagnostic criteria for identifying the labral tears are intrasubstance contrast material, labra with irregular margins with and without labral detachments. Labral detachment is identified by contrast material interposed at the labral-acetabular interface with or without displacement.

4B.7 BIOMECHANICS OF HIP (Q73–75)

73. Discuss biomechanics of hip. Also discuss Trendelenburg gait and sign.

Ans: Biomechanics **(Fig. 4B.7.1)**:

Axes and center of gravity:
- Mechanical axis line passes between center of hip joint and center of ankle joint.
- Anatomic axis line is between the tip of greater trochanter and center of knee joint.
- Angle formed between these two is around 7°.
- Weight of any object acts through center of gravity, in humans, the center of gravity passes just anterior to second sacral vertebra.

Forces transmitted across hip joint: The hip joint is never fully unloaded during daily activities and, even though, it may not be bearing weight (says during swing phase of gait); there is a residual compressive force across the joint from muscle action approximating the body weight (BW). Pauwels described the "*balancing moments*" across the hip joint. Moment is the effective force and is simply a product of force times the distance from which it acts (M = F × D). For balancing the weight moment, the hip acts like a class-1 lever where the fulcrum is the hip joint that lies in the center, balancing the forces applied on either side of it. The abductors act to balance the force moments to maintain level pelvis. The joint reactive force is primarily a compressive force at femoroacetabular articulation, resulting from pull of abductors, and balancing the moment of arms to maintain a level pelvis.

Abductor force of contraction must balance the resultant forces on head of femur to balance the pelvis, else it will drop (Trendelenburg sign). The joint reaction force is sum of BW and the abductor contraction force. It is not a moment but a pure force depicted with the units of Newton (N). The equation is not as simple and the muscle force is not just abductors but a combined muscular activity across the joint, and the BW is also "effective BW".

For analytical purpose, let us say that "effective BW (K)" exerts a turning moment on femoral head through its moment arm "b". The combined muscular activity "M" balances the moment K × b through the moment arm "a". This arm acts approximately at 30° (θ) to the center of femoral head.

So, $M \times a = K \times b$

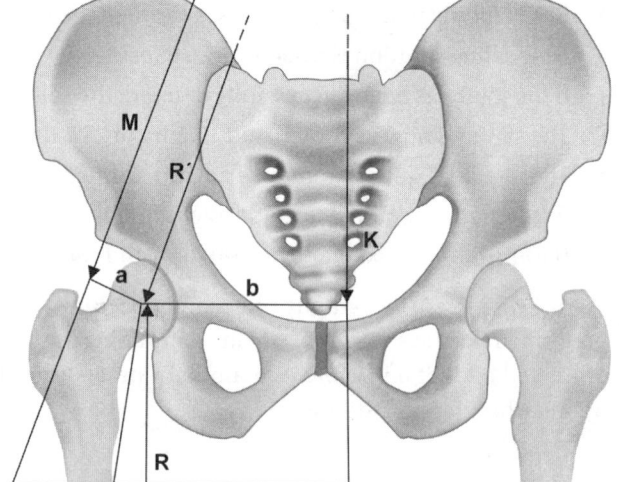

Fig. 4B.7.1: Hip biomechanics.

The lever arm ratio (a:b) typically decides the magnitude of forces. As b > a so, from above, "M" > "K". This analytic estimate typically reveals joint forces range of 2.3–4.6 BW (for a short-statured female to heavy muscular male) for one-legged stance.

Complexity of measurements: The hip joint supports the BW (minus weight of lower limbs during standing, minus weight of one limb during walk) presented to it with vectorial disposition generating resultant forces (vectorial summation of BW, joint reaction forces and lever vectors).

We know that lower limbs constitute 2/6 (1/6 + 1/6) of BW, while the upper limb and trunk constitute 4/6 of the total BW. In a two-leg stance, as there is no muscular contraction so no force is needed to maintain equilibrium. The BW is equally distributed across both hips. Each hip carries one-third of BW (6/6–1/6–1/6 = 4/6 ≡ 2/3 → 1/3 + 1/3).

In the free body diagram analysis for single-leg stance, hip is assumed to be in the resting position at one-legged stance and only abductors acting at 30° are active. It should be noted that it is impossible to determine instant center of rotation of hip joint, as movements occur simultaneously in all three planes. Core assumptions here include position of center of gravity minus one leg (so, effective body weight = 5/6 BW; approximately 81% of BW), the muscles active in position of the test (abductors for single leg stance), and lastly that the forces in a system of mechanical links of various lengths and areas in the test will correspond to the forces developed in the muscles of living body (difficult to approximate).

Now considering a = 5 cm and b = 12.5 cm (a:b will be 1:2.5) and the moments of forces to be balanced, the muscle forces acting at 30° to trochanter are around 2.5 BW. For hip to remain static, the sum of forces should be zero, so » R′ – (M + K) = 0 (R′ is joint reaction force acting at 30°):

- R′ = 3.5 K
- R = R′/cos θ = R′/cos 30° (R is joint reaction force)
- R = 4K ≈ 4 BW

From above, it can be seen that joint reaction force can be reduced by shifting BW over the hip (reducing "a") as in Trendelenburg gait, by tilting toward the affected hip. Holding cane in other hand reduces the "K" partially as the weight is supported also on the cane; here, the "R" will be dependent on how much force passes through cane moment (usually

60%). People with shorter necks have higher hip forces, more so people with wider pelvis have higher forces due to far away distance of hip center from line of BW. Conceivably, females (wider pelvis—higher "b" and smaller "a" due to shorter neck) are at mechanical disadvantage with respect to hip forces (and hence more hip fractures, arthritis, and athletic activities) though this does not translate always to clinical effects.

Direct measurements of resultant joint forces using endoprosthesis instrumented with transducers by various authors provided variable records. The peak forces varied 2.1–4.3 times BW during gait, 2.3–5.5 BW during stair climbing to exceeding 8 BW during stumbling.

Torsional forces are higher by 23% during stair climbing compared to normal walking. The magnitudes of forces experienced in hip during walking are biphasic, with a zenith reached at heel strike and terminal stance of the gait cycle. A slower unassisted gait produces higher peak forces compared to brisk walk and similar association has been found between being overweight and higher hip moments for obvious reasons predisposing to injury and joint dysfunction.

For a Moore type endoprosthesis, maximum forces (measured in MPa) transmitted across hip joint during gait were found to occur between heel strike and early midstance.

Trendelenburg gait *(abduction lurch gait)*: It may be unilateral or bilateral. It depends upon the abductor lever arm, any abnormality of which leads to Trendelenburg gait. When present unilaterally, the patient lurches on the affected side and the pelvis drops on the opposite hip. Bilateral Trendelenburg gait is also known as *waddling gait*.

Any condition in which there is deficit in abduction mechanism of the hip joint, medial deviation of mechanical axis of lower limb and gross costo-pelvic impingement (e.g., congenital dysplasia of hip, fracture of femoral neck, and polioparalysis) will cause this.

Trendelenburg sign: Friedrich Trendelenburg described this test in year 1895 for assessment of congenital dislocation of hip. This test is done while the patient is standing. Basically, a positive Trendelenburg test indicates weakness of the gluteus medius muscle, which may also reveal hip joint pathology.

Principle: It assesses the integrity of the abductor mechanism of the hip (the fulcrum, lever arm, and power). Intact abductor mechanism ensures stability of the hip joint. With affection of any of the above, the normal mechanism of weight bearing is disrupted and gluteal or Trendelenburg lurch develops.

The test: In a normal test when one stands on one leg, opposite part of the body, pelvis (represented on the surface by anterior–superior iliac spine), and the lower limb are lifted up to clear the ground. This is affected by the force of contraction of the ipsilateral gluteus medius with an intact lever arm and fulcrum, working from below and pulling the upper part of the pelvis down. Therefore, the opposite pelvis is lifted up. Clinically, it is visualized by elevation of the gluteal fold, the iliac crest, the level of the scapula, and the shoulder top on the other side observed by standing behind the patient. It can also be palpated by keeping your thumbs on the iliac crests, by which it will be easy to access the dipping down of the pelvis. 5° drop of pelvis or gluteal fold may be normal. More than 5° is definitely abnormal.

Failure of gluteal mechanism causes opposite pelvis to sag down as indicated by lowering down of the gluteal fold (iliac crest, scapula/shoulder top) on that side. This is Trendelenburg positive test indicating trouble with any or all or part of the three, namely fulcrum, lever, and power as in congenital dislocation of hip, fracture neck femur, abductor paralysis due to poliomyelitis, etc.

Fallacies:
- The intact quadratus lumborum muscle plays its role in affecting the normal gluteal mechanism. The ipsilateral muscle working from below pulls down that side of the trunk, while the opposite muscle working from above lifts up the iliac crest, i.e., pelvis. Hence, affection of this muscle can also give a positive test.
- In certain congenital dislocations, where there is dissociation of coordination of different groups of controlling muscles of joints (even other than the hip), there may be affection of these mechanism, e.g., cerebral palsy and congenital dysplasia of hip.
- Affections of sacroiliac joints by virtue of producing pain may produce a pseudo-positive Trendelenburg test.

- The medial shift of the mechanical axis of leg below the hip (e.g., in bow knee, bow leg, malunited fracture of femur, or tibia)—the test may be pseudo positive.
- In obese and bulky persons, the test may be pseudo positive.

74. Describe hip biomechanics along with a diagram. Explain how a stick in the opposite hand decreases the load on the hip along with a diagram.

Ans: For hip biomechanics see above.

Cane reducing hip joint reaction forces (JRFs):
When we walk or stand on one leg (e.g., during the stance phase of gait), the hip abductors (mainly *gluteus medius and minimus*) contract to keep the pelvis level.
- This contraction produces a large abductor muscle force on the hip.
- The hip JRF is the sum of:
  - Body weight (BW) acting downward.
  - Abductor muscle force acting upward from the greater trochanter side.

In normal single-leg stance, JRF can be 3–4 × BW.

When a stick (cane) is used in the opposite hand (**Fig. 4B.7.2**):
- The stick presses down on the ground.
- The ground pushes up on the stick with an equal upward force.
- This creates an upward moment around the hip on the stance side.
- This upward moment assists the abductors in balancing the pelvis.
- The abductors now exert less force → JRF decreases.

Mechanics:
- *Without stick*:
  - Abductor muscle force ≈ 2.5 × BW → JRF ≈ 3–4 × BW.
- *With stick (opposite hand)*:
  - Abductor muscle force reduced by ~30–40% → JRF ≈ 2–2.5 × BW.
  - *Opposite hand*: Stick pushes down away from the stance hip, creating a longer moment arm and thus a greater torque to assist abductors.
  - *Same side*: Minimal mechanical advantage—does not effectively reduce abductor force.

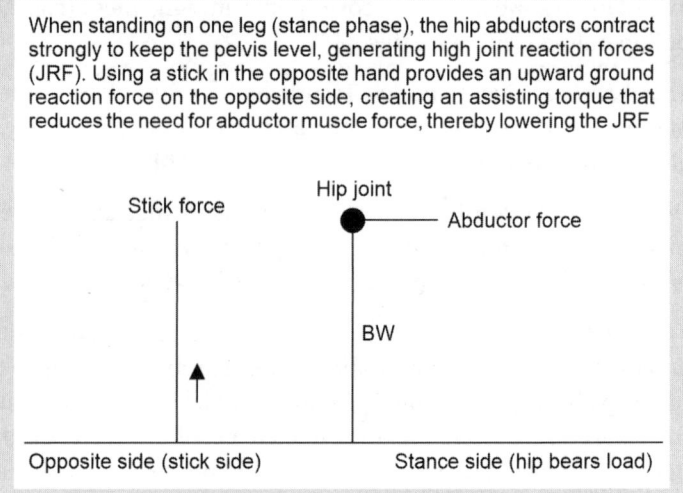

Fig. 4B.7.2: How using a stick in the opposite hand reduces hip load.

75. What are the factors which affect joint reaction force?

Ans: Factors may increase or decrease joint reaction force (JRF) as follows:

Factors decreasing JRF:
- *Hip arthroplasty*:
  1. *Acetabular side*: Medial, inferior and anterior shifting of joint center during arthroplasty, i.e., by deepening the acetabulum.
  2. *Femoral side*: Increasing offset of femoral component or by using increased offset neck, optimally (not excessively) advancing the trochanter distally. Varus neck shaft angulation
- Joint reaction force can be reduced by shifting body weight over the hip as in Trendelenburg gait, by tilting toward the affected hip. Holding cane in other hand reduces the effective body weight partially as the weight is supported also on the cane, here the JRF will be dependent on how much force passes through cane moment (usually 60%).
- Weight loss decreases JRF.

Factors increasing JRF:
- Valgus neck shaft angulation
- People with shorter necks have higher hip forces, more so people with wider pelvis have higher forces due to far away distance of hip center from line of body weight. Conceivably females (wider pelvis and shorter neck) are at mechanical disadvantage with respect to hip forces. Decreasing the horizontal offset increases JRF.

4B.8 FEMOROACETABULAR IMPINGEMENT (Q76)

76. Describe femoroacetabular impingement (FAI).

Ans: The term is itself descriptive of an early pathological contact between the bony prominences of the acetabulum and femur that mechanically limits the physiologic movements of hip producing pain at the extremes of hip range of motion. The most readily identifiable FAI is the pathological early contact of anterior acetabular rim with femoral neck causing "anterior impingement" that typically restricts hip flexion and internal rotation movements. In fact, there are various other forms of impingement that can be also appraised from definition, which does not limit itself to only the anterior impingement. So, anteroinferior FAI is commonly seen in a valgus hip, superior impingement is seen in varus hip, likewise global impingement results in protrusio hip, and so on. This entails the fact that FAI is by itself not an entity (it is a disorder of hip movements) rather a conglomerate of various "modes" that restrict the complete hip range of movement ultimately leading to painful arthritis in a common pathomechanism.

The concept of FAI has been proposed by Ganz and others, so it was quite known to the orthopedic population. Per se, the phenomenon of impingement was first recognized as an iatrogenic complication seen with overcorrection of aggressive periacetabular osteotomy (PAO) performed for dysplasia. Only the disorder (FAI) as a native cause of osteoarthritis was linked later and is quite in vogue now. Clinically and radiologically, two types of FAI have been classified, though most patients have a mixture of both:

- *Cam FAI impingement* is due to femoral cause and is due to an aspherical portion of the femoral head-neck junction. This asphericity of femoral head may arise from various causes like growth disturbance, LCPD (Legg-Calve-Perthes disease), missed SUFE (Slipped-upper femoral epiphysis), or subsequent to trauma. There are two prominent morphological features of femoral head that can produce a cam impingement:
  - Commonly cam impingement is due to a "pistol grip" deformity (decreased femoral head-neck offset on the superior or anterolateral region of the femoral neck). The reduced offset of head-neck junction in the anterolateral region hampers joint clearance.
  - The other significant cause of cam impingement is due to bony abnormalities of the anterior and lateral femoral head or neck junction. Commonly, this morphological aberration expresses itself as a variable thickness "bump" or exuberant bone that arises in the anterosuperior region of the femoral neck producing the classic anterior impingement. As this aspherical portion squeezes itself in the acetabulum the motion is slowed and hence a subtle stop is appreciated clinically. The pathological bump stretches out and pushes the labrum peripherally while the articular cartilage is pushed centrally producing "chondrolabral separation".
- *Pincer impingement* is due to acetabular cause (commonly a retroverted acetabulum)—characterized by focal (anterior) or general overcoverage (as in protrusio hip) of the femoral head as in retroverted acetabulum.

Etiology, Pathophysiology, and Natural History of Disease
Several theories exist to explain FAI but the inciting event is elusive.
- Cam impingement:
  - Pistol-grip neck deformity
  - Nonspherical head.
- Pincer impingement:
  - Deep socket-coxa profunda, protrusio acetabuli, bony buildup of the anterior acetabular rim, high center-edge (CE) angle, low sourcil angle, or a more complex acetabular retroversion seen constitutionally in some individuals.
  - Dynamic pincer impingement occurs in dancers and gymnasts.

- *Sagittal plane deformities* of proximal femur produce coxa valga or vara.
- *Torsional deformity of proximal femur*: The FAI due to torsional deformities is complicated to understand at least due to the compensatory or supplementary effect of acetabular torsion.

Clinical features: Femoroacetabular impingement usually affects patient in active middle years and is more commonly seen in athletic individuals. The usual complaint is a deep groin pain often accompanying activity appearing with or after it. Typically, the pain is exacerbated by activities requiring hip flexion (cam impingement) and internal rotation. Initially, the sporting (sprinting or kicking sports) and strenuous activities (ascending hills or stairs) requiring large movements of hip (prolonged sitting in low-lying chairs) cause symptoms, but later even simple acts like walking, driving, or getting in and out of low vehicles may produce them. Symptoms could range from mild to severe and are often intermittent but in advanced cases may also come up with sitting. Pain often is seen radiating to anterior thigh, or in the region of symphysis pubis or even to the ipsilateral testicle in men. The groin pain could be activity limiting for athletes.

Pincer impingement anteriorly presents complaints similar to cam impingement while posterior impingement produces buttock or sacroiliac pain.

Posterior impingement produces pain in hyperextension activities like fast walking and walking downhill and during intercourse. Pincer impingement is more common in middle-aged women, occurring at an average age of 40 years, and can occur with various disorders. Labral tears additionally produces catching, clicking, and a feeling of giving way.

On examination, patients have characteristic finding of reduced internal rotation and adduction both while the hip is positioned in flexion. This maneuver exacerbates pain if already present or produces pain, if asymptomatic during presentation.

Impingement test: Passively flexing the adducted hip and gradually internally rotating will often elicit anterior groin pain.

Fitzgerald's acetabular labral tests: The test has been described to identify anterior or posterior labral tear.

Investigations: Plain hip radiographs are usually normal, but subtle abnormalities could be present that should be suspected, especially for symptomatic patients. These are better detailed by anteroposterior (AP) radiograph of pelvis with both legs in 15° of internal rotation that gives a gross comparison of both proximal femurs, with particular attention to head-neck offset. Avoid gonadal shielding. Some characteristic features are seen in radiographs that indicate cam-type or pincer-type impingement; kindly also see the radiographic features described above for acetabular labral tears.

Cam impingement: Cross-table lateral radiograph (Dunn/Rippstein view) illustrates the cam lesions as a bump disrupting the normal concave arc. Quantification of the amount of asphericity is commonly done by:

- *Measuring the angle* α: Angle α is the angle between the femoral neck axis and a line connecting the head center with the point of beginning asphericity of the head-neck contour. It can be measured on radiographs but better done on a CT film. Angle α exceeding 500 indicates an abnormally shaped femoral head-neck junction most commonly a cam lesion.
- *Anterior offset*: It is the difference in radius between the anterior femoral head and the anterior femoral neck on a Dunn or Rippstein projection of the proximal femur. Normal hips have anterior offset of 11.6 ± 0.7 mm while value less than 10 mm strongly indicates cam lesion.
- *Offset ratio*: It is the ratio between the anterior offset and the diameter of the head. It has been observed that for smaller hips, the measurement of anterior offset may overestimate cam lesion. The problem can be resolved by taking head of femur as a reference. The offset ratio is 0.21 ± 0.03 in asymptomatic patients and ≤0.13 ± 0.05 in hips with cam impingement.

Pincer impingement: Acetabular features for *pincer impingement* on the AP film include the presence of a deep (coxa profunda, protrusio) or shallow socket (dysplasia) and an alteration of acetabular version (anteverted or retroverted that may be focal or global).

Pincer lesion radiographic findings: General acetabular overcoverage—
- The acetabular fossa line lies in a normal hip lateral to the ilioischial line on AP pelvic radiograph.
- *In coxa profunda*: The floor of the acetabular fossa touches or just overlaps the ilioischial line medially.
- *In a higher grade of deformity*: The protrusio acetabuli; the femoral head itself overlaps the ilioischial line medially, obviously the floor of acetabular fossa lies medially.
- Femoral head overcoverage is quantified by:
  - Lateral CE angle
  - The acetabular index "acetabular roof angle"
- Femoral coverage can also be quantified by femoral head extrusion index
- Focal femoral head overcoverage:
  - Cross-over sign
  - Posterior wall sign
  - Impingement between the posteroinferior acetabulum and posteromedial aspect of femoral head due to posteroinferior subluxation from anterior impingement.

Management: **Structural abnormality** often does not improve with *conservative treatment*. Nearly all patients failed on conservative management have to be operated and the modality is determined by the location of the pathology that dictates the ultimate treatment plan. The deformity has to be corrected surgically and both hip arthroscopy and open surgery have their proponents. The *operative management* of these lesions gives two prime benefits:
- Pain relief by virtue of removal of the structural abnormality
- Early recognition and addressal of this entity may curb or halt the unfortunate progression to osteoarthritis in these younger patients.

The technical goals of surgery for FAI are:
- Precise deformity correction (intra-articular and extra-articular)
- Consistent deformity correction
- Comprehensive deformity correction
- Treatment of soft tissue abnormalities (labrum, articular cartilage, etc.)
- Dynamic exam to assess all potential sources of FAI.

The various surgical tools for management of FAI include:
- Femoral osteochondroplasty
- Proximal femoral osteotomy
- Labral repair or refixation, resection, or replacement
- Reshaping of the acetabular rim
- Acetabular chondral debridement
- Acetabular realignment (periacetabular osteotomy).

Cam impingement due to aberrations in femoral neck anatomy is usually amenable to arthroscopic debridement or correction. Once corrected and if the head-neck offset is correct then repetitive impingement will not occur. Open techniques (and modifications like surgical dislocation of hip–Ganz osteotomy, etc.) have been the traditional approach to address most of FAI abnormalities that can be used to treat nearly all abnormalities whether femoral or acetabular.

For pincer impingement—the anterior acetabulum is simply recontoured (acetabuloplasty) to eliminate the impingement in "focal retroversions". The retroversion may be severe and global needing correction with reverse PAO, but the risk of destabilizing the joint is very high.

(Further details can be gathered from the Chapter 36 of Essential Orthopedics: Principles and Practice, 2nd edition.)

4B.9 OSTEOTOMIES AROUND HIP JOINT (Q77–81)

77. List osteotomies around hip. Write briefly about principles of each osteotomy.

Ans: There are three groups of osteotomies that can be done around the hip joint:

1. *Periacetabular osteotomies*:
   - Innominate osteotomy (Salter)
   - Acetabuloplasty (Pemberton)
   - Osteotomies that free the acetabulum (steel triple innominate or Ganz acetabular osteotomy), Shelf operation (Staheli), and
   - Innominate osteotomy with medial displacement of the acetabulum (Chiari).
2. *Proximal femoral osteotomies*:
   - *Depending on the functional correction that osteotomy achieves, it can be classified as*:
     - *Lineal*: When it is performed to correct shortening or lengthening.
     - *Torsional*: When performed to correct internal or external rotation deformity.
     - *Translational*: When the fragments are displaced medially or laterally, e.g., McMurray's osteotomy.
     - *Angular*: When performed to correct the angular deformities, e.g., Blount osteotomy and Schanz osteotomy.
   - *Depending on the type of bone cut, osteotomy can be grouped into following types*:
     - *Transverse osteotomy*: This is ideal for correction of rotation and is performed in metaphyseal or diaphyseal region. It is easy to perform but is unstable and not ideally suited for interfragmentary compression.
     - Angular corrections are difficult to control by this osteotomy, so not indicated.
     - *Oblique osteotomy*: Gives superior bending and rotational stability as it is easily compressed with interfragmentary lag-screw. Oblique osteotomy is especially useful in metaphyseal or diaphyseometaphyseal area.
     - *Crescentic osteotomy (dome or reverse dome-shaped)*: This osteotomy maintains good bony contact and preserve length while correcting angulations and rotational deformity. It is difficult to plan and is technically difficult to perform. It is a very good option (preferable) to correct varus or valgus deformity close to joint, if one is experienced in performing crescentic osteotomies.
   - *Depending on the relative position of two fragments after bone cuts*:
     - *Displacement or transpositional osteotomy*: Usually, a transverse metaphyseal osteotomy and one of the fragments (usually distal) is shifted or rotated so that the corner of fragment is impacted into medullary canal of the other fragment. Longitudinal axis of distal fragment remains parallel to the longitudinal terminal axis of proximal fragment. This osteotomy relies on biological changes induced and preserves or improves the joint forces and physiology. By specific translation of fragments, the bending and loading force are converted into compressive load. The osteotomy preserves length and joint alignment, e.g., McMurray's osteotomy, Dimon-Hughston osteotomy, etc.
     - *Angulation osteotomy*: Most other osteotomies fall into this category where the longitudinal axis of distal fragment forms an angle with that of proximal fragment. This is done to reorient the joint and/or realign the limb to maintain proper mechanical axis or improve load transmission across the joint. Extra-articular deformities are commonly corrected by this method. Today the majority of osteotomies include displacement and angulation both to achieve a multiplanar correction. In addition to alterations in the frontal plane, rotation, and sagittal plane corrections are also combined together.
   - *Depending on the location of proximal osteotomy, it can be referred to as*:
     - *Intertrochanteric osteotomy*: It is of various types and depending on the use it has been variedly described by authors:
       - Pauwels' osteotomy (this is a valgus or varus repositioning osteotomy)
       - McMurray's osteotomy (for osteoarthrosis and also used for nonunion neck femur; it is a pelvic support medial displacement intertrochanteric osteotomy)

- Modified osteotomy of Muller
- Ball and socket osteotomy
- Dimon and Hughston osteotomy are for improving the stability of intertrochanteric fractures.
  - *Trochanteric displacement osteotomy*: These are done to reposition the trochanter for either:
    - An abnormal pathologic position of the greater trochanter compromising abductor function; or
    - Short femoral neck and elevated greater trochanter.
- *Subtrochanteric osteotomy*: These are mainly done either as a part of pelvic support osteotomy or to correct rotational deformity:
  - Milch-bachelor type—improves stability of the hip; for nonunion of femoral neck fracture and unstable hip with positive telescopy test and Trendelenburg limp
  - Blount osteotomy
  - Schanz osteotomy similar to Milch osteotomy.
- *Femoral neck osteotomy*: These are done for—
  - Slipped capital femoral epiphysis
  - Sugioka osteotomy (avascular necrosis of head of femur).

3. *Combined type*:

(Kindly read details from the Chapter 65 of the book Essential Orthopedics: Principles and Practice, 2nd edition.)

78. What is pelvic support osteotomy? Outline principles and operative technique.

Ans: *Pelvic support osteotomy*: The pelvic support osteotomy (PSO) is a double level femoral osteotomy with the objective of eliminating a Trendelenburg and short limb gait in young patients with unstable hips. It can also be done to stabilize the hips after resection arthroplasty or infected prosthesis removal to stabilize the hip. The surgery is performed at two levels in femur:

1. The proximal valgus-extension osteotomy is performed with the femur in maximum adduction and at a level where the femoral shaft is seen to about the pelvis.
2. The second distal osteotomy restores the limb alignment by bringing the knee and ankle joint lines in the coronal plane.

Principles:
- Lateralize greater trochanter
- Distally displace greater trochanter—improve abductor strength
- Eliminate adduction between femur and pelvis preventing pelvic drop
- Reduce limp by abolishing Trendelenburg lurch
- Equalize limb length by stabilizing the hemipelvis
- Produce energy efficient gait.

Technique—Milch bachelor type pelvic support osteotomy (PSO). The site of osteotomy is predetermined by radiological planning on radiographs. It is at the level of ischial tuberosity. There is a limit to which the pelvis can tilt for compensation. Usually, the upper limit of pelvic tilt is 20–25° so the degree to which the postosteotomy angle can be permitted to exceed the determined angulation of lateral pelvic wall should not be more than 15–20°. His tilt permits correction of disparity up to 5 cm, for any more deformity, it is better to use shoe-raise than increasing the angle, else problems mentioned above will come.

The osteotomy is performed through a lateral iliofemoral approach extending from anterior superior iliac spine to the base of trochanter and downward along the lateral aspect of femur. The nerve to tensor fascia lata is usually sacrificed. The plane between the gluteus medius and tensor fascia is developed and neck is resected at the intertrochanteric line. Subtrochanteric osteotomy is performed at the predetermined level and distal fragment is abducted and internally rotated to 20–25°. Internal rotation is done to compensate for the external rotation that is produced due to loss of pelvic support.

79. What is Schanz osteotomy?

Ans: This is a type of pelvic support osteotomy aimed at eliminating Trendelenburg gait and compensating limb shortening in young patients for treatment of destroyed hip joint (most commonly sequel of septic arthritis). Schanz osteotomy is a low subtrochanteric angular osteotomy. The osteotomy is similar to Milch osteotomy but no angle β is calculated.

The major emphasis is providing stability to the pelvis through malformed or absent hip joint. The corrections in flexion, adduction, and external rotation are made by making the osteotomy at ischial tuberosity level by introducing a valgus, and sometimes extension, position to the distal femoral segment. This osteotomy differed from Lorenz osteotomy as no proximal shift displacement was done to the distal femoral segment **(Fig. 4B.9.1)**.

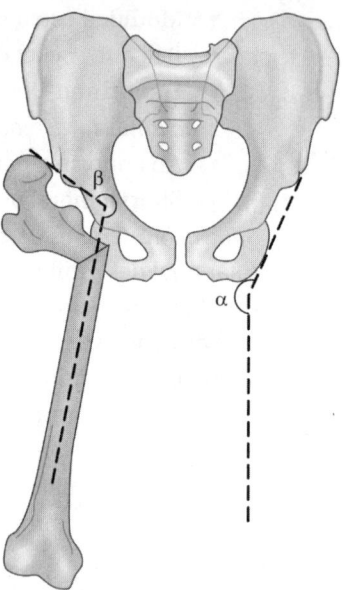

Fig. 4B.9.1: Schanz osteotomy.

Advantages
- Lurching gait will be diminished
- The depression of the trochanter also improves the leverage of the glutei.

Contraindication: Before 15 years of age, because loss of angulation occurs during growth period later.

(Details of surgical procedure and general steps can be read from Chapter 65 of the book Essential Orthopedics: Principles and Practice, 2nd edition.)

80. Describe indications of valgus osteotomy for fracture neck femur. Discuss preoperative planning, implant choice, advantages, and disadvantages of the procedure.

Ans:

Indications:
- *Nonunion fracture neck of femur*: The aim of surgery is to achieve Pauwels' angle at fracture site from 25° to 30° to bring the fracture site under compression to achieve sound union of the fractures.

Other indications:
- *Osteonecrosis*: To unload anterolateral head—usually valgus-flexion combined osteotomy
- Severe osteoarthritis (OA) with medial osteophytes—the capital-drop osteophyte (inferomedial femoral head osteophyte):
  - Acts as fulcrum against acetabular osteophyte
  - Widens the superolateral joint surface.
- *Coxa vara*:
  - Congenital or developmental
  - Fibrous dysplasia.
- Protrusio in young patient
- Fixed abduction contracture.

Preoperative planning: Preserved ROM of hip joint—90° flexion and 15° adduction or abduction, normal contralateral hip is needed. Body forces subtend an angle of 16° at hip joint. The anatomical axis is at an angle of 8–10° to body forces, so the pseudarthrosis site is subjected to forces at around 25°. Subtract this from the pseudarthrosis angle (vide Pauwel's classification). This gives the wedge angle to be resected at osteotomy site.

Implant choice—double angle blade plate and instrumentation used with it.

Advantages:
- Limb length equality can be achieved
- Lateralization can be achieved to prevent genu valgum

- Osteotomy can be fixed and patient can mobilized at the earliest
- Subsequent total hip replacement (THR) can be performed.

Disadvantages:
- Stresses per unit area of femoral head increased
- Reduced abductor efficiency (reduced offset) though this is compensated by increased length of abductor muscles. Still limp may be persistent due to abductor weakness.

81. Steps of valgus osteotomy in hip.

Ans: The following are the surgical steps of performing valgus osteotomy of proximal femur:
- Stabilize the femoral neck fracture with a 6.5-mm cancellous screw prior to insertion of the seating chisel.
- Entry point for chisel is made in the anterior half of the greater trochanter to locate the chisel/blade in the center of the femoral neck.
- The seating chisel is inserted into the femoral neck along the wire k3 (the chisel is not parallel to this k-wire) with its vertical flap 'i' set at an angle of 100° (the angle is made with the hammering side of chisel). The chisel in this instance will hence be seated at an angle of 80° to the femoral shaft (=120°—osteotomy angle). The flap is always kept parallel to the vertical axis (If one uses 130° blade plate then seating angle would be 90°).
- With the chisel in situ in the femoral head, the 35° intertrochanteric wedge of bone "k"-based laterally is excised. The distal osteotomy cut is made first followed by proximal complete cut to protect come calcar medially to act as a hinge. There are two ways of calculating the size of wedge:
  a. *Approximation method*: It is generally considered that 1° of angle corresponds to 1 mm of wedge size (which is really crude but very easy). This means that for angle of correction of 40° we need a wedge of 40 mm. The approximation method is often incorrect but if one sees practically up to 3–4 mm error in the correct direction will not make much difference, if still performed meticulously.
  b. *Geometric method*: This relies on the tangent to the angle of correction and diameter of the bone at osteotomy site. The size of wedge is given by the formula:
   - Wedge in mm = Tangent to angle of correction × angle of correction × diameter of bone
   - This is a bit difficult for general calculation purposes so a simpler version is as follows:
   Wedge in mm = 0.02 × angle of correction × diameter of bone at the osteotomy
   - Remove the chisel and insert the osteotomy blade plate into the slot.
   - Abduct the limb to close the osteotomy by inserting screws from distal to proximal direction one by one.

4B.10 FRACTURE NECK OF FEMUR COMPLICATIONS AND MANAGEMENT (Q82–91)

82. Describe management of failed osteosynthesis of fracture neck femur in a young adult.

Ans: *Investigation*: Plain X-rays are the initial modality to assess and diagnose fracture nonunion. One can estimate the nonunion angle (very crudely), assess osteopenia (Singh's index), bone loss and resorption, length of remaining proximal fragment, presence of osteonecrosis (discernible by 2 months but evident clearly by 6 months), calcar comminution, and angulation at nonunion. Radiographs of contralateral hips with proximal femur are also needed to plan the treatment especially calculation of wedge size in case of osteotomy and estimation of neck resorption ratio. Magnetic resonance imaging (MRI) has become the investigation of choice for assessing osteonecrosis.

Additionally, one may evaluate for infection (if suspected) using hematological investigation ± aspiration of the joint.

Treatment: The treatment of nonunion is highly influenced by the age at presentation, presence of osteonecrosis, and functional demands of patient. Other factors that may have additional bearing on planning treatment include presence of degenerative joint disease (tilt to arthroplasty), smoking, liver, or renal disease (reduces chances of success of union).

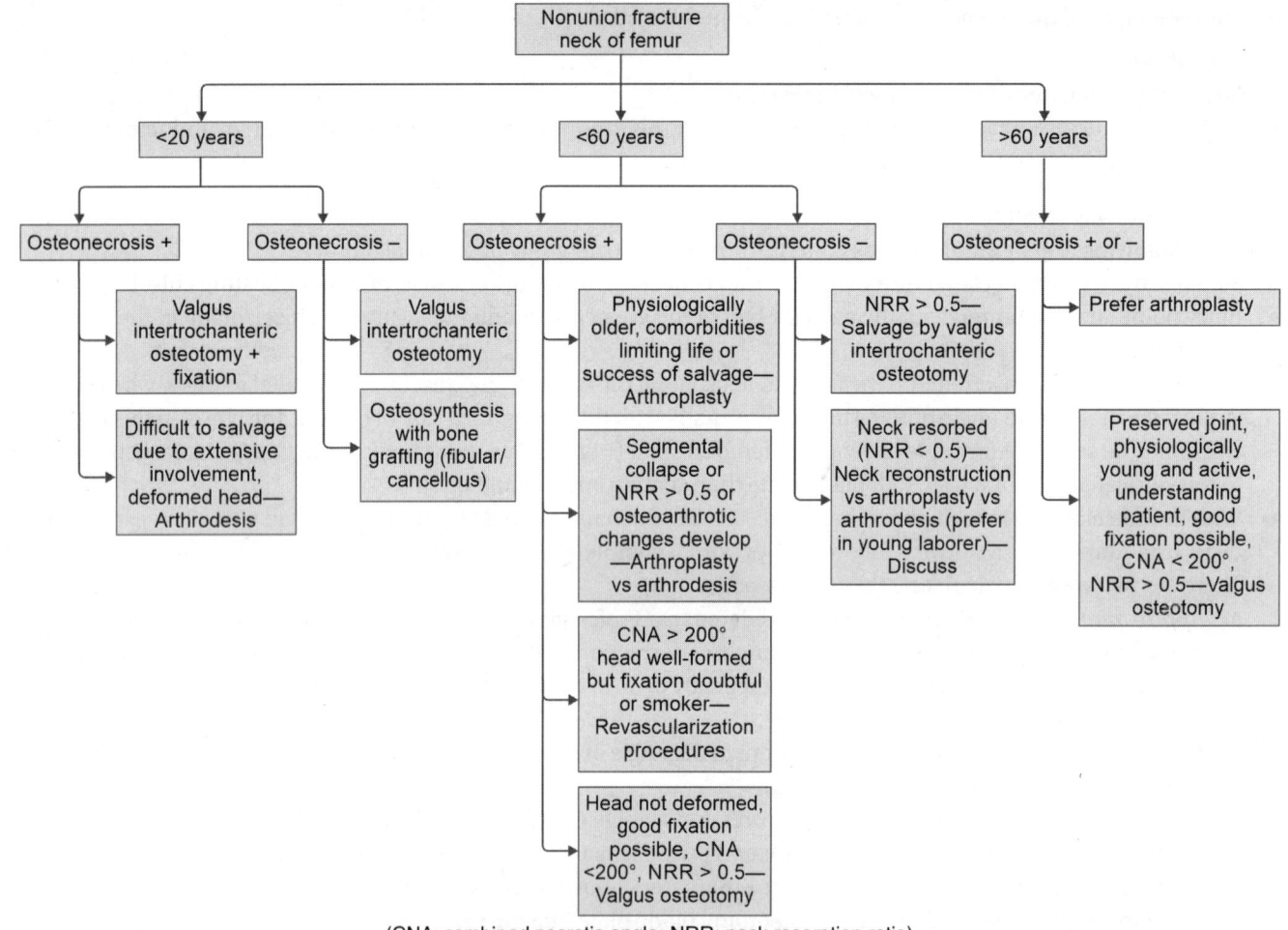

Flowchart 4B.10.1: Treatment for nonunion fracture neck of femur.

(CNA: combined necrotic angle; NRR: neck resorption ratio)

Adjoining **Flowchart 4B.10.1** gives a broad outline of the available options. While prosthetic replacement is considered best choice for the treatment of displaced fractures in patients above 60 years of age or even in some younger patients with physiologically higher age or whose life expectancy is limited by associated comorbidities, efforts are focused on preserving the femoral head in physiologically younger patients. We have three broad categories of surgical options.

1. *Head-preserving procedures*: These are most suitable for patients aged less than 60 years and physiologically younger patients, if femoral head is viable and adequate neck length is left over.
   - *Fixation alone*: This is an option only for late presenters or untreated fractures that report within 3 weeks of injury
   - Open reduction and internal fixation (ORIF) with cortical (fibular) or corticocancellous bone grafting—ORIF or closed reduction and internal fixation (CRIF) with fibular grafting
   - *Open reduction and internal fixation with cancellous bone grafting*: The nonunion site is grafted anteriorly by carving out a window across the nonunion.
   - *"Triple attack technique" for femoral neck nonunion*: Here three techniques are combined to reduce the chances of femoral neck shortening. Iliac autogenous cancellous bone grafting is done after excising nonunion using open technique combined with static fixation across nonunion, followed by valgus intertrochanteric osteotomy.
   - *Open reduction and internal fixation with various revascularization procedures*: The procedure additionally addresses the issue of osteonecrosis as revascularization is deemed not only to hasten osteogenesis at the fracture but also provide vascularity to the femoral head.

- *Proximal femoral osteotomy ± fixation*: The proximal femoral osteotomies work on the principle of converting shearing displacing forces to compressive forces by realigning the fracture site.
    - Pauwels osteotomy
    - Dickson high geometric osteotomy
    - McMurray's osteotomy
    - Schanz angulation osteotomy
    - Combination of osteotomy and bone grafting
    - Neck reconstruction.
2. *Head-sacrificing procedures*: These are indicated in patients with chronological age more than 60 years, physiologically older patients, and those with comorbidities
    - Hemiarthroplasty
    - *Total hip arthroplasty*: This is the preferred option in the head-sacrificing group.
3. *Salvage procedures*: These are rarely offered but have their own specific place in the management of nonunion fracture neck femur.
    - Arthrodesis of hip
    - Girdlestone arthroplasty.

83. **A. Classify neglected femoral neck fracture in adults.**
B. Treatment with rationale in each type of neglected femoral neck fracture.
C. Management of nonunion of neck femur fracture with viable head in a 40-year-old patient.

Ans: A. Sandhu et al., classification—based on the various parameters evaluated on plain radiographs, MRI, and computed tomography (CT) scan, the fractures are allocated into one of the three stages along with suggested guidelines of management.
1. Stage I—(authors of classification suggested closed reduction with fibular graft or closed reduction with muscle pedicle bone graft, valgus osteotomy, or McMurray's osteotomy with POP spica).
    - Irregular fracture surfaces (fresh).
    - Size of proximal fragment (measured from upper margin of fovea centralis to the midpoint of fracture margin) more than or equal to 2.5 cm.
    - Gap between the fragments less than or equal to 1 cm.
    - Viable femoral head—no sign of osteonecrosis on MRI or CT.
2. Stage II—(CRIF with screw + fibula, open reduction freshening of nonunion and screw fixation with fibula, ORIF with muscle pedicle bone grafting, McMurray's osteotomy, Bachelor's procedure, or Girdlestone procedure):
    - Smoothened fracture surfaces
    - Proximal fragment more than or equal to 2.5 cm
    - Gap between fragments more than 1 cm, but less than 2.5 cm
    - Viable femoral head.

    If either of features Ist or 3rd is present, the nonunion is classified as stage II.
3. Stage III—(hip arthroplasty, McMurray's osteotomy, subtrochanteric osteotomy with internal fixation, Girdlestone procedure, or Bachelor procedure):
    - Smoothened fracture surfaces
    - Proximal fragment size less than 2.5 cm
    - Gap between fragments more than 2.5 cm
    - Head shows signs of osteonecrosis.

    If any of the features of 2nd, 3rd, or 4th is present, it is classified as stage III.

B. This patient requires head preserving procedure. I will go ahead with osteosynthesis and vascularized graft for enhancing union or preserving vascularity although surgeons have also successfully treated these nonunions with osteotomy. ORIF or CRIF with fibular grafting has been reported by various authors from India with limited to moderate success in achieving union and is individually popular among believers. Inserting fibula along with two to three partially threaded cancellous screws has been portended to initiate or hasten osteogenesis by somehow modifying vascularity but defies logic of how the biological factors really change by just inserting fibula across the nonunion, which also is a weak mechanical fixation.

Proximal femoral osteotomy ± fixation-orientation of the fracture line is possibly the most important contributory factor for development of nonunion apart from the primary biological factors. Reorientation of this nonunion line to more horizontal has been intrigued by various surgeons in turn developing their methods of achieving the same. The proximal femoral osteotomies work on the principle of converting shearing displacing forces to compressive forces by realigning the fracture site.

C. Kindly see Answer to Question 82 above.

(For details of procedures and discussion on methods kindly refer Chapter 15 of the book Essential Orthopedics: Principles and Practice, 2nd edition.)

84. Investigations in an old neglected neck of femur fracture.

Ans: A high-quality radiographic examination (skiagram) of the pelvis, which includes both hips positioned as identically as possible from a distance of 1 meter, should be conducted. Specific parameters that require evaluation include fracture surfaces, the size of the proximal fragment, the gap between the fragments, the level of the greater trochanter, and any indications of avascular necrosis (AVN) or osteoporosis. In instances where it is feasible, computed tomography (CT) or magnetic resonance imaging (MRI) can provide more precise measurements and facilitate the early detection of AVN.

For plain MRI assessments, T1-weighted (T1W) and T2-weighted (T2W) coronal and axial images are utilized, with most measurements typically taken in the coronal plane. The section corresponding to the level of the fovea centralis is selected to ascertain the size of the proximal fragment, defined as the maximum distance at the midpoint between the fracture margin and the fovea. Concurrently, the maximum distance between the fracture margins is also measured within the same section.

Avascular necrosis changes in the proximal fragment are evaluated and are characterized by subchondral hypointense areas on T1W images and a double-line sign on T2W images, along with alterations related to the Mitchell staging system. While multislice CT can also be employed for these measurements, its sensitivity in detecting avascular necrosis is lower compared to MRI, with the proximal fragment potentially appearing normal in Ficat stages I and II of avascular necrosis.

Imaging, particularly MRI, is critical in the staging of neglected fractures, as plain radiographs alone may not reveal early changes associated with avascular necrosis. The accuracy of measurements regarding the femoral head and fracture gap is significantly enhanced with MRI compared to conventional X-ray techniques. These imaging findings are integral in guiding the selection of appropriate surgical interventions.

Multislice CT may also be employed for these measurements; however, its sensitivity in detecting AVN is inferior to that of MRI. Notably, the proximal fragment may appear normal during Ficat stages I and II of AVN. Imaging modalities, particularly MRI, are instrumental in staging neglected fractures, as plain skiagrams are insufficient in revealing early signs of AVN. Furthermore, MRI provides greater accuracy in measuring the femoral head and fracture gap compared to traditional X-ray imaging. The findings derived from these assessments are paramount in guiding the selection of the appropriate surgical intervention.

85. What is neglected neck of femur fracture?

Ans: As classically defined a neglected femoral neck fracture is one where there has been a delay of more than 30 days to seek medical help (poverty, ignorance, lack of facility) or medical management being given (quacks ignorant to injury, missed injury in coma patient or polytrauma) from the time of the original injury. Osteonecrosis is the most prominent complication (≈15%; range 0–67%) followed by nonunion. The patients present with shortening, upriding greater trochanter, external rotation deformity at hip with restricted movements due to pain and mechanical obstruction. Mostly the mobile patients tend to present later than bedridden patients. Sandhu classification may be used to assess this injury as follows:

- Fracture site irregular or smooth
- Size of proximal fragment >2.5 cm or <2.5 cm

- Gap between fragments (<1 cm, 1 cm–2.5 cm or >2.5 cm)
- Signs of AVN

(Kindly read further details from the 3rd Edition of Essential Orthopedics: Principles and Practice, Chapter 37)

86. Enumerate causes of avascular necrosis (AVN) and nonarthroplasty surgical methods of AVN of femoral head. Describe core decompression.

Ans: Causes: Trauma, corticosteroid use, alcohol abuse, smoking, hemoglobinopathies (e.g., sickle cell anemia), coagulation disorders, myeloproliferative disorders (Gaucher disease, leukemia), caisson disease, human immunodeficiency virus infection, and pregnancy. In many cases, a cause cannot be identified, and these patients are designated as having idiopathic osteonecrosis.

Nonarthroplasty surgical methods:
- Core decompression
- Vascularized and nonvascularized bone grafting and revascularization procedures
- Osteotomies of proximal femur
- Application of various osteogenic strategies like growth factors with and without delivery systems
- Osteochondral reconstruction.

- *Osteotomies*:
  - *Angular osteotomies*: That changes the angle in a given two-dimensional plane taking away the head from the weight-bearing acetabular dome. Typically, the varus or valgus osteotomies are done in subtrochanteric region that may be combined with flexion or extension component for "offset" defects. These are relatively easier to perform and commonly used, if osteotomy is the planned method.
  - *Rotational osteotomy*: Done at the transtrochanteric region that moves the head three-dimensionally anteriorly or posteriorly. These are difficult to perform and have not produced consistent results despite logical superiority.
    - Arthrodesis
    - Resection arthroplasty
    - Porous tantalum rod insertion.

Core decompression

Indications:
- Stage 1 or 2 ON (ARCO system, i.e., precollapse)
- Initial procedure for deemed intralesional bone marrow, stem cell injection
- Initial procedure for vascularized or nonvascular fibula grafting
- Patients less than 50 years.

Contraindications
- Advanced disease (stage 3 or 4 ARCO)
- Patients medically unfit for surgery
- Relative contraindication is a patient more than 50 years of age as the advancements in arthroplasty have improved the quality of life and management perspective beyond this age.

Specific procedure details are as follows:
- On a fracture table or in the supine position hip draped free. Image intensifier positioned for anteroposterior and lateral views
- Keep the leg internally rotated about 15° so that the entry point into lateral metaphysis is not too anterior
- 1–2 cm incision on lateral thigh beginning 5–6 cm distal to tip of trochanter
- Entry point is also just proximal to the insertion of the gluteus maximus into the proximal femur on the lateral metaphyseal flare
- Later cortical window is made a bit larger than the drill size (Ficat and Arlet used 8–10 mm diameter Michele Trephine, Hungerford used 12 mm Jewett starter) so that the drill can be maneuvered to necrotic lesion. A coring device will help obtain core for additional histopathological evaluation.

87. Medical and surgical management of osteonecrosis of femoral head.

Ans: *Medical management*:
- *Analgesics*: They should be judiciously used while reinforcing the need of definitive management.
- *Bisphosphonates*: They have been found to give symptomatic relief from pain and improved quality of life. The rate of collapse has been found lower with the therapy but the effect does not seem to provide critical level of cure enough to replace surgical management. It is interesting to note that bisphosphonates themselves cause ON (BRONJ) of jaw. They probably protect the bone from resorption during healing phase but how sound a bone will form in healing then is unclear without resorption. The effect is akin to homeopathic treatment where the poison of a disease is itself the cure for it!
- *Patients with hyperlipidemias*:
  - Lipid-lowering agents and stanozolol have been found to provide symptomatic benefit and curative effect.
- *Patients with coagulopathies*:
  - Warfarin, low-molecular-weight heparin, stanozolol have been found to be effective to some extent.
- Transplant patients have been found to get relief from calcium channel blockers but the mechanism is not clear. Nifedipine has by itself also been reported to give symptomatic relief in patients of ON.
- Injectable prostacyclin analogue iloprost has reported relief in isolated study on ON femoral head due to its vasoactive effects.

Surgical management:
The surgical treatment options can be divided into hip preserving and hip sacrificing methods:
- *Hip preserving methods*: They are aimed to relieve patient's pain and to prevent progression of the disease:
  - Core decompression
  - Vascularized and nonvascularized bone grafting and revascularization procedures
  - Osteotomies of proximal femur
  - Application of various osteogenic strategies like growth factors with and without delivery systems
  - Osteochondral reconstruction
- *Hip sacrificing*:
  - Hip arthroplasty
  - Hip arthrodesis
  - Excisional (Girdlestone) arthroplasty.

88. Describe sectoral sign in clinical examination of hip joint and its clinical significance.

Ans: *Sectoral sign*: Seen in osteonecrosis—reduced internal rotation in extension that improves when checked in flexion.

Clinically, it indicates segmental involvement of the femoral head rather than global involvement. Also, it helps in guiding rotational osteotomy to move away the diseased portion of femoral head from 'block-producing' zone thus improving hip function and movements.

89. Describe pathology of AVN of femoral head and outline principles of management in Ficat 3 stage of femoral head in a 30-year-old man.

Ans: *Pathology*: Bone cells are highly sensitive to hypoxia and die within 12–48 hours, but structural integrity and macroscopic appearance is maintained for days or even weeks. Bone marrow shows the most conspicuous changes → there is loss of fat cell outlines, inflammatory cell infiltration, marrow edema, the appearance of tissue histiocytes, and eventual replacement of necrotic marrow by undifferentiated mesenchymal tissue.

Features of bone repair and regeneration are also seen simultaneously within a few weeks—there is growth and regeneration of new blood vessels within the necrotic region and osteoblastic proliferation at the interface between ischemic and live bone. This forms a boundary along the necrotic sector. The vascular granulation tissue advances from the surviving trabeculae and new bone is laid down upon the dead. As the old necrotic bone fails to resorb it is this increase in mineral mass that later produces the radiographic appearance of increased density or "sclerosis".

Reparative new bone formation is very slow and does not advance for more than 8–10 mm into the necrotic zone. With time the necrotic bone gets weak and is crushed under the weight-bearing portion of the acetabulum causing structural failure that usually takes the form of a linear tangential fracture close to the articular surface, possibly due to shearing stress. The articular cartilage retains its thickness and viability till the very final stages of osteonecrosis as it derives its nutrition from synovial fluid mostly.

Principles of management:
- *Age > 50 years*: It is better to choose an arthroplasty procedure with a lasting bearing surface
- *Age < 50 years* with well-preserved head overall (necrotic angle <240°)—choose proximal femoral derotational or angular osteotomy to take the collapse part away from line of weight bearing. Vascularized bone graft may be chosen in some where necrotic angle is less than 150°.
    - If combined necrotic angle is >240° then choose arthroplasty even in younger age.

(Details of the specific procedures can be read from Chapter 6 of the book Essential Orthopedics: Principles and Practice, 2nd edition.)

90. Discuss diagnosis and stage wise management of AVN hip.
Ans:
Diagnosis

Radiographs
The bones are radiologically silent in early stages. After a lag of 3–4 months from the onset of symptoms they progressively demonstrate radiologically:
- Osteopenia is seen early in the course of disease due to hypervascularity
- Sclerosis (diffuse) and density changes of the involved region which is invariably the proximal region of the involved bone. This represents gross loss of vascularity, and hence suspended remodeling process. The sclerosis results from initially increased osteoblastic activity suspended remodeling and bone resorption and relative osteopenia of the surrounding bone due to hyperemia
- Cystic changes and development of irregular dense areas. This represents the attempt at repair by the body resorbing the bone irregularly with unresorbed areas in between
- Development of subchondral lucencies (crescent sign) and impending collapse
- "Half-moon sign" on radiographs represent subchondral fracture and collapse. It should be understood that collapse is not due to reduced vascularity or bone necrosis but mainly due to reparative activity of the regenerative tissue that absorbs the bone and causes weakness and collapse. Thus, collapse comes late otherwise it should have been present from start if it was due to bone necrosis itself. There are two types of reparative mechanisms that get activated in the femoral head of ON patients. First is the appositional bone formation initiated by osteoblast like cells around necrotic trabeculae that produces reparative osteogenesis, the other one is the destructive repair that is creeping of granulation tissue along the necrotic trabeculae to cause increased bone resorption. The latter form predominates in most patients causing collapse.
- Loss of shape, form and flattening of the bone then follows.
- Secondary arthritis of the joint develops as a result.

Scintigraphic scanning
In the initial radiographically silent but clinically painful stage, there is increased vascularity of the affected bone. This is also supplemented with increased osteoblastic activity. Thus, the disease process can be picked up by scintigraphic scan that depends on the metabolic activity of bone.

Magnetic resonance imaging (MRI)
This is the most sensitive (nearly 100%) and specific (90%) investigation to evaluate occurrence of ON or differentiating the disease process from other related disorders.
- There is decreased signal intensity in the subchondral region on both T1- and T2-weighted images in early stage localized to medial aspect of femoral head causing appearance of cortical thickening (false).

- In next stage of reparative process, the reactive zone shows ring or band of low signal intensity on T1-weighted scans in subchondral bone appearing high signal intensity on T2-weighted scans due to edema of reparative or granulation tissue (double-line sign)—diagnostic for ON.

Necrotic lesions are classified into four types, based on their location on T1-weighted images or X-ray images.
1. Type A lesions occupy the medial one-third or less of the weight-bearing portion.
2. Type B lesions occupy the medial two-thirds or less of the weight-bearing portion.
3. Type C1 lesions occupy more than the medial two-thirds of the weight-bearing portion but do not extend laterally to the acetabular edge.
4. Type C2 lesions occupy more than the medial two-thirds of the weight-bearing portion and extend laterally to the acetabular edge.

Stage wise management **(Flowchart 4B.10.2)**

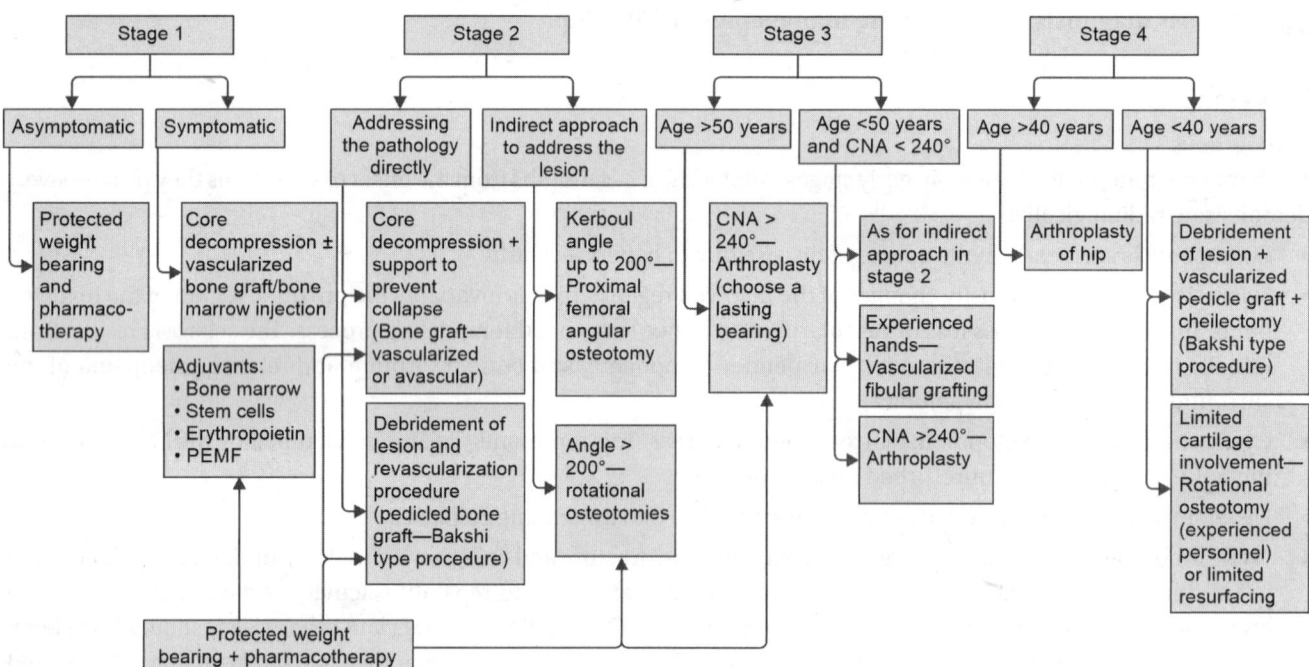

Flowchart 4B.10.2: Treatment algorithm for ONFH.

(ONFH: osteonecrosis of the femoral head; CNA: combined necrotic angle; PEMF: pulsed electromagnetic fields.)

91. Discuss classification of osteonecrosis of the femoral head (ONFH). Discuss clinical features.

Ans: Classification:
Ficat and Arlet classification of ONFH is given in **Table 4B.10.1**.

TABLE 4B.10.1: Ficat and Arlet classification of osteonecrosis of the femoral head (ONFH).					
Stage	Symptoms	Radiography	Bone scan	Pathological findings	Biopsy
0	None	Normal	Decreased uptake?		
1	None/mild	Normal	Cold spot on femoral head	Infarction of weight bearing portion of head	Abundant dead marrow cells, osteoblasts, osteogenic cells
2	Mild	Density change in femoral head	Increased uptake	Spontaneous repair of infarcted area	New bone deposited between necrotic trabeculae
2A		Sclerosis or cysts, normal joint line, normal head contour	Increased uptake		

Contd...

Contd...

Stage	Symptoms	Radiography	Bone scan	Pathological findings	Biopsy
2B		Flattening (crescent sign)			
3	Mild to moderate	Loss of sphericity, collapse	Increased uptake	Subchondral fracture, collapse, compaction and fragmentation of necrotic segment	Dead bone trabeculae and marrow cells on both sides of fracture line
4	Moderate to severe	Joint space narrowing, acetabular changes	Increased uptake	Osteoarthritic changes	Degenerative changes in acetabular cartilage

Steinberg classification is given in **Table 4B.10.2**.

TABLE 4B.10.2: Steinberg classification.

Stage	Clinical and laboratory findings
0	• Asymptomatic • Radiography or magnetic resonance imaging (MRI) or scintigraphy normal • Histology or intraosseous pressure measurement only demonstrates osteonecrosis (ON) • Used for staging the other normal hip in a diagnosed case of ON hip

1	• Symptoms ±
	• Radiography and computed tomography (CT) scan commonly unremarkable
	• Histology findings are abnormal
	• Avascular necrosis diagnosed on MRI (or bone scan) and subclassified as percentage of area involved (MRI only):
	  – *IA*: <15% (minimal)
	  – *IB*: 15–30% (moderate)
	  – *IC*: >30% (severe)

2	• Patient is symptomatic • Radiographs may show osteopenia, osteosclerosis, or cysts • Subchondral radiolucency is absent • MRI findings are diagnostic and subclassified as for stage I

3 (critical stage)	• Patient is symptomatic
	• Radiographic findings include subchondral lucency (crescent sign) and subchondral collapse. The shape and form of the head is maintained
	• The stage is critical as treatment for restoration surgeries are helpful
	• Subclassification depends on the extent of crescent on (MRI or radiographs):
	  – *Stage IIIa*: <15% of the articular surface
	  – *Stage IIIb*: 15–30% of the articular surface
	  – *Stage IIIc*: >30% of the articular surface

4	• Flattening or collapse of femoral head is present
	• Joint space may be irregular
	• CT scanning is more sensitive than radiography
	• Subclassification depends on the extent of collapsed surface (radiographs only):
	  – *Stage IVa*: <15% of surface is collapsed
	  – *Stage IVb*: Approximately 15–30% of surface is collapsed
	  – *Stage IVc*: >30% of surface is collapsed

5	• Radiography findings show changes of secondary osteoarthritis (narrowing of joint space, sclerosis of acetabulum, and marginal osteophytes) • Subclassification is done on X-ray for region of narrowing joint space: Medial, central, lateral
6	Findings include extensive osteoarthritic changes and destruction of the femoral head and joint

The Association Research Circulation Osseous classification (ARCO) staging is given in **Table 4B.10.3**.

TABLE 4B.10.3: The Association Research Circulation Osseous classification (ARCO) staging.

Stage	Radiological features
0	• All present diagnostic techniques are normal or nondiagnostic • Only pressure measurements would reveal increased intraosseous pressure, at this stage patient is asymptomatic • This could be the stage of normal contralateral hip (Future diagnostic techniques such as measurement of resistance to flow may help diagnosing this stage)

1	• Plain X-ray and computed tomography (CT) scan are normal
	• At least one of the scintigraphy or magnetic resonance imaging (MRI) is positive
	• An open biopsy will confirm the diagnosis
	• This stage is subdivided in three categories according to the *location* (MRI only) of the lesion and the extension of the lesion under WB dome of the acetabulum
	  1. Medial
	  2. Central
	  3. Lateral
	• For further study and follow-up on the results of different forms of treatment and the development of the disease, *quantitation* (MRI only) can be added. This quantitation is a calculation of the area of femoral head involvement
	  – *Minimal*: <15%
	  – *Moderate*: 15–30%
	  – *Extensive*: >30%

2	• Radiographs show areas of abnormalities: Porosis, sclerosis, osteolysis, and focal lysis • The femoral head remains spherical on anteroposterior and lateral views on X-ray and CT-scan. Again scintigraphy and MRI are positive. There is no subchondral fracture or *crescent sign* or flattening. Subclassification is important, as described in stage 1

3	• *Crescent sign* is visible on the X-ray. The femoral head fails mechanically
	• The X-ray (usually more prominent on lateral film) shows a fine radiolucent subchondral fracture line, usually referred to as the "crescent sign". Progressive flattening of the femoral dome will occur. Late radiographs show the articular surface of the femoral head to be flattened, but there is no evidence of joint line narrowing or acetabular involvement
	• Subclassification and quantitation (X-ray or CT-scan) is added, but quantitation can also be done by the calculation of the amount of flattening of the femoral dome
	• First, it is determined whether the crescent sign appears more prominent in the anteroposterior (AP) or lateral view. After selection of the most prominent view, the length of the crescent is expressed as a percentage of the entire articular surface
	  – *Minimal*: <15% involvement or a depression of <2 mm
	  – *Moderate*: 15–30% involvement or a depression of 2–4 mm
	  – *Extensive*: >30% involvement or a depression of >4 mm

4	• Appearance of osteoarthritis • The joint-space starts narrowing • This is progressively associated with changes on the acetabular side of the joint and with signs of a beginning osteoarthritis with areas of sclerosis, cysts, and marginal osteophytes. Later on, the radiographic examinations show advanced degenerative changes, and finally a complete joint destruction is seen

Clinical features: The process of bone infarction is usually asymptomatic and patient hardly ever notices it in early stages, especially the traumatic cases, as the trauma overshadows other disease processes. Pain in the affected joint is typically the presenting symptom of ON and is true for nearly all nontraumatic causes of ON. The pain appears with mobilization and is usually more on standing and walking. Continuous pain is uncommon. Some patients may have night pains also.

Frequently the ON is recognized on radiographs done for other purposes. The patient notices gradual increase in pain and slowly developing limp that initially subsides with analgesics to only worsen and become nonresponsive later. With collapse of femoral head, the movements of the hip diminish, especially the flexion, abduction and internal rotation. In any case, the attending physician should have high index of suspicion for ON as there are no pathognomonic signs for early disease. It is imperative to realize that in nontraumatic causes the *other hip* should be given due attention. Only a few cases may spontaneously regress with resolution of the symptoms, but in them, the diagnosis could hardly ever be established. With progression to deformity, the pain is present at rest and ultimately the symptoms and signs of OA develop in the joint.

4B.11 TOTAL HIP ARTHROPLASTY: CONCEPTS, PROCEDURE, EVOLUTION, AND COMPLICATIONS (Q92–113)

92. A. Role of templating in total hip arthroplasty (THA).
B. Outline steps of templating in protrusio acetabuli and a lateralized hip with suitable diagrams.

Ans: A. Templating allows the surgeon to anticipate potential difficulties in advance that can be addressed intraoperatively, the hip biomechanics is more accurately reproduced as in fact the surgery is double checked and also discrepancy in leg length is minimized. The goals of templating are:
- Analyze hip anatomy and variations
- Determine anatomic hip center that needs to be restored also for correcting the leg length and femoral offset
- Determine implant size and position: This reduces inventory by and large, and one is clear as to what is to be done in the operation theater
- Rehearse surgery in mind as one is clear he can communicate to the staff and assistants better so the speed of surgery also increases
- Identify problems in advance and correct them for smooth surgery.

B. *Steps*:
- *Mark the following references on the radiographs*:
  - Ilioischial (Kohler's) line for protrusio assessment
  - Interischial line for determining leg lengths
  - *Interteardrop line*: Teardrop is the most accurate landmark from a conventional radiograph. The teardrop represents an actual anatomic landmark of the inferomedial acetabulum rather than a radiographic image. Make a line joining the base of the tear drops
  - *Vertical teardrop line*: These lines bisect the tear drop and are perpendicular to the intertear drop line
  - *Femoral head center*: Use circular templates to mark the center of femoral head
  - *Femoral offset*: The perpendicular distance from the neutral long axis of the femur and the center of rotation of the hip
  - *Femoral neck-shaft angle*: The angle between the central axis of the femur and the axis of the femoral neck
  - Lesser trochanter
  - *Saddle point*: The junction of superior aspect of femoral neck and the greater trochanter.
- *Identify*:
  - Acetabular dysplasia
  - Leg length discrepancy.
- *Procedure*:
  - Template the acetabulum. Place acetabular template adjacent to lateral edge of teardrop at 40–45° angle relative to interteardrop line and adjust component size to maximize cup coverage and avoid excessive bone resection. In case of protrusio, it is imperative to lateralize the template adjacent to the lateral edge of the teardrop to increase offset and reduce cup-neck impingement.
  - Template the femur based on the chosen stem type (cemented versus noncemented) or proximal versus distal filling stem. The stem size is best determined on AP film.

93. Explain Charnley's low friction arthroplasty concept.
B. Explain different generations of stem cementing in total hip replacement (THR) (in tabular form).
C. Explain the concept of antibiotic bone cement and which antibiotics can be added in bone cement and at what dosage.

Ans: A. Charnley's Low Friction Arthroplasty Concept

Overview:
Charnley's low friction arthroplasty, pioneered by Sir John Charnley in the 1960s, is a foundational concept for modern THR. It aims to minimize friction and wear in artificial hip joints, improving longevity and function. The concept revolutionized orthopedic surgery by introducing a durable, low-friction bearing surface for hip arthroplasty.

Key principles:
- *Low friction bearing*:
  - Uses a small-diameter femoral head (initially 22.225 mm) articulating with a polyethylene acetabular cup to reduce frictional torque and wear.
  - Smaller head size decreases the surface area, minimizing wear debris compared to larger metal-on-metal designs.
- *Materials*:
  - *Femoral component*: Stainless steel (later cobalt-chromium) for strength and biocompatibility.
  - *Acetabular component*: High-density polyethylene (HDPE), chosen for its low friction and wear resistance when paired with metal.
  - This combination mimics cartilage-like low-friction articulation.
- *Cemented fixation*:
  - Polymethylmethacrylate (PMMA) bone cement anchors both components to bone, ensuring immediate stability and load transfer.
  - Allows fixation in osteoporotic or irregular bone surfaces.
- *Design goals*:
  - Reduce wear and aseptic loosening by minimizing frictional forces.
  - Restore hip biomechanics with stable, durable components.
  - Enable pain-free mobility with long-term implant survival.

Salient features:
- *Small femoral head*: Reduces wear but may increase dislocation risk compared to larger heads used today (e.g., 28–36 mm).
- *Polyethylene cup*: Provides a low-friction interface; modern ultra-high-molecular-weight polyethylene (UHMWPE) improves durability.
- *Cemented technique*: Ensures rigid fixation but may fail over time due to cement fatigue or bone-cement interface breakdown.
- *Clinical success*: Achieved 90–95% implant survival at 10–15 years in early studies, setting the standard for hip arthroplasty.

B. Different generations of stem cementing in THR **(Table 4B.11.1)**.

TABLE 4B.11.1: Generations of stem cementing in total hip replacement.

Generation	Time Period/ Evolution	Key features	Advantages	Limitations
1st generation	1960s–early 1970s	• Hand mixing of cement • Finger-packing into canal • No canal preparation • No pressurization	Simple, quick technique	• High incidence of loosening • Poor cement penetration • Voids and porosity due to air entrapment
2nd generation	Mid-1970s–1980s	• Improved canal preparation with brushes and pulsatile lavage • Retrograde cement insertion using cement gun • Pressurization with proximal seal • Distal cement restrictor introduced	• Better cement penetration • Improved fixation	• Still manual mixing (porosity) • Cement creep over time
3rd generation	Late 1980s–1990s	• Vacuum mixing to reduce porosity • Centralizers to maintain stem position • Pulsatile lavage • Pressurization maintained throughout • Distal restrictor used routinely	• Lower cement porosity • Improved stem alignment • Longer survivorship	• More complex instrumentation • Higher cost

Contd...

Contd...

Generation	Time Period/ Evolution	Key features	Advantages	Limitations
4th generation	2000s–present	• All 3rd generation features • Modern stem designs (polished tapered stems for controlled subsidence) • Modern cement formulations • Computer-assisted techniques in some centers	• Optimal cement mantle and fixation • Further improved longevity	• High cost • Requires experienced surgical team

C. Antibiotics Added to Bone Cement and Dosages.

Antibiotics used in bone cement must be heat-stable (to withstand cement curing at ~70–90°C), water-soluble, and effective against common orthopedic pathogens (e.g., *Staphylococcus aureus*, coagulase-negative staphylococci). Below are commonly used antibiotics and their typical dosages per 40 g of PMMA cement:

- *Gentamicin*:
  - *Dosage*: 0.5–1 g (low-dose, prophylactic); 2–4 g (high-dose, therapeutic for PJI).
  - *Features*: Broad-spectrum, effective against gram-negative bacteria and some gram-positive organisms (e.g., *S. aureus*). Commonly used in primary and revision arthroplasty.
- *Tobramycin*:
  - *Dosage*: 1–2.4 g (prophylactic); 3.6–4.8 g (therapeutic).
  - *Features*: Similar spectrum to gentamicin; effective against *Pseudomonas aeruginosa*. Often used in North America.
- *Vancomycin*:
  - *Dosage*: 1–2 g (prophylactic); 2–4 g (therapeutic).
  - *Features*: Effective against methicillin-resistant *S. aureus* (MRSA) and gram-positive organisms. Often combined with gentamicin/tobramycin for synergistic effect.
- *Cefuroxime*:
  - *Dosage*: 1–1.5 g (prophylactic).
  - *Features*: Broad-spectrum cephalosporin, effective against gram-positive and some gram-negative bacteria. Less common than aminoglycosides.
- *Clindamycin*:
  - *Dosage*: 1–2 g (prophylactic or therapeutic).
  - *Features*: Effective against anaerobes and gram-positive bacteria; used in penicillin-allergic patients or for specific infections.
- *Other antibiotics (less common)*:
  - *Erythromycin*: 0.5–1 g; used for specific gram-positive infections.
  - *Ceftazidime*: 1–2 g; targets gram-negative bacteria (e.g., *Pseudomonas*).
  - *Amphotericin B*: 50–200 mg; for fungal infections in rare cases.

94. Describe the combined angle of anteversion during THR.

Ans: It has been considered that version of the acetabular cup is the most common cause of recurrent instability after THR. Though other factors like soft tissue balance across hip and femoral anteversion are also important, cup anteversion is the commonly fraught abnormality that can be meticulously corrected or compensated during surgery. Accurate femoral and acetabular cup anteversion ensures prosthetic position in such a construct as to avoid impingement throughout ROM. Instead of maintaining the femoral and acetabular anteversion separately it has been argued that combined version of cup and stem is more important than either individually. This combination compensates for the error in one of the component (stem/cup) by increasing/decreasing version in other component.

McKibbin first introduced the term in a study of infant cadavers and defined 30–40° combined anteversion as being normal, with 15° anteversion of the femur. Men had lower combined anteversion than women. Clinically, it has been found that the range be 25–45° lower for men.

During cementless THA, this concept of combined anteversion becomes highly relevant as the femoral stem has to be fit according to bony anatomy to achieve initial stability. This may distort achieved anteversion to neutral rotation or sometimes even retroversion. The issue is much less common with cemented stems as the stem can be rotated manually in the cement mantle so that it does not go into retroversion. In such a situation where femoral stem version could not be changed (as in cementless stem), the cup needs to be anteverted more according to the stem anteversion to give a combined anteversion between 25° and 50°. Normally, the acetabulum has anteversion of 15–20° (lesser in arthritic hips due to remodeling). In any case making the THA prosthesis construct to have a combined anteversion of 30–40° often optimizes the "static" position of implant. Dynamic variables still have a play and may still cause THA instability (as in ankylosing spondylosis, where due to spine stiffness this anteversion may be too high!).

95. **A. What is Lewinnek safe zone concept in THA?**

B. Role of altered spinopelvic kinematics in hip instability and functional acetabular position.

Ans: A. Cup position correlates somewhat with dislocation risk so optimized cup positioning in THR is a strongly searched issue. Lewinnek et al. proposed some guidelines 'safe range' for acetabular cup placement with regards optimal cup position after reviewing radiographs of 300 total hip replacements as follows:

- 15 ± 10° anteversion
- Inclination of 40 ± 10°

Since publication they were greatly hyped but have been now consistently challenged with development in understanding the 'dynamic' hip position during movements rather than the static measures proposed by Lewinnek. In particular, the spinopelvic relationship and imbalance may require cup positioning outside of the Lewinnek zone to achieve 'functional' hip stability.

B. Movements at lower spine supplement or complement the movements at hip joint so the inclination and version of native acetabulum keeps changing throughout the ROM of hip joint. Most of the hip dislocations reviewed in studies were found to be implanted within the Lewinnek safe zones conversely significant number of stable hips when reviewed were 'outside' the proposed safe zones of Lewinnek. The following spinopelvic relation should be borne in mind:

- *Reduction in anterior hip impingement*: When moving from standing to sitting position, the pelvis tilts posteriorly to accommodate flexion of the hip joint. For each 1° of increased pelvic tilt, acetabular anteversion increases from 0.7 to 0.8°. This translates to a change of acetabular anteversion of approximately 15.6° when moving from standing to sitting position.
- Acetabular inclination also increases with pelvic tilt and may be protective of anterior impingement with hip flexion.
- Deformity and stiffness of the lumbar spine from degenerative processes or lumbar fusion can prevent this normal accommodation and lead to excessive anterior impingement with sitting or posterior impingement when standing. Spinopelvic stiffness is defined as a change in sacral slope of ≤10°. When this is the case, the hip joint must flex further to assume a seated position, with a greater risk of anterior impingement. In these patients, more anteversion of the acetabular component will be needed to compensate for the reduced posterior pelvic tilt imposed by the stiff spine.

If the cup is excessively anteverted, then anterior dislocation can occur during hip extension, adduction, and external rotation. If the cup is overly retroverted, dislocation occurs posteriorly with flexion, adduction, and internal rotation. Excessive inclination of the cup can lead to superior dislocation with adduction. Conversely, if the cup is inclined almost horizontally, impingement occurs early in flexion and the hip dislocates posteriorly. All this complexity hence entails finding 'functional stable position' of acetabular cup during planning of THR. The following is a generalization for easier understanding:

- A stiff lumbosacral junction requires relatively increased inclination and combined anteversion.
- Kyphotic or hypermobile patients are better served with lesser degrees of inclination and anteversion.

(*Details can be read further from the 3rd edition of the book, Essential Orthopedics*: Principles and Practice. More lucid and detailed explanation is provided by the author in video lecture on YouTube channel—Myths, Mysteries, and Practicalities)

96. Principle of dual mobility hips.

Ans: *Design and mechanism*: The dual mobility hip system features a mobile polyethylene liner articulating with a femoral head inside a metal acetabular cup. This creates two points of motion, increasing the jump distance (displacement needed for dislocation) and reducing dislocation risk compared to traditional single-mobility designs.

Biomechanical benefits:
- Greater range of motion (flexion/abduction) without instability.
- Higher dislocation resistance, especially against rotational forces.
- Reduced wear due to load distribution across a larger surface area.

Clinical advantages:
- Lower dislocation rates, particularly in high-risk patients (elderly, neuromuscular disorders, revisions).
- Improved functional outcomes, enabling confident mobility and daily activities.
- Long-term durability, with studies supporting its efficacy in complex cases.

Conclusion: Dual mobility hips offer superior stability, motion, and patient satisfaction, making them ideal for high-risk arthroplasty patients.

97. A. What is spinopelvic relationship? Enumerate common radiological parameters pertinent to discussion of spinopelvic tilt.
B. Discuss hip arthroplasty in presence of spinopelvic pathology.

Ans: A. The spinopelvic relationship represents a critical biomechanical and postural concept, describing the intricate kinematic chain that links the vertebral column to the pelvis. Its quantitative assessment relies on a suite of standardized radiological parameters derived from full-length standing radiographs, which allow for the objective analysis of pelvic orientation and spinal alignment.

1. **The concept of spinopelvic relationship**: The human upright posture is maintained through a complex interplay between spinal curvatures and pelvic position. The spine, a semi-rigid column, is biomechanically coupled to the pelvis, which functions as its base. This spinopelvic complex operates under the principle of sagittal balance, a state where the body's center of mass is aligned over its base of support, minimizing the need for compensatory muscle activation.

   The pelvis serves as the foundational regulator of this balance. Its orientation dictates the alignment of the sacrum, which in turn sets the positional requirements for the lumbar lordosis (LL) and the subsequent spinal segments. A harmonious relationship ensures that the gravitational line falls within a narrow physiological range. Conversely, a pathological disruption—whether from degenerative change, deformity, or iatrogenic causes—triggers a cascade of compensatory mechanisms. These often include pelvic retroversion, knee flexion, and thoracic hypokyphosis, which are quantifiable indicators of imbalance and increased energy cost.

2. **Key radiological parameters of spinopelvic tilt and alignment**: The assessment of spinopelvic alignment is predicated on the precise measurement of angular and linear parameters, categorized as follows:

   2.1. Pelvic parameters (the foundation)
   - *Pelvic incidence (PI):* A fundamental morphological (invariant) parameter defined as the angle between the line perpendicular to the sacral plate at its midpoint and the line connecting this point to the bicoxofemoral axis. It is a patient-specific anatomic constant that dictates the degree of lumbar lordosis required for optimal balance. A higher PI necessitates a greater LL.
   - *Pelvic tilt (PT):* A positional parameter measuring the inclination of the pelvis. It is the angle between the vertical reference line and the line from the femoral head center to the sacral plate midpoint. An elevated PT signifies pelvic retroversion, a primary compensatory mechanism for positive sagittal imbalance. It is intrinsically linked to other parameters by the formula: PI = PT + Sacral Slope (SS).
   - *Sacral slope (SS):* The angle between the superior endplate of S1 and the horizontal plane. It describes the sacral inclination and correlates positively with lumbar lordosis.

2.2. Spinal parameters (the superstructure)
- *Lumbar lordosis (LL):* Measured as the Cobb angle between the superior endplates of L1 and S1. The critical relationship is the PI-LL mismatch; a mismatch of >10° is a principal driver of sagittal imbalance and a key preoperative planning metric in deformity surgery.
- *Thoracic kyphosis (TK):* Measured as the Cobb angle between the superior endplate of T4/T5 and the inferior endplate of T12. It exhibits an inverse relationship with LL, and its alteration is a common compensatory mechanism.

2.3. Global alignment parameters (the composite measure)
- *Sagittal vertical axis (SVA):* A linear measure of global balance, representing the horizontal offset between the C7 plumb line and the posterosuperior corner of S1. A positive SVA > 5 cm is a hallmark of significant sagittal malalignment and correlates strongly with clinical disability.
- *T1 pelvic angle (TPA):* A composite angle between lines from the femoral head center to the center of T1 and to the center of S1. TPA elegantly incorporates both spinal malalignment and pelvic compensation (PT) into a single, robust measure that is less susceptible to measurement error and is highly predictive of health-related quality-of-life outcomes.

B. The patterns of spinopelvic mobility abnormalities are divided into two types:
1. *Hypermobility*: It is defined as pelvic motion (change in SS) of ≥ 30° between standing and sitting. It may be normal also and is advantageous to the patients because it reduces required hip motion and minimizes impingement. Hypermobility is considered to be unbalanced when it is a result of the lumbar spine tilting into kyphosis (flexible and unbalanced type of Phan et al.) with sitting (seated sacral tilt of < 10° and is considered severe when < 5°). This is associated with three conditions:
    i. Stiff hips that have flexion range of motion (ROM) of ≤ 50°, which forces increased posterior tilt of the pelvis during sitting.
    ii. Patients with a body mass index (BMI) of > 40 kg/m^2, who have a large trunk mass that forces increased posterior tilt of the pelvis with sitting to balance their body.
    iii. Patients with neuromuscular imbalance (Parkinson's disease).
2. *Spinopelvic stiffness*: It is defined as ≤ 10° change in sacral tilt between standing and sitting positions (as may occur in lumbar degenerative disk disease, facet spondylosis of the lumbar spine, lumbar fusion, or ankylosing spondylitis). Stiffness can occur in three patterns (Stefl et al.):
    i. The pelvis tilts posteriorly from standing to sitting.
    ii. ≤ 10°, such that the sacral tilt crosses a value of 30°—decreased pelvic motion but is not fixed anteriorly or posteriorly.
    iii. Stuck standing—loss of posterior tilt when sitting so that the pelvis is fixed in anterior tilt (sitting sacral tilt is >30°) (Phan et al. rigid and balanced, see table below).
    iv. Stuck sitting—the pelvis is fixed in posterior tilt and never tilts anteriorly with standing (standing sacral tilt is <30°) (Phan et al. rigid and unbalanced, see table below).

Recommendations for hip arthroplasty in presence of spinopelvic pathology **(Table 4B.11.2)**.

TABLE 4B.11.2: The recommendations on altering acetabular cup version based on spinopelvic imbalance as proposed by Phan et al.

Parameter	Balanced	Unbalanced
Flexible	Cup version from 5–25°	Spinal realignment followed by THA—component anteversion from 15 to 25° Or Primary THA with decreased component anteversion.
Rigid	Cup version from 15–25°	Spinal realignment followed by THA—component anteversion from 15 to 25° Or Primary THA with decreased component anteversion.

98. A. Clinical and radiological features of aseptic loosening after cementless THA.
B. Classification of cavus deformity.

Ans: A. *Cementless femoral components*: The radiographic evaluation of cementless femoral components for loosening is poorly defined. Engh and Bobyn proposed a simple classification system for implant fixation based on radiographic inspection alone. Fixation is classified as: (1) bone ingrowth, (2) stable fibrous fixation, or (3) unstable.

Fixation by bone ingrowth is defined as an implant with no subsidence and minimal or no radiopaque line formation around the stem. Most of the bone-implant interface seems stable. Cortical hypertrophy may be present at the distal end of the porous surface, and "spot welds" may be evident between the stem and endosteum.

An implant is considered to have a stable fibrous ingrowth when no progressive migration occurs, but an extensive radiopaque line forms around the stem. These lines surround the stem in parallel fashion and are separated from the stem by a radiolucent space 1 mm wide. The femoral cortex shows no signs of local hypertrophy, suggesting that the surrounding shell of bone has a uniform load-carrying function.

An unstable implant is defined as one with definite evidence of progressive subsidence or migration within the canal and is at least partially surrounded by divergent radiopaque lines that are more widely separated from the stem at its extremities. Increased cortical density and thickening typically occur beneath the collar and at the end of the stem, indicating regions of local loading and lack of uniform stress transfer. These criteria were developed to describe only a stem design with extensive porous coating and are not applicable to designs with more limited proximal porous coating or nonporous stems.

Cementless Acetabular Components
On the acetabular side, socket migration, screw breakage, fracture of the metal shell, and shedding of the porous surface are clear evidence of loosening. A continuous radiolucent line may indicate stable fibrous ingrowth rather than loosening and may be compatible with a successful clinical result.

Clinical features: Loosening usually produces pain on weight-bearing, which may be present in the thigh or groin. So-called start-up pain refers to pain that is worst with the first few steps and improves to some degree with further ambulation. This pain suggests a loose implant that moves but settles into a relatively stable position with weight bearing. Usually, the pain is relieved by rest and aggravated by rotation of the hip. An antalgic gait may develop, and sometimes a patient volunteers that the limb is becoming shorter and is turning outward. Although most patients with loosening have an asymptomatic period postoperatively, some complain of pain from the time of surgery. Early postoperative pain should suggest that an infection has developed, that one or both components were not fixed securely, or that the pain is referred from a source extraneous to the hip joint.

B. *Classification of cavus deformity*: There are various classification schemes of cavus foot depending on severity of the deformity (mild, moderate, and severe/rigid), severity of cavus itself, etiological, etc.
A simple format based on pathogenesis of the deformity is as follows:
- *Idiopathic*:
  - Most common
  - Develops after 3 years of age
  - Males and females are equally affected
  - Often associated with spina bifida occulta.
- *Secondary*:
  - *Neurologic disease*:
    - Spinocerebellar hereditary degeneration of Mollaret
    - Friedreich's ataxia
    - Poliomyelitis
    - Diseases of conus medullaris or cauda equina—diastematomyelia, cauda equina tumor
    - Pyramidal or extrapyramidal syndromes, cerebral palsy
    - Progressive peroneal palsy, Charcot-Marie-Tooth disease.
  - Direct trauma to foot
  - Myopathies, for example, muscular dystrophy
  - Plantar fibromatosis
  - Congenital talipes equinovarus.

99. Describe current concepts in mechanism of osteolysis after arthroplasty. What is role of bone grafting in such patients without performing a revision arthroplasty?

Ans: Osteolysis causes aseptic loosening of the implanted prosthesis and is the biggest cause of revision surgery and failure of arthroplasty. Osteolysis results from resorption of bone as a result of biological reaction to wear particles and is seen more commonly around the acetabular component of hip arthroplasty, though femur is also involved in many cases. For obvious reasons, osteolysis is seen more commonly in patients with high wear of their implants and resulting biological reactions are not simply defined by mere wear quantification but comprehensively, they are defined by combination of:

- *Size of wear particles*: The size of the wear particles is of equal importance to their number. Nanometer particulate wear debris as seen in ceramic bearings does not appear to affect the osteoblasts or osteoclasts.
- Morphology of wear particles
- Volumetric concentration of wear particles
- Wear volume as such

Polyethylene linear wear rate of 0.10 mm^3/year is the threshold for the development of osteolysis that corresponds to 38.8 mm^3/year volumetric wear. Ceramic-on-ceramic (COC) articulations produce much less wear particles and in microseparation conditions COC bearings have 50 times less osteolytic potential as compared to highly cross-linked ultrahigh molecular weight polyethylene (UHMPE).

Radiology of osteolysis:

Osteolysis radiologically is seen as lucency around the prosthetic implant and often appears several years after the index procedure. The lysis varies in intensity and extent around the prosthesis with most common areas in acetabulum, located in the superior WB dome and around screws used to fix an uncemented cup. In femoral regions, the regions of stress like the calcar are usually the first to show lysis and in advanced cases, areas all around the stem would be osteolytic. The osteolysis around the cemented implants is seen as a uniform gap at the cement–bone interface. Cementless implants typically the acetabular socket show an expansile cavitary pattern of radiolucency. The CT better defines, identifies, and localizes the osteolysis region. The lesions around acetabulum are recorded with respect to the location—anterior, posterior, medial, and superior regions involvement. On the femoral side, lysis is commonly seen in medial, lateral, or circumferential regions.

Biology of osteolysis:

The osteolytic-inducing wear particles migrate to the third space (periprosthetic space) by slow convection currents or suction compression mechanisms and induce biological response locally. The primary cellular mediator is the monocyte/macrophage cell line. They phagocytose the debris particles and produce a number of cytokines and inflammatory mediators [macrophage colony-stimulating factor (M-CSF), granulocyte macrophage colony-stimulating factor (GM-CSF), interleukin (IL)-1, IL-6, IL-10, tumor necrosis factor alpha (TNF-α), NO, macrophage migration inhibitory factor, matrix metalloproteinase (MMP)-inducer (emmprin) and prostaglandin E2], especially in the regenerating interface tissues. These stimulate increased osteoclast activity and differentiation causing excessive bone resorption.

Bone grafting for managing osteolysis without revision:

For well-fixed implants, particulate bone grafting has been reported by investigating groups. This is based on the premises that for well-fixed implants if the osteolysis lesions are filled with bone (eaten away by occurring osteolysis), then there may be a possibility to improve the bone stock with reversal of the lysis. The bone graft will additionally plug the areas from where the wear material percolates and induces osteolysis. This reduces the "effective joint space" where the wear particles would circulate and cause progression of osteolysis. The added bone would also serve as bone stock for later reconstructions.

This concept, however, interesting and reported some success in late 90s, has not been very intuitive for various reasons:

- The periacetabular area can be difficult to access when the acetabular shell is well fixed, and osteolytic lesions can be difficult to identify and debride at the time of surgery

- Osteolytic lesions may be lined with a pseudomembrane that may prevent bone graft incorporation. If the membrane is not completely excised, healing can be compromised by the lack of direct contact between graft material and host bone.
- This method does not address the issue of biological aspects of osteolysis that is an ongoing process and not being addressed at all with this technique.

The "generator" of wear particles is not being addressed with this technique.

So, just bone grafting or trying to bone graft the osteolytic areas only is not adequate. One has to combine it with exchange of polyethylene and femoral head. Also one needs CT scan to evaluate the adequacy of bone grafting rather than just plain X-rays that overestimate the grafting. The procedure may be a little simpler on femoral side but very less feasible on the acetabular side due to volumetric 3D distribution that cannot be surgically accessed.

In total knee replacement, the issue of bone grafting is less pertinent because the implants are used often cemented. Bone grafting in these cases will not cause cement–bone bonding as cementing is also not intended for this purpose. If the total knee arthroplasty (TKA) prosthesis is uncemented, then isolated bone grafting may be deployed on femoral side after adequate debridement (posterior condylar regions may still not be assessable). On tibial side, trap-door procedure may be used. I suggest a liner exchange in all these cases also.

100. Discuss causes of aseptic loosening after THR. Discuss its clinical features, diagnosis, and management.

Ans: Aseptic loosening implies implant loosening as a result of noninfective osteolysis resulting from various factors primarily the inflammatory reaction to wear particles. The main reason for aseptic loosening had been poly [ultra-high-molecular-weight polyethylene (UHMWPE)] wear. Polyethylene wear debris starts a subtle chronic granulomatous inflammatory response, which becomes more pronounced as osteolysis progresses. Polyethylene particles above a critical size of about 0.2–0.8 μm can be phagocytosed by macrophages and initiate a series of physiological reactions, which finally lead to osteolysis, and aseptic loosening of the implant. This particle-induced periprosthetic osteolysis may affect both the acetabular and the femoral prostheses' components.

Polyethylene debris is created with a typical size of 0.2–5 μm, whereas metallic debris released from MoM prosthesis (no longer in use) exhibits typically a size of 50 nm. Debris particles can also be generated and released from surfaces not designed for tribological applications, such as conical taper junctions or in case of micromotion between stem and bone or stem and cement along the stem surface and analogously on interfaces on the acetabular side that should not be subjected to movements under normal conditions.

(For further detail also see Answer to Question 98)

101. A. Outline technical steps to achieve desired degree of version of acetabular and femoral components during THR.
   B. What is combined angle of anteversion?
   C. How will you modify your version in a case of fixed lumbar lordosis or flat back?

Ans: A. *Steps to achieve target version*:
- In navigated cup position, the version is quite easily determined by the system.
- In non-navigated hips—reaming should be done using a jig to guide the version and angular placement of cup (it is however only a rough guide). A digital protractor on the inserter handle improves accuracy of insertion angles.
- Transverse acetabular ligament is the most important landmark for determining cup version intraoperatively (even better than the jig).
- Cup position intraoperatively is also guided by the acetabular notch or the psoas groove. The anterior margin of the cup should be sunk well below the notch so that there is no psoas irritation.
- Last is using combined anteversion angle—after trialing the femur once the cup is prepared insert the trial and reduce hip using proper head and offset. If using posterior approach then lift the ankle up until the femoral head diameter and acetabular shell are coplanar. The angle subtended by the leg (tibia-fibula) to the plane parallel to floor gives the combined anteversion of hip. This should be maintained between 25° and 45° (lesser in males).

B. *See Answer to Question 94.*

C. In case of stiff spine or flat back as in ankylosing spondylosis the angle of anteversion has to be reduced, sometimes in convex posterior lumbar spine one may need acetabular retroversion to get a stable hip (rare).

102. A. Enumerate bearing surfaces in THR.
   B. Advantages and disadvantages of each bearing surfaces.

Ans: The various bearing surfaces along with their advantages and disadvantages are as follows:

- *Ceramic-on-ceramic (CoC)*: Ceramic bearings are among the most exciting bearings of today for their evolution and reported lowest in vivo wear rates. This is due to the hydrophilic nature permitting better wettability of the surface by adsorption. These bearings are also scratch resistant due to hardness and the fact that they can be polished to a much lower surface roughness. Ceramic bearing combination achieves fluid-film lubrication. Importantly ceramic is highly biocompatible (compared to metal or poly bearings). The CoC bearings are however susceptible to rapid wear, if they are suboptimally positioned in situ.

  Surgical grade CoC bearings are of three types:
  1. *Alumina ceramics*: These are inorganic nonmetallic materials formed by compounding of a non-metal and a metal. In particular, alumina is a monophasic, but polycrystalline structure imparting hardness and stability. It has low bending stress and low resilience but to make it brittle and may break due to low fracture toughness.
  2. *Zirconia ceramics*: Zirconia has comparatively higher fracture toughness than alumina ceramic and is a newer introduction in the field. The bending strength is also higher but pure zirconia is unstable in its phasic structure. Zirconia exhibits large volume changes and decreased mechanical properties because of cracking on cooling. Best mechanical properties are seen for yttrium-stabilized tetragonal polycrystalline zirconia (Y-TZP) that effectively reduces grain size.
  3. *Alumina-matrix-composite ceramics, ceramic-on-alumina (mixture of 75% aluminum oxide, 25% zirconia with less than 1% chromium and strontium oxides)*: This is the newest generation of CoC bearings quite popular nowadays. It incorporates nano-sized, yttria-stabilized tetragonal zirconia particles into alumina producing alumina-matrix-composite. For very obvious reasons, one would combine the above two ceramics as both have disadvantages that can be compensated by the other. Alumina is brittle while zirconia is hydrothermally unstable. Logically combining them into a composite is believed to improve the mechanical properties. These alumina-zirconia nanocomposites have relatively low zirconia content so the hardness is similar to alumina but the susceptibility to hydrothermal instability is drastically reduced. This delta ceramic composite bearing surface has shown high survivorship resulting from improved mechanical properties especially preventing the initiation and propagation of cracks that was significant with previously prevailing alumina ceramics.

  Ceramic-on-ceramic bearing is not a widely preferred bearing though good in many characteristics. It is the preferred bearing surface for replacement in a young female. It may also be preferred in young patients with renal disease or those with renal transplants.

  Advantages of mechanical properties of ceramics:
  – Most importantly minimal wear (COC bearings) and virtually no osteolysis due to inert nature of alumina wear particles.
  – Because alumina ceramics are highly oxidized, they cannot be further oxidized, so are biologically inert.
  – The hardness imparts resistance to surface damage. The hardness of alumina makes it very abrasive and wear resistant increasing its resistance to scratching.

  Disadvantages of mechanical properties of ceramics:
  – Very precise production techniques are needed in order to ensure proper fit of the head within the socket—else accelerated wear would result in COC bearings.
  – The lack of ceramic deformation reduces the contact areas between the head and socket increasing contact stress. To counter this disadvantage clearance must be optimized.
  – *Incompatibility with cement fixation*: Alumina is more than 300 times stiffer than cancellous bone and nearly 200 times stiffer than polymethylmethacrylate (PMMA) due to modulus mismatch.

- *Fracture susceptibility*: Previously used alumina is very brittle and hence susceptible to fracture. The risk factors for fractures are:
  - Short neck femoral heads
  - Long neck femoral heads (less supported)
  - Malpositioning the acetabulum
  - Presence of noise
  - Trauma and fall
  - Poor surgical technique.

- *Metal-on-metal bearings (MoM)*: The steady-state wear rates of these designs were very low. The MoM bearings implants also have ingenious property of "self-healing" by virtue of reduction in asperites. This is the ability to polish-out isolated surface scratches in the MoM bearings. On a wider analysis, the long-term survival had been comparable to metal on poly designs. Laboratory studies suggest that MoM bearings exhibit 10–20 times greater wear during first 1–2 years of use called the "run-in wear" period. These then reduce by virtue of self-heal. The improvement in the surface finish facilitates lubricating fluid film (elastohydrodynamic films) by coherence and causing reduction in wear rate. The first-generation MoM hips were fabricated by casting, whereas contemporary second-generation implants are manufactured from wrought cobalt-chromium (Co-Cr) alloys. This significantly improves the properties of hardness, yield and ultimate strength of the MoM bearings. Chromium is used specifically in these alloys to enhance mechanical properties; it also promotes the formation of a passive oxide layer. Addition of molybdenum improves its corrosion resistance.

Disadvantages of MoM bearings:
- *Metal ions*: Metal ions from MoM prosthesis include an array of titanium, chromium, cobalt, vanadium, and molybdenum. There is a corresponding decrease in cytotoxic CD8+ T-lymphocytes. These cells are involved in defense against intracellular pathogens and cancerous cells. In the initial run-in period volumetric wear rate and average particle size estimation suggested that 6.7×10^{12}–2.5×10^{14} metal particles are produced per year. This is much higher than standard metal-on-polyethylene (MoP) bearing by 13–50 times and for newer MoP articulation by 500 times approximately. The most important cause of failure leading to a blow on the use of MoM implants in last decade came from systemic dissemination of soluble and particulate corrosion products from modular junctions like trunnion of head and morse taper on femoral stem.
- *Biological response*: Not just a higher failure rates of 2–3-fold higher than contemporary THA using MoP bearings as noted above but also the adverse tissue reactions (ARMD—adverse reaction to metal debris) gradually emerged around the hip joint to be an important reason for their (MoM bearing) ultimate withdrawal. The following manifestations of adverse local tissue reaction (ALTR) are seen:
  - Effusions
  - Soft-tissue masses (pseudotumors)—associated with increased metal ion concentrations and edge loading of the implant. The pseudotumors are characterized by an extensive necrosis of dense connective tissue, a locally heavy macrophage and lymphocytic infiltration as well as the presence of plasma cells and eosinophils.
  - Early osteolysis and failure.
  - *Late osteolysis*: Osteolysis following MoM implant could be due to production of potentially osteolytic cytokines rather than recruitment of inflammatory cells (as is common mechanism with MoP bearings). These immunological responses may be triggered by metal ions that act as antigens and stimulate an allergic (hypersensitivity) reaction by forming organometallic complexes with proteins.
  - *Local and systemic effects and cancer risk*: T-cell lymphopenia due to raised levels of Co and Cr ions may be associated with increased cancer risk.

The tissue response can be inflammatory or immunological in nature.
- *The aseptic, lymphocyte-dominated vasculitis-associated lesion (ALVAL) reaction*: When comparing tissues surrounding MoP and MoM THAs more lymphocytes are found histologically in the MoM THAs. This could be due to delayed-type hypersensitivity response to the metal wear products but pattern of inflammatory reaction

and cellular distribution distinguishes this from classical type IV delayed-type hypersensitivity reaction. The presence of B-lymphocytes, plasma cells, and massive fibrin exudation point to a vasculitis-like lesion instead. Thus, descriptive term of ALVAL or as a lymphocyte-dominated immunologic answer (LYDIA) has been named for the histological finding.

- *Metal-on-polyethylene bearings*: The metal bearings used with PE include—
  - *Stainless steel*—used if patient is allergic to cobalt or chrome.
  - *Cobalt-chromium alloy (in the vast majority)*—most preferred bearing setting gold standard against which other couples are tested. The average wear rate of the cobalt-chrome-poly bearing is 0.1–0.2 mm/year. Improvements in surface characteristics by ion implanting and other surface-hardening techniques have been applied to Co-Cr alloy but the clinical effect on wear rate in vivo is undetermined.
  - *Titanium alloy*—not much favored due to high wear in presence of third-body particles (run-away wear). This susceptibility to surface abrasion is partly reduced by hardening with techniques such as gas nitriding, solution nitriding, or ion implantation. This improvement has produced better 10-year results by increasing resistance to abrasion from third-body particles. But if the hardened surface is penetrated say by a scratch then severe wear of the underlying alloy gets triggered.

- *Ceramic-on-polyethylene bearings*: Alumina and zirconia femoral balls have since introduction been increasingly used as bearing surfaces against poly based on reported substantially lower poly wear rates as compared to metal balls (the wear ratios of 0.25–0.75). Oxidized zirconium (Oxinium®, Smith and Nephew) has been specifically produced for this articulation but wear properties are not very impressive (compared to available materials). The oxinium improves the wear characteristics of zirconium while simultaneously utilizing the hardness and its fracture resistance. This has also allowed the use of large heads as the volumetric wear would be less ultimately while increasing stability. Alumina seems to have outpaced zirconia in the race against wear as it has reduced wear rates than the latter.

  Disadvantages:
  - Imperative need of hardened poly as a safety measure to be used against harder femoral head bearings (hence preferring highly cross-linked poly).
  - Contamination by metal particles in a ceramic ball effectively roughens the ceramic ball because the metal particles can adhere to the surface of the ceramic increasing abrasion of the PE.

- *Ceramic-on-metal (CoM) articulation*: The wear for alumina CoM articulations is very favorable, no run-in period is observed with the CoM bearings and a volumetric wear rate of 0.01 mm^3 per 1 million cycles is reported.

  Advantages:
  - There is a reduction in serum metal ions in the patients at 6 months postoperatively.
  - In addition, this bearing also appears to produce less stripe wear with edge loading than MoM or CoC implants.
  - The potential advantage of this novel CoM bearing is thus lower wear and the production of significantly reduced metal particles quantitatively.
  - This bearing combination also allows for the use of large femoral heads (due to low wear) thus improving the stability and jump distance.

  Disadvantages:
  - All said concerns of metal wear particles always remain.
  - In addition larger ceramic heads reduce the fracture risk and an increased number of femoral head options are made available increasing modularity.
  - The clinical performance is unknown.

103. A. Bearing surfaces in THR.
   B. Investigation and management of dislocation of hip after THR.

Ans:

A. *Kindly see Answer to Question 91.*

B. *Investigation*: During reduction of hip, assess the stability as to easily dislocatable or lax hip vs. normal or tight hip. Try to assess the combined anteversion angle under fluoroscopy (rough measure only). Impingement of components or cement can also be assessed dynamically under c-arm. CT scans are done to objectively see for version of femoral and acetabular components.

Management: If the components are in satisfactory position, closed reduction is followed by a period of bed rest. Immobilization for 6 weeks to 3 months is recommended preferably with knee in extension. Mobilization is accomplished in a prefabricated abduction orthosis that maintains the hip in 20° of abduction and prevents hip flexion past 60°.

If one or both components are malaligned, or hip is to lax to remain stable even after reduction or dislocated easily in flexion and neutral rotation and dislocation becomes or is deemed to be recurrent, revision surgery usually is required. Specific causes for instability should be sought and specifically corrected.

- *Impingement*: Retained osteophytes and cement can be easily removed.
- Malpositioned component(s) should be revised and repositioned as follows:
  - Minor malposition of the acetabular component → replace with an elevated rim liner or changing the position of the one already present
  - Malposition >10° → revise the component
  - Inadequate neck length changes offsets so exchange a modular head or revise femoral component (non-modular). Revision of the femoral component for malrotation alone rarely is required.
- No component malposition or impingement → distal advancement of the greater trochanter to tighten soft-tissue.
- If instability is compounded by neurological deficit or abductor insufficiency → use a bipolar prosthesis.
- As a last resort, a constrained socket design can be used in which the femoral head is locked into the socket.
- Finally, some patients are not candidates for reconstruction. Noncompliant individuals, alcohol and drug abusers, elderly debilitated patients, and patients with several previous failed attempts to stop recurrent dislocation are best treated by girdlestone type procedure.

104. Describe trabecular metal used in THR.

Ans: Trabecular metal is a unique, highly porous biomaterial made from elemental tantalum with structural, functional, and physiological properties similar to that of bone. The material features are 100% open, engineered, and interconnected pore structure to support bony ingrowth and vascularization. The material has over 20 years of demonstrated clinical use in a variety of orthopedic applications.

Structure: It is made from commercially pure elemental tantalum and designed to withstand physiologic loads. The architecture shows up to 80% porosity allowing good bone ingrowth.

Function: The trabecular metal has low modulus of elasticity similar to cancellous bone for more normal physiological loading which has the potential to reduce stress shielding when used in a monoblock or monolithic application. It has high coefficient of friction compared to cancellous bone for stable initial fixation.

Physiology: Chemically stable and biocompatible material which creates very little adverse biological response.

105. Write briefly about principle, advantages and disadvantages of hip resurface arthroplasty.

Ans: Hip resurfacing arthroplasty is a metal-on-metal arthroplasty of the hip where the diseased surfaces are resurfaced aimed to preserving the bone stock as much as possible. Younger, larger-built, male patients were better candidates for hip resurfacing arthroplasty.

Principles:
- *Preservation of femoral head*: The femoral head is not removed, only the diseased portion of femoral head and acetabulum is excised.
- Restoration of hip biomechanics—because the offset of hip is minimally changed so the biomechanics is better restored than conventional head sacrificing arthroplasty.

- Compromise to the blood flow using posterior approach was one of the factors for failure, so using anterior approach or trochanteric flip approach would be better.

Advantages:
- *Easier to revise*: Due to preservation of bone in primary resurfacing procedure, the revision arthroplasty is easier to perform and will most likely not require long stem implants.
- *Reduced risk of hip dislocation*: Due to large bearing surfaces, the jump distance of bearing increases significantly. Also, the range of movements is higher before limits of movement or implant-implant/bone impingement occurs, so risk of dislocation is reduced.
- *More normal gait*: It was found that hip resurfacing disturbed the anatomy to a much lesser extent than conventional head sacrificing arthroplasty, so gait pattern was better.

Disadvantages:
- *Femoral neck fracture*: The femoral head is preserved so implant fits over the resurfaced articular surface and stress is passed on to the neck that may fracture.
- Could not be done if the femoral head is significantly osteonecrotic— poor bone to support the femoral head prosthesis.
- All complications of metal-on-metal arthroplasty—ALVAL, ALTR, etc. *(See Answer to Question 91 above)*

106. Define protrusio acetabuli. Discuss its etiology, classification, clinical features, and management.

Ans: Definition: Protrusio acetabuli is a radiological diagnosis on AP radiographs of the pelvis where the acetabular line projects medial to the ilioischial line.

Etiology and Classification:
Primary (idiopathic)
Secondary (known pathology that causes protrusio)
- *Genetic*:
  - Trichorhinophalangeal syndrome
  - Stickler syndrome
  - Trisomy 18
  - Ehlers–Danlos syndrome
  - Marfan's syndrome
  - Sickle cell disease
- *Inflammatory*:
  - Rheumatoid arthritis
  - Juvenile rheumatoid arthritis
  - Psoriatic arthritis
  - Ankylosing spondylitis
  - Reiter's syndrome
  - Acute idiopathic chondrolysis
  - Osteolysis following hip replacement
- *Infectious*:
  - *Gonococcus*
  - *Syphilis*
  - *Echinococcus*
  - *Staphylococcus*
  - *Streptococcus*
  - *Mycobacterium tuberculosis*
- *Metabolic*:
  - Paget's disease
  - Osteogenesis imperfecta

- Osteomalacia
- Hyperparathyroidism
- Ochronosis
- Acrodysostosis
- *Neoplastic*:
  - Hemangioma
  - Metastatic carcinoma (breast, prostate)
  - Neurofibromatosis
  - Radiation-induced ON
- *Traumatic*:
  - Sequelae of acetabular fracture
  - Surgical error during hip replacement

Clinical features:
- The condition is most prominently seen in the middle age group between 35 and 50 years of age; however, patients in their teens and those between 51 and 85 years of age also show higher prevalence than other age groups. The condition is female preponderant and also has racial distribution. The Bantu females in Natal have high prevalence of the Otto pelvis with as many as one-fourth of them are affected.
- Typically, patients with primary protrusio acetabuli present with activity-related increasing stiffness rather than pain. Often, stiffness has been noticed in adolescence as the OA is not prominent in this age group, so pain is less reported. The deepening effect of acetabulum relatively shortens the femoral neck and reduces offset. Arising from a seated position frequently exacerbates the symptoms. Pain is reported in the groin with some patients reporting radiating pain to the knee. There is impingement during hip movements of abduction and flexion. This causes labral tears and repetitive attacks of synovitis. The changes degrade the cartilage, and hence, progression to OA is very prominent. Secondary changes due to limitation of hip movements are seen in the form of increased lumbar lordosis
- Family history should be obtained as the genetic associations have been found and also metabolic defects may affect the siblings altogether. Past history of hip trauma and surgery should also be obtained.
- On examination, there is often global limitation of active and passive movements with terminal pain.
- Impingement signs are often positive. Pain is also reproduced in active straight leg raise. Trendelenburg sign may be positive due to reduced offset, and hence abductor effectiveness. The gait is a combination of antalgic and Trendelenburg gait.

Management:
Conservative management is mostly supportive and utilizes approaches such as strengthening exercises, maintaining mobility and relieving pain by appropriate medications. Ultimately, surgery is needed and conservative management serves only as an interim measure. Primary pathology should always be looked for and treated, as this may prevent progression and reduce the amount/extent of surgical intervention later.

The surgical management broadly falls into two measures:
1. *Joint compromising methods*: These disturb the normal anatomy and/or function of joint.
   - *Total joint arthroplasty*: Quite popular and the bias toward this procedure has reduced tremendously.
     - The procedure is first choice in patients past their middle age and obvious arthritic changes in the hip joint. Most important concern is anatomical repositioning of the cup. Cemented cups placed
     - 1 cm away from the anatomical position resulted in failure in all the three zones. Higher medial stresses are produced with medial placement of the cup. Methods to circumvent this are use of morselized bone graft, use of protrusio cage, lateralization of cup by using metal-backed implants or protrusion-cup itself. Augmenting the medial wall by bone graft only has little benefit as the stresses are ultimately transmitted to it. Still successful results have been reported by the use of "concavoconvex" femoral head graft for filling medial acetabular defect and cementing the acetabular cup.
   - Hip arthrodesis
   - Excision arthroplasty

2. *Joint preservation methods*:
   - *Hanging hip of Voss (not used at all today)*: This was based on premises that gravity will distract the joint and resultant forces will be reduced. I am unaware of any current indications for this procedure.
   - *Acetabuloplasty (rimectomy of Smith-Peterson)*: This may be appropriate for mild-to-moderate protrusio in a middle-aged patient where the symptoms are more of pincer type impingement.
   - *Valgus intertrochanteric osteotomy (ITO) (Pauwel's)*: This is known to reorient the resultant forces of the hip to a more cranial position, thus controlling the superomedial migration of the femoral head. Correction of 20–30° is desirable; overcorrection causes abductor contracture. The added advantage of the procedure is reduced impingement at the superior acetabular margin. If correction is greater than 40°, then abductor tension should be released by opening wedge osteotomy of trochanter, and limb-shortening may also need to be performed. This procedure should not be performed on patients over 40 years of age or in whom significant degenerative changes were evident on plain radiographs.
   - *Surgical closure of triradiate cartilage*: This is indicated in skeletally immature patients with open triradiate cartilage and absence of inflammatory pathology. It is, however, difficult to determine which protrusio will progress as opposed to those where there is more likelihood of indolent course (not needing surgery). This procedure is, hence recommended for Marfan's syndrome and genetic causes of protrusio.

107 **A. Principles of cementless acetabular implantation.**

B. What are the important steps in cementless implantation in protrusio acetabuli?

Ans: A. In a cementless acetabular component, the liner is locked in the shell. Here, the acetabular shell provides the outer face of the acetabular cup, which must be fixed into the pelvis, either by bone cement or by press-fitting. The fixation can be enhanced by use of screws. Uncemented components present porous surface finishing (e.g., sintered titanium beads) or hydroxyapatite coatings to foster improved bone integration. Three generations of acetabular cups have been described according to their evolution:

1. *First-generation cementless acetabular cups*: These were porous ingrowth acetabular components aimed to provide long-term biologic fixation to bone. Most designs offered cementless monoblock component, however, some were modular too, providing reasonably satisfactory fixation. The typical cause of failure was result of ultrahigh molecular weight polyethylene (UHMWPE) wear or dissociation between the liner and metal shell. Dissociation was associated with deformation or fracture of the UHMWPE at the liner-locking mechanism.
2. *Second-generation cups with highly cross-linked UHMWPE*: This began with the use of highly crosslinked UHMWPEs in combination with the clinically successful second-generation modular acetabular components since early 2000s. The wear rates were improved but unique problem creep up of edge impingement with increased use of larger femoral heads that have greater range of motion (ROM). To use a large-diameter head in a relatively small acetabular shell and to maintain adequate thickness of UHMWPE at the weight-bearing region of the dome, thicker poly has to be used lateralizing the head. This eccentric relation of head center to acetabular shell center causes peripheral impingement, especially at the elevated liner margin. This further leads to liner fracture.
3. *Third-generation cementless modular acetabular cups*: Third-generation modular acetabular cups have been developed to reduce the risk of fracture of the liner rim when large-diameter femoral head are used with highly crosslinked UHMWPE. The following design changes have been incorporated:
   - Eliminating UHMWPE protruding above the rim
   - Minimizing sharp corners at the liner-locking mechanism
   - Recessing the locking mechanism into the interior of the metal shell.

B. *Lots of methods are needed to fill defects or augment acetabulum*: Use of morselized bone graft, use of protrusio cage, lateralization of cup by using metal-backed implants or protrusion cup itself are commonly used. Augmenting the medial wall by bone graft only has little benefit as the stresses are ultimately transmitted to it. Still successful results have been reported by the use of "concavoconvex" femoral head graft for filling medial acetabular defect and cementing the acetabular cup. The femoral head articular cartilage was denuded using reverse reamer, and the center of head was scooped of the bone resulting in typical concavoconvex graft that was impacted in the protrusio defect and augmented with the retrieved bone graft from center of femoral head. I prefer medial morcelized bone graft and using a porous coated metal-backed cup. Rim augments (antiprotrusio rings) have also been used that transmit the stress on acetabular rim rather than the center. In general, as recommended by Ranawat and Zahn, protrusio up to 5 mm does not require any bone graft, protrusio greater than 5 mm and intact medial wall need bone graft but augmentation devices may not be needed. Gross deficiency would need above described methods.

108. What are the indications and principles of revision THR? Discuss different types of acetabular defects and management.

Ans: Indications: Revisions have been done for: (1) painful, aseptic loosening of one or both components; (2) progressive loss of bone; (3) fracture or mechanical failure of the implant; (4) recurrent or irreducible dislocation; (5) infected THR as a one-stage or two-stage procedure; and (6) treatment of a periprosthetic fracture.

Principles: The overall principles are more or less similar to primary hip arthroplasty, viz., normalizing hip center, reconstructing a stable mobile hip articulation providing adequate (or ideally complete) pain relief. For revision arthroplasty, additionally one should maximize bone preservation, fill all bone defects, enhance bone mass as much as possible to provide good fixation of the prosthesis. All this should try to reconstruct the hip anatomy as close to normal as possible.

The principles of acetabular reconstruction include:
- Creation of a stable acetabular bed
- Secure prosthetic fixation with freedom of orientation
- Bony reconstitution (impaction bone grafting)
- Restoration of a normal hip center of rotation with acceptable biomechanics

The principles for femoral reconstruction broadly are:
- Enhancing the bone mass and stability to provide as good a fixation of femoral stem as possible (impaction bone grafting/onlay bone splinters)
- Bypassing the femoral defects maximally to avoid further periprosthetic fracture
- Adequate fixation to prevent subsidence of stem—if calcar fixing stem, then reconstruct the calcar or use calcar replacing stem, else go for diaphyseal/distal fixing stem.
- Proper horizontal and vertical offsetting to resolve the abductor function

Management of acetabular defects:

Types of acetabular defects: The American Academy of Orthopedic Surgeons (AAOS) classification of acetabular bone defects:
- *Type I*: Segmental deficiency:
  - Peripheral (rim defect)
    - Superior
    - Anterior
    - Posterior
  - Central (medial-wall defect)
- *Type II*: Cavitary deficiencies
  - Peripheral
    - Superior
    - Anterior
    - Posterior
  - Central (medial-wall intact)
- *Type III*: Combined deficiencies
- *Type IV*: Pelvic discontinuity
- *Type V*: Arthrodesis

Paprosky classification for acetabular defects is given in **Table 4B.11.3**.

TABLE 4B.11.3: Paprosky classification of acetabular defects.					
Defect	Rim	Walls/Dome	Columns	Migration	Teardrop lysis
Type 1	Intact	Intact	Intact/supportive	None	
Type 2	Distorted	Distorted	Intact/supportive	<2 cm	
2-A	Distorted	Intact	Intact/supportive	Superomedial	Minimal
2-B	Missing	Distorted	Intact/supportive	Superolateral	Minimal
2-C	Distorted	Intact	Intact/supportive	Medial	Severe
Type 3	Missing	Compromised	Nonsupportive	>2 cm	
3-A	Missing	Compromised	Nonsupportive	Superolateral	Moderate
3-B	Missing	Compromised	Nonsupportive	Superomedial	Severe

Management: Some reconstruction options for acetabular defects are as follows:
- *Jumbo cup*: Minimum diameter of 60–70 mm; these were suggested as a more reliable alternative to structural allograft in treating cavernous acetabular deficiencies but have been also successfully applied for segmental loss of the anterior column and medial wall.
- *High hip center*: For bone deficiency, i.e., most pronounced superiorly resulting in oblong acetabulum. The high hip center is defined at a minimum of 35 mm proximal to the interteardrop line. Because of nonanatomic location, cemented fixations have higher failure rates. Dislocation rates are not higher than conventional hips.
- Oblong cup/double bubble
- Impaction grafting
- Bulk allograft and reinforcement rings—for severe acetabular deficiency.

109. Classify femoral bone stock deficiency in THR. Describe broad principles of management.
Ans:
Classification: The AAOS classification of the femoral bone defects:
- *Type I*: Segmental deficiency
    - Proximal
    - Partial
    - Complete
    - Intercalary
    - Greater trochanter
- *Type II*: Cavitary deficiencies
    - Cancellous
    - Cortical
    - Ectasia
- *Type III*: Combined deficiencies
- *Type IV*: Malalignment
    - Rotational
    - Angular
- *Type V*: Femoral stenosis
- *Type VI*: Femoral discontinuity

Chandler–Penenberg classification
Femoral defects
- Calcar deficiency
    - IM
    - Total

- Trochanteric deficiency
  - Cortical thinning
  - Cortical perforation
- Femoral fractures about or below the stem of a femoral component
  - Fractures of the patient's femur
  - Fatigue fracture of an allograft
- Circumferential deficiency of the metaphysis and proximal diaphysis
  - Loss of the trochanter and metaphysis with a thin shell of the diaphysis remaining
  - Total loss of the proximal femur

Paprosky classification for femoral defects is given in **Table 4B.11.4**.

TABLE 4B.11.4: Femoral defects.

Type	Femoral defect
1	Minimal metaphyseal and diaphyseal bone loss
2-A	Absent calcar extending just below the intertrochanteric level
2-B	Anterolateral metaphyseal bone loss
2-C	Absent calcar with posteromedial metaphyseal bone loss
3-A	2-A plus diaphyseal bone loss
3-B	2-B plus diaphyseal bone loss
3-C	2-C plus diaphyseal bone loss

Principles: Kindly see the Answers to Questions above.

110. Describe the common surgical factors affecting early outcome of THR.

Ans: The factors that influence early outcome after THR include:
- Hospital stay—shorter supposed to be better psychologically
- Postoperative pain and duration—painless postoperative period best for rehabilitation
- Preoperative functional status—higher the preoperative function better is postoperative
- Younger age—lesser the age better is outcome
- Accelerated rehabilitation protocol—may have positive effect (unproven)
- Preconditioning the patient about future events and possibilities with knowledge of rehabilitation and physiotherapy has positive effect
- Weight of patient—lesser the better
- Opposite hip condition—normal other hip is good for early rehabilitation
- Minimally invasive surgery, type of surgical approach, has minimal or controversial effect on early outcome.

111. Discuss in brief various complications of THA.

Ans: Various complications are associated with THA that can be summarized by dividing them into early and late as follows:

Early complications:
- *Cardiopulmonary*:
  - Chest pain
  - Palpitations
  - Dyspnea
  - Pulmonary embolism
  - Congestive heart failure
  - Atelectasis
  - Fat embolism
  - Blood loss

- *Neuropsychotic*:
  - Altered sensorium
  - Postsurgical psychosis
  - Hyponatremia
  - Delirium
- *Nonspecific*:
  - Fever
  - Nausea
  - Abdominal pain
- *Renal*:
  - Oliguria
  - Chronic renal failure
  - Urinary retention
  - Urinary tract infection
- *Wound complications*:
  - Superficial infection
  - Wound necrosis
- Instability and dislocation
- Neurovascular injury

Late complications:
- Aseptic loosening
- Heterotopic ossification
- Malignancy
- Metal hypersensitivity
- Late instability
- Stress fractures
- Periprosthetic fractures

112. Discuss patient-specific instrumentation (PSI) in arthroplasty.

Ans: Patient-specific instrumentation is an alternative to both navigation and robotic surgical guidance for implant positioning. They are custom-made on a case-to-case basis, specific to both the anatomy of the patient and the surgical plan made by the surgeon.

TKR: PSI is a modern technique in TKR aiming to facilitate implantation of the prosthesis. The customized cutting blocks of PSI are generated from preoperative 3D model, using CT or MRI imaging. The PSI guide takes into account any slight deformities or osteophytes and applies preoperative planning for bone resection using the predetermined implant size, position, and rotation. Apparent benefits of technology are that neutral postoperative alignment is more reproducible, surgical time is decreased and the entire procedure results more efficient and cost effective. Use of PSI is indicated in advanced OA, severe pain, limited function/walking ability.

Also, it can be used when IM guides cannot be used, e.g., post-traumatic femoral deficiency. In cases where prior femoral and tibial fractures that have healed with a malalignment; preoperative planning may not be accurate and intraoperative technical difficulties may arise, such as during the use of IM rod. In these selected patients, PSI may be very useful to avoid errors in alignment and planning.

THR: Acetabular PSI system is used to optimize the cup size, medialization, and orientation (anteversion and inclination). Femoral PSI is used to optimize the stem size, position, offset, version, and leg length of the patient. These are small block jigs which are designed dependent on the surgical approach. These fit to the anatomy of the femoral head and neck to guide the angle and position of femoral neck cut.

Patients undergo a low-dose CT scan of pelvis and hip. Scan creates a virtual 3D model which is used to plan the size and position of implant. The PSI guides and jigs are then manufactured.

Alongside guides, physical 3D models of pelvis and proximal femur are produced, sterilized, and used intraoperatively. These allow for visualization of patient's own bony anatomy and demonstration of how the guide will fit prior to use on patient. They help in osteophyte removal, soft-tissue dissection.

113. Describe the principles of Charnley's low friction arthroplasty.

Ans: Charnley's low friction arthroplasty (LFA) aims to enhance the longevity of total hip replacements (THRs). The primary principles include:

- *Minimizing shear forces*: High shear forces at bearing surfaces increase loosening risk. The low friction-torque arthroplasty concept emphasizes minimizing these forces.
- *Reducing wear debris*: Frictional shear generates wear debris that can lead to tissue reactions and loosening.

This is achieved by combining:

- *Small femoral head (22.225 mm = 7/8 inch) diameter*: This has low volumetric wear, allows for a larger poly to be placed.
- *Thick poly*: This provides good support at the acetabular side and favors socket to remain stationary due to larger difference in radii of curvature of the femoral head and the poly. Charnley proposed that with small radius of curvature of the femoral head (11.1125 mm) and long radius of curvature of the poly, movement is more likely to occur at the interface between metal and poly rather than straining the poly-bone interface.
- *Maintain optimal offset for femoral stem*—to optimize the vectorial distribution of forces and avoid undue stress.
- *Distributing the load* on a larger surface of bone uniformly by using cement interface between the acetabular cup and bone.

4B.12 HIP ARTHROSCOPY (Q114–117)

114. A. Indications, positioning, portals, and techniques of hip arthroscopy.
B. How do you manage an incongruous reduction after a reduced hip dislocation because of a loose body with hip arthroscopy?
C. What is an absolute contraindication to manage such a case with conventional hip arthroscopy?

Ans: *(Kindly see Chapter 36 of the book Essential Orthopedics: Principles and Practice, 2nd edition for details and illustrations.)*

A. *Indications*:
- *Loose bodies and osteochondromatosis*: This is probably the best indication as arthrotomy for same has significant morbidity and limited exposure.
- *Labral tears and femoroacetabular impingement (FAI)*: Both cam and pincer type. Labral tears are often elusive and not fully characterized on even advanced diagnostic investigations. Arthroscopy serves in localization, debridement, confirming, and repairing the tears. In addition, the chondral injuries can also be simultaneously addressed.
- *Chondral injuries*: For a badly damaged surface that is bound to still damage more of the articular surface, it is better to remove the cartilage by debridement.
- *Synovial disease*: Synovial debridement is quite adequately performed arthroscopically.
- Joint sepsis.
- Osteonecrosis.
- *Early osteoarthritis (one may call this as advanced FAI)*: The pathology involves thickened labrum synovitis, labral degeneration, osteophytes, articular cartilage damage, geodes formation, loose bodies in the joint, etc.; arthroscopy in this context may at best be considered an interim measure (bridge technique). Patients undergoing this procedure must have 50% range of motion and must have greater than 50% normal cartilage. The arthroscopic procedure comprises of partial capsulectomy (T-type along neck and rim for most patients or H-type for capsular plication) or capsulotomy only, acetabular rim trimming and cystectomy, notch osteophytectomy, labral refixation or grafting, microfracture for cartilage regeneration, head-neck osteoplasty, bone grafting defects, and capsular repair or plication.

- Ruptured ligamentum teres.
- Unresolved hip pain.
- *Greater trochanteric pain syndrome*: This involves a mix of unrelated entities like external hip snapping, trochanteric bursitis (arthroscopy is indicated for refractory cases not responding to medical treatment), gluteus medius or/and minimus tears. Release of the iliotibial band endoscopically is an effective procedure for management of external snapping and trochanteric bursitis causing resolution in nearly 100% cases.
- *Deep gluteal syndrome*: This is due to sciatic nerve entrapment from any of the structures in the gluteal region (including piriformis—part of piriformis syndrome).
- *Ischiofemoral impingement*: It is caused by abnormal contact between the lesser trochanter and ischium causing compression of the quadriceps femoris muscle.
- *Internal snapping*: Internal snapping of iliopsoas can be managed by endoscopic partial or complete iliopsoas release ± subtendinous bursectomy.
- Arthroscopically assisted computer-guided pelvic acetabular osteotomy is another option in future.

Positioning: The procedure can be done in supine (preferred) or lateral position.
- *Supine*: Use a fracture table with lateralized perineal post to provide a transverse component to traction. Abduct hip 25° for proper traction vector. Adduction is used to improve path for screw fixation, if needed. Flexion of hip is avoided as it brings sciatic nerve near and vulnerable to injury. Vacuum effect is seen in the joint with distraction that gets released with fluid insufflation.
- *Lateral position*: Here, the standard table is used with a custom distractor attached. Necessary changes are made in the position of monitor and instrument table to accommodate for this position.

Portals: Commonly for hip joint, two standard portals are enough, if the distraction is adequate else three portals are needed:
1. *Anterior portal*: Made at intersection of vertical line through anterior superior iliac spine (ASIS) and horizontal line across proximal margin of greater trochanter (skin incision is 4–6 cm distal to the ASIS). It passes through sartorius and rectus femoris. Protect lateral femoral cutaneous nerve and femoral nerve.
2. *Anterolateral portal*: The skin incision for this portal lies about 2 cm anterior to the anterosuperior edge of the greater trochanter. The path of this portal is not straight but instead the needle is directed about 10–20° cranially and 20–30° posteriorly. The portal is thus made through the gluteus medius and then at the anterior margin, if femoral head protect the superior gluteal nerve. This is the first portal to be made as it lies in the "safe zone" and usually homes the scope.
3. *Posterolateral portal*: Penetrates gluteus medius and minimus anterosuperior to piriformis tendon. Protect the sciatic nerve.

Techniques: Supine position arthroscopy—
- After establishing the three portals, place the outflow in the posterolateral portal.
- To view the acetabulum, labrum, and femoral head from each of the three portals, alternate the 70° scope and 30° scope between the anterolateral and anterior portals. Rotate the lens, and internally and externally rotate the hip. The 70° degree scope is best for viewing the labrum and the periphery of the acetabulum and femoral head, and the 30° scope is used for viewing of the central portion of the acetabulum, femoral head, and superior portion of the acetabular fossa.

B. Loose body causing incongruous reduction after reduction of a dislocated hip needs to be removed by either open or arthroscopic methods. Standard hip arthroscopy is planned and loose body can be removed by above described technique. If facilities or expertise of arthroscopy are not available, then safe surgical dislocation of the hip joint can be done to remove the loose body.
C. Open injury violating the space for portal creation, associated major acetabular or femoral side fractures (fracture neck/head) are absolute contraindications for arthroscopic technique. Presence of protrusio acetabuli, advanced osteoarthritis, or heterotopic ossification are relative contraindications. For conventional surgical dislocation, compromised vascularity to femoral head is an absolute contraindication.

115. What are the potential complications of hip arthroscopy?

Ans: *Complications of hip arthroscopy*:
- Iatrogenic articular cartilage/soft-tissue injury
- Undercorrection/overcorrection of FAI
- *Neurologic/vascular complications*: Injury to lateral femoral cutaneous nerve during portal making. Traction injury to sciatic nerve, femoral nerve, common peroneal nerve. Injury to inferior gluteal artery from laceration, pseudoaneurysm is rare but can occur.
- *AVN femoral head*: Injury to lateral epiphyseal branch of medial femoral circumflex artery can occur during femoral osteoplasty and may result in AVN. Other causes leading to AVN are excessive traction, increased intra-articular hip pressure, partial capsulectomy.
- *Postoperative hip instability*: Due to excessive rim trimming, capsulotomy or capsular resection, inadequate labral repair.
- *Miscellaneous*: Heterotropic ossification, deep vein thrombosis (DVT), pulmonary embolism, septic arthritis, wound infection, abdominal compartment syndrome, complex regional pain syndrome (CRPS).

116. A. Discuss the current status of hip arthroscopy.
B. Indications in contemporary orthopedic practice.
C. Explain important steps of procedure.

Ans: Kindly see Answer to Question 114.

117. Discuss outcomes of hip arthroscopy.

Ans: Hip arthroscopy is a growing technique that has reached fair level of maturity and duration where outcomes can be measured. The reported outcomes vary decently in different studies but the most commonly reported ones are as follows:
1. Compared with open surgical dislocation, arthroscopy resulted in significant improvements in nonarthritic hip scores (NAHS—measure for level of pain and stiffness in a patient's hips) at 3- and 12-month follow-ups.
2. Hip arthroscopy resulted in a significantly lower reoperation rate.
3. Hip arthroscopy for labral pathology and FAI leads to both short- and long-term return improved function using patient reported outcomes, as well as showed a successful return to daily activity and sport.
4. Patients undergoing hip arthroscopy within the last 20 years with Tönnis grade <1 and labral repair experienced greater than 90% survivorship.
5. There is a low conversion rate to THA in patients undergoing hip arthroscopy in mid to long term follow-up. Advanced age at index procedure and higher grade of cartilage damage were the important predictors for conversion to THA or revision surgery.

4B.13 TUBERCULOSIS OF HIP (Q118–120)

118. A. Describe the stage of TB hip.
B. Differentiating clinical features, treatment, and prognosis of each stage.

Ans: A. The stages of TB hip have been described in **Table 4B.13.1**.

TABLE 4B.13.1: Modified staging system from Tuli.

Stage	Pathology	Clinical findings	Movements	Radiologic features
I (Stage of apparent lengthening)	Synovitis	Abduction deformity (pelvic tilt), no true shortening. FABER (flexion, abduction and external rotation). Limp is the earliest and commonest symptom. Muscle spasm can be appreciated in the lower abdominal muscles, and in the adductors of the thigh on attempting sudden abduction-external rotation at the hip joint	>75% preserved	Osteopenia + haziness of articular margins

Contd...

Contd...

Stage	Pathology	Clinical findings	Movements	Radiologic features
II (Stage of apparent shortening)	Early arthritis	Shortening <1 cm, adduction deformity. Flexion, adduction, external rotation (FADER). Appreciable muscle wasting, and restriction of movements, due to pain and muscle spasm, in all directions	>50–75% preserved	Osteopenia + haziness of articular margins + marginal erosions
III (Stage of true shortening)	Advanced arthritis	True shortening >1 cm. FADER + shortening. Restriction of movements, muscle wasting, true and apparent shortenings are exaggerated	Loss of >75% movements	Above + reduced joint space + joint destruction
IV (Arthritis)	Advanced arthritis ± pathological dislocation or subluxation	Shortening usually >2.5 cm Usually FADER	Loss of >75% movements	Gross destruction and reduction of joint space, wandering acetabulum
V (Joint destruction—either ankylosis or "disintegrated tuberculous hip"—wandering acetabulum, pathological dislocation, destruction of head)	Terminal arthritis	Shortening variable. Depending on condition of joint and compensation. If ankylosed then usually FADER	Ankylosis and gross deformity	All above findings with joint degeneration

B. *Treatment*: All patients during active stage are treated by multidrug therapy. In acute symptomatic stage give traction to the limb. Traction reduces pain, counters and relaxes spasm by reducing pain, prevents deformity, maintains joint space, minimizes chances of wandering acetabulum and corrects deformity. A weight of 0.45 kg/year of age is used given bilaterally (to prevent pelvic tilt and increase in abduction deformity). Abduction in the affected limb is given to compensate for the shortening and counter tendency for adduction. Any palpable cold abscess may be aspirated with instillation of streptomycin with or without isoniazid. If there is favorable clinical response the same treatment should be continued. In cases which do not have gross ankylosis, active assisted movements of the hip are started as soon as the pain has subsided. The hip mobilization exercises are gradually increased to 5–10 minutes every hour during the period the patient is awake, and within the limits of tolerable pain. Usually, after 4–6 months of treatment the patient may be permitted ambulation with suitable orthosis and crutches. The ambulation should be non-weight bearing for first 12 weeks and partial weight bearing for the next 12 weeks.

Surgery is indicated, if there is inadequate response to conservative treatment or outcome of conservative treatment is not good (painful or deformed joint). Also if there is advanced disease with unstable hip joint (stage 4 or 5) surgery will be primarily indicated. In poor response to conservative treatment often the disease load is too high to respond to chemotherapy and joint debridement with excision of focus helps, this is however very infrequently required as an isolated procedure. The advantage is that material for reconfirmation or initial confirmation of diagnosis can be done. With gross joint destruction in healing phase surgical management to provide mobile or fixed painless joint is required. Arthrodesis of hip joint is preferred in a young adult patient with painful hip and doing laborious job for earning his living. In resistant TB cases that fail to respond to chemotherapy multiple debridements to clear disease and sequestra from joint (excision of focus) and obtain tissue for culture sensitivity may be required. It is preferable to do simultaneous arthrodesis in such cases for possible resurgence of disease following joint arthroplasty. Arthroplasty and joint replacement to provide painless mobile hip is increasing in use for a well-controlled disease but painful hip. Prerequisites for performing replacement include a quiescent joint both clinically and radiologically (increase bone density and thickness of trabeculae) with stable serology (normal ESR and CRP). Previous recommendation of 10 years of quiescent disease possibly does not hold true with current treatment regimens and drugs. Antitubercular chemotherapy is given for 4–6 weeks before surgery and is continued prophylactically as full course following arthroplasty (apparently an over treatment). Large head prosthesis is preferred but metal on metal implants have been out of favor especially in young patients.

Stage of disease and operative procedure:
- *Synovitis*—arthrotomy and synovectomy.
- *Early arthritis*—removal of loose bodies/rice bodies, debris, pannus covering the articular cartilage, loose articular cartilage, and careful curettage of osseous juxta-articular foci.
- *Advanced arthritis* arthrodesis vs. joint replacement vs. girdlestone type arthroplasty.

Prognosis: The outcome of prognosis with modern antitubercular drugs depends essentially on the stage of the disease when the treatment is initiated.
- Early disease (synovitis or early arthritis) may heal leaving a normal or nearly normal hip joint.
- Healing in the state of advanced arthritis generally results in fibrous ankylosis.
- Active disease during growing age may interfere with the blood supply of the epiphysis of femoral head giving rise to radiological picture resembling Perthes' disease.

119. Describe clinical features, diagnosis, and management of TB hip in children.

Ans: *Clinical features*: Pain, limping, deformity, and fullness around the hip are the presenting symptoms when the disease is active. Pain is often referred to the medial aspect of the knee and is maximum toward the end of the day. A child may wake from sleep due to night cries. Few patients show clinically palpable cold abscesses with or without sinuses (10%), and nearly equal number present with varying degrees of pathological subluxation or dislocation of the hip.

The limp (antalgic gait) is the earliest and most common symptom. Physical examination reveals tenderness by direct pressure on the hip in the femoral triangle, or medial to the greater trochanter posteriorly or indirectly by bitrochanteric pressure or thumping. Muscle spasm is prominent in thigh muscles and may even involve lower abdominal muscles. This increases with sudden abduction-external rotation at the hip joint.

A cold abscess usually forms within the joint, the inferior weaker part of capsule or may migrate after capsular perforation to anywhere around the hip joint such as femoral triangle, medial, lateral or posterior aspects of thigh, ischiorectal fossa, or pelvis. The abscess tracks away from the hip joint mostly along the neighboring vessels and nerves to reach the surface. The intrapelvic abscess above the attachments of the levator ani muscle tracks upward to point in the inguinal region; whereas those below this muscle track into the ischiorectal fossa.

Radiologically, the presentation varies on pathogenesis:
- Chronic hyperemia would lead to enlargement of femoral head epiphysis and metaphysis (coxa magna)
- Thromboembolic phenomenon of selective terminal vasculature may create the changes resembling Perthes' disease
- Gross decrease in the blood supply of the femoral head and its physis due to thromboembolic phenomenon or due to rapidly developing tense intracapsular effusion (tamponade effect) may be responsible for reduction in the size of femoral head and neck (coxa breva)
- Restricted growth of capital femoral epiphysial plate in the presence of normal growth of trochanteric growth-plate would lead to coxa vara
- Restricted growth of trochanteric physis in the presence of normal growth of femoral head physis would result in coxa valga
- Vascular changes can also occur due to destructive osseous cavities (affecting intraosseous circulation) in the upper end of femur-causing pathological dislocation or wandering acetabulum
- Rarely simultaneous damage to the trochanteric physis and femoral head physis would result in generalized hypoplasia of upper end of femur (coxa breva).

Diagnosis

Blood: A relative lymphocytosis, low hemoglobin, and raised erythrocyte sedimentation rate are often found in the active stage of disease.

Radiographs: Anteroposterior and lateral views of the part, and an X-ray of the chest are mandatory. Localized osteoporosis is the first radiological sign of active disease. The articular margins and bony cortices become hazy, (giving a "washed-out" appearance) and other findings may be present as detailed above.

Magnetic resonance imaging additionally shows—increased synovial fluid, thickened synovium, capsule and pericapsular tissues that also cause a soft tissue swelling. Bone edema is prominent. There may be cartilage destruction and destruction of epiphyseal growth plate.

Computed tomography scans may demonstrate small destroyed areas (lytic cavities) in the bone and marginal erosions much before evident in X-rays. Swelling in the soft tissues caused by tissue edema, granulations, exudations, or abscess formation can also be demonstrated much earlier.

Biopsy: Whenever there is doubt (particularly in early stages), it is mandatory to prove the diagnosis by obtaining the diseased tissue (granulations and/or synovium and/or bone and/or lymph nodes).

Management: In children with arthritis, the deformity and subluxation/dislocation is corrected or minimized by employing traction. Rarely one may require correction of the deformity by applying plaster under general anesthesia with or without adductor tenotomy. Failure of conservative treatment or severe deformities or subluxation or dislocation in children would need open arthrotomy, synovectomy, and debridement of the diseased joint and improvement of displacement.

Arthrodesis or excisional arthroplasty in children should be deferred till the completion of growth potential of the proximal femur. Children presenting with disease healed with gross deformity (flexion more than 30°, adduction more than 10° or abduction more than 10°) require an extra-articular corrective osteotomy to enable them to walk better till they reach skeletal maturity. In some children, the disease may heal with gross fibrous ankylosis. If there is no gross distortion of anatomy of the hip joint subtotal excision of the contracted fibrous capsule (arthrolysis) followed by traction and repetitive exercises may restore a useful range of movement for a few years.

120. Enumerate radiological types of TB hip. How does it help in prognostication.

Ans: *Shanmugasundaram divided the TB hip into seven clinicoradiological types*:

1. Normal hip—minimal or initial disease, only synovial involvement minimal, if any bony disease, no subchondral bone involvement.
2. Traveling acetabulum—gradual destruction of bony acetabulum due to preferential location of disease here, weight-bearing part of bone eroded, so that femoral head migrates proximally.
3. Dislocating hip—partially, destroyed head and acetabulum with constant adductor and flexor spasm pushing the head posterosuperiorly out of acetabulum. The capsule is also weakened or ruptured by chronic inflammation.
4. Perthes type—superolateral disease and destruction of head. Sclerosis makes distinguishing the disease from Perthes difficult, presence of cyst and acetabular osteopenia may help in making diagnosis.
5. Mortar and pestle type—gross destruction of head thin bone left and acetabulum acquiring saucer-like shape.
6. Atrophic type—in stage of destruction the disease burns out due to minimal infection.
7. Protrusio acetabula—due to softening of medial wall of acetabulum.

Prognostication: The first four types are commonly seen in children and have better prognosis with the normal type often becoming normal after treatment. The other three are seen in adults and have poor prognosis often needing joint reconstruction or salvage procedures.

If the disease occurs during childhood (growing period) chronic hyperemia would lead to enlargement of femoral head epiphysis and metaphysis (coxa magna), thromboembolic phenomenon of selective terminal vasculature may create the changes resembling Perthes' disease, gross decrease in the blood supply of the femoral head and its physis due to intracapsular effusion (tamponade effect) may be responsible for reduction in the size of femoral head and neck (coxa breva), restricted growth of capital femoral epiphysial plate in the presence of normal growth of trochanteric growth-plate would lead to coxa vara, and restricted growth of trochanteric physis in the presence of normal growth of femoral head physis would result in coxa valga. Vascular changes can also occur due to destructive osseous cavities (affecting intraosseous circulation) in the upper end of femur, by a sudden pathological dislocation, or as a complication of operative intervention.

4B.14 TRANSIENT OSTEOPOROSIS OF HIP (Q121–122)

121. A. Clinical features of transient migratory osteoporosis (TMO) of hip.
B. Tabulate differences between osteonecrosis and TMO.
C. Enumerate steps of managing TMO.

Ans:

A. Transient osteoporosis is an idiopathic condition mostly affecting young and middle-aged males and rarely females in third trimester or immediate postpartum period. Transient osteoporosis involves only the lower extremities, especially the hip joint and, less frequently, the knee, ankle, and foot. Transient osteoporosis of hip and other local osteoporosis syndromes are subtypes of transient osteoporosis. There is sudden onset, spontaneous pain of the affected joint, which increases on weight bearing and is associated with limping and disability. These symptoms gradually subside within 4–9 months. Recurrence may involve the same or adjacent joints. Physical examination is quite unremarkable and there is minimal restriction of range of movement and pain only at the extremes of range. The disjunction between physical examination and disability may help in diagnosing this self-limiting condition, avoiding unnecessary diagnostic, and therapeutic measures.

B. Differences between osteonecrosis and TMO has been described in **Table 4B.14.1**.

TABLE 4B.14.1: Differences between osteonecrosis and TMO.

Feature	Osteonecrosis	TMO
M:F	1:1	M>F
Predisposing factors	Trauma, steroids, etc.	Unknown
Onset	Gradual	Acute
Course	Progressive	Self-limiting
X-ray	Increased bone density	Demineralization
Bone scan	Decreased activity	Increased activity
MRI	Focal changes	Diffuse changes
Histology	Marrow and bone necrosis	Marrow edema

(MRI: magnetic resonance imaging; TMO: transient migratory osteoporosis)

C. Transient osteoporosis is a self-limiting disease and treatment is mainly supportive primarily aimed to reduce pain and protect the bone due to reduced mechanical strength. Protected weight bearing, mild analgesics and administration of nonsteroidal anti-inflammatory drugs are main therapeutic approaches. Glucocorticoids are not found to be effective for remineralization though they improve pain symptoms. Sympathetic blockade provided no improvement of results in the treatment of transient osteoporosis. Bisphosphonates (especially intravenous) may help in reducing pain and improving bone strength. Calcium and corrective doses of vitamin D should be started. Iloprost, a prostacyclin analog, has shown pain relief in patients with transient osteoporosis of hip and bone marrow edema syndrome by possibly dilating the vessels and reducing permeability.

122. Differential diagnosis of transient osteoporosis of hip joint.

Ans:
- Osteonecrosis
- Infective conditions like tuberculosis of hip
- Transient synovitis of hip joint
- Inflammatory conditions such as rheumatoid arthritis, crystal arthropathy and sero-negative arthritis
- Metastatic disease to hip joint

4B.15 SACROILIITIS (Q123)

123. Discuss etiology and management of sacroiliitis.

Ans: *Etiology*: The joint is involved in 5–10% of cases of low back pain (LBP). Various pathologies can involve the joint causing pain:
- Spondyloarthropathy
- Crystal arthritis
- Infection [(tuberculosis of sacroiliac joint (SIJ)]
- Sacral and pelvis fracture
- Ligament laxity and joint dysfunction during pregnancy.

Management: The SIJ has been implicated as the primary source of pain in 16–30% cases. Pain from the SIJ is generally localized in the gluteal region. Referred pain may be perceived in lower limb lumbar region, groin, or abdomen. There are many provocative tests to diagnose SIJ pain clinically and they are positive when they reproduce a patient's typical pain. Seven most important clinical tests to identify SIJ as a pain source are listed below:

- *Compression test (approximation test)*: The patient lies in lateral position with the affected side up. Patient's hips are flexed 45°, and the knees are flexed 90°. The examiner stands behind the patient then exerts downward medial pressure with both hands on the front side of the iliac crest.
- *Distraction test (gapping test)*: The patient rests in supine position and the examiner stands on the affected side. Then pressure in the dorsolateral direction is applied by examiner keeping hands on anterior superior iliac spine of the affected side.
- *Patrick's sign (flexion abduction external rotation test)*: The patient is in supine position and examiner stands on affected side. The foot of affected side is positioned under the opposite knee and then downward pressure is applied to the knee of the affected side.
- *Gaenslen's test (pelvic torsion test)*: Affected side is kept on the edge of the examination table while patient lies in a supine position. The unaffected leg flexed until the knee is pushed against the abdomen. The affected side is brought into hyperextension by applying light pressure to that knee.
- *Thigh thrust test (posterior shear test)*: The patient lies in the supine position with unaffected leg in extension and examiner stands on affected side. Examiner flexes the extremity on the affected side at the hip approximately 90° with slight adduction while applying light pressure to the bent knee.
- *Fortin's finger test*: Consistently, patient indicates the location of the pain with one finger just inferior and medial to the posterior superior iliac spine.
- *Gillet's test*: The patient stands on one leg and pulls the knee of other leg up to his or her chest.

Radiological imaging is important to exclude "red flags"; however, it does not contribute much in the diagnosis. Diagnostic blocks are the gold standard for diagnosis. Multidisciplinary approach is required to treat pain of SIJ. Intra-articular SIJ infiltrations with local anesthetic and corticosteroids are effective to treat SIJ pain and have highest evidence of success. If steroid injection provides only short-term relief then cooled radiofrequency (RF) treatment of the lateral branches of S1–S3 (S4) is recommended. Pulsed RF procedures targeted at L5 dorsal ramus and lateral branches of S1–S3 may be considered, if cooled RF is not available. Percutaneous RF neurotomy of SIJ provides long-term relief; however, cooled RF neurotomy of lateral branch has better evidence over conventional RF.

Technique of Sacroiliac Joint Injection

The patient is positioned prone and under fluoroscopy lower end of posterior SIJ is identified and marker is placed. A 25- or 22-gauge, 3.5-inch spinal needle is directed into the SIJ using a posterior approach. Once the needle has entered the joint space, intra-articular placement is confirmed with an injection of contrast medium. If the needle has been correctly placed, injection of the contrast medium will outline the joint space.

Only a minimum volume of contrast medium (0.3–0.5 mL) is required to establish intra-articular injection.

4B.16 FEMORAL SHAFT NONUNION (Q124)

124. A. Classify infected nonunion.

B. Infected fracture shaft of femur after surgery, and discuss principles and management.

Ans: A. Classification: Umiarov divided infected nonunions into four types based on the viability of bone ends, the presence of limb shortening, the presence of bone, and soft tissue defect.

1. *Type I*: Normotrophic without shortening
2. *Type II*: Hypertrophic with shortening
3. *Type III*: Atrophic with shortening
4. *Type IV*: Atrophic with bone and soft tissue defect usually with shortening.

B. Principles:
- Infected and noninfected nonunions can both be managed with compression distraction method commonly provided with Ilizarov method.
- For infected nonunion with active infection and discharging pus initially thorough debridement should be done followed by second stage stabilization ± bone grafting when the infection settles.
- For infected nonunion with quiescent infection single stage debridement with Ilizarov fixation ± bone grafting may suffice.

Investigations

Radiographs: Radiographs show some characteristic features:
- *Nonunion*:
  - Marked sclerosis of ends with rounding off appearance
  - Medullary canal closed
  - Diffuse osteoporosis of both fragments
  - Fracture gap persists and widened due to unsuccessful bridging
  - Proximal end convex and distal end concave (pseudoarthrosis).

Computed tomography

Magnetic resonance imaging: Bone scan—
- Used to detect the presence of synovial pseudoarthrosis—a cold cleft is seen between two areas of high uptake.
- Scintigraphy is employed to assess nonunion biological activity and infection.
- Scintigraphy is a particularly useful technique to distinguish hypervascular active nonunion and nonresponsive avascular nonunions.
- Indium scans are more sensitive and specific for diagnosing infections.

Positron emission tomography scan: *Positron emission tomography scan* increases the sensitivity and specificity when combined with bone scan and MRI for diagnosing infection and vascularity but cost is a prohibiting factor. *Laboratory investigations* are aimed to find infection at the nonunion site and include erythrocyte sedimentation rare (ESR), C-reactive protein (CRP), and total leucocyte count (TLC). Renal and liver functions are other investigations that can be done to find risk factors. For choosing surgical treatment, nutritional status of the patient should also be evaluated. Bone biopsy is rarely if ever employed to diagnose nonunion.

Treatment: Infected nonunion with implant in situ—
- Infected nail should be removed and either reaming alone in first stage or a masala nail be used to control infection. Renailing is an option once infection subsides after 6 weeks to 3 months.
- Infected plate needs to be removed thorough debridement done and either Ilizarov fixator or masala nail can be done. Usually nailing is avoided till infection heals.

Infected nonunion without any implant:
- Do staged procedure by first infection control and debridements followed by internal fixation or Ilizarov fixator application.
- Gap nonunion with unstable fracture can be treated by Ilizarov preferably or masquelet technique.

4B.17 KNEE: TRIPLE DEFORMITY, TRAUMATIC ARTHROTOMY (Q125–127)

125. A. What is triple deformity of knee?
B. What are its causes?
C. Its management in TB arthritis of knee.

Ans: A. Triple deformity of knee

Deformity components:

- *Flexion deformity at knee* (due to chronic nature of diseases and synovial effusion knee is commonly kept in position of maximum joint space–30° which persists to produce flexion deformity of knee).
- *Posterolateral subluxation of tibia* (most of chronic destructive diseases joint subluxates laterally—reasons are not clear; one explanation could be that in rheumatoid disease which commonly affects females there is already more physiological valgus which leads to increased stresses over lateral joint compartment, other more plausible one is that in destructive diseases there is exaggeration of the physiological alignment—remember there is a physiological valgus and posterior tibial slope in a normal knee joint).
- *External rotation of tibia over femoral condyles*–various reasons; quadriceps pull, popliteus action, iliotibial band (ITB), etc.

B. Classically, triple deformity of knee (above) is described for tuberculosis of knee. However, it is also found in various long-standing chronic diseases like rheumatoid arthritis and in ITB contracture.

C. *Management*

Children: The deformity and subluxation is initially corrected by double traction (for deformities above 60° flexion) or rarely by corrective plasters (for lesser degree of deformity). Residual deformity (<20°) can be corrected by orthosis and mobilization of the patient. Arthrodesis of the grossly destroyed knee in children should be deferred till the completion of growth potential of the distal femur and proximal tibia.

Adults: Initial debridement of joint (arthroscopic or open) should be done to remove hypertrophied synovium, removal of loose or rice bodies, debris, pannus, loose articular cartilage. If possible and needed careful curettage of osseous juxta-articular foci should be carried out under standard antitubercular chemotherapy cover. Maintenance is done by traction, intermittent active, and assisted exercises and later (2–3 weeks postoperative) suitable brace ambulation should be continued.

Arthrodesis as primary procedure can be performed in advanced arthritis or in cases which resulted in painful fibrous ankylosis during the process of healing. This is aimed to provide a painless stable knee and simultaneous correction of deformity. If done appropriately the disease load is markedly reduced to prevent recrudescence, and the patients can do long hours of standing and walking. Proper aggressive antitubercular treatment (ATT) is imperative as often advanced fulgurant disease shows wound dehiscence and sinus formation. This is because in advanced disease overlying capsule, subcutaneous tissue, and skin may be scarred, and may also be affected by the disease process. Compression arthrodesis of Charnley has limited role, if any and intra-articular procedure with excision of focus is mostly preferred.

126. What is triple deformity of knee?
Ans: Kindly see Answer to Question 125.

127. What is traumatic arthrotomy of knee joint? What is fluid challenge test? Outline principles of management.
Ans: Traumatic arthrotomy refers to opening up of joint externally or internally due to trauma and is more serious than a simple laceration. The articular cartilage undergoes irreversibly damaged by infection, and the joint has limited ability to fight infection. Therefore, all traumatic arthrotomies should be treated urgently. The injury is usually an "outside-in" injury but can be "inside-out" (i.e., periarticular bone pieces piercing the capsule and skin or joint dislocation).

Etiology: Trauma as above, needles, knives, thorns, nails, bullets, and animal or human bites have all been cited. There could be a puncture wound, bite, or laceration near a joint; or an open fracture into or adjacent to a joint. One should always look for the possibility of joint contamination and breach of sterility—as a thumb rule the joint is considered unsterile and contaminated unless proved otherwise, so appropriate treatment should be initiated.

Diagnosis: To determine whether a joint communicate with a laceration or open fracture, saline load test is performed. Saline (150 cc) with methylene blue is injected aseptically into the joint from an uninjured area. The presence of dye at the laceration site indicated that the sterility of the joint has been compromised. For individuals allergic to methylene blue or patients taking monoamine oxidase (MAO) inhibitors or other serotonergic drugs (methylene blue potentiates serotonin release in brain), either indigo carmine (1:100 dilution) or fluorescein dye should be used. The amount of saline required varies with the size of laceration, site of injection of fluid, etc. It is found that to detect 95% of 1 cm communicating lacerations around 150 mL of saline needs to be injected. There is a high incidence of false negatives in small joint lacerations (31–99% reported sensitivity) for this reason, joint sterility should mostly be considered to be compromised unless proven otherwise. The saline load test needs not to be done in patients whose radiographs show obvious intra-articular air or a foreign body.

Treatment:
- The treatment is formal arthrotomy. The traumatic arthrotomy site can be used for debridement, if it is in a convenient place and allows adequate access to the joint. Otherwise a convenient standard incision should be made to expose the joint adequately.
- In smaller traumatic arthrotomies, arthroscopy or a standard incision may be used to debride the joint. Antiseptics, surfactants, and saponifying agents used in open fractures are avoided for washing the hyaline cartilage.
- If infection is subacute or chronic, include a thorough synovectomy in the surgical debridement.
- It is a very good opportunity to confirm the suspected ligament injuries during the debridement. Ligament injuries, if present simultaneously, should be thoroughly assessed in operating room to formulate a plan for later reconstruction.

4B.18 DISCOID MENISCUS AND MENISCAL INJURIES (Q128–130)

128. Discuss the clinical features and management of discoid meniscus.

Ans: *Clinical features*: Discoid meniscus (3–5% population) is oval- or disc-shaped (instead of regular kidney bean shape), is thicker than normal meniscus, and has a posterior meniscal attachment. Discoid medial menisci are much less common than discoid lateral menisci, 25% are bilateral. Both complete (type II) and incomplete (type I) forms are described. Third variant (Wrisberg type, type III) does not have a posterior meniscal attachment. Being larger than normal they are more prone to injury. These types usually are asymptomatic, with no abnormal motion of the meniscus during knee flexion or extension. In type III, as the meniscus is relatively free (absent Wrisberg ligament), a popping sound is heard every time the knee is flex-extended and is frequently injured. This type is not disc shaped. Wrisberg-type discoid menisci often occur at a younger age than complete or incomplete types and are unassociated with trauma. Abnormal motion of this type of discoid meniscus results in a popping sound during knee flexion and extension (snapping knee syndrome).

If discoid meniscus is injured, symptoms are similar to those of any other meniscal tear: lateral joint line tenderness, clicking, and effusion.

Radiology: Plain radiographs demonstrate a widened joint space and squaring of lateral femoral condyle. The tibial plateau may show excessive cupping. The lateral tibial spine may be hypoplastic in complete types. MRI is the investigation of choice and demonstrates bow-tie sign with an abnormally thick and flat meniscus that covers entire lateral compartment on coronal images.

Management: An intact, discoid meniscus seen incidentally during arthroscopy or arthrotomy done for unrelated purpose does not necessarily require treatment. The proper treatment must be selected for each patient, and unless a stable, complete, or incomplete discoid meniscus has caused grooving, chondromalacia changes, or other pathological conditions within the compartment, meniscal balancing is possibly not needed.

Tears of complete or incomplete discoid menisci that cause pain, popping, and snapping within the knee and that show a hypermobile medial segment but intact peripheral attachments are best treated by saucerization of the mobile fragment. This can be done either by arthroscopic techniques or through an arthrotomy.

For a Wrisberg-type discoid meniscus, the treatment generally is total meniscectomy, either open or arthroscopic. Subtotal meniscectomy of type III discoid meniscus would certainly fail as it leaves an unstable rim of meniscus that is frequently caught between femoral and tibial condyles causing recurrent tears. Progressive osteoarthrosis after complete menisectomy is slow to develop in discoid cases.

129. Describe discoid meniscus.
Ans: Kindly see Answer to Question 128.

130. A. Describe, classify, and explain management of RAMP lesion of meniscus.
B. Explain indications and salient features of the different methods of meniscal repair.

Ans: Ramp lesions are longitudinal tears at the posterior horn of the medial meniscus, affecting the meniscocapsular junction or meniscotibial ligament, often associated with anterior cruciate ligament (ACL) injuries (15–42% prevalence). They contribute to knee instability.

Classification (Thaunat/Greif):
- *Type 1*: Stable meniscocapsular tear.
- *Type 2*: Stable partial superior tear.
- *Type 3A/B*: Unstable partial inferior tear or meniscotibial ligament tear.
- *Type 4*: Unstable complete meniscocapsular tear.
- *Type 5*: Unstable double tear.

Management:
- *Diagnosis*: MRI (48–86% sensitivity; fluid signal at meniscocapsular junction) and arthroscopy (trans-notch or posteromedial portal).
- *Stable lesions (types 1–2)*: Conservative; monitor during ACL reconstruction (high healing potential in red-red zone).
- *Unstable lesions (types 3–5)*: Arthroscopic suture hook repair via posteromedial portal; all-inside repair for smaller lesions. Combine with ACL reconstruction to restore stability.
- *Rehabilitation*: Limited weight-bearing (4–6 weeks), avoid deep flexion, return to sport at 6–9 months.

Indications and Salient Features of Meniscal Repair Methods

Indications for meniscal repair:
- Peripheral tears in red-red or red-white zones (vascular, within 5 mm of meniscocapsular junction).
- Longitudinal, bucket-handle, or ramp lesions (*especially Thaunat Types 3–5*: unstable).
- Younger patients (< 40 years), active individuals, or concomitant ACL reconstruction.
- *Contraindications*: Avascular (white-white) tears, degenerative tears, or osteoarthritis.

Methods of meniscal repair:
- *Inside-out repair*:
    - *Indications*: Longitudinal or bucket-handle tears in red-red/red-white zones; posterior horn tears.
    - *Features*:
        - Sutures passed from inside joint to outside, tied over capsule.
        - Precise, strong repair; high healing rate (80–90%).
        - Technically demanding; risks neurovascular injury.
        - *Rehab*: Nonweight-bearing 4–6 weeks, return to sport 6–9 months.
- *All-inside repair*:
    - *Indications*: Peripheral longitudinal tears; smaller ramp lesions (types 1–3).
    - *Features*:
        - Uses arthroscopic suture anchors (e.g., fast-fix) within joint.
        - Minimally invasive, faster; healing rate ~75–85%.
        - Higher failure rate (15–20%) for posterior tears.
        - *Rehab*: Similar to inside-out; earlier weight-bearing possible.

- *Outside-in repair*:
  - *Indications*: Anterior horn or mid-body tears.
  - *Features*:
    - Sutures passed from outside capsule into meniscus, tied externally.
    - Effective for anterior tears; lower neurovascular risk.
    - Limited for posterior horn/ramp lesions.
    - *Rehab*: Tailored to tear stability, 4–6 weeks limited weight-bearing.
- *Suture hook repair (posteromedial portal)*:
  - *Indications*: Unstable ramp lesions (types 3–5); posterior horn tears with ACL injury.
  - *Features*:
    - Sutures placed via posteromedial portal for precise repair.
    - Low failure rate (5–10%), high healing rate (80–90%).
    - Requires technical skill; risk of saphenous nerve injury.
    - *Rehab*: Nonweight-bearing 4–6 weeks, avoid deep flexion 6–8 weeks.
- *Meniscal root repair*:
  - *Indications*: Posterior/anterior root tears or avulsions mimicking ramp lesions.
  - *Features*:
    - Transosseous sutures/anchors reattach root to tibia.
    - Restores hoop stresses; healing rate ~85%.
    - Technically complex; longer rehab (6–12 months).
    - *Rehab*: Nonweight-bearing 6 weeks, return to sport 9–12 months.

4B.19 KNEE ARTHROSCOPY: UTILITY, LIGAMENT INJURIES AROUND KNEE DIAGNOSIS AND MANAGEMENT (Q131–149)

131. Enumerate portals for arthroscopy of knee joint. Describe various arthroscopies, their accessories, and indication of arthroscopy of knee joint.

Ans: *Portals*:
- *Standard portals*: Anterolateral, anteromedial, posteromedial, and superolateral
- *Optional portals*: Posterolateral portal, proximal midpatellar medial and lateral portals, accessory far medial and lateral portals, and central transpatellar tendon (Gillquist) portal.

Various types:
Following types of knee arthroscopy are described:
- Diagnostic knee arthroscopy
- *Therapeutic knee arthroscopy*: This can be further divided into two types—
  1. Therapeutic arthroscopy without implants (e.g., meniscectomy, chondroplasty, microfractures, etc.)
  2. Therapeutic arthroscopy with use of implants, e.g., anterior cruciate ligament (ACL) reconstruction.
- *Assistive arthroscopy*: Here the arthroscopy is done to assist another procedure, e.g., arthroscopic-assisted tibial plateau fracture fixation.

Indications:
- Meniscal tears
- Loose bodies in the knee joint
- Synovial plicae of the knee
- Osteochondritis dissecans of the femoral condyles and patella
- Crucial ligament tear
- Chondromalacia of the patella syndrome
- Fractures around the knee

- Arthrofibrosis
- Evaluation before proximal tibial osteotomies
- Débridement of osteoarthritis and abrasion arthroplasty.

Accessories: I do not really know what this part of question means, but may be they are asking for instrumentation or set-up accessories apart from standard. Mostly this includes arthroscopic pump, radiofrequency or VAPR probe, high-speed burr, recording facility, etc.

132. Describe etiology of loose bodies in knee. How will you manage a case of 30-year-old sportsman who presents with locked knee?

Ans: *Etiology*:
- Injury (a chip of bone or cartilage)
- Osteochondritis dissecans (which may produce one or two fragments)
- Osteoarthritis (pieces of cartilage or osteophyte)
- Charcot's disease (large osteocartilaginous bodies)
- Synovial chondromatosis (cartilage metaplasia in the synovium, sometimes producing hundreds of loose bodies).

Management of locked knee:
Differentiate between true and pseudo locking. Pseudo locking of knee may be caused by:
- A fracture
- Dislocation or subluxation, especially of the patella
- Bursitis
- Tendonitis
- Tendon tears.

These factors need to be individually assessed and corrected. (*Detailed reading of plica syndrome, patellar instability, and tendonitis needs to be read from Chapter 34 of the book Essential Orthopedics*: *Principles and Practice, 2nd edition.*)

True locking due to loose body or meniscal tears needs to be specifically corrected. Manipulation of knee has no documented role though many studies suggest good initial relief with the method. There are concerns of further joint damage due to manipulation that could extend the injury or produce secondary joint damage. Evaluate using X-ray and MRI for the offending cause of locking and true locking can usually be addressed arthroscopically in most of the cases. This also gives opportunity to inspect the joint and correct other pathologies, if present simultaneously.

133. Classify loose bodies.

Ans: Loose bodies can be classified into the following types:
- *Osteocartilaginous*: These loose bodies are composed of bone and cartilage and are detectable radiographically. Osteocartilaginous loose bodies may originate from several sources, the most common being osteochondritis dissecans, osteochondral fractures, osteophytes, and synovial osteochondromatosis.
- *Cartilaginous*: These radiolucent loose bodies usually are traumatic and originate from the articular surfaces of the patella or the femoral or tibial condyle.
- *Fibrous*: These radiolucent loose bodies occur less frequently and result from hyalinized reactions originating usually from the synovium secondary to trauma or, more commonly, from chronic inflammatory conditions. Synovial villi become thickened and fibrotic, may become pedunculated, and may detach and fall into the joint as loose bodies. Chronic inflammations, such as tuberculosis, may produce multiple fibrinous loose bodies known as "rice bodies."
- *Others*: Intra-articular tumors, such as lipomas, and localized nodular synovitis may be pedunculated and by palpation feel like loose bodies or, in rare instances, drop free into the joint. Bullets, needles, and broken arthroscopic instruments also may appear as foreign loose bodies within the knee.

134. Describe various clinical tests for evaluation of ligamentous injuries of knee.

Ans: Clinical tests:

Valgus and varus stress test: Though considered to test the collateral ligaments primarily these also test the additional stabilizing structures (secondary restraints) to varus and valgus stability including even the cruciates.

Method: The patient lies supine with the leg extended. To test the medial side, hold the ankle firmly with one hand while placing the other hand over the head of the fibula gripping the knee firmly. Push with an inward force in an attempt to open the side of the knee at 0° and at 30° of flexion.
- At 0° it tests the TCL, posteromedial capsule, and cruciates.
- At 30° of flexion, the TCL is isolated for testing its integrity.

For varus instability, the hand positions are reversed to test the lateral side with a varus force at 0° and then with 30° of flexion.
- At 0° the LCL and posterolateral capsule are tested.
- At 30° of flexion, the LCL is isolated for testing its integrity.

Apley's distraction test: The examiner applies distraction force to the leg to separate the tibia and femur and moves it back and forth. If the capsule or ligaments are injured pain will occur. This test distinguishes if the pain in knee is coming from meniscus injury or extra-articular structures. Torn meniscus pain will be relieved in distraction test.

Next the examiner applies compression and repeats the maneuver if the pain is due to meniscus tears then distraction test will be negative while pain will occur on compression test.

Anterior drawer test at 90° of flexion (sensitivity of 9-93%, mean 62%): The patient lies supine on table with knee flexed. The examiner holds upper tibia or leg with both hands encircling it immediately below the knee joint. Fingers are placed in the popliteal space and they ensure that the hamstrings are adequately relaxed as they lie on the tendons. The thumbs are placed on the medial and lateral joint lines. Examiner tries to pull the tibia forward, if the tibia slides forward from under the femur and there is no sudden "hard or firm" stop to translation this is considered a positive anterior drawer sign (the stop in ACL tears is often "mushy or soft").
- Grade 1 = translation of half inch (1.25 cm)
- Grade 2 = translation of half to three-fourths inch (1.25-1.9 cm)
- Grade 3 = translation of three-fourths inch or more (1.9 cm or more).

Slocum anterior rotary drawer test is basically anterior drawer test performed in both external as well as internal rotation of 30°.
- Excessive anterior translation with externally rotated tibia indicates—injury to posteromedial aspect of the joint capsule, the ACL or possibly the TCL.
- Anterior translation when the leg is internally rotated indicates that the ACL and posterolateral capsule may be torn.

Feagin modification—performing the test in sitting position with the legs hanging down the edge of table (relaxed muscles) and avoids the effect of meniscus.

Weather wax modification—placing the lower leg in examiner's axilla.

Lachman test (sensitivity of 60-100%; mean 84%): The Lachman test is preferred over drawer test. The Lachman test is done in approximately 30° of knee flexion. An attempt is made at translating the tibia anteriorly by holding on the proximal end of tibia with one hand and at the same time stabilizing the distal thigh by the other hand. For large thighs or small examiner hands following alternatives help:
- Place a tightly rolled towel or other support under the femur and use one hand to stabilize the femur and the other to anteriorly translate the tibia.
- Slide the lower leg off the edge of the examining table with the knee and femur supported by the edge of the table. Now stabilize the femur with one hand and use the other to anteriorly translate the tibia.
- *Prone Lachman test:* The patient lies prone with the knee and lower leg just off the edge of the table. This position minimizes any posterior sag of the tibia that can mask a positive test. Examiner then tries to translate the tibia.

The grading for Lachman test is performed as follows:
- Grade 1+ has 0-5 mm displacement with a firm end point.
- Grade 2+ has 5-10 mm displacement with no end point.
- Grade 3+ has greater than 10 mm displacement.

Pivot shift test of MacIntosh (sensitivity of 27-95%, mean 62%, specificity of 35-99% in chronic tears): The pivot shift test specifically elicits anterolateral rotary instability of which ACL injury is a part. It is used in chronic conditions and is a sensitive test when the ACL has been torn. Even in an ACL deficient knee, the capsule maintains reduction of tibia on femur in extension. This phenomenon is possibly attributed to anterolateral ligament (ALL) of Segond. Loss or deficiency of ALL is supposed to produce higher grades of pivot shift test. With the patient lying supine, the hip of the patient is flexed to 30°, knee is flexed to 20° and the leg is internally rotated by holding at the ankle to unlock knee. Internal rotation of tibial condyle is necessary to reverse the screw home mechanism (see earlier) and begin knee flexion. Unlocking the tibia this way relaxes the collaterals so that examiner can then flex knee. Examiner also keeps thumb of one hand over fibular head (pivot) while supporting the knee by fingers from behind. The knee is then further flexed and a simultaneous valgus force is applied by one hand at the level of proximal fibula (pivot) and an axial force is applied by the other hand holding ankle. In patients with damaged ACL and lateral knee structures, the lateral tibial plateau subluxates anteriorly producing a palpable shift of pivot (fibular head) or clunk when the knee is in 20–40° of flexion. With further flexion the knee is again reduced by the iliotibial band (ITB) that pulls back the tibia posteriorly.

The pivot shift is graded subjectively:
- Grade 1+ is pivot glide
- Grade 2+ is a pivot shift
- Grade 3+ is a gross pivot shift with feeling that the condyles will dislocate.

With grade 3+ pivot shift test it is assumed that the ALL is also torn or deficient so it should also be reconstructed.

Jerk test: The jerk test is pivot shift test begun in flexion and the knee is then extended. If there is anterior cruciate insufficiency the tibia will subluxate at about 20° of flexion as the knee moves into extension; producing a palpable shift or clunk.

Flexion-rotation drawer test of Noyes: Here the lower leg is held with the knee flexed between 15° and 30°. At 15°, the tibia is subluxated anteriorly with the femur externally rotated in an ACL deficient knee. As the knee is flexed to 30°, the tibia reduces posteriorly and the femur rotates internally.
- *Losee test* is similar to the flexion-rotation drawer test, but it is done in a side lying position.

Posterior drawer test: The posterior drawer test is performed in a position similar to the anterior drawer test, but in this test instead of anteriorly directed force, the proximal tibial plateau is pushed posteriorly. A positive posterior drawer test is indicated by posterior tibial translation and is due to damage to the posterior cruciate ligament (PCL).

External rotation recurvatum test: The athletic trainer grasps the great toe and lifts the leg off the table. In a PCL deficient knee the tibia externally rotates and slides posteriorly, an associated injury to the posterolateral joint capsule makes the test more conspicuous, due to posterolateral instability.

Posterior sag test of Godfrey: An apparent posterior sag in the PCL deficient knee when both the knees, which are placed in 90° flexion with the patient lying supine, are observed from the lateral aspect.

135. Describe mechanics of injury of unhappy triad of O'Donoghue.
Ans: Please read Chapter no. 3.

136. Describe Ober test.
Ans: Ober's test is performed to check for contracture of ITB. The test may also be used to evaluate inflamed tensor fasciae latae.

Iliotibial band is a broad ribbon-shaped band that tapers distally present on the lateral aspect of thigh. It receives attachment from tensor fasciae lata and gluteus maximus. It originates from iliac crest and inserts over Gerdy's tubercle of tibia.

The ITB provides stability to the extended knee joint and is synergistic to the hip abductors.

Test: Patient lies in lateral decubitus position [the non-test leg (lower leg) should be kept flexed at knee and hip to obliterate lumbar curve]. Stand behind the patient and stabilize elvis with left hand over iliac crest. With right hand hold the ankle of patient and bring test knee in flexion to 90°. Now produce hip abduction of 40° and then extend the hip as permitted. Now produce gentle hip adduction by lowering the leg preventing any internal rotation or flexion at the hip. If the ITB is shortened or tight the hip will not adduct. Patient may additionally feel lateral knee pain. In case of TFL inflammation lateral upper thigh pain will be observed over the muscle belly.

137. Outline management of chronic ACL insufficiency in a young athlete.

Ans: High-performance athletes invariably need an intact ACL. Arthroscopic ACL reconstruction using different graft choices has become the standard of care, the controversy here though is to choose between conventional vs anatomic; single-bundle reconstruction vs. double-bundle reconstruction. The latter requires higher level of training and experience but the results possibly are comparable to single-bundle anatomic reconstructions. Due to recent concerns raised for suboptimal results after ACL reconstruction it has been proposed that one should also carefully evaluate ALL patency especially in high grade pivot shift positive patients and those with anteromedial rotatory instability. There is often an ALL deficiency that negatively influences the results of ACL reconstruction so ALL should be additionally reconstructed in such cases. Lots of grafts have been proposed in the literature, however, the commonly used grafts for ACL reconstruction involve:

- *Autograft tissue*:
  - Bone–patellar tendon–bone graft—described by Jones in 1960, popularized by Erickson in 1970s.
  - Four-strand (quadruple) hamstring tendon (semitendinosus and gracilis)
  - Quadriceps tendon.
- *Allograft tissue*:
  - Patellar tendon
  - Achilles tendon
  - Tibialis anterior tendon
  - Posterior tibialis tendon.
- Synthetic—high failure rates and difficult revision so not used mostly.

Goals of surgical reconstruction: Restore knee stability; maintain normal knee motion, minimum donor site complications and return of patient to desired level of activity.

[Kindly also see Question 85 and Chapter 34 of the book *Essential Orthopedics: Principles and Practice*, 2nd edition, for details.]

138. A. Describe ACL injuries in female athletes.
B. Role of meniscal repair in knee joint.

Ans:

A. Female athletes are more prone to have ACL injuries due to anatomical and hormonal factors.
  - Narrower intercondylar notch and small ACL size
  - Wider pelvis
  - Ligaments laxer than in men
  - Slower reflex time
  - Changes in estrogen levels
  - Greater quadriceps or hamstring strength ratio
  - Flat foot landing.

B. The knee may function well without the meniscus, sometimes for the rest of a patient's life, but late degenerative changes within the joint do occur and now-a-days there is increasing tilt towards restoring the meniscus. Loss of meniscus even partial has been shown to cause:
  - Development of an anteroposterior ridge that projected distally from the margin of the femoral condyle
  - Flattening of the peripheral half of the articular surface of the condyle
  - Narrowing of the joint space.

These changes have been reported in 40–90% of patients with meniscectomy in ACL-deficient knees.

Patients who had any degree of meniscal resection reported significantly more subjective complaints and activity limitations than did those with intact menisci. Considerable evidence indicates that meniscectomy often is followed by degenerative changes within the joint, but whether the injury restoring normal (or near normal) anatomy is considered better than mutilation of joint. So meniscus repair should be done unless the torn fragment is fragile or is too interior to repair. For massive tear that cannot be repaired, meniscus allografting is an option.

(For details of meniscal repair kindly refer to Chapter 34 of the book Essential Orthopedics: Principles and Practice, 2nd edition.)

139. Describe all-inside technique for meniscal repair. What are its advantages and disadvantages?

Ans: Various meniscal repair devices that can be placed arthroscopically across the tear and tethering the same. The technique is truly arthroscopic, easier, quicker, and needs minimal assistance. Nearly all of the devices are based on reverse-barbed fish-hook design using bioabsorbable polylactic or polyglycolic acid copolymers. The tear are freshened and its distance from periphery is measured. Appropriate-sized fixator device is chosen and passed perpendicular to the tear so vertical longitudinal tears are most amenable to this method.

The fixators are best utilized for peripheral capsular detachments and meniscal allografts tethering. The head should be countersunk so that articular cartilage is not damaged. The various fixator devices available are either first-generation (meniscus arrow®, staple®, SD sorb staple®, biostinger®, fastener®, dart®, creafix screw®, etc.) or second-generation (RapidLoc®, FasT-Fix®, etc.).

The advantages of all-inside repair technique are:
- Quick
- Easy insertion
- Minimal or no assistance
- All arthroscopic
- Bioresorbable

The disadvantages of technique are:
- Limited compression, reduced strength
- Hydrolysis of implant is undefined and has variable course
- Breakage
- Chondral injury from prominent implant.

140. Meniscal transplantation.

Ans: Because not all meniscal tears can be repaired and arthritic changes may develop in the involved knee compartment in young patients; meniscal allografts, autograft fascial material, and synthetic menisci scaffolds have been developed. Meniscal transplantation is aimed to provide pain relief, improved function, lack of meniscal symptoms, lack of rejection, and peripheral healing of the graft. Long-term studies are missing so prevention of arthritis with this technique is unknown.

Meniscal allografts can be preserved in one of four ways: fresh, fresh frozen (deep freezing), freeze-dried (lyophilization), and cryopreserved but only cryopreservation maintains a substantially viable cell population (10–40%). On the other hand, deep-freezing or freeze-drying of meniscal tissue tends to decrease immunogenicity but cryopreservation maintains the content of donor human leukocyte antigen—encoded antigens and is more sensitizing to the host. The clinical significance of GVH disease for meniscus transplant is not fully known. With regards to disease transmission cryopreservation does not ensure sterilization but freeze-drying and gamma irradiation effectively eliminate the risk of viral transmission, however, the latter techniques cause graft shrinkage; irradiation >3 Mrad of gamma irradiation to kill HIV virus negatively affects the mechanical properties of collagen-containing tissues.

Meniscal allograft replacement using bone-plug technique is most preferred. Biologic tissue scaffolds for partial or complete meniscal replacement are under study. Sizing is best done on anteroposterior radiographs, and MRI may be used to determine meniscal coverage. The technique is divided into four parts: graft preparation, tunnel placement, graft insertion, and graft fixation.

Indications and prerequisites:
- Skeletally mature young patient with absent or nonfunctioning meniscus (previous meniscectomy) who is primary failure for management of knee pain and improving function. All other options for medical management of pain, including a thorough trial of conservative therapy and bracing techniques have failed.
- Meniscal damage is mechanical, not degenerative, and must not be caused by synovial disease. For a nonmechanical disease state the allograft fails.

- The pain should be localized to the affected compartment with activities of daily living or sports.
- The patient should have normal mechanical alignment, a stable knee, and only outer bridge grade I or grade II articular cartilage changes.
- A joint space of 2 mm or greater on standing posteroanterior view is necessary.

Contraindications:
- Knee instability
- Varus valgus malalignment (≡ Asymmetry of 2–4° or more compared with the contralateral knee or the weight-bearing line on long-leg alignment radiographs falls into the affected meniscus-deficient compartment).
- Advanced osteoarthritis.
- Chondromalacia greater than grade III
- Previous joint infection
- Relative contraindications are in patient needing simultaneous osteochondral allograft transplantations, ACL reconstructions, and realignment procedures.

141. Discuss current status of management of meniscal injuries of knee.

Ans: Kindly read and combine the Answers to Questions above.

142. A. What are the various types of grafts used to reconstruct ACL?
B. What is double bundle ACL reconstruction? Postoperative rehabilitation in ACL repair patients.
C. Steps to reconstruct multiligamentous injury around knee. D. Tests for clinical diagnosis of ACL injury?

Ans: A. The commonly used grafts for ACL reconstruction involve:
- *Autograft tissue*:
  - Bone–patellar tendon–bone graft—described by Jones in 1960, popularized by Erickson in 1970s.
  - Four-strand (quadruple) hamstring tendon (semitendinosus and gracilis)
  - Quadriceps tendon.
- *Allograft tissue*:
  - Patellar tendon
  - Achilles tendon
  - Tibialis anterior tendon
  - Posterior tibialis tendon.
- Synthetic—high failure rates and difficult revision so not used mostly (GoreTex, Leeds-Keho, LARS, etc.). These synthetic ligaments are now into their third generation having a knitted extra-articular portion with intra-articular free longitudinal fibers.

B. *Double bundle ACL reconstruction*: Considering the two-bundle anatomy of the native ACL. The technique usually involves making two femoral tunnels with one tibial tunnel, but some are also using two tibial tunnels. Biomechanical testing demonstrated improved ability to restore ACL function with reconstruction by two femoral tunnels, but improved clinical results have not yet been reported.

Postoperative rehabilitation:
- *For first 2 weeks*: Continuous passive motion (CPM) is started the next day and done for 5–10 hours/day. Dressing is done after 2 days and replaced with disposable or waterproof dressings. Cryotherapy should be given and continued for 5–7 days. Braces are often prescribed though there is no rationale to its use. They are used as protective methods and support to knee initially making the patient deliberately conscious and follow the mandatory precautions. Movements should be gained fast following surgery to allow 90° knee flexion by 5–7 days and full knee movements should be gained by 2–3 weeks. It is imperative to gain full extension by 7–10 days. For patellar tendon graft full weight-bearing is allowed immediately, but some physicians prescribe partial weight-bearing walk for hamstring graft.
- *2–6 weeks*: Brace is continued to protect the knee but movements should be gained fully by 3 weeks. Usually, knee brace is locked in full extension for 6 weeks while weight-bearing, if meniscus is also repaired concomitantly. Stationary bicycle is started for 5–7 days/weeks. Strengthening exercises are prescribed for quadriceps training and hamstring rehabilitation. Exercises remain closed chain.

- *6-12 weeks*: The braces are discontinued. Additional hip or trunk exercises are begun. Wall slides and chair squats to stretch the quadriceps are allowed. Open chain exercises are begun. Running, jumping, pivoting, and knee extension with weight-lifting machine are prohibited.
- *12-16 weeks*: Continue above exercises. Begin cardiovascular conditioning. Jump and plyometric training is begun. Progressive knee strengthening program is begun. Sports specific training is begun at 20-24 weeks.

C. For active individuals, the management is often a staged or single sitting reconstruction. Arthroscopic reconstruction for intra-articular ligaments is preferred; however, due to associated capsular injury, the reconstruction should be delayed by 3-6 weeks. Also they have often associated chondral injuries that need to be taken care of. Delay in reconstruction also helps reduce chances of arthrofibrosis. Nerve injuries are managed after reconstruction procedures. Electromyography (EMG) or nerve conduction velocity (NCV), if do not show any progress then neurolysis or nerve grafting is done as indicated. Posterolateral corner (PLC) injury is the most common association and should always be repaired, reconstructed or augmented with autograft or allograft.

D. The following tests help evaluate ACL tear:
- *Anterior drawer test at 90° of flexion (sensitivity of 9-93%, mean 62%)*: The patient lies supine on table with knee flexed. The examiner holds upper tibia or leg with both hands encircling it immediately below the knee joint. Fingers are placed in the popliteal space and they ensure that the hamstrings are adequately relaxed as they lie on the tendons. The thumbs are placed on the medial and lateral joint lines. Examiner tries to pull the tibia forward if the tibia slides forward from under the femur and there is no sudden "hard or firm" stop to translation this is considered a positive anterior drawer sign (the stop in ACL tears is often "mushy or soft").
    - Grade 1 = translation of half inch (1.25 cm)
    - Grade 2 = translation of half to three-fourths inch (1.25-1.9 cm)
    - Grade 3 = translation of three-fourths inch or more (1.9 cm or more).
- Slocum anterior rotary drawer test is basically anterior drawer test performed in both external as well as internal rotation of 30°.
- Feagin modification—performing the test in sitting position with the legs hanging down the edge of table (relaxed muscles) and avoids the effect of meniscus.
- Weatherwax modification—placing the lower leg in examiner's axilla.
- *Lachman test (sensitivity of 60-100%; mean 84%)*: The Lachman test is preferred over drawer test. The advantages are:
    - Can be performed in an injured knee without eliciting too much pain
    - Eliminates the hamstring tightness
    - No restriction from menisci.

  The Lachman test is done in approximately 30° of knee flexion. An attempt is made at translating the tibia anteriorly by holding on the proximal end of tibia with one hand and at the same time stabilizing the distal thigh by the other hand. For large thighs or small examiner hands following alternatives help:

  The grading for Lachman test is performed as follows:
    - Grade 1+ has 0-5 mm displacement with a firm end point
    - Grade 2+ has 5-10 mm displacement with no end point
    - Grade 3+ has greater than 10 mm displacement.
- *Pivot shift test of MacIntosh (sensitivity of 27-95%, mean 62%, specificity of 35-99% in chronic tears)*: The pivot shift test specifically elicits anterolateral rotary instability of which ACL injury is a part. It is used in chronic conditions and is a sensitive test when the ACL has been torn. With the patient lying supine, the hip of the patient is flexed to 30°, knee is flexed to 20° and the leg is internally rotated by holding at the ankle to unlock knee. Internal rotation of tibial condyle is necessary to reverse the screw home mechanism (see earlier) and begin knee flexion. Unlocking the tibia this way relaxes the collaterals so that examiner can then flex knee. Examiner also keeps thumb of one hand over fibular head (pivot) while supporting the knee by fingers from behind. The knee is then further flexed and a simultaneous valgus force is applied by one hand at the level of proximal fibula (pivot) and an axial force is applied by the other hand holding ankle. In patients with damaged ACL and lateral knee structures, the lateral tibial plateau subluxates anteriorly

producing a palpable shift of pivot (fibular head) or clunk when the knee is in 20–40° of flexion. With further flexion the knee is again reduced by the iliotibial band that pulls back the tibia posteriorly.

The pivot shift is graded subjectively:
- Grade 1+ is pivot glide
- Grade 2+ is a pivot shift
- Grade 3+ is a gross pivot shift with feeling that the condyles will dislocate. With grade 3+ pivot shift test it is assumed that the ALL is also torn or deficient so it should also be reconstructed.

- *Jerk test*: The jerk test is pivot shift test begun in flexion and the knee is then extended. If there is anterior cruciate insufficiency the tibia will subluxate at about 20° of flexion as the knee moves into extension; producing a palpable shift or clunk.
- *Flexion-rotation drawer test of Noyes*: Here the lower leg is held with the knee flexed between 15° and 30°. At 15°, the tibia is subluxated anteriorly with the femur externally rotated in an ACL deficient knee. As the knee is flexed to 30°, the tibia reduces posteriorly and the femur rotates internally.
- *Losee test* is similar to the flexion-rotation drawer test, but it is done in a sidelying position.

143. A. Mention briefly the intraoperative factors leading to failure of primary ACL reconstruction.
B. Discuss in short, the factors to be considered during revision ACL surgery.

Ans: The four most commonly cited technical errors that can lead to graft failure include improper tunnel placement, graft impingement, inappropriate graft tensioning, and poor graft fixation.

- *Improper tunnel placement*: The placement of bone tunnels in a nonanatomic position is the most common reason for graft failure. Inaccurate bone tunnels on the femur, tibia, or both, can subject the graft to abnormal forces even before the patient leaves the operating room. Malpositioned tibial tunnels, particularly those that are placed too anterior, lead to excessive graft lengthening during knee flexion or loss of flexion secondary to a tethering effect. Tibial tunnels that are positioned excessively posterior will result in a vertically oriented graft that is lax in flexion and unable to adequately resist anterior translational forces. Accurate tunnel placement is even more critical on the femoral side, because the femoral origin is close to the axis of rotation of the knee. Anterior femoral tunnels are created when the surgeon fails to appreciate the "over-the-top" position, and when tensioned between 0 and 30° of extension, the ACL will either lengthen during flexion or prohibit full knee flexion.
- *Graft impingement*: Graft impingement can result when tunnel placement in the sagittal plane is incorrect, or the surgeon fails to perform an adequate notchplasty. Bone tunnels that are either too far medial or lateral can impinge on the posterior cruciate ligament (PCL) or medial aspect of the lateral femoral condyle, respectively.
- *Graft tensioning*: Rough guidelines suggest that most grafts should be fixed with 5–10 lbs of tension while the knee is flexed between 10 and 15°, whereas higher loads may be applied with the knee in extension and axially loaded.
- *Graft fixation*: Newer screws with blunted threads have also helped to decrease the incidence of graft laceration, a rare complication that can result from interference screw placement. Bone plug fracture is another complication that has been reported in BTB ACL reconstructions.

B. *Factors to be considered during revision ACL surgery*:
- *Primary surgery details*: Drilling technique and fixation methods, and graft used. This will help guiding the revision surgery and graft choice
- *Clinical examination*: Gait examination for painful gait vs stiff knee gait vs varus thrust gait helps in clinical diagnosis. Cyclops lesion causes loss of extension while loss of flexion occurs in arthrofibrosis. Infection/inflammation is suggested by synovial proliferation, effusion, rise in temperature and possible sinus. Knee hyperextension should be carefully evaluated as also any rotatory instability of knee that remained uncorrected.
- Serology—CBC, ESR, CRP for assessment of infection
- *Imaging*: AP standing, lateral, Rosenberg and Merchant views for bone tunnel and patellar tracking assessment. Stress X-rays may be done for dynamic assessment. MRI is needed to look for synovitis, impingement, meniscal injury, other ligament injury and status of cartilage. CT scan better delineate the bony anatomy—tunnel position/dilatation/bone erosion.

144. **A.** Describe the surface marking of the arthroscopic portals for "Anatomic anterior cruciate ligament (ACL) reconstruction" with a 30° arthroscope.
B. Enumerate the risk factors for failure of a well-placed "Anatomic ACL reconstruction".
C. Describe the pros and cons of hamstring, soft tissue quadriceps, bone patellar tendon, and peroneal autograft for ACL reconstruction in a tabular form.

Ans: A. Surface Marking of Arthroscopic Portals for Anatomic ACL Reconstruction (30° Arthroscope)

Anatomic ACL reconstruction aims to restore the native ACL footprint using arthroscopic techniques. A 30° arthroscope is standard for visualization. Below is a brief description of the surface markings for the main arthroscopic portals, focusing on their anatomical locations and roles.

Anterolateral portal (viewing portal):
- *Surface marking:*
  - Located ~1 cm lateral to the patellar tendon, just inferior to the distal pole of the patella.
  - Approximately 1–2 cm above the lateral joint line, near the lateral border of the patella.
- *Purpose:* Primary portal for the 30° arthroscope to visualize the intercondylar notch, femoral and tibial footprints, and menisci.
- *Salient features:*
  - Positioned high and lateral to avoid fat pad impingement and optimize notch view.
  - Allows trans-notch visualization of posterior structures (e.g., ramp lesions).

Anteromedial portal (working portal):
- *Surface marking:*
  - Located ~1 cm medial to the patellar tendon, at or slightly below the level of the inferior patellar pole.
  - Approximately 1–2 cm above the medial joint line.
- *Purpose:* Primary working portal for instrumentation (e.g., femoral tunnel drilling, graft passage).
- *Salient features:*
  - Placed under arthroscopic guidance to ensure access to the femoral ACL footprint (anatomic position on lateral femoral condyle).
  - Adjustable to avoid cartilage damage or fat pad interference.

Accessory anteromedial portal (optional):
- *Surface marking:*
  - Located 1–2 cm medial and slightly distal (1–2 cm) to the standard anteromedial portal, closer to the medial joint line.
  - Marked with a spinal needle under arthroscopic visualization to confirm trajectory.
- *Purpose:* Facilitates femoral tunnel drilling at the anatomic footprint, especially in single-bundle or double-bundle reconstructions.
- *Salient features:*
  - Enhances access to the lateral femoral condyle without crowding the anteromedial portal.
  - Critical for precise tunnel placement in anatomic ACL reconstruction.

Posteromedial portal (optional for ramp lesions):
- *Surface marking:*
  - Located ~1 cm posterior to the medial femoral condyle, just above the posterior joint line.
  - Identified with trans-illumination or a spinal needle to avoid saphenous nerve/vein (~1 cm posterior to the nerve).
- *Purpose:* Used for visualization or repair of posterior horn meniscal tears (e.g., ramp lesions) with the 30° arthroscope.
- *Salient features:*
  - Requires careful placement to avoid neurovascular structures.
  - Provides direct access to the posterior compartment for suture hook repair.

B. Risk Factors for Failure of a Well-Placed Anatomic ACL Reconstruction

Despite optimal tunnel placement and surgical technique in anatomic ACL reconstruction, failure can occur due to various patient, surgical, and postoperative factors. Failure is typically defined as recurrent instability, graft rupture, or inability to return to preinjury activity levels. Below is a concise enumeration of the key risk factors:

- *Patient-related factors*:
  - *Young age (< 25 years)*: Higher activity levels and risk-taking behavior increase graft stress.
  - *High activity level*: Return to high-demand pivoting sports (e.g., soccer, basketball) increases re-rupture risk.
  - *Male sex*: Slightly higher failure rates due to greater muscle mass and forces on the graft.
  - *Obesity (BMI > 30)*: Increased joint loading and altered biomechanics.
  - *Generalized ligamentous laxity*: Compromises knee stability, stressing the graft.
  - *Meniscal deficiency*: Loss of meniscal tissue (especially posterior horn) increases anterior and rotational instability.
  - *Concomitant injuries*: Unaddressed injuries (e.g., posterolateral corner, ramp lesions) lead to persistent laxity.
  - *Smoking*: Impairs graft healing and vascularization.
- *Surgical factors*:
  - *Graft type*:
    - Allografts have higher failure rates (~2–3x) than autografts (e.g., hamstring, patellar tendon) in young, active patients.
    - Smaller graft diameter (< 8 mm for hamstring autografts) increases risk.
  - *Inadequate fixation*: Suboptimal graft fixation (e.g., loose screws, poor interference fit) leads to micromotion and failure.
  - *Missed associated injuries*: Failure to address ramp lesions, meniscal tears, or collateral ligament injuries increases graft stress.
  - *Suboptimal tunnel placement*: Even in "anatomic" reconstruction, minor deviations from the native footprint can alter biomechanics.
- *Postoperative factors*:
  - *Noncompliance with rehabilitation*:
    - Premature return to sport (< 6–9 months) before graft maturation.
    - Inadequate strength or neuromuscular control (e.g., weak quadriceps/hamstrings).
  - *Infection*: Septic arthritis compromises graft integrity (rare, < 1%).
  - *Trauma*: Early or late reinjury (e.g., pivot-shift mechanism) can cause graft rupture.
  - *Inadequate healing*: Poor graft incorporation due to biological factors (e.g., low vascularity, inflammation).
- *Biomechanical factors*:
  - *Increased tibial slope (> 12°)*: Elevates anterior tibial translation, stressing the graft.
  - *Persistent rotational instability*: Unaddressed anterolateral ligament (ALL) or capsular laxity increases failure risk.
  - *Malalignment*: Varus or valgus knee alignment overloads the graft.

Pros and cons of hamstring, soft tissue quadriceps, bone patellar tendon, and peroneal autograft for ACL reconstruction (**Table 4B.19.1**).

Graft type	Pros	Cons
Hamstring tendon (Semitendinosus ± Gracilis)	• Smaller incision, less anterior knee pain • Good tensile strength • Lower donor site morbidity than BPTB • Easier rehabilitation	• Tendon-to-bone healing (slower than bone-to-bone) • Potential hamstring weakness • Risk of graft elongation/stretch • Difficult to fix in small tunnels
Soft tissue quadriceps tendon	• Large cross-sectional area (good for large patients) • Can harvest with or without patellar bone plug • Lower anterior knee pain than BPTB • Strong and versatile	• Less familiarity among surgeons • Possible quadriceps weakness • Scar more visible (larger incision)

TABLE 4B.19.1: Comparison table of the four commonly used autografts for ACL reconstruction.

Contd...

Contd...

Graft type	Pros	Cons
Bone–patellar tendon–bone (BPTB)	• Bone-to-bone healing (fast and strong) • High initial fixation strength • Gold standard in many competitive athletes • Long-term stability data available	• Higher risk of anterior knee pain, kneeling pain • Patellar fracture/tendon rupture risk • Donor site morbidity • Risk of patellar tendinitis
Peroneus longus tendon	• Preserves hamstring and quadriceps strength • Long graft length, good tensile strength • Minimal functional loss (redundant ankle plantarflexion contributors) • Small incision at donor site	• Newer technique, less long-term data • Possible altered foot biomechanics in some patients • Requires careful harvesting to avoid nerve injury

145. **A. Describe the concept of "flexible guide wire and flexible reamer based femoral tunnel creation in arthroscopic anterior cruciate ligament (ACL) reconstruction."**
B. Describe its indications, advantages, and disadvantages.

Ans: In arthroscopic anterior cruciate ligament (ACL) reconstruction, the flexible guide wire and flexible reamer system enables anatomic femoral tunnel placement at the native ACL footprint without requiring extreme knee hyperflexion (> 20°), which is needed with traditional rigid systems. Using a curved, nitinol guide wire and flexible reamers, this technique allows precise tunnel drilling through the anteromedial portal at ~90° knee flexion, improving safety and accuracy.

Key features:
- *Flexible guide wire*: A nitinol wire with a curved tip navigates the femoral footprint independently of knee position, inserted via the anteromedial portal under arthroscopic visualization (30° scope).
- *Flexible reamer*: A bendable reamer follows the wire's path, creating a longer, anatomic tunnel (25–35 mm) through the lateral femoral cortex, avoiding medial condyle damage.
- *Purpose*: Ensures anatomic graft placement, optimizes tunnel length for suspensory fixation (e.g., cortical buttons), and reduces complications associated with rigid systems.

Indications:
- *Primary ACL reconstruction*: For anatomic single- or double-bundle ACL reconstruction, aiming to place the femoral tunnel at the native ACL footprint (lateral femoral condyle).
- *Revision ACL surgery*: When precise tunnel placement is needed, especially with prior nonanatomic tunnels.
- *Patients with anatomical challenges*: Narrow intercondylar notch or difficult knee hyperflexion, where rigid systems risk cartilage damage or nonanatomic tunnels.
- *Suspensory fixation preference*: When longer femoral tunnels (25–35 mm) are desired for cortical button fixation.

Advantages:
- Eliminates need for hyperflexion, reducing medial condyle scuffing.
- Longer tunnels (e.g., 30–35 mm) improve suspensory fixation stability.
- Anatomic placement enhances biomechanical outcomes (e.g., rotational stability).
- Comparable tunnel geometry to rigid systems with lower risk of cartilage damage.

Disadvantages:
- Requires specialized equipment and surgeon familiarity.
- Learning curve for precise wire/reamer handling.
- Potential cost increase due to flexible instruments.
- Limited evidence on long-term outcomes compared to rigid systems.

146. **What are closed and open chain exercises and discuss ACL rehabilitation protocol?**
Ans: *ACL Rehabilitation*:
- *For first 2 weeks*: CPM is started the next day and done for 5–10 hours/day. Dressing is done after 2 days and replaced with disposable or waterproof dressings. Cryotherapy should be given and continued for 5–7 days. Braces are often

prescribed though there is no rationale to its use. They are used as protective methods and support to knee initially making the patient deliberately conscious and follow the mandatory precautions. Movements should be gained fast following surgery to allow 90° knee flexion by 5–7 days and full knee movements should be gained by 2–3 weeks. It is imperative to gain full extension by 7–10 days. For patellar tendon graft full weight-bearing is allowed immediately, but some physicians prescribe partial weight-bearing walk for hamstring graft.

- *2–6 weeks*: Brace is continued to protect the knee but movements should be gained fully by 3 weeks. Usually, knee brace is locked in full extension for 6 weeks while weight-bearing, if meniscus is also repaired concomitantly. Stationary bicycle is started for 5–7 days/weeks. Strengthening exercises are prescribed for quadriceps training and hamstring rehabilitation. Exercises remain closed chain—means the foot is mandatorily kept in contact with the couch during course of exercise and should not be lifted in air or hang freely. Closed chain means there is a continuous loop made by hip knee leg foot and couch back to hip and this loop should not be disrupted.
- *6–12 weeks*: The braces are discontinued. Additional hip or trunk exercises are begun. Wall slides and chair squats to stretch the quadriceps are allowed. Open chain exercises are begun. Running, jumping, pivoting, and knee extension with weight lifting machine are prohibited.
- *12–16 weeks*: Continue above exercises. Begin cardiovascular conditioning. Jump and plyometric training is begun. Progressive knee strengthening program is begun. Sports-specific training is begun at 20–24 weeks.

147. **A. Describe the management of postoperative knee stiffness.**

B. Anatomy of posterolateral corner of knee and various patterns of injuries in this area.

Ans: A. Identify if the stiffness is due to bony irregularity or in soft tissue as after surgery poor reduction or implants may be the mechanical obstruction to movements. Soft tissues may get contracted due to prolonged immobilization or tenting over implants or may get adhered to bone surface that became raw during surgery. Also note if the stiffness is due to CRPS. The established stiffness has usually two components unless identified early in its course.

Intra-articular—dense intra-articular adhesions, extensive proliferation of fibrous scar tissue, retraction of periarticular soft-tissues, and bony impingement.

Extra-articular—quadriceps adhesions, muscle retraction due to scar tissue, skin adhesions to deeper tissue, and Hamstring tendon contractures.

Management options include a variety of open and arthroscopic surgical treatments; however, failure is eminent if all pathologies are not addressed by the utilized method or its combination. Manipulation under anesthesia is usually never employed these days due to too frequent complications and high recurrence rate. Any bony impingements must be treated before soft tissue release is performed.

Intra-articular stiff knees with a loss of flexion can be treated by an anterior arthroscopic arthrolysis. This is the preferred method of treatment of intra-articular soft-tissue causes of knee stiffness. This should be done early to have better outcome. Clear the lateral gutters and suprapatellar pouch that are most common sites of adhesion formation. Other adhesions should be released as indicated usually in the following order: release of patellar retinaculum→ lateral retinaculum release→ infrapatellar fat pad and tibial adhesions.

Extra-articular pathology causing a flexion contracture can be treated by open or endoscopic quadriceps release. Extension contractures can be treated by arthroscopic or open posterior arthrolysis. Open quadriceps release is the most common method deployed for correction of extra-articular contractures. For patella baja—lengthening of patellar tendon, allograft reconstruction, and proximalization of tibial tubercle may be done.

B. *Posterolateral corner of knee* represents large aponeurotic expansion of the lateral hamstrings **(Fig. 4B.19.1)**. Capsular ligaments form the central portion of this expansion and help in tibiofemoral stability. This expansion spans from the muscle belly to (and including) the meniscus (the meniscocapsular ligament-musculotendinous unit complex) **(Fig. 4B.19.2)**.

- The anterolateral ligament (ALL, Vieira and Vincent) or mid-third lateral capsular ligament of Hughston and Johnson has recently caught the interest of anatomists and orthopedic surgeons (while intriguing the less than complete results of ACL reconstruction). It is also known as "capsulo-osseous layer of the iliotibial band", "anterior oblique ligament", etc. Orthopedicians have found incompetence of the ALL to negatively influence the results of ACL reconstruction and recommend simultaneous reconstruction of ALL to optimize the results.

- The popliteal tendon inserts at lateral epicondyle slightly anterior to the origin of fibular collateral ligament. The popliteal muscle belly takes its origin from the proximal posterior fibula coursing obliquely and proximally continuing with the tendon. It is attached to the lateral meniscus through anteroinferior, posterosuperior, and posteroinferior popliteal meniscal fascicles. The functions of the popliteus muscle include stabilizing the knee during flexion and protecting the lateral meniscus by pulling it posteriorly while contracting. The popliteus is also a secondary restraint to posterior tibial translation. It also plays role in screw home mechanism.
- The fibular collateral ligament is a round, fibrous cord and courses distally to insert just anterior to the lateral aspect of the fibular head. It is taut during knee extension, but relaxed during flexion. It is the primary static varus restraint for the knee (especially at 30° of flexion) and limits external rotation at 30° of flexion.
- The popliteal fibular ligament originates at the popliteal musculotendinous junction and courses distally to attach to the medial aspect of the fibular styloid.
- Both the popliteus and popliteal fibular ligament provide restraint against tibial external rotation at higher flexion angles (≈ 60° of flexion).
- The fabellofibular ligament originates from the lateral aspect of fabella and inserts lateral to the tip of the fibular styloid just lateral to the insertion of the popliteal fibular ligament.
- The arcuate ligament is formed by thickening in the posterior joint capsule and has three components:
    - The lateral portion borders mid-third capsular ligament.
    - The medial portion lies deep to the lateral gastrocnemius head.
    - Posterior component merges with the oblique popliteal ligament.

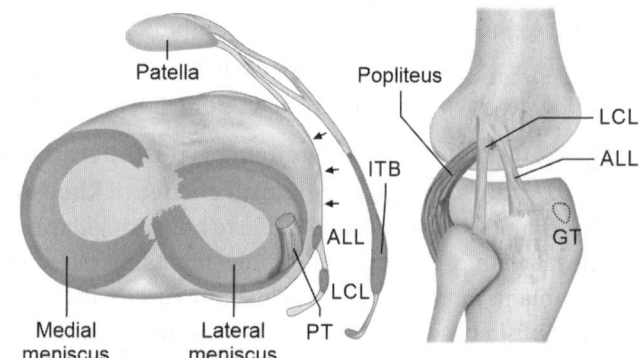

Fig. 4B.19.1: Anatomy of posterolateral corner of knee.

    The arcuate complex comprises of the fibular collateral ligament, popliteus, lateral head of the gastrocnemius muscle, and arcuate ligament.

    Injuries of the PLC are far less common than collateral or cruciate ligament damage, but they rarely occur isolated also.
- Isolated PLC injuries account for only 1.6% of all knee ligament injuries. Associated ligamentous injuries are common ranging from 43% to 80% of cases.
- Anterior cruciate ligament or PCL injury is most commonly associated.
- Posterolateral corner injuries are seen in association with tibial plateau fractures significantly (68%).
- Neglected PLC injury can render isolated anterior or posterior cruciate reconstructive surgery unsuccessful.

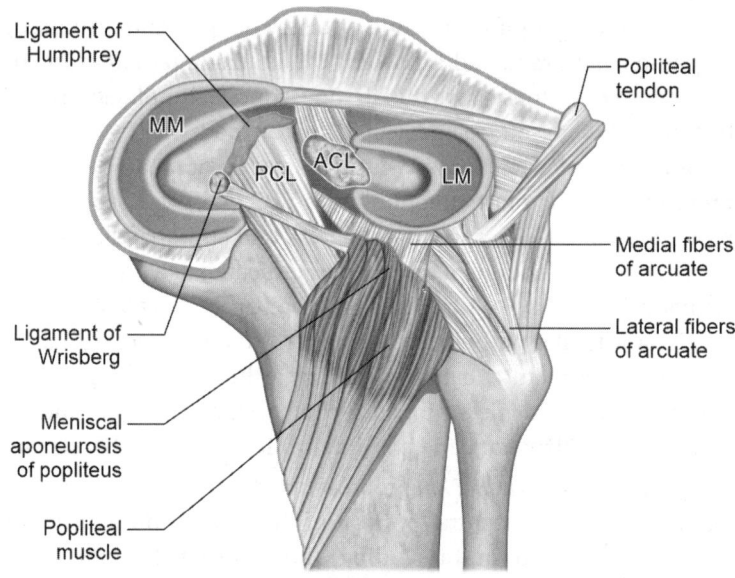

Fig. 4B.19.2: Anatomy of posterolateral corner of knee as in profile view.

148. Discuss clinical tests, diagnosis, and management of posterolateral corner (PLC) injury.

Ans: Clinical tests for diagnosing PLC injury:

- *External rotation recurvatum test (Hughston and Norwood, discussed above)*: The examiner holds onto both of the patient's great toes with knee in extension and lifts their heels off of the examination table at the same time. The affected knee hyperextends and the tibia rotates externally.
- *Posterolateral drawer test (Hughston and Norwood)*: With the knee in 90° of flexion, the foot is rotated externally by 15°. Posteriorly directed force is applied to the proximal tibia and degree of subluxation is compared to normal leg. A positive posterolateral drawer test usually indicates a popliteal tendon or popliteofibular ligament (PFL) injury.
- Varus stress testing
- *Dial test*: Performed at 30 and 90° of knee flexion. Positive test at 30° knee flexion suggest PLC injury, while at 90° knee flexion indicates combined posterior cruciate ligament (PCL) and PLC injury.
- *Reverse pivot shift test (Jakob, 1981)*: With knee at 70–80° of flexion and foot externally rotated, posterior sag of tibia is noted due to posterior subluxation. The leg is then slowly brought into full extension as a valgus force is applied. With this maneuver performed slowly, the knee is felt to reduce at about 20° of flexion.

Grading PLC injury (this is arbitrary grading based on varus stress test and posterolateral drawer test, not validated, it helps in differentiating severe injuries from milder ones):

- Grade I injuries have minimal instability (either varus 0–5 mm opening or rotational instability 0–5°).
- Grade II injuries have moderate instability (6–10 mm or 6–10°).
- Grade III injuries have significant instability (> 10 mm or > 10°).

Diagnosis:

Radiographs: May show a variable combination of:

- Segond lateral capsular avulsion fracture [seen also with anterior cruciate ligament (ACL) injuries]
- Medial segond fracture (usually with combined PCL and PLC injuries).
- Arcuate sign (fibular styloid fracture)—pathognomonic sign for PLC injury. It is better seen in lateral radiographs in slight external rotation.
- Gerdy tubercle avulsion fracture
- Abnormal widening of lateral joint space.

Magnetic resonance imaging (MRI): Grade 1 injuries are visualized as increased signal intensity on T2-weighted images superficial to ligament; grade 2 injuries are seen as increased signal intensity within the ligament, but ligament is in continuity; grade 3 injuries are visualized as complete disruption of the ligament with deep and superficial edema.

Management of PLC injury:

Nonoperative: For milder grade 1 injuries and minimal disability to patient:

- Hinged knee brace × 6 weeks
- Locked in extension for ambulation
- Progressive ROM, WB and strengthening with return to activity at 3–4 months.

Operative care is acceptable in avulsion fractures, multiligament injuries and grade 3 injuries. For grade 2 injuries, meticulous reconstruction gives good results, particularly in active individuals and sports persons.

- Acute ligament repair (<3–4 weeks) is indicated with sutures and anchors or bioscrews fixing the avulsed fragments with attached ligamentous structures. Acute repair is always better than late reconstruction.
- *Reconstruction of the PLC*: Mainly following techniques are used:
- *Nonanatomical*: Biceps tenodesis, proximal bone block advancements, extracapsular iliotibial (ITB) sling, and arcuate complex reconstruction
- Anatomical reconstructions of prominent ligaments, such as the Laprade style anatomic reconstruction or fibular-based Larson type reconstruction, are commonly preferred. These aim to reconstruct the functionally predominant components of PLC like, the fibular collateral ligament, PFL and popliteus tendon.

- Larson procedure aimed at reconstructing the lateral collateral ligament (LCL) and PFL with distal insertion sites located at the fibula. It was one of the first fibular-based techniques. It is less technically demanding with good clinical results. The anatomical reconstructions are more cumbersome and detailed with potential for overconstraining PLC if force distribution between LCL and PFL is not balanced.

149. Describe the symptoms of posterolateral corner (PLC) injury. Briefly discuss principles of its surgical reconstruction.

Ans: *Symptoms*:

Symptoms of PLC injury:
- *Instability*: The patient may experience a feeling of instability in the knee, especially during activities that require pivoting or changing direction.
- *Lateral knee pain*: There is often localized pain along the outer side of the knee, which can be exacerbated by weight-bearing activities.
- *Swelling*: Swelling around the knee may occur due to internal bleeding or inflammation resulting from the injury.
- *Difficulty with movement*: Patients may have difficulty fully extending or flexing the knee due to pain or mechanical instability.
- *"Giving way" episodes*: The knee may "give way" during activities, leading to unpredictable loss of control.
- *Bruising*: There may be bruising on the outer aspect of the knee, often seen after an acute injury. Patients with chronic instability have activity limitation secondary to instability. Running is difficult because of a varus thrust gait. Knee gives-way during extension maneuvers requiring absolute stability posteriorly (preventing posterior subluxation of femur) as in climbing stairs. Pivoting maneuvers cause the lateral tibial plateau to rotate externally and this produces symptoms of instability—especially in football.

Principles:

The principles of surgical reconstruction for a PLC injury focus on restoring knee stability and function. Here is a brief overview:
- *Accurate diagnosis*: A thorough assessment using physical examination and imaging (like MRI) is essential to determine the extent of the injury and plan the surgical approach.
- *Reconstruction of ligaments*: The primary goal is to repair or reconstruct key ligamentous structures, including:
    - *Lateral collateral ligament (LCL)*: Often reconstructed using autografts (e.g., hamstring or quadriceps) or allografts.
    - Popliteofibular ligament (PFL) and popliteus tendon may also require repair or reconstruction to restore full PLC function.
- *Anatomical restoration*: The surgical technique should aim to restore the ligaments to their anatomic positions, ensuring proper tensioning of grafts to maintain stability while allowing for normal knee movement.
- *Addressing concurrent injuries*: If there are associated injuries, such as to the ACL or PCL, these should be managed simultaneously to ensure comprehensive knee stabilization.
- *Postoperative rehabilitation*: A carefully designed rehabilitation program is critical for recovery. This includes range of motion exercises, strengthening, balance training, and eventually returning to sports and high-impact activities.

4B.20 MANAGEMENT OF CARTILAGE DEFECT IN KNEE (Q150–155)

150. What is osteochondritis dissecans (OCD) of femoral condyles? Discuss its classification, clinical features, and diagnosis.

Ans: Osteochondritis dissecans is a pathological destruction of the subchondral bone following necrosis that eventually separates as an osteochondral fragment with disease progression, the overlying articular cartilage, however, often survives for considerable time due to nourishment from synovial fluid.

Classification:
- The Harding classification for localizing the osteochondritis lesion on lateral projection dividing into three zones. Zone A is in front of the Blumensaat line. Zone C is behind the tangential line to the posterior cortex of the femoral diaphysis. Zone B is between zones A and C.

- The Cahill and Berg classification for localization of OCD lesion on AP projection of knee dividing into five zones. Zone 1: medial condyle (internal half). Zone 2: Medial condyle (external half). Zone 3: Femoral notch. Zone 4: Lateral condyle (internal half). Zone 5: Lateral condyle (external half)

Staging/grading of OCD is given in **Table 4B.20.1**.

TABLE 4B.20.1: Staging/grading of osteochondritis dissecans (OCD).

Radiological staging of OCD (Bedouelle)	Magnetic resonance imaging (MRI) grading of OCD	Arthroscopic grading of OCD	Surgical staging of OCD
Stage 1: Incomplete lesion with well-defined image (1a) with more or fewer calcifications within (1b)	Grade 1: Thickening of cartilage, no break in cartilage. Low signal changes	Stage 1: Irregularity and softening of cartilage. No definite fragment is seen	Stage 1: Stable lesion in continuity with host bone, intact articular cartilage
Stage 2: Presence of a nodule (2a) with more or less shrinkage of nodule in relation to condyle (2b)	Grade 2: Fissure in cartilage. Low signal rim behind fragment indicating fibrous attachment	Stage 2: Fissure in cartilage, definite fragment seen, but fragment not displaceable	Stage 2: Stable lesion on probing, partly discontinuous from parent bone
Stage 3: Sleigh Bells aspect—the fragment dangling from a thin pedicle and is shaped like a small Christmas bell	Grade 3: Cartilage breached, high signal on T2 behind fragment indicating synovial fluid between fragment and underlying bone	Stage 3: Discrete fragment, displaceable, but still attached by fibrous attachment or by overlying cartilage	Stage 3: Unstable lesion on probing, but fragment in position. Fragment separated from bone completely
Stage 4: Free fragment in the joint with empty bed	Grade 4: Loose body	Stage 4: Loose fragment and osteochondral defect	Stage 4: Dislocated free fragment in the joint

Clinical features: Vague and poorly localized pain of insidious onset is the usual complaint. Later with fragment separation clicking, popping or locking may be reported. The symptoms are often associated with activity. On examination, mild-to-moderate effusion with muscle atrophy is observed. The lesion may be tender to palpation. For knee, Wilson's test may be helpful. Subtle restriction of movements (like loss of terminal extension of knee or elbow) is quite characteristic and should caution one to investigate the lesions thoroughly.

Diagnosis:
- Radiographs are less sensitive and specific to diagnose early lesions. The two-dimensional imaging is liable to miss the lesions with overlapping bony structures of bones in joints. Special views to demonstrate the suspected articular surface should be done like tunnel views for knee and special views for capitellum and talar dome. If radiographs are normal, usually further evaluation is not required, unless very high suspicion remains or if the symptoms are escalating.
- MRI seems to be the modality of choice for investigating the lesion, especially staging them once demonstrated on radiographs. For a large number of possible bilateral lesions, the contralateral joint should be examined on identifying pathology in one joint. The MRI staging is also helpful for differentiating the stable lesions from unstable ones (Grade II vs. Grade III) as the latter require definite surgical intervention. Further help can be obtained from arthroscopy.
- Arthroscopy of the joint, quite commonly recommended, is a good therapeutic modality, but may miss initial lesions as the articular cartilage is frequently normal till quite late. The arthroscopic staging closely matches the MRI staging system.
- Technetium bone scans have been proposed to partly determine the possible success of conservative management. If a significantly increased uptake is observed, then it suggests marked osteoblastic activity, so that the conservative management would be successful.
- Ultrasonography is highly user dependent and may be useful in evaluating lesions of elbow if done by an experienced person.

151. **A. Describe the arthroscopic management of osteochondral lesions of knee.**
B. Discuss the etiology of osteochondritis dissecans.

Ans: A. Arthroscopic evaluation and treatment are indicated in all patients who are 12 years old or older as determined by bone age radiographs, and who have lesions larger than 1 cm in diameter located primarily in a weight-bearing area.

Treatment of the lesion is based on the arthroscopic examination. The lesions are classified into one of the following groups: (1) intact lesions, (2) lesions showing signs of early separation, (3) partially detached lesions, and (4) craters with loose bodies (salvageable or unsalvageable). Arthroscopic procedures usually undertaken in knee are:
- Removal of loose bodies in osteochondritis dissecans for bodies that are already completely detached and floating free within the joint usually are not suitable for reduction and fixation or bone grafting.
- Facilitation of regeneration by "microfracture" technique
- Pinning or refixation of salvageable fragment for large osteochondritis dissecans (>2.5 cm). Screw fixation devices are preferable as they allow compression and better stabilization of the lesion than the absorbable pin fixation.

B. The etiology of osteochondritis dissecans is controversial and remains unclear. Theories include ischemia, repetitive microtrauma, familial predisposition, endocrine imbalance, epiphyseal abnormalities, accessory centers of ossification, growth disorders, osteochondral fracture, repetitive microtrauma with subsequent interruption of interosseous blood supply to the subchondral area of the epiphysis, anatomic variations in the knee, and congenitally abnormal subchondral bone. Duthie and Houghton proposed a model of development of osteochondrosis:
- Normal epiphysis subjected to extreme trauma, for example, "pitcher's elbow" with osteochondritis dissecans of capitellum
- Mildly dyschondrotic epiphysis subjected to more than usual stress, for example, Perthes disease
- Severely affected dyschondrotic epiphysis subjected to normal stress, for example, capital femoral epiphysis in Gaucher's disease.

The differences in the clinical pictures of osteochondritis dissecans between a skeletally mature patient and a child with open physes have led some to conclude that osteochondritis dissecans in a young patient simply may be a variant of normal growth. Biochemical abnormalities in the form of altered expression of matrix metalloproteinases (MMP-1, 3, 13), altered collagen to proteoglycan ratio, glycosaminoglycans and aggrecan overexpression consequent upon altered mechanics furthering cartilage damage are all proposed but need further assertion by concrete evidence.

152. Describe pathogenesis and clinical features of medial compartment osteoarthritis.

Ans: *Pathogenesis*: There are two major mechanisms of osteoarthritis development. The first one involves failure of defective cartilage (genetic or otherwise) to sustain normal joint loading causing joint damage. The other one involves normal cartilage that is injured by repeated microtrauma or a single traumatic event. A genetic basis appears possible for polyarticular small joint nodal arthritis in women. Traumatic insult and increased IL1 stimulate chondrocytes to undergo cell division (cloning) and start repair, producing increased quantities of collagen, metalloproteinases and proteoglycans. This leads to thickening of cartilage in the very early stages of osteoarthritis (because of increased proteoglycan accumulation) but the repaired tissue has qualitatively inferior type 1 collagen and has increased fibronectin. Patchy sclerosis and osteophytes, however, reduce bone elasticity transferring increasing loads to the cartilage causing further damage.

Joint instability and/or mechanical derangement is the most important factor for development of unicompartmental osteoarthritis in lower limbs. Even 5° of varus at knee increases 70–90% loading of the medial knee compartment increasing the risk of osteoarthritis fourfold while 5° of valgus increases similar risk in lateral compartment by five times.

Clinical features:
- Pain is undoubtedly the most important symptom of osteoarthritis, especially activity related or mechanical pain.
- Stiffness of short duration ("gelling" of joints) often described as a short-lived stiffness seen after inactivity localized to the joint region.
- Joint instability—This is a feeling of instability or buckling (shifting of bone surfaces without actually giving way).

The *physical findings* of osteoarthritis include:
- Joint line tenderness due to myofascial trigger points, adjacent bursitis or tendonitis, and ligament enthesopathy.
- Crepitus on joint movement—palpable cracking or crunching sound.
- Bony enlargement often felt along the joint line
- Restricted joint ROM—Caused by variable contribution of pain, effusion, capsular contractures, muscle spasm or weakness, loose bodies, joint malalignment and altered center of rotation.
- Painful ROM especially terminal in early disease that increases in arc with disease progression.

- Joint deformity—varus and fixed flexion deformity at knee
- Muscle atrophy.

153. Describe treatment options of focal cartilage defect over medial femoral condyle in a 40-year-old man.

Ans: The surgical repair strategies for focal cartilage defects in a young patient broadly fall into the following groups:
- *Palliative*:
    - Neglect
    - Arthroscopic lavage
    - Radiofrequency ablation (RFA).
- Marrow (subchondral) stimulation
- *Reconstruction using direct tissue transfer*:
    - Mosaicplasty
    - Osteochondral autograft transfer system (OATS)
    - Allograft implantation.
- *Newer strategies aiming to obtain hyaline cartilage*:
    - Cell-based repair
    - Scaffold-based repair
    - Cell + scaffold based repair
    - Cell + scaffold + growth factors.

(Kindly refer to Chapter 10 of the book Essential Orthopedics: Principles and Practice, 2nd edition, for details of each of the methods.)

154. Describe the principles of chondroplasty in osteoarthritis of knee joint.

Ans: Chondroplasty (arthroscopic debridement) is arthroscopic cartilage preserving procedure for degenerative disease of the knee. The method is based on preserving the remaining cartilage by minimizing mechanical damage to it. The procedure is not aimed at promoting regeneration of the cartilage. It is expected to give relief from pain, recurrent effusions, and mechanical symptoms in patients with focal cartilage defects that can be reformed or smoothened. The surgical technique is variable and depending on surgeon or center it can be one of the following:
- *Radiofrequency thermal ablation*: Monopolar and bipolar RFA are both used. Its efficacy for articular cartilage lesion treatment has remained controversial due to the risk of normal tissue damage and osteonecrosis. The greatest limitation is that this is a technique only for "partial thickness defects"; one cannot expect cartilage formation at bald surfaces using radiofrequency energy (RFE). The biggest advantage of RFE is that it is a simple tool that can be delivered arthroscopically under direct vision; it is inexpensive and safe for operating room personnel.
- *Mechanical chondroplasty*: This is done using a regular arthroscopic shaver system however problems of accessibility to all lesions and precision is a major limitation.
- *Abrasion chondroplasty*: This is done using laser [Holmium:Yag (Ho:YAG)]. Laser has been expected to be helpful for preventing damage to the intact cartilage and articular cartilage roughening, which can occur during mechanical shaving. However, severe abrasion on the intact cartilage, osteonecrosis, risk to operating room personnel and high cost are increasingly recognized as problems of the use of laser.

(Details on arthroscopic lavage and radiofrequency are available in Chapter 10 of the book Essential Orthopedics: Principles and Practice, 2nd edition.)

155. A. Cartilage grafting
B. Focal resurfacing implants

Ans: A. Cartilage Grafting in Orthopedics

Definition and purpose: Cartilage grafting is a surgical technique used to repair localized articular cartilage defects, typically in weight-bearing joints (knee, ankle, and hip). It aims to restore joint function, reduce pain, and delay or prevent osteoarthritis progression.

Types of cartilage grafting:
Autografts (patient's own tissue):
- Osteochondral autograft transfer (OATS/mosaicplasty):
  - *Method*: Harvests cylindrical plugs of healthy cartilage + subchondral bone from nonweight-bearing areas (e.g., femoral trochlea) → implants into the defect.
  - *Best for*: Small defects (1–2 cm^2).
  - *Pros*: Single-stage procedure, high integration rate.
  - *Cons*: Donor-site morbidity (knee pain in 10–20% of cases).
- Autologous chondrocyte implantation/matrix-Induced autologous chondrocyte implantation (ACI/MACI):
  - *Method*:
    1. *Stage 1*: Arthroscopic cartilage biopsy → lab expansion of chondrocytes.
    2. *Stage 2*: Implantation under a periosteal patch (ACI) or scaffold (MACI).
  - *Best for*: Larger defects (2–5 cm^2).
  - *Pros*: Hyaline-like cartilage regeneration.
  - *Cons*: Two surgeries, longer rehab (9–12 months).

Allografts (donor tissue):
- Osteochondral allograft transplantation:
  - *Method*: Uses cadaveric cartilage-bone grafts for large defects (> 2 cm^2).
  - *Best for*: Young patients with extensive lesions or failed prior grafts.
  - *Pros*: No donor-site morbidity, good for irregular defects.
  - *Cons*: Limited availability, risk of immune rejection (rare).

Synthetic/bioengineered grafts:
- *Examples*: Hyaluronan scaffolds, collagen matrices (e.g., Chondro-Gide®).
- *Best for*: Adjuvant to microfracture or ACI.

Indications:
- *Ideal candidate*:
  - Age < 50, focal defect [International Cartilage Repair Society (ICRS) Grade III–IV], stable joint, minimal osteoarthritis.
- *Common sites*:
  - Knee (femoral condyles, trochlea, and patella), talus, hip.

Outcomes of various techniques for management of cartilage defect **(Table 4B.20.2)**.

TABLE 4B.20.2: The reported outcome of various cartilage grafting techniques.

Metric	OATS	ACI/MACI	Allograft
Success rate	85–90% (10 years)	75–85% (10 years)	80–90% (5 years)
Rehab time	4–6 months	9–12 months	6–9 months
Return to sport	60–70%	50–60%	50–70%

(ACI: autologous chondrocyte implantation; MACI: matrix-Induced autologous chondrocyte implantation; OATS: osteochondral autograft transfer)

Key advantages:
- Preserves native joint, delays arthroplasty.
- Better long-term outcomes versus microfracture (fibrocartilage formation).

Limitations:
- Not suitable for diffuse arthritis.
- Complex rehab [nonweight bearing (NWB) phases, continuous passive motion (CPM) required].

Focal Resurfacing Implants in Orthopedics

Definition and purpose: Focal resurfacing implants are localized, bone-preserving prostheses designed to treat isolated chondral or osteochondral defects in joints (typically knee, hip, or ankle). Unlike total joint replacements, they replace only the damaged area, preserving healthy bone and cartilage.

Types of Focal Resurfacing Implants
Metal/polymer implants:
- *Examples*: HemiCAP® (shoulder/knee), Episealer® (knee)
- *Design*:
  - Metal (cobalt-chrome) cap anchored into the defect.
  - Polyethylene (PE) liner in some designs for articulation.
- *Best for*: Medium to large focal defects (1–5 cm²) in older patients (50+ years) or failed prior cartilage repair.

Biopolymer hydrogel implants:
- *Example*: BioPoly RS® (partial knee resurfacing)
- *Design*:
  - Metal base + hydrogel (polyurethane) surface mimics cartilage.
  - *Advantage*: Shock absorption, low wear rates.

Custom 3D-printed implants:
- *Emerging tech*: Patient-specific designs based on CT/MRI.

Indications:
- Focal chondral/osteochondral defects (ICRS Grade III-IV)
- Early osteoarthritis (OA) in one compartment (not diffuse OA)
- Failed prior cartilage repair (OATS, ACI)

Contraindication: Inflammatory arthritis, infections, or severe malalignment.

Surgical technique:
- *Preoperative planning*: 3D imaging for implant sizing.
- *Approach*: Mini-arthrotomy or arthroscopy-assisted.
- *Implantation*: Ream defect → press-fit or screw-fixated implant.
- *Recovery*:
  - *Weight-bearing*: Immediate (vs. 6–12 weeks for grafts).
  - *Rehab*: 6–8 weeks to full activity.

Outcomes and comparisons **(Table 4B.20.3)**.

TABLE 4B.20.3: The comparison of focal implant to cartilage grafting technique.

Factor	Focal implant	Cartilage graft (OATS/ACI)
Defect Size	1–5 cm²	1–4 cm² (autograft)
Age	>50 years	<50 years
Recovery	6–8 weeks	6–12 months
Durability	5–10 years	10–15 years (biological)
Pros	Fast recovery, simple	Biologic integration
Cons	Wear/loosening risk	Long rehab, donor-site issues

(ACI: autologous chondrocyte implantation; OATS: osteochondral autograft transfer)

Clinical data:
- 85% survival at 8 years (HemiCAP® knee).
- 75% patient satisfaction (BioPoly RS®).

Advantages over grafts:
- Faster rehab (return to sports in 3–6 months vs. 9–12 months for ACI).
- No donor-site morbidity (unlike OATS).
- Salvage option after failed cartilage repair.

Limitations:
- Off-label use for some designs.
- Risk of progression to total knee arthroplasty (TKA) if osteoarthritis (OA) spreads.
- Cost

4B.21 MANAGEMENT OF DEGENERATIVE/INFLAMMATORY ARTHRITIS OF KNEE JOINT (Q156–165)

156. What is unicompartmental osteoarthritis of knee joint? Discuss pathology, clinical features and principles of management.

Ans: The knee has functionally three important compartments—Medial, lateral and patellofemoral compartments. Osteoarthritis of the knee that affects only the medial or only the lateral compartment is commonly called unicompartmental arthritis. Technically patellofemoral arthritis is also unicompartmental, but it is not so common, and surgeons refer to it discretely as patellofemoral arthritis rather than unicompartmental disease. Here I will restrict myself to the medial compartment disease and its description and management, students aiming for comprehensive complete answer may additionally describe patellofemoral disease and patellofemoral arthroplasty (not very successful clinically)

Pathology: The osteoarthritic changes are found to progress in following stages:
- *Stage 1*: Proteolytic breakdown of the cartilage matrix along with altered chondrocyte metabolism. The chondrocytes produce increased amount of catabolic enzymes (metalloproteinases like collagenase and stromelysin) destroying the cartilage matrix. The production of protease inhibitors [tissue inhibitors of metalloproteinases (TIMP) 1 and 2] is reduced.
- *Stage 2*: Fibrillation and erosion of the cartilage, releasing the degenerated and altered proteoglycan and collagen fragments into synovial fluid producing inflammatory reaction.
- *Stage 3*: Chronic inflammatory reaction in the synovium. Production of metalloproteinases, IL1, and TNFα by synovial macrophages. Other proinflammatory molecules like free radicals may also be a factor.
- *Stage 4*: Alteration in the joint architecture and compensatory bone overgrowth further irritate the synovium and a vicious cycle gets laid down.

Clinical features:
- Pain is undoubtedly the most important symptom of osteoarthritis, especially activity related or mechanical pain. Young patients often have maximal pain several hours after the physical activities. Pain at night could be present in patients with mild osteoarthritis who have used joints for several hours (sports person), patients with advanced osteoarthritis with severe destructive changes in bone and cartilage breakdown and in acute inflammatory exacerbation of the disease.
- Stiffness of short duration ("gelling" of joints) is often described as a short-lived stiffness seen after inactivity localized to the joint region.
- Reduced movements (knee flexion) and crepitus

Physical findings
- Joint line tenderness—medial or lateral depending on compartment involved.
- Crepitus on joint movement
- Restricted joint ROM
- Joint deformity varus at knee for medial compartment osteoarthritis

Principles of management: Better reflected by the common methods used to manage unicompartmental osteoarthritis of knee:
- High tibial osteotomy unloads the affected part of knee joint by correcting malalignment and redistributing stresses hence relieves pain and restores function.

- Unicompartmental knee arthroplasty removes the diseased painful portion (replacement procedure) of the knee and is a resurfacing arthroplasty (joint preserving) reconstructing the bearing surfaces. It restores natural alignment of the joint and restores ligament tension and joint line.

Both the treatment methods are discussed in detail in the following answers.

157. Describe management of unicompartmental osteoarthritis of knee.

Ans: *Osteotomies*: The following are the commonly used osteotomies for knee isolated compartment osteoarthritis—

- Varus-producing distal femoral osteotomy is indicated in patients with valgus gonarthrosis and isolated lateral compartment arthritis.
- Valgus-producing high tibial osteotomy is indicated in patients with varus gonarthrosis and isolated medial compartment arthritis.

High tibial osteotomy (HTO) unloads the affected part of knee joint by correcting malalignment and redistributing stresses hence relieves pain and restores function. Though popular and commonly used in past, proximal tibial osteotomy (HTO) is losing popularity as a reconstructive procedure, however HTO was first described by Lagenback in 1854.

Indications of HTO:
- Pain and disability from unicompartmental involvement (usually medial) osteoarthritis <grade 4 (Ahlback grading) documented on radiographs (or better arthroscopically) in a high demand young individual. Patella femoral osteoarthritis should be less than grade 3 (Ahlback).
- Age less than 60 years and varus (or valgus) of less than 15° at the knee with full extension.
- Motivated patient who can use assistive devices and understands activity limitation for significant period of time.
- In menisectomized knees HTO is indicated for prevention of long-term overload or as additional procedure to meniscal transplantation.
- As a protective procedure for chondral resurfacing or various cartilage reconstructive procedures.
- Anterior cruciate ligament (ACL), posterior cruciate ligament (PCL) or posterolateral complex insufficiency with varus alignment or thrust.

Patient selection: Ideal patient—40–60 years old active male with varus of less than 15° having isolated medial activity and no patellofemoral symptoms. Patients should have full extension and more than 100° of flexion, nonsmoker, BMI less than 30 kg/m^2 and lateral compartment arthrosis of less than grade 3.

(*The topic is vast kindly refer to Answers to Questions 90 and 92 and Chapter 11 of the Essential Orthopedics: Principles and Practice, 2nd edition, for details of the procedure.*)

Unicompartmental Knee Arthroplasty

The term "Unicondylar" refers to a device with two components that resurface the tibiofemoral articulation. "Unicompartmental" refers to the philosophy of resurfacing only one compartment, with a specific implant; this can be medial, lateral or patellofemoral. They should not be used interchangeably. Unicompartmental knee arthroplasty (UKA) restores the kinematics without significantly altering the natural alignment or ligament balance.

Principle: UKA removes the diseased painful portion (replacement procedure) of the knee and is a resurfacing arthroplasty (joint preserving) reconstructing the bearing surfaces. It restores natural alignment of the joint and restores ligament tension and joint line.

Indications: Classically, UKA is indicated in unicompartmental osteoarthritis of the knee in a low-demand, elderly, thin patient (>55 years) with competent cruciates and collateral ligaments.

Patient selection:
- Patients > 55 years
- BMI < 30 kg/m^2
- Low level of activity
- Minimal rest pain
- ROM-minimum arc of 90°:
  - Flexion contracture < 5°
  - Passively correctible angular deformity less than or equal to 10° varus or 15° valgus.

Contraindications:
- Age < 60 years
- Weight > 95 kg
- High activity level
- Patellofemoral pain
- Contralateral tibiofemoral joint arthritis
- Menisectomized patient (other compartment)
- Inflammatory arthritis
- Symptomatic ACL insufficiency
- PCL insufficiency
- Collateral ligament insufficiency
- Varus > 15°; valgus > 15°; flexion contracture > 10°.

Preoperative planning: Standard anteroposterior (AP) and lateral radiographs to identify damage to compartments (especially patellofemoral) and possible cruciate damage. Long-leg films to assess alignment. Patellofemoral and stress views to better assess patellofemoral compartment and ligament laxity respectively.

Prosthetic designs and rationale: Two basic designs are available with their advantages and limitations, the clinical results with them seem to be similar:
1. A fixed femoral and fixed tibial component with low conformity between the two articular surfaces. This allows relatively unconstrained movement between the femoral and tibial articulations. The ligaments control the movement. Disadvantage is that the limited conformity results in high stresses in the tibial component, which produces excessive polyethylene wear and possible early component loosening especially if the polyethylene is thin.
2. A free mobile bearing with absolute congruency between the metal femoral and metal tibial articulating surfaces maintained through the full range of movement.

Disadvantage of this design is the possibility of a dislocation of the mobile articulating surface. The components should be placed in such a way that the tibial and femoral components are parallel and in maximum congruency in both flexion and extension. The components should be placed in the center of the compartment as an offset placement will result in weak fixation and early loosening. The posterior slope should be restored as close as possible to avoid strain on ACL. In contrast to HTO undercorrection is recommended in UKA. Minimum 6 mm of poly thickness is recommended.

Performance and results: The cumulative benefits of UKA over TKA and HTO are short hospital stay, full RoM, speedy recovery and unaided walk, able to sit cross-legged on floor, reciprocal stair climbing, brisk walking, jogging allowed, joint preserving, not compromising future surgery and joint preserving. Postoperative morbidity and infection after UKA is less than TKA. The long-term failure rates for UKA are some 1.8 times than TKA. The cumulative revision rates for TKA have reduced, however, remain same for UKA.

Component loosening due to malpositioning and various other factors is the most common cause of failure. Disease progression in the other compartments is the second most common cause followed by polyethylene wear. In conclusion, prefer UKA in older, light, sedentary patient or middle-aged female with unicompartmental osteoarthritis.

158. What are the advantages and disadvantages unicompartmental knee arthroplasty (UKA)?

Ans: *Advantages*:
- It restores the kinematics without significantly altering the natural alignment or ligament balance.
- Faster recovery time with minimal invasiveness
- Revising UKA to TKA later is probably easier than after HTO.
- Short hospital stay
- Full ROM
- Unaided walk
- Able to sit cross-legged on floor, reciprocal stair climbing, brisk walking, jogging

Disadvantages:
- The long-term failure rates for UKA are some 1.8 times than TKA.
- The cumulative revision rates for TKA have reduced; however, remain same for UKA.
- Component loosening due to malpositioning and various other factors is the most common cause of failure. Disease progression in the other compartments is the second most common cause followed by polyethylene wear.
- It has steep learning curve and is not good in the hands of inexperienced surgeons

159. Discuss role of HTO in osteoarthritis of knee. Compare its outcome, advantages and disadvantages with unicompartmental knee arthroplasty in medial compartment osteoarthritis of knee.

Ans:
Role: HTO is done in patients of malalignment with concomitant osteoarthritis aimed to correct angular deformities of the knee to prevent development or progression of unicompartmental osteoarthritis. This procedure finds its primary relevance in varus knee with medial compartment osteoarthritis but can also be done in valgus knee with lateral compartment osteoarthritis (infrequently).

Outcome: The outcomes of HTO are comparable to unicompartmental knee replacement as studied by various investigators and in systematic reviews provided proper patient selection is done. Importantly the HTO patients achieve higher ROM of knee and is better suited for patients with high activity requirements but overall patient satisfaction (pain) and survival (w.r.t. revision rates, complications) appears to be bit higher with unicompartmental knee arthroplasty **(Table 4b.21.1)**.

Advantages: HTO offers pain relief for around 8–10 years. HTO has been shown to have improved results in ACL-deficient knees. This may be related to HTO improving the stability of the knee.

Disadvantages: All HTOs have been shown to *alter the slope of the tibia*.

Main concerns following HTO for performing arthroplasty arises from retropatellar fibrosis, patella baja, deformed proximal tibia and offset tibial shaft (implant placement, probability of varus cut), altered slope, altered joint line, implant-related complications, lateral soft tissue scarring and prior incision.

TABLE 4B.21.1: Comparison of unicompartmental knee arthroplasty (UKA) to high tibial osteotomy (HTO).

Feature	UKA	HTO
Age	>55 years	<60 years
Activity level	Low demand	Active person
Weight	<30	Obese can undergo
Ideal alignment	<10° and passively correctable	5–15°
ROM	Flexion >90°, <5° flexion contracture	Flexion arc 120°, <5° flexion contracture
Arthrosis severity	Any	Ahlback <3
Joint instability	None tolerated (?ACL deficiency can be tolerated)	Some amount of ACL/PCL deficiency acceptable
Multiplanar deformity	No	Can be corrected
Corrective goal	Undercorrection	Overcorrection
Complications	Less	More
Conversion to TKA	• Bone stock loss on both femoral and tibial side • Results UKA → TKA inferior than primary	Tibial component alignment, exposure difficulties. Results HTO → TKA better

160. Discuss differential diagnosis in a 25-year-old male presenting with monoarticular arthritis of knee joint. Tabulate the management in algorithmic manner.

Ans: Monoarticular rheumatoid arthritis (MARA) is a presentation of rheumatoid arthritis (RA) and not a disease entity in itself. Nearly all of the patients of MARA develop RA over 4–5 years down the disease duration. Only difference is that patients with MARA have large joint affection initially (usually knee or hip) and then the disease migrates/presents in other joints of the body.

Differential diagnosis:
- Gout
- Pseudogout
- Trauma
- Infection.

Management (Flowchart 4B.21.1):
Careful history and general physical examination should be the standard protocol. Send joint fluid for examination and guiding for diagnosis. Examination of joint fluid should include leukocyte counts, culture and Gram staining, light and polarized microscopy.

(The details of synovial fluid examination and characteristics need to be read in detail from Chapter 8 of the book Essential Orthopedics: Principles and Practice, 2nd edition.)

Flowchart 4B.21.1: Management of monoarticular arthritis of knee joint.

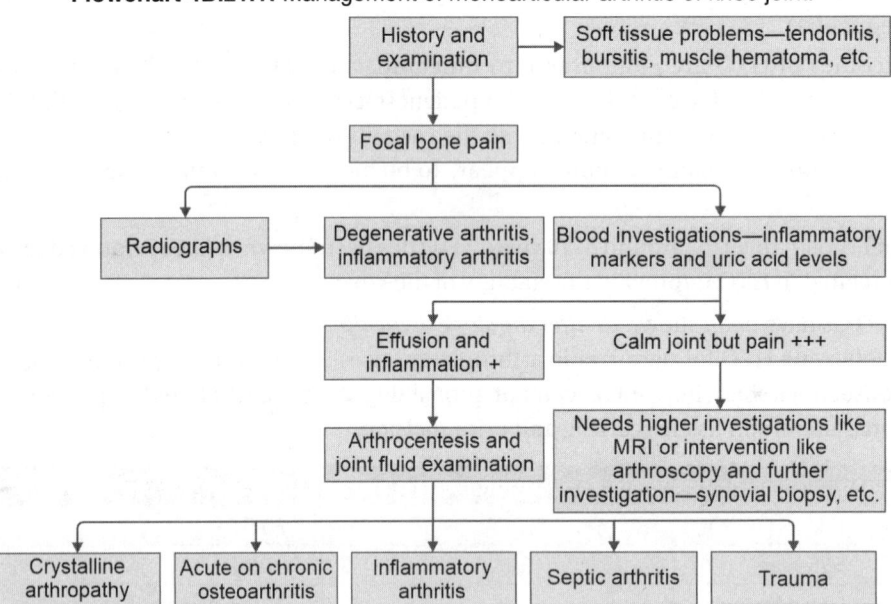

161. Explain the following:
A. Management of degenerative arthritis of knee in the young patients.
B. Viscosupplementation for knee arthritis.

Ans: A. Following are the measures used for *management of degenerative knee arthritis*:

Topical analgesics: Topical nonsteroidal anti-inflammatory drugs (NSAIDs) and capsaicin may be used as alternative to those having contraindications to their systemic use. Topical capsaicin works by depleting the neuropeptide substance P and must be used for more than 3–4 weeks for optimal benefit.

Exercise, weight loss and lifestyle modifications: Exercise improves flexibility and strengthening muscles supports the affected joints for want of ligament stability, increases aerobic capacity and endurance and facilitates weight loss. Strengthening the muscles improves joint stability and reduces pain. Low-impact isokinetic and isotonic strengthening exercises (swimming, biking and walking) are preferable but initially isometric exercises should be introduced gradually escalating to isotonic and resistive exercises.

Weight loss reduces the symptoms of osteoarthritis in weight-bearing joints. Each kilogram of weight loss results in a sixfold to eightfold reduction in the load exerted on the knee per step during daily activities.

To improve symptoms of medial joint compartment knee osteoarthritis, lateral wedge orthotics or knee bracing for more muscular, younger patients may provide symptomatic improvement.

The use of transcutaneous electrical nerve stimulation (TENS) has been recommended by National Institute for Health and Care Excellence (NICE).

Oral analgesics and anti-inflammatory drugs: Nonsteroidal anti-inflammatory drugs effectively relieve pain in patients with osteoarthritis. They reduce inflammation associated with osteoarthritis by inhibiting the production of prostaglandins. Acetaminophen at doses of up to 4 g/day also gives good pain relief with lesser side effects.

Selective COX-2 enzyme inhibitors are as effective as the nonspecific NSAIDs in treating osteoarthritis with decreased incidence of gastric toxicity. It is important to note that still all NSAIDs and COX-2 inhibitors may cause cardiovascular and renal side effects to varying degrees.

Tramadol and combination of tramadol with acetaminophen can provide improved pain relief in patients that cannot tolerate NSAIDs or are contraindicated.

Recently, prostaglandin-sparing anti-inflammatory drugs (PSAIDs) have been introduced typified by *oxaceprol* (N-Acetyl-L-Hydroxyproline). These are atypical inhibitors of inflammation and joint damage by inhibiting granulocyte infiltration of the arthritic joint without inhibiting prostaglandin synthesis. They also have chondroprotective effect.

Natural inhibitors of neovascularization like *curcumin* and *resveratrol* have been found effective in inhibiting metastatic tumor cell homing and angiogenesis. They are now available and also being used for treatment of osteoarthritis.

Injectable corticosteroid: Localized osteoarthritis to a joint or acute inflammatory exacerbation can be managed with depot preparations of steroids. Effects last 4–6 weeks then wane-off fast. It should not be used more frequently than once in 4 months as cartilage damage and disease progression occurs.

Avocado and soybean unsaponifiables: Avocado and soybean unsaponifiables may have potential as slow-acting symptom-relieving drugs for osteoarthritis. They do not have any structure modifying action but regular use has been found to reduce the need of NSAIDs.

Harpagoside (Devil's claw extract): This is an iridoid glycoside that has shown anti-inflammatory, antirheumatic and antioxidant effects. The medicine has shown promising relief from osteoarthritic pain and fewer side effects compared to diacerein.

Estrogens: Estrogen replacement therapy has been found to lower the prevalence of osteoarthritis of knee. The side effects possibly limit their use as regular therapy.

Disease Modifying Drugs for Osteoarthritis
Symptomatic slow acting drugs for osteoarthritis (SYSADOA), glucosamine and chondroitin sulfate (Chondroprotective): The term chondroprotective is a misnomer as no such concrete effect on preservation or regeneration of cartilage has been demonstrated.

Glucosamine sulfate is the monosaccharide precursor to glycosaminoglycans. Chondroitin sulfate is composed of repeating units of galactosamine sulfate and glucuronic acid. Oral supplementation with glucosamine and/or chondroitin sulfate is thought to stimulate synthesis of glycosaminoglycan and proteoglycans and inhibiting degradative proteolytic enzymes. The results have been mixed and not very encouraging. Only in early disease do we require medication to relieve patient of pain. Another interesting finding is that in most of the randomized controlled trials (RCTs) done to evaluate the efficacy of drugs where a placebo is used the "placebo effect" is itself very high around 60% and therapeutic drugs find it difficult to surpass this high efficacy to produce a significant difference.

Glycosamine polysulfuric acid, glycosaminoglycan peptide complex, and pentosan sulfate are available for animal use and act variously by inhibiting collagenase and having trophic action on cartilage. Human trials have not been impressive.

S-adenosylmethionine (SAM): It is a methyl group donor and oxygen radical scavenger supposed to prevent cartilage damage due to peroxidation and inflammation. The results have been mixed and possibly require prolonged administration.

Diacerein: Diacerein and its active metabolite rhein are anthraquinones related to senna compounds. They inhibit the synthesis of interleukin (IL)-1β in human osteoarthritis synovium in vitro, as well as the expression of IL-1 receptors on chondrocytes. Effects have not been consistent in all reported studies.

Doxycycline: Tetracyclines appear to inhibit tissue metalloproteinases (collagenase and gelatinase). This could be due to their ability to chelate calcium and zinc ions. They also prevent proteoglycan loss, cell death, and deposition of Type X collagen matrix.

Newer agents:
- *Use of autologous blood product*: These blood products are usually fractionated fragments of blood highly rich in platelet content. The platelets have the capability to release chemokines from β-granules positively influencing the tissues with low healing potential. Intra-articular injection of activated platelet concentrate may enhance cartilage healing and remodeling.
- *Univestin*: This is a combination of plant extracts obtained from *Scutellaria baicalensis* and *Acacia catechu* that helps in alleviating pain and stiffness. The proposed mechanism is through inhibition of both cyclooxygenase (COX) and lipoxygenase (LOX) though dedicated trials are not available.
- *Interleukin-1 receptor and tumor necrosis factor (TNF)-β antagonist*: IL-1 receptor antagonist (IL-1Ra) has shown reduced expression of collagenase in cartilage and prevents osteoarthritis progression in animal studies. IL-1Ra (Orthokine, Anakinra) is an example of approaches that inhibit activity of catabolic cytokines. It inhibits the signaling of IL-1 and has been studied in equine knees. Additional inhibition of TNF-β is associated with cartilage preservation by decreasing release of glycosaminoglycans and increasing lubricin production. Tocilizumab and infliximab plus methotrexate (MTX) have shown reduction in synovial VEGF and inflammation.
- *Mitogen-activated protein (MAP) kinase inhibitors*: Mitogen-activated protein kinase regulates production and activity of multiple mediators of joint tissue destruction. Inhibition of this pathway can slow disease progression in osteoarthritis.
- Angiogenic inhibitors like angiostatin and endostatin are being evaluated for inhibition of βVB3-mediated angiogenesis.
- *Nuclear factor (NF-kβ) inhibitors*: NF-kβ transcription factors are triggered by a host of inflammatory cytokines and can be targeted to reduce the disease progression.
- Vitamin E, N-acetyl-L-cysteine (NAC), and superoxide dismutase have the potential to protect the chondrocyte from reactive oxygen species (ROS) released during traumatic insult.
- Rotenone inhibits the secretion of superoxide from mitochondria and may have a therapeutic role.
- *Inducible nitric oxide synthase (iNOS) inhibitors*: Substances like N-Nitro-L-arginine methyl ester (L-NAME) and N-iminoethyl-L-Lysine (L-NIL) have been found to reduce the progression of post-traumatic osteoarthritis in animals.
- Pan Caspase inhibitors like Z-VAD-FMK [benzyloxycarbonyl-Val-Ala-Asp(OMe) fluoromethylketone], a cell permeable fluoromethylketone that inhibit caspase enzyme in a broad-spectrum prevent apoptosis may benefit when injected intra-articularly.
- *Poloxamer 188 (P188)*: The compound acts via direct inhibition of IL-6-mediated pathway inhibiting the phosphorylation of Stat1, Stat3, and p38. This prevents their migration to nucleus and hence synthesis of catabolic products is not initiated.

Surgical management: Various surgical options exist for relieving pain and improving the function of involved joint(s). *Arthroscopic lavage* has shown no better lasting results than analgesic therapy. It provides temporary pain relief (similar to injectable steroids and viscosupplementation) by washing away the painful metabolites from synovial fluid full of catabolic mediators and worn fragments of cartilage to relieve inflammation.

Osteotomy: This corrects the resultant or causative misalignment of joint and additionally unloads the pathological side of joint involvement. Osteotomies have been previously used for hip osteoarthritis (like the classical McMurray osteotomy) but now hardly anyone uses them for this indication. Knee is still an area for practice of osteotomy for specific indications and patients. The following are the commonly used osteotomies for knee isolated compartment osteoarthritis:
- Varus-producing distal femoral osteotomy is indicated in patients with valgus gonarthrosis and isolated lateral compartment arthritis.
- Valgus-producing high tibial osteotomy is indicated in patients with varus gonarthrosis and isolated medial compartment arthritis.

Though popular and commonly used in past, proximal tibial osteotomy [high tibial osteotomy (HTO)] is losing popularity as a reconstructive procedure, however HTO was first described by Lagenback in 1854.

Principle: HTO unloads the affected part of knee joint by correcting malalignment and redistributing stresses hence relieves pain and restores function.

Rationale of doing HTO (realignment procedure):
- *Role of alignment*: Severity of varus directly correlated to radiologic progression. Varus worsens the problem and odds for radiological progression increased fourfold with a varus malalignment.
- *Baseline stage of disease*: Varus affects damaged knees more. In a Kellgren-Lawrence score 3 knee with varus alignment the risk of progression of osteoarthritis is tenfold.
- *Dynamic loading*: With a varus knee, the adductor moment leads to progression of osteoarthritis by dynamically loading the deformed joint.

Indications of HTO:
- Pain and disability from unicompartmental involvement (usually medial) osteoarthritis <grade 4 (Ahlback grading) documented on radiographs (or better arthroscopically) in a high demand young individual. Patella femoral osteoarthritis should be less than grade 3 (Ahlback).
- Age less than 60 years and varus (or valgus) of less than 15° at the knee with full extension.
- Motivated patient who can use assistive devices and understands activity limitation for significant period of time.
- In menisectomized knees HTO is indicated for prevention of long-term overload or as additional procedure to meniscal transplantation.
- As a protective procedure for chondral resurfacing or various cartilage reconstructive procedures.
- Anterior cruciate ligament, PCL or posterolateral complex insufficiency with varus alignment or thrust.

Patient selection: Ideal patient—40–60 years old active male with varus of less than 15° having isolated medial activity and no patellofemoral symptoms. Patients should have full extension and more than 100° of flexion, nonsmoker, BMI less than 30 and lateral compartment arthrosis of less than grade 3.

B. *Intra-articular hyaluronans (viscosupplementation)*: At low load speed, hyaluronic acid acts as a lubricant and during faster movements as a shock absorber. In osteoarthritis, the concentration of hyaluronic acid is reduced by one-half to one-third of normal. Hyaluronic acid injections (high or low molecular weight) appear to moderately improve short-term pain not seen with other analgesics (NSAIDs) though their recommendation for use is dwindling slowly. Adverse reactions are rare; however, "pseudoseptic" reactions in 1–1.5% patients have been reported.

162. Explain the management of knee osteoarthritis in elderly.

Ans: *Investigations*: Radiographic investigations are the most common investigations performed.

The radiopathologic correlations of osteoarthritis are presented below:
- Cartilage fibrillation and erosion = joint space narrowing (may be localized)
- Subchondral new bone formation = subchondral sclerosis
- Myxoid degeneration = subchondral cysts (geodes formation)
- Trabecular compression = bone collapse/attrition
- Fragmentation of osteochondral surface = loose bodies.

Radiological staging is important for further management of the disease:

Kellgren and Lawrence (KL) system
- *Grade 0*: No discernible radiographic features of osteoarthritis present
- *Grade 1*: "Doubtful" joint space narrowing and possible osteophytic lipping
- *Grade 2*: Definite osteophyte(s) and possible joint space narrowing ("minimal") on AP weight-bearing radiograph
- *Grade 3*: Multiple osteophytes, definite JSN ("moderate"), sclerosis, and minimal bony deformity
- *Grade 4 (severe)*: Large osteophytes, marked joint space narrowing, severe sclerosis and definite bony deformity disturbing the bony contour or joint alignment.

Arthroscopy may be used for confirmation in specific situations (unicompartmental osteoarthritis of knee) or sometimes to stage arthritis, which can show cartilage and synovial membrane abnormalities and also detect osteophytes. CT scan, MRI, and ultrasonography are not recommended for diagnostic purpose.

*Treatment (**Flowchart 4B.21.2**)*: The *goal* in osteoarthritis or degenerative joint disorder is to maintain a *painless active life* with objectives of control of pain and swelling, minimizing disability. Initially reducing inflammation with NSAIDs and pain control beginning with acetaminophen are appropriate. Exercises to strengthen the muscles and improve flexibility, as well as weight loss, should be stressed immediately. Before prescribing surgery which is the ultimate modality, education, exercises, weight loss, physical therapy, braces, and orthotics should be given due admission as they all have definite role in improving the quality of life and alleviating symptoms.

Flowchart 4B.21.2: Algorithm for osteoarthritis management.

KL grade 1:	KL grade 2:	KL grade 3:	KL grade 4:
• Regular exercise (all stages, throughout treatment) • Weight reduction (all stages, throughout treatment) • Topical analgesics • Acetaminophen ± oxaceprol • ± Harpagoside/doxycycline	• Oxaceprol • Acetaminophen/ intermittent NSAIDs • ± SYSADOA • I/A hyaluronic acid • If traumatic then intra-articular autologous blood	• NSAIDs ± Opioids • Intra-articular corticosteroids for acute flareups • Intra-articular hyaluronic acid • Footwear modification (lateral shoe raise) • HTO for unicompartmental OA • Persistent symptoms – IL-1Ra/TNF-α antagonist	• Joint debridement (only as interim measure to joint replacement) • Joint replacement • Surgery contraindicated– manage pain with IL-1Ra/TNF-α antagonist +NSAIDs ± opioids/ oxaceprol

(HTO: high tibial osteotomy; IL: interleukin; NSAIDs: nonsteroidal anti-inflammatory drugs; OA: osteoarthritis; TNF: tumor necrosis factor)

163. Describe pathogenesis of primary osteoarthritis of knee.

Ans: The following are the proposed mechanisms for development of "primary" osteoarthritis of knee:

A *genetic basis* appears possible for polyarticular small joint nodal arthritis in women. The following are some putative targets for genetic linkage of osteoarthritis:

- Mutations in the *COL2A1* gene (Type II procollagen) have been inflicted; however, mechanisms are not clear.
- *Asporin* gene (ASPN) has yielded significant interest. Its codes for the small leucine-rich proteoglycan subfamily of proteins that binds to transforming growth factor-β (TGF-β) and to collagen and aggrecan. There is a functional link among ECM proteins, TGF-β activity, and disease. ASPN containing 14 aspartic acid repeats (D14) was significantly associated with osteoarthritis knee.
- There is an imbalance between the catabolic and anabolic pathways of cartilage metabolism in osteoarthritis. The catabolic pathways are commonly associated with proinflammatory proteins, including IL-1β, tumor necrosis factor-β (TNF-β), IL-17, macrophage inflammatory protein-1β (MIP), etc. Proteinases (such as cysteine proteinases, metalloproteinases, and serine proteinases) are upregulated in response to stress on cartilage. There is impairment of production of new extracellular matrix proteins by chondrocytes under the influence of cytokines while increased degradation of the products already present. Matrix metalloproteinases (MMPs) have been linked to development of osteoarthritis due to their effect on cartilage degradation. Members of MMP include ADAM and ADAMTS (alpha-disintegrin and metalloproteinase with thrombospondin motifs), a haplotype of the *ADAM12* gene polymorphism is associated with osteoarthritis knee (seven-fold increased risk in females).
- Alteration in the canonical Wnt signalling pathway—single nucleotide polymorphism in the FRZB (strong association) and possibly LRP5 (indefinite) is associated with osteoarthritis hip.
- BMP2 is associated with development of osteoarthritis of knee while GDF5 (required for formation of bones and joints in the limbs, skull, and axial skeleton) has been associated with hip osteoarthritis in Asian population (Chinese and Japanese).

Angiogenesis and osteoarthritis: Angiogenesis is related to synovial inflammation and is an intermediary pathway for development of osteoarthritis. Angiogenesis is responsible for immigration of inflammatory cells and release of inflammatory mediators into the joint. The angiogenic factors are released by synovial macrophages, endothelial cells and synoviocytes with possible interaction of VEGF. Metabolic changes in the synovial membrane lead to decreased concentration and viscosity of the synovial fluid and poor lubrication characteristics. Endogenous production of growth factors such as TGF-β and BMPs have been implicated in driving osteophyte formation and synovial thickening associated with osteoarthritis.

164. Discuss proximal fibular osteotomy.

Ans: Osteoarthritis is the most common cause of disability in the older population. Disability is caused by pain and limitations in mobility. TKA, which aims to relieve pain and improve joint function and mobility, is the main surgical alternative in this patient population. However, TKA is expensive and complex, and some patients need a second knee revision after the first surgery. Although HTO is the first-choice treatment for young patients with OA of the medial compartment of the knee, there are some potential disadvantages after surgery. In 2015, Zhang et al., reported that proximal fibular osteotomy (PFO) relieves pain and improves joint function in human knee OA. This new surgery is simple, safe, and affordable. Pain relief after surgery occurs in almost all patients. PFO may delay or replace TKA in a subpopulation of patients with knee OA. The most striking finding is medial pain relief and an increase in the medial joint space. The majority of patients have significant pain relief immediately after PFO, although the mechanism was unclear.

Interestingly, the pain relief continued to improve, and some patients even report no pain at all in subsequent follow-up visits. Postoperative ambulation (i.e., walking) is also obviously improved when compared with the preoperative state. PFO also improves the axial alignment of the lower extremity in some patients, especially in those with severe genu varus.

Compared with TKA or HTO, PFO is a simple, safe, fast, and affordable surgery that does not require insertion of additional implants. As such, PFO is a suitable surgical option in most developing countries that lack financial and medical resources.

Procedure: The patients were placed in the supine position after administration of anesthesia. An approximately 5-cm longitudinal incision was made over the lateral skin of the proximal fibula, and the fibula was exposed between the peroneus muscle and soleus muscle. PFO was performed by removing a 2–3-cm length of fibula at a site 6–10 cm from the caput fibulae. Full WB and free mobilization were allowed postoperatively.

Theories about the possibilities in which PFO works:
- Mechanical axis realignment of knee, shifting loads from medial to lateral. Possible mechanism how PFO relieves pain and improves the joint space is that it removes the fibula support that may cause genu varus. The fibula supports one sixth of the body weight; thus, PFO may rebalance or redistribute the load on the lateral and medial tibia plateau after surgery.
- Another possible mechanism is nonuniform settlement. It states that the lateral support provided to the osteoporotic tibia by the fibula—soft-tissue complex may lead to nonuniform settlement and degeneration of the plateau bilaterally, which may cause the load from the normal distribution to shift farther medially to the medial plateau, consequently leading to knee varus and aggravating the progression of medial compartment OA of the knee joint.

Complications:
Common peroneal nerve palsy: It is seen in various forms as mentioned below. All these happen due to retraction and pull, with small incisions.
- Transient foot drop recovering in 3 days
- Extensor hallucis longus (EHL) weakness lasting for over 3 weeks
- Paresthesia, on dorsum of foot for 6 weeks
- Permanent neurological damage

165. Effects of different high tibia osteotomy (HTO) types on tibial slope and patellar height.

Ans: A closing wedge osteotomy has been found to increase patellar height while opening wedge osteotomy reduces it.

All HTOs have been shown to *alter the slope of the tibia*. Lateral closing wedge osteotomies tend to decrease posterior tibial slope, translate the tibia in posterior direction stabilizing knees with anterior instability (ACL deficient) while medial opening wedge osteotomies increase posterior tibial slope and translate tibia in anterior direction stabilizing knees with posterior instability (PCL deficient knees).

4B.22 HIGH TIBIAL OSTEOTOMY (Q166–167)

166. Describe the types and principles of high tibial osteotomy for osteoarthrosis.

Ans: *Types*: Various techniques have been described for realigning the joint by high tibial osteotomy (HTO), oldest one and most popular is the lateral closing wedge, valgus-producing osteotomy, described by Jackson and Waugh (1961) popularized by Coventry (1965). The different techniques of performing HTO (with or without navigation) are:
- Lateral closing wedge, valgus producing osteotomy
- Medial opening wedge osteotomy with bone graft (Debeyre and Patte in 1951)
- Dual osteotomy
- Dome (barrel vault) osteotomy of Macquet
- Chevron osteotomy (oblique)
- *Opening wedge osteotomy using external fixators (hemicallotasis)*:
  – Ilizarov
  – External fixators.

Principles: HTO unloads the affected part of knee joint by correcting malalignment and redistributing stresses hence relieves pain and restores function.

Rationale of doing HTO (realignment procedure):
- *Role of alignment*: Severity of varus directly correlated to radiologic progression. Varus worsens the problem and odds for radiological progression increased fourfold with a varus malalignment.
- *Baseline stage of disease*: Varus affects damaged knees more. In a Kellgren-Lawrence score 3 knee with varus alignment, the risk of progression of osteoarthritis is tenfold.
- *Dynamic loading*: With a varus knee, the adductor moment leads to progression of osteoarthritis by dynamically loading the deformed joint.

167. What are the types of proximal tibial osteotomies in children and adults? What are the contraindications of HTO for OA knees?

Ans: Proximal tibial osteotomies in children (used for deformity correction):
- Closed-wedge medial/lateral tibial osteotomy
- Opening-wedge medial/lateral tibial osteotomy
- Opening-wedge medial oblique tibial osteotomy
- Barrel vault (dome) tibial osteotomy with fibular osteotomy
- Chevron osteotomy

Proximal tibial osteotomies for adults:
- Valgus-producing high tibial osteotomy is indicated in patients with varus gonarthrosis and isolated medial compartment arthritis.
- Lateral closing wedge, valgus producing osteotomy
- Medial opening-wedge osteotomy with bone graft (Debeyre and Patte in 1951)
- Dual osteotomy
- Dome (barrel vault) osteotomy of Maquet
- Chevron osteotomy (oblique)
- Opening wedge osteotomy using external fixators (hemicallotasis):
  – Ilizarov
  – External fixators

Contraindications of HTO for OA knees

Absolute:
- Age > 65 years (the risk of failure increases 7.6% per year of age, and in patients over 65 years the relative risk is 1.5 times that of younger patients)
- Diffuse OA

- Tibiofemoral subluxation—lateral subluxation of tibia >1 cm
- Medial compartment bone loss >2-3 mm
- Medial compartment OA grade ≥ 4 (Ahlback)
- Flexion contracture > 15°.
- Inflammatory arthritis
- Meniscectomy in the compartment or other compartment
- Rheumatoid arthritis
- Mediolateral insufficiency
- Unrealistic patient

Relative:
- Obese [body mass index (BMI) > 40]
- Poor ROM <90° knee flexion
- Nonspecific knee pain
- >20° of correction needed.
- Peripheral vascular disease
- Smoker >15 cigarettes/day
- Osteoporosis
- Extra-articular deformity

Technique of HTO: Coventry recommended a lateral closing wedge osteotomy for varus deformity in osteoarthritic knee and medial closing wedge tibial osteotomy for valgus deformity but suggested supracondylar femoral medial closing wedge osteotomy if deformity exceeds 12°. In closing wedge osteotomy, the proximal osteotomy line is located in parallel with the articular surface and 2-2.5 cm inferior to the joint line. The distal osteotomy line is determined referring to the α angle and the wedge of bone between the osteotomy lines is removed. The proximal tibiofibular joint has to be frequently disrupted for proper wedge (lateral closing wedge for varus deformity) or else inferomedial portion of fibular head can be partially removed. It is helpful to preserve a posteromedial beak of proximal fragment that overrides the distal fragment on closure of osteotomy and provides added support and stability. It is better to use L-plates with compression (preferred) or simply cast immobilization or Steinman pin fixation (avoid). For opening wedge HTO, the proximal osteotomy line is drawn from a point 3.5-4 cm inferior to the medial knee joint line to the tip of the fibular head from which another same length line is drawn obliquely by the α angle.

Various fixation methods are available all in common to avoid collapse of osteotomy gap. Puddu plate with predefined metal blocks, Tomofix (Synthes, Pennsylvania) with synthetic bone graft wedges, locked plate constructs

Barrel vault osteotomies (though it is technically difficult and involves creation of inverted "U" osteotomy followed by fragment rotation into desired plane) and hemicallotasis are preferable for larger corrections.

4B.23 TOTAL KNEE ARTHROPLASTY: PRINCIPLES, COMPLICATIONS, AND MANAGEMENT (Q168-177)

168. **A. Outline the biomechanical principles of total knee replacement (TKR) and complications of TKR.**
B. Discuss gap balancing technique.

Ans: **A. Biomechanical principles:** Successful total TKR requires strict adherence to two guiding principles—

1. *Alignment*: It has been shown in multiple studies that the femoral and the tibial components have to be implanted in such a manner that the mechanical axis of the lower extremity is restored. The mechanical axis of the limb is defined by a straight line passing through the center of the hip joint, center of the knee joint and the center of the ankle joint. In a replaced knee, when a straight line is drawn from the center of the hip to the center of the ankle, ideally it should pass through the center of the knee joint. Restoration of this axis equilibrates the load distribution in the medial and the lateral compartment, going by the recommendation of Insall. Hungerford and Kenna have challenged this concept of mechanical alignment by stating that restoring the prearthritic anatomy of the patient will lead to better patient satisfaction and better joint kinematics. They recommend placing the femoral component in 9-10° of anatomic valgus

and the tibial component in 3° of anatomic varus thereby recreating 6–7° of valgus at the knee joint. This concept is known as the concept of anatomical alignment. Although the concept looks appealing, it has not found many takers simply because of the fact that if the surgeon is inexperienced; cutting the tibia in varus intentionally may actually cause an excessive varus, leading to early failure.

2. *Gap balance*: The gaps have to be balanced both in coronal (mediolateral) and sagittal plane (flexion-extension gaps). The coronal plane balancing is mostly achieved by ligament releases and proper component rotation. For balancing the knee in sagittal plane, a complex combination of capsular releases, variation of component sizes and extra cuts need to be performed. If the knee is left unbalanced excessive load transfer through one compartment will lead to early loosening and failure. Also, tight compartments will cause the knee to become painful and reduce the range of motion.

Complications:
Systemic complications
- Thromboembolism
- Fat embolism.

Local complications
- Wound drainage and delayed wound healing
- Vascular complications
- Neurological complications.

TKR-specific complications
- Instability
- Arthrofibrosis
- Component loosening
- Patellar complications:
  – *Patellar clunk syndrome*
  – *Synovial entrapment/hyperplasia*—less well-defined condition. Patient complains of pain and crepitus on knee extension from 90° flexed position
  – *Treatment of both clunk and hyperplasia*
  – *Patellar subluxation/dislocation.*

B. **Gap balancing technique:** This technique was developed for implanting the PS knees. The main focus of this technique was on the restoration of flexion and extension gap balance, which was achieved by varying the depth of the distal femur cut. Varying femoral distal cut was necessitated by the fact that the restricted sizes of the femoral component often led the surgeon to choose a smaller femoral component in relation to the actual size of the femur. This led to an increase in the flexion gap, which required to be balanced, by increasing the distal femoral cut. Classic gap balancing technique had the following steps:
- Initial ligament releases to bring the knee in approximate alignment before bone cuts
- Tibia cut perpendicular to the mechanical axis with varying posterior slope. The tibial cut was conservative to prevent creating a large flexion gap
- Knee flexed and distracted—anteroposterior (AP) cutting block rotated to make it parallel to the tibial cut and fixed to the femur and flexion gap created
- Knee extended and distracted. The depth of distal cut determined by the spacer block, which filled the flexion space most appropriately.

Varying distal cut in "gap balancing technique" often led to the elevation of joint line which at times could be detrimental.

169. Describe concept of metaphyseal sleeve and cone in TKR.
Ans: Revision total knee arthroplasty (rTKA) and rarely primary TKA requires management of severe bone defects. This can be done by using allografts but due to scarce supply and difficulty obtaining them using a tantalum cone or/and a titanium sleeve is commonly resorted to. Tantalum cones and titanium sleeves have been known to provide a better

satisfactory meta-diaphyseal fixation to reduce the mechanical stress and the need for high levels of constraint. Severe bone defects (Anderson Orthopedic Research Institute classification (AORI) type II and III) managed during revision TKA using cones and sleeves have fared better than allografts. The cones and sleeves are two distinct reconstruction systems with their pros and cons:

- *Highly porous tantalum cones*: These were developed to address structural allograft weaknesses and have been used in revision arthroplasty. The high porosity of tantalum and its scaffolding abilities for osteoblastic activity enable bone ingrowth and incorporation. Tantalum cones are often inserted with short- or intermediate-length cemented stems to ensure adequate initial stability. Cement interface between the cone and the implant is a site of junctional mechanical failure.
- A titanium sleeve is also designed to fill large contained cavitary and combined cavitary-segmental metaphyseal defects in the femur and tibia. Metaphyseal sleeves limits bony ingrowth and requires long and uncemented diaphyseal stems that are often undersized (thin) to minimize stem pain. The most common complication from the use of metaphyseal sleeve is fracture when broaching the sleeves or impacting the final stem-sleeve in the tibia or femur.

170. What is medial collateral ligament (MCL) injury in TKR?

Ans: MCL injury is an uncommon complication. The incidence is reported to be around 2%. Injury patterns include intrasubstance tears as well as femoral and tibial avulsion injuries.

The three major risk factors for MCL injury are morbid obesity, osteopenia, and varus alignment. The MCL is most at risk for sharp injury during preparation of the tibial plateau and when making the tibial cuts. As soft tissue is released medially, especially when the medial-sided structures are tight due to varus alignment, care must be taken to protect the superficial MCL. When the medial-sided tibial cut is made, the medial border of the tibial plateau should be well visualized and a retractor should be in place to protect the MCL. Avulsion injuries are usually due to excessive anterior subluxation of the tibia. It is important to adequately release the deep medial soft tissue prior to subluxating the tibia, and the tibia should only be brought forward with gentle traction. If the MCL has been insufficiently released and the tibia is forced forward, this can lead to a traumatic intrasubstance tear. Avulsion injuries are usually obvious when they occur. A pop is heard, and in an instant, a difficult exposure becomes easy.

There are two accepted treatment options once an MCL injury is recognized. The "standard teaching" is to implant a condylar constrained knee (CCK). These constrained implants provide greater stability by having a large polyethylene post that prevents varus and valgus movement of the knee. The CCK, however, is believed to increase the stress on the implant and lead to higher rates of aseptic loosening. IM rods should be added to the CCK to provide better fixation of the components, which makes the TKA significantly more invasive.

Another option is fixing MCL injuries either primarily for mid-substance tears or via suture anchors when the injuries are avulsion injuries followed by up to 6 weeks of postoperative bracing. An avulsion off the tibia can also be fixed to the tibial bone with a single staple in the tibia.

MCL injury should be repaired in all patients. The younger, healthier, higher-demand patients have a higher likelihood of healing the repair and will benefit more from the theoretical lower rates of loosening by avoiding a constrained knee. They should be treated with a hinged brace for 8 weeks. Older, lower-demand, less healthy patients who have a less likely chance of healing the repair can be treated with a CCK implant to supplement the MCL repair. They will benefit less from avoiding a constrained knee. They do not require bracing since the knee is inherently more stable in the valgus direction.

171. A. Explain the role of navigation in TKA.
B. What precautions you will take while doing TKA with fixed flexion and valgus deformity in knee?

Ans: A. *Role of navigation*: Efforts to improve the accuracy of bone preparation and implant alignment have been attempted using computer-assisted techniques. Regardless of the technique used, improved alignment has been documented by multiple authors compared with conventional alignment methods. Although complications attributable to the computer-assisted technique have been infrequent, increased operative time and increased cost have limited its widespread acceptance. Long-term studies also are necessary to document improved outcomes as a result of more reproducible implant positioning. The navigation systems have several cameras to track surgical instrumentation, bony geometry, and alignment. The cameras are positioned above the patient and communicate with instruments and bony landmarks through light-emitting diodes (LEDs)/infrared rays. In each and every surgery and individualized computer-assisted orthopedic surgery (CAOS) system has to be established through coactions of navigator, theraputic object (TO), and virtual object (VO) that is done through three key procedural steps:

1. The first is the calibration of end-effectors (EEs) (describe the EEs' geometry and shape) in the 3-D coordinate system of the navigator. When an optical tracker is used, this is done via rigid attachment of three or more optical markers onto each EE.
2. The second process is registration, which aims to provide a geometrical transformation between the TO and the VO in order to display the end-effect's spatial and geometric localization with respect to the virtual representation on display. Registration is automatic in robotic systems but in most of CAOS, it has to be done as a separate step. The geometrical transformation could be rigid or nonrigid. This registration is an algorithm-based process that differs in different systems making them unique.
3. The third key ingredient is referencing. Referencing compensates for the relative motion of the navigator and/or the TO during the surgical actions. This is controlled by either attaching a so-called "dynamic reference bases (DRB)" holding three or more optical markers to the TO (like the tibial reference pins in older systems) or immobilizing the TO with respect to the navigator.

Advantages:
- Restore accurate limb alignment.
- Increase the survival of implanted joint (may be related to better placement).
- Constant guidance and monitoring during surgery.
- Reduce the risk of complications related to implant fitting.
- Secondary assistance/confirmation during minimally invasive spine surgery (MISS) procedures.
- Decreased hospital stay—only later in the course when one is well-versed with the system and is performing MISS surgeries.
- Record keeping of the surgery for later analysis.
- No radiation during surgery.
- Intraoperative range of motion analysis to achieve maximum function.

Disadvantages:
- Increased blood loss
- Increased operative time
- Increased risk of general complications like fat embolism, infection, atelectasis, etc. due to prolonged surgery.

B. *Precautions*: Fixed flexion deformity—Depending on deformity surgical planning should be done—
- <15°—regular TKA with good posterior release
- 15–45°—gap balancing by additional distal femoral cut, posterior release. Preoperative manipulation casts are better for bringing deformity to less than 30°
- 45–60°—preoperative serial cast correction to reduce deformity to minimum of 45° or better 30°. Intraoperative osteophyte removal, posterior capsule separation, additional distal femoral resection, tibial posterior slope adjustment, and posterior cruciate ligament (PCL) resection. Always prefer PCL-substituting implant
- ≥60°—preoperative manipulation and serial casting, use extension rods and stabilized insert with higher cam engagement like total condylar–III or LCCK type implant as there will definitely be gap mismatch with flexion laxity whatever technique is deployed.

It is a general recommendation that complete deformity correction is not necessary intraoperatively and some suggest "rule of one third" for flexion contracture greater than 40° identified preoperatively under anesthesia in patients with inflammatory arthritis. This rule states that intraoperative correction must be limited to one-third of the flexion contracture assessed preoperatively under anesthesia. This is because the residual two-thirds will resolve satisfactorily with postoperative physical therapy, sometimes supplemented by serial casting or the use of a dynamic splint. In degenerative arthritis one may aim for correction of half to two-thirds of the deformity and rest will correct over time.

Valgus deformity: Determine if the deformity is correctible (Ranawat grade I and II) or noncorrectible/fixed (Ranawat grade III). In a fixed deformity, the lateral structures are tight and require release. Additionally, if the medial collateral ligament (MCL) is suboptimal then constrained prosthesis would be needed.
- Radiographic patella femoral subluxation would indicate need of lateral release intraoperatively to correct patellar tracking.
- Posterolateral release is a must for knee balancing.
- Popliteus tendon should be preserved unless absolutely necessary to be released. If it is released, then choose constrained prosthesis or a hinged knee.
- Distal femoral cut be taken in less than routine valgus angle cut.

172. **A. Enumerate causes of painful stiff knee after TKR.**
B. How will you investigate and manage such a case?

Ans: A. *The following can be causes of stiff knee after TKA*:
- Excessive pain sensitivity/inadequate pain control
- Preoperative knee stiffness and excessive flexion/varus deformity that is not adequately corrected during knee balancing
- Arthrofibrosis and capsular contracture
- Excessive keloid formation and scar shrinkage
- *Implant malpositioning*:
  - Mismatch in flexion and extension gap (usually causes painful instability instead of painful stiffness)
  - Excessively tight flexion or extension gap
  - Overstuffing patella-femoral articulation
  - Tight PCL—in cruciate retaining designs
  - Femoral and/or tibial malrotation
  - Highly conforming design that limits bearing excursion
  - Wrong size of implant
- *CRPS*: Complex regional pain syndrome
- Infection—overt or subclinical
- Patella baja or alta due to alteration of joint line
- Extensor mechanism scarring and/or patellar tendon adherence to tibia
- Neurological causes—rigidity
- Heterotopic ossification
- Kinesiophobia.

B. *Investigation and Management*

Clinical evaluation: Evaluate RoM. Determine if the stiffness is intra-articular or extra-articular. Evaluate neurological cause and also look for clinical signs of CRPS. Loosening at the knee joint and positive drawer test are indicators of unequal gaps during balancing. For flexion deformity, also assess the hamstring tendons for stiffness. Additionally, evaluate hips and spine for associated pathologies as hip pathology may also cause pain at knee and hamstring tightness. Spine pathology may produce whole lower limb pain limiting mobilization and exacerbating knee pains (sort of double-crush).

Radiological evaluation:
- Evaluate for component rotation using cross-section imaging
- Plain radiographs demonstrate heterotopic ossification, osteophytes, and gross malposition of implants
- A metal suppression MRI assists in quantifying the extent of fibrosis and its location in the anterior or posterior compartment of the knee.

Aspirate knee and obtain prolonged liquid medium culture and Gram staining for evaluation of infection. Also send for atypical infections like acid-fast bacillus (AFB).

Treatment:
- Medical management for CRPS, neurological causes, and superficial scarring
- Aggressive physiotherapy and manipulation under anesthesia within 3 months if other factors (implant position/infection) are normal
- Arthroscopic arthrolysis ± quadriceps tendon lengthening
- Open arthrolysis
- Component revision for identified malrotation
- Revision arthroplasty for infection.

173. **A. Classify periprosthetic fractures around TKR.**
B. Discuss principles and management of each type.
Ans: Please read Chapter no. 3.

174. **A. Role of PCL in knee arthroplasty.**
B. Benefits of PCL retention versus substitution.
Ans: A. *Role of PCL*: PCL retention (CR) achieves an increased potential range of motion by effective femoral rollback and a relatively flat tibial articular surface. As a design feature, the PCL retaining designs conserve bone loss during primary arthroplasty as there is no box cut.

B. *Advantages of PCL retention*:
- *Increased RoM (especially flexion)*: This has not been proven well as substituting designs also achieve similar ROM.
- *Improved knee kinematics*: This is expected as one of the cruciate ligaments is retained, however there is also some debate as to altered rollback and deterioration of knee kinematics.
- PCL substitution (PS) puts stress on cement-bone interface as the cam of femur contacts tibial post to achieve roll-back so there is higher chance of loosening (survival rates of both CR and PS designs have been however similar).
- Individuals with PCL-retaining prostheses have a more symmetrical gait, especially during stair climbing, than do individuals with either PCL-sacrificing or PCL-substituting designs. Other studies however suggest contradictory findings like paradoxical forward translation of the femorotibial contact point during weight-bearing flexion in PCL-retaining knees whereas PCL-substituting knees studies showed more uniform femoral rollback.
- Posterior cruciate ligament-retaining designs do not tolerate much alteration in the level of the preoperative joint line while balancing the flexion and extension gaps, whereas PCL-substituting designs frequently balance with some mild elevation of the joint line.
- *Bone conserving*: This is the only proven advantage of CR design as in PS designs; femoral components have a cutout for a cam mechanism that begins just below the trochlea of the patellofemoral joint. Additional bone is removed from the femur when PCL-substituting designs are used to accommodate this box-and-cam mechanism.
- No patellar clunk syndrome—due to absent box cut in CR knee, the patella and hypertrophic synovium on the undersurface of the quadriceps tendon has no binding restriction in box cuts seen exclusively in PS designs.

175. **A. Explain the concept of constraint in total knee replacement design and their indications.**
B. Describe the characteristics and reasons for catastrophic poly failure in total knee replacement.
Ans: Constraint in total knee replacement (TKR) design refers to the degree to which the implant restricts knee motion to provide stability, compensating for ligament deficiencies or bone loss. It is achieved through implant geometry (e.g., conforming surfaces, posts, and hinges) that counteract varus-valgus, anteroposterior, or rotational forces, balancing mobility with stability to prevent instability or loosening. Designs range from unconstrained (minimal restriction, relying on native ligaments) to highly constrained (maximum restriction via mechanical links), selected based on patient anatomy, ligament status, and surgical needs.
- *Unconstrained (posterior cruciate ligament retaining, CR)*:
  - *Description*: Minimal constraint; preserves PCL for anteroposterior stability, with shallow tibial insert allowing natural rollback.
  - *Indications*: Intact PCL and collaterals; primary TKR in active patients with minimal deformity or instability.

- *Semiconstrained (Posterior stabilized, PS)*:
  - *Description*: Moderate constraint; cam-post mechanism substitutes for PCL, providing anteroposterior stability and femoral rollback.
  - *Indications*: PCL deficiency or sacrifice; moderate instability or deformity; common in primary TKR for better kinematics.
- *Constrained nonhinged (varus-valgus constrained, VVC)*:
  - *Description*: Higher constraint; deep-dish insert or condylar stabilization restricts varus-valgus and rotation without a hinge.
  - *Indications*: Collateral ligament deficiency, moderate bone loss, or valgus deformity; revision TKR or primary in unstable knees.
- *Constrained hinged (rotating or fixed hinge)*:
  - *Description*: Maximum constraint; linked femoral-tibial components (hinge) allow flexion-extension while restricting other motions; rotating hinges reduce stress.
  - *Indications*: Severe instability, global ligament deficiency, massive bone loss, or hyperextension; salvage in revisions or complex primaries.

B. *Catastrophic failure* refers to gross, rapid, and complete mechanical breakdown of the polyethylene tibial insert in a total knee prosthesis—often with fragmentation, deformation, or total wear-through to metal.

Characteristics:
- Gross fracture of polyethylene insert
- Delamination (layer separation) and pitting
- Chipping or fragmentation into loose bodies
- Complete wear-through exposing underlying metal tray
- Often asymmetric (more medial or lateral)
- Associated with osteolysis and component loosening
- May occur in younger, active, high-BMI patients or in older designs

Reasons:
- Poor-quality polyethylene (low-grade UHMWPE)
- Inadequate sterilization (γ irradiation in air → oxidation → brittleness)
- Poor processing → internal defects
- Thin insert (< 8 mm) → high contact stress
- Incongruent articular geometry (flat-on-flat) → point loading
- Poor locking mechanism between insert and tibial tray → micromotion, fretting
- Malalignment (varus/valgus) → uneven load
- Malrotation → abnormal shear forces
- Inadequate ligament balancing → instability, increased edge loading
- Over-resection → use of thin insert
- High BMI → high repetitive loads
- High activity level → accelerated wear
- Postoperative trauma or instability episodes
- γ sterilization in air → free radicals + oxygen → embrittlement over time

176. Discuss the causes of maltracking of patella.
Ans:
- *Lower extremity malalignment*:
  - Increased Q angle—genu valgum, external tibial torsion, internal femoral torsion, and coxa vara
  - Pes planus
  - Subtalar pronation
  - Dynamic malalignment—altered mechanics during motion, altered firing of vastus medialis oblique (VMO) and quadriceps, and quadriceps weakness.

- *Anatomical abnormalities*:
  - Small patella
  - Hypoplastic lateral femoral condyle
  - Hypoplastic trochlea
  - Patella alta
  - Hypoplastic medial patellar facet.
- *Muscle dysfunction*: VMO weakness or weakness of hip adductors to which VMO is attached
- *Tight lateral structures*: ITB tightness and tight lateral retinaculum
- Hamstring or gastrocnemius tightness
- Patellar hypermobility
- Overuse of patella
- Trauma.

177. Discuss septic complications of total knee replacement and their treatment.

Ans: Septic complications following total knee replacement (TKR).

Introduction: Periprosthetic joint infection (PJI) remains a serious complication following TKR, contributing to significant morbidity, prolonged hospitalization, and increased healthcare costs. The incidence of PJI ranges between 1% and 2%, though certain high-risk populations face a substantially elevated risk. Early recognition, accurate diagnosis, and timely intervention are crucial to optimizing patient outcomes.

Classification of Septic Complications:

Septic complications following TKR can be categorized based on the timing of symptom onset:
- *Early Infection (≤ 3 months postoperatively)*: Typically results from intraoperative contamination or hematogenous seeding from a distant infection. Common pathogens include *Staphylococcus aureus* and gram-negative organisms.
- *Delayed infection (3–12 months postoperatively)*: Often caused by indolent organisms such as Propionibacterium acnes or coagulase-negative staphylococci, presenting with subtle symptoms.
- *Late infection (> 12 months postoperatively)*: Usually hematogenous in origin, secondary to bacteremia from urinary tract infections, dental procedures, or skin infections.

Risk Factors:

Patient-specific factors increasing PJI risk include:
- *Systemic comorbidities*: Diabetes mellitus, obesity, rheumatoid arthritis, and immunosuppression.
- *Procedural factors*: Prolonged operative time, revision surgery, and prior joint infection.
- *Lifestyle factors*: Smoking, poor nutritional status.

Diagnostic Approach:

A multimodal diagnostic strategy is essential for confirming PJI:
- Clinical evaluation:
  - *Local signs*: Persistent pain, joint effusion, erythema, warmth, and wound drainage.
  - *Systemic symptoms*: Fever, chills, and malaise (less common in chronic infections).
- Laboratory investigations:
  - *Serum markers*: Elevated CRP (> 10 mg/L) and ESR (> 30 mm/hour) suggest infection but lack specificity.
  - *Synovial fluid analysis*:
    - Leukocyte count > 1,100 cells/µL (or > 3,000 cells/µL in chronic infections).
    - Neutrophil percentage > 80%.
    - Elevated synovial CRP or α-defensin (where available).
  - *Microbiological workup*:
    - *Synovial fluid culture*: Critical for pathogen identification; prolonged incubation may be needed for slow-growing organisms.
    - *Intraoperative tissue cultures*: At least three to five samples should be obtained during revision surgery to improve sensitivity.
    - *Molecular techniques*: PCR or next-generation sequencing (NGS) may aid in culture-negative cases.

- Imaging Modalities:
  - *Radiographs*: Assess for loosening, osteolysis, or periosteal reaction.
  - *Advanced imaging*:
    - *MRI (with metal artifact reduction sequences)*: Evaluates soft tissue abscesses/sinus tracts.
    - *CT*: Useful for assessing bone defects prior to revision.
    - *Nuclear imaging [e.g., WBC scintigraphy, fluorodeoxyglucose-positron emission tomography (FDG-PET)]*: May help differentiate infection from aseptic failure.

Management Strategies:
Treatment selection depends on infection chronicity, implant stability, and patient factors.
- Early acute infection (≤ 4 weeks, stable implant):
  - Debridement, antibiotics, and implant retention (DAIR):
  - Aggressive surgical debridement with polyethylene exchange.
  - Culture-directed intravenous (IV) antibiotics (4-6 weeks) followed by oral suppression in select cases.
  - *Success rates*: ~50-70% if performed within 2-4 weeks of symptom onset.
- Chronic/late infection (> 4 weeks or unstable implant):
  - *Two-stage revision (gold standard)*:
    - *Stage 1*: Explantation, radical debridement, antibiotic-loaded spacer placement (static or articulating).
    - *Stage 2*: Reimplantation after 6+ weeks of IV antibiotics and confirmed infection clearance (normalized CRP, negative aspiration).
  - *Single-stage revision*: Considered in low-virulence infections with soft tissue viability, though long-term data remain limited.
- Antibiotic therapy:
  - *Empirical coverage*: Vancomycin + piperacillin-tazobactam (adjusted based on local antibiogram).
  - *Definitive therapy*: Tailored to culture results; duration typically 4-6 weeks IV followed by oral suppression in high-risk patients.
- Salvage options for uncontrolled infection:
  - *Resection arthroplasty (Girdlestone procedure)*: For medically frail patients or recurrent infections.
  - *Amputation*: Rarely required, reserved for life-threatening sepsis or extensive bone loss.

Adjunctive therapies:
- *Negative pressure wound therapy (NPWT)*: For wound management after debridement.
- *Hyperbaric oxygen therapy (HBOT)*: May aid in refractory osteomyelitis cases.
- *Biofilm-disrupting agents*: Investigational (e.g., topical rifampin, bacteriophages).

Long-term monitoring and prevention:
- *Surveillance*: Regular clinical and laboratory follow-up for 1-2 years posttreatment.
- *Prophylaxis*: Antibiotic prophylaxis before invasive procedures in high-risk patients.
- *Multidisciplinary care*: Collaboration between orthopedic surgeons, infectious disease specialists, and microbiologists is essential.

4B.24 SPONTANEOUS OSTEONECROSIS OF KNEE AND OSTEOCHONDRITIS DISSECANS OF ANKLE (Q178)

 Describe the following:
  A. Osteochondritis dissecans of ankle.
  B. SPONK (spontaneous osteonecrosis of knee).

Ans:

A. *Osteochondritis dissecans of ankle*: In 1922, Kappis described osteochondritis dissecans in the ankle joint. Osteochondritis dissecans is a localized injury or condition affecting an articular surface that involves separation of a segment of cartilage and subchondral bone. Osteochondritis dissecans of the talus account for 4% of all osteochondral lesions in the body.

Etiology and natural history of disease: Although thought originally to be avascular now it is considered mostly traumatic origin. The osteochondral fragment is usually separated from the parent bone. If the fragment is stable new capillaries may cross fracture and revascularize it while, if unstable or displaced osteonecrosis (ON) fragmentation occurs and the fragment becomes separated and behaves like a loose body. Lesions are located, either posteromedial or anterolateral on the talus.

- *Posteromedial lesions*: Often asymptomatic, with no history of trauma. There is less risk of osteoarthritis
- *Anterolateral lesions*: Usually symptomatic, associated with trauma 98% of lateral lesions, and 70% of medial lesions are associated with trauma.

Mechanism of injury: It is mainly caused by inversion injuries of the foot. Mechanisms of injuries for various commonly occurring lesions are as follows:

Anterolateral lesions
- Result from inversion and dorsiflexion forces, which cause the anterolateral aspect of the talar dome to impact the fibula
- These lesions are usually shallower and more wafer shaped than medial lesions, possibly because of a more tangential force vector, that results in shearing type forces.

Posteromedial lesions: Result from a combination of inversion, plantar flexion and external rotation forces, which cause the posteromedial talar dome to impact the tibial articular surface with a relatively more perpendicular force vector.

Clinical features:
- Ankle pain usually localized to the side of the talar lesion
- Intermittent swelling
- Patient may complaint of catching or grinding, instability and frequent giving way
- History of ankle sprain is common
- May have crepitus with movements
- Joint effusion is common
- Tender along tibiotalar joint line either anterolaterally or posteromedially depending on lesion location.

Investigations

X-rays:
- Lesions appear as a well-circumscribed area of sclerotic subchondral bone separated from the remainder of the epiphysis by a radiolucent line
- Nontraumatic lesions should be radiographed for other ankle as disease is bilateral in 10–25% of cases
- Stress radiographs are indicated, if instability detected, on examination.

Magnetic resonance imaging: Magnetic resonance imaging allows determination of location of lesion as well as integrity of articular cartilage.

Computed tomography scan: Computed tomography (CT) provides best definition of bone fragments seen on plain X-ray, but not as helpful at detecting subtle lesions.

Bone scan: Bone scan can identify lesions, but is not helpful in determining integrity of articular cartilage.

Classification or staging: Berndt and Harty proposed staging system in 1959 based on progressive involvement of structures with ongoing stress on joint. However, newer MRI and arthroscopic systems are more popular.

Hepple et al. MRI staging
- *Stage 1*: Only articular cartilage is damaged
- *Stage 2*: Cartilage injury with underlying fracture. This stage can further be divided into following substages as follows:
  - *Stage 2A*: Cartilage injury with underlying fracture and edema
  - *Stage 2B*: Cartilage injury with underlying fracture but no edema
- *Stage 3*: Detached (rim signal) but not displaced fragment
- *Stage 4*: Displaced fragment
- *Stage 5*: Subchondral cyst formation.

Cheng et al. Arthroscopic staging system
- *Stage A*: Smooth, intact but soft or ballotable lesion, stable.
- *Stage B*: Rough surface but stable fragment.
- *Stage C*: Fibrillation of cartilage seen, but is stable.
- *Stage D*: Flap present or bone exposed and is unstable.
- *Stage E*: Loose, undisplaced fragment and is unstable.
- *Stage F*: Displaced fragment and is unstable.

Treatment

Conservative management:
- Conservative management of osteochondral lesions of the talus (OLT) should be attempted first
- Symptomatic patients with negative findings on plain radiographs (but MRI positive) should undergo an initial period of immobilization, followed by physical therapy.

Surgical management:
Surgical treatment depends on a variety of factors, including:
- Patient's profile (activity level, age, degenerative changes)
- Lesion characteristic (location, size, and chronicity of lesion).

Principles of surgery
- Loose body removal, with stimulation of fibrocartilage growth (microfracture, curettage, abrasion or transarticular drilling). Drilling can be accomplished, using existing arthroscopic portals, a curved meniscus repair needle guide and transmalleolar drill holes.
- Securing lesion to the talar dome, through retrograde drilling, bone grafting or internal fixation.
- Stimulating the development of hyaline cartilage through osteochondral autografts, [osteochondral autograft transfer system (OATS) mosaicplasty], allografts or cell culture.

Treatment for different stages (Based on MRI) of OLT
- *Stage 1*: Posteromedial and anterolateral lesions—conservative (an initial period of nonweight bearing with cast immobilization, followed by progressive weight bearing and mobilization to full ambulation by 12-16 weeks).
- *Stage 2A*: Conservative as above for both locations. Further treatment depends on restaging.
- *Stage 2B*: Large lesions more than 1 cm in diameter with recalcitrant symptoms may be treated with open OATS or mosaicplasty. Anterolateral lesions are managed with arthroscopic debridement and stimulation technique.
- *Stage 3*: Posteromedial lesions treated with immobilization and nonweight bearing for 3-6 months. Lateral lesions are treated with arthroscopy (stimulation/OATS/refixation of the fragment). Screw fixation typically is used only for anterolateral lesions because of the difficulty in gaining good exposure for posteromedial lesions and inadvertent damage to the articular cartilage.
- *Stage 4*: Displaced fragment is unstable and should be removed. For large lesions (>5 mm anterolateral or >1 cm posteromedial) the defect is covered with OATS or allograft.
- *Stage 5*: Arthroscopically excise the lesion fill the cyst with bone graft and OATS. Retrograde (transtalar) drilling can facilitate bone grafting, which is ideal for large subchondral cystic lesions, with intact articular cartilage.

Postoperative care: Rehabilitation can generally begin after healing is demonstrated, which may occur after 6-7 weeks of nonweight bearing. Ankle active and passive RoM exercises, strength development, and proprioceptive training are main pillars for treatment. Patient should be informed that pain following operative treatment is common for up to a year. After 6 months, a persistent effusion, a catching sensation or severe pain, signifies that healing is not progressing as intended and further investigation and management is indicated. Salvage in the form of ankle arthrodesis or ankle arthroplasty may be proposed.

Complications:
- Ankle arthritis
- Chronic pain

- Stiffness
- Resorption of grafts
- Infection
- Transmission of viral diseases in allograft transplants.

B. SPONK: *Synonyms*—Ahlback disease, spontaneous ON of knee, osteonecrosis of distal femoral condyles. This is the second most common site of ON after ONFH and accounts for 10% of all ON diagnosis. Spontaneous ON of the knee was described by Ahlback in 1968.

Etiology: As is the case with other forms of ON, the etiology for ON of distal femur is unsettled and most are proposals as causative agents based on isolated or clustered reports.

- Multiple repetitive trauma and osteoporosis may be a causative factor in spontaneous osteonecrosis of the knee (SPONK)
- *Other risk factors (secondary ON)*:
    - Alcohol abuse
    - Corticosteroid use
    - Sickle cell disease and other hemoglobinopathies
    - Systemic lupus erythematosus
    - Gaucher's disease
    - Renal transplantation
    - Microvascular embolism or thrombosis
    - HIV and hepatitis B infection
    - Caisson's decompression disease
    - *Iatrogenic*: Posterior cruciate ligament (PCL) reconstruction and arthroscopy.

Clinical Features and Classification

Osteonecrosis of knee has been classified (Patel et al.) into two forms based on etiopathogenesis, clinical presentation, and extent of bone involvement:

1. Spontaneous or idiopathic form—localized disease, usually unilateral in elderly age group more than 55 years
2. Secondary ON—more extensive disease, known primary cause, and is bilateral in 80% patients aged 40–55 years commonly. One should also look for other joint involvement in these patients.

Females are affected three times more than males in both forms. The symptoms relate less to the ON per se but for the development of subchondral collapse of necrotic segment, which results in development of incongruity of the articular surfaces and painful secondary arthritis. The collapse of necrotic bone produces sudden localized pain that increases with weight bearing and stair climbing. The pain is also felt more at night, especially in the secondary ON group where dull aching, diffuse pain may be present for months preceding the collapse of bone. In SPONK, the disease is limited to one knee usually with a predominance of medial femoral condyle involvement. This is more limited to subchondral bone and epiphysis. The secondary form is on the contrary more extensive and often involves metadiaphysis also.

Lotke et al. classified the ON of medial condyle into three groups based on the relative size of lesion with respect to the width of medial femoral condyle.

1. *Group 1*: Radiographs normal. Bone scan is positive. Patients may be asymptomatic for up to 15 months.
2. *Group 2*: Lesions measuring less than 50% of the femoral condyle.
3. *Group 3*: Lesions larger than 50% of femoral condyle and produce rapid collapse. These should be treated early before development of fixed deformity.

This classification based on size gained importance to prognosticate the patients and possibly guide timing of intervention. It is suggested that lesions that are more than 40% the size of condyle have a poor prognosis. In absolute terms, lesions more than 5 cm^2 are associated with bad prognosis. This size can be estimated by multiplying the width of lesion (AP projection) to the length obtained from lateral radiographs.

Pathophysiology: For secondary ON, the mechanisms of development of the disease are similar to those explained in above sections. Interestingly, the development of SPONK has been partly linked to osteoporosis. These weak bones sustain multiple insufficiency fractures even with normal weight-bearing processes. The injury-healing mechanisms produce intraosseous edema, hence increased pressure. This may lead to development of ON due to ischemia of subchondral bone whose vascularity may also get cut-off from this process.

Investigations: Laboratory investigations should be done to rule out hemoglobinopathies and various coagulopathies. Screening for viral infection is a routine for surgical procedure. Anteroposterior, lateral knee radiographs and tunnel views should be obtained. Radiolucent area is seen in the subchondral region followed by collapse and development of deformity. The advanced disease is accompanied by arthritic changes in the knee. MRI is a sensitive investigation and lesions are visible on MRI before appearance in the knee. The disease extent and localization are more precise on an MRI and is the investigation of choice. Bone scans are preferred modality to identify lesions at other locations in cases of secondary ON of distal femur.

Staging and treatment: Spontaneous osteonecrosis of the knee of femoral condyles have been staged for progression of disease by Koshino, which is modified into five stages by Aglietti **(Table 4B.24.1)**. Based on the Ficat and Arlet system of staging of the ONFH radiographic staging of distal femoral ON was proposed by Mont et al. **(Table 4B.24.2)**. The treatment is commonly based on general guidelines as prescribed for ONFH.

TABLE 4B.24.1: The Koshino and Aglietti staging systems.

Stage	Koshino system	Aglietti system
Stage 1	*Incipient*: Pain (+). Normal radiographs. Positive bone scans	Radiographs normal. If disease does not progress for 6 months then will remain static more likely
Stage 2	*Avascular*: Subchondral radiolucency in weight-bearing area. Distal sclerosis. Minimal articular change at arthroscopy	Area of slight flattening of femoral condyle
Stage 3	*Collapse*: Calcified plate with radiolucency surrounded by sclerotic halo. Collapse of subchondral bone	Crescent sign: Radiolucency with distal sclerosis and halo of bony reaction
Stage 4	*Degenerative*: Osteoarthritic changes including joint space narrowing, osteophyte formation, and sclerosis	Calcified plate, sequestrum with radiolucency and sclerotic halo
Stage 5	NA	Osteoarthritis

TABLE 4B.24.2: Mont et al. classification based on modified Ficat and Arlet radiographic staging of distal femoral ON.

Stage 1	Normal joint space, normal joint contour, areas of mottled osteoporosis
Stage 2	Normal joint space, normal joint contour, wedge sclerosis
Stage 3	Slightly decreased joint space, subchondral collapse, sequestrum appearance
Stage 4	Decreased joint space, collapse, destruction of trabecular pattern

Conservative management: This is based on the premises that smaller and limited disease may resolve completely over time due to repair and revascularization of the lesion, especially with SPONK. An attempt for supporting the ongoing revascularization should be done along with symptomatic control of the disease. Ahlback et al. found lesions less than 0.24 cm^2 often resolve taking months. The conservative treatment should be associated with regular follow-up to identify nonresponders so that early intervention could be undertaken. Following are the usual components of a standard conservative protocol varying in duration of submission:
- Protected weight-bearing in a splint or patella tendon bearing (PTB) cast or better rest for 4–6 weeks followed by gradual weight bearing on splint
- Use of lateral wedge insole in the footwear for affected limb
- Analgesics
- Physical therapy with quadriceps and hamstring strengthening exercises.

Operative treatment

- *Arthroscopy*: This procedure has been used primarily for debridement of the intra-articular pathologies resulting from disease like cartilage flaps, osteochondral fragments, meniscal tear and possibly managing the wear on cartilage by creating microfracture simultaneously.
- *High tibial osteotomy*: The osteotomy is based to unload the femoral condyle and enhance revascularization. Osteotomy can be done only if one of the condyles is affected so more appropriate for SPONK variety as the usually progressive other form of secondary ON has larger span of disease within the bone and may pose future complications to HTO (contraindicated). A valgus osteotomy is done for medial femoral condyle while varus osteotomy is done for lateral femoral condyle involvement. The indications for high tibial osteotomy for ON distal femur are:
    - Localized disease or disease limited to one femoral condyle
    - Stage less than 3 (Koshino system), or stage 3 with less than 50% of condyle involvement
    - Age less than 60 years (else prefer replacement)
    - Willing patient.
- *Core decompression*: Based on the philosophy for development of disease due to primary increased intraosseous pressure and hence possible improvement by decompression of bone in ONFH by attempting to increase vascularity, the procedure has been used quite commonly for distal femur also. This procedure has, however, not been recommended by Lotke et al. The core decompression achieves early symptom relief (pain), however, once flattening occurs the procedure is ineffective.
- *Autologous bone grafting*: Use of osteoperiosteal graft into the femoral defect has been described with reasonable symptomatic relief. This is useful for stage 3 (flattened femoral condyle). The only positive aspect of this surgery is that it maintains the bone stock even, if future surgeries are required.
- *Osteochondral allograft*: Where facilities are available for procurement and storage of osteochondral allograft, this is a promising surgery to restore the articular surface and subchondral bone in younger patients.
- *Arthroplasty*: Unicondylar knee arthroplasty (UKA) is preferred for spontaneous disease localized to one compartment in elderly age group. With gross malalignments total knee arthroplasty (TKA) should be done.
- *Total knee arthroplasty* is the ultimate modality to treat the patients with advanced disease. It remains the most predictable surgical treatment modality, particularly in the elderly patient with ON and those with secondary ON of knee.

4B.25 TIBIALIZATION OF FIBULA AND DISORDERS OF ACHILLES TENDON (Q179–181)

179. A. Describe clinical signs and symptoms of a neglected tendo-Achilles in a middle-aged man.

B. Discuss management of neglected tendo-Achilles (same case as in "a").

Ans: A. *Clinical examination*:
- Scar mark, tenderness may be present
- Palpable gap/irregularity on posterior aspect of lower leg in the region of tendo-Achilles
- Inability to toe-walk.

Tests:
- Weakness of gastrocsoleus and painful plantar flexion (especially when resisted).
- *Thompson-Simmonds-Doherty test*: patient prone: Squeeze the calf muscle of patient—passive plantar flexion of foot demonstrates continuous tendon [*after 7 days (neglected cases) due to intervening scar formation the test may be falsely negative*].
- *Needle test of O'Brien*: Insert a hypodermic needle 10 cm above the insertion of tendo-Achilles so that its tip is just inside the tendon. Alternately plantar and dorsiflex foot. If the outer portion of needle points cranially on dorsiflexion the tendon is supposed to be intact.
- *Sphygmomanometer test*: Wrap the cuff around calf region and inflate it to 100 mm Hg, if then on dorsiflexion of foot pressure rises to 140 mm Hg then it indicates intact tendon.
- *Knee flexion test*: With patient prone ask the patient to flex knee to 90°, neutral position or dorsiflexion of ankle suggests torn tendon.

- *Reverse Silfverskiold test (not very popular)*: With knee in full extension (ankle dorsiflexion here is solely restricted by tendo-Achilles) measure the range of dorsiflexion at ankle (more on injured side compared to the normal side).
- *Single leg heel raise test*: Ask the patient to stand on injured leg with heel raised (not possible with torn Achilles tendon).

B. *Management*: After confirming complete rupture of Achilles tendon a symptomatic patient with disability needs surgical reconstruction, mobilize the gastrocnemius and soleal components of the complex and after flexion of knee and plantar flexing the ankle, try to approximate the ends without tension and do an augmentation with plantaris tendon (or turn down of two flaps of gastrocnemius aponeurosis). If the ends cannot be approximated, then use the peroneus brevis dynamic tendon transfer (rather "splint") of White and Kraynick for reconstruction of tendon.

Guidelines as per classification:
- *Myerson's classification*:
  - *Type-1 defect*: 1–2 cm long → End to end repair and posterior compartment fasciotomy.
  - *Type-2 defect*: 2–5 cm → V-Y lengthening with or without tendon transfer.
  - *Type-3 defect*: > 5 cm →Tendon transfer alone or combined with V-Y advancement and augmentation.
- *Kuwada's classification*:
  - *Type-I*: Partial tear → Conservative management
  - *Type-II*: Complete tear → <3 cm defect → end to end repair
  - *Type-III*: 3–6 cm defect → debride + tendon transfer ± augmentation
  - *Type-IV*: >6 cm defect → debride + tendon graft ± augmentation.

180. **Explain:**
   A. Tibialization of fibula.
   B. Pathoanatomy, clinical features of Achilles tendon rupture, and treatment of a fresh rupture in a 60-year-old patient.

Ans: A. *Huntington's procedure (ipsilateral fibula transfer, tibialization of fibula)*: The concept was first used by Kahn in 1884 for pseudarthrosis of tibia. Huntington described the procedure for treating the tibial defect using the ipsilateral fibula transposition in 1903. This method has been used to treat post-traumatic tibial defects; OM produced defects, pseudarthrosis and congenital deformities. The original procedure was described as having two steps (now often performed in one step). In the first stage, the distal part of fibula is osteotomized and inserted into medullary canal of tibia or into a trough created on surface for fibula. The construct may be stabilized with cortical screws or K-wires. The second stage is done at 2–4 months where the proximal portion of the fibula is cut and approximated to tibial surface in a slot created for the same. This can also be stabilized with screws. The bone union occurs at around 6 months. Till then some protection is legible in the form of plaster cast or fixator. It is imperative to preserve the blood supply to bone. Advantages of the procedure include:
- Requires less expertise than free microvascular fibula transfer
- Bone remodels with weight bearing and hypertrophies
- Union and bone uptake are more certain that avascular fibula transplant as the graft is vascular here
- Union bypasses the stage of creeping substitution.

B. *Pathoanatomy*: The pathological changes that have been proposed to cause weakness and hence rupture of tendon are tendinosis, paratendinitis, and paratendinitis with tendinosis. The term tendinosis describes various degenerative changes within tendon (hyaline, mucoid, myxoid, fatty, fibrofatty, etc.) that may arise out of various above listed causes. Often tendinosis is not symptomatic and is realized only on rupture of tendon. Repetitive trauma or inflammatory conditions produce paratendinitis, which may be later accompanied with tendinosis and is often painful before rupture. This when combined with eccentric loading/sudden loading with incomplete synergism of agonist muscles leads to rupture of tendon in an "unexpected" manner. Steroid injection(s) at the site of insertion have also been suggested to induce degenerative changes in the tendon by halting collagen remodeling and weakening fibers making it susceptible to rupture. Rupture of gastrocnemius musculotendinous junction is specifically called tennis leg.

Clinical features: See answer above.

Treatment: There is still no consensus as to the best treatment.

Nonoperative treatment involves functional bracing and an aggressive rehabilitation. Some surgeons use ultrasound-based criteria for choosing nonoperative treatment as follows:
- Gap of less than 5 mm with maximal plantar flexion
- Gap of less than 10 mm with the foot in neutral position and
- More than 75% tendon apposition with the foot in 20° of plantar flexion.

Operative treatment: A variety of techniques and modifications have been described for repair of acute Achilles tendon ruptures, including open repair, with or without augmentation (tendon transfer, local fascial turndown, allograft, the plantaris and peroneus brevis tendons, and biologic or synthetic scaffolds) and percutaneous or minimally invasive repair, with or without the use of a device or endoscopy. In addition, numerous suture materials and configurations have been used for repair, including single and double Bunnell, Kessler, and Krackow (locking-loop) techniques and various modifications of these. There are described benefits and specific advantages of each technique but none has been firmly proved to be superior.

181. Explain:
A. Clinical features of chronic painful mid portion tendinopathy of Achilles tendon.
B. Role of plantaris tendon in the pathogenesis of this condition, with special emphasis on anatomy of plantaris tendon.

Ans: A. *Clinical features*:
- Exercise-induced pain
- Swelling located typically at 2–7 cm from the insertion onto the calcaneus
- Impaired function due to pain
- Swelling moves with plantar and dorsiflexion of ankle
- Pain on resisted plantarflexion.

B. It has been demonstrated that in many cases with Achilles tendinopathy the plantaris tendon is affixed onto the Achilles tendon on the medial side at the level of pain. The swelling in Achilles tendon is also more prominent on posteromedial aspect where plantaris tendon runs closely parallel to the Achilles tendon. Normally, the plantaris and Achilles tendon move independent of each other but in chronic tendinopathy there is a marked element of paratenon involvement that leads to adhesion between these tendons.

Plantaris has a small triangularly muscle belly proximally with a long thin tendon that descends through the leg and joins the calcaneal tendon. The muscle takes origin superiorly from the lower part of the lateral supracondylar ridge of the femur and from the oblique popliteal ligament associated with the knee joint. It lies posterior to the knee joint, originating from the inferior part of the lateral supracondylar line of the femur and the short spindle-shaped muscle body of plantaris descends medially, deep to the lateral head of gastrocnemius. The thin long tendon passes between the gastrocnemius and soleus muscles and eventually fuses with the medial side of the calcaneal tendon near its attachment to the calcaneus. Plantaris contributes to plantarflexion of foot, ankle inversion and flexion of the leg at the knee joint, and is innervated by the tibial nerve.

4B.26 BLOOD SUPPLY OF TALUS (Q182–186)

182. Describe the blood supply of talus.
Ans: The three major arteries of the leg contribute to a rich, extraosseous, anastomotic plexus, supplying blood to the head, neck, and body of the talus. The head and neck regions are richly supplied by the superior neck vessels, branching off the dorsalis pedis artery and the artery of the sinus tarsi. Osteonecrosis of these areas is extremely rare. The tarsal canal is formed by the sulcus on the inferior surface of the talus and the superior sulcus of the calcaneus and contains the artery of the tarsal canal and the talocalcaneal intraosseous ligament. The tarsal canal runs from posteromedial to anterolateral, where it opens into the tarsal sinus. The talar body is vulnerable because of its blood supply. Related primarily to the degree of displacement of the body, osteonecrosis rates can be 100%.

The artery of the tarsal canal, which branches off the posterior tibial artery approximately 1 cm proximal to the division into medial and lateral plantar arteries, is the most consistent major supplier of blood to the body of the talus. In the tarsal canal, it sends four to six direct vessels into the body of the talus.

The deltoid artery, which branches off the artery of the tarsal canal and directly supplies blood to the medial one-fourth to one half of the talar body, is the second major blood supply to the talar body. Through intraosseous anastomoses, it has the potential to supply blood to a much greater area.

The artery of the sinus tarsi, which is more variable in its size and origin, supplies the lateral one eighth to one fourth of the talar body. It is formed by branches of the perforating peroneal artery, the dorsalis pedis (or anterior tibial) artery, or anastomoses between the two. The artery of the sinus tarsi forms an anastomosis with the artery of the tarsal canal and has the potential to supply blood to more of the talus.

The posterior tubercle of the talus is supplied by direct branches from the posterior tibial artery (most common) or the peroneal artery. Although quite small, because of intraosseous anastomoses, this region also has the potential to supply blood to more of the body.

183. Describe biomechanics of ankle joint. Describe current status of total ankle arthroplasty.

Ans:

Biomechanics:
- The ankle joint is a complex hinge. The main movements at the joint are plantar and dorsiflexion and secondary movements are inversion/eversion and rotation.
- The ankle joint axis of rotation keeps on changing with ankle motion. Majority of the ankle motion takes place in the sagittal plane but there is subtle amount of motion taking place in the longitudinal and vertical axis. The plane of ankle plantar and dorsiflexion passes nearly 5 mm from the tip of medial malleolus distally and 3 mm distal and 8 mm anterior to the lateral malleolus. The concept of a single axis may be helpful in understanding the basic biomechanics and simplifying the concepts. With dorsiflexion, the axis inclination is downward and laterally, whereas in plantar flexion, the axis inclined downward and medially.
- The differential contouring of the talar head and trochlea may explain the changing axes of rotation; this is also responsible for mortise widening with dorsiflexion. There is approximately 1.5 mm increment in the intermalleolar distance during dorsiflexion of ankle because of external rotation of the fibula and lateral rotation of the talus as an attempt to match the wedge contour of the talus in the mortise.
- The deltoid ligament imparts rotational stability to talus in the ankle mortise and also maintains its closed pack configuration in the ankle mortise while dorsiflexion of ankle in the stance phase of gait cycle. Also the syndesmosis firmly binds the tibia to the fibula, preventing any additional movements.
- About five times the body weight is transmitted by the ankle joint while walking. Most of the stability of the joint is imparted by the articular congruity. The mortise view is taken with the patient's leg internally rotated approximately 15°, so the beam of the X-ray is perpendicular to the transmalleolar axis. The articular surface of the talus should be congruous with the distal tibia and the clear space between the talus and the medial malleolus, distal tibia, and lateral malleolus should be equal.
- The talocrural angle is the angle subtended by a line drawn parallel to the articular surfaces of the distal tibia and one connecting the tips of both malleoli. Normally, range of talocrural angle is from 83° ± 4°. It is used to judge the anatomical restoration of the ankle by comparing to other side. Fibular shortening is indicated by a difference greater than 2–3°. Medial clear space is the distance between the lateral border of the medial malleolus and the medial border of the talus. It should be equal to the superior clear space between the talus and the distal tibia. A space > 4 mm is considered abnormal and indicates a lateral shift of the talus.
- The radiological distance between the medial wall of the fibula and the incisural surface of the tibia, the tibiofibular clear space should be less than 6 mm

    Current status: Following success of hip and knee arthroplasty, the ankle prosthesis introduced in 1970s met with failure and disappointing results. The first-generation designs were cemented and bulky with large IM stems. These often also required subtalar fusion at the index operation and the results were very disappointing. With design changes, the results improved quite substantially and were not that dismal, though some patients did require amputations. These

amputations were actually ultimate measures to relieve pain in patients and were not a sole complication of ankle arthroplasty. The failure is attributed to various causes that were not recognized at the time of designing the implant:
- The ankle joint is a relatively small joint bearing the weight of whole body so forces acting per unit area of bone or joint are large. This results in higher moment and higher compressive forces. The quality of bone in the distal tibia frequently may be questionable and the bone strength is not uniform across the distal tibia.
- The soft tissues about the ankle are thin and frequently compromised by previous trauma, surgery, systemic disease, and steroid use. The vascularity of these thin soft-tissue flaps can be easily impaired with hematoma formation.
- Delayed wound healing has been reported to occur in as many as 40% of patients and most long-term series cite rates of deep infection of 3–5%.
- Subsidence, wear, and loosening occurred within a few years due to poor quality of articular bearings.

The high incidence of nonunion, secondary degeneration at adjacent joints, loss of physiological movement of foot and ambulation, development of equinus deformity of feet and the concern that patients may need other procedures for lower limb that may add to disability in future have regained the interest in ankle arthroplasty. With improved understanding and studies on anatomical design and biomechanics of the native ankle joint, the second-generation designs have become popular. The main constrains to use are financial and that the patient often have had multiple prolonged treatment that they are averse to ankle arthroplasty. The current indications can be maximally expanded to:
- Primary degenerative arthritis after explaining all the pros and cons of procedure and arthrodesis as alternative
- Systemic arthritis [e.g., rheumatoid arthritis, systemic lupus erythematosus (SLE), mixed connective tissue disorders]
- Patients who would require subtalar fusion or triple arthrodesis in future or has bilateral arthritis requiring treatment—the results of bilateral arthrodesis and pantalar fusion have been dismal.
- Secondary OA:
  - ON talus (< one-third talus involved)
  - Posttraumatic (if the malalignment and instability are manageable)
- Salvage of malunion and nonunion after ankle arthrodesis
- Low-demand patients who are not likely to go for aggressive laborious jobs

[For details, kindly refer to chapter 6 of the book, Essential Orthopedics under Discussion for Osteonecrosis of Talus]

184. Briefly describe Broström procedure in ankle joint and its indications.

Ans: *Repair of acute rupture of the lateral ligaments*: The technique described for Broström repair is commonly followed and is appropriate. Through a curved incision beginning 5 cm proximal to the distal tip of the fibula and 1.5 cm anterior to its margin to end distal to the fibula, the superficial peroneal nerve and its branches anteriorly and the sural nerve posteriorly and distally are identified and protected. The immediate structure below the incision is the ankle joint and tibiofibular joint capsule with their aponeurotic covering, the aponeurotic covering is incised and with blunt dissection the tear is exposed. To expose the calcaneofibular and the anterior portion of posterior tibiofibular ligament the peroneal sheath is incised and the tendons are retracted. The lateral ligaments are stressed for stability of the ankle and the subtalar joint. The torn ends of the ligaments are approximated and if there is any bony avulsion, suture anchor are used. For talocalcaneal ligament tear with subtalar instability, the subtalar joint is stabilized by suturing the calcaneofibular ligament. Wound is then closed in layers over drain and joint protected in a cast. Commonly, the ligament ends are friable so it is recommended to augment the repair by pulling up and suturing the transverse portion of extensor retinaculum (Gould technique) onto the Broström repair.

185. What are the indications and contraindications of tibiotalarcalcaneal (TTC) nail? What are the advantages of TTC nail over other methods of ankle arthrodesis?

Ans:
Indications:
- Painful arthritis following posttraumatic arthritis, rheumatoid arthritis, infection, neuromuscular conditions, neuropathic joints, chronic instability, AVN of talus, primary OA, tumor resection
- Salvage of failed total ankle arthroplasty, failed ORIF
- As a salvage procedure for failure of ankle fusion by other modalities

Contraindications:
- Stiffness of other joints of the lower limbs
- Severe OA of other joints of lower limbs
- Severe malalignment of tibia
- Severe vascular disease of lower limb
- Loss of calcaneal body height

Advantages of TTC nail over other methods of ankle arthrodesis:

Hindfoot nail is a good option as it is an intra-articular compression device giving:
- Relative stability and earlier return to function with bone grafting increasing chances of a solid fusion.
- The procedure is less time consuming.
- Results cosmetically superior than other modalities
- There is minimal soft-tissue stripping.
- Lesser chances of malunion/nonunion/loss of reduction

186. Discuss briefly principle and indications of hindfoot nail in acute and neglected trauma.

Ans: *Principle*: Retrograde intramedullary nailing provides a load-sharing fixation device with superior biomechanical properties and is an excellent choice for use in tibiotalocalcaneal arthrodesis. It provides good primary stability and cause limited soft-tissue damage and compression. They are capable of generating compression and thereby accelerate bone healing, increasing fusion rates especially in debilitated patients with poor bone quality. The common goal of the procedure is to achieve a painless solid arthrodesis with a biomechanically stable plantigrade foot.

Indications:
- Complex hindfoot deformity
- Failed ankle arthroplasty
- Primary or secondary osteoarthritis of ankle
- Failed ankle joint arthrodesis with subsequent subtalar arthritis
- The other common general indications include arthrodesis in Charcot foot arthropathy, rheumatoid arthritis affecting the ankle joint.

4B.27 ARCHES OF FOOT AND PRINCIPLES OF FOOT STABILIZATION (Q187–189)

187. Describe the arches of foot.

Ans: The foot as a segmented structure is capable of bearing weight, as it is in the form of arch. The foot has three arches maintained by the bony anatomy, muscular activity, and the ligaments. They are present at birth.
- *Medial longitudinal arch*: The medial margin of the foot, from the heel to the first metatarsal head, is arched above the ground because of the important medial longitudinal arch. This part is missing from the wet footprints as it is too tall and does not normally touches the floor.
- *Lateral longitudinal arch*: This is formed by the lateral margin of foot to the lateral two toes and bears most of the weight during ambulation. The pressure exerted on the ground by the lateral margin of the foot is greatest at the heel and the fifth metatarsal head and least between these areas because of the presence of the low-lying lateral longitudinal arch.
- *Transverse arch*: The transverse arch involves the bases of the five metatarsals and the cuboid and cuneiform bones. This is, in fact only half an arch (the other half being provided by the other foot when placed together), with its base on the lateral border of the foot and its summit on the foot's medial border.

Bones of the arches:
- *Medial longitudinal arch*: The calcaneum, the talus, the navicular bone, the three cuneiform bones, and the first three metatarsal bones.
- *Lateral longitudinal arch*: This consists of the calcaneum, the cuboid, and the fourth and fifth metatarsal bones.
- *Transverse arch*: This consists of the bases of the metatarsal bones, the cuboid, and the three cuneiform bones.

Mechanism of arch support (Masonry concept)
- *The shape of the stones*: The stones are wedge shaped, with the thin edge of the wedge lying inferiorly preventing it from slipping. This applies particularly to the important stone that occupies the center of the arch and is referred to as the "keystone".
- *Cementing the stones*: This is accomplished by interlocking the stones (bones) or binding their lower edges together with strong cords (ligaments). This method binds the lower edges of the stones together, when the arch is weight bearing.
- *The use of the tie beams*: They connect the distant pillars of long arches by preventing their separation. This is especially useful when the foundations at either end are shallow or base insecure, a tie beam effectively prevents sagging of the arch in such cases.
- *Suspension mechanism*: The structure of the arch is maintained by suspension cables from above to prevent from sagging or collapsing.

Maintenance of medial longitudinal arch:
- *Shape of the bones*: The rounded head of the talus is the keystone in the center of the arch. The sustentaculum tali holds up the talus, the concave proximal surface of the navicular bone receives the rounded head of the talus and it itself fits into the proximal surface of the medial cuneiform bone. The medial longitudinal arch is supported by the spring ligament, which shoulders the head of the talus.
- *Interosseous ties (cement and staples)*: The inferior edges of the bones are tied together by the plantar ligaments, which are larger and stronger than the dorsal ligaments. The most important ligament is the plantar calcaneonavicular ligament. The tendinous extensions of the insertion of the tibialis posterior muscle also hold the small bones together.
- The tie beams for medial longitudinal arch are the plantar aponeurosis, the medial part of the flexor digitorum brevis, the abductor hallucis, the flexor hallucis longus, the medial part of the flexor digitorum longus, and the flexor hallucis brevis.
- *Arch suspension*: Suspending the arch from above are the tibialis anterior and posterior and the medial ligament of the ankle joint. Though previously considered very important structure for static maintenance of the arches the tibialis anterior, the peroneus longus, and the small muscles of the foot have been now found to play no important role in the normal static support of the arches. They provide support only while, walking, and running.

Maintenance of lateral longitudinal arch:
- *Shape of the bones*: The cuboid is the keystone.
- The inferior edges of the bones are tied together by the long and short plantar ligaments and the origins of the short muscles from the forepart of the foot.
- *Tie beams*: The plantar aponeurosis, the abductor digiti minimi, and the lateral part of the flexor digitorum longus and brevis.
- *Arch suspension*: The peroneus longus and the brevis.

Maintenance of transverse arch:
- *Shape of the bones*: The marked wedge shaping of the cuneiform bones and the bases of the metatarsal bones.
- The inferior edges of the bones are tied together by the deep transverse ligaments, the strong plantar ligaments and the origins of the plantar muscles from the forepart of the foot, the dorsal interossei, and the transverse head of the adductor hallucis are particularly important in this respect.
- *Tie beam*: The peroneus longus tendon.
- *Arch suspension*: The peroneus longus tendon and the peroneus brevis.

188. What is pes cavus? Discuss classification of pes cavus. What are the causes of pes cavus? Discuss Coleman block test and its interpretation in pes cavus.

Ans: Cavus foot is a deformity of the foot characterized by an excessively high longitudinal plantar arch (sagittal plane deformity, with either a plantarflexion of the forefoot on the rearfoot, or dorsiflexion of the rearfoot on the forefoot).

Classification:
Kindly see Answer to *Question 98B above.*

Etiology: The following are the causes of pes cavus:
- Idiopathic or postural deformity
- Paralytic foot
  - Contracture during acute stage, e.g., poliomyelitis
  - Charcot–Marie–Tooth disease
  - Muscle imbalance during growth period
- In association with certain neurological diseases or developmental deformity of spine

Coleman block test:
Coleman's block test is also called Coleman lateral block test. This test is used to determine the flexibility of hindfoot in a patient with pes cavus and heel varus and ultimately guide treatment. Principle of test is that in some cases the hindfoot varus is produced by excessive plantar flexion of the first metatarsal (metatarsal drop), and if that is eliminated, then the varus corrects. The test is performed by asking the patient to stand on a wooden block in such a way that the heel and lateral edge of forefoot (fifth metatarsal) rests on the block but the first metatarsal is off the block. Usually the block is 1 inch in height. The examiner observes from rear side of patient. Standing in such a way allows the first metatarsal to drop to the floor (plantarflex) without driving the rest of the foot.
  - If the heel varus corrects and returns to neutral position (or even valgus), it indicates that the deformity is due to first metatarsal plantarflexion and the foot would be correctable by reducing the plantarflexion of the first ray and/or balancing the dynamic cause (peroneus longus overdrive).
  - If the hindfoot remains in varus, then it indicates rigid hindfoot deformity and pes cavus is due to tripod effect of fixed varus. This deformity will not correct with correction of first metatarsal flexion. This may also arise from tibialis posterior spasticity.

189. Describe the principles of stabilization of foot.

Ans: This is an incomplete question and as is the case with most of DNB theory questions, one has no idea as to what should be written as answer so students often write anything to fill pages (there is also no other alternative as such)—typical example of GIGO (garbage in garbage out).

The question can be completed if one asks *the principles of foot stabilization by arthrodesis.*

These principles are as follows:
- Proceed from proximal to distal reconstruction if multiple deformities are to be corrected (hip → knee → ankle)
- Intra-articular arthrodesis is preferable to extra-articular procedure
- Prepare wide cancellous apposing surfaces for bony arthrodesis to be successful
- Remove all devitalized bone in osteonecrosis for good bone deposition
- In microvascular diseases (like diabetes): Immobilization and skin flaps need more importance
- Fluoroscopic guided anesthetic injections are best to guide the target joint for arthrodesis
- Ask patient to stop smoking for at least 2 weeks before surgery and until bone union
- Perform two-stage arthrodesis in cases of infection—first stage to ameliorate infection and excision of focus
- Increase surface area of arthrodesis by fish-scaling or feathering
- Put the joints in most optimal position of function before coaptation
- Achieve adequate compression at the apposing surfaces
- Soft tissues must be respected else whole purpose of surgery is defeated.

PES PLANUS, CALCANEOVALGUS DEFORMITY, AND POSTERIOR TIBIAL TENDON DYSFUNCTION (Q190–195)

190. Explain pes planus.

Ans: Flatfoot is a frequently-encountered pathology in the adult population affecting females more than males peaking at 55 years of age. It refers to partial or complete loss of the normal medial longitudinal arch that develops after skeletal

maturity. Pes planus may arise out of various osseous, ligamentous, muscular-paralytic, spastic or postural causes resulting from mostly a benign process reflecting continuation of a congenital problem, trauma, or a condition associated with systemic pathology:
- Osseous—trauma (run-over fracture, fracture of navicular or calcaneus) or from osseous diseases
- Ligamentous variety develops from rupture or avulsion of plantar ligaments
- Paralytic and spastic muscular types—the flattening of the arch is secondary to altered muscle balance. Posterior tibial tendon dysfunction/insufficiency is the most common cause of adult acquired flatfoot.

Pathomechanism:
- There are two main pathological mechanisms for development of pes planus or loss of longitudinal arch:
  - Calcaneus may be at fault and heel gets drawn up resulting in equinus deformity.
  - The medial anterior pillar may be pulled up keeping the big toe off the ground as a result of the varus deformity.
- The common causes of flatfoot resulting from muscular causes are excessive fatigue of normal muscles as in:
  - Occupations which require standing or working for long hours
  - Rapid gain in weight (e.g., menopause)
  - Shoe wear
  - Severe trauma.

Symptoms:
- Feet feel tired after activity.
- Tendency to walk with feet everted.
- Tenderness is felt over navicular, inferior calcaneonavicular ligament, sole of the foot, and below the first metatarsal head.
- Gait is inelastic and clumsy, rising of the heel is avoided, to prevent strain on tarsal and metatarsal ligaments.
- Patient carefully lifts ball and heel of the foot together. The toes are turned outward.
- Medial parts of shoe wear-out more quickly.
- Skin, along the medial border of the heel and foot, is thickened and painful. Callosities may form in weight-bearing areas, and over little toe.

Physical examination:
- Depression of the medial longitudinal arch
- Everted or valgus heel in relaxed stance
- Abduction of the forefoot relative to the rearfoot
- Localized tenderness at posterior tibial tendon, plantar fascia, and lateral rearfoot
- *Assess*:
  - Range of motion at various components
  - Flexibility and reducibility of deformity by the Hubscher maneuver (Jack test)
  - Single heel rise and double heel rise test (reducibility of rearfoot valgus).

Radiology:
- Calcaneal pitch is decreased in a flatfoot deformity and becomes negative in the presence of a rocker-bottom deformity.
- Talocalcaneal angle is formed by the long axis of the rearfoot and the midtalar line. This angle is increased in pronated feet on both the anteroposterior (AP) and lateral views.
- Increased talar-first metatarsal angle.

Stages:
- Foot strain or incipient flatfoot. It is the earliest stage and corresponds to the period, when foot is undergoing deformation and bearing pressure. The ligaments absorb the pressure and undergo stretching and lengthening changes. There is no evident deformity.
- Mobile or flexible flatfoot.
- Rigid flatfoot.

Flexible pes planus
The arch may not develop fully until the child is 7–10 years old. Even then once the child is made to stand on toes, the arch appears. Generally adult flexible pes planus is a progression of a pediatric condition unilateral or, more commonly, as bilateral frequently associated with a short or contracted TA. In its late stages of progression, degenerative arthritis may occur, leading to loss of flexibility or ankylosis ± peroneal spasm due to arthritis produces pronation of rearfoot causing long arch collapse.

Etiology: The following conditions are commonly implicated in the development of flexible pes planus—
- Faulty postural activity of the muscles
- Short tendo-Achilles
- Varus deformity of forefoot (skewfoot)
- Spinal dysraphism (e.g., spina bifida, diastematomyelia, and lumbosacral lipomata).

Clinical examination of flexible flatfoot:
- When the child stands, there is a flattening of the longitudinal arches, which disappears on standing on toes.
- Short tendo-Achilles is apparent when the foot is correctly aligned and equinus is revealed.
- Valgus deformities of the knees.
- *Tender areas may be seen at*:
  - Sinus tarsi—suggestive of lateral subtalar impingement
  - Talonavicular joint
  - Plantar arch and heel
  - Posterior tibial tendon
  - Anterior tibial tendon
  - Anterior or posterior tibia
  - Subfibular impingement pain.

Conservative
- *Shoe modification*: An arch support is placed in shoe with a firm heel counter, an extended medial counter, a steel shank, a Thomas heel and a medial heel wedge. Continuous use of a molded orthosis over an extended period can result in an improved arch radiographically and clinically.
- Analgesics.
- Orthotic management [ankle-foot orthosis (AFO)] and activity modification.

Surgical management: Surgical management is done for controlling disabling pain (and disability) after exhausting every means of conservative management (symptomatic nonresponder). It should not be performed for cosmetic reasons only. The surgeon should explain the loss of inversion and eversion of the foot resulting from surgical correction for the relief of pain and disability. The commonly used techniques are as follows:

Osteotomy:
- *Evans lateral column lengthening*: The Evans procedure involves lengthening the lateral column, by placing a bone graft from the tibia into the anterior process of the calcaneus. Medial and lateral columns are equalized in length. This procedure preserves the calcaneocuboid joint and pushes the navicular bone medially in relation to the talus. This procedure reduces forefoot abduction and realigns midtarsal joints. The first metatarsal is plantarflexed and also talocalcaneal subluxation is reduced.
- Posterior calcaneal displacement osteotomy (Koutsogiannis)—restores the inverter capability of gastrocsoleus and decreases medial arch load. In a symptomatic patient with flexible pes planus and excessive heel valgus, this calcaneal osteotomy is intended to displace the posterior part of the calcaneus medially to restore normal weight-bearing alignment.
- Double calcaneal osteotomy (evans + posterior calcaneal displacement osteotomy).
- Plantar flexion osteotomy of medial cuneiform (Hirose and Johnson).
- Cotton medial cuneiform opening wedge osteotomy.
- Anterior calcaneal lengthening-distraction wedge osteotomy (Mosca).

Arthrodesis:
- Medial column—naviculocuneiform joint(s) and/or metatarsocuneiform joint when medial column collapse is noted. Durham pes planus plasty (Caldwell Coleman) combines advancement of the posterior tibial tendon and osteoperiosteal flap with arthrodesis of the navicular-first cuneiform joint.
- Talonavicular—corrects talar head subluxation.
- Calcaneocuboid distraction—similar to Evans procedure.
- Double (midtarsal joint)—talonavicular and calcaneocuboid joints. These produce lesser subtalar joint arthrosis than isolated talonavicular arthrodesis.
- Subtalar—better done for flatfoot with a reducible deformity without midtarsal joint arthrosis or fixed forefoot varus.
- Triple—more suitable for rigid flatfoot. The patient's bone age should be 12 years or older. Arthrodesis for relieving painful pes planus has been most successful when subtalar joint is included, although midtarsal arthrodesis without inclusion of the subtalar joint has gained popularity.

Soft tissue procedure:
- Kidner posterior tibial tendon advancement
- FDL transfer
- Spring ligament reconstruction + medial arch reconstruction.

Rigid pes planus

The rigid pes planus deformity results from bony abnormality such as tarsal coalition or congenital vertical talus or arthritis (subtalar or midtarsal). Posterior tibial tendon dysfunction is the most common cause of adult acquired flatfoot. Other causes like Charcot's/post-traumatic are less common.

Clinical examination: In rigid flatfoot deformity in adults: There may be medial pain from posterior tibial tendonitis, lateral pain from talocalcaneal impingement or fibulocalcaneal impingement.

Patients examined from behind revealing medial flatness of arch and heel valgus. In advanced deformities "too many toes" are visible laterally but is not pathognomonic. Ankle range of motion should be evaluated that may be limited due to tendo-Achilles tightness. Tender areas may be seen at:
- Sinus tarsi
- Talonavicular joint
- Plantar arch and heel
- Posterior tibial tendon
- Anterior tibial tendon
- Anterior or posterior tibia
- Subfibular impingement pain.

Radiographic examination: One should obtain weight-bearing AP, lateral foot and ankle AP radiographs. Measure the Meary's angle, forefoot abduction, talar head uncoverage and talar tilt. Talar head uncoverage may be calculated as percentage or may be alternatively assessed by lateral talonavicular in congruency angle that indirectly indicates 30% or more talar head uncoverage.

Radiographs also help in identifying arthritic changes that develop in advanced deformities.

Nonsurgical treatment: Cast (cam type or removable boot), AFO.

Surgical treatment: Brace wear is quite cumbersome and so the compliance rate is low. Obesity is also a contributory factor for failure of conservative treatment. This entails frequent need for operative management.
- *Stage 1*: Synovectomy if noninvasive method ineffective. Conservative management is attempted for 3 months initially.
- *Stage 2A*: Synovectomy or tendon debridement is done. Posterior calcaneal displacement osteotomy or Evans procedure may be required in some cases as above. This is often combined with flexor digitorum longus (FDL) transfer to navicular with/without tendo-Achilles/gastrocnemius lengthening. For elevated medial column precluding the tripod function of foot, one can do open dorsal medial cuneiform osteotomy (cotton osteotomy) to bring down 1st metatarsal if TMT joint is stable. For arthritis/unstable joint arthrodesis of the joint is better.

- *Stage 2B*: Synovectomy or tendon repair and tendon transfer. Realignment procedures as osteotomy for stage 2A may be required. Medial column arthrodesis, calcaneocuboid interpositional bone block as isolated procedures have also been recommended. Lateral column lengthening such as Evans-like procedure or calcaneocuboid distraction are commonly performed to improve foot arch by correcting talonavicular joint abduction.
- *Stage 3* requires triple arthrodesis for whole foot involvement. It is commonly prescribed but attempt should be made to preserve calcaneocuboid joint as far as possible. Heel valgus should be corrected to less than 5° and if this is not possible during arthrodesis then calcaneal osteotomy is an option. The forefoot should be neither in pronation or supination.
- *Stage 4* deformity (valgus deformity without arthrosis) correction need triple arthrodesis in combination with deltoid ligament repair and a medializing calcaneal osteotomy. Pantalar arthrodesis/ankle replacement is needed for involvement of foot and ankle joint arthrosis.

191. Describe muscular dynamics in calcaneovalgus deformity. Describe management in patients before and after skeletal maturity.

Ans: Calcaneovalgus deformity produces flat foot and exaggeration of same deformity over time. Flexible flat foot is the precursor that becomes rigid if not corrected later. The muscular dynamics is mostly centered around posterior tibial tendon dysfunction as follows:

Posterior tibial tendon insufficiency is central to development of adult flatfoot in most of the cases. This is however associated with failure of both capsular and ligamentous structures at midfoot region for complete expression of the deformity. Peritalar subluxation defines the pathologic malalignment of the talus about the subtalar and midtarsal joints resulting from the combined ligamentous, capsular and tendon insufficiency.

- As the calcaneonavicular ligament yields, the head of the talus is pressed forward, downward, and medially.
- The calcaneum may deviate medially and its anterior end is depressed, resulting in sustentaculum tali and head of the talus and tuberosity of navicular forming prominences on the medial side of foot.
- The long and short plantar ligaments yield, followed by yielding of deltoid ligament. Dysfunction of the deltoid ligament results in medial ankle instability with development of ankle and foot deformity occurring in the most advanced cases of flatfoot deformity.

(*For management of flexible and rigid deformities, kindly vide Answer to Question 190*)

192. Anatomy of tibialis posterior tendon. What is tibialis posterior dysfunction? Describe management of such cases.

Ans: *Anatomy (Fig. 4B.28.1)*:

Origin: Lateral side of posterior aspect of tibia, upper two-thirds of medial surface of fibula, interosseous membrane.

Insertion: Tuberosity of navicular and via ligaments to all cuneiforms; second, third, and fourth metatarsals; and cuboid and sustentaculum tali.

Action: Plantar flexor and invertor of foot.

Nerve supply: Tibial nerve.

Dysfunction and management: The posterior tibial tendon is the primary dynamic stabilizer of the medial longitudinal arch. The tendon inserts mainly on the navicular, but has minor additional attachments to the cuneiforms and metatarsal bases. Insufficiency of tendon is caused by an elongated or degenerative tendon over the course of its watershed area from the tip of the medial malleolus to 2 cm distal. Over a course of evolution other structures also get involved like the spring ligament, talonavicular capsule, and deltoid ligament exacerbating the pathology. The superior medial portion of spring ligament combines with the deltoid ligament and is frequently initially involved. In rare instances, isolated spring ligament

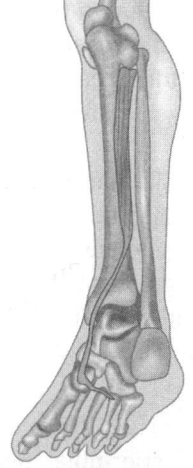

Fig. 4B.28.1: Anatomical disposition of tibialis posterior tendon.

rupture may initiate the pathology of adult acquired flatfoot deformity (AAFD). With the progressing insufficiency of posterior tibial tendon unopposed peroneus brevis causes further attenuation of the spring ligament.

This causes plantar flexion and downward tilt of the talar head and the Achilles or gastrocnemius-soleus complex develops a contracture. The forefoot then abducts, creating talonavicular uncoverage. With advanced disease, flexible deformities can become rigid, limiting treatment options.

The following are the common features of posterior tibial tendon dysfunction:
- Typically unilateral
- Usually progressive flexible to rigid flatfoot depending on stage
- Common in women 45–65 years of age
- Family history common.

Classification—modified Johnson Strom

The classification basically represents the stages of progression of adult flatfoot deformity over time if uninterrupted. A patient may present with any of the stage depending on the severity at seeking consultation. Following are the clinical features of different stages that can be identified at presentation.
- *Stage 1*:
  - Pain and edema along the medial aspect of the rearfoot indicating tenosynovitis or early tendinosis
  - Increased warmth, edema, and tenderness along the course of the tendon. Spondyloarthropathy has also been associated with stage I AAFD in a subgroup of patients.
  - The patient is able to complete single heel rise with ease.
- *Stage 2A*:
  - Medial rearfoot pain, edema, and tenderness along the course of the posterior tibial tendon, and mild valgus of the heel, with or without lowering of the medial longitudinal arch
  - Abduction of the forefoot on the rearfoot (too many toes sign)
  - Complete single heel rise with difficulty
  - Increased talo-first metatarsal angle, peritalar subluxation on radiographs. There is less than 30% talonavicular uncoverage on a standing AP radiograph of the foot.
- *Stage 2B*: Stage 2A + lateral pain (sinus tarsi, subfibular, cuboid), more severe valgus, medial arch collapse. There is more than 30% talonavicular uncoverage on AP radiographs representing higher grade failure of spring ligament and other midfoot restraints. Lateral subtalar joint impingement will also come under stage IIb.
- *Stage 3*:
  - More severe and fixed deformities. The rigidity classically arises at the triple joint complex (talonavicular, subtalar, and calcaneocuboid joints) leading to fixed hindfoot valgus and abduction through the midfoot
  - Loss of subtalar joint motion
  - Posterior muscle group contracture
  - Unable to perform single heel raise test
  - Rearfoot remains everted with double heel eversion
  - Degenerative changes in rearfoot, increased angular deformities.
- *Stage 4*:
  - Medial soft tissue restraints become weak. The deformity at foot is basically aggravated by valgus deformity at ankle joint. There is valgus tilt of talus in AP view on radiographs.
  - Degenerative changes in ankle joint also. The deformity is further divided into two stages—4A is characterized by hindfoot valgus, flexible ankle valgus without significant ankle arthritis. Stage 4B refers to hindfoot valgus with rigid or flexible ankle valgus with significant arthritis.

Nonsurgical treatment
- *Stage 1*:
  - Cast (Cam type cast or removable boot) or brace for 4 weeks→ physiotherapy [strengthening exercises for the posterior tibial, peroneals, anterior tibial, and gastrocnemius and soleus muscles. Also incorporate isokinetic exercises, exercise band, heel rises (double and single support), and toe walking]
  - Nonsteroidal anti-inflammatory drugs.

- *Stage 2*:
  - Orthosis with deep heel cup
  - Extended medial counter and medial heel wedge
  - Immobilization for painful foot.
- *Stage 3*: Short articulated AFO or custom brace (viz. Arizone brace).
- *Stage 4*: Nonarticulated AFO.

Surgical treatment: Brace wear is quite cumbersome and so the compliance rate is low. Obesity is also a contributory factor for failure of conservative treatment. This entails frequent need for operative management.
- *Stage 1*: Synovectomy if noninvasive method ineffective. Some recommend additional medializing calcaneal osteotomy to correct heel valgus.
- *Stage 2A*: Synovectomy or tendon debridement is done. Posterior calcaneal displacement osteotomy or Evans procedure may be required in some cases as above. This is often combined with FDL transfer to navicular with/without tendo-Achilles/gastrocnemius lengthening. For arthritis/unstable joint arthrodesis of the joint is better.
- Blocking the movement at subtalar joint (hindfoot valgus) and reorienting the calcaneus vertically using implant (usually screw-like spacer) at sinus tarsi often ameliorates the symptoms but pain may not subside until screw removal. Arthroereisis also dorsiflexes the talus and corrects talonavicular subluxation.
- *Stage 2B*: Synovectomy or tendon repair and tendon transfer. Realignment procedures as osteotomy for stage 2A may be required. Medial column arthrodesis, calcaneocuboid interpositional bone block as isolated procedures have also been recommended. Lateral column lengthening such as Evans-like procedure or calcaneocuboid distraction are commonly performed to improve foot arch by correcting talonavicular joint abduction.
- *Stage 3* requires one of the arthrodesis procedures. Triple arthrodesis for whole foot involvement is commonly prescribed but attempt should be made to preserve calcaneocuboid joint as far as possible. Heel valgus should be corrected to less than 5° and if this is not possible during arthrodesis then calcaneal osteotomy is an option.
- *Stage 4* deformity (valgus deformity without arthrosis) correction need triple arthrodesis in combination with deltoid ligament repair and a medializing calcaneal osteotomy. Pantalar arthrodesis/ankle replacement is needed for involvement of foot and ankle joint arthrosis.

193. Discuss causes, diagnosis, treatment of peroneal tendon disorders.
Ans:

Causes:
Peroneal tendon disease secondary to trauma or stenosis is very common. Traumatic include overuse with microrupture or calcification, dislocation or subluxation, lateral malleolar fractures, calcaneal fractures, and inversion ankle injuries. Nontraumatic entities include inflammatory arthritis, infection, os peroneum, congenital enlarged peroneal tubercle, or very rarely local tumors.

Diagnosis:
Peroneal tendon disorders typically involve issues with the peroneal tendons, which include the peroneus longus and peroneus brevis. Diagnosis of peroneal tendon disorders involves a combination of clinical evaluation, imaging studies, and sometimes special tests. Here are the steps commonly involved in the diagnosis:

Clinical Evaluation:
- *History taking*:
  - Patient's symptoms (pain, swelling, and tenderness).
  - Duration and onset of symptoms.
  - Any history of trauma or overuse activities (e.g., running, dancing).
  - Any previous ankle injuries or surgeries.
- *Physical examination*:
  - Inspection for swelling, deformities, or discoloration.
  - Palpation to identify tender areas along the course of the peroneal tendons.

- Range of motion assessment to evaluate ankle mobility.
- Assessment for swelling or crepitus (a crackling or grating sound) during movement.
- Strength tests to check for weakness in foot eversion and plantarflexion.

Special tests:
- Resisted eversion test: Pain during resisted eversion indicates potential peroneal tendon involvement.
- Tendon stability test: Assessing for any subluxation of the tendons during ankle motion.

Imaging studies:
- *X-rays*: To rule out fractures or bony abnormalities, especially if there is a history of trauma.
- *Ultrasound*: Can assess tendon thickness and detect tears or inflammation (tendinosis).
- *MRI*: The most comprehensive imaging modality, providing detailed images of soft tissues to identify tendon tears, degeneration, or any associated conditions like tenosynovitis.
- *CT scan*: Rarely used but can help assess bony structures and possible impingements.

Differential diagnosis:
Differentiate peroneal tendon disorders from other conditions such as:
- Lateral ankle sprains
- Peroneal tendon subluxation
- Tarsal tunnel syndrome
- Ankle impingement
- Other tendon pathologies

Management:
Once a diagnosis is made, management may include conservative treatments (rest, ice, physical therapy, orthotics) or surgical intervention, depending on the severity of the disorder.

Treatment:
- Activity modification (cast immobilization for a short period if necessary), PRICE (protection, rest, ice, compression, elevation), NSAIDs
- Orthotics and shoe wear modifications (decreasing calcaneal fibular impingement with a medial heel wedge)
- Physiotherapy directed at muscle strengthening and improving mobility should be instituted.
- Surgery is reserved for resistant cases and mostly comprises of debridement of the diseased tendon. Often peroneal instability contributes to the diseased peroneals, and therefore strong consideration should be given to a peroneal stabilization procedure concurrent with a debridement. An acute rupture may benefit from early surgical intervention to promote rehabilitation and prevent re-rupture as with other tendons. With respect to partial or chronic tears, a debridement and repair or reconstruction of the tendon is indicated.

194. What is tibialis posterior dysfunction? Describe the management of such cases.
Ans: Kindly see Answer to Question 171.

195. What is calcaneoplasty? What are its indications, advantages and shortcomings?
Ans: Calcaneoplasty is a surgical treatment of Haglund's syndrome posterior calcaneal exostosis involving dorsal closing wedge osteotomy of the posterosuperior aspect of calcaneal tuberosity with saw followed by smoothening of the resultant osteotomized surface. The procedure can now be performed in a minimal invasive manner using arthroscope (osteotomy is not performed).

Indications: Failed conservative treatment for Haglund's deformity

Advantages:
- Removal of impinging calcaneal bone causing tendinopathy
- Removal of diseased tendon and replacement by healthier tendon
- Endoscopic procedure can be performed in an outpatient manner with shorter recovery time

Shortcomings:
- Pain for prolonged periods of time
- Wound dehiscence
- Secondary calcaneal impingement due to insertional tendon enlargement.

4B.29 PERONEAL NERVE AND ITS DISORDER: FOOT DROP (Q196–200)

196. **Explain the anatomy of common peroneal nerve (CPN). Name the muscles supplied by it and tendon transfer in CPN palsy.**

Ans: The common peroneal nerve originates from the sciatic nerve in the posterior compartment of thigh or in the popliteal fossa, and follows the medial margin of the biceps femoris tendon over the lateral head of the gastrocnemius muscle and toward the fibula **(Fig. 4B.29.1)**. Here it gives origin to two cutaneous branches, which descend in the leg:

- The *sural communicating nerve,* which joins the sural branch of the tibial nerve and contributes to innervation of skin over the lower posterolateral side of the leg
- The *lateral sural cutaneous nerve,* which innervates skin over the upper lateral leg.

The CPN continues around the neck of the fibula and enters the lateral compartment by passing between the attachments of the fibularis longus muscle to the head and shaft of fibula. Here the common fibular nerve divides into its two terminal branches:

- The superficial fibular nerve
- The deep fibular nerve.

The superficial fibular nerve descends in the lateral compartment deep to fibularis longus and innervates fibularis longus and fibularis brevis. It then penetrates deep fascia in the lower leg and enters the foot where it divides into medial and lateral branches, which supply dorsal areas of the foot and toes except for:

- The web space between the great and second toes, which is supplied by the deep fibular nerve
- The lateral side of the little toe, which is supplied by the sural branch of the tibial nerve.

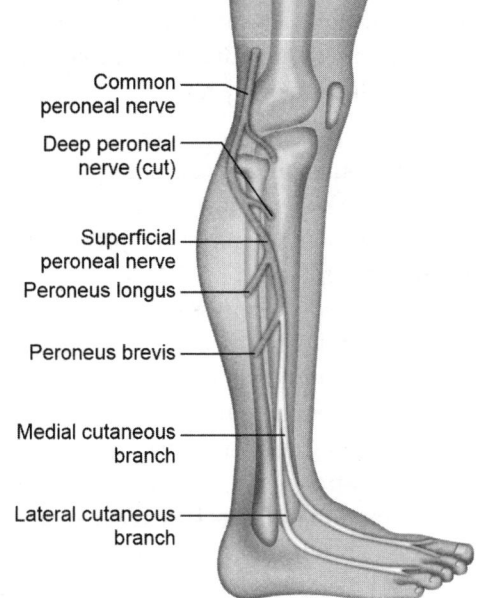

Fig. 4B.29.1: Branches of the common peroneal nerve.

The deep fibular nerve passes anteromedially through the intermuscular septum into the anterior compartment of leg.

Muscles supplied:

Deep peroneal—
- Tibialis anterior (TA)
- Extensor hallucis longus
- Extensor digitorum longus
- Peroneus tertius.

Superficial peroneal—
- Peroneus longus
- Peroneus brevis.

Tendon transfer: In surgical correction for foot drop, tendon transfer procedures involve a transfer of a tendon that is still working in place of the tendon that is not functioning. Mostly, it involves transfer of the posterior tibial tendon.

- *Bridle procedure*: It is called so because in this procedure, three tendons are attached in bridle configuration, namely posterior tibial tendon, tibialis anterior, and peroneus longus tendon. Normally, tibialis posterior tendon is inserted

on the navicular bone from which it is taken off and attached to second cuneiform bone, and it is attached to anterior tibial tendon and anteriorly transferred peroneus longus tendon in bridle configuration. Now, the posterior tibial muscle will pull the foot up when it contracts, and thus balance the foot in dorsiflexion.
- In neurotendinous transposition, the lateral head of the gastrocnemius is transposed along with the proximal end of the deep peroneal nerve to the tendons of the anterior muscle group. The nerve is neurotized to the motor nerve of the lateral head of the gastrocnemius. This restores active voluntary dorsiflexion of the foot and automatic walking.

197. Common peroneal nerve injury: early and delayed management after hip dislocation.

Ans: Early-sciatic nerve palsy complicates simple posterior hip dislocation in 13% of patients. No neurologic sequelae have been reported after anterior hip dislocation. The peroneal portion of the sciatic nerve is more commonly affected than the tibial branch. The relationship of the peroneal distribution to the piriformis muscle, tethering of the nerve at the sciatic notch and fibular neck, and the overall morphology of the peroneal division are possible explanations for its relatively increased risk. At least partial recovery of nerve function can be expected in approximately two-thirds of patients. Significant controversy exists regarding the merits and timing of surgical exploration of the sciatic nerve after hip dislocation if closed reduction has been successfully performed and nerve function does not improve. Tornetta and Mostafavi recommended nerve exploration only if sciatic function was normal before reduction and deteriorated after closed reduction of the hip.

Delayed Management (> 6 weeks):
- Persistent neurological deficit:
  - Repeat electromyography (EMG)/nerve conduction studies (NCS) at 3 months to assess recovery.
  - MRI neurography if compressive lesion suspected.
- Surgical options:
  - Nerve decompression:
    - Indicated if fibular head compression or neuroma present.
    - Common peroneal nerve (CPN) release at fibular neck.
  - Nerve repair/grafting:
    - For complete transection (rare in hip dislocation).
    - Sural nerve autograft if gap present.
  - Tendon transfers (late reconstruction):
    - Bridle procedure (post. tibialis transfer to dorsum) for permanent foot drop.
    - Peroneus longus to tibialis anterior transfer.
  - Arthrodesis (last resort):
    - Ankle fusion in severe, nonrecoverable cases.
- Rehabilitation:
  - Strengthening exercises for residual motor function.
  - Gait training with ankle-foot orthosis (AFO).

198. Describe foot drop and equinus deformity.

Ans: *Foot drop*: Foot drop is a crippling and complex problem that can be defined as a significant weakness of ankle and toe dorsiflexion so that the foot takes-up a plantarflexed position. There are many conditions that can lead to foot drop. Some of the associated conditions are stroke, trauma to foot or lower limb, nerve damage, diabetes, adverse drug reaction, alcoholic neuropathy, Parkinson's, multiple sclerosis, etc.

Generally, foot drop can be categorized into three groups:
1. *Neurologic [peripheral (commonly) or central]*:
   - Injury or neuropathy of deep peroneal, common peroneal of sciatic nerve
   - Prolapsed intervertebral disk (PIVD) (mainly L4-L5), injury to lumbar or sacral segments of spinal cord
   - Cerebral lesions involving motor area of foot (parasagittal region) or motor neuron disease
   - Compression of common peroneal or deep peroneal nerve at the fibular head is the most common compressive neuropathy in the lower extremity seen as a result of varied pathology. Peroneal nerve injury may arise iatrogenically due to ischemia, mechanical irritation, and traction, crush injury, laceration intraoperatively during total knee or hip

arthroplasty, proximal tibial osteotomy, correction of a severe valgus or flexion deformity at knee or postoperatively by hematoma or constrictive dressings
- In patients having rapid weight loss after operation (e.g., bariatric surgery), neuropathy leading to foot drop may occur. Vitamin B12 deficiency may be an involved factor
- Central causes include stroke, multiple sclerosis, Charcot-Marie-Tooth disease, etc.

2. *Muscular*:
   - Direct injury to the dorsiflexors, subcutaneous tendon (tibialis anterior) rupture
   - Muscular dystrophy, polio, amyotrophic lateral sclerosis (Lou Gehrig's disease).
3. *Anatomic*:
   - Compartment syndromes (anterior leg compartment syndrome resulting in weakness of the dorsiflexors, deep posterior compartment Volkmann ischemic contracture causing tethering of the foot in plantar flexion, chronic compartment syndrome slowly causing the symptoms especially in the soldiers—march gangrene
   - Habitual crossed leg sitting
   - Charcot's joints.

Pathophysiology: Axoplasmic flow is necessary for functional integrity of an axon (basic unit to transmit the electric impulse in a nerve) and its target. A laceration interrupts the anatomical axon unit. Axoplasmic flow may also be compromised by crush injury. It may also be diminished by an injury proximally in nerve root, rendering it more susceptible to subsequent injury (double-crush phenomenon). Foot drop occurs when distal lesion occurs resulting in clinical palsy. Double-crush phenomenon may be the cause for increased prevalence of foot drop in spinal stenosis patients undergoing total hip joint replacement. The proximal insult occurs by spinal stenosis and the distal insult may result from sciatic nerve stretch during the surgery.

Clinical features: Patient stands with the foot everted and has some loss of dorsiflexion, when attempting to heel-walk.

Gait: Patients have a steppage gait or a high stepping gait like that of soldiers in paretic foot drop. In paralytic foot drop, the foot slaps on the ground after heel makes the initial contact as the dorsiflexors are unable to hold the foot during heel strike. This produces "slapping foot gait".

Diagnosis

Laboratory studies: Work-up of foot drop proceeds according to the suspected cause. Investigation of metabolic cause includes—
- Fasting blood sugar
- Hemoglobin A1c
- Liver function test (alcoholic)
- Erythrocyte sedimentation rate
- C-reactive protein
- Serum protein electrophoresis
- Renal function test
- Vitamin B_{12} levels.

Imaging studies

Plain films: To look for exostosis or Charcot's joint.

Ultrasonography: If bleeding is suspected in a patient with a hip or knee prosthesis.

Nerve conduction studies (NCS): To assess the regeneration of nerve fibers, site of lesion and document the damage to nerve. Electromyogram additionally helps to identify peripheral neuropathy, myopathy, nerve radiculopathy, motor neuron disease, peripheral nerve compression (peroneal of CPN), etc.

Treatment

Conservative and medical therapy

The condition is commonly managed conservatively at detection for establishing diagnosis and preventing contracture. An ankle-foot orthosis (AFO) is used to control the position of ankle and toes during swing and stance phase, to compensate for ankle dorsiflexors, to minimize abnormal gait pattern and to increase the efficiency of walking. Foot stretch and isometric dorsiflexion are encouraged continuously. Sympathetic blocks help to control painful paresthesia. Managing metabolic etiologies like diabetes, alcohol liver damage, and neuropathies with supplements of B1, B6 or B12 can also be useful. Peroneal nerve stimulation can help faster recovery of neuropathy (especially successful for stroke and multiple sclerosis patients).

Depending on the cause of foot drop that is finally identified the surgical intervention is planned.

- Foot drop secondary to lumbar disk herniation needs discectomy
- Decompression of sciatic nerve may be necessary after foot drop following hip arthroplasty, especially following hematoma collection compressing the nerve is suspected and the nerve has not been surgically damaged
- Direct damage to the peroneal nerve needs neural repair
- In acute foot drop due to deep peroneal nerve injuries (less than 1-year duration); tibial or superficial peroneal nerve fascicle transfer can be done
- For chronic foot drop, contracture needs to be corrected by Achilles tendon lengthening
- Foot drop due to polio or Charcot's joint cannot be corrected by above-mentioned modalities and these patients require arthrodesis of ankle joint. Along with arthrodesis, if there is severe contracture, Achilles tendon lengthening needs to be done
- *Tendon transfers*: In surgical correction for foot drop, tendon transfer procedures involve a transfer of a tendon that is still working in place of the tendon that is not functioning. Mostly, it involves transfer of the posterior tibial tendon
    - *Bridle procedure*: It is called so because in this procedure, three tendons are attached in bridle configuration, namely posterior tibial tendon, tibialis anterior and peroneus longus tendon.
    - In neurotendinous transposition, the lateral head of the gastrocnemius is transposed along with the proximal end of the deep peroneal nerve to the tendons of the anterior muscle group. The nerve is neurotized to the motor nerve of the lateral head of the gastrocnemius. This restores active voluntary dorsiflexion of the foot and automatic walking.
- *Bone-block procedures for foot drop*: Gill, Campbell or Inclan posterior bone block were preferred methods of management of paralytic foot drops that resulted from polio in children who specifically had a limited involvement. The posterior bone block serve as an interim measure till a pantalar arthrodesis or Lambrinudi triple fusion could be undertaken on a skeletally mature foot.
- For the sheer reasons of uncommon post-polio feet in children and creation of nonanatomical deformity the procedure is less commonly followed if at all.
- *Arthrodesis*: For patients with unacceptable power in peroneals and a flail foot that cannot be managed by reconstruction of adequate dorsiflexion power, ankle or pantalar arthrodesis is a good option. The former is preferred for limited damage done to bone unless there are arthritic changes in the tarsal bones where latter is preferable.

Equinus foot: It is a deformity where the patient cannot dorsiflex ankle actively or passively.

Causes:
- Congenital talipes equinovarus (CTEV)
- Compensation for limb length discrepancy
- Polio
- Tendo-Achilles contracture
- Long-standing cases of foot drop.

Clinical examination: If patient is able to stand then make him stand on ground with knee in extension otherwise passively dorsiflex the foot to maximum possible. A normal patient will stand with plantigrade foot (ball of great toe and heel simultaneously touching the ground). In equines deformity the patient will not be able to touch the heel or the heel and great toe ball are not in the same horizontal plane. For quantification measure the distance between center of heel and great toe, else measure the angle foot makes with perpendicular to long axis of foot.

[Grading (*subjective*—*I*: cannot walk on heel, *II*: smaller heel with appearance of cavus, *III*: splaying of forefoot with exaggeration of II, *IV*: clawing of toes with III)]

Silfverskiold test: This test assesses passive dorsiflexion with knee extended and flexed (*In isolated gastrocnemius contracture, more dorsiflexion is possible with knee flexed as it relaxes muscle arising above knee. In isolated soleus contracture, knee position does not affect range of dorsiflexion. If both muscles are involved, slight increase in passive dorsiflexion is noted with knee flexed but still it is not within normal range*).

199. Explain the surgical reconstruction of 1.5-year-old common peroneal nerve palsy.

Ans: Kindly see the tendon transfers in Answer to Question 198.

200. Discuss pathoanatomy of sciatic nerve with special considerations in nerve injuries.

Ans: The *sciatic nerve*, which is formed by roots from the lumbosacral plexus (L4, L5, S1, S2, S3), appears in the buttock from beneath the lower border of the piriformis, just lateral to the inferior gluteal and pudendal nerves and vessels. It is usually surrounded by fat and is often easier to feel than to see. It passes vertically down the buttock together with its artery, lying on the short external rotator muscles of the inner muscular sleeve, the obturator internus, the two gemelli, and the quadratus femoris. Distally, it passes deep (anterior) to the biceps femoris and disappears from view, lying on the adductor magnus.

The sciatic nerve is safe during posterior approaches unless surgeon makes careless dissection or in conditions where there will be inevitable stretch on the nerve like significant lengthening done during the surgery. It can be injured if it is trapped in the posterior blade of the self-retaining retractor that holds the fascial edge. It also can be damaged if it is not protected during reduction of the prosthetic head into the acetabulum.

The tibial portion of the sciatic nerve supplies all the hamstring muscles, except the short head of the biceps femoris and the extensor portion of the adductor magnus in the thigh. All its branches arise from the medial side of the nerve. Dissections around the sciatic nerve in the thigh therefore should remain on the lateral (safe) side, since the only branch coming off that side runs to the short head of the biceps, a muscle that causes few clinical problems if its nerve supply is damaged.

The *common peroneal and tibial nerves*, the terminal branches of the sciatic nerve, supply all the muscles below the knee. In addition, they (and other sciatic branches) supply skin over the sole of the foot, the dorsum of the foot (except for its medial side), and the calf and lateral side of the lower leg.

Damage to the sciatic nerve at the level of the hip joint injures both tibial and common peroneal elements, resulting in a balanced flaccid paralysis below the knee, together with paralysis of the hamstring muscles. Complete sciatic nerve lesions are relatively rare; more often, the damage seems to affect either the tibial or the common peroneal components. Hence, neurologic findings may vary, regardless of the level of the lesion.

Common peroneal nerve palsies do occur after posterior approaches to the hip.

The question then arises as to whether the nerve was damaged at the operative site or whether it was compressed by external pressure on the nerve as it winds around the neck of the fibula. The differential diagnosis can be made by doing an electromyogram (EMG) of the short head of the biceps, the only muscle of the thigh that is supplied by the common peroneal division of the sciatic nerve. Lesions in the pelvis or at the level of the hip joint denervate this muscle. Lesions at the level of the fibular head leave it unaffected.

Only 20% of the cross section of the sciatic nerve at the hip joint is formed by nerve fibers. The remaining 80% is made up of connective tissue. Nerve repairs in this area are often unsuccessful, because bundle-to-bundle contact is difficult to achieve.

4B.30 TARSAL TUNNEL SYNDROME (Q201)

201. Discuss tarsal tunnel syndrome.

Ans: The term "tarsal tunnel syndrome" embraces entrapment neuropathy of posterior tibial nerve or its associated branches as it passes through the porta pedis (tarsal tunnel) deep to flexor retinaculum (laciniate ligament).

The individual neural components may also get compressed so their distribution should be known:
- Calcaneal branch—supplies the sensations to heel in medial and posterior distribution.
- Medial plantar branch—provides sensation to the medial aspect of sole of foot including the hallux and three toes and gives motor branches to the abductor hallucis (while traversing through it) and flexor digitorum brevis muscles.
- Lateral plantar branch—gives cutaneous sensation to the fifth digit and gives motor supply to the abductor digiti quinti and quadratus plantae muscles.

Etiology: Any condition that compromises the volume of tarsal tunnel will produce the syndrome, so tibial nerve may get constricted by either external pressure or lesions constricting space within the tunnel. The common causes include:
- *Fractures and malunion*: Bone fragments from displaced calcaneal fracture fragments (commonly), medial malleolus or talus
- *Inflammatory conditions*: Tenosynovitis and rheumatoid arthritis
- *Space occupying lesions*: Lipoma, ganglia, amyloidosis, schwannoma or exostosis
- *Double crush syndrome*: In case of lumbar spondylosis or prolapsed intervertebral disk at S1 the tibial nerve may be more susceptible to compression at the flexor retinaculum
- Varicosities
- *Intrinsic*: Neural tumor (neurilemmoma) and perineural fibrosis
- Valgus deformity of hindfoot may stretch the tibial nerve and cause perineural fibrosis by increasing tensile load on the nerve.

Clinical features:
- Patients report a nonspecific vague pain in the foot and sole often confusing with plantar fasciitis
- Pain, paresthesia, and numbness are not uncommon. The paresthesia and pain are normally referred distal to the site of compression but in one-third of patients, the pain may also radiate proximally into the midcalf (Valleix phenomenon)
- Tenderness may occur over the posterior tibial nerve causing local pain and paresthesia in the foot
- In patients with leprosy and amyloid neuropathy perineural thickening may be palpable
- Tapping over the posterior tibial nerve (Tinel's test) may give rise to paresthesias in the sole of the foot, medial heel, the instep of the sole and the toes
- In late cases, one may note atrophy of the intrinsic foot muscles
- In long-standing cases, neuropathic changes may be noted including deformity like pes cavus, and atrophic changes like loss of hair and skin ulceration.
- *The dorsiflexion-eversion test (Kinoshita et al.)*: Maximally dorsiflex the ankle and the metatarsophalangeal (MP) joints of all three toes, firmly evert the foot and hold this position. In a positive case, the patient's symptoms will be reproduced. Look also for increased local tenderness, accompanying the maneuver.
- The tourniquet test.

Investigations: Standard radiographs of the ankle and foot may demonstrate the fracture fragment protruding into the canal, exostosis, and bony deformities. Magnetic resonance imaging (MRI) may demonstrate the soft tissue causes of compression neuropathy. Nerve conduction studies (NCS) are the best and reliable diagnostic modalities to demonstrate the site of compression, type (sensory, motor, both), pathophysiology (axonal versus demyelinating), and changes in the muscles if performed by experienced person. Hematological investigations include evaluation for diabetes mellitus and long-term glycemic control (HbA1C), erythrocyte sedimentation rate (ESR), blood urea nitrogen (BUN), creatinine, and vitamin B12 levels.

Treatment

Medical treatment: This is indicated in the absence of demonstrable nerve compression.
- Initially the nonsteroidal anti-inflammatory drugs, oral steroids, and neurotropic vitamins are commonly tried for mild to moderate symptoms
- For nonresponsive patients, local injection of steroids into the tarsal canal may give temporary to permanent relief in some
- Correction of planovalgus deformity with physiotherapy or orthosis may also relieve symptoms in specific patients

- Use of night splints to maintain plantar flexion and inversion may also be tried for symptomatic relief (similar to carpal tunnel extension splint).

Surgical treatment: Surgical treatment is done in patients unresponsive to conservative therapy or if there is identified pathology on MRI or clinically or a deformity is present. Also, surgical release of the nerve is required in Ehlers-Danlos syndrome (EDS)-demonstrable nerve compression. Predictors of failed nonsurgical treatment included longer motor nerve conduction latency (7.4 ms or greater) and greater predominance of foot comorbidities. Tarsal tunnel release is the commonly performed surgery. Tunnel release and septum excision greatly reduce canal pressures. Additionally, one or more of the following may be required.

- External neurolysis is an acceptable procedure especially if on surgical exploration there are adhesions or scar tissue formation causing the nerve impingement.
- Space-occupying masses require specific removal. Also, correction of deformity of feet as needed for planovalgus correction, calcaneal malunion, bone spurs, etc. should be done.
- Decompression of the nerve should be attempted by those versed with anatomy. Expose the nerve through incision made posterior to the tibia. Release the retinaculum in entirety and identify the tibial nerve. Leave it undisturbed unless there is fibrosis for which neurolysis is required. Neuroma or compressing lesions should be identified and removed.

4B.31 DIABETIC AND CHARCOT'S FOOT (Q202–207)

202. **Explain lesions of the diabetic foot and outline its management.**

Ans: *Lesions*: Diabetic ulcers are most common in the forefoot beneath one of the metatarsal heads or the interphalangeal joint of the hallux.

The Wagner classification of diabetic (and dysvascular and insensitive) ulcers is given in **Box 4B.31.1**.

Box 4B.31.1: Wagner classification of diabetic ulcers.
Grade 0—skin intact, but bony deformities produce a "foot at risk"
Grade 1—localized, superficial ulcer
Grade 2—deep ulcer to tendon, bone, ligament, or joint
Grade 3—deep abscess, osteomyelitis
Grade 4—gangrene of toes or forefoot
Grade 5—gangrene of entire foot

Management

Antibiotic therapy: The use of antibiotics in diabetic ulcers may or may not be indicated. Localized ulcers without cellulitis, abscess, osteomyelitis, or pyarthrosis heal in an occlusive weight bearing cast or with prolonged nonweight bearing, *provided that* adequate vascularity is present. Even small, contiguous, localized areas of osteomyelitis involving one bone may heal by immobilizing the part and removing shear stress. Antibiotics should be used if an abscess is drained, if cellulitis is present, or in conjunction with surgical debridement of an area of osteomyelitis or pyarthrosis. Aerobic and anaerobic cultures should be obtained before initiation of antibiotic treatment. A broad-spectrum antibiotic is begun, covering gram-positive and gram-negative organisms until sensitivities return and appropriate antibiotic choices are made. An infectious disease consultation, if available, is helpful. The length of treatment usually depends on the tissue involved (soft tissue or soft tissue and bone or joint).

Nonoperative treatment:
- *Total contact casting* is the standard of care, because it reduces plantar loads better than a well-molded shoe cast and, by extrapolation, better than shoes with custom insoles.
- *Removable diabetic boots* have been shown to be as efficacious as total contact casting in some studies;

- *Negative pressure wound treatment* with vacuum-assisted closure can improve wound healing. Immediate abscess evacuation with debridement or partial amputation as needed, followed by placement of negative pressure wound therapy, along with vascular intervention as required, can be successful for limb salvage in patients with severe diabetic foot infections. Negative pressure wound therapy also can be beneficial for diabetic ulcer healing, with higher healing rates and lower amputation rates than advanced moist wound therapy.
- *Hyperbaric oxygen treatment* has been shown in multiple studies to have some efficacy in diabetic wound healing, with an overall healing rate of 76% compared with 48% without the use of hyperbaric oxygen and an amputation rate of 19% compared with 45% without hyperbaric oxygen. It also can be helpful in wound healing when infection is involved.
- *Extracorporeal shockwave treatment* can be helpful for healing of chronic ulcers.

Operative treatment: The indications for urgent surgical intervention include necrotizing infections and gangrene or deep abscesses. Less urgent surgery may be required if there is a substantially compromised soft tissue envelope, loss of mechanical function of the foot, or bone involvement that is limb threatening or if the patient prefers to avoid prolonged antibiotic therapy. Surgical debridement of osteomyelitis is not always required. For severe infections with abscess formation, incision and drainage with thorough debridement may be required. In cases of chronic osteomyelitis that has failed to respond to intravenous antibiotics, surgical debridement may be necessary.

Infected bone should be completely excised; however, every effort should be made to preserve as much bone as possible. For osteomyelitis in the toes, amputation may be required. Preservation of part of the proximal phalanx may help keep the adjacent toes from drifting. Metatarsal head resection may be indicated. If multiple metatarsal heads are involved, resection of all lesser metatarsal heads or transmetatarsal amputation may be required. Ray resection may be needed if the osteomyelitis involves more than the metatarsal head. Midfoot osteomyelitis can be treated with exostectomy if stability can be preserved. Hindfoot infections occasionally can be treated with amputation at that level, but a below-knee amputation often is more functional. Partial calcanectomy may be attempted if osteomyelitis affects the calcaneus secondary to a heel ulcer and can avoid a below-knee amputation.

Modified resection arthroplasty after debridement of infected tissue can avoid toe amputation in patients with chronically infected ulcers and claw toe deformities, and toe flexor tenotomies can lead to healing of ulcers at the tip of the toe if the claw toe deformity is flexible and wounds are Wagner grade 1, 2, or 3.

Achilles lengthening can decrease plantar pressures and can help ulcer healing. Healing of forefoot ulcers can be helped by tendon lengthenings using gastrocsoleus recession for all forefoot ulcers and adding an intramuscular lengthening of the posterior tibial tendon for fifth metatarsal head ulcers and Z-type lengthenings of the peroneus longus tendon for first metatarsal head ulcers.

203. Diabetic foot: Etiopathogenesis and clinical features.

Ans: Etiopathogenesis
- *Neuropathic component* (most significant factor):
  - *Sensory neuropathy*: Loss of protective sensation → unrecognized trauma
  - *Motor neuropathy*: Muscle atrophy → foot deformities (hammer toes, Charcot foot)
  - *Autonomic neuropathy*: Reduced sweating → dry, cracked skin
- *Vascular insufficiency*:
  - *Macroangiopathy*: Atherosclerosis of leg arteries
  - *Microangiopathy*: Capillary basement membrane thickening
  - Impaired circulation → poor wound healing
- *Immunological factors*:
  - Hyperglycemia impairs leukocyte function
  - Reduced inflammatory response → silent infections
- *Biomechanical factors*:
  - Abnormal foot architecture

- Increased plantar pressures
- Repetitive stress on insensate foot

Clinical Features:
The diabetic foot triad consists of neuropathy, ischemia, and infection—often coexisting to create a complex clinical picture. Early recognition of these features is crucial to prevent limb-threatening complications.
- *Neuropathic foot (most common)*:
  - Painless foot ulcers (typically plantar surface)
  - Callus formation around pressure points
  - Loss of vibration, light touch, temperature sensation
  - Intact pulses with warm foot
- *Ischemic foot*:
  - Painful ulcers (often toes or heels)
  - Cold, pale foot with shiny skin
  - Absent/diminished pulses
  - Delayed capillary refill
- *Infectious manifestations*:
  - Malodorous discharge
  - Surrounding cellulitis
  - Creptus (gas gangrene)
  - Deep abscess formation
- *Charcot neuroarthropathy*:
  - Swollen, warm, erythematous foot
  - Progressive deformity (rocker-bottom foot)
  - Joint instability
  - Often mistaken for infection

204. What are the indications and advantages of total contact casts in orthopedics?

Ans: Total contact casts are a method of wound management in diabetic patients where the limb is fitted with nonremovable cast that is in contact with the foot (diabetic foot ulcers) and the leg—below knee cast. The cast serves to protect the diseased limb and promote wound healing.

Indications:
- Diabetic foot ulcers—enhanced healing due to protection, offloading of forces and limiting the use of foot
- Charcot arthropathy with uneven distribution of forces—the total contact cast offloads the limb and more evenly distributes forces preventing new lesions from formation.
- Diabetic neuropathy—the patients are at increased risk of injury due to reduced sensation so need protection
- Foot deformity—toe clawing and bony deformity cause callus formation producing pressure points and ulcer formation.

Advantages:
- Optimizes wound healing by relieving undue pressure/forces on the wound. This is not possible with surgical or medical management.
- It offers protection to the limb in addition to promoting healing.

205. Define neuropathic joint.

Ans: Neuropathic arthritis is an extreme form of post-traumatic osteoarthritis. It is a progressive condition of the musculoskeletal system that is characterized by continued bony destruction of a WB joint, joint dislocations, pathologic fractures, and debilitating deformities. Charcot neuroarthropathy involves progressive destruction of the joints, most commonly in the feet and ankles. The condition is named after Jean Martin Charcot who noted the occurrence of mutilated feet in syphilis (1868), and was later related to diabetes in 1936. It is characterized by pathologic fractures, joint dislocation, and overt loss of normal joint architecture. Diabetes mellitus is the most common cause while others being syphilis, alcoholism, leprosy, and idiopathic neuropathy.

[For further details and stages of progression, reader is encouraged to read Chapter 11 and Chapter 76 of the book Essential Orthopedics Principles and Practice.]

206. What is diagnosis of neuropathic joint?

Ans: *Radiology*: The radiographic hallmark of neuropathic arthritis is one of "osteoarthritis with a vengeance". Predominantly there are two types of presentations—the "atrophic form" and "hypertrophic form". In the latter not only will affected joints show narrowing, sclerosis, and osteophytes but also they will show these with such exuberance that the appearance is one of marked increased (Yochum and Rowe's 6 "D"):

1. Density about the joint
2. Disorganization of the joint structures
3. Debris surrounding and within the joint
4. Destruction of the joint surfaces
5. Dislocation of the joint
6. Distended joint.

This collection of "D" word descriptors should bring the diagnosis to mind. Thus, the viewer must be vigilant to make the diagnosis, especially since neuropathic arthritis may have a wide range from the purely productive arthropathy to one that resembles an aggressively destructive process.

The atrophic form is less common and has typical radiological appearance of:
- "Licked candy stick" appearance of distal aspect of bones
- Osteopenia
- Osteolysis

The radiographic staging for Charcot's arthropathy (especially as related to Charcot foot):

Stage I: Developmental or acute:
- Hyperemia due to autonomic neuropathy weakens bone and ligaments.
- Diffuse swelling, joint laxity, subluxation, frank dislocation, fine periarticular fragmentation and debris formation.

Stage II: Coalescence or Quiescent:
- Absorption of osseous debris, fusion of larger fragments
- Dramatic sclerosis
- Joints become less mobile and more stable
- Aptly known as the "hypertrophic" or "subacute" phase of Charcot.

Stage III: Consolidation or resolution:
- Osseous remodeling
- For clinical purposes, stage I is regarded as the acute phase, while stages II and III are regarded as the chronic or quiescent phase.

Magnetic resonance imaging is not very useful and early images are nonspecific for Charcot's arthropathy (CA) and can be seen in reflex sympathetic dystrophy (RSD), osteomyelitis, etc. There is a significant signal intensity overlap for infection and edema. The greater the signal from marrow in T2-weighted images the more likely the bone is infected. Gadolinium enhancement does not differentiate infection from edema. MRI can be of use possibly in preoperative assessment and monitoring disease progression. PET scan may be better in patients with metallic implants and has been shown to differentiate infection from CA. Bone scan is a sensitive but nonspecific investigation. Three-phase bone scan is positive in all three phases. A four-phase bone scan (taken at 24 hours) can depict woven bone but cannot differentiate CA from fractures, tumors, advanced degeneration.[333] In-labelled scan complemented alongside with Tc-nanocolloid marrow scanning can indicate absence of infection if the scan reports are congruent.

207. **Describe the etiology, pathology, clinical features, and the principles of management of Charcot joints.**

Ans: *Etiology*:
- Diabetes
- Charcot-Marie-Tooth (CMT) disease
- Syringomyelia (in the shoulder)
- Amyloid
- Alcoholic neuropathies
- Leprosy
- Neurosyphilis (in the knee)
- Congenital insensitivity to pain
- Renal dialysis
- Sensory and autonomic neuropathy
- Spinal cord injury
- Cerebral palsy
- Intra-articular steroid injections
- Traumatic denervation of a limb—spinal cord or peripheral nerve injury.

Pathology: Pathological findings in neuropathic arthropathy include severe degeneration and fragmentation of the joint surfaces with extensive dendritic synovitis, resulting from particles of bone and cartilage embedded in the synovium.

Clinical features: Individuals have varied presentations; the onset is usually insidious.

Acute presentation is a common diagnostic dilemma and can present like septic arthritis.
- These individuals almost always present with signs of inflammation.
- Profound unilateral swelling, an increase in local skin temperature (generally, an increase of 3–7° above the unaffected foot's skin temperature), erythema, joint effusion, and bone resorption in an insensate foot are present. These characteristics, in the presence of intact skin and a loss of protective sensation, are often pathognomonic of acute Charcot arthropathy.
- Painless swollen lax and deformed joint is a misconception as pain is present in more than 75% of patients; however, pain severity is significantly less than expected.
- The joint may reveal erythema, edema, "loose bag of bones" kind of appearance.
- Significant number of patients (40%) has skin ulceration complicating diagnosis to osteomyelitis as primary pathology, which is actually incorrect. Bone and synovial biopsy may settle the confusion.

Principles of management:
- Upon diagnosis immobilization in total contact casts or brace [Charcot resistant orthotic walker (CROW)] helps prevent accelerated joint destruction. Patellar tendon-bearing brace is used to transfer weight-bearing forces from the orthosis through the patellar tendon, thereby decreasing weight-bearing forces through the foot and ankle.
- Joint edema and swelling may take 6–9 months to subside. Average healing times vary from 55 days to 97 days depending on location. Up to 1–2 years may be required for complete healing.
- Bisphosphonates have been used in a few patients particularly the injectable ones for possible role of osteoclasts in bone destruction. Though not approved the response to therapy is moderately acceptable with reduction in alkaline phosphatase levels and local temperature accompanied with clinical improvement.
- Calcitonin has also shown improvement (faster healing) in sporadic studies with calcium supplementation.
- Future therapies pointing and attacking the RANKL-TNFα pathway may provide targeted pharmacotherapy.

The role of low intensity ultrasound is controversial. Surgery is warranted in less than one-fourth of patients and is predominantly preventive. Surgery is specifically contraindicated in active inflammation.

4B.32 HALLUX VALGUS, TRIPLE ARTHRODESIS, AND TALECTOMY (Q208–212)

208. Explain the following:
   A. Hallux valgus deformity
   B. Role of triple arthrodesis

Ans: A. Bunion is a bump on the side of the big toe. The deformity is often seen and referred to as hallux valgus. The hallux valgus deformity is characterized by lateral (fibular) deviation (away from midline of body or towards midline of foot) of the proximal phalanx on the metatarsal head. This is often associated with disorders of lesser toes. In describing hallux valgus, it is still uncertain as to which is the primary deformity metatarsus primus varus or lateral deviation of the great toe, though considering the pathogenesis, it appears that the latter is primary.

Etiology
- Metatarsophalangeal (MTP) joint arthritis (inflammatory, metabolic conditions, connective tissue disorders):
  - Rheumatoid arthritis
  - Psoriatic arthritis
  - Gouty arthritis
  - Ehlers-Danlos syndrome, Marfan syndrome, Down syndrome, and ligamentous laxity.
- Traumatic:
  - Dislocations
  - Malunions
  - Intra-articular damage
  - Soft-tissue sprains.
- Neuromuscular disease
  - Charcot-Marie Tooth disease
  - Cerebral palsy
  - Multiple sclerosis.
- Primary structural deformity
  - Metatarsus primus elevates
  - External tibial torsion
  - Malalignment of articular surface or metatarsal shaft
  - Abnormal metatarsal length
  - Genu varum or valgum
  - Femoral retroversion.

Pathogenesis

Biomechanical instability: This involves a complex interplay of disorders of bones, articular surfaces, and the capsule-ligamentous structures. The angle between the first and second metatarsals is normally up to 10°, more than this is pathological. The valgus angle of the first MTP joint angle measured up to 20° is normal. Following are some of the pathogenic mechanisms explaining development of this progressive deformity:

- Excess lateral pull results from the unopposed pull of the adductor hallucis that is only countered by medial capsular ligament along with the capsule-sesamoid portion
- The first ray is pulled laterally by the flexor hallucis brevis, flexor hallucis longus, adductor hallucis and extensor hallucis longus all of which have a medially directed moment along with their primary action, increasing the valgus deformity.
- Attenuation of the sesamoid ridge under the first metatarsal head.

Some associated factors contribute to progression of the deformity and if present they may exacerbate it. These include:
- Equinus due to gastrocnemius or gastrocsoleus complex involvement (dynamic)
- Flatfoot (pes planovalgus, flexible or rigid)
- Rigid or flexible forefoot varus.

Pathoanatomy: The following deformations are commonly seen in a hallux valgus deformity (so it is called a complex deformity). As a result of this lateral subluxation of the proximal phalanx (which is now considered as a primary deformity) on the metatarsal head, several secondary changes occur.
- Medial deviation of the first metatarsal, giving rise to an increase in the intermetatarsal angle (first metatarsal varus), great toe valgus, bunion formation
- Hammer toe-like deformity of the second toe due to overlapping of the second toe on valgus great toe underneath
- Contracture of the lateral joint capsule
- Attenuation of the medial joint capsule
- First MTP joint degenerative arthritis
- Corns, calluses, and metatarsalgia
- Pronation of the hallux, as the deformity becomes more severe
- Formation of the medial eminence (may actually represent hypertrophic component or from the medial deviation of the metatarsal head itself).

Clinical and radiological features: Note any pain about the MTP joint, synovial thickening or crepitation. The foot should be examined for mentioned etiological conditions.

Radiographic examination:
- Measure the first MTP joint angle, which should be less than 15°.
- The intermetatarsal angle should be less than 8°.
- Look for arthrosis in the first MTP joint and assess whether the joint is congruent or incongruent.
- Measure the distal metatarsal articular angle (DMAA), which is the relationship of the articular surface to the long axis of the metatarsal.
- Normally, this should be less than 10° of lateral deviation.

Treatment

Conservative management: For initial deformities and patients unwilling for surgery, conservative management is tried that provides symptomatic relief often and retards the progression of deformity. In any case, deformity being progressive surgery is needed at the end. Broad, soft-soled shoes, preferably with a low heel that provides adequate room for the great toe and the medial eminence are prescribed. Silicon spacer for abducting the great toe are also worn the whole day and can be taken off at night or better worn even then.

Principles of surgical correction: In general, any chosen surgical procedure must correct the following structural components of deformity for optimal outcome:
- Hallux valgus deformity per se: Valgus deviation of the great toe
- First metatarsal varus
- Pronation deformity of hallux, first metatarsal or both
- The medial eminence (bunion)
- First MTP arthritis and stiffness
- Maintaining length of short first metatarsal
- The displacement of the sesamoid apparatus
- Pathology (Excessive mobility or obliquity) at first metatarsomedial cuneiform joint
- Muscle-tendon imbalance at the MTP.

B. *Role of arthrodesis*: If the deformity is severe (hallux valgus angle of >40° and the intermetatarsal is >16°) use a distal soft-tissue procedure with proximal osteotomy (arthrosis should be minimal). These severe deformities usually quickly develop arthrosis so threshold for arthrodesis should be low.
- The second consideration is of arthrosis which if present or the deformity is too severe and then consider an arthrodesis. If there is significant arthrosis of the MTP joint, an arthrodesis is probably the procedure of choice.

209. Indications and disadvantages of pan talar arthrodesis.

Ans: *Indications*:
- Equinus or calcaneus with lateral instability of foot and whose leg and foot muscles are not strong enough to control foot and ankle when only foot is stabilized.
- Recurrence after Lambrinudi or Campbell's procedure.
- The various pathologies leading to the need of pantalar arthrodesis include:
    - Charcot arthropathy
    - Post-traumatic arthritis
    - End-stage posterior tibial tendon dysfunction
    - Clubfoot—neglected or failed multiple treatments with deformities persisting
    - Failed total ankle replacement
    - Rheumatoid arthritis
    - Paralytic foot like in polio or spine disorders

Disadvantages: Restrictions, problems and disabilities occur after pantalar arthrodesis that may impair activities of daily living. These include:
- Development of ipsilateral knee pain
- Climbing a hill or walking on a steep ramp
- Restrictions in athletic activities
- Difficulties in four-wheeler and two-wheeler driving
- Difficulties in riding bicycle
- Need to wear shoes of different sizes
- Development of calluses and late subtalar and knee arthritis.

210. Discuss the indications, merits, and demerits of talectomy.

Ans: *Indications*:
- Severe, rigid, resistant clubfoot deformity
- Arthrogryposis multiplex congenita
- Myelomeningocele, tuberculosis
- Tumors.

Adults—salvage procedure:
- Nonunion of ankle fusions
- Failed total ankle arthroplasty
- Inflammatory arthropathy
- Neuroarthropathy
- Failed talar prostheses
- Failed pantalar fusions
- Adult neglected clubfoot
- Post-traumatic avascular necrosis talus
- Deformities that are due to sciatic nerve palsy and compartment syndrome.

Advantages:
- Achieving stable joint without ankylosis
- Improved limb function
- Mechanical support to limb
- Walking without support
- Single stage surgery.

Disadvantages:
- Nonphysiological joint creation
- Mutilating surgery
- Severe arthritis development and pain in longer term.

211. How will you diagnose a case of hallux valgus?
Ans: Kindly see Answers to Questions above.

212. Discuss causes, clinical features, investigations, and treatment of posterior heel pain.
Ans: Posterior heel pain is a prevalent clinical complaint that may emerge from a variety of underlying etiologies.

Etiologies:
- *Achilles tendinopathy*: This pathology represents the most common etiology of posterior heel pain, characterized by degenerative changes in the Achilles tendon resulting from chronic overuse.
- *Achilles tendon rupture*: Acute ruptures occur frequently in athletes engaged in sports that demand jumping or rapid acceleration, leading to sudden onset pain.
- *Retrocalcaneal bursitis*: Inflammation of the retrocalcaneal bursa, situated between the Achilles tendon and the calcaneus, can provoke localized pain and tenderness.
- *Sever's disease*: Primarily affecting growing adolescents, especially those participating in sports, this condition involves inflammation of the growth plate in the heel.
- *Haglund's deformity*: This structural abnormality, characterized by a bony enlargement on the posterior aspect of the heel, can irritate both the Achilles tendon and the retrocalcaneal bursa.
- *Calcaneal fracture or stress fracture*: Although infrequent, these injuries can also present as posterior heel pain.
- *Systemic conditions*: Various systemic illnesses, such as rheumatoid arthritis, ankylosing spondylitis, or gout, may manifest with heel pain as a significant symptom.

Clinical features:
The clinical presentation of posterior heel pain typically includes:
- *Localized pain*: Discomfort is commonly centralized around the posterior heel, particularly near the Achilles tendon, though it may radiate.
- *Onset*: Pain may manifest gradually, particularly in cases of tendinopathy, or may present acutely in instances of tendon rupture.
- *Pain characteristics*: Symptoms often intensify with activity—especially during running or walking—and tend to improve with rest. Patients frequently report increased pain upon waking or following periods of inactivity.
- *Swelling and tenderness*: The affected area may exhibit swelling and tenderness upon palpation.
- *Limited range of motion*: Notable restrictions in dorsiflexion or stiffness in the ankle joint may be observed.
- *Deformity*: In cases of Haglund's deformity, a prominent bony enlargement may be evident.

Investigations:
A multi-faceted approach to diagnosis is critical:
- *Physical examination*: A comprehensive clinical assessment is paramount, emphasizing pain response, range of motion, and palpation of the affected structures.
- *Imaging studies*:
  - *X-rays*: These are instrumental in excluding fractures and identifying bony deformities such as Haglund's deformity. An enlarged calcaneal tuberosity or spur may also be visible.
  - *Ultrasound*: This modality is beneficial for assessing the Achilles tendon for signs of tendinosis, tears, or bursitis.
  - *MRI*: When suspicion of tendon rupture exists or if conservative measures are unsuccessful, MRI provides detailed images of soft tissue structures, facilitating accurate diagnosis.
- *Blood tests*: These may be indicated in cases where systemic conditions are suspected or to eliminate inflammatory processes (e.g., rheumatoid factor, uric acid levels).

Treatment:

Treatment strategies for posterior heel pain can be categorized as follows:

- *Conservative management*:
  - *Rest*: Temporarily abstaining from aggravating activities promotes healing.
  - *Ice therapy*: Cryotherapy serves to mitigate swelling and alleviate pain.
  - *Physiotherapy*: Implementing targeted stretching and strengthening exercises, along with modalities such as ultrasound and massage, can yield positive outcomes.
  - *Orthotics/cushioning*: The use of custom-made or over-the-counter orthotics can provide essential foot support and pressure redistribution.
  - *Nonsteroidal anti-inflammatory drugs (NSAIDs)*: These agents are effective for pain relief and inflammation reduction.
- *Invasive treatments*:
  - *Corticosteroid injections*: While useful for managing acute inflammatory conditions, these should be administered with caution near tendons due to the risk of rupture.
  - *Platelet-rich plasma (PRP) therapy*: This emerging treatment option holds promise for chronic tendon pathologies.
  - *Surgery*: Persistent cases may necessitate surgical intervention, including debridement of degenerated tendon tissue, repair of ruptured tendons, or excision of prominent bony deformities.
  - *Rehabilitation*: Following recovery, a structured rehabilitation program focusing on strength and flexibility is imperative to mitigate the risk of recurrent injuries.

4C. SPINE

4C.1 TUBERCULAR AFFECTION OF SPINE (Q1–21)

1. What is a tubercle? Discuss pathoanatomy, diagnosis, and principles of management of cold abscess.

Ans: *Tubercle*: Following the insemination of infection, the initial response is in the reticuloendothelial depots of the skeletal tissues. This is characterized by accumulation of polymorphonuclear cells which are rapidly replaced by macrophages and monocytes (mononuclears), the highly phagocytic members of the reticuloendothelial system **(Fig. 4C.1.1)**. The tubercle bacilli are phagocytosed and broken down and their lipid is dispersed throughout the cytoplasm of the mononuclears thus transforming them into epithelioid cells. Epithelioid cells are the characteristic feature of the tuberculous reaction. These are large pale cells with a large vesicular nucleus, abundant cytoplasm, indistinct margins, and processes which form an epithelioid reticulum. Langhans giant cells are probably formed by fusion of a number of epithelioid cells, these are formed only if caseation necrosis has occurred in the lesion, and often they contain tubercle bacilli.

Their main function is to digest and remove necrosed tissue. After about a week lymphocytes appear and form a ring around the peripheral part of the lesion. This mass formed by the reactive cells of the reticuloendothelial tissues constitutes a nodule popularly known as the tubercle.

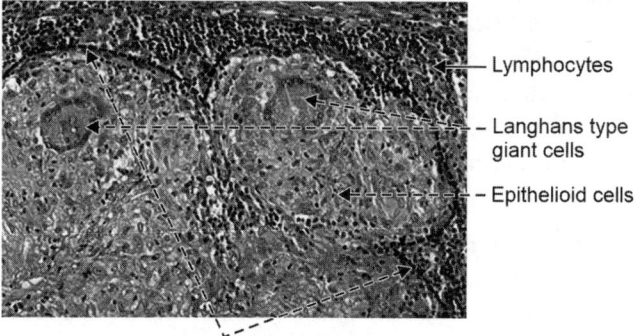

Fig. 4C.1.1: The microscopic appearance of tubercle. The image demonstrates inner caseating necrosis (outlined by dashed line) with formation of Langhans type giant cells. The central area is surrounded by mononuclear infiltrate.

Cold Abscess

Pathoanatomy: Marked exudative reaction is a common feature in tuberculous infection of the skeletal system. A cold abscess is formed by a collection of products of liquefaction and the reactive exudation. The cold abscess is mostly composed of serum, leukocytes, caseous material, bone debris, and tubercle bacilli. The abscess penetrates the ligaments in articular disease, bone, and periosteum in osseous disease and migrates in various directions following the facial planes and along the vessels and nerves. The "cold abscess" feels warm, though the temperature is not raised as high as in acute pyogenic infections. A superficial abscess may get secondarily infected and clinically behave like pyogenic abscess; it may burst to form a sinus or an ulcer. The walls of an abscess, sinus or ulcer are covered with tuberculous granulations.

Diagnosis: Clinical examination (soft swelling with no signs of inflammation)

Delineation of the shape, extent and the route of spread of a cold abscess can also be very well visualized by CT scan.

Principles of Management

Palpable or peripheral cold abscesses: Repeated aspiration and instillation of streptomycin was sufficient to heal 95% of abscesses, 5% healed by surgical evacuation. Majority of the abscesses were healed within 6 months. There were a few (less than 2%) abscesses which were not fully controlled in spite of surgical drainage and continuous treatment. These cases were probably having resistant strains. They presented with recurrence after a quiescent period varying between 6 months and 12 months. Modern antitubercular drugs in conjunction with surgery were able to heal recurring cases.

Operative treatment of cold abscess: The palpable (peripheral) cold abscess if needed can be drained by standard surgical approaches. Iliopsoas abscess may be drained by anterior approach by making an 8–10 cm incision on the iliac crest one cm behind the anterior superior iliac spine. Cut external and internal obliquus abdominis muscles from the iliac crest and reach the inner surface of iliac bone. Palpate abscess and drain extraperitoneally. If the abscess (essentially contained in psoas sheath) is pointing more posteriorly drain through the floor of the Petit's triangle. The floor is covered by obliquus internus abdominis muscle which requires to be incised (4–6 cm) between latissimus dorsi posteriorly, obliquus externus abdominis anteriorly and iliac crest inferiorly. Ludloff's approach is used for an abscess pointing on the medial side of thigh. Make a 2–3 cm incision distal to pubic tubercle longitudinally between gracilis and adductor longus muscle. Develop plane between adductor longus and brevis anteriorly and the gracilis and adductor magnus posteriorly. Protect the posterior branch of obturator nerve and neurovascular bundle to gracilis. The abscess can be easily drained through the wound by developing a plane toward the lesser trochanter. Cold abscess in the cervical spine is drained by making a transverse or longitudinal skin incision anterior or posterior to the sternocleidomastoid muscle depending upon the site of presentation of the abscess. It is wise to use suction drainage for nearly 72 hours after the surgery. If the size of the abscess is large (draining more than 300 mL in an adult) fluid must be replaced by intravenous route.

2. **What is tuberculoma? Discuss primary drugs used to treat tuberculosis (TB) of spine. Enumerate complications of isoniazid, streptomycin and ethambutol.**

Ans: Tuberculoma is extradural extraosseous spinal TB. It is a tumor-like TB lesion formed of inspissated caseating material surrounded by fibrous capsule. The sites are lung, brain, kidney, and spinal cord.

Very rarely, a small tuberculoma of the spinal cord or diffuse extradural granuloma of the cord may be responsible for neurological complications without any radiological evidence of tuberculous involvement of the vertebrae. Such cases present as a "spinal tumor syndrome".

Primary Drugs used in Antitubercular Chemotherapy

Isoniazid: It was discovered by Fox in 1951 (Krantz and Carr 1958), and became available for clinical use in late 1951. It is bactericidal and has two phase action on bacteria, one reversible and occurring even when cell growth is inhibited; the other irreversible, requiring growth. The enzyme peroxidase transfers isoniazid into the cell where it (INH) inhibits the synthesis of phospholipid fraction, insoluble carbohydrate containing fraction and nucleic acid, which are essential for the growth and viability of mycobacterium.

Rifampicin: It is a potent semisynthetic antibiotic, like pyrazinamide it has the ability to kill so-called "persisters"—mycobacteria that lie dormant, often within the cells. Absorption is complete and rapid after administration on an empty stomach. The presence of food causes marked variation in serum concentrations, though it does not seem to interfere with the efficacy of the drug. The distribution of rifampicin is extensive and the patient should be warned about red-brown coloration of body fluids like sweat, tears, urine, feces, etc. It is subject to hepatic metabolism and transferred to bile. The metabolism is principally by deacetylation. The deacetylated metabolite is active. The excretion of rifampicin is both biliary and renal, and modification in dosage is required in patients with hepatobiliary or hepatorenal insufficiency.

Pyrazinamide: This drug is especially bactericidal to mycobacteria multiplying intracellularly at low pH levels. It is well absorbed after oral administration and is eliminated principally by hepatic metabolism. Only about 3% of an oral dose is excreted unchanged in the urine in the first 24 hours. Like isoniazid, pyrazinamide penetrates well into cerebrospinal fluid (CSF), and it may, therefore, be specially indicated in tuberculous meningitis, and paraplegia.

Ethambutol: It suppresses the growth of bacteria by inhibiting arabinosyl transferase involved in cell wall synthesis. It is a bacteriostatic drug. Dose adjustment needed in renal impairment. It is not recommended for children below 5 years of age due to inability to check their visual acuity and color-related symptoms.

Complications

Isoniazid: The most important complications are the neurotoxic effects of isoniazid due to depletion of vitamin B factors. Neurotoxic complications may take the form of peripheral neuritis, muscular twitching, paresthesiae, and psychological disturbances. They should be treated by administration of 50 mg of pyridoxine, 100 mg of nicotinamide and other B complex factors daily. Rarely skin rashes or gastrointestinal symptoms or hepatitis may develop. Behavior disorders, convulsions, hepatitis, hypersensitivity are other uncommon adverse effects.

Streptomycin: Eighth nerve damage is reported due to streptomycin toxicity. Streptomycin sulfate is more likely to affect the labyrinthine division leading to vertigo, and dihydrostreptomycin is more likely to damage the acoustic division thus causing deafness. Other rare complications are aplastic anemia, neutropenia, drug rashes, drug hypersensitivity, nausea, and vomiting. In patients above the age of 45 years, streptomycin may enhance respiratory paralysis by interacting with neuromuscular blocking agents especially while giving anesthesia.

Ethambutol: Most important complication is retrobulbar neuritis and optic neuritis which fortunately recover on stopping the drug. Therefore, during ethambutol administration visual acuity, red-green color vision and gross peripheral visual fields must be frequently examined. Special care must be taken if this drug is to be administered to a child. It is metabolized by oxidation in the liver. Hepatic and renal dysfunction may increase the risk of toxicity.

3. Describe etiopathogenesis and clinical features of a cold abscess.

Ans: Cold abscess develops around the lesion of variable sizes. Cold abscess is a collection of tubercular debris, disintegrated bone lamellae, serum, caseous material, granulation tissue, bone marrow, and tubercular bacilli. It has all the features of infective abscess due to collection of pus (swelling, fluctuation, etc.) but is minimally inflamed so temperature is not raised on examination. Due to continued development of cold abscess and migration of the pus, the abscess may track into different planes. The spread occurs beneath the anterior longitudinal ligament to variable distance then it takes one of the following courses:

- *Tracking posteriorly into vertebral canal*: This is a dreadful complication as it causes compression and development of neurological complications.
- Tracking to skin through line of least resistance.

In cervical spine:
- Cold abscess collects behind the prevertebral fascia forming retropharyngeal abscess that might be large enough to interfere with deglutition.
- The abscess may track posterolaterally to posterior triangle of neck and present behind the posterior border or sternocleidomastoid muscle.
- Abscess may track down into mediastinum and may even cause mediastinal syndrome.
- Laterally, the pus may track along the brachial sheath into axilla or even cubital fossa.

In dorsal spine:
- Cold abscess of thoracic disease often forms paravertebral abscess in extrapleural space. The abscess may burst into intrapleural space causing pseudoempyema thoracis or may track along the intercostal nerves and vessels to point anteriorly.
- The cold abscess may track along the rectus sheath or lower abdominal wall.

In lumbar spine:
- Cold abscess in lumbar lesions (typically the psoas abscess) may track to form paravertebral abscess palpable posteriorly on one side of spine or may travel along the intercostal, ilioinguinal, and iliohypogastric nerves.
- It may go to Petit's triangle along the flat muscles of abdominal wall or in the ischiorectal fossa along the internal pudendal nerve.
- Posteriorly, it may track to buttock along the gluteal nerve.
- Anteriorly, it may form typical psoas abscess that may point anywhere from abdomen to groin to thigh to even popliteal region.
- If it develops a connection in the inferior abdominal wall, it may form an inverted horseshoe abscess also (uncommon presentation).

4. A. Discuss pathophysiology of Pott's spine; and
B. Routes through which TB abscess can travel to far off regions in the body based on anatomical facts.

Ans: A. Pathophysiology:

Spinal involvement is usually a result of hematogenous spread of *Mycobacterium tuberculosis* into the dense vasculature of cancellous bone of the vertebral bodies.

Primary infection site is either a pulmonary lesion or an infection of the genitourinary system

- *Arterial*: An arterial arcade, in the subchondral region of each vertebra, is derived from anterior and posterior spinal arteries; this arcade forms a rich vascular plexus. This vascular plexus facilitates hematogenous spread of the infection in the paradiskal regions.
- *Venous*: Batson's paravertebral venous plexus in the vertebra is a valveless system that allows free flow of blood in both directions depending upon the pressure generated by the intra-abdominal and intrathoracic cavities following

strenuous activities like coughing. Spread of the infection via the intraosseous venous system may be responsible for central vertebral body lesions. Spread by venous system could be discontiguous and involve vertebrae at a distance explaining noncontiguous vertebral TB.

- The "central type" of vertebral body involvement, "skipped lesions" in the vertebral column, and vertebral disease associated with tubercular meningitis as due to spread of infection along Batson's perivertebral plexus of veins.
- Typical paradiskal lesions and vertebral lesions associated with tubercular foci in the extremities are considered due to spread by way of arteries.
- "Anterior type" of involvement of vertebral bodies seems to be due to extension of an abscess beneath the anterior longitudinal ligaments and the periosteum.

The infection may spread up and down stripping the anterior or posterior longitudinal ligaments and the periosteum from the front and the sides of the vertebral bodies. This results in loss of periosteal blood supply and destruction of the anterolateral surface of many contiguous vertebral bodies. All these modes of spread of infection play their role in different patients or in the same patient. The knowledge of the bacillemic nature of the spread of infection is essential for a true assessment of the problem presented by such patients. This information should be a safeguard against the folly of believing that a patient would be cured by some local operation irrespective of the systemic treatment.

B. Routes of Spread of the Cold Abscess (Fig. 4C.1.2)

Cervical lesions:
- *Retropharyngeal abscess*: Collection behind prevertebral fascia
- Spread lateral to posterior triangle of neck and present at posterior border of sternocleidomastoid muscle
- Mediastinum → mediastinitis (may be life threatening)
- Axilla/cubital fossa (along brachial plexus).

Dorsal lesions:
- Paravertebral abscess (*upper dorsal spine—squaring of mediastinum, mid-dorsal spine—fusiform swelling*)
- Extrapleural space
- Intrapleural space → empyema thoracis
- Along intercostal nerves and vessels.

Lumbar lesions:
- Psoas abscess
- Petit's triangle/lumbar triangle
- Scarpa's triangle
- Posterior aspect of thigh/popliteal region.

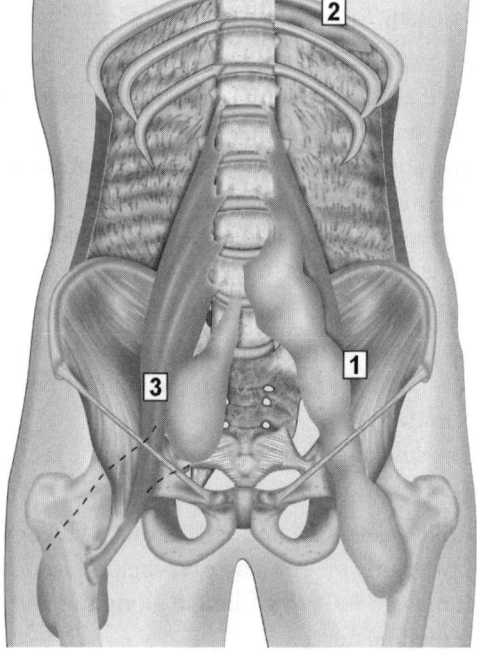

Fig. 4C.1.2: Psoas abscess and routes of spread—The different routes of spread of the abscess—(1) Spread to groin and thigh, (2) Spread to lumbar region and Petit's triangle, (3) Spread to gluteal region.

Psoas abscess is as a rule associated with detectable tuberculous disease of the vertebral column from dorsal 10th vertebra to the sacrum, or disease of sacroiliac joint, pelvic bones and hip joint.

5. Describe the various types of abscesses seen in Pott's spine and its significance on the disease outcome.

Ans: *(Refer Chapter on Vertebral Discitis and Osteomyelitis and other Spinal Infections in the 3rd Edition of Essential Orthopedics: Principles and Practice)*

Cold abscess develops around the lesion of variable sizes. Cold abscess is a collection of tubercular debris, disintegrated bone lamellae, serum, caseous material, granulation tissue, bone marrow and tubercular bacilli. The spread occurs beneath the anterior longitudinal ligament to variable distance then it takes one of the following course:

- *Tracking posteriorly into vertebral canal*: This is a dreadful complication as it causes compression and development of neurological complications.
- Tracking to skin through line of least resistance.

Cervical spine tuberculosis:
- Cold abscess collects behind the prevertebral fascia forming retropharyngeal abscess that might be large enough to interfere with deglutition.
- The abscess may track posterolaterally to posterior triangle of neck and present behind the posterior border or sternocleidomastoid muscle.
- Abscess may track down into mediastinum and may even cause mediastinal syndrome.
- Laterally, the pus may track along the brachial sheath into axilla or even cubital fossa.

Dorsal spine:
- Cold abscess of thoracic disease often forms paravertebral abscess in extrapleural space. The abscess may burst into intrapleural space causing pseudoempyema thoracis or may track along the intercostal nerves and vessels to point anteriorly.
- The cold abscess may track along the rectus sheath or lower abdominal wall.

Lumbar spine tuberculosis:
- Cold abscess in lumbar lesions (typically the psoas abscess) may track to form paravertebral abscess palpable posteriorly on one side of spine or may travel along the intercostal, ilioinguinal, and iliohypogastric nerves.
- It may go to petit's triangle along the flat muscles of abdominal wall or in the ischiorectal fossa along the internal pudendal nerve. Posteriorly, it may track to buttock along the gluteal nerve.
- Anteriorly, it may form typical psoas abscess that may point anywhere from abdomen to groin to thigh to even popliteal region.
- If it develops a connection in the inferior abdominal wall it may form an inverted horseshoe abscess also (uncommon presentation).

These abscesses do not influence the disease outcome at all, the examiner possibly confused with the types of vertebral involvement (anterior, paradiscal, complete, central, posterior, skip lesion, spinal tumor syndrome and tubercular arthritis) in tuberculosis spine and its influence on disease outcome.

6. Discuss neurological deficit in caries spine, types, pathogenesis, and prognostic factors.

Ans: Pott's paraplegia (neurological complication of spinal TB) is estimated to occur in 10–43% cases. The exact prevalence and incidence in endemic nations appears to be under-reported and is not well calculated that can also be partially attributed to increasing prevalence of multidrug resistant (MDR) and extensively drug resistant (XDR) cases and increasing prevalence of HIV infection in the population. Age incidence of tuberculous paraplegia follows closely the incidence of the tuberculous disease of the vertebral column itself, being more common during first 3 decades of life. Paraplegia most commonly results from interference with the function of the cord, thus disease below the level of first lumbar vertebra rarely causes paraplegia due to compression of cauda equina. Above the level of first lumbar vertebra, the highest incidence of paraplegia is associated with tuberculous disease of the lower thoracic region. Twenty-four percent patients of cervical spine TB showed varying degree of neural deficit. Involvement of cervical and upper dorsal region of cord leads to quadriparesis or quadriplegia.

Girdlestone classification of onset of paraplegia (**Table 4C.1.1**):
- Early-onset paraplegia (develops within 2 years of disease onset).
- Late-onset paraplegia (develops after 2 years of disease may even develop 2–3 decades after active infection).
- Hodgson's classification is more detailed differentiating the causes and types of paraplegia:
  - *Paraplegia of active disease*: These develop mainly in response to the ongoing inflammation during active phase of disease, so respond favorably to conservative management and often subsiding with successful chemotherapy.
  - *Paraplegia of healed disease*: Here the mechanism is mechanical so chemotherapy or conservative management is likely to fail producing a guarded prognosis.

TABLE 4C.1.1: Classification of tuberculous paraplegia/tetraplegia (Predominantly based upon motor weakness).

Stage		Clinical features
1	Negligible	Patient unaware of neural deficit, physician detects plantar extensor and/or ankle clonus
2	Mild	Patient aware of deficit but manages to walk with support
3	Moderate	Nonambulatory because of paralysis (in extension), sensory deficit less than 50%
4	Moderate	III + Flexor spasms/paralysis in flexion/flaccid/sensory deficit more than 50%/sphincters involved

The prognosis is better if there is only partial cord involvement, the neural complications are of short duration, there is "early onset" cord involvement, the neural complications developed slowly, the patient is young and his general condition is good.

Pathogenesis: Pott's paraplegia is more common in dorsal and cervicodorsal lesions as the spinal canal is narrower and there is propensity toward kyphosis and retropulsion. In the lumbar lesions, it is less common as the canal is wider and cord ends at lower border of L1.

Motor functions are almost always affected before and to a greater extent than the sensory functions because the diseased area in the spine lies anterior to the cord thus being nearer to the motor tracts. Besides, probably the motor tracts are more sensitive to compression of the cord. The paralysis may pass with varying rapidity through the following stages: Spastic motor paraparesis, spastic paraplegia in extension and later on spastic paraplegia in flexion. As the cord is increasingly compressed the patient develops uncontrollable flexor spasms which in later stages remain established in flexion, this indicates complete loss of conductivity in the pyramidal and extrapyramidal tracts. In very advanced cases of compression, bladder and anal sphincters may be involved and there may be a varying degree of sensory deficit. Sense of position and vibration are the last to disappear. In extremely severe cases, all spasticity disappears and the paralysis becomes flaccid (areflexic paraplegia) with anesthesia and loss of sphincter control.

7. Discuss radiological features for the diagnosis of TB spine.

Ans: *Anterior inferior portion of the vertebral body*: These are more common in thoracic spine region. Infection spreads under anterior longitudinal ligament. Shallow erosion of anterior surface of vertebral bodies occurs. Collapse and decreased disk space are uncommon and late if at all.

Paradiskal: The infection spreads through epiphyseal arteries. Disk destruction occurs through loss of nutrition. The infection begins from the anterior vertebral body adjacent to the anterior end plate. With continued destruction anterior wedging of vertebra occurs, causing kyphosis. Intraosseous and extraosseous abscess formation are often found in this type of lesions which is major risk of cord damage due to pressure effect by the abscess, displaced bone, or ischemia from spinal artery thrombosis.

Complete lesion: Destruction of one or two vertebrae. This type is seen in children less than 10 years of age, possibly associated with poor nutrition and lack of immunity. There is severe anterior column defect. They are prone to late onset paraplegia.

Central lesions: These are again common in children. The infection spreads through Batson's venous plexus and posterior vertebral artery. Radiograph shows patchy destruction and loss of bony trabeculae. Initially, there is expansion of the vertebral body and later in advanced lesions, there is vertebra plana due to concentric type of collapse.

Posterior lesions (appendiceal lesions/apophyseal TB): This is characterized by involvement of partially or wholly pedicle, lamina, transverse process and spinous process. Spread via the posterior external venous plexus of vertebral veins or direct spread. The lamina was most commonly involved followed by pedicles, articular processes, spinous processes, and transverse processes. The radiographs show destruction of one (winking owl) or both pedicles, loss of spinous process (beakless owl) or other processes. There is lateral translation and/or rotational deformities. There is increased chance of neurological deficit due to proximity to spinal canal and often delayed diagnosis.

Skip lesion: Poor general health in children with compromised immunological status is the predominant cause. MDR TB also presents in this manner.

Spinal tumor syndrome: The lesion starts at the posterior margin of vertebral body with proliferation of the granulation tissue in canal causing cord compression.

True tubercular arthritis: This is seen in occipito-atlanto-axial type involvement.

8. Discuss diagnosis and management of Pott's paraplegia.

Ans: Paraplegia is the most unfortunate complication of spinal disease. The tubercular abscess or granulation tissue can directly compress the neuraxis leading to symptoms of cranial nerve involvement or spinal nerve root compression. The inflammatory exudates in CSF can cause clumping of the nerve root leading to arachnoiditis. Children are more prone to late onset paraplegia. The neurological complications can arise early in the disease or develop later as has been classified by Girdlestone or Hodgson.

- *Girdlestone classification of onset of paraplegia*:
    - Early-onset paraplegia (develops within 2 years of disease onset)
    - Late-onset paraplegia (develops after 2 years of disease may even develop 23 decades after active infection).

Diagnosis: The level of cord compression can be deciphered from clinical, neurological, radiological, and MRI examination. Myelography may be done in "spinal tumor syndrome" additionally for diagnosis confirmation, or in cases with multiple vertebral lesions myelography is helpful in determining the level of obstruction. Another situation when myelography is indicated and useful is when a patient has not recovered after decompression operation.

Management: Management in a specialized spine care center is recommended. The treatment is directed to control the disease and performing a mechanical decompression of the cord by removing the diseased tissues without compromising stability in cases who need surgery. In these cases, multidrug therapy and rest is given for 3–6 weeks. If there is progressive neurological recovery, then medication is continued and walking allowed after recovery is complete.

If no recovery, then surgical decompression is done. If recovery occurs after surgery, then medication is continued but if neurology does not improve, then MRI or myelogram is done. If no cord compression or block is demonstrated, then it indicates intrinsic damage to cord → give medication and start rehab in these cases.

If mechanical block is demonstrated, then perform repeat decompression followed by continued medication and permit walking when recovery is complete.

In the usual paradiskal lesion, the compression of the cord takes place primarily and maximally anteriorly. Therefore, it is absolutely rational to adequately decompress the cord anteriorly by anterior approach or through an anterolateral approach. Laminectomy for decompression is contraindicated as this procedure is inadequate for decompression of the anterior part of the cord; besides it removes the healthy areas of the vertebrae thus rendering the vertebral column unstable and liable to pathological dislocation in the usual tuberculous lesion of the spine.

Development of severe kyphotic deformity should be minimized by performing posterior spinal fusion for extensive spinal disease during childhood, because kyphosis of 60° or more as a rule produces delayed neural complications 10–15 years after the onset of disease and deformity. In cases of paraplegia with kyphosis of 60° or more, removal of the "internal gibbus" (even if comprised by healthy bones) is mandatory permitting the cord complete freedom anteriorly. This may produce some relief in the neural deficit though seldom complete recovery is observed.

Evoked potential studies have been suggested for objective documentation of sensory and motor deficits in patients with tuberculous paraplegia. This may be of some value in very advanced cases of neurological deficit, however, there are many cases who would exhibit false positive or false negative results.

The above is the classical middle path regime followed. The commonly followed indications for surgical decompression in clinical practice are as follows:
- Failure of clinical improvement after 6–10 weeks of treatment
- Recurrence of disease
- Primary drug resistance or history of irregular chemotherapy
- *To prevent deformity*:
    - *Adults*: Vertebral body loss of greater than 1 in dorsal and dorsolumbar regions and greater than 1.5 in lumbar region.

- *Children*:
  - "Spine at-risk signs" score of greater than 2.
  - Vertebral body loss of greater than 0.75 in dorsal and dorsolumbar region and loss of greater than 1 in lumbar region.
  - Children who present with a kyphus greater than 30° before start of chemotherapy.

9. **A. Explain the basis of the middle path regime for spinal tuberculosis (TB) management.**
B. Write current national guidelines on antitubercular treatment (ATT) for Pott's spine.
C. Enumerate the indications for decompression surgery in a case of Pott's spine.
D. Enumerate the indications for additional stabilization surgery in a case of Pott's spine.
E. Explain the concept of "paradoxical reaction (PR) in bone and joint tuberculosis treatment" versus clinical suspicion of "multidrug resistant bone and joint tuberculosis."

Ans: Current National Guidelines on Antitubercular Treatment (ATT) for Pott's spine (India, 2025)

In India, the management of Pott's spine follows the National Tuberculosis Elimination Programme (NTEP) guidelines, updated in alignment with the World Health Organization (WHO) recommendations. Below is a concise summary of the current (2025) national guidelines for ATT of Pott's spine, based on NTEP and related sources.

Indications for Antitubercular Treatment
- *Confirmed diagnosis*: Positive microbiology [e.g., GeneXpert *Mycobacterium Tuberculosis* (MTB)/Rifampicin (RIF), acid-fast bacilli (AFB) smear, culture] or histopathological evidence of TB from spinal tissue/biopsy.
- *Presumptive diagnosis*: Clinical and radiological findings (e.g., vertebral destruction, paravertebral abscess, gibbus deformity) in high TB burden settings, with or without neurological deficits.
- *High-risk groups*: Patients with human immunodeficiency virus (HIV), diabetes, malnutrition, or other immunosuppressive conditions.

Antitubercular Treatment Regimen
- *Standard regimen (drug-sensitive TB)*:
  - *Duration*: 9–12 months total:
    - *Intensive phase (2 months)*: Daily oral regimen of HRZE [Isoniazid (H), Rifampicin (R), Pyrazinamide (Z), Ethambutol (E)].
    - *Continuation phase (7–10 months)*: Daily HR (Isoniazid + Rifampicin).
  - *Dosage* (adult, weight-based, per NTEP):
    - *Isoniazid*: 5 mg/kg (max 300 mg/day).
    - *Rifampicin*: 10 mg/kg (max 600 mg/day).
    - *Pyrazinamide*: 25–35 mg/kg (max 2,000 mg/day).
    - *Ethambutol*: 15–20 mg/kg (max 1,600 mg/day).
  - *Fixed-dose combinations (FDCs)*: Preferred to improve adherence (e.g., four-drug FDC in intensive phase, two-drug FDC in continuation phase).
- *Drug-resistant TB (MDR-TB)*:
  - *Diagnosis*: Confirmed by GeneXpert MTB/RIF or line probe assay showing rifampicin resistance.
    - *Regimen*: Individualized based on drug susceptibility testing (DST):
    - *Shorter oral regimen (9–11 months)*: Includes bedaquiline, levofloxacin, clofazimine, linezolid, and others (per WHO/NTEP guidelines).
    - *Longer regimen (18–20 months)*: For complex cases, including pre-XDR/XDR-TB, with drugs such as bedaquiline, delamanid, or pretomanid.
  - *Dosage*: As per NTEP MDR-TB guidelines, weight-based (e.g., bedaquiline 400 mg daily for 2 weeks, then 200 mg thrice weekly).
- *Special populations*:
  - *HIV coinfection*: Same ATT regimen; initiate antiretroviral therapy (ART) within 2–8 weeks of ATT. Adjust rifampicin interactions (e.g., use rifabutin if needed).

- *Pediatric*: Weight-based dosing; HRZE for 2 months, HR for 7-10 months; avoid ethambutol in young children unless necessary.
- *Pregnancy*: HRZE safe; avoid streptomycin (ototoxic); consult for second-line drugs.

Paradoxical Reaction versus Clinical Suspicion of Multidrug-Resistant Bone and Joint Tuberculosis
Paradoxical Reaction in Bone and Joint Tuberculosis Treatment
- *Definition*: A paradoxical reaction is a transient worsening or new onset of symptoms, signs, or radiological findings during effective ATT for bone and joint TB, despite microbiological evidence of response (e.g., negative cultures). It is an immune-mediated phenomenon, not treatment failure.
- *Mechanism*:
  - Enhanced immune response after starting ATT, likely due to the release of mycobacterial antigens from dying bacteria, triggering inflammation.
  - Common in extrapulmonary TB, including Pott's spine, due to high antigen load in bone/joint tissues.
- *Clinical features*:
  - Worsening pain, swelling, or deformity (e.g., kyphosis) within 2-12 weeks of ATT initiation.
  - New or enlarging abscesses, sinuses, or neurological deficits (e.g., paresis).
  - Radiological progression (e.g., increased vertebral destruction, soft tissue mass) despite negative TB tests.
- *Indications of PR*:
  - Occurs early in treatment (typically within 3 months).
  - Negative repeat cultures or GeneXpert MTB/RIF, ruling out active TB progression.
  - Improvement with conservative management (e.g., corticosteroids) without changing ATT.
- *Management*:
  - Continue standard ATT (*HRZE*: Isoniazid, rifampicin, pyrazinamide, ethambutol).
  - Corticosteroids (e.g., prednisolone 0.5-1 mg/kg/day, tapered over 4-8 weeks) to reduce inflammation.
  - Aspiration/drainage of large abscesses if symptomatic.
  - Reassurance and close monitoring [clinical, imaging, inflammatory markers like erythrocyte sedimentation rate (ESR)/C-reactive protein (CRP)].

Clinical Suspicion of Multidrug-Resistant Bone and Joint Tuberculosis
- *Definition*: Multidrug-resistant (MDR) bone and joint TB is suspected when TB is resistant to at least isoniazid and rifampicin, confirmed by DST, or when clinical/radiological deterioration persists despite adequate ATT.
- *Mechanism*:
  - Resistance arises from mutations in *Mycobacterium tuberculosis* genes (e.g., rpoB for rifampicin), often due to prior inadequate treatment, nonadherence, or exposure to resistant strains.
  - Bone and joint TB (e.g., Pott's spine) have poor drug penetration, increasing resistance risk.
- *Clinical features*:
  - Persistent or worsening symptoms (pain, deformity, neurological deficits) beyond 3-6 months of ATT.
  - Nonhealing sinuses, persistent abscesses, or progressive bone destruction on imaging.
  - Positive TB cultures or GeneXpert MTB/RIF showing rifampicin resistance.
- *Indications of MDR-TB*:
  - History of prior TB treatment, nonadherence, or contact with MDR-TB cases.
  - Positive microbiological tests (e.g., GeneXpert, culture) despite prolonged ATT.
  - Lack of response to standard HRZE regimen after 3-6 months.
- *Management*:
  - Confirm MDR-TB with DST (GeneXpert MTB/RIF, line probe assay).
  - Initiate MDR-TB regimen per NTEP or WHO:
    - *Shorter regimen (9-11 months)*: Bedaquiline, levofloxacin, clofazimine, linezolid, etc.
    - *Longer regimen (18-20 months)*: For pre-XDR/XDR-TB, with bedaquiline, delamanid, or pretomanid.
  - Surgical intervention (e.g., debridement, stabilization) for extensive destruction or neurological compromise.
  - Monitor with monthly cultures, imaging, and clinical assessment.
- *Key note*: MDR-TB indicates true treatment failure requiring regimen change and prolonged therapy.

PR versus MDR TB
- *Cause*: PR is immune-mediated; MDR-TB is due to resistant bacteria.
- *Timing*: PR occurs early (2–12 weeks); MDR-TB manifests later (3–6 months).
- *Microbiology*: PR has negative cultures/DST; MDR-TB shows positive cultures with resistance.
- *Management*: PR managed with corticosteroids and continued ATT; MDR-TB requires second-line drugs and possible surgery.

10. Describe indications of surgery in TB spine.

Ans: *Indications for patients on middle path regimen*:
- No neurological recovery even after 4 weeks of chemotherapy
- Development of neurologic complications during chemotherapy
- Recurrence of neurological complications during chemotherapy
- Worsening of neurological complications during chemotherapy
- Advanced cases of neurologic involvement (stage 4)
- Rapidly advancing paresis which is advancing daily
- Common indications (whether or not neurological complications present):
  - Patients with prevertebral cervical abscess and difficulty in deglutition
  - Dorsal spine involvement with spasmodic respiration,
  - Older patients in whom one would like to avoid complications of prolonged recumbency.

Indications of surgery in a patient who does not have neurological complications:
- Failure of clinical improvement after 6–10 weeks of ATT (modified from original middle path regimen that observes for 3–6 months—most examiner observe for up to 3 months)
- Recurrence of disease
- Primary drug resistance or history of irregular chemotherapy
- To prevent deformity:
  - *Adult*: Vertebral body loss >1 in dorsal and D-L regions and >1.5 in lumbar region.
  - Children who present with a kyphus >30° before start of treatment.
- Rare indications:
  - To establish diagnosis (only when CT-guided biopsy inconclusive)
  - In patients with persistent sinuses and abscess
  - Tuberculosis of cervical spine with paravertebral abscess causing difficulty in deglutition and respiration.

11. What are the indications and contraindications for surgical decompression in TB spine?

Ans: *Indications*:
- Progressive bone destruction producing instability in spite of chemotherapeutic regime
- Failure to respond to conservative therapy
- Uncertainty in diagnosis—need to prove disease through biopsy/tissue diagnosis.
- Large abscess/increasing paravertebral abscess despite chemotherapeutic regime—threatening neurological status of causing compressive symptoms
- Recrudescence of the local disease
- Development of neural complications on chemotherapy or later
- Uncontrollable pain in the spine due to mechanical instability

Absolute indications for operative decompression in patients with neural complications:
- Neurological complications which do not start showing signs of progressive recovery to a satisfactory level after a fair trial of conservative therapy (3–4 weeks).
- Patients with spinal caries in whom neurological complications develop during the conservative treatment.
- Patients with neurological complications which become worse while they are undergoing therapy with anti-tuberculous drugs and bedrest.

- Patients who have a recurrence of neurological complication.
- Patients with prevertebral cervical abscesses, neurological signs and difficulty in deglutition and respiration.
- Advanced cases of neurological involvement such as marked sensory and sphincter disturbances, flaccid paralysis or severe flexor spasms.

Contraindications:
- Mild disease
- Stable spine
- Neurology intact and recovering
- Relief in symptoms (pain) with chemotherapy
- Resolving abscess
- Morbid/moribund patient with disease unfit for surgery

12. **Describe TB dorsal spine with paraplegia. Briefly discuss clinical features, investigations, differential diagnosis, and principles of management.**

Ans: Clinical features:
Symptoms of TB of the spine are commonly insidious but sometimes these may be acute. The usual clinical symptoms in active stage of the disease are malaise, loss of weight, loss of appetite, night sweats and evening rise of temperature. The spine is stiff and painful on movement with localized kyphotic deformity which would be tender on percussion. Spasm of the vertebral muscles is present. During sleep, the muscle spasm relaxes permitting movement between the inflamed surfaces resulting in the typical night cries. A cold abscess may be present clinically. A history of TB in the patient or his family should raise suspicion of tubercular nature of the spinal disease. Careful neurological examination will reveal paraplegia. If the clinician makes it a routine to palpate the spinous processes by sliding his fingertips from the cervical spine to the sacrum he would be able to detect even a small knuckle kyphosis by palpation of a step or a prominence thus diagnosing a case before gross destruction has taken place.

Rarely paraplegia may be the presenting symptom of TB of the spine. Commonly this is associated with a known lesion of the vertebral column. In a paraplegia of slow onset, the first signs of interference with the conduction of cord may be spontaneous twitching of muscles in the lower limbs and clumsiness while walking, extensor plantar response and exaggerated reflexes. Sustained clonus of ankle and patella may be present. Exceptionally the damage to the cord may be so sudden and complete that the patient presents with sudden, complete flaccid paralysis like the clinical picture of "spinal shock". This may later gradually change into spasticity. Sudden complete paralysis may be caused by ischemia of the cord due to thromboembolic phenomenon or transection of the cord due to pathological dislocation or extremely rarely due to rapid accumulation of infected material.

On rare occasions paraplegia of tuberculous etiology may present like a "spinal tumor syndrome" due to a localized tuberculoma or a diffuse granuloma or due to peridural fibrosis.

Investigations:
- CBC, ESR, CRP, Genexpert
- X-ray of dorsal spine
- CT scan for assessing destructive lesions
- MRI extremely useful in diagnosis of TB and an excellent modality to judge the health of spinal cord
- Myelography rarely is needed and only in special cases (multiple vertebral lesions, spinal tumor syndrome).

Differential diagnosis:
- Trauma
- Metastasis to spine
- Spinal tumors
- PIVD.

Principles of management:
- Treatment should start with multidrug antitubercular therapy and supervision, rest in recumbency for 3–6 weeks and then the future course should be decided.

- The treatment of tuberculous paraplegia is the treatment of TB of the spine with the added aim of performing a mechanical decompression of the cord by removing the diseased tissues without compromising stability in cases who need surgery.
- Laminectomy for decompression is contraindicated as this procedure is inadequate for decompression of the anterior part of the cord; besides it removes the healthy areas of the vertebrae thus rendering the vertebral column unstable and liable to pathological dislocation in the usual tuberculous lesion of the spine.
- Development of severe kyphotic deformity should be minimized by performing posterior spinal fusion for extensive spinal disease during childhood.
- Every case of neurological complication with TB of the spine warrants immediate admission and care by a suitable orthopedic center where all facilities for spinal surgery are available.

13. Discuss the indications of surgery in TB spine with or without neurological complications.
Ans: Kindly see Answer to Question 11.

14. Discuss anterolateral decompression of TB spine of D5–D6 spine.
Ans: *Anterolateral decompression (ALD)*: In 1933, Norman Capener devised lateral rachiotomy where decompression was obtained anterior to theca. He excised a part of the lamina and pedicle from one side to enter the spinal canal anteriorly. This procedure was modified by Dott and Alexander into *anterolateral decompression*, in which the spine is opened more anteriorly by removal of part of the body of the vertebra to gain access to the spinal canal. Lamina remains untouched. This affords access to the front and side of the cord, permitting decompression by the removal of bony spurs, granulation tissue, and sequestra or the evacuation of abscesses. Because the procedure entails resection of one or more pedicles, it is contraindicated if the spine is unstable. Steps of procedure are as follow:
- *Position*: The right lateral position is used (avoids venous congestion and excessive bleeding, and permits freer respiration also the lung and mediastinal contents easily fall anteriorly). Approach the spine from the left side.
- Begin the incision in the midline at a point 10 cm proximal to the lesion, gently curve it laterally a distance of 7.5 cm, and return to the midline at a point 10 cm distal to the lesion. Reflect the skin and superficial and deep fasciae as a thick flap.
- Retract the trapezius muscle laterally, cut and retract the erector spinae muscles to expose underlying rib.
- Resect rib from its angle to the transverse process.
- Separate the intercostal nerve from its accompanying vessels, and divide it using the proximal end as a guide to further dissection and later for traction on the cord.
- Retract the pleura along with the intercostal vessels, and remove the medial end of the rib and the transverse process and pedicle of the vertebra.
- Visualize the dura using traction on the intercostal nerve following anterior decompression.
- Gently remove diseased bone with curet and also the impinging tissues. Thoroughly evacuate the paravertebral abscess.

15. What are the surgical approaches for Pott's paraplegia?
Ans: Pott's paraplegia occurs for tubercular affection of the spine in dorsal region and uncommonly in cervical spine or rarely in lumbar spine. So surgical intervention is needed for dorsal spine tubercular disease and ensuing compression of the neural structures.

Transthoracic transpleural approach for spine D1 to L1:
The chest is usually opened on the left side where it is easier to handle aorta. On the right side, the inferior vena cava being more delicate is liable to be damaged while exposing the vertebral bodies. One may approach through the right thoracotomy where X-rays show an unusually large abscess on the right side with little or negligible bulge on the left side, or when left thoracotomy is difficult because of pulmonary complications or prior operation.

For the left thoracotomy approach, the patient is placed in the right lateral position and the surgeon stands on the dorsal side of the patient. An incision is made along the rib which in the mid-axillary line, opposite the center of the lesion. This is usually two ribs higher than the center of the vertebral lesion. In patients with severe kyphosis, an operative view is better if a rib is removed along the line of incision and a sandbag or a bridge is used under the involved vertebrae to spread the ribs apart. A J-shaped parascapular incision is required for lesions from C7 to D8 so that the scapula can be lifted off the chest wall and the appropriate rib can be selected for opening the chest. The muscles and the periosteum are cut over the selected rib from the costochondral junction to the posterior part of the rib. The selected rib is resected subperiosteally. In the bed of the rib, a small incision is made in the parietal pleura, in the absence of adhesions, the lung falls away from the parieties.

However, when adhesions are present, by gentle blunt dissection, the parietal and visceral pleura are separated. Through the incision in the bed of the rib, index and middle fingers are introduced in the pleural cavity (which also help identifying the underlying adhesions) and the opening is extended by cutting the parietal pleura with the help of scissors over these fingers and the wound edges are retracted by a self-retaining retractor. The lung is freed from the parieties as completely as possible.

There may be adhesions between paravertebral abscess and the lung and/or aorta. Thick adhesions require cutting with cautery and careful hemostasis. Having freed the lung, it is retracted anteriorly displaying the aorta and any paravertebral bulge or the diseased area of the vertebral column. A plane is to be developed now between the descending aorta and the paravertebral abscess/diseased vertebral bodies. For these intercostal vessels and branches of hemiazygos veins present opposite the site of disease have to be identified through the parietal pleura, dissected and cut between two ligatures. Now mobilize the aorta for displacement forward and to the right by making a longitudinal incision in the parietal pleura lateral to the aorta between the two ligatures. Use blunt dissection to retract the aorta and the contents of the mediastinum to the right and anteriorly. Opposite to D5–D10 vertebral bodies, the whole of (descending) aorta, after cutting the intercostal arteries between two ligatures, cannot only be reflected to the right side with the help of spatulas but also lifted up on two loops. This permits extensive space to work on the front and left surface of vertebral bodies and disks. In the presence of a severe kyphotic deformity, one is obliged to work in the depth of a depression—a very tedious job.

If a paravertebral abscess is present, it is opened by a T-shaped incision with the vertical limb of the T placed horizontally at the center of the diseased bodies and the horizontal limb of the T placed vertically medial to the lateral parts of the divided intercostal vessels. Two triangular flaps are then raised and retracted to expose the diseased vertebral bodies. The diseased area is then dealt as required by performing debridement or decompression with or without bone grafting.

Anterolateral decompression (D2 to L1):
Kindly see Answer to Question 14 above.

16. Discuss instrumentation in spinal TB—rationale and its indications.

Ans: *Rationale*: Implant-associated infections are related to altered local environment and bacterial thriving around implants due to relative inadequacy and ineffectiveness of host defenses and antibiotics, respectively. Biofilm formation plays a significant role in evading defense mechanisms and safeguarding bacteria from chemotherapy. Biomaterial centered infections are related to preferential bacterial colonization of inert surfaces and production of biofilm (glycocalyx) protecting them from host defenses and chemotherapy. As mycobacterial adhesiveness is less and there is decreased tendency to biofilm production so risk of persistence of infection is minimal. Due to limited tendency of biofilm production of *Mycobacterium tuberculosis* risk of persistent infection is smaller. This has led to now an increasingly popular use of instrumentation. Anterior surgery alone is ineffective, additional posterior instrumentation is often required. Adjuvant posterior stabilization hastens early mobilization and rehabilitation.

Radical anterior debridement clears the diseased focus while simultaneously restoring the anterior column by cage. Healing of the disease and fusion of the graft across the affected vertebrae is improved. The incidence of graft related problems and the progression of the kyphosis are significantly less by the combined approach when compared with anterior surgery alone. The postoperative loss of correction is insignificant for combined anterior and posterior surgery.

Indications:
- Pan vertebral disease, in which all 3 columns are involved
- Long segment disease
- Kyphosis correction
- Spine at risk, signs are present.

17. Discuss antituberculous therapy (ATT) in osteoarticular TB in terms of doses, regimen and duration of ATT.

Ans: Doses as daily administration–

First-line drugs:
- Isoniazid: 5 mg/kg
- Rifampicin: 10 mg/kg
- Pyrazinamide: 25 mg/kg
- Ethambutol: 15 mg/kg
- Streptomycin: 15 mg/kg

Second-line drugs:
- Fluoroquinolones: 400–600 mg/day
- PAS: 12 g
- Thioacetazone: 150 mg
- Ethionamide: 1 g
- Cycloserine: 1 g
- Capreomycin: 15 mg/kg
- Kanamycin: 15 mg/kg
- Clofazimine: 100–200 mg
- Amikacin: 15 mg/kg
- Minocycline: 100–200 mg

Regimen (middle path regimen): Start with "intensive phase" treatment comprising daily dosage of isoniazid 300–400 mg, rifampicin 450–600 mg, and fluoroquinolones 400–600 mg for 5–6 months. All replicating sensitive mycobacteria are likely to be killed by this bactericidal regime.

The "continuation phase" treatment should last for 9–10 months where the aim is to attack the persisters, slow-growing or intermittently growing or dormant or intracellular mycobacteria. It comprises isoniazid and pyrazinamide (1,500 mg/day) for 4–5 months (pyrazinamide is considered to have maximum penetrability to kill intracellular mycobacteria) to be followed by isoniazid and rifampicin for another 4–5 months. The slow-growing mycobacteria by this phase of treatment hopefully would be in their "state of replication," the combination of isoniazid and rifampicin is considered the safest and most effective treatment to eliminate such organisms.

The "prophylactic phase" consists of isoniazid and ethambutol (1,200 mg) for 3–4 months. This is the time when the treated patient is back to his normal-working environments.

My preference and practice should receive at least 6 months treatment with 2HRZE/4HR (intensive/continuation phase) that can be extended to 9 months (2HRZE/7HR) as by some experts. The combination HE in continuation phase has been withdrawn (high failure rate) similarly omission of ethambutol from intensive phase is being contemplated.

Under DOTS (difficult for all osteoarticular patients as they have difficulty being mobile) thrice weekly intermittent regimens [2HRZE/4(HR)3] and [2(HRZE)3/4(HR)3] extended to 9 months are acceptable.

Duration: Hodgson and Stock (1956–60) and other workers advocate antituberculous drugs for 18 months to 2 years along with the radical excisional surgery for the osteoarticular lesion. Dutt et al. (1986) reported that a short-course chemotherapy (9 months) with INH and rifampicin was as effective in newly diagnosed and drug-susceptible cases as the conventional therapy for 18–24 months in extrapulmonary TB.

18. Enumerate names of 1st, 2nd and 3rd line drugs of ATT.

Ans: {I have no idea about third-line anti-tubercular therapeutic drugs – possibly there is also no such term!!}

First-line drugs:
- *Essential*:
  – Isoniazid
  – Rifampicin

- Pyrazinamide
- Ethambutol
- *Supplementary*:
  - Streptomycin
  - Rifabutin
  - Rifapentine

Second-line drugs:
- Thiacetazone
- Para-aminosalicylic acid
- Ethionamide
- Cycloserine
- Kanamycin
- Capreomycin
- Amikacin
- Fluoroquinolones
- Linezolid
- Bedaquiline + Delamanid
- Prothionamide
- Terizidone
- Reserved drugs unknown use (meropenem, pretomanid, sutezolid, etc.)

19. **Differentiate paraplegia with active disease (early onset paraplegia) and paraplegia with healed disease (late onset paraplegia). Also discuss causes and management of late onset paraplegia.**

Ans: Difference has been shown in **Table 4C.1.2**.

TABLE 4C.1.2: Difference between paraplegia with active disease and late-onset paraplegia.

Feature	Paraplegia with active disease	Late-onset paraplegia
Cord involvement	Better prognosis	Relatively poor prognosis
Degree of paraplegia	Partial (stage I, II)	Complete (stage IV)
Duration	Shorter	Longer (>12 months)
Type	"Early onset"	"Late onset"
Speed of onset	Slow	Rapid
Age	Younger	Older
General condition	Good	Poor
Vertebral disease	Active	Healed
Kyphotic deformity	<60°	>60°
Cord on MRI	Normal	Myelomalacia/Syrinx
Peroperative	Wet lesion	Dry lesion

Causes: Neurological complications may be associated with recrudescence of the disease or due to mechanical pressure on the cord. Underlying pathology in most of the cases of later variety is tuberculous caseous tissue, tubercular debris, sequestra from vertebral body and disk, internal gibbus, stenosis of the vertebral canal or severe deformity.

Management: In the cases who started showing progressive recovery of neurological complications on triple drug therapy between 3 weeks and 4 weeks and progressed to complete recovery, surgical decompression was considered unnecessary. Decompression of the cord for neurological complication should be performed for those cases who did not show progressive recovery after a fair trial of conservative therapy for a few weeks, or cases in which the patients developed the neurological complications during the conservative therapy, or in cases where the neurological status became worse while the patient was undergoing treatment with antitubercular drugs and bedrest, or cases who had a history of recurrence of neurological complication. In advanced cases with motor, sensory, and sphincter involvement or those having severe flexor spasms as well as in elderly patients' decompression should not be delayed unduly.

20. Describe spine at risk sign.

Ans: Rajasekaran (2007) suggested radiographic signs to assess "spine-at risk" for kyphotic deformity in children. These signs seen in lateral X-rays included points A, B, D, and point C on AP X-ray:

A. *Separation of the facet joint*: The facet joint dislocates at the level of the apex of the curve, causing instability and loss of alignment.

B. *Posterior retropulsion*: This is identified by drawing two lines along the posterior surface of the first upper and lower normal vertebrae. The diseased segments are found to project posterior to the intersection of the lines.

C. *Lateral translation*: This is confirmed when a vertical line drawn through the middle of the pedicle of the first lower normal vertebra does not touch the pedicle of the first upper normal vertebra.

D. *Toppling sign*: Often in the initial stages, a line drawn along the anterior surface of immediate lower normal vertebra intersects the inferior surface of the first upper normal vertebra usually. "Tilt" or "toppling" occurs when this line intersects higher than the middle of the anterior surface of the first normal upper vertebra.

21. Tuberculosis of subaxial spine: Pathology, clinical features, investigations, and treatment.

Ans: Tuberculosis of the Subaxial Spine (Cervical, Thoracic, and Lumbar Spine)

Tuberculosis of the subaxial spine (vertebrae below C2) is a form of spinal TB (Pott's disease), caused by *Mycobacterium tuberculosis*. It primarily affects the vertebral bodies and intervertebral discs, leading to bone destruction, deformity, and potential neurological deficits.

Pathology:
- *Route of infection*: Hematogenous spread from a primary focus (lungs, lymph nodes, or other organs).
- *Site of involvement*:
  - Lower thoracic and lumbar spine are most commonly affected (due to high vascularity).
  - Cervical spine involvement is less common but can be more severe due to spinal cord compression.
- *Pathological stages*:
  - *Predestructive stage*: Granulomatous inflammation without bone destruction.
  - *Early destructive stage*: Bone and disc destruction, leading to vertebral collapse and kyphosis.
  - *Advanced stage*: Abscess formation (cold abscess), spinal deformity, and neurological deficits.

Clinical features:
- *Constitutional symptoms*:
  - Fever, night sweats, weight loss, fatigue.
- *Local symptoms*:
  - Back pain (most common symptom, worse at night).
  - Stiffness and restricted movement.
  - Tenderness over the affected vertebrae.
- *Neurological deficits (in advanced cases)*:
  - Radiculopathy (nerve root compression).
  - Myelopathy (cord compression) → weakness, sensory loss, bladder/bowel dysfunction.
  - Paraplegia (in severe cases).
- *Cold abscess formation*:
  - May track along tissue planes (e.g., psoas abscess in lumbar TB).
  - Cervical TB can present as a retropharyngeal abscess or neck swelling.

Investigations:
- *Imaging*:
  - X-ray spine [anteroposterior (AP) and lateral]:
    - *Early*: Narrowing of disc space, osteopenia
    - *Late*: Vertebral collapse, kyphosis, paravertebral shadow (abscess)
  - *MRI spine (gold standard)*:
    - Detects early bone edema, abscesses, and spinal cord compression
    - Shows skip lesions (multiple noncontiguous vertebrae)
  - *CT spine*: Better for assessing bone destruction
  - *Positron emission tomography (PET)-CT (if needed)*: To detect occult TB lesions
- *Laboratory tests*:
  - *ESR and CRP*: Elevated (nonspecific)
  - *Tuberculin skin test (Mantoux)/interferon-γ release assay (IGRA)*: Positive in most cases.
  - *Microbiological confirmation*:
    - AFB staining and culture (sputum, abscess aspirate, or biopsy).
    - *Cartridge-based nucleic acid amplification test (CBNAAT), e.g., GeneXpert MTB/RIF*: Rapid diagnosis + rifampicin resistance detection.
  - Biopsy (CT/USG-guided): Histopathology shows caseating granulomas.

Treatment:
- *Antitubercular therapy*:
  - Standard regimen (WHO guidelines):
    - *Intensive phase (2 months)*: Rifampicin, isoniazid, pyrazinamide, ethambutol (HRZE)
    - *Continuation phase (7–10 months)*: Rifampicin + Isoniazid (HR)
  - *Total duration*: 9–12 months (longer if drug resistance or extensive disease)
  - *Drug-resistant TB*: Modified regimen based on DST (e.g., bedaquiline, linezolid).
- *Immobilization (if needed)*:
  - *Cervical spine*: Minerva jacket or halo vest (if instability)
  - *Thoracolumbar spine*: Brace (for pain relief and deformity prevention)
- *Surgery (indications)*:
  - Neurological deficits (cord compression)
  - Spinal instability (severe deformity)
  - Abscess drainage (if large or causing compression)
  - Failed medical therapy/drug resistance.
- *Surgical options*:
  - Anterior decompression and fusion (most common for cervical/thoracic spine)
  - Posterior stabilization (if severe kyphosis)
  - Drainage of abscess (percutaneous or open)

4C.2 URINARY BLADDER ANATOMY AND ITS INVOLVEMENT IN SPINAL CORD LESIONS (Q22–25)

22. A. Describe nerve supply of urinary bladder.

B. Discuss pathophysiology and management of autonomous bladder.

Ans:

A. *Nerve supply of urinary bladder*: There are two differently innervated muscles in bladder control. Parasympathetic fibers arising from S2–S4 cord segments innervate the urinary bladder via pelvic splanchnic nerves and the inferior hypogastric and vesical plexuses. This bladder motor (detrusor) is under local spinal control S2–S4, whereby any stimulus that arises due to bladder filling leads to contraction of bladder and emptying being inhibitory to the internal urethral sphincter. Sympathetic fibers arising from the T11 to L3 cord segments innervate the neck and trigone via lumbar splanchnic nerves. Their stimulation allows for bladder neck closure required for bladder filling. The external urethral sphincter is controlled by somatic fibers arising from motor neurons in the S2-S4 cord segments via the pudendal nerve. When micturition is initiated via cortical signals and the internal sphincter opens, the external sphincter relaxes reflexively but still can be contracted voluntarily **(Fig. 4C.2.1)**.

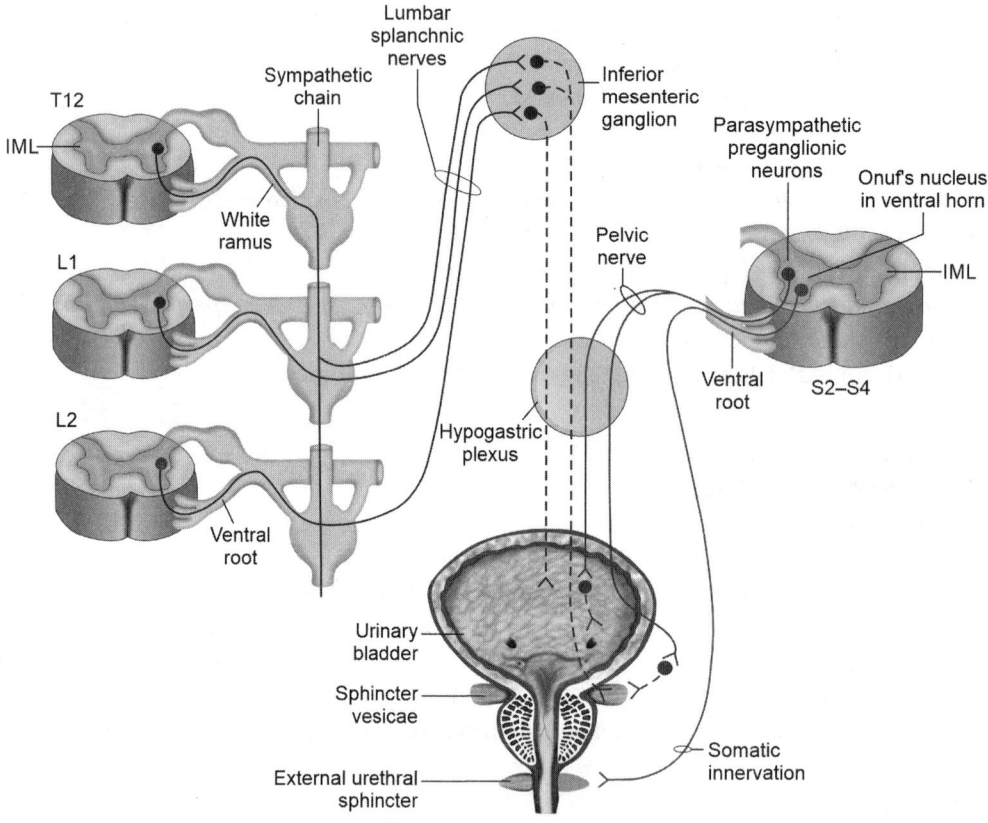

Fig. 4C.2.1: Nerve supply of urinary bladder.

B. *Pathophysiology*: If this local reflex is lost [as will happen in S2-S4 lesions like cauda equina syndrome—lower motor neuron (LMN) lesion] the bladder will not be able to contract due to its lost motor supply and also the sympathetic (L1-L2) reflex is still activating the sphincters that additionally prevent emptying. This type of bladder keeps filling till the capacity is exceeded when the urine dribbles due to exceeded competency of sphincters—"atonic bladder". With time, however intramural reflexes develop whence with overfilling the bladder may contract due to direct detrusor stimulation—the so called *"Autonomous bladder"*.

For management, kindly see Answer to Question 23.

23. Describe neurogenic bladder.

Ans: A dysfunctional urinary bladder caused by an injury to the central or peripheral nerves controlling urination is called a neurogenic bladder.

Pathophysiology and etiology: Voiding cycle is affected when any part of the nervous system is affected. It may result in overactive bladder (spastic bladder) or urinary retention or a combination of both. Bladder overactivity is associated with stress incontinence while sphincter underactivity is associated with urge incontinence. A combination of both may also occur.

Brain lesions: Lesions above the pons destroy the master control center and entire control over the voiding is lost. Patients develop urge incontinence, the bladder empties too quickly and too often. They rush to bathroom and can leak urine on their way to the bathroom. Some common causes are stroke, hydrocephalus, brain tumor, Parkinson disease, cerebral palsy, and Shy-Drager syndrome.

Spinal cord lesions: Diseases or injuries to the spinal cord result in overactive or spastic bladder and patients develop urge incontinence.

Sacral cord injury: Sacral cord injury can cause a sensory neurogenic bladder where the patient cannot sense that the bladder is full, or motor neurogenic bladder where the patient senses the bladder is full but detrusor does not contract, a condition known as detrusor areflexia causing overflow incontinence.

Examples:
- Sacral cord tumors
- Herniated disk
- Pelvic crush injuries
- Following lumbar laminectomy, radical hysterectomy or abdominal perineal resection
- Tethered cord syndrome (TCS) in teenagers.

Peripheral nerve injury: Destruction of the nerves to the bladder results in silent, painless distension of bladder with urinary retention. Causes are diabetes mellitus, Guillain-Barré syndrome, herpes in genital area, acquired immunodeficiency syndrome (AIDS) and poliomyelitis, and neurosyphilis (tabes dorsalis).

Classification: The Lapides classification is the most commonly used classification.
- The *sensory neurogenic bladder* with lesion in posterior columns of the spinal cord or in the afferent tracts leading from the bladder.
- The *motor paralytic bladder* with damage to motor neurons of the bladder.
- The *uninhibited neurogenic bladder* in which there is an incomplete spinal cord lesion above S2 or a cerebral cortex or cerebellopontine axis lesion.
- The *reflex neurogenic bladder* with a complete spinal cord lesion above S2 showing a pine cone bladder on cystogram.
- The *autonomous neurogenic bladder* seen in cauda equina or conus lesions.

Investigations:
- Laboratory studies
- Urinalysis and urine culture
- Urine cytology
- Chemical profile

Other tests:
- Voiding diary
- Pad test

Diagnostic procedures:
- Postvoid residual urine (PVR)
- Uroflow rate
- Filling cystometrogram
- Voiding cystometrogram (pressure flow study)
- Cystogram
- Electromyography
- Cystoscopy
- Videourodynamics.

Treatment: Treatment may be nonsurgical or surgical. Nonsurgical treatment measures include medications and other measures.

Treatment of urinary incontinence varies by types, such as:
- Treatment of urge incontinence is done with behavioral modification or with bladder-relaxing agents.
- Treatment of stress incontinence is done with surgical and nonsurgical means.

- Mixed incontinence also requires a combination of medications as well as surgery.
- Catheter regimen is used for overflow incontinence.
- Functional incontinence is treated by correcting the underlying cause (e.g. urinary tract infection, constipation) or changing medications.

Nonsurgical treatment measures
Nonmedical measures:
- Absorbent products
- Urethral occlusive devices
- Catheters
- Diet
- Pelvic floor exercises (Kegel exercises)
- Vaginal weights
- Biofeedback
- Electrical stimulation
- Bladder training.

Medications:
- *Anticholinergic drugs*
- *Estrogen derivatives*
- *Antispasmodic drugs*
- *Tricyclic antidepressant drugs.*

Surgical measures: Surgical care for stress incontinence involves procedures that improve urethral outlet resistance. Some such procedures are bladder neck suspension, sling procedures, periurethral bulking therapy, and artificial urinary sphincter.

Some surgical procedures work by improving bladder compliance or bladder capacity like sacral neuromodulation, bladder augmentation, botulinum toxin injections, and detrusor myomectomy.

24. **Discuss ASIA score. Classify bladder paralysis in spinal cord injury with salient features.**
Ans: *For ASIA scoring, kindly refer the Answer to Question 30.*

Bladder paralysis: There are two differently innervated muscles in bladder control. One is the bladder motor (detrusor) which is under local spinal control S2–S4, whereby any stimulus that arises due to bladder filling leads to contraction of bladder and emptying. The other one is the innervations of sphincters which is inhibited (relaxed) by local reflex (S2–S4) and stimulated by sympathetic system (L1–L2). Now secondly there is a higher control which has an inhibitory influence on local reflex (S2–S4). Now if local reflex is released from all upper inhibitions (as happens in UMN lesion) the bladder becomes an *"Automatic bladder"* which will contract as soon as it fills up and there will be detrusor hypertrophy due to hyperactive local reflex (S2–S4).

If the local reflex is lost (as will happen in S2–S4 lesions like cauda equina syndrome—LMN lesion), the bladder will not be able to contract due to its lost motor supply and also the sympathetic (L1–L2) reflex is still activating the sphincters that additionally prevent emptying. This type of bladder keeps filling till the capacity is exceeded when the urine dribbles due to exceeded competency of sphincters— "atonic bladder". With time, however intramural reflexes develop whence with overfilling the bladder may contract due to direct detrusor stimulation—the so called *"Autonomous bladder".*

25. **Describe automatic bladder.**
Ans: Kindly see Answer to Question 24.

4C.3 AUTONOMOUS DYSREFLEXIA AND REHABILITATION IN SPINAL CORD INJURY (Q26–29)

26. **Discuss autonomous dysreflexia in spinal cord injury.**
Ans: Please read Chapter no. 3.

27. **Discuss the sexual and bladder rehabilitation of a 30-year-old male following a complete spinal injury at D12 vertebral level.**

Ans: *For sexual rehabilitation, kindly see Answer to Question 29 below.*
Bladder rehabilitation is of utmost importance from day 1 of spinal cord injury (SCI). Usually, till the spinal shock subsides indwelling catheter is used but depending on expected prognosis, rehabilitation can be begun early. The following are recommended methods/medications for bladder rehabilitation:

- *Intermittent catheterization [clean intermittent catheterization (CIC) is commonly practiced and preferred]*: This provides complete bladder emptying and an easy practical method of management of atonic bladder. It can also be used in spinal shock and does not depend on intact sacral micturition reflex. Intermittent catheterization is a method by which the patient with SCI or a caregiver, empty the bladder at a specified time interval by inserting a clean catheter into the bladder and removing it.
    - Patient should be willing and trainable especially with regard to technique and maintaining asepsis.
    - *Avoid CIC in*:
        - Inability to catheterize themselves.
        - A caregiver who is unwilling to perform catheterization.
        - Abnormal urethral anatomy, such as stricture, false passages, and bladder neck obstruction.
        - Bladder capacity less than 200 mL.
        - Poor cognition, little motivation, or inability or unwillingness to adhere to the catheterization time schedule.
        - High fluid intake regimen.
        - Adverse reaction to passing a catheter into the genital area multiple times a day.
        - Tendency to develop autonomic dysreflexia with bladder filling despite treatment.
- *Credé and Valsalva*: These methods are usually suitable for patients with LMN injuries producing low outlet resistance or those having a sphincterotomy but should not be used as primary method in patients. Credé is a method of applying suprapubic pressure to express urine from the bladder. Credé is usually used when the bladder is flaccid or a bladder contraction needs to be augmented. So sphincter function is the main determining factor for use of Crede. Valsalva is a method in which an individual uses the abdominal muscles and the diaphragm to empty the bladder. Valsalva is used when the bladder is flaccid from SCI affecting the sacral reflex arc or when the bladder contracts but does not empty completely. Both the measures do not ensure complete bladder emptying. These methods are relatively contraindicated in:
    - Detrusor sphincter dyssynergia
    - Bladder outlet obstruction
    - Vesicoureteral reflux
    - Hydronephrosis
- *Indwelling catheterization*: Here a catheter is kept inserted in the urinary tract providing a continuous conduit (unless obstructed) to urinary drainage. Though considered an "easy" method, it is associated with many complications in short and long run. It may be useful in polytrauma patients initially for input/output monitoring but for rehabilitation CIC (see above) is preferred. Indwelling catheterization is considered for rehabilitation in patents with:
    - Poor hand skills
    - High fluid intake
    - Cognitive impairment or active substance abuse
    - Elevated detrusor pressures managed with anticholinergic medications or other means
    - Lack of success with other, less invasive bladder management methods
    - Need for temporary management of vesicoureteral reflux
    - Limited assistance from a caregiver, making another type of bladder management not feasible
    - *Avoid indwelling catheters in patients with*:
        - Immediately following acute SCI if urethral injury is suspected, especially after pelvic trauma (blood at the urethral meatus and perineal and scrotal hematomas may be indicative of urethral trauma).
        - If bladder capacity is small, with forceful uninhibited contractions despite treatment.

Consider using suprapubic catheterization for individuals with:
- Urethral abnormalities, such as stricture, false passages, bladder neck obstruction, or urethral fistula.
- Urethral discomfort.
- Recurrent urethral catheter obstruction.
- Difficulty with urethral catheter insertion.
- Perineal skin breakdown due to urine leakage secondary to urethral incompetence.
- Psychological considerations, such as body image or personal preference.
- A desire to improve sexual genital function.
- Prostatitis, urethritis, or epididymo-orchitis.

- *Reflex voiding*: It depends on an intact sacral micturition reflex. With bladder filling, the sacral efferents responsible for voiding get activated and urine starts dribbling but because of loss of central coordination, complete voiding does not happen and elevated pressures result causing complications to upper tract. The detrusor sphincter dyssynergia usually needs additional measures like suprapubic bladder tapping, alpha-blockers, botulinum toxin injection, urethral stents, or sphincterotomy for effective bladder emptying and preventing complications. Consider reflex voiding in patients with adequate bladder contractions and:
  - Sufficient hand skills to put on a condom catheter and empty the leg bag or have a willing caregiver.
  - Poor compliance with fluid restriction.
  - Small bladder capacity.
  - Small postvoid residual volumes.
  - Ability to maintain a condom catheter in place.

  Avoid reflex voiding in:
  - Have insufficient hand skills or caregiver assistance.
  - Are unable to maintain a condom catheter in place.
  - Are female.
  - Have incomplete bladder emptying despite treatment to facilitate voiding.
  - Have high-pressure voiding despite treatment to facilitate voiding.
  - Develop autonomic dysreflexia despite treatment to facilitate voiding.

- *Medications*:
  - *Alpha-blockers*: Alpha adrenergic blockers have been found to lower urethral resistance and improve voiding as α-receptors are found in proximal urethra, prostate, and bladder neck.
  - *Botulinum toxin injection*: Transurethral or transperineal injection of botulinum toxin into the urinary sphincter mechanism controls detrusor sphincter dyssynergia. Botulinum can also be used to treat the neurogenic overactive bladder, by injecting it directly into the bladder wall proper.

- *Mechanical methods*: Urethral stents help improve detrusor-external sphincter dyssynergia by preventing sphincter closure while detrusor is contracting aiding bladder emptying. This method however needs a continuous collecting device such as an external condom catheter. This can be considered in patients that:
  - Have insufficient hand skills or caregiver assistance to perform intermittent catheterization.
  - Have a repeated history of autonomic dysreflexia.
  - Experience difficult catheterization due to false passages in the urethra or secondary bladder neck obstruction.
  - Have inadequate bladder drainage with severe bladder wall changes, drop in renal function, vesicoureteral reflux, and/or stone disease.
  - Have prostate-ejaculatory reflux with the potential for repeated epididymo-orchitis.
  - Experience failure with or intolerance to anticholinergic medications for intermittent catheterization.
  - Experience failure with or intolerance to alpha-blockers with reflex voiding.

- *Transurethral sphincterotomy*: The principles are similar to urethral stenting.
- *Electrical stimulation and posterior sacral rhizotomy*: Stimulating the sacral parasympathetic nerves (S2–S4) causes detrusor (bladder) contraction. These also however produce sphincter (smooth muscles) contraction. This difficulty can be circumvented by intermittent pattern of stimulation taking advantage of the different rates of smooth and striated muscle contractions. Thus, an effective void is obtained. The electrodes are surgically implanted on the sacral

nerve (roots preferred) and connected to a subcutaneous stimulator device placed in abdomen. The stimulator can be radio-controlled by the user when voiding is desired.

Sacral rhizotomy is an option to abolish the detrusor hyper-reflexia. It is usually combined with electrical stimulation implant to reduce reflex incontinence, increase bladder capacity and compliance, protect the upper tracts, and reduce autonomic dysreflexia. One must understand that this procedure will lead to loss of erection, reflex ejaculation and loss of sacral sensation. This procedure also reduces reflex defecation.

- *Bladder augmentation*: This technique is basically aimed to reduce intravesical pressure by increasing the bladder capacity. It restores urinary continence and preserves upper urinary tracts by alleviating reflux and hydronephrosis.
- *Urinary diversion*: This is sort of an end measure deployed when other methods have all failed. The ureters are transected just above the bladder and connected to a segment of intestine (usually terminal ilium), which is in turn brought to the skin of the lower abdominal wall. It may also be used as an alternative to augmentation cystoplasty.
- Cutaneous ileovesicostomy.

28. Bladder rehab in paraplegics.

Ans: Goals of Rehabilitation
- *Prevent complications*: Urinary tract infections (UTIs), renal damage, bladder stones
- *Achieve continence*: Social dignity and quality of life
- *Preserve renal function*: Avoid high-pressure bladder damage
- *Optimize independence*: Self-catheterization when possible

Types of neurogenic bladder dysfunction in paraplegia are given in **Table 4C.3.1**.

TABLE 4C.3.1: Types of bladder dysfunction in paraplegia.

Type	Cause	Characteristics
Areflexic bladder	Lower motor neuron (LMN) injury	Flaccid, overdistention, overflow incontinence
Spastic bladder	Upper motor neuron (UMN) injury	Hyperreflexic, detrusor-sphincter dyssynergia (DSD)
Mixed dysfunction	Incomplete spinal cord injury	Combination of storage/emptying issues

Bladder Management Strategies:
- *Initial postinjury phase (spinal shock)*:
  – Indwelling Foley catheter (2–6 weeks)
  – Transition to intermittent catheterization (IC) once reflex activity returns
- *Long-term management options*:
  – *Intermittent catheterization (gold standard)*:
    - Every 4–6 hours (adjust based on bladder capacity)
    - Sterile technique → clean technique for home management
    - *Advantages*: Low infection risk, preserves bladder anatomy
  – *Indwelling catheters*:
    - Suprapubic (preferred over urethral for long-term use)
    - *Urethral Foley*: Higher UTI/stricture risk
  – *Reflex voiding (condom catheter)*:
    - For upper motor neuron (UMN) injuries with detrusor hyperactivity
    - Requires α-blockers (tamsulosin) for sphincter relaxation
    - Risk of high-pressure bladder → hydronephrosis
  – *Pharmacological management*:
    - *Anticholinergics (oxybutynin, solifenacin)*: Reduce detrusor overactivity
    - *Botulinum toxin (intradetrusor injections)*: For refractory spasticity
    - *Alpha-blockers*: Improve bladder outlet resistance (for DSD)
  – *Surgical options*:
    - *Augmentation cystoplasty (ileal/colonic segment)*: For low-capacity bladder
    - Sphincterotomy (for severe DSD)
    - *Urinary diversion (ileal conduit)*: Last-resort option

- *Monitoring and complications prevention*:
  - *Annual urodynamics*: Assess bladder pressure, capacity, and DSD
  - *Renal ultrasound*: Screen for hydronephrosis
  - *Urine cultures*: Only if symptomatic (fever, odor, sediment)
  - *Bladder stones prevention*: Adequate hydration, citrates
- *Lifestyle and education*:
  - *Fluid management*: 1.5–2 L/day, spaced intake
  - *Timed voiding*: Scheduled catheterization
  - *Skin care*: Prevent pressure ulcers from incontinence
  - *Autonomic dysreflexia awareness*: Emergency protocol for bladder overdistention

29. Discuss principles of sexual rehabilitation of a paraplegic patient.

Ans: Sexual and reproductive health is an important component for maintaining quality of life in longer term rehabilitation in patients of SCI and improving patient satisfaction. Approximately 10–20% of erectile dysfunction (ED) is of neurological origin where nearly 50% of neurogenic ED cases result from SCI. The neurogenic ED is classified into three groups, as supraspinal, spinal (sacral and suprasacral), and peripheral.

There are four components associated with erection:
1. *Neurological*: It is controlled by central nervous system (CNS) and spinal cord from T10 and above for transmission of the stimulatory and control pathways. Stroke, Alzheimer's disease, and SCI up to T10 level are responsible for ED resulting from neurological-central involvement.
2. *The sympathetic center (T11–L2 segments)*: It is responsible for psychogenic erection controlled by CNS. Trauma, deformity, spinal cord lesions/surgery, and degenerative disease processes may lead to damage this region.
3. *The parasympathetic center (spinal cord segments S2–S4)*: It is responsible for reflexogenic erection. Trauma, deformity, spinal cord lesions/surgery, and degenerative disease processes may lead to damage this region.
4. Peripheral pelvic splanchnic plexus pudendal nerves and organ itself. Pelvic injury, pelvic surgery, diabetic neuropathy, and multiple sclerosis are responsible for ED here.

Erectile dysfunction following SCI may be classified in three sections, due to the level of the spinal centers playing role in sexual function.
- *T10 and above*: Local stimulation of the genital organs may still cause erection due to intact reflex pathway (especially in incomplete UMN lesions). However, erection will not occur in response to psychogenic stimulus.
- *From T11–L2*: Erection can be expected from genital stimulation as well as with psychogenic stimulation.
- *Conus-cauda (parasympathetic)*: Usually, any type of erection does not occur.
  - *Conus terminalis*: Injury here usually preserves the psychogenic pathway more than the cauda equine type.
  - *The cauda equine*: Dismal injury.

Psychogenic erection is possible according to the site of neurological damage (lateral or medial) both incomplete upper and incomplete lower motor neuron lesion.

Evaluation: Evaluate the physiological (spinal cord damage/injury, stroke, Alzheimer's disease, pelvic injury, pelvic surgery, diabetic neuropathy and multiple sclerosis vs. psychological causes) (social, existential, and emotional factors) of sexual dysfunction.

Treatment/management: The following are some of the used modalities (often in combination) to treat ED in men:
- *PDE-5 inhibitors*: Daily use of tadalafil induces regular erections and increases penile blood flow that may prevent fibrosis development.
- *Topical pharmacotherapy*: Some of vasoactive drugs (2% nitroglycerine, 15–20% papaverine gel and 2% minoxidil solution or gel) are used for topical application to the penis.
- *Intracavernous injection agent—Alprostadil*: It can also be used intraurethrally as sacral stimulator.
- *Mechanical devices*:
  - *Vacuum constriction devices*: They provide passive pooling to the blood in the corpora cavernosa.
  - *Penile implants*: The patients who do not respond to pharmacotherapy or want a permanent solving to be considered by the penile prosthesis implantation.

4C.4 ASIA SCORING AND RELATED QUESTIONS ON SPINAL CORD INJURY (Q30–32)

30. Describe ASIA score.

Ans: According to American Spinal Injury Association (ASIA) definitions, the neurologic injury level is the most caudal segment of the spinal cord with normal motor and sensory function on both sides: Right and left sensation and right and left motor function. For functional scoring **(Fig. 4C.4.1)**, 10 key muscle segments corresponding to innervation by C5, C6, C7, C8, T1, L2, L3, L4, L5, and S1 are each given a functional score of 0–5 out of 5. For sensory scoring, both right and left sides are graded for a total of 100 points. For the 28 sensory dermatomes on each side of the body, sensory levels are scored on a zero- to two-point scale, yielding a maximum possible pinprick score of 112 points for a patient with normal sensation.

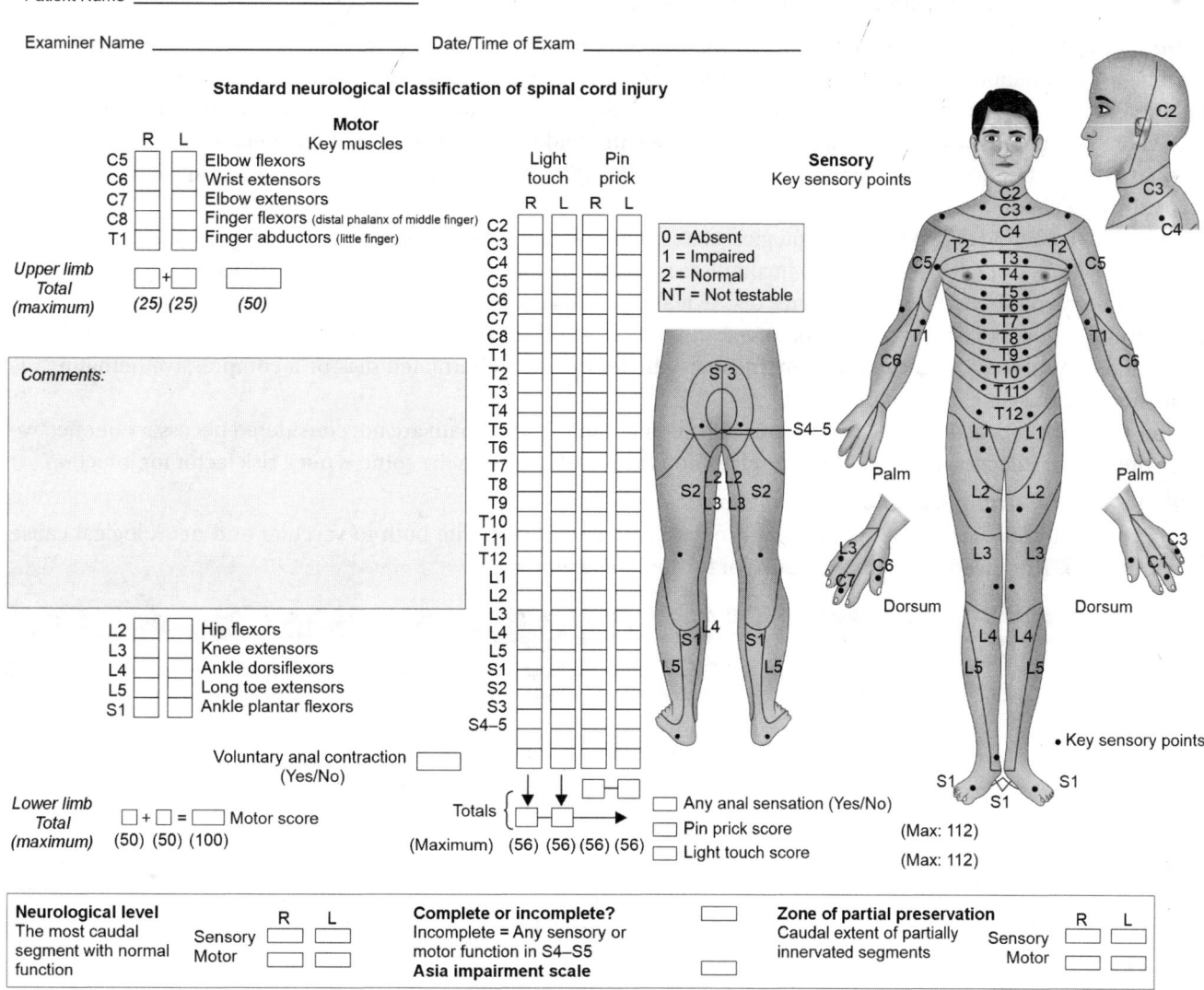

Fig. 4C.4.1: ASIA scoring for spinal cord injury.

31. What are the various protocols which have been used for pharmacological intervention in spinal cord injuries? What is the current opinion on pharmacological intervention?

Ans: Please read Chapter no. 3.

32. Discuss the role of injectable methyl prednisolone in post-traumatic spinal injuries.

Ans: Please read Chapter no. 3.

4C.5 CLAUDICATION AND SPINAL CANAL STENOSIS (Q33–39)

33. Enumerate various spinal cord syndromes. Describe salient features of each syndrome with mechanism of each.

Ans: Please read Chapter no. 3.

34. What is ballistics? Briefly describe current management of ballistic injuries of the spine.

Ans: Wound ballistics is the science that studies the effects of penetrating projectiles on the body (most of it involved concepts of physics as studied in laboratory simulated environment). It studies the reaction of body to projectiles, the interaction of wounding agents (such as bullets and fragments from explosive weapons) with tissue.

Ballistic trauma is the term used to describe the pathophysiological reaction of the body to the physical process and includes blood loss, shock, wound infection and death.

Management: Follow the ATLS (Advanced Trauma Life Support) guidelines and immobilize the patient. A complete neurologic examination must be performed and repeat it regularly to document deterioration. Give tetanus prophylaxis and broad-spectrum antibiotics (extended for 10–14 days). Steroids have no documented role and should be avoided.

- Obtain radiographs with radiopaque markers at the entry and exit wounds. Also obtain detailed CT scan and MRI scan to assess bullet fragments and associated soft tissue injury. MRI has been reported a safe study despite metallic nature of bullet.
- Decision to operate depends on neurological status, spinal stability, level of injury and location of bullet.
- Progressive neurological deficit, or an incomplete injury in an unstable spine is a definite indication of surgery.
- Lower thoracolumbar injury or presence of CSF leak is also taken for surgery urgently.
- Complete injury to cervical or cervicothoracic injury may be observed in a stable spine.
- Emergency surgery is indicated if bone fragment, bullet fragment, herniated disk or a compressive hematoma is identified as causing neurological deficit.
- The surgical removal of the bullet and bone debridement in the spine path are not considered necessary or effective in preventing infectious complications, and leaving the bullet lodged in the spine is not a risk factor for infection.

35. Describe neurological and vascular claudication.

Ans: Claudication is development of leg pains on walking and is seen due both to vascular and neurological cause **(Table 4C.5.1)**. They need to be differentiated for further management.

TABLE 4C.5.1: Difference between vascular and neurological claudication.

Parameter	Vascular	Neurogenic
Walking distance	Constant (the patient cannot walk beyond a fixed distance)	Variable (distance varies with respect to uphill (spine bent) or downhill climb)
Palliative factors	Standing for few minutes	Sitting/bending, just standing does not relieve pain as nerve remains stretched
Walking uphill	Painful as work of muscles increases	Symptoms come after delay as the nerve is a bit relaxed with spine flexed forward and knee bent
Bicycle test	Positive (painful)	Negative
Pulses	Absent/reduced	Present
Skin	Loss of hair; shiny	Normal
Muscle weakness	Rarely	Not usually at rest but after long walk, the nerve stretch tests are positive and muscles power may be felt weak
Low back pain	Occasionally	Commonly
Spine movements	Normal	Limited
Pain character	Cramping—distal to proximal	Numbness, aching—proximal to distal

Vascular symptoms typically felt in the upper calf are relieved after a short rest (5 minutes) while still standing, do not require sitting or bending, and worsen despite walking uphill or riding a stationary bicycle. Neurogenic claudication improves with trunk flexion, stooping, or lying, but may require 20 minutes to improve. Patients often report better endurance walking uphill or up steps and tolerate riding a bicycle better than walking on a treadmill because of the flexed posture that occurs. Pushing a grocery cart also allows spinal flexion, which enhances endurance in most patients with neurogenic claudication.

36. Describe spinal canal stenosis. What is differentiating feature between vascular and neurogenic claudication with management?

Ans: Spinal stenosis can be categorized according to the anatomical area of the spine affected, the region of each vertebral segment affected, and the specific pathological entity involved. Stenosis can be generalized or localized to specific anatomical areas of the cervical, thoracic, or lumbar spine **(Table 4C.5.2)**. It is most common in the lumbar region, but cervical stenosis also occurs frequently. It has been reported rarely in the thoracic spine. Spinal stenosis can be localized or diffused, affecting multiple levels as in congenital stenosis. Degeneration of the disk occurs with disk narrowing and subsequent ligamentous redundancy, which compromises the spinal canal area. Instability may ensue. This relative hypermobility precipitates the formation of facet overgrowth and ligamentous hypertrophy. The ligamentum flavum may be markedly thickened into the lateral recess where it attaches to the facet capsule causing nerve root compression. These phenomena occur alone or in combination to create the symptom complex characteristic of spinal stenosis.

TABLE 4C.5.2: Anatomical classification of spinal canal stenosis.

Anatomical area	Anatomical region
Cervical	Central
	Foraminal
Thoracic	Central
Lumbar	Central
	Lateral recess
	Foraminal
	Extraforaminal (far-out)

Pathological classification
- *Congenital*:
  - Achondroplastic (dwarfism)
  - Congenital forms of spondylolisthesis
  - Scoliosis
  - Kyphosis.
- Idiopathic
- Degenerative and inflammatory
  - Osteoarthritis
  - Inflammatory arthritis
  - Diffuse idiopathic skeletal hyperostosis
  - Scoliosis
  - Kyphosis
  - Degenerative forms of spondylolisthesis.
- Metabolic
  - Paget disease
  - Fluorosis

Central spinal stenosis denotes involvement of the area between the facet joints, which is occupied by the dura and its contents. Stenosis in this region usually is caused by protrusion of a disk, bulging annulus, osteophyte formation, or buckled or thickened ligamentum flavum. Symptomatic central spinal stenosis results in neurogenic claudication. Lateral to the dura is the lateral canal, which contains the nerve roots; compression in this region results in radiculopathy. The *lateral recess,* also known as "Lee's entrance zone", begins at the lateral border of the dura and extends to the medial border of the pedicle. This is where the nerve root exits the dura and courses distally and laterally under the superior articular facet. The borders of the lateral recess are the pedicle laterally, the superior articular facet dorsally, the disk and posterior ligamentous complex ventrally, and the central canal medially.

"Lee's midzone" describes the *foraminal region,* which lies ventral to the pars. Its borders are the lateral recess medially, the posterior vertebral body and disk ventrally, the pars dorsally, and the lateral border of the pedicle laterally. The dorsal root ganglion and ventral motor root occupy 30% of this space. This also is the point where the dura becomes confluent with the nerve root as epineurium. Causes of stenosis in this area are pars fracture with proliferative fibrocartilage or a lateral disk herniation.

The *exit zone* is identified as the area lateral to the facet joint. The nerve root is present in this location and can be compressed by a "far-lateral" disk, spondylolisthesis and associated subluxation, or facet arthritis.

The *radiographic identification* and confirmation of lumbar spinal stenosis have improved with the development of new imaging techniques. Currently, axial imaging has supplanted standard radiographs in the diagnosis of spinal stenosis. MRI is helpful in identifying other disease processes, such as tumors and infections, and is a good noninvasive study for patients with persistent lower extremity complaints after radiographic screening evaluation. MRI should be confirmatory in patients with a consistent history of neurogenic claudication or radiculopathy, but it should not be used as a screening examination because of the high rate of asymptomatic disease.

Despite the prevalence of MRI, myelography followed by CT scanning is still accepted and widely used for operative planning in patients with spinal stenosis. Because of the dynamic nature of the study, stenosis not visible on MRI with the patient recumbent may be identified on standing flexion and extension lateral views. CT scanning after myelography characterizes the bony anatomy better than MRI, which helps the surgeon plan decompression surgery.

Treatment: Symptoms of spinal stenosis usually respond favorably to nonoperative management. Despite symptoms of back pain, radiculopathy, or neurogenic claudication, conservative management is successful in most patients. Conservative measures should include rest not exceeding 2 days, pain management with anti-inflammatory medications or acetaminophen, and participation in a trunk-stabilization exercise program, along with good aerobic fitness. For a patient with unremitting symptoms of radiculopathy or neurogenic claudication, epidural steroid injections may be useful in alleviating symptoms to allow better participation in physical therapy. Epidural steroids can give significant symptomatic relief.

A patient's inability to tolerate the restricted lifestyle necessitated by the disease and the failure of a good conservative treatment regimen should be the primary determining factors for surgery in a well-informed patient. The patient should understand the potential for the operation to fail to relieve pain or to worsen it, especially with regard to the axial component of the symptoms. In addition to the general risks of spinal surgery, the severity of symptoms and lifestyle modifications should be considered.

Decompression by laminectomy or a fenestration procedure is the treatment of choice for lumbar spinal stenosis. Fusion is required if excessive bony resection compromises stability or if isthmic or degenerative spondylolisthesis, scoliosis, or kyphosis is present.

Vascular and neurogenic claudication have been differentiated in Answer to Question 35.

37. Etiology, clinical features, investigations and diagnosis of lumbar canal stenosis.

Ans: *Etiology*:
- *Congenital/Developmental*:
  - Degenerative-age related
  - Achondroplasia
  - Congenital small spinal canal
  - Congenital meningeal cysts
  - Osteoporosis
- *Acquired*:
  - Degenerative-age related
  - Degenerative spondylolytic/spondylolisthesis
  - Degenerative scoliosis
  - Ankylosing spondylitis

- Rheumatoid arthritis
- Pseudogout
- Acromegaly
- Diffuse idiopathic skeletal hyperostosis (DISH)
- Iatrogenic—Postdiscectomy/laminectomy/fusion, scarring/fibrosis postchemonucleolysis
- Malunited vertebral fractures
- Spinal infections with abscess bone collapse
- Paget's disease
- Fluorosis
- Pseudogout
• Combined

Clinical features: Patients are usually older than 50 years of age. Low back pain and stiffness are commonly reported as a baseline pain along with neurogenic claudication—refers to buttock and leg pain that worsens with lumbar extension and ambulation and is relieved by lumbar flexion and/or rest. The neurogenic claudication must be differentiated from vascular claudication and degenerative disk disease. Over the years, the patients develop lower extremity weakness, persistent radiculopathy and symptoms compounded by concomitant cervical stenosis causing cervical myelopathy. The prevalence of combined cervical and lumbar, or tandem spinal stenosis (TSS) is reportedly 5–25%.

Physical Examination:
- Reduced lumbar extension
- Muscle atrophy
- Difficulty in toe/heel walking
- Absent long tract signs
- Sensations and motor examination are usually normal except in advanced cases
- Patients walk with lumbar flexion and avoid lying flat or standing straight. The manifestations of central and lateral canal stenosis are not easily distinguished.
- Unilateral radicular pain from foraminal stenosis is worsened by extension to the painful side (Kemp sign)
- Presence of paresthesia indicates dorsal root compression in foramen.

Diagnostic imaging:
Plain radiographs: Upright anteroposterior, lateral and flexion/extension radiographs.
- Delineate the amount of lumbar degeneration:
  - Disk space narrowing and degenerative disk disease
  - Endplate osteophytes and sclerosis
  - Facet enlargement and osteophyte formation
  - Narrowed neuroforaminal canal
  - Loss of lumbar lordosis
- Evaluate for congenital stenosis
- Evaluate associated scoliosis and spondylolisthesis; and rule out trauma, infection, or malignancy as a potential source of symptoms.

Magnetic resonance imaging is currently the recommended advanced imaging modality to evaluate LSS. MRI is as accurate as computed tomography myelography and is noninvasive. Contrast is needed only in postoperative cases. Obtain both axial and sagittal—coronal cuts. Evaluate the following on MRI scan:
- Spinal and lateral recess stenosis
- Disk bulge and herniations
- Facet changes (degeneration, osteophyte, hypertrophy, cyst formation)
- Evidence of obliteration of perineural fat on images is an early indicator of foraminal stenosis
- Ligamentum flavum hypertrophy
- Tumors, lysis, infection, etc.

Electrodiagnostic testing using electromyography has high specificity for diagnosing LSS (and in differentiating LSS from other neuromuscular disorders including peripheral or diabetic neuropathy, myopathy, and inflammatory neuropathies). In combination with MRI, it reduces the high false-positive rate associated with the former.

38. Discuss the various types of lumbar canal stenosis based on magnetic resonance imaging (MRI).

Ans: Lumbar canal stenosis (LCS) is a condition characterized by the narrowing of the spinal canal in the lumbar region, which can compress the spinal cord or nerve roots, leading to symptoms like pain, numbness, or weakness in the lower back and legs. Magnetic resonance imaging (MRI) is the gold standard for diagnosing and classifying lumbar canal stenosis due to its ability to visualize soft tissues, neural structures, and bony anatomy in detail. Based on MRI findings, LCS can be classified by:

- Anatomical location
- Etiology
- Severity

Classification by anatomical location: MRI allows precise visualization of the spinal canal and surrounding structures, enabling classification based on the specific region of narrowing within the lumbar spine. The main anatomical types of LCS are:

- *Central canal stenosis*: Narrowing of the central spinal canal, which houses the thecal sac and spinal cord (or cauda equina in the lumbar region).
  - *MRI findings*:
    - Reduced anteroposterior (AP) diameter of the spinal canal (typically < 10 mm is considered stenotic).
    - Compression of the thecal sac, with loss of cerebrospinal fluid (CSF) signal surrounding the cauda equina on T2-weighted images.
    - "Hourglass" or "trefoil" appearance of the canal on axial images due to compression.
    - Potential obliteration of epidural fat around the thecal sac.
  - *Causes*:
    - Degenerative changes (e.g., disc bulging, facet joint hypertrophy, ligamentum flavum thickening).
    - Congenital narrowing (e.g., short pedicles or achondroplasia).
    - Spondylolisthesis or other structural deformities.
  - *Clinical implications*: Central canal stenosis often leads to neurogenic claudication, characterized by leg pain, numbness, or weakness exacerbated by walking or standing and relieved by sitting or flexing the spine.
- *Lateral recess stenosis*: Narrowing of the lateral recess (subarticular zone), the area where nerve roots exit the thecal sac before entering the neural foramen.
  - *MRI findings*:
    - Compression of the nerve root in the lateral recess, often seen on axial T2-weighted images.
    - Hypertrophy of facet joints or ligamentum flavum encroaching into the lateral recess.
    - Reduced space around the nerve root, with loss of surrounding CSF signal.
  - *Causes*:
    - Facet joint arthropathy
    - Disc protrusion or extrusion into the lateral recess
    - Synovial cysts or osteophytes
  - *Clinical implications*: Lateral recess stenosis typically causes radicular pain or symptoms specific to the compressed nerve root (e.g., L5 or S1 radiculopathy).
- *Foraminal (neural foraminal) stenosis*: Narrowing of the neural foramen, the bony canal through which nerve roots exit the spinal canal.
  - *MRI findings*:
    - Obliteration of perineural fat surrounding the exiting nerve root on sagittal or axial T1- and T2-weighted images.
    - Nerve root compression or displacement within the foramen.
    - Foraminal height reduction or osteophyte formation.

- *Causes*:
    - Disc herniation extending into the foramen.
    - Facet joint hypertrophy or osteophytes.
    - Spondylolisthesis or lateral disc bulge.
- *Clinical implications*: Foraminal stenosis often results in radicular symptoms, such as pain, numbness, or weakness radiating along the distribution of the affected nerve root.
- *Extraforaminal (far-lateral) stenosis*: Compression of the nerve root outside the neural foramen, in the extraforaminal zone.
    - *MRI findings*:
        - Compression of the nerve root beyond the foramen, often seen on coronal or sagittal MRI.
        - Loss of perineural fat and nerve root displacement.
        - Disc protrusion or osteophytes extending laterally.
    - *Causes*:
        - Far-lateral disc herniation
        - Osteophytes from the vertebral body or facet joint.
        - Spondylolisthesis or scoliosis.
    - *Clinical implications*: Like foraminal stenosis, but symptoms may be less common or harder to localize due to the extraforaminal location.
    - *Classification by etiology*: The underlying cause of lumbar canal stenosis can also be classified based on MRI findings, which reveal the pathological processes contributing to the narrowing.
- *Congenital/developmental stenosis*: Narrowing of the spinal canal present at birth or due to developmental anomalies.
    - *MRI findings*:
        - Short pedicles or a congenitally narrow canal (AP diameter < 10 mm).
        - Trefoil-shaped canal due to thickened laminae or short pedicles.
        - Associated anomalies like achondroplasia or hypochondroplasia.
    - *Clinical implications*: Symptoms may manifest earlier in life, especially when combined with degenerative changes later.
- *Degenerative stenosis*: The most common type, caused by age-related degenerative changes in the spine.
    - *MRI findings*:
        - Disc bulging or herniation reducing canal or foraminal space.
        - Facet joint hypertrophy or synovial cysts compressing the canal or nerve roots.
        - Thickening or buckling of the ligamentum flavum, often seen on T2-weighted axial images.
        - Osteophyte formation from vertebral endplates or facet joints.
        - Spondylolisthesis (anterior or posterior displacement of vertebrae).
    - *Clinical implications*: Symptoms typically develop in older adults and are progressive, often presenting as neurogenic claudication or radiculopathy.
- *Iatrogenic stenosis*: Stenosis caused by surgical interventions or medical procedures.
    - *MRI findings*:
        - Scar tissue or epidural fibrosis postsurgery, seen as abnormal soft tissue on T1- and T2-weighted images.
        - Hardware (e.g., screws, rods) or bone grafts encroaching on the canal or foramen.
        - Altered anatomy due to laminectomy or fusion procedures.
    - *Clinical Implications*: Symptoms may mimic those of degenerative stenosis but are often related to prior surgical history.
- *Traumatic stenosis*: Stenosis resulting from spinal trauma or fractures.
    - *MRI findings*:
        - Fractures of vertebral bodies, pedicles, or laminae causing canal narrowing.
        - Hematoma or soft tissue swelling compressing the canal or nerve roots.
        - Displaced bone fragments or traumatic disc herniation.
    - *Clinical implications*: Acute onset of symptoms, often with associated neurological deficits.

- *Pathological stenosis*: Stenosis caused by tumors, infections, or metabolic conditions.
  - *MRI findings*:
    - Tumors (e.g., metastasis, meningioma, or schwannoma) causing mass effect on the canal or nerve roots.
    - Epidural abscess or granulation tissue in infections, often with abnormal enhancement on postcontrast T1-weighted images.
    - Paget's disease or other metabolic bone disorders causing bony overgrowth.
  - *Clinical implications*: Symptoms may be accompanied by systemic signs (e.g., fever in infections or weight loss in malignancy).
  - *Classification by severity*: MRI can also help grade the severity of lumbar canal stenosis, which is critical for treatment planning. A commonly used grading system based on MRI findings is the "Lee et al. classification" for central canal stenosis, which assesses the degree of thecal sac compression on axial T2-weighted images:
    - *Grade 0 (no stenosis)*: No narrowing of the central canal; normal CSF signal surrounds the cauda equina.
    - *Grade 1 (mild stenosis)*: Mild narrowing with partial obliteration of CSF signal but no significant thecal sac compression.
    - *Grade 2 (moderate stenosis)*: Moderate narrowing with significant reduction in CSF signal and some compression of the thecal sac, but nerve roots remain distinguishable.
    - *Grade 3 (severe stenosis)*: Severe narrowing with complete obliteration of CSF signal and marked compression of the thecal sac, where nerve roots are indistinguishable (crowding or clumping).

For foraminal stenosis, severity is often described qualitatively (mild, moderate, and severe) based on the degree of nerve root compression and loss of perineural fat.

39. How will you clinically differentiate central from lateral lumbar canal stenosis? Briefly discuss the management.

Ans: *Clinical difference*: In patients with central spinal stenosis, symptoms usually are bilateral and involve the buttocks and posterior thighs in a nondermatomal distribution. With lateral recess stenosis, symptoms usually are dermatomal because they are related to a specific nerve being compressed. Patients with lateral recess stenosis may have more pain during rest and at night, but more walking tolerance than patients with central stenosis.

Kindly see Answer to Question 36 for further details.

4C.6 SPONDYLOLISTHESIS (Q40–41)

40. A. Define spondylolisthesis.
   B. Its classification in adults.
   C. Its clinical features and radiological signs.
   D. Outline its management.

Ans:

A. "Spondylolisthesis" means forward translation of one segment of the spine upon another.

B. *Classification*: Modified Wiltse, Newman and McNab classification of spondylolisthesis:
   - *Dysplastic (20%)*: The superior sacral facets are congenitally defective; slow but inexorable forward slip leads to severe displacement. Associated anomalies (usually spina bifida occulta) are common.
   - *Lytic or isthmic (50%)*: In this, the most common variety, there are defects in the pars interarticularis (spondylolysis), or repeated breaking and healing may lead to elongation of the pars. The defect (which occurs in about 5% of people) is usually present by the age of 7, but the slip may appear only some years later. It is difficult to exclude a genetic factor because spondylolisthesis often runs in families, and is more common in certain races, notably Eskimos; but the incidence increases with age up to the late teenage years, although clinical presentation with pain can continue into late middle age. An acquired factor probably supervenes to produce what is essentially an ununited stress fracture. The condition is more common than usual in those whose spines are subjected to extraordinary stresses (e.g. competitive gymnasts and weight-lifters).

- *Degenerative (25%)*: Degenerative changes in the facet joints and the disks permit forward slip (nearly always at L4/5 and mainly in women of middle age) despite intact laminae. Many of these patients have generalized osteoarthritis and pyrophosphate crystal arthropathy.
- *Post-traumatic*: Unusual fractures may result in destabilization of the lumbar spine.
- *Pathological*: Bone destruction (e.g. due to TB or neoplasm) may lead to vertebral slipping.
- *Postoperative (iatrogenic)*: Occasionally, excessive operative removal of bone in decompression operations results in progressive spondylolisthesis.

C. *Clinical features*: There is a dull aching pain in the back, buttocks, or thighs beginning during the adolescent growth spurt and exacerbated by activity. There is no relation of pain to the degree of slip or development of lysis. So most patients with spondylolysis or even low-grade slips are asymptomatic. This makes it imperative to search for other causes of the pain (infection, neoplasm, fracture, or disk herniation) before attributing symptoms to the spondylolisthesis. Of symptomatic children, 92% complain of recurrence during adulthood; 55% complain of sciatica at the affected nerve root or roots. True radicular symptoms are rare but if present, are often restricted to L5 root distribution (irritation, compression or tension due to L5–S1 listhesis). In *adults* backache is the usual presenting symptom; it is often intermittent, coming on after exercise or strain. Sciatica may occur in one or both legs. *Patients aged over 50 years* are usually women with degenerative spondylolisthesis. They always have backache, some have sciatica and some present because of claudication due to spinal stenosis.

On examination the buttocks look flat, the sacrum appears to extend to the waist and transverse loin creases are seen. The lumbar spine is on a plane in front of the sacrum and looks too short. Sometimes there is a scoliosis.

A "step" can often be felt when the fingers are run down the spine. Eighty percent have spasm and foreshortening of the paraspinal and hamstring muscles. Movements are usually normal in the younger patients but there may be "hamstring tightness"; in the degenerative group the spine is often stiff.

Radiological signs: Lateral views show the forward shift of the upper part of the spinal column on the stable vertebra below; elongation of the arch or defective facets may be seen. The gap in the pars interarticularis is best seen in the oblique views. Classically, the defect in the pars interarticularis is seen as a collar on the "Scottie dog's neck with collar" on oblique views. Measure the slip angle, lumbar index, sacral inclination, and lumbar lordosis. In doubtful cases, single-photon emission computed tomography (SPECT) or reversed gantry CT may be helpful, while MRI is the investigation of choice to diagnose spinal stenosis.

D. *Management*: Most patients are asymptomatic with an incidental finding of a pars interarticularis defect without a slip. They can be followed on an as-needed basis if symptoms develop. With a listhesis serial radiographs on a 3–6 months basis may be done to determine the stability of the slip until skeletal maturity. In the pediatric and adolescent population, spondylolisthesis is the predominant cause of low-back pain and sciatica. In them also conservative management is quite successful.

Nonoperative treatment

Activity modification: Restriction of high-risk athletics, avoiding repetitive extension maneuvers, physical therapy and graded strengthening exercises, selective nerve/pars injections, and brace therapy are the conservative management tools. Positive bone scan or SPECT scan in a young child or adolescent implies the potential for possible healing at the pars interarticularis defect with external immobilization lysis heals well so immobilization should be considered.

Operative treatment: The accepted criteria for surgical intervention include—
- Persistence of pain or neurological symptoms despite an adequate course of nonoperative treatment
- Progression of slippage greater than 30%
- Presentation with greater than Grade II subluxation
- Cosmetic deformity secondary to postural and gait difficulties.

Goals of surgery include reduction in pain, prevention of further slip, stabilization of the spine, restoration of normal posture and gait, reversal and prevention of neurological deficit, and improved cosmetic appearance.

In adults either posterior or anterior fusion is suitable. However, in the "degenerative" group, where neurological symptoms predominate, decompression without fusion may suffice.

41. **A. Describe the clinical and radiological features of spinopelvic sagittal balance.**
B. Discuss its clinical and management implications in lumbar spondylolisthesis.

Ans: Spinopelvic sagittal balance refers to the alignment of the spine and pelvis in the sagittal plane, which is critical for maintaining an energy-efficient posture, minimizing mechanical stress, and preventing spinal disorders.

Clinical Features of Spinopelvic Sagittal Balance

The clinical presentation of spinopelvic sagittal balance (or imbalance) is often related to compensatory mechanisms and symptoms arising from altered biomechanics. Key clinical features include:

- *Postural abnormalities*:
  - *Normal balance*: Patients with good sagittal balance typically maintain an upright posture with minimal effort, a neutral head position, and a vertical line of gravity passing through key anatomical landmarks (e.g., C7 plumb line near the sacral promontory).
  - *Imbalance*: Patients with sagittal imbalance may present with:
    - Forward head posture or stooping (common in positive sagittal imbalance, where the trunk leans forward).
    - Increased thoracic kyphosis (hunchback appearance) or loss of lumbar lordosis (flat back syndrome).
    - Pelvic retroversion (posterior tilt of the pelvis), leading to a compensatory flexed posture at the hips or knees to maintain balance.
- *Pain and discomfort*:
  - Low back pain
  - Neck pain
  - Fatigue
- *Functional limitations*:
  - Difficulty walking or standing for prolonged periods
  - Compensatory mechanisms
  - Knee flexion or hip extension to shift the center of gravity backward.
  - Retroversion of the pelvis, leading to a crouched or leaning posture.
- *Neurological symptoms (in severe cases)*: Radiculopathy (radiating leg pain), neurogenic claudication, or, rarely, myelopathy.

Radiological Features of Spinopelvic Sagittal Balance

Radiological assessment is critical for evaluating spinopelvic sagittal balance. Full-length standing lateral radiographs (spine and pelvis) are the gold standard for measuring key parameters. The main radiological features and parameters are:

- *Key Radiographic Parameters*:
  - *Sagittal vertical axis (SVA)*: The horizontal distance between a plumb line dropped from the C7 vertebral body and the posterior-superior corner of S1.
    - *Normal*: SVA < 5 cm (ideally close to 0 cm in balanced individuals).
  - *Pelvic incidence (PI)*: A fixed anatomical parameter, measured as the angle between a line perpendicular to the sacral endplate and a line from the sacral endplate midpoint to the center of the femoral heads.
    - *Normal range*: 40–60° (varies by individual, constant after skeletal maturity).
  - *Lumbar lordosis (LL)*: The angle between the superior endplate of L1 and the superior endplate of S1.
    - *Normal*: LL should be within 10° of PI (PI ≈ LL ± 10° for optimal balance).
  - *Pelvic tilt (PT)*: The angle between a vertical line and a line from the sacral endplate midpoint to the center of the femoral heads.
    - *Normal*: PT < 20°.
  - *Sacral slope (SS)*: The angle between the sacral endplate and the horizontal plane.
    - *Normal*: SS typically ranges from 30 to 50°, closely related to PI (PI = PT + SS).
  - *Thoracic kyphosis (TK)*: The angle between the superior endplate of T1 (or T4) and the inferior endplate of T12.
    - *Normal*: 20–40° (increases slightly with age).
- *Global alignment*:
  - *C7 plumb line*: A vertical line dropped from the center of the C7 vertebra should ideally pass through or near the posterior-superior corner of S1 in a balanced spine.

- *T1 pelvic angle (TPA)*: Definition: The angle between a line from the T1 centroid to the femoral head axis and a line from the femoral head axis to the sacral endplate midpoint.
  - *Normal*: TPA < 15°.

Spinopelvic Sagittal Balance in Lumbar Spondylolisthesis: Clinical and Management Implications
Clinical Implications
- *Pathogenesis and progression*:
  - Increased PI has been identified as a predisposing factor for the development and progression of degenerative spondylolisthesis (DS). A higher PI correlates with increased SS and PT, leading to compensatory mechanisms such as increased LL to maintain sagittal balance. Over time, these compensations may become insufficient, resulting in sagittal imbalance and progression of vertebral slippage.
- *Compensatory mechanisms*:
  - Patients with DS often develop compensatory strategies to maintain balance. These include increasing LL and retroverting the pelvis (increasing PT) to offset the anterior displacement of the vertebra. However, when these mechanisms fail, patients may experience increased pain and functional disability.
- *Impact on clinical outcomes*:
  - Restoration of sagittal balance is associated with improved clinical outcomes. Studies have shown that adequate correction of sagittal alignment parameters, such as LL and PT, leads to significant reductions in persistent low back pain (PLBP) and improvements in functional scores like the Oswestry disability index (ODI).

Management Implications
- *Preoperative assessment*:
  - Comprehensive evaluation of spinopelvic parameters is essential in the preoperative planning for patients with lumbar spondylolisthesis. Understanding individual sagittal alignment helps in predicting surgical outcomes and tailoring surgical interventions to restore optimal balance.
- *Surgical strategies*:
  - Surgical approaches aim to correct the vertebral slip and restore sagittal balance. Techniques such as posterior lumbar interbody fusion (PLIF) or transforaminal lumbar interbody fusion (TLIF) are commonly employed. These procedures focus on reducing the vertebral slip, correcting segmental lordosis, and restoring intervertebral disc height.
- *Postoperative management*:
  - Postoperative monitoring of sagittal alignment is crucial to ensure the maintenance of corrected balance. Failure to maintain sagittal balance postoperatively can lead to adjacent segment degeneration and persistent low back pain

4C.7 PROLAPSED INTERVERTEBRAL DISK, DISKECTOMY, AND ROOT ANOMALIES (Q42–47)

42. Discuss pathology, clinical features, diagnosis, and treatment of L4–L5 intervertebral disk prolapsed.

Ans: *Pathology*: A lot of factors take part in degeneration of the disk.

Loss of proteoglycan: This is the most significant biochemical change to occur in disk degeneration. The aggrecan molecules become smaller and get leached from the tissue more readily than larger portions. This reduces glycosaminoglycans and water holding capacity and thus there is fall in the osmotic pressure of the disk matrix. The amount of decorin and biglycan is elevated in degenerated human disks to fill the space as compared with normal ones.

Loss of collagen fibers: The absolute quantity of collagen does not change much but the types and distribution of collagens get altered. The fibrillar collagens such as type II collagen become more denatured and get replaced by type 1 collagen.

Increase in fibronectin: Fibronectin content increases with increasing degeneration and it becomes more fragmented. They down-regulate aggrecan synthesis and also simultaneously up-regulate the production of some MMPs in in vitro systems.

Enzymatic activity: Increased fragmentation of the collagen, proteoglycan, and fibronectin is mediated by increased enzymatic activity including cathepsins, MMPs, and aggrecanases.

Cathepsins have maximal activity in acid conditions (seen in degenerative disks).

Functional changes of the disk due to degeneration: The normal mechanics of the disk in response to axial compression and shear forces is disrupted due to the molecular disorganization mentioned above, chief among which is the loss of proteoglycans in nucleus pulpous.

Reduced proteoglycan in degenerated disks alters the disk's load-bearing behavior.
- The osmotic pressure of the disk falls → the disk is less able to maintain hydration under load → when loaded they lose height and fluid more rapidly → the disks tend to bulge.
- Loss of hydration → degenerated disks develop nonhydrostatic loads and inappropriate stress concentrations along the endplate or in the annulus → annular tear → discogenic pain produced during discography.
- Rapid loss of disk height under load in degenerate disks → Z-joint osteoarthritis, reduced tensional forces on the ligamentum flavum causing remodeling and thickening → the ligament tends to bulge into the spinal canal → all three leading to spinal stenosis.
- Fall in concentration of aggrecan in degeneration → allow increased penetration of large molecules such as growth factor complexes and cytokines into the disk → progression of degeneration.
- Aggrecan is an inhibitor of neural growth, its loss hence allows pathological neural ingrowth seen in degenerate disks and hence causing chronic back pain.
- Pressure from a disk bulge is asymptomatic in normal individuals but in those with degenerated disks the increased migration of cytokines like PGE2, thromboxane, phospholipase A2, tumor necrosis factor-α, the interleukins (see above) and increased neural density (see above) would predispose to development of pain by sensitizing these new dense nerves in close vicinity. Thus even slight pressure would be painful in them.

Nutritional pathways of disk degeneration: The activity of disk cells is very sensitive to extracellular oxygen and pH, with matrix synthesis rates falling steeply at acidic pH and at low oxygen concentrations and the cells do not survive prolonged exposure to low pH or glucose concentrations.
- A fall in nutrient supply → lowering of oxygen tension and/or pH (arising from raised lactic acid concentrations) → reduced ability to synthesize and maintain the disk's ECM → disk degeneration.

Clinical features: Patient has had intermittent episodes of back pain for many months or even years before the onset of severe leg pain. In many instances, the back pain is relatively fleeting and is relieved by rest. This pain often is brought on by heavy exertion, repetitive bending, twisting, or heavy lifting. In other instances, an inciting event cannot be elicited. Radicular pain usually extends below the knee and follows the dermatome of the involved nerve root. There is mostly associated a marked paraspinal spasm. A Lasègue sign usually is positive on the involved side. A positive Lasègue sign or straight leg raising should elicit buttock and leg pain distal to the knee. Occasionally, if leg pain is significant, the patient leans back from an upright sitting position and assumes the tripod position to relieve the pain. This is referred to as the "flip sign". Contralateral leg pain produced by straight leg raising should be regarded as pathognomonic of a herniated intervertebral disk.

Unilateral disk herniation between L4 and L5 results in compression of the L5 root. L5 root radiculopathy should produce pain in the dermatomal pattern. Numbness, when present, follows the L5 dermatome along the anterolateral aspect of the leg and the dorsum of the foot, including the great toe. The autonomous zone for this nerve is the dorsal first web of the foot and the dorsum of the third toe. Weakness may involve the extensor hallucis longus (L5), gluteus medius (L5), or extensor digitorum longus and brevis (L5). Reflex change usually is not found. A diminished posterior tibial reflex is possible, but difficult to elicit.

A far lateral disk leads to L4 nerve root involvement.

Diagnosis: History and clinical examination. Currently, the most useful test for diagnosing a herniated lumbar disk is MRI. Since the advent of MRI, myelography is used much less frequently, although in some situations it may help to show subtle lesions. When myelography is used, it should be followed with a CT scan. Plain radiographs are of limited use in the diagnosis because they do not show disk herniations.

Treatment
Nonoperative: The number and variety of nonoperative therapies for back and leg pain are diverse and overwhelming. Treatments range from simple rest to expensive traction apparatus. The simplest treatment for acute back pain is rest for 2–3 days. Lying in a semi-Fowler position with a pillow between the legs should relieve most pressure on the disk

and nerve roots. Muscle spasm can be controlled by the application of ice, preferably with a massage over the muscles in spasm. Pain relief and anti-inflammatory effect can be achieved with NSAIDs. Some patients respond to the use of transcutaneous electrical nerve stimulation. Others do well with traction varying from skin traction in bed with 5–8 lb to body inversion with forces of more than 100 lb. Back braces or corsets may be helpful to other patients. Ultrasound and diathermy are other treatments used in acute back pain. The scientific efficacy of many of these treatments has not been proved.

Operative treatment: Surgical disk removal is mandatory and urgent only in cauda equina syndrome. All other disk excisions should be considered elective. The elective status of surgery should allow a thorough evaluation to confirm the diagnosis, level of involvement, and physical and psychological status of the patient. The patient should be aware that the procedure is predominantly for the symptomatic relief of leg pain. Patients with predominantly back pain may not be relieved of their major complaint—back pain.

Microlumbar disk excision has replaced the standard open laminectomy as the procedure of choice for herniated lumbar disk. This procedure can be done on an outpatient basis and allows better lighting, magnification, and angle of view with a much smaller exposure. Because of the limited dissection required, there is less postoperative pain and a shorter postoperative stay.

43. Interpretation of straight leg raising test (SLRT) in patients with acute low backache.

Ans: The straight leg raising test can be done in the following manners:

- The passive straight-leg raise test (Lasègue test) defined as production of ipsilateral, concordant leg pain at 35–70° of leg elevation in supine or sitting positions, has demonstrated a high sensitivity, but low specificity for L4-5 and L5-S1 disk herniations. The test is sensitive (true positive in 72–97% of patients), but not specific (false positive in 11–66% of patients). The straight leg raise will not produce pain, if nerve root pathology is cephalad to the L5 nerve root because the straight-leg raise test maneuver tensions lower nerve roots (L5-S1). The nerve is stretched only during 35–70° range of movement in SLRT (A typical L5 or S1 nerve is deformed by 2–6 mm in SLRT). In the first 35° the slack in the nerve is taken up and beyond 70° the deformation of sciatic nerve occurs beyond spine and is not sensitive for radicular pathology. So a stretch test for being positive should elicit pain during this range. Sometimes with intense acute inflammatory reaction it may not at all be possible to lift the leg. This can be taken as positive with other findings but should prompt for an urgent search for pathology. A mere feeling of 'posterior stretch' is not a positive SLRT and is common between 70–90° ranges.
- The contralateral or crossed straight leg raise test or crossed Lasègue or well-leg raise test (production of concordant leg pain with contralateral leg elevation) has a lower sensitivity (true positive in 23–42%) of patients, but higher specificity (false positive in 85–100% of patients). This test signifies that the disk is central or that there is a large lateral recess herniation and it is more specific for a "free" disk fragment.
- *Femoral nerve stretch test (reverse SLRT)*: For L2-L4—prone patient then lift the thigh keeping buttocks stable.

44. A. Describe endoscopic spinal surgery technique.
B. What is sacral nutation and its role in chronic low backache?

Ans: A. *Endoscopic spinal surgery technique*: Dorsal and lumbar spines are commonly approached endoscopically for treatment of various lesions. Video-assisted thoracoscopic surgery (VATS) procedure is a minimally invasive technique that allows adequate specimens to be obtained and decompression of various lesions. Some excisions can also be performed. Advantages include minimum blood loss, less tissue damage, less pain in the postoperative period, and short hospital stay.

Endoscopic thoracic diskectomy:
- *Position*: Left lateral decubitus position (right-sided approach)—this placement further displaces the aorta and heart to the left.
- Insert four trocars in a triangular fashion along the middle axillary line converging on the disk space. Introduce a rigid endoscope with a 30° optic angle attached to a video camera into one of the trocars, leaving the other three as working channels.
- Deflate the lung.

- Split the parietal pleura starting at the medial part of the intervertebral space and extending up to the costovertebral process.
- Preserve and mobilize the segmental arteries and sympathetic nerve out of the operating field.
- Drill away the rib head and lateral portion of the pedicle. Remove the remaining pedicle with Kerrison rongeurs to improve exposure to the spinal canal. Removing the superior posterior portion of the vertebra caudal to the disk space allows safer removal of the disk material.
- Remove the disk posteriorly restricting bone and disk removal to the posterior third of the intervertebral space to maintain stability.
- Insert chest tubes in the standard fashion, and set them to water suction; close the portals.

In the lumbar spine, endoscopic techniques have been developed with the purported advantage of shortened hospital stay and faster return to activity. These techniques generally are variations of the microdiskectomy technique using an endoscope rather than the microscope and different types of retractors. This remains another alternative technique. Each system is unique. The basic principles remain the same as with microdiskectomy. Less-invasive tubular retractors also have been used in a transmuscular fashion, allowing disk excision with less soft tissue damage because of the more precise exposure; however, better objective clinical results have not been shown with this technique.

B. *Sacral nutation*: Nutation refers to the sagittal plane movement at the sacroiliac joint where the movement of sacrum resembles a "nod" thus instead of flexion or extension this reciprocating movement is referred to nutation. Nutation is defined as a relative anterior tilt of the sacral promontory in relation to the ilium. Counternutation is the movement in other direction. This movement is hardly 3–5 mm in total but is significant. Excessive movement would produce sacroiliac pain due to strain on the ligaments and may produce sacroiliitis. One way to control sacroiliac pain is hence by reducing the sacral nutation with muscle strengthening. Specifically, erector spinae and rectus abdominis (cause nutation) and hamstring muscles (counternutation) should be balanced to stabilize the sacroiliac joint dynamically.

45. Describe various types of lumbar root anomalies. List down complications of lumbar disk surgery.

Ans: The congenital anomalies predispose to poor results from lumbar disk surgery because the abnormal and unrecognized roots may be injured or actually involved and remain untreated. This risk increases with minimally invasive techniques where direct nerve visualization is often less than optimal. The following are some commonly described anomalies in anatomic studies:

- *Conjoined nerve roots*: It is the most common anomaly (14–17% of cadavers). Conjoined roots have been classified anatomically into three classes.
    - *Type 1*: Two roots exit the dura with one common sheath.
        - *Type 1A anomalies*: The cephalad root departs the conjoined stalk at an acute angle to exit below the pedicle, and the caudal root travels within the canal to exit also below the appropriate pedicle.
        - *Type 1B anomaly*: The cephalad root exits at 90° from the conjoined portion.
    - Type 2 anomalies occur when two roots exit through a single foramen.
        - Type 2A anomalies have one vacant foramen.
        - Type 2B anomalies have a portion of one of the roots exits via the other foramen that may be cephalad to the foramen occupied by the two nerve roots.
    - Type 3 anomalies have an anastomosing branch between two adjacent nerve roots. This branch crosses the disk space and can easily be injured during diskectomy.

Complications of lumbar disk surgery:
- Cauda equina syndrome
- Thrombophlebitis
- Pulmonary embolism
- Wound infection
- Pyogenic spondylitis
- Postoperative diskitis

- Dural tears
- Nerve root injury
- CSF fistula
- Laceration of abdominal vessels
- Injury to abdominal viscera.

46. Briefly describe double crush syndrome and its pathophysiology.

Ans: This is not a syndrome but a general phenomenon that is common to various compression neuropathies such as radial nerve compression at elbow and cervical spondylosis, sciatic nerve compression near piriformis muscle and lumbar spondylosis, etc. A double-crush phenomenon occurs when a proximal nerve root pathology diminishes axoplasmic flow, making it more susceptible to injury. Double-crush phenomenon is based on the work of Upton and McComas (1973) who summarized their findings that "local damage to a nerve at one site along its course may sufficiently impair the overall functioning of the nerve cells (axonal flow), such that the nerve cells become more susceptible to compression trauma at distal sites than would normally be the case". So, in case of lumbar spondylosis or prolapsed intervertebral disc at S1 the tibial nerve may be more susceptible to compression at the flexor retinaculum. Double-crush phenomenon may be seen in up to three-fourths of the patients with compression neuropathy.

47. Discuss lumbar discectomy: indications, surgical approach and complications.

Ans: Lumbar discectomy is the standard procedure for herniated disc causing severe or progressive compression of the nerve roots resulting in neurological intractable symptoms.

Indications
- Progressing neurological deficit
- Cauda equina syndrome (CES)
- Severe peripheral neurological deficit, viz. foot drop
- Failure of conservative treatment to relieve pain and neurological signs and symptoms
- Severe persistent pain and disability for more than 1 year (6 months is probably a better guide as there is some concern of an inferior result after 1 year).

Surgical approach
- Verify the level (C-arm).
- Make the incision from the mid spinous process of the upper vertebra to the superior margin of the spinous process of the lower vertebra at the involved level.
- Incise the fascia at the midline using electrocautery. Elevate the deep fascia and muscle subperiosteally from the spinous processes and lamina, on the involved side only.
- Re-verify the level.
- Using a Cobb elevator, gently sweep the remaining muscular attachments off in a lateral direction exposing the interlaminar space and the edge of each lamina. Secure bleeding.
- Identify the ligamentum flavum and lamina.
- Detach the lateral portion of the ligamentum flavum from the caudal edge of the superior lamina and the cephalad edge of the inferior lamina. Remove some bone from the superior lamina.
- The lamina, facet, and facet capsule should remain intact. Dissect away the ligamentum flavum and bone from the lamina using Kerrison rongeur as needed to identify the nerve root clearly.
- Carefully mobilize the root medially, the disc now is visible as a white, fibrous, avascular structure.
- Enlarge the annular tear with a Penfield No. 4 dissector and remove the disc material with the microdisc forceps.
- Remove the exposed disc material. Remove additional loose disc or cartilage fragments. Inspect the root and adjacent dura for disc fragments. Irrigate the disc space well.
- Close the fascia and the skin.

Complications
- Cauda equina syndrome
- Thrombophlebitis
  Pulmonary embolism
- Wound infection
- Pyogenic spondylitis
- Postoperative discitis
- Dural tears
- Nerve root injury
- Cerebrospinal fluid fistula
- Laceration of abdominal vessels
- Injury to abdominal viscera

4C.8 SCOLIOSIS AND RELATED QUESTIONS (Q48–61)

48. **Classify scoliosis. Briefly discuss safety measures in scoliotic surgery.**

Ans: Classification according to age given by Scoliosis Research Society is shown in **Table 4C.8.1**.

TABLE 4C.8.1: Classification of scoliosis.			
	Infantile	*Juvenile*	*Adolescent*
Usual age at presentation	Birth to 3 years	4–9 years	10–20 years
Male:female	1:1–2:1	<6 years: 1:3 >6 years: 1:6	1:6
Incidence	United States: 2–3% Great Britain: 30%	United States: 12–15% Great Britain: 12–15%	United States: 85% Great Britain: 55%
Curve types	Left thoracic L:R (2:1) Left thoracic/right lumbar	Right thoracic R:L (6:1)	Right thoracic R:L (8:1)
Associated findings	Mental deficiency, CDH, plagiocephaly, congenital heart defects	None	None
Risk of cardiopulmonary compromise	High	Intermediate	Low
Risk of curve progression	<6 months: low >1 year: high	67%	23%
Rate of curve progression	Gradual progression: 2–3° per year Malignant progression: 10° per year	Progression at puberty: 6° per year Malignant progression: 10° per year	1–2° per month during puberty
Curve resolution	<1 year: 90% >1 year: 20%	20%	Rare
Curve magnitude and maturity	Gradual progression: 70–90° Malignant progression: >90°	Progression at puberty: 50–90° Malignant progression: > 90°	Curves >90° are rare
Orthotic management	Effective at delaying and slowing rate of progression Ultimate progression: 100%	Decreases rate of progression until puberty (failure rate: 30–80%)	Effectively controls curves <40° (success rate: 75–80%)
Surgical treatment	Instrumentation without fusion <8 years After 8 years: ASF-PSF After 11 years: PSF	Instrumentation without fusion <8 years After 8 years: ASF-PSF After 1 year: PSF	PSF with instrumentation ASF if younger than 11 years with open triradiate cartilage
Risk of crankshaft	High	High	Low

Safety measures: Neurological injury is the most dreaded complication that may occur intraoperatively. One must be thorough with the instrumentation and curve correction should undertake the risk of traction cord injury that can be checked intraoperatively by neurophysiological monitoring. Kindly see Answer to Question 40 for stagnara wake-up test. (*Kindly refer to Chapter 90 of the book Essential Orthopedics: Principles and Practices, 2nd edition, for detailed discussion on intraoperative neurological monitoring.*)

49. Discuss the classification of congenital scoliosis.

Ans: The classification proposed by MacEwen et al. and later modified by Winter, Moe, and Eilers is the one most uniformly accepted.

1. *Group 1*: Failure of formation
   - Partial failure of formation (wedge vertebra)
   - Complete failure of formation (hemivertebra)
2. *Failure of segmentation*:
   - Unilateral failure of segmentation (unilateral segmented bar)
   - Bilateral failure of segmentation (block vertebra)
3. *Miscellaneous*:

   The congenital curve also should be classified according to the area of the spine involved because this is indicative of the prognosis of the specific deformity. The areas generally distinguished are the cervicothoracic spine, thoracic spine, thoracolumbar spine, and lumbosacral spine.

50. How will you differentiate structural scoliosis from nonstructural scoliosis? Describe infantile idiopathic scoliosis. What is the importance of rib vertebral angle?

Ans: *Structural scoliosis*: The structural defect lies in the curve which shows fixed rotation of vertebra and spinous process (and ribs). This rotation is persistent on clinical examination (The Adam's forward bending test reveals rotation that is accentuated on forward flexion. The rib hump becomes more prominent and needs intervention to correct.

Nonstructural scoliosis: A curve that corrects totally on bending forward/lying down/traction or other maneuvers. Clinically there is no rotation of vertebrae, there is no structural change.

For infantile idiopathic scoliosis, kindly refer to Q38.

Rib vertebral angle (RVA): A method to prognosticate idiopathic thoracic curves in infancy described by Mehta. The measurement is done at the apical vertebra—draw lines along the neck of ribs adjoining apical vertebra and measure the angle they subtend with vertical drawn at the center of vertebra. The angles measured on two sides are subtracted and if the difference (RVAD) is more than 20°; the curve is likely to progress **(Fig. 4C.8.1)**.

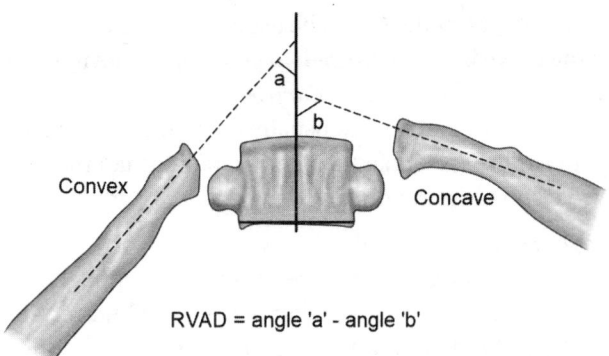

Fig. 4C.8.1: Rib vertebral angle difference (RVAD).

51. Nonstructural scoliosis.

Ans: *Nonstructural curve/scoliosis (functional scoliosis)*: It has no structural component, it corrects on supine side bending films. The curves correct passively and possibly arise from without the loss of osteoligamentous continuity, which develops over a segment or over the entire length of the spine. The most common causes of functional scoliosis are lower limb length differences, unilateral paravertebral muscle contracture, torticollis, etc. This type of scoliosis is classified into three types by Stagnara:

1. *Reducible scoliotic curvatures*: Reversible lateral curvature without rotation that usually arise out of painful spasms of muscles caused by vertebral and juxtavertebral abnormalities.

2. Compensatory curvatures develop due to defects located at a distance from the vertebral column, lower limb length differences, hip adduction or abduction fixed deformities, irreducible muscle retraction.
3. *Postural defects are scoliotic postures without an obvious cause (often seen during childhood)*:
   - They can be intermittent or permanent
   - Not accompanied by vertebral rotation
   - Do not evolve into structural scoliosis
   - Disappear during the pubertal growth spurt.

52. Define end vertebra and apical vertebra in adolescent idiopathic scoliosis.
Describe two radiological methods to measure curve in adolescent idiopathic scoliosis.
Explain fusionless technique of correction in idiopathic scoliosis.

Ans: Definitions:

- *A superior end vertebra* is the vertebra at the upper limit of the curve, whose upper-end plate has the greatest inclination toward the concavity of the curve.
- *An inferior end vertebra* is the vertebra at the lower limit of the curve, whose lower-end plate has the greatest inclination toward the concavity of the curve.
- An apical vertebra is the central vertebra within a curve.

The end vertebra are typically the least rotated and least horizontally displaced vertebra within the curve.
Apical vertebra is typically the least tilted, most rotated and most horizontally displaced vertebra within a curve.

Radiological methods to measure curve in adolescent idiopathic scoliosis:

The Cobb method of measurement consists of three steps:
1. Locating the superior end vertebra
2. Locating the inferior end vertebra
3. Drawing intersecting perpendicular lines from the superior surface of the superior end vertebra and from the inferior surface of the inferior end vertebra.

The angle of deviation of these perpendicular lines from a straight line is the angle of the curve. If the end plates are obscured, the pedicles can be used instead. The end vertebra of the curve is the one that tilts the most into the concavity of the curve being measured. In general, on moving away from the apex of the curve, the next intervertebral space below the inferior end vertebra or above the superior end vertebra is wider on the concave side of the curve. Within the curve, the intervertebral spaces usually are wider on the convex side and narrower on the concave side. When significantly wedged, the vertebrae themselves, rather than the intervertebral disk spaces, may be wider on the convex side of the curve and narrower on the concave side.

Risser-Ferguson method:
- First line originating at the center of the upper end vertebra
- Second line from the center of the lower end vertebra
- Angle formed by the intersection of two lines at the center of the apical vertebra gives the degree of curvature.

Fusionless technique of correction in idiopathic scoliosis:
Traditionally, the surgical management of scoliosis has been focused on correcting the curvature and obtaining a solid fusion of the growing spine thus halting further progression of deformity.

Important considerations in the operative treatment of patients with juvenile idiopathic scoliosis are the expected loss of spinal height and the limited chest wall growth and lung development after spinal fusion.

To overcome these unwanted effects, fusionless corrective techniques are used namely:
- Growing rods
- Vertical expandable prosthetic titanium rib (VEPTR)
- Shilla procedure
- Vertebral stapling
- Vertebral tethering

Growing rods: Growing rod instrumentation is a technique of posterior instrumentation that is sequentially lengthened to allow longitudinal growth while still attempting to control progressive spinal deformity. The growing rod techniques should be considered in a cooperative patient with a stable family unit. This procedure usually is considered for patients younger than 10 years of age who have a curve of 60°. Surgery is required every 6 months to lengthen the construct. A thoracic lumbar sacral orthosis (TLSO) often is necessary for at least the first 6 months to protect the upper and lower levels of the instrumentation. Dual growing rods have been found to be effective in controlling severe spinal deformities and allowing spinal growth. With the use of dual rods, an apical fusion does not appear to be necessary during the course of treatment.

Vertical expandable prosthetic titanium rib is already described in Question 50.

The Luque trolley and Shilla procedure: The Luque trolley consists of sublaminar wires and rods without fusion. The Shilla technique consists of a nonlocking pedicle screw implant. The apex of the deformity is fixed and fused with pedicle screws while the ends of the construct are instrumented with screws that are not locked to the rod. This theoretically allows for apical control of the deformity and continued axial lengthening of the spine with growth.

Vertebral stapling: Intervertebral stapling is used to produce a tethering effect on the convex side of the spine. This tether theoretically will allow for continued growth on the concave side of the spine deformity and gradual correction of the deformity with growth. Devices that have been used for this growth modulation are a flexible titanium clip, a nitinol staple, and an anterior spinal tether using anterior vertebral body screws and a polypropylene cord. Current indications for vertebral body stapling for scoliosis include age younger than 13 years in girls and 15 years in boys, skeletal maturity of Risser grade 0 or 1, with 1 year of growth remaining by wrist bone age, minimal rotation of both the thoracic and lumbar curves of 45° and flexibility to <20°, and a sagittal thoracic curve of 40° or less. If the thoracic coronal curve is between 35° and 45° and does not correct on bending films to <20°, adding a posterior rib-to-spine hybrid construct may be considered. If the first erect radiograph does not measure 20° or less after vertebral body stapling, recommendation is having the patient wear a corrective brace until the curve measures less than 20°. Children younger than 8 years of age may not be ideal candidates for this surgery because of the possibility of overcorrection with growth.

Vertebral tethering: Purported advantages of anterior vertebral tethering include that it allows the spine to grow and remain flexible, it is one-time surgery, and a later fusion can be done if needed. The indications for this technique have not been well established, but it is most likely beneficial for patients with enough growth remaining to substantially alter the shape of the spine and is most suited for primary thoracic curves with typical hypokyphotic apices.

53. Discuss various techniques including recent advances in management of adolescent idiopathic scoliosis (AIS).

Ans: Adolescent idiopathic scoliosis is a common spinal deformity characterized by a lateral curvature of the spine that often manifests during the growth spurts of adolescence. The management of AIS depends on the severity of the curve, the age of the patient, and the degree of skeletal maturity. Various techniques and recent advances have emerged for the management of AIS, which can be grouped into nonsurgical and surgical options.

Nonsurgical Management
- *Observation*: For mild scoliosis (curves < 20°), the most common approach is "watchful waiting". Regular follow-ups are scheduled to monitor the curve's progression, particularly during periods of rapid growth.
- *Bracing*: Bracing is indicated for moderate spinal curves (20–40°) in skeletally immature patients (typically under 14 years old). The goal is to prevent further progression of the curve.
  Recent advances:
  - *3D printed braces*: Custom-fit braces employing 3D printing technology allow for better fit and comfort, potentially improving compliance.
  - *Dynamic bracing*: Newer designs focus on allowing certain movements while still providing corrective forces to the curve.
- *Physical therapy and exercise programs*: Although not universally effective, tailored physical therapy programs and exercise regimens can help improve posture, flexibility, and strength.
  - *Schroth method*: A specialized physical therapy technique that focuses on scoliosis-specific exercises to improve deformity and postural alignment.

Surgical Management
- *Spinal fusion*: The traditional approach for severe curves (>45°) or progressive curves is spinal fusion surgery. This involves stabilizing the spine using rods and screws, which can prevent further curvature.
  Recent advances:
  - *Minimally invasive surgery (MIS)*: Techniques that use less invasive approaches reduce muscle damage and improve recovery times.
  - *Alternative fusion techniques*: Newer fusion materials and techniques (e.g., expandable cages, biologics) may enhance healing and reduce complications.
  - *Intraoperative neuromonitoring*: Real-time monitoring of spinal cord function during surgery to decrease the risk of postoperative complications.

Growth Modulation Techniques
- For young patients with moderate curves, growth modulation methods, such as "vertebral body tethering (VBT)," is being explored. This technique uses screws and tension bands to adjust the spine's growth direction.
- *Magnetic controlled growing rods (MCGR)*: For children with progressive scoliosis who are still growing, MCGR allows noninvasive lengthening of the rods via magnetism, accommodating spinal growth without additional surgeries.

Osteotomies and deformity correction: In complex cases, surgical techniques may involve osteotomies to correct spinal deformity completely. Techniques are continuously evolving to optimize outcomes and reduce recurrence.

Emerging Technologies and Innovations
- *Robotics and navigation*:
  - Surgical robotics and computer-assisted navigation systems are increasingly used to enhance precision in spinal deformity correction and improve surgical outcomes.
  - These technologies help in better screw placement, which can reduce complication rates and improve overall alignment.
- *Bioprinting and regenerative medicine*:
  - Research into bioprinting of spinal tissues and the use of stem cells aims to improve healing and potentially reduce the need for extensive fusion procedures.
- *Artificial intelligence (AI) in diagnosis and treatment planning*:
  - AI-driven tools are being developed for better classification of scoliosis severity and predicting progression, facilitating more personalized management plans.

54. Discuss wake-up test.

Ans: *Stagnara wake-up test*: This is considered often the gold standard for monitoring spinal cord injury. The test consists of waking the patient up during the surgery and asking to move their feet. The test does not require any sophisticated apparatus or method but needs a skilled anesthetist who can quickly reverse the effect of anesthesia with return of enough cognitive function for patient to understand. Often short acting and fast reversing drugs are used like the desflurane and remifentanil. The method is however crude and does not tell the level of injury or mode of injury like direct nerve injury or cord injury due to ischemia/distraction, etc. So the basic purpose of removing or reversing the offending factor is not fulfilled and only the surgeon gets tense from cord injury!

Contraindications to test include:
- Mental retardation
- Psychological problems
- Pre-existing neurological damage
- Language problem.

If a neurological complication is suspected based on an abnormal wake-up test result, immediate correction of hypotension and release of distraction should be undertaken.

If the wake-up test continues to indicate abnormality, removal of the instrumentation is recommended. If a neurological complication is suspected based on an abnormal wake-up test result, immediate correction of hypotension and release of distraction should be undertaken. If the wake-up test continues to indicate abnormality, removal of the instrumentation is recommended.

55. Describe factors influencing spinal curve progression in congenital scoliosis.

Ans: Rate of deterioration and the severity of final deformity are predictable according to the type of anomaly and curve location.

- *Type of anomaly/defect*: Vertebral anomalies in decreasing order of risk progression:
  - Unilateral (U/L) unsegmented bar with contralateral hemivertebrae >U/L unregimented bar > Unilateral unsegmented bar combined with single or multiple contralateral convex hemivertebrae — fastest progression up to 10° per year.
- *Patient's age at the time of diagnosis*: Younger the age the higher is the rate and degree of deformity at maturity. Curve progression (caused by unbalanced growth of one side of the spine relative to the other) occurs more rapidly during the first 5 years of life and during puberty.
- *Site of defect (junctional regions)*: Both thoracolumbar and thoracic curves are more progressive than cervicothoracic and lumbar types. Upper thoracic curves tend to be less severe than thoracolumbar curves (these are most severe). For example, thoracic hemivertebra have a higher rate of progression.

56. Describe the management of congenital scoliosis.

Ans: Observation and bracing has no known definitive role in management of congenital scoliosis. Either the curve will progress or need surgical treatment or it will not and will never require deformity correction. Observation (till skeletal maturity) is strictly done only for:
- Incarcerated hemivertebrae
- Nonsegmental hemivertebrae
- Some partially segmented hemivertebrae.

Bracing has no role in management of congenital scoliosis either for prevention of curve progression or correction as it universally fails for these inflexible curves. The only known role of bracing is to control the supple compensatory curves if they develop [Milwaukee for upper curves, TLSO (thoracic/lumbar/sacral orthosis) brace for lumbar curves].

Surgical management: Congenital spinal deformities are rigid and correction is generally achieved through the mobile segments above and below the anomaly. Instrumentation is the preferred modality these days compared to the cast management done previously. Instrumentation maintains or improves correction but the postoperative risk of neurological impairment is the highest in this group due to the following reasons:
- Small spinal canal size
- Severe deformities
- Frequent presence of intraspinal anomalies such as diastematomyelia or tethering.

Ideally for early deformities surgical fusion is performed to prevent deformity progression and for patients presenting late with severe deformity correction of deformity becomes the goal. The goals of surgical management include in general:
- Achieve a straight spine
- Maintain a physiological sagittal profile while maintaining flexibility
- To arrest progression of the curve
- Short fusion segment preserving as much normal spinal growth as possible.

The principles of surgery include:
- Early and aggressive treatment of deformities
- In surgical planning, the superior/inferior endpoints of instrumentation are so chosen that the head is centered over the pelvis in both the frontal and sagittal planes.

The compensatory curve need not be included in the fusion, unless it is anticipated that the structural component of the compensatory curve is the main cause of trunk decompensation. These compensatory curves must be however closely monitored.
- Posterior instrumentation is reserved for the thoracic and lumbar deformities in adolescents or in cases where spinal instability or unacceptable truncal shortening will result from combined anterior-posterior procedures/osteotomies.
- Preventing lengthening the spinal cord intraoperatively.
- Routine use of MRI evaluation.
- Tethered cords and diastematomyelia must be corrected before deformity correction.

- instrumentation appropriate to the patient's size must be chosen.
- Monitored use of controlled hypotension.
- Monitoring intraoperative neurology and postoperative neurological status.

As mentioned, the surgery is done either to prevent deformity from occurring or correcting the deformity so they are corresponding two broad forms of surgical procedures. Out of the various surgical options posterior fusion (including in situ fusion), anterior fusion, combined anterior-posterior fusion, hemivertebra excision, and spinal osteotomy and fusion some are used for preventing deformity while others for correction of deformity.

Procedures preventing deformity in future

In situ fusion: Posterior spinal fusion is the gold standard for both congenital scoliosis and kyphosis. To be successful, the posterior fusion must include the entire curve, from stable vertebra to stable vertebra. It is ideally suited for short curves like those with unilateral failure of segmentation (unilateral bar) with a curve less than 40°. Also deformities at the lumbosacral and cervicothoracic junction should be fused very early as they are cosmetically most disfiguring. The crankshaft phenomenon or bending of the posterior fusion mass may occur in some very young patients (<5 years of age) with congenital scoliosis and hence the major controversy is whether combined anterior and posterior fusion should be done routinely. It has been argued that there is less potential for anterior growth in a spine with congenital scoliosis because the growth plates may not be properly formed. So currently it is deemed that when thoracic lordosis is part of the deformity, anterior diskectomy and fusion is preferable to prevent any crankshaft phenomenon and also to avoid progressive thoracic encroachment. Some recommend that for unilateral bars and contralateral hemivertebra the curve progression potential is high and should be managed by combined anterior and posterior procedures. In mild cases of congenital kyphosis, spontaneous correction after posterior fusion alone can occur in young patients (<5 years of age) with kyphotic deformity less than 50°.

Convex hemiepiphysiodesis (Roaf, 1955): The common indication is a unilateral formation failure (hemivertebra). There should be potential for growth on the concave side so definite exclusion of contralateral bar should be made before the procedure. In convex hemiepiphysiodesis, the convex lateral half of disks adjacent to the hemivertebra are removed without touching the concave side and thus potentiate correction by preferential concave growth. This procedure should be reserved (Winter, et al.) for patients younger than 5 years of age, with a progressive curve of less than 70° (ideally < 40°) involving five segments or less (ideally < 3) without any kyphosis or lordosis modifier. Hemivertebra excision or wedge resection is more predictable procedures than hemiepiphysiodesis.

Hemivertebra excision: Here the culprit vertebra is removed by wedge resection where in situ fusion (or convex hemiepiphysiodesis) will not work as in kyphotic deformities and truncal imbalance. Ideally this procedure is reserved for an L-5 lumbosacral junction hemivertebra causing trunk decompensation. Excision of hemivertebrae at other levels is typically reserved for cases of severe kyphotic deformities, which may or may not be associated with neurological defects. Excision of hemivertebra decompresses the spinal cord tented over the apex of kyphosis. It is best done at and before 2 years of age as cast is less easily tolerated by patients older than this age. After excision compression instrumentation is mandatory. The procedure can be accomplished by posterior only or a combined anterior and posterior approach, having their individual pros and cons:
- Posterior only approach—using pedicle screw instrumentation to correct deformity has been preferred for less operative time and morbidity and lesser risk to anterior vascular and visceral structures.
- Combined approach is advocated by some for its capability to achieve higher correction including sagittal plane deformity correction. The growth plates can be removed and reduce the chances of development of crankshaft phenomenon.

Procedures Done to Correct the Deformity

Gradual correction techniques—include hemiepiphysiodesis and hemiarthrodesis: Used for failure of formation (there is no growth potential left in segmentation failure). Curves with limited growth potential on the concave side like the convex hemivertebra will not be benefitted by the procedure. The procedure is aimed to arrest growth on the convex side and relies on continued growth on the concave side for curve correction.

Growing rods (see also in the management of early onset scoliosis): For management of cases in early years of life (2-3 years of age), it is imperative to understand that sitting height reaches the adult height by the age of 5 years. So long fusions will result in stunted growth. Also the thoracic volumes reach 30% of adult volumes by 5 years of age and similarly the fusion surgeries will produce a loss in the thoracic volume and thoracic insufficiency.

Growing rods (Akbarnia and Mccarthy system) permit growth of the spine and curve correction and apical fusion to correct the congenital anomaly (especially failure of segmentation) may be needed.

Acute correction techniques—include correction and fusion with instrumentation: The aim is to obtain a balanced spine in the safest way possible. High thoracic and lumbar spines need particular care as they cause maximum imbalance. The best curves for these procedures are those with relatively preserved segmentation, partially flexible and less severe truncal deformity. If the disk spaces are well preserved then anterior fusion is combined. One should ensure by preoperative MRI that there is no cord tethering or diastematomyelia.

Hemivertebra Excision

Reconstructive osteotomy: Fixed curves are not amenable to manipulative correction either acute or gradual. The nonflexible curves with truncal decompensation need to be repositioned by corrective osteotomies. Other indications are pelvic obliquity and developing neurological deficit. The corrective osteotomies can be combined with hemivertebra resection or "fusion with instrumentation" procedures described above.

Vertical expandable prosthetic titanium rib and expansion thoracoplasty: Thoracic insufficiency (introduced by Campbell, et al.) refers to poor thoracic and lung parenchymal development that produces poor lung function resulting from restricted growth of the thoracic cavity. Tethering of the ribs is also responsible for curve progression that in turn reduces thoracic cavity exacerbating the insufficiency in pulmonary function with growth (contrary to the expectation of improving lung function with growth). The poor lung function primarily results from reduced height and volume of the thoracic cavity that precludes lung expansion and alveolar development that get arrested to infancy maturity. Both the numbers and size of alveoli are diminished. The growth of the lung and alveoli multiplication is the greatest in the first 8 years of life reaching 50% of the adult thoracic volume. Early fusions will hence restrict not only the development of spine but also the thoracic height and volume.

Children who have borderline lung function at maturity are at high risk for developing respiratory insufficiency in late adulthood due to the following reasons:
- Approximately 400 cc's of vital capacity is lost in aging process.
- Development of COPD will reduce the available lung volume.
- Acute respiratory infections and pneumonia will reduce the lung function to critical survival levels. Thoracic insufficiency is a lately recognized complication of total growth inhibition of thoracic spine by combined anterior and posterior spinal fusion, convex anterior epiphysiodesis or arthrodesis performed with the ideology of having a "short straight spine instead of long crooked one". VEPTR technique challenged the above concept by showing an increase in length of the unilateral unsegmented bars and equal increases in length of the concave and convex sides in congenital scoliosis. VEPTR expands thorax by rib distraction on the concave side of the curve achieving indirect correction.

When the focal kyphosis exceeds 50°, correction requires anterior release followed by posterior fusion. If the anterior release is not performed, the pseudarthrosis rate may be as high as 54% compared with 13% when combining anterior and posterior fusion. Winter et al. recommended routine re-exploration of the posterior bone graft 6 months after a posterior surgery if anterior fusion was not performed. In their series, however, instrumentation was not used.

57. Investigations in congenital scoliosis.

Ans: The following investigations are legible in management of congenital scoliosis:
- Renal ultrasonography, cardiac consultation (and echocardiogram), and MRI of the entire brainstem and spinal cord are essential for complete evaluation. Systemic deficiencies are evaluated for anesthesia and general wellbeing of the patient to bear surgery. The predominant congenital deformity usually exists as a scoliosis, kyphosis, or lordosis in a multiplanar distribution.
- Radiographic description of deformity should include the involved area of the spine, type of vertebral anomaly, and configuration of the deformity. CT scan should be judiciously used to detail the deformity and for classification.
- The specific indications for MRI include:
  - The presence of neurological defects such as weakness, sensory loss, bowel or bladder dysfunction
  - Associated skin abnormality over the spine such as a dimple, hairy patches, or nevi

- Complaints of back or leg pain
- Patients with lumbosacral kyphosis
- Radiographic evidence of interpedicular widening
- Diastematomyelia
- Presence of a unilateral congenital bar with a contralateral hemivertebra
- Any patient who is to undergo spinal stabilization surgery [rule out (r/o) tethered cord, syringomyelia intradural lipoma, etc.]
- Pulmonary evaluation includes obtaining vital capacity and if it is <60% of normal then a full spirometry workup.

58. **Discuss principles of application of Milwaukee brace. What are the clinical features of idiopathic kyphoscoliosis? Enumerate indications of surgical intervention.**

Ans: *The orthosis consists of three basic components*:
1. Pelvic section
2. The superstructure
3. The pads.

1. *The pelvic section*: It is carved from patient cast and is made of thermoplastics lined with foam interface (now prefabricated modules are commercially available). Custom molding of the pelvic component is needed especially with pelvic obliquity or atypical spinal deformity. It should be a snug fit to provide stable foundation from which pads gain a mechanical advantage.
2. *Superstructure*: It is composed of neck-ring and three metal bars that attach the pelvic structure to neck ring. The anterior bar is made of aluminum to give adequate radiolucency and posterior bars are made of steel to provide strength and rigidity. The chin attachment has been removed from the neck ring which was originally used due to concerns of malocclusion. The superstructure provides traction force and means of pad suspension to permit force application to body. The other function is to provide superior end point of control. In the high profile design the neck ring is placed with the throat mold just inferior to mandible. In the low-profile design the neck ring is placed at the level of sternal notch that makes it inconspicuous and more acceptable.
3. *Pads*: These are the most important parts of brace as they provide the corrective forces to the deformity. They need to be carefully and tactfully placed to provide benefit to the patient. The pads are made of rigid material like aluminum back with foam back and covered with vinyl. The pads must be stiff enough to impart forces onto bone but prevent skin breakdown. Lumbar pads are incorporated in the "foundation" (pelvic section). Axilla slings and rings provide counterforce against the thoracic pads and permit maximal force to be applied.

The force of thoracic pads can be altered by adjusting the axilla strap. Pads are "floating" when they are suspended from superstructure by straps. Gradually increasing pad forces applied produce decent correction provided brace is worn as scheduled.

Assessing the fit of brace:
- In the pelvic component after wear, even finger should not pass inside [say to palpate anterior superior iliac spine (ASIS)] to maintain a snug fit. If snug fit is not obtained then it will not serve as a strong foundation and control of forces will not be achieved. This entails use of custom-made component (plaster mold cast) rather than commercial or measurement derived build.
- The width of the posterior opening should be of magnitude equal to or slightly larger than that of the largest lumbar vertebral body. This ensures lateral counter rotation force exerted by the lumbar pad instead of central force.
- Superstructure should contour to the body walls.
- Thoracic pads are positioned posterolaterally so as to provide both a derotating force as well as a laterally directed force which can act in the coronal plane for correction of thoracic scoliosis.
- Lumbar pad should be positioned at the level of the apex of the lumbar curve "Null point".
- Axillary pad should be placed as superior as possible without patient experiencing pain or paresthesias.

The basic concept was that the lumbar lordosis needs correction for correction of scoliosis. This designed the "foundation" of brace which remains in contact with the iliac crest and lumbar spine. From this base foundation three uprights are erected one anterior and two posterior connecting to the neck ring above the shoulders (chin rest was removed from brace due to production of malocclusion). The brace has an occipital pad or rest posteriorly to care for the occipital portion of the skull.

Biomechanics of brace: Following are the general biomechanical principles as applied for various braces:
- Prevention of asymmetric compressive forces related to passive posture
- Reduction of secondary muscle imbalance
- Prevention of lordosing reactive forces
- Prevention of asymmetric torsional forces from gait
- Production of dynamic detorsional forces involving breathing mechanics.
- The brace applies external corrective forces to the trunk with the aim to halt the curve progression or to correct it during growth or to avoid further progression of an already established pathological curve in adulthood.

Clinical features of idiopathic kyphoscoliosis:

Pain: It occurs in 30% of patients with adolescent idiopathic scoliosis (AIS) but is never bothering or prominent (virtually AIS has been described as a painless condition). Pain often arises due to associated muscular weakness, spasm due to imbalance or stretching of ligaments due to rapid change in curve.

Age at onset: Patients may present symptoms in the adolescent period; however, they may have had earlier onset. It is important to determine the etiology—it may be juvenile or infantile onset. The presence of an important thoracic deformity before the age of 5 years increases the risk of altered pulmonary function and secondarily, cardiac function (cor pulmonale).

Assessment of deformity:
- The extent of spinal curvature generally guides the treatment. The extent of spinal curvature and angle of trunk rotation (ATR) determine the severity of scoliosis.
- Coronal imbalance assessment: Plumb line to judge balance of curve.
- Coronal curve assessment: Thoracic/thoracolumbar/lumbar curve with convexity to right/left side.
- Shoulder height or asymmetry.

Forward protrusion of chest wall on affected side:
- Increased flank creases on opposite (concave side).
- Higher anterior superior iliac spines (ASIS) and posterior superior iliac spines (PSIS) on concave side.

Indications of surgical intervention: Surgery is aimed most importantly to halt curve progression with fusion (primary goal) and also to reduce deformity using instrumentation (secondary goal). In general curves greater than 45–50° should be treated by surgery. The specific indications for operative treatment are as follows:
- *Thoracic curves*:
  - *Skeletally immature patients*: Curve magnitude greater than 40–50°.
  - *Mature patients*: Curve magnitude greater than 50° (as they have high chances of progression even after maturity).
- *Thoracolumbar/lumbar curves*: Curve magnitude greater than 40° with significant coronal decompensation.

59. What is the lateral mass fixation technique?

Ans: The technique for lateral mass screw placement is that of Magerl, as modified by Anderson:
- If the patient is already in traction, maintain traction and alignment. Coordinate with the anesthesiologist for an awake intubation or manually maintain head position and use a GlideScope. If the patient has a spinal cord injury, maintain a mean arterial pressure of 85–90 mm Hg throughout the procedure. Use a turning frame such as the Jackson table to position the patient prone.
- Radiographically verify injury reduction; if pedicle screws are to be used, make sure imaging can adequately be accomplished before preparation and draping.
- Incise the skin over the area of exposure. Infiltrate the subcutaneous tissue and muscle with 1 mg epinephrine in 500 mL normal saline.
- Expose the posterior cervical spine subperiosteally to the far lateral border of the facet joints after verifying levels.

- Remove any facet capsules in the area to be fused and identify the boundaries of the lateral mass, which consist of the superior joint line, the inferior joint line, the lateral border, and the medial sulcus at the junction with the lamina.
- If a laminectomy or laminoplasty is planned, do not perform it until the screw holes are completed so the bony landmarks can be used.
- Select an entry portal 1 mm medial to the center of the lateral mass and penetrate only the cortex with a burr.
- Drilling of the lateral mass should be directed 25–35° laterally and 25° cephalad (parallel to the plane of the facet joint) for C3–C6. This trajectory can reliably be accomplished by placing the drill guide against the midpoint of the posterior tip (remove large osteophytes if present) of the spinous process of the vertebra caudal to the level being drilled. Use a hand drill set to a depth of 14 mm that will provide unicortical fixation in most patients.
- If bicortical fixation is planned, use a drill of preset length and drill in 2-mm increments. Use a ball-tipped wire to sound the drill hole after each advance of the drill and feel the far cortex. Ideally, the drill will exit just lateral to the vertebral artery, but the artery is at risk if the drill is too medially directed.
- Place each screw. Decorticate the lateral mass and lamina, and burr each joint. Cut and contour the rod, and secure the rod to the screws with the blockers.
- Pack the bone graft into place.
- Close the wound in layers over a drain.

60. What are the indications of spinal osteotomy in a young patient of ankylosing spondylitis? Enumerate osteotomy techniques and their principles. What are the potential complications of spinal osteotomy?

Ans: *Lumbar osteotomy*: To correct the flexion deformity that often develops in ankylosing spondylitis.
- Restricted field of vision is limited to a small area near the feet.
- Extremely difficult walking.
- Gastrointestinal symptoms resulting from pressure of the costal margin on the contents of the upper abdomen.
- Dysphagia or choking.

Cervical osteotomy may be indicated:
- To elevate the chin from the sternum, improving the appearance, the ability to eat, and the ability to see ahead.
- To prevent atlantoaxial and cervical subluxations and dislocations, which result from the weight of the head being carried forward by gravity.
- To relieve tracheal and esophageal distortion, which causes dyspnea and dysphagia.
- To prevent irritation of the spinal cord tracts or excessive traction on the nerve roots, which causes neurological disturbances.

Osteotomy techniques and their principles:

Lumbar osteotomy: The osteotomy usually is made at the upper lumbar level because the spinal canal here is large, and the osteotomy is distal to the end of the cord. A lumbar lordosis is created to compensate for the thoracic kyphosis; motion of the spine is not increased.

Osteotomy methods include resection of the spinous processes from the laminae to the pedicles, simple wedge resection of the spinous processes into the neural foramina, chevron excision of the laminae and spinous processes, and combined anterior opening wedge osteotomy after posterior resection of the spinous processes and laminae:
- *Smith–Petersen osteotomy*: The Smith–Petersen osteotomy is an excellent option for correction of smaller degrees of spinal deformity. Bone is removed through the pars and facet joints. If a previous fusion has been done, care should be taken to thin the fusion mass gradually until the ligamentum flavum or dura is exposed. Symmetrical resection is necessary to prevent creating a coronal deformity. Removal of the underlying ligament is also is helpful in preventing buckling of the dura or iatrogenic spinal stenosis. Approximately 10° of correction can be obtained with each 10 mm of resection. Excessive resection should be avoided because it may result in foraminal stenosis. In patients with degenerative disks, decreased flexibility may limit the amount of correction that can be obtained. The osteotomy is closed with compression or with in situ rod contouring, and bone graft is applied.

- *Pedicle subtraction osteotomy*: Pedicle subtraction osteotomy is best suited for patients who have significant sagittal imbalance of 4 cm or more and immobile or fused disks. Pedicle subtraction osteotomy is inherently safer than the Smith-Petersen osteotomy because it avoids multiple osteotomies. Typically, 30° or more of correction can be obtained with a single posterior osteotomy, preferably at the level of the deformity. If the deformity is at the spinal cord level, pedicle subtraction osteotomy can be used, but manipulation of the cord must be avoided. Care must be taken to avoid compression of the dura or creation of a coronal deformity. A wake-up test is done after correction and cancellous bone grafting have been completed.
- *Eggshell osteotomy*: The eggshell osteotomy requires anterior and posterior approaches and usually is reserved for severe sagittal or coronal imbalance of >10 cm from the midline. This is a spinal shortening procedure with anterior decancellization followed by removal of posterior elements, instrumentation, deformity correction, and fusion.

Cervical osteotomy:
The appropriate level for osteotomy is determined by the deformity and the degree of ossification of the anterior longitudinal ligament.
- Law successfully performed osteotomies at the levels of C3 and C4, C5 and C6, and C6 and C7. He fixed the spine internally with the plates devised by Wilson and Straub for use in lumbosacral arthrodesis. Wiring of the spinal processes, or use of a halo alone, also should be effective.
- In the osteotomy technique described by Simmons, decompression is done first and is extended into the neural foramina. After decompression and resection of the inferior aspect of the pedicles, extension manipulation is done.

Potential complications of spinal osteotomy:

Lumbar osteotomy:
- Danger of damaging the aorta, the inferior vena cava, and the major nerves to the lower extremities.
- If average correction from 80° to 44°, then hypertension, gastrointestinal problems, neurological defects, urinary tract infections, psychological problems, dural tears with leakage, and retrograde ejaculation can occur.
- Iatrogenic spinal stenosis
- Mortality

Cervical osteotomy:
- Overcorrection of the deformity leading to overstretching of trachea and esophagus that may become obstructed.
- If internal fixation is used for more postoperative stability, reoperation is required for adjustment of correction.

61. What is MISS surgery?
Ans: MISS stands for *M*inimally *I*nvasive *S*pine *S*urgery.
Please read Chapters no. 2 and 4C.

4C.9 SCHEUERMANN DISEASE (Q62-63)

62. Describe Scheuermann disease.
Ans: This is the most common cause of adolescent kyphosis (incidence as low as 0.4% to as high as 10%, varying with region). It is a rigid juvenile kyphosis associated with a growth disturbance of the vertebral endplates. The condition arises in prepubertal growth spurt becoming apparent by 10-12 years of age. The deformity is most commonly located in the thoracic spine (called type 1 with apex between T7 and T9) but could well be found in thoracolumbar (called type 2, apex between T10 and T12) and lumbar (L1 and below) region. The type 2 deformity is uncommon and was specifically referred to by Sorenson as "apprentice's spine".

The etiopathogenesis has not been fully understood (the universal histological finding has been abnormal vertebral endplate cartilage, irregular mineralization and disorders in vertebral ossification) but the following causes of the disease have been proposed:
- Osteonecrosis of the ring apophysis of vertebral body (Scheuermann, 1921).
- Herniation of the disk material into vertebral body (Schmorl nodes) causing disturbance of endochondral bone formation with subsequent wedging (Schmorl, 1930).

- Osteochondroses.
- Persistence of anterior vascular grooves in vertebral bodies creating a point of structural weakness (Ferguson, 1956).
- Transient osteoporosis (Bradford, 1976)—refuted.
- Hereditary (pattern still not established).
- Mechanical stress causing tightness of the anterior longitudinal ligament (Lambrinudi, 1934).
- Malabsorption, infection or endocrine disorders (growth hormone hypersecretion).
- Abnormal collagen and matrix of vertebral endplate cartilage, including decreased ratio between collagen and proteoglycan (Auf Der Maur, 1981).
- Biomechanical theory—vertebral body wedging is secondary to the increased anterior forces due to the first occurring kyphosis. Bilateral hamstring tension is a common finding resulting in focused bending stresses on the thoracic spine causing kyphosis consequent to Hueter-Volkmann law.

Natural history of disease: Ponte, et al. demonstrated that all curves greater than 45° progressed during the adolescent growth spurt and continued to increase after the age of 30 years. Bradford, et al. reported a higher incidence of disabling thoracic and lumbar back pain in untreated adults. There is often unremitting and incapacitating pain that is seen in 50% of patients during the adolescent growth spurt. These patients were more likely to have thoracic pain, had higher pain intensity readings, were more likely to work in sedentary jobs, and were more likely to be unmarried. There is usually no significant interference with the ADL.

Clinical presentation: Patients consult for their cosmetic deformity and back pain. The low back pain is due to lumbar hyperkyphosis compensation and consequent facet joint involvement. The pain may radiate to buttocks and lower extremities. It may awaken them from sleep in night.

Physical examination
- Thoracic kyphosis with sloping shoulders
- Forward posturing of the head and neck due to cervical hyperlordosis
- Adam's forward bend test: Slight truncal asymmetry associated with mild scoliosis:
  - When viewed from side, it shows posterior angulation of the thoracic spine.
- The deformity is not correctible by manipulation or postural changes
- Protuberant abdomen due to hyperlordosis in lumbar region
- Loss of lumbar lordosis (in lumbar kyphosis)—Flattened lumbar region.

Radiology: Obtain large 36 inch films.
- AP films may show scoliosis not exceeding 25°. It also helps in assessing skeletal maturity—Risser's sign.
- Lateral projection demonstrates kyphosis greater than 40°. There are various ways Scheuermann's kyphosis is defined on a lateral projection.

Sorenson's criteria (1964)—more than 5° of anterior wedging of minimum of three consecutive adjacent vertebral bodies at the apex of the kyphosis.

Drummond's criterion is minimum of two vertebral body wedging more than 5°.

Bradford criteria for diagnosis of Scheuermann's disease on lateral radiographs:
- The presence of a hyperkyphosis greater than 40°
- Irregular upper and lower vertebral endplates
- Wedging of more than 10° in one or more vertebrae
- The apparent loss of disk space height
- Irregular, flattened and wedged vertebral apophyseal lines
- Narrowing of the intervertebral disk spaces
- Variable presence of Schmorl's nodes.

Lumbar Scheuermann's will show—decreased lumbar lordosis or even a kyphotic deformity, the involved vertebrae have increased anteroposterior dimension than the uninvolved vertebrae. The lumbar vertebrae are scalloped with lucent defects at the anterosuperior corners.

Magnetic resonance imaging is needed in rapidly progressive cases of Scheuermann's disease as there may be thoracic spine stenosis. Also any neurological symptom mandates an evaluation of the spine by MRI. Preoperative evaluation by MRI is necessary for missing the neurology.

Management: *Conservative management* is aimed to control deformity progression and improve vertebral height by applying hyperextension force (Hueter-Volkman law). It has been envisaged that any amount of deformity can be corrected by conservative management in skeletally immature patients (Risser stage 2 or less), but this seems to be an overstatement. There is finding that deformities large to begin with bracing (>70°) loose correction quickly after removal of brace, so there is little ultimate correction in the end. Thus, ideally bracing will be indicated for immature spine with enough growth potential (Risser 2 or less) with curves around 60°.

Bracing the spine: Milwaukee brace is recommended for thoracic apex at T8 or above. There is also secondary impact on the lumbar curve and sagittal imbalance with the use of this brace. For curve apex below T9 a TLSO (thoracolumbosacral orthosis) is used with anterior sterna and infraclavicular outriggers to avoid extension moment superior to apex. Bracing should be done full time initially removing only for hygiene maintenance and exercises.

There are two distinct radiological types of patients: One is the Sorenson type with multiple small wedging of vertebra distributed over few segments. These patients respond well to bracing and achieve faster correction so bracing is given full-time to them for 9–18 months (depending on individual correction). The other type is the Bradford type with single apical edging that is quite remarkable. These patients respond late and it is recommended to continue bracing in them full-time till apical remodeling is done (5° remaining wedge only). Programed reduction in wearing time (2–4 hours intervals) can be advocated with deformity correction gradually; however, the bracing is continued till skeletal maturity in part-time (say night-time) application.

Risser casts: Passive correction on lateral bolster radiograph is less than 40%, brace treatment is not likely to be effective. Risser casts can be applied in a serial fashion to produce more correction of the kyphosis. Two or three casts (changed every 2–3 months) are applied to progressively correct the deformity. They provide better long-term angular correction, with lower loss of correction and lesser deterioration despite less initial correction. The cast correction is then maintained by brace application.

Surgical treatment: Considering the limited functional loss and if there is no self-image distortion with the rounded back, surgical treatment was fraught with caution in these patients, particularly due to high complication rates. Now with newer implant systems and segmental fixation techniques interest has risen in improving the deformity and function of these patients.

The typical indications for a Scheuermann's kyphosis are:
- Patients with pain
- Rigid deformity
- Curve more than 70–75° or progressive deformity: In immature patients, the lower value is the indication (despite brace treatment) while in adults curves higher than larger value need surgery.
- Unacceptable cosmetic appearance.

The management principles for deformity correction in Scheuermann's kyphosis have been anterior column lengthening and posterior column shortening so a standard two-stage corrective procedure comprising anterior release and fusion is commonly performed.

Further, there was observed a frequent loss of initial correction with previously practiced posterior only techniques and increased rigidity of large curves in adults often mandates anterior release. There is a concern that attempt to correct deformity more than 50% of the preoperative deformity may lead to development of junctional kyphosis, so commonly up to 50% of the deformity magnitude is corrected.

Fusion should include the proximal most tilted vertebral body into the kyphosis while distally the caudal extent of fusion should include the first lordotic disk space. Stable vertebra (till where the fusion should usually extend) can be defined for fusion. It is the lumbar vertebra most closely bisected by the posterior sacral line. The vertebra just proximal to the stable vertebra can be used for distal fusion level if the proximal disk is lordotic. In case the disk above the stable vertebra is kyphotic then fusion has to be extended to one level below.

63. Discuss pathology, differential diagnosis of Scheuermann's disease.

Ans: Scheuermann proposed that the kyphosis resulted from osteonecrosis of the ring apophysis of the vertebral body. The results of clinical and genetic investigation suggest that Scheuermann's disease is a genetically dependent pathology inherited in autosomal dominant manner resulting in discordant vertebral endplate mineralization and ossification during growth, causing disproportional vertebral body growth with the resultant classic wedge-shaped vertebral bodies that lead to kyphosis.

Differential diagnosis:
- Postural kyphosis
- Scoliosis
- Ankylosing spondylitis
- Postsurgical kyphosis

4C.10 DIFFUSE IDIOPATHIC SKELETAL HYPEROSTOSIS (Q64)

64. Describe clinical features, pathology, and radiological features of DISH.

Ans: DISH stands for diffuse idiopathic skeletal hyperostosis.

Clinical features:

Spinal: The usual presentation is a middle-aged or older patient with mild, chronic back pain in the middle to lower spine and stiffness. For extraspinal manifestations, bilateral involvement is characteristic.

- *Thoracic spine*:
  - The thoracic spine is the most commonly involved segment.
  - Thoracic myelopathy has been reported but is rare.
- *Cervical spine*:
  - Pain and stiffness of the neck may be prominent symptoms but are rarely, if ever, the presenting complaints. Involvement of the cervical spine is less reported than involvement of the lumbar or thoracic spine.
  - Dysphagia may result from large cervical syndesmophytes, which are present in as many as 28% of patients with DISH.
  - Hoarseness, sleep apnea, stridor, aspiration pneumonia, thoracic outlet syndrome and difficulty with intubation have all been reported due to syndesmophytes.
  - Ossification of the posterior longitudinal ligament (PLL) not uncommon in DISH and cervical cord compression from osteophytes can cause cervical myelopathy, as well as C1–C2 atlantoaxial pseudarthrosis and subluxation.
- *Lumbar spine*:
  - Patients often complain of low back pain or stiffness but without the presence of changes on lumbar radiographs, so association of back pain with DISH is not established.
  - Significant compression of the inferior vena cava due to large anterior osteophytic excrescences has been reported.
- *Traumatic changes*:
  - Patients with DISH are vulnerable for fracture from even minor trauma (hyperextension injury) to the fused spine that may result in pseudarthrosis. The increased incidence of fracture instability in these patients is due to long lever arm of fused vertebral segments proximal and distal to the fracture even in low-energy injuries.

Concerns with these injuries include:
- Delay in diagnosis and a high rate of immediate and delayed neurologic consequences.
- They occur in the middle or at the ends of ankylosed segments so difficult to visualize and fix.
- Must be carefully evaluated for occult fracture with computed tomography or magnetic resonance imaging.

Extraspinal: Tendinitis and enthesophytes (osseous outgrowths at the sites of attachment of tendon, ligament or capsule to bone) are the most common findings but their association with symptoms is unclear. Subtle periostitis at the site of ligament or tendon insertion is also common. The characteristic findings associated with DISH are usually bilateral and symmetrical.

Pelvis
- Enthesophytes are seen in the iliac wing and ischial tuberosity along with calcification of the sacrotuberous and iliolumbar ligaments.
- Periarticular osteophytes about the hip, sacroiliac joints, and symphysis pubis can often be found.
- Bone proliferation (whiskering) can be seen at sites of ligament and tendon attachment.
- To differentiate from ankylosing spondylitis, bone erosions in the sacroiliac joints and at the sites of ligament attachment are generally absent in DISH, but bridging or nonbridging osteophytes about the sacroiliac joint have been seen.

Hip
- Hip involvement is variable, with some patients having few or no pathologic changes.
- Those with signs and symptoms may have periarticular bone proliferation with an intact joint space, hyperostosis with a narrowed joint space, or osteonecrosis, none of these findings are solely attributed to DISH and can be seen at any stage as due to age-related changes.

Knee
- Patients with DISH have a much higher prevalence (nearly 30%) of knee changes, compared to normal population.
- Tendinous ossification is seen in quadriceps mechanism associated with often patellar hyperostosis and large osseous excrescences on the poles.
- A prominent tibial spine is the most common finding but incidence of symptomatic osteoarthritis of the knee is not higher than other population.

Foot and ankle
- Most of the DISH patients (more than three-fourth) have manifestations involving the foot and ankle.
- Any bone in the foot may exhibit hyperostosis due to numerous sites of ligament and tendon attachment that make spur formation frequent.
- Achilles tendinitis is common.
- Calcaneal spurs are frequent (seen in three-fourths of DISH patient population compared to around one-fifth of normal population).
- The cortex of the calcaneus may be thickened.
- Calcification of the Achilles tendon or plantar fascia may be seen but have no definite relation with symptoms.
- The presence of large calcaneal spurs in the setting of Achilles tendinitis or plantar fasciitis should lead one to consider DISH as an underlying diagnosis.
- Talar beaking due to enthesophytes may be seen, other sites for spur formation include medial navicular, lateral and plantar cuboid, and the base of the fifth metatarsal.

Shoulder
- Irregular osseous excrescences can occur at the deltoid tubercle, the greater and lesser tuberosities, inferior glenoid, distal clavicle, as well as at the sites of attachment of the coracoclavicular ligaments. These changes are variably associated with pain, stiffness, and loss of motion.

Elbow
- Enthesophytes around elbow contrary to other places are frequently symptomatic.
- Spurs on the olecranon are frequently seen in DISH.
- Hyperostosis can occur along the distal medial humerus.

Hand and wrist
- Similar to feet, cortical thickening may be seen in the tubular bones, along with hyperostosis and spur formation in periarticular sites.
- The distal phalangeal tufts may appear pointed ("arrow-heading"). Soft-tissue and cartilage hypertrophy are present in acromegaly but not in DISH.

Ribs
- Hyperostosis of the ribs also has been noted in patients with DISH. Typically, it affects the posteromedial aspect of the rib (no definite clinical significance).

Pathology: Focal and diffuse calcification and ossification of anterior longitudinal ligament, degeneration of peripheral annulus fibrosus fibers, anterolateral extension of fibrous tissue, hypervascularity, chronic inflammatory cellular infiltration, periosteal new bone formation on anterior surface of vertebral bodies.

Radiological features: Diffuse idiopathic skeletal hyperostosis radiological changes in axial skeleton are thoracic spine centric, so much so that changes are most prominent in this region, and with cervical spine affection, the lower vertebrae, and for lumbar spine, the upper lumbar vertebrae are commonly affected.

The characteristic features seen in axial skeleton are:
- *Thoracic spine*: Large syndesmophytes and flowing, laminated new-bone formation along the anterolateral margins of vertebral bodies.
- The syndesmophytes project horizontally from the vertebral bodies with the classic appearance of flowing candle wax, becoming confluent to form an extra-articular ankylosis (*cf.* vertically oriented "bamboo spine" outgrowths in ankylosing spondylitis).
- The syndesmophytes are more prominent on the right side (they are reduced to left side due to effect of pulsatile aorta), whereas they are commonly symmetrical in the cervical and lumbar spine.
- Hyperostosis of posterior elements is rare, although hyperostosis of costovertebral joints may be present. Osteopenia (commonly seen in ankylosing spondylitis) is not a feature of DISH. Patients with DISH are quite protected against osteoporosis also.
- Facet articulations and disk spaces are generally preserved and their involvement goes in favor of age-related spine changes rather DISH.
- In *cervical spine,* radiographic findings are most common in the lower segments and less prevalent at the more cephalad levels. Ossification and loss of elasticity occur along the anterior paravertebral tissues, such as the anterior longitudinal ligament.
- In the cervical spine, the changes in canal diameter, alignment, and mobility of motion segments not only cause neck pain and stiffness but put patients with DISH at risk for severe neurologic injury.
- Ligamentum flavum hypertrophy, dystrophic calcification of spinal ligaments (including ossification of the PLL), and mild cervical kyphosis can occur, occasionally resulting in cervical spinal stenosis and myelopathy.
- Lumbar spine: Radiographic evidence of DISH in the lumbar spine is most frequently seen in the upper levels and is less common caudally (thoracic centric disease); the syndesmophytes are more confluent and may take appearance of "parrot beak".
- Degenerative changes are common between the fourth lumbar and first sacral vertebrae due to the exacerbated stress imposed on the lumbosacral area by a stiff spine superiorly.
- Technetium bone scanning can show increased uptake in areas of involvement, which may be confused with evidence of periarticular metastatic disease.

4C.11 FILUM TERMINALE SYNDROME (Q65)

65. Discuss filum terminale syndrome.

Ans: Also known as tethered cord syndrome. It refers to a low-lying conus medullaris with a thickened (>2 mm diameter) filum. It may also include fibrolipomatous infiltration and, rarely, abnormal extension of the central canal. The cord reaches up to lower lumbar and the sacral vertebrae. Though generally associated with a low lying conus (the "classic" type), TCS is also seen in a normally positioned conus (dorsal or ventral tethering of the cord).

Pathogenesis: The mechanism of development of TCS is obscure. Tethering of cord is theoretically possible at two points—one at the site where an extrinsic lesion such as a dermal sinus tract traverses through the dura and another at the caudal attachment of the conus to a taut or fatty filum.

Either or both tethers may be present in any given case and they need to be individually addressed. Filum terminale normally anchors the conus to the sacral bony vertebral canal and suspends the entire lower cord in the buoyant CSF. A taut (short fibrous) or a thick (fat infiltrated) filum is inelastic and results in tension on the conus. Not only the filum abnormalities but the cord movement may also be limited by anomalous fixity to a dorsal (e.g., lumbosacral lipoma, dermal sinus tracts, congenital inclusion tumors like dermoids and epidermoids) or ventral structure (e.g., bony diastema, neurenteric cyst). There is a high likelihood of reduced blood supply to stretched cord due to diminished microcirculation producing ischemia, hypoxia, and impaired oxidative metabolism at cellular level. Traction injury probably results due to an altered growth rate between the spinal cord and column, combined with traction forces implied by contraction of the tissue within the abnormal filum. The process of tethering is more dynamic than this. Mechanisms additionally suggested that may finally culminate into tethering include:

- Hemorrhage and inflammation in the developing caudal cord in early fetal life
- Non-neoplastic growth of fat in the fatty filum
- Lumbosacral cord lipomata
- Progressive accumulation of putty material in congenital inclusion tumors and ensuing chemical meningitis
- Exogenous infection tracking along a dermal sinus tract.

These are mostly a combination of these results in evolution of fibrous intradural bands which tether the cord. However, none explains the ectatic dural sac, the bifid vertebrae, and the associated cutaneous and subcutaneous lesions.

Clinical features: The functional deficits in TCS may result from traction, compression or a combination of these. The lower motor neuron (LMN) symptoms are considered to be an effect of mechanical compression while the upper motor neuron (UMN) symptoms apparently result from ischemia and traction injury. The large fibers of the tracts cranial to the site of tethering are the most susceptible to injury.

Neurological deficits: Often a patchy, asymmetric combination of UMN (spasticity, hyper-reflexia) and LMN (atrophy, hyporeflexia) symptoms referable to the conus and the lumbosacral nerves occurs.

Motor deficits are more evident than sensory aberrations.

Orthopedic manifestations: These are trophic ulcers (painless) and deformities (foot deformities most commonly pes cavus, limb length discrepancies, scoliosis, gluteal asymmetry, gait disturbances).

Urological abnormalities: These are frequency, urgency, incontinence, and urinary infections. Cutaneous stigmata are often multiple and they occur in 50–70% of all. These neurocutaneous markers can be classified into:
- *High-risk category*—atypical midline lumbosacral dimples (larger than 5 mm, located more than 25 mm cranial to the anal verge, directed cranially), hemangiomas, protruding lesions (masses, hairy patch, tails), and multiple cutaneous stigmata. These require further investigations to evaluate underlying TCS or occult spinal dysraphism.
- *Low-risk category* markers include coccygeal pits, simple dimples, discolorations, and deviated gluteal fold.

Investigations: Plain radiographs—these are too insensitive to detect spinal cord malformations to merit any use. Occasional L5–S1 bifid spine or scoliosis may even be a normal finding. Ultrasonography is a useful investigation but quite operator dependent:
- Pulsations are reduced in tethered cord
- Level of conus can be easily documented
- Detailed images of meninges and cord can be documented along within the filum terminale till 4–5 months of gestation after which the acoustic window is dampened and details are not very prominent.
- MRI—modality of choice for anatomical detailing
- Sagittal T1- and T2-weighted images demonstrate the level of the conus.
- T1-weighted axial images illustrate the fat in the terminal filum and facilitate measuring its diameter.

Voiding cystourethrogram and urodynamic studies—the earliest features of subclinical neurovesical dysfunction are detrusor hyper-reflexia and detrusor sphincter dyssynergia resulting in vesicoureteral reflux.

Treatment: Operative treatment is preferred in many and is essential in symptomatic patients. Only in asymptomatic patients, the views of surgeons regarding surgical release of tether are controversial. The aim of surgical management is

restoring the normal mobility of spinal cord by eliminating the tethering structures and resuspending the freed conus and spinal nerves in the CSF. The following are some of the commonly performed surgical procedures:
- Sectioning of the filum reverses clinical and urodynamic deficits in a subset of the symptomatic tight or fatty filum terminale
- Laminectomy and detethering of the cord
- Excision/debulking of cord lipoma/dermoid or epidermoid
- Excision of the bony/fibrous diastema.

4C.12 KLIPPEL-FEIL SYNDROME (Q66)

66. Describe Klippel-Feil syndrome.

Ans: Klippel-Feil syndrome is a congenital fusion of the cervical vertebrae that may involve two segments, a congenital block vertebra, or the entire cervical spine. Congenital cervical fusion is a result of failure of normal segmentation of the cervical somites during the third to eighth week of life. The skeletal system may not be the only system affected during this time; cardiorespiratory, genitourinary, and auditory systems frequently are involved. In most patients, the exact cause is unknown. One proposed cause is a primary vascular disruption during embryonic development that results in fusion of the cervical vertebrae and other associated anomalies.

The classic features of Klippel-Feil syndrome are a short neck, low posterior hairline, and limited range of neck motion. Patients may consult an orthopedist because of neurological problems, because of signs of instability of the cervical spine, or for cosmetic reasons. Because many patients are asymptomatic, the actual incidence of this condition is unknown, but estimates in the literature range from 1 in 42,400 births to 3 in 700. There is a slight male predominance (1.5:1).

Feil classified the syndrome into three types: type I, block fusion of all cervical and upper thoracic vertebrae; type II, fusion of one or two pairs of cervical vertebrae; and type III, cervical fusion in combination with lower thoracic or lumbar fusion. Minimally involved patients with Klippel-Feil syndrome lead normal, active lives with no significant restrictions or symptoms. More severely involved patients have a good prognosis if genitourinary, cardiopulmonary, and auditory problems are treated early.

In patients with Klippel-Feil syndrome, neurological compromise, ranging from radiculopathy to quadriplegia to death, can occur. The neurological symptoms are caused by occipitocervical anomalies, instability, or degenerative joint and disk disease. Instability and degenerative joint diseases are common when two fused areas are separated by a single open interspace. Patients with multiple short areas of fusion (three or more vertebrae) separated by more than one open interspace do not develop instability or degenerative joint disease as frequently, possibly because of a more equal distribution of stress in the cervical spine.

Associated conditions: Scoliosis, renal anomalies, cardiovascular anomalies, deafness, synkinesis, respiratory anomalies, sprengel deformity, and cervical ribs.

Clinical features: The classic clinical presentation of Klippel-Feil syndrome is the triad of a low posterior hairline, a short neck, and limited neck motion. Many patients with Klippel-Feil syndrome have a normal appearance, and the syndrome is diagnosed through incidental radiographs. Shortening of the neck and a low posterior hairline are not constant findings and may be overlooked; webbing of the neck (pterygium colli) is seen in severe involvement. The most constant clinical finding is limitation of neck motion. Rotation and lateral bending are affected more than flexion and extension. If fewer than three vertebrae are fused or if the lower cervical vertebrae are fused, motion is only slightly limited.

Radiographs: Routine radiographs, tomograms, cineradiograms, CT scans, and MRI may be useful in the evaluation of Klippel-Feil syndrome. Adequate radiographs can be difficult to obtain in severely involved children, but initial examination should include anteroposterior, odontoid, and lateral flexion and extension views of the cervical spine. Lateral flexion-extension views are the most important to identify atlantoaxial instability or instability near an open segment between two congenitally fused areas. If routine lateral radiographs are difficult to interpret, lateral flexion-extension tomograms can be obtained. Spinal canal narrowing can occur from degenerative osteophytes or from congenital spinal stenosis. If enlargement of the spinal canal is evident on radiographs, syringomyelia, hydromyelia, or Arnold-Chiari malformation should be suspected. In young patients with Klippel-Feil syndrome, serial lateral flexion-extension views should be obtained to evaluate instability at the atlantoaxial joint or at an open interspace between fused areas. Development of congenital or idiopathic scoliosis should be documented by radiographic examination of the entire spine.

Treatment: Mechanical symptoms caused by degenerative joint disease usually respond to traction, a cervical collar, and analgesics. Neurological symptoms should be evaluated carefully to locate the exact pathological condition; surgical stabilization with or without decompression may be required. Prophylactic fusion of a hypermobile segment is controversial. The risk of neurological compromise must be weighed against the further reduction in neck motion, and this decision must be made for each patient individually. Cosmetic improvement after surgery has been limited, but surgical correction of Sprengel deformity can significantly improve appearance, and occasionally soft-tissue procedures such as Z-plasty and muscle resection improve cosmesis. Partial thoracoplasty is performed as a two-stage procedure: removal of the upper four ribs on one side and, after the patient has recovered from the first surgery, removal of the upper four ribs on the other side.

CHAPTER 5

Neoplasia

5.1 SKELETAL METASTASIS AND MANAGEMENT (Q1–6)

1. Explain clinical workup and laboratory diagnosis of metastatic bone tumors. Outline the management of these in long bones.

Ans:

Clinical Workup
The patient with a metastatic disease usually presents in one of the following ways:
- Pathological fracture or neurological compromise (spine lesions may even have cauda equina syndrome)
- Referral from oncologist/surgeon/radiologist
- Referral for unexplained generalized musculoskeletal pain.

Pain: The most common but most inconsistent symptom in presentation. Pain may range from a dull ache to deep intense pain. It usually gets exacerbated by weight-bearing and is often worse at night or at rest. Ironically the pain is usually partially improved with activity unless associated with pathological fracture. A progressive and unrelenting pain nonresponsive to symptomatic treatment usually indicates invasion of adjacent tissues or pathological fracture. There is associated loss of appetite, weight loss, and fatigue with loss of interest in usual activities.

Hypercalcemia [mediated by parathyroid hormone-related protein (PTHrp) from tumor cells] is seen in some 10% of patients with metastatic disease commonly with breast cancer, multiple myeloma (MM), and squamous lung cancer.

Bone loss (osteopenia/porosis) is multifactorial and may not solely result from primary metastatic lesions. Treatment of primary cancer also is associated with bone loss. Aromatase inhibitors (used for breast and ovarian cancers), oophorectomy (for ovarian cancers and breast cancer), and orchiectomy (for prostate cancer) and use of gonadotropin-releasing hormone (GnRH) analogs that produce hypogonadism lead to bone loss. Use of corticosteroids and radiation therapy has direct effect on bone strength.

Pathological fractures: Bone loss predispose to development of pathological fractures in metastatic bone disease.

The following history should be elucidated in these patients as part of evaluation:
- Use of or change in assistive devices for ambulation—loss of ambulatory ability is a poor prognostic factor
- Personal history—smoking, alcohol, and other drug abuse
- Professional history—exposure to asbestos/aerosols
- Details of noticing any shortness of breath, chest pain, pleuritic pain, hemoptysis (pulmonary), hematemesis (esophageal/gastric), gastritis, alteration in urinary (increased frequency or pain) or bowel habits (alternating constipation/diarrhea), rectal bleeding, blood in urine or at end of micturition, heat or cold intolerance (thyroid neoplasm). Changes or appearance of soft tissue swelling(s), changes in appearance of skin spots (melanoma) should also be inquired.
- Enquire about the documentation of screening tests—Pap smear, mammogram, prostate examination, colonoscopy, etc.
- Past history of cancer or related treatment (radiotherapy/chemotherapy)
- Family history of cancer.

Physical Examination
Accurate note of tender spots, bones, joints, and swellings should be made. Spine tenderness, range of motion (ROM) of involved joints and spine, and deformity should be noted. Presence of limp, sensory—motor deficit should be recorded.

Additionally per abdomen, per rectal examination, examination of breast, and thyroid should be thoroughly done for evaluation of any clinically identifiable primary. One should evaluate costovertebral angle (renal lesion) and examine the lymph node chains for localization or lymphoma.

Laboratory Diagnosis

A complete hemogram and blood count along with erythrocyte sedimentation rate, urinalysis, and blood chemistry for liver and renal function should be obtained. For suspected myeloma, urine and serum electrophoresis with immunofixation should be done. B2-microglobulin levels should be measured for staging. Based on clinical suspicion, specific blood tests or markers can be done that include carcinoembryonic antigen (colon and pancreas), thyroid function tests, prostate-specific antigen, and cancer antigen-125 (ovarian tumor). Urinary N-telopeptide of type I collagen (urinary NTX) correlate with occurrence of skeletal-related events (SREs) and are being increasingly under focus **(Flowchart 5.1.1)**.

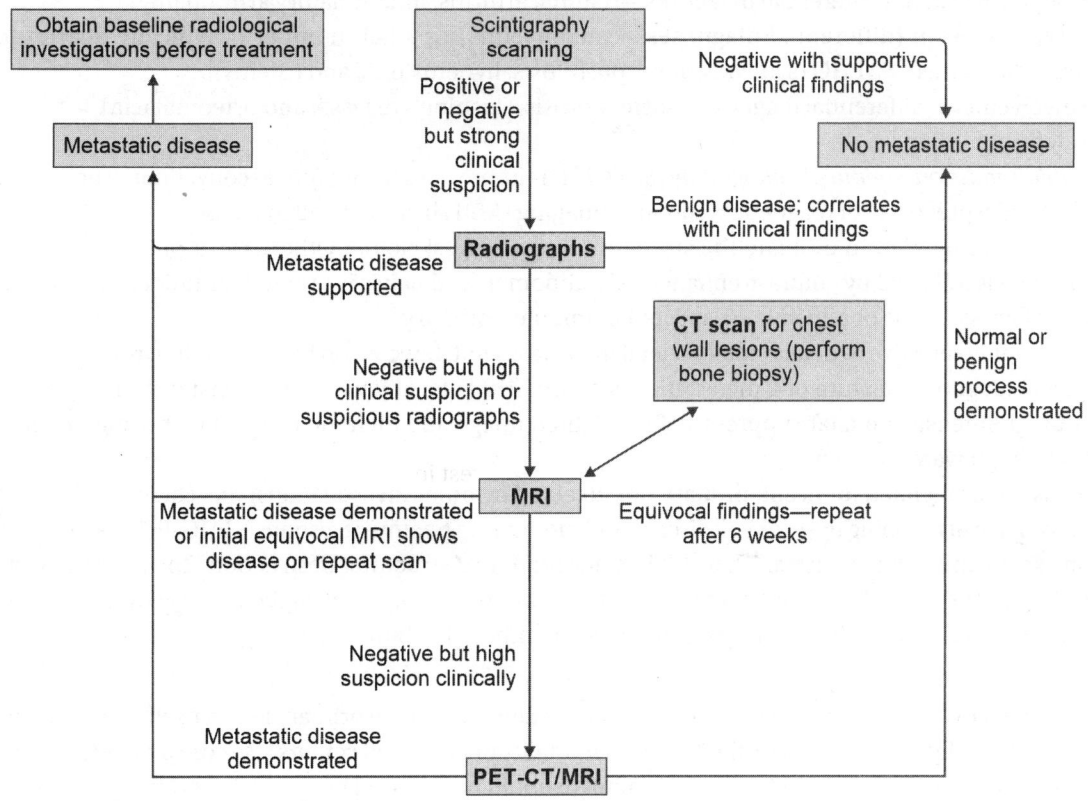

Flowchart 5.1.1: Laboratory diagnosis of metastatic bone tumor.

Imaging and Radiological Workup

To identify primary the following battery of test is currently recommended. Plain radiographs of the whole bone involved by the lesion, computed tomography (CT) scan of the chest, abdomen and pelvis with contrast, and bone scan. Biopsy of the lesion is then done for pathological correlation. This strategy reveals primary in 85% patients. Completion of staging is also done with identification of the primary. This is important if a sarcoma is found then an inappropriate biopsy may preclude limb salvage, if a renal cell carcinoma is found then preoperative embolization is preferred.

There is great deal of confusion on evaluation of treatment response—while most physicians utilize sophisticated investigations for evaluation of bone metastasis the criteria have not till recently included these in treatment evaluation. The diagnostic algorithm commonly practiced for evaluation is given in adjacent table.

Plain X-rays reveal a solitary or multiple, localized or diffuse, small or large usually lytic lesion(s). Skeletal survey should be ordered as a preliminary investigation that includes radiographs of pelvis, long bones, chest, skull, and spine (dorsolumbar region). The lytic lesions are common with metastasis from lung, kidney, thyroid, and colonic malignancies and MM and lymphomas are also osteolytic. Lytic lesions are identified on X-ray with 25–50% loss of bone mineral at the site, hence radiographs are quite insensitive and probably the stage for pathological fracture is already set by then. Metastasis from lung neoplasia may be located to cortical regions of bone. Osteoblastic lesions are seen with prostate and breast malignancy metastasis, but lytic lesions are seen with advanced prostate lesions and mixed appearance is common with breast malignancies.

Technetium Tc-99 bone scan identifies the bone lesion(s) avidly and is quite sensitive. Additionally, it has the advantage of scanning all the skeletal sites at reasonable cost. It can also be used as a guide to identify "easier" site for bone biopsy. It is recommended as the initial modality for investigating bone metastasis. The lesions appear hot on scan unless the metastasis is from pure osteolytic aggressive lesion that has minimal or no osteoblastic activity (few renal cell carcinomas, multiple myeloma). Fluorodeoxyglucose-positron emission tomography (FDG-PET) may be used to identify such bone scan negative lesions. Positive scan is defined by:
- Multiple focal typically distributed lesions (random distribution)—obtain radiographs definitely for future assessment of treatment response and SREs
- Multiple atypical lesions (differential diagnoses—trauma, arthritis, inflammatory arthropathy)
- Solitary typical lesion (differential diagnoses—osteomyelitis) or small number of typically distributed lesions [differential diagnoses—SAPHO (synovitis, acne, pustulosis, hyperostosis, and osteitis)]
- Diffuse involvement (differential diagnoses—osteoporosis, Cushing's disease, and osteomalacia)
- Photon-deficient lesions.

Single-photon emission computed tomography (SPECT) has improved sensitivity over conventional bone scan for small metastasis but widespread use of magnetic resonance imaging (MRI) has superseded its use.

CT scan is recommended to evaluate the structural integrity of skeleton. Otherwise, a preliminary ultrasound of abdomen and pelvis followed by contrast-enhanced CT abdomen and pelvis is ordered for unidentified primary. High-resolution CT of chest can be obtained for suspected pulmonary primary.

MRI scan is highly sensitive to detect small skeletal metastases not detected on bone scans as it reveals abnormal bone marrow. Typical diagnostic feature of a metastatic lesion on MRI is focal low-signal intensity on a T1-weighted image and a mix-to-high intensity on a fat-suppressed T1-weighted image and high intensity on a T2-weighted image due to marrow edema (high water content).

FDG-PET is recommended for occult primary not detected by other investigations; this can be ordered and has the additional advantage of mapping the extent of disease and monitoring treatment response. FDG-PET detects metabolically active lesions so it can detect metastasis that still has not produced structural destruction. The sensitivity of FDG-PET varies according to the type of metastasis, and for this reason, the sensitivity is higher for osteolytic lesions (multiple myeloma) but less for osteoblastic lesions (prostate) when compared to bone scan.

Bone Biopsy
Biopsy is performed to confirm the suspicion of primary or to know about the primary lesion itself. Fine needle aspiration cytology (FNAC) (usually image guided) is the preferred modality in dedicated centers else core biopsy (preferred) or even open biopsy can be done. Principles of bone tumor biopsy should be followed but most importantly it should be done at a center (or at least guided by it) that is going to manage the patient finally. Site errors of biopsy have caused patients to lose their limb in past. Most of the spinal lesions require image guidance in the form of ultrasound or better a CT scan. For a blastic lesion, multiple samples should be obtained to increase yield of biopsy for representative tissue.

Management: Kindly refer Answer to Question 2.

2. Explain the management of skeletal metastasis.
Ans: Bone metastasis is a systemic disease. Currently, the standard of care for skeletal metastasis is a combined multimodality approach that includes pain management, systemic therapy (bone modifying agents, chemotherapy, hormone therapy), radiation therapy, and radiopharmaceuticals, and surgery depending on patient factors (fragility, prognosis of tumor), tumor factors (aggressive lesion vs moderate, extensive vs limited disease, sensitivity to chemotherapeutic agents, etc.), site factors (single vs multiple lesion, location of lesion in skeleton—periarticular, diaphyseal, metaphyseal, etc.). Recently image-guided percutaneous cryoablation, radiofrequency ablation, focused ultrasound (MRI-guided high-intensity focused ultrasound), and cementoplasty have been variably used and recommended for isolated or limited metastasis. Some of these claim immediate and lasting pain relief but large trials are required for definite indications and

recommendations. In all, early and aggressive management yields better quality of life and functional independence. A simple algorithm is provided in the **Flowchart 5.1.2**.

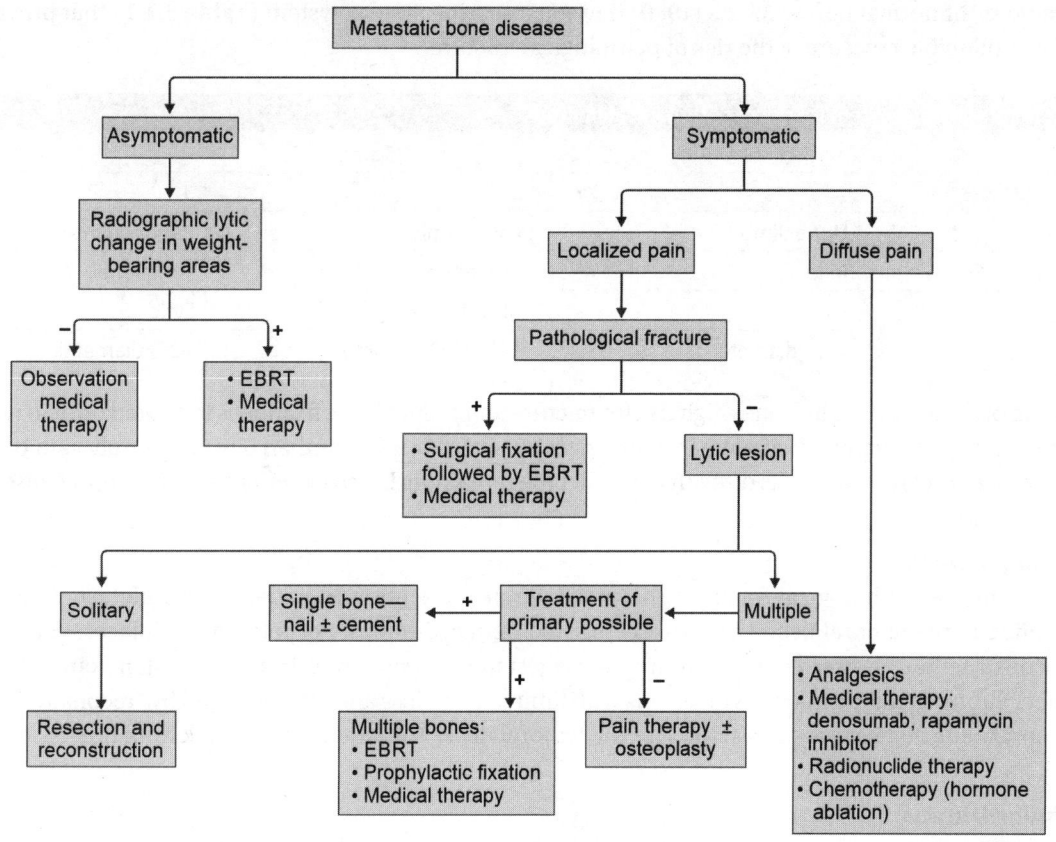

Flowchart 5.1.2: Management of bone metastasis.

The need of the orthopedic surgery
The common needs of surgical intervention include:
- Maximize pain control and tumor control locally
- Prophylactic fixation of bones with a risk of pathological fracture due to metastasis
- Stabilization of pathological fracture
- Reconstruction of periarticular metastasis
- Management of spinal instability and neurological symptoms due to cord/nerve compression.

The primary *aim of surgical intervention* is to relieve pain and restore function of the limb. The *orthopedic principles* followed for management of pathological fractures occurring in metastatic bone disease include:
- Providing immediate stability, allowing weight bearing
- Treatment is done assuming that the fracture may not unite
- The fixation should aim to last the lifetime of the patient
- To stabilize all the affected parts of bone and all "necessary" bones (as required to achieve above aim).

Fracture Risk Assessment

Plain radiographs are neither sensitive nor reliable to measure cortical destruction and loss of bone strength due to lack of three-dimensional evaluation. Fidler (1973) suggested that a long bone lesion with more than 50% cortical destruction should be prophylactically stabilized.

Harrington (1982) recommended prophylactic surgery to femur if there is:
- Destruction of 50% of a single cortex of any long bone (in any radiological view)
- Avulsion of the lesser trochanter

- Lesion in proximal femur that is more than or equal to 2.5 cm in any dimension
- Pain with weight bearing that persists, increases or recurs following radiotherapy.

Weakened bone produces an "open section" defect where stress gets concentrated and fracture occurs with minor trauma/twisting movement. These fractures are low-energy and soft tissue injury is minor compared conventional traumatic fractures of normal bones. *Mirels* (1989) devised a scoring system system **(Table 5.1.1)** that provides a more reliable and reproducible measure of the risk of pathological fracture.

TABLE 5.1.1: Mirel's scoring system for risk of pathological fracture.

Variable	Score		
	1	2	3
Site	Upper limb	Lower limb	Peritrochanter
Pain	Mild	Moderate	Functional
Lesion	Blastic	Mixed	Lytic
Size	<1/3 diameter	1/3 to 2/3 diameter	>2/3 diameter

Mirel's score of eight or above indicates high risk for fracture and prophylactic fixation is indicated prior to radiotherapy. It is imperative but to understand that patients with short life expectancy (less than 6 weeks) rarely gain useful benefit from surgical procedures; however, it is difficult to predict the remaining life so experience and thorough discussion with family should preside.

Fractures Around the Hip
It is the most common pathological fractures that need surgical attention in patients with metastatic bone disease. For lesion limited to the femoral neck or head, a cemented hemiarthroplasty or total joint replacement is modality of choice for reconstruction. Short stem implants are the biggest mistake surgeons do and long-stem femoral implants are recommended. Subtrochanteric fractures or lesions with limited bone loss are best stabilized by "reconstruction" nails or proximal femoral nails that have locking screws up the femoral neck. This also protects neck from the risk of subsequent femoral neck fracture.

Pelviacetabular Disease
This region is difficult to approach surgically and prophylactic palliative radiotherapy is commonly used to control symptoms. Periacetabular lesions have tendency for central migration of the femoral head due to soft acetabular floor. Such lesions could be reconstructed with massive (composite) allograft and special implants with antiprotrusio reconstruction cage, multi hole cups, threaded rods, pins, elastic nails (cut and shaped into the defect), and reinforcement rings. Bone cement is often used to augment the construction strength. Extensive radiotherapy to this region has high chances of radiation osteonecrosis of the femoral head and subsequent pain.

Shoulder Girdle and Upper Limb
Metastatic lesions of shoulder girdle usually managed with radiotherapy alone. Humeral head lesions are best treated by hemiarthroplasty. Limited glenoid involvement can be managed with total shoulder or reverse shoulder replacement. For forearm bones (acral metastasis), the lesions are limited in size and stresses are low; it is effectively managed with plate fixation and cement augmentation. Elastic nailing with cement augmentation is another option.

Shafts of Major Long Bones (Humerus, Femur, and Tibia)
Reamed interlocked intramedullary nailing (preferably unreamed for renal metastasis) is the modality of choice for treatment of cortical breach or pathological fractures through metastatic lesions of long bones. This prevents telescoping and locked nail gives torsional stability. It is imperative that following reaming the tumor cells that spread through the medullary canal are "controlled" or "killed" by postoperative radiotherapy. The entire bone and operative site should be included in the postoperative radiotherapy field. The benefits of reaming outwit the intramedullary contamination for a palliative therapy, unlike for a primary bone tumor where reaming could be disaster and nailing may spread the tumor throughout the canal ("rodding" a sarcoma) precluding a potentially limb salvaging surgery (thus biopsy confirmation is a must). Ideally load-bearing implants are suited for palliation (for immediate mobilization); however, plating will provide limited length coverage and bones may get weaker in proximal or distal unprotected region with spread of the

disease. Large diameter nails (preferably solid, need customization) are a better option that circumvent these problems and give good stability. Some large bone defects can be packed/reconstructed with stainless steel mesh and bone cement in addition to stabilization with an intramedullary nail. It should be remembered that the chosen implant takes care of all the lesions of the bone and none is left through which a fracture can occur. Isolated lesions in diaphysis that are amenable to resection can be excised and filled with "segmental spacers". For lesions of distal humerus and distal tibia the surgical treatment has to be customized and often is not easy. Functional cast brace as external support with radiation therapy is the recommendation for such nonreconstructable lesions. For "limited lesions" (isolated lesions at these sites viz. the elbow, ankle, and possibly the knee) a viable option is curettage, cementation, and internal fixation. Distal and proximal tibial isolated lesions are also managed this way. A further method for managing the distal tibial and distal humeral lesions that encroach articular cartilage is endoprosthetic reconstruction especially if the primary can be controlled (better cured) and patient has good prognosis.

Endoprosthetic Surgery

Developed for primary bone tumors, the use of endoprosthesis is increasingly getting popular for metastatic bone lesions. For metaphyseal lesions that are difficult to reconstruct using conventional methods because of extensive bone destruction, it is possible to provide a functional limb with custom-made or modular endoprosthetic systems (sometimes called "megaprostheses"). This is successfully used for the proximal femur and distal femur, proximal tibia and proximal or distal humerus. Though uncommon but lesions around ankle are also amenable to this (currently many think that below-knee amputations and prosthetic fitting provide a good functional outcome and is the standard practice). They are highly effective in maintaining function having a low failure rate (primarily due to limited patient survival) but cost is a prohibiting factor in the developing nations where health insurance penetration is low. Also, dedicated centers regularly treating such patients are missing. The high success rate for any arthroplasty primarily depends on the volume of treated cases, and hence the expertise developed through experience.

3. Explain the management of metastasis to spine.

Ans: Spinal metastasis is usually extensive and that is the common reason for frequent "conservative" management of the disease. Also, extensive surgical decompression or stabilization was logically not supported for a compromised patient. Extensive decompression destabilizes spine and fixation methods were cumbersome and quite conventional. However, with changing perspective and advances in cancer therapy, this approach is fast changing. Also, the availability of newer pedicle screws and rod systems and cages has improved surgical stabilization. For isolated compression fractures of vertebral kyphoplasty and vertebroplasty achieve good pain relief. A patient with persistent severe pain or having partial neurological deficit is deemed to have unstable spine amenable for surgical treatment unless extensive imaging suggests structural integrity. Such patients should be kept on spinal beds/ripple mattress (to prevent bed sores); a Philadelphia collar should be given for cervical spine lesions.

Few oncological, neurological, systemic, and mechanical factors should be considered before ultimate management plan is fabricated.

Oncologic factors:
- Histological type and responsiveness of tumor to radiation, chemotherapy, and hormonal manipulation. Hematological, small cell lung cancer, choriocarcinoma, and breast carcinoma are radiosensitive; colon and non-small cell lung cancer are moderately resistant; and renal cell and melanoma are radioresistant.
- Tumor type—high-grade malignant lesion with rapid and progressive destruction (require early surgery).

Neurological considerations:
- Extent of involvement (limited/extensive)
- Duration of compression
- Exact level and direction of compression (for limited involvement)
- Compression with fracture or isolated compression of cord only
- *Staging of epidural extension:* Weinstein–Boriani–Biagini system and Spine Oncology Study Group.

Mechanical factors:
- Spine is unstable if (Fisher et al.):
  – Movement-related pain

- Symptomatic or progressive deformity
- Neurological compromise under physiological loads.
• Radiological involvement of bilateral facet joints and pedicles.

Systemic considerations and patient factors:
• Biological age
• Systemic tumor burden
• Life expectancy (generally should be >3 months)
• General medical condition
• Motivation and understanding of the patient.

The most common tumors that involve the spine are breast, lung, renal, prostate, thyroid, melanoma, myeloma, lymphoma, and colorectal cancer.

The advancements in chemotherapy, radiotherapy, and hormonal therapy have improved patient survival. Classical surgical decompression without stabilization had put surgical intervention into disfavor and radiotherapy used to be classically relied upon intervention. With greater realization of improved mechanical stability and opportunity to surgically decompress spine using anterior and posterolateral combined approaches, the role of surgery has again been emphasized. Surgery is now the preferred treatment for spinal metastasis although role and indications of various techniques need to be better defined. The most important consideration is maintaining the quality of remaining life of the patient which is already compromised by choosing appropriate "aggressiveness" in surgical intervention. So, it is imperative to avoid complications (especially with complex en bloc resections) and gather the maximum benefits of intervention to improve remaining life. A simplified surgical planning based on the various evaluation systems available is presented in **Flowchart 5.1.3**.

Flowchart 5.1.3: Metastatic disease of spine.

The classification and prognosticating systems vary a lot and are based on institutional experiences provide a useful guide. Staging is the first step to guide future treatment however for planning a surgical intervention functional status, expected life remaining, tumor load, and anatomical extent of tumor need to be primarily defined. The scoring systems (Tomita, Tokuhashi, North, and Harrington) avidly define the mentioned criteria barring the anatomical extent. The revised Tokuhashi system is based on six individual scores for the primary site of cancer, presence or absence of paralysis, Karnofsky's performance status, number of extraspinal bone metastases, vertebral body metastases, and visceral metastases, producing a total score in the range 0–15 **(Table 5.1.2)**.

TABLE 5.1.2: Revised Tokuhashi prognostic score.

Criteria	Score = 0	Score = 1	Score = 2	Score = 3	Score = 4	Score = 5
Karnofsky's performance	10–40	50–70	80–100	–	–	–
Extraspinal bone metastasis	≥3	1–2	0			
Vertebral metastasis	≥3	2	1			
Visceral metastasis	Unremovable	Removable	None			
Primary site	Lung	Liver	Other	Kidney	Rectum	Breast
Palsy	Frankel A and B	Frankel C and D	Frankel D			

For a score of 12–15, excisional surgery is recommended with good prognosis, while palliative surgery is suitable for patients with intermediate score (9–11) and patients with score less than or equal to 8 should undergo only conservative treatment.

The Weinstein–Boriani–Biagini staging system initially devised for primary vertebral tumors (an improvement over the McLain and Weinstein and Enneking system) is a useful guide to anatomically define the extent of spinal metastasis. This system divides the axial plane of the vertebral body into 5 concentric and 12 radiating segments and defines the axial tumor involvement of spine comprehensively. The Spine Oncology Study Group uses a 6-point scale to describe metastatic spinal tumors as follows:

- Grade 0 defines tumors confined to bone only without epidural extension.
- Grade 1 is tumor extension up to epidural space but there is no spinal cord abutment (further divided into three categories depending on deformation of epidural fat or thecal sac).
- Grade 2 is spinal cord abutment or even deformation due to pressure but the cerebrospinal fluid remains around the cord.
- Grade 3 is spinal cord compression with obliteration of any fluid around it.
- Grade 2 and 3 tumors are likely to result in neurologic deficits and most likely require surgical decompression (unless radiosensitive).

After these evaluations, the primary interventions can be chosen as follows:

Primary radiotherapy is indicated for a multiple level disease in a stable spine with a radiosensitive tumor. The neurological condition should be stable or slowly progressive. Radiotherapy is also done primarily in a patient with poor prognosis and low general condition precluding surgery or as adjuvant to surgical treatment.

Surgical intervention is done with the following goals in mind and planning should be directed to achieve these objectives:

- Decompress the spinal cord or root causing symptoms and restore function
- Stabilize spine
- Preserve the normal motion segments.

Primary surgical intervention is required in patients with grade 2 or 3 tumors, Tokuhashi score of more than or equal to 9, progressive or severe neurological deficit, fast advancing deficit, progressive deformity (with or without neurological deficit), and in patients with neural compression predominantly by bone. Patients having metastatic tumor insensitive to radiotherapy or chemotherapy with intractable symptoms, and in those patients, where the radiotherapy dose has reached cord tolerance limits, surgical intervention is relatively indicated due to absence of other effective methods. Intractable pain in patients unresponsive to nonoperative methods may also be another relative indication for surgical decompression.

Despite the low threshold for surgical intervention nowadays due to higher acceptability of error and already compromised and limited life of patient, a surgeon should follow some underlying principles:
- Foremost to bear in mind is that the magnitude of surgical procedure should not exceed (or compromise) patient's ability to survive it or the surgeon's level of competence.
- The surgeon should be familiar with various approaches to spine. Thoracolumbar or cervicodorsal regions require specialized approaches.
- If life expectancy of patient is deemed to exceed the probable stress bearing capability of implant (usually assumed to be 6 months), fusion should be additionally considered.
- It is better to choose titanium implants for possible future need of MRI.
- The planned construct should provide immediate stability for quick functional gain.

In patients with malignant extradural spinal cord compression, the following guidelines apply:
- Give steroids (8–10 mg bolus dexamethasone followed by 16 mg daily) if neurological deficit is suspected or confirmed.
- Patients with compression caused by bone alone and those whose neurological symptoms have developed slowly and not resulted in complete deficits for more than 12–24 hours are the most likely to benefit from surgery. This should be supplemented with radiotherapy.
- Patients treated with radiotherapy alone may be treated with single 8 Gy dose if there is poor life expectancy or with multiple fractionated dose for patients expected to live longer.

4. Discuss approach to find out a primary tumor in a 65-year-old man presenting with vertebral metastasis and low backache.

Ans: Kindly see the Answer to Question above.

5. Discuss spinal metastasis: list causes, discuss clinical presentation and investigations.

Ans: Spinal metastasis: Causes, clinical presentation, and investigations

1. Causes (Primary Tumors Leading to Spinal Metastasis)
Spinal metastases most commonly arise from hematogenous spread of cancer. The primary tumors most frequently involved include:
- *Breast cancer* (most common in women)
- *Prostate cancer* (most common in men)
- *Lung cancer* (highly aggressive, often thoracic spine)
- *Renal cell carcinoma* (hypervascular, may cause bleeding)
- *Thyroid cancer* (especially follicular carcinoma)
- *Multiple myeloma* (lytic lesions, pathological fractures)
- *Melanoma* (rare but aggressive)
- *Colorectal cancer*
- *Lymphoma*

The thoracic spine is the most commonly affected region (70%), followed by the lumbar spine (20%) and cervical spine (10%).

2. Clinical Presentation
Symptoms depend on the location, extent of spinal involvement, and degree of spinal cord/nerve compression.

A. Pain (Most Common Symptom)
- *Local pain:* Dull, constant, worse at night, not relieved by rest.
- *Mechanical pain:* Worsens with movement (suggests spinal instability).
- *Radicular pain:* Sharp, shooting pain along nerve distribution (e.g., sciatica if lumbosacral)

B. Neurological Deficits (Red Flags for Cord Compression)
- *Weakness* (limbs, depending on level: paraparesis vs. quadriparesis)
- *Sensory loss* (numbness, paresthesia below the level of compression)

- *Bowel/bladder dysfunction* (urinary retention, incontinence – late sign)
- *Hyperreflexia, spasticity, Babinski sign* (upper motor neuron signs)

C. Spinal Instability and Deformity
- Pathological fractures → kyphosis and scoliosis.

3. Investigations
A. Imaging
- MRI Spine (Gold Standard)
    - Best for soft tissue (tumor, cord compression, and epidural extension)
    - Whole-spine MRI, if multiple levels suspected
    - *T1-weighted:* Hypointense tumor (replaces marrow fat)
    - *T2-weighted:* Hyperintense (edema and tumor)
    - Postcontrast: Enhances with gadolinium.
- CT spine
    - Assesses bony destruction, fractures, and spinal stability.
    - Useful, if MRI contraindicated.
- X-rays
    - May show lytic/sclerotic lesions, vertebral collapse, or pedicle destruction ("winking owl sign", if pedicle erosion).
- Bone scan (Tc-99m)
    - Detects osteoblastic activity (e.g., prostate metastases).
    - Less sensitive for purely lytic lesions (e.g., myeloma)
- PET-CT
    - Helps to identify primary tumor and other metastases.

B. Laboratory tests
- Tumor markers: PSA (prostate), CA-15-3 (breast), and CEA (colorectal)
- Serum protein electrophoresis (if myeloma suspected)
- Calcium (hypercalcemia due to bone destruction)
- ALP (elevated in bone turnover)

C. Biopsy
- CT-guided biopsy for histopathological confirmation if primary is unknown.

6. Explain the role of injectable bisphosphonates in the management of bone metastasis.

Ans: Hypercalcemia (serum calcium > 14 mg/dL) of malignancy affects up to 20% cancer patients during the course of their disease. The most common neoplasia involved is lymphomas and myelomas. Lytic metastasis (20% of cases) from neoplasia of breast, kidney or squamous cell carcinoma are other major group that in particular produce prolific bone resorption by activation of osteoclasts and cause excessive calcium to be released in the blood-producing hypercalcemia. The majority of cases are humoral in etiology and related to PTHrP but direct lysis of bone tissue and in a very few cases extrarenal 1,25-dihydroxyvitamin D (calcitriol) and ectopic parathyroid hormone production may contribute to the same.

Bisphosphonates have a tendency to bind specially at place where active bone resorption is going on and hence controls to some extent bone resorption by inhibiting osteoclast recruitment and activation. Bisphosphonates are the drug of choice for all patients with multiple myeloma and radiologically confirmed bone metastases from breast cancer. Bisphosphonates are to be started in these cases immediately as soon as the diagnosis is made and are continued indefinitely. Other bone metastasis should also be treated with bisphosphonates for management of malignant hypercalcemia. Injectable pamidronic acid was used previously but has been mostly superseded by zoledronic acid which is now considered the most effective compound and controls not only the hypercalcemia but also has shown to lower the incidence of SREs and delay their onset. Injectable bisphosphonates [particularly the zoledronic acid (4 mg given every 3 weeks)] has been found effective in breast, renal, and pulmonary metastasis. Zoledronate is nearly one thousand times more potent than pamidronate owing to its superior inhibition of both farnesyl diphosphate and geranylgeranyl diphosphate synthase, enzymes essential for osteoclast activity. The effects of bisphosphonates have been two-fold:
- Reducing pain
- Prevention of pathological fractures. It should be remembered that they are approved only for cancer with metastasis.

It should be remembered however that bisphosphonates only reduce extraction of calcium out of bone; circulating excessive calcium has to be removed and countered through other medical measures like aggressive hydration, calcitonin, and corticosteroids etc. For refractory hypercalcemia one may have to resort to denosumab or calcimimetic cinacalcet, or even hemodialysis.

5.2 STAGING AND LIMB SALVAGE SURGERY (Q7–11)

7. Describe in detail:
   A. Staging of bone tumors.
   B. Principles, indications, and contraindications of limb salvage surgery (LSS).
   C. Limb salvage in osteosarcoma of distal femur.

Ans:

A. Staging of Bone Tumors

This is the first and most important step to learn as much about the pathology clinically and its possible differential diagnosis *before* performing biopsy. This avoids wrong decisions that may be otherwise made and likely worsen the eventual outcome of management. A comprehensive routine for staging needs skeletal survey, a total body scan (to look for other bony lesions or metastasis), a high-resolution computed tomography (HRCT) scan of the chest, and an MRI of the primary lesion and most importantly thorough clinical examination.

Staging systems recognize a neoplasia in terms of size, site, grade, and metastasis. The staging systems of the Musculoskeletal Tumor Society (also called the Enneking system) and the American Joint Commission on Cancer (AJCC) are quite popular. Both are useful for tumor evaluation planning strategies and predicting prognosis.

Enneking System

Enneking system is based on knowing the histologic grade of the lesion (G), tumor site (T, intracompartmental or extracompartmental), and metastases (M). Enneking system is simple and the three broad categories based on low grade (I), high-grade lesion (II), and metastatic lesion (III) are further divided into subgroups based on intracompartmental (IIIA) or extracompartmental (IIIB) location **(Table 5.2.1)**.

TABLE 5.2.1: Enneking system.		
Stage	**Grade [G, low (1), high (2)], tumor location [intracompartmental (1), extracompartmental (2)], and metastasis [absent (0), present (1)]**	**Description**
IA	G1 T0, T1 M0	Low grade Intracompartmental No metastasis
IB	G1 T2 M0	Low grade Extracompartmental No metastasis
IIA	G2 T0, T1 M0	High grade Intracompartmental No metastasis
IIB	G2 T2 M0	High grade Extracompartmental No metastasis
IIIA	Any G T1 M1	Any grade Intracompartmental Metastasis
IIIB	Any G T2 M1	Any grade Extracompartmental Metastasis

"T" defines tumor located within the bone compartment. Tumor that remains bounded by "natural barriers" to extension such as bone, fascia, cartilage, muscle aponeurosis, and synovium is called intracompartmental (T1) while those extending beyond the confines of the bone or "natural barriers" are extracompartmental (T2). The location of the tumor is established using a combination of specialized procedures, including radiography, tomography, nuclear studies, CT, and MRI. Compartments are specified to describe the tumor site. Compartments are defined on the basis of fascial borders in the extremities.

For any intra-articular tumor (T1), any soft tissue extension is extracompartmental (T2). Similarly, a paraosseous (T1) tumor will become extracompartmental (T2) if it extends into bone or extends through fascia.

T0 lesions are confined within the tumor capsule and within its compartment of origin. T1 tumors have extracapsular extension into the reactive zone around it, but both the tumor and the reactive zone are confined within the compartment of origin. T2 lesions extend beyond the anatomic compartment of origin by direct extension or some other means (e.g., trauma, surgical seeding). Most bone sarcomas are bicompartmental at presentation (have violated the bone cortex migrating into the soft tissues). Sometimes the tumor may remain within the compartment but break through the pseudocapsule to form *"skip" metastasis* (within same anatomical compartment). *"Satellite" nodules* form "within" the pseudocapsule separated from the main mass by intervening normal tissue of pseudocapsule.

Defining "G" and "M"
Intermediate grade, high grade, and undifferentiated lesions are all included in *G2*. Low-grade and well-differentiated tumors are kept in G1 lesions. Both locoregional and distal metastases are grouped under M1 as any metastasis (whether to nearby tissues or nodes or too far away organs) has poor prognosis and changes management.

AJCC System
The American Joint Committee on Cancer system has become more popular recently for its similarity to various TNM classifications (for other neoplasms) popular amongst medical oncologists and many orthopedic oncologists. To use this system, the clinician must know the grade, the size, the presence or absence of discontinuous tumor (skip metastases), and the absence or presence of systemic metastases. Unlike the Enneking system, involvement of regional nodes is a separate category for staging. The variables in the AJCC staging system have differing importance: stage of tumor is most important followed by metastases, discontinuous tumor, grade, and size in that order. AJCC system differentiates: G1, well-differentiated (low grade); G2, moderately differentiated (low grade); G3, poorly differentiated (high grade); G4, undifferentiated (high grade) tumors as opposed to Enneking system. Metastasis has also been segregated into: M0, no distant metastasis; M1a, metastasis to lung, and M1b, metastasis to other distant sites. Tumor is assessed primarily based on the size. Tx defines primary tumor that cannot be assessed following previous surgery; T0, no evidence of primary tumor; T1, tumor 8 cm or less in greatest dimension (note that the "T" for soft tissue tumors is 5 cm, but for bone tumors is 8 cm); T2, tumor >8 cm in the greatest dimension; T3, discontinuous tumors in the primary bone **(Table 5.2.2)**.

TABLE 5.2.2: The American Joint Committee on Cancer system.				
Stage	Grade	Primary tumor	Regional lymph nodes	Distant metastasis
IA	G1 or G2	T1a or T1b	N0	M0
IB	G1 or G2	T2a	N0	M0
IIA	G1 or G2	T2b	N0	M0
IIB	G3 or G4	T1a or T1b	N0	M0
IIC	G3 or G4	T2a	N0	M0
III	G3 or G4	T2b	N0	M0
IV	Any G	Any T	N1	M0
	Any G	Any T	Any N	M1

Involvement of regional/contiguous lymph nodes is N1; N0, no regional lymph node, discontinuous lymph node involvement is M1b.

B. Principles of Limbs Salvage Surgery
The primary goal of LSS is acceptable degree of function in reconstructed limb. Secondary objectives being durability, sustained remission of disease, painless limb, and cosmetic appearance. Decision to reconstruct is individualized based on the tumor location and extent, experience, support available, and the psychosocial characteristics of the patient. Most of the time in developing nation, the LSS is precluded due to delayed presentation.

"Three-strike rule" is quite efficient in quickly screening is a patient is suitable for limb salvage. Access the status of bone, nerves, vessels, and soft tissue envelop. If any three of the structures are involved at the planned site for LSS, then probably it is not worth considering. Even with advancements in surgical technique and reconstruction procedures, the morbidity is unacceptably high, limiting the possibility of functional reconstruction. LSS is contraindicated in following conditions:

Inability to achieve wide surgical margins due to any or combination of:
- Invasion of major neurovascular structures whose resection will compromise either the viability or functionality of limb terminally
- Involvement or contamination of multiple compartments with extensive muscle involvement
- Patients with extensive skin involvement
- Pathologic fractures where the risk of recurrence increases several folds
- Sepsis jeopardizing the effectiveness of adjuvant chemotherapy
- Inappropriate or improper biopsy contaminating normal tissue planes and compartments

The various modalities for limb reconstruction used are:
- Arthrodesis
- Mobile joint reconstruction:
  - Autoclaved tumor bone
  - Allograft bone including osteoarticular allograft
  - Turn-o-plasty
  - Bone transfer (ulna and fibula to reconstruct radius and tibia respectively), Huntington's procedure
  - Endoprosthetic reconstruction
  - Allograft endoprosthetic reconstruction
  - Custom-made prosthesis

Surgical margins for performing LSS are classified into four types (Fig. 5.2.1):
1. Intralesional margins (excision) have plane of dissection within the tumor mass removing only a portion of the lesion. Gross tumor and its pseudocapsule (containing satellites), and skip lesions in the surrounding normal tissues are all left behind. This is usually suited for benign bone lesions such as simple bone cyst (SBC), aneurysmal bone cysts (ABCs), and enchondroma. Depending on intent for surgery, most metastatic lesions operated for palliative surgery are treated with intralesional excision (but for curative excision, such as removing solitary metastasis, a wide margin is preferred).
2. Marginal excision margins have dissection plan through the pseudocapsule aiming to remove the lesion en bloc, but leaves behind the skip lesions and possibly microscopic satellite lesions. This is also suited for less aggressive lesions such as ABC, and giant cell tumor (GCT).
3. Wide margin is the en-bloc excision of the lesion where the plane of dissection passes outside the reactive zone of the lesion through the normal tissue removing the tumor with its pseudocapsule and cuff of normal tissue. This is the desired margin for most primary bone sarcomas, but it leaves behind the skip foci. The distance away from the tumor required to achieve this margin is usually 1–2 cm and depends on type of tissue involved. Lesser of normal tissue is removed with "resistant" tissue to tumor spread like cartilage, bone, and thick fascia but some liberal margin is needed for "soft tissue" like the loose areolar tissue or fat. Also, a high grade or aggressive tumor that poorly responds to chemotherapy requires wide margin of normal tissue. With advances in imaging, the margins can be shrunk in future preserving the normal tissue as much.
4. Radical margins involve removing the entire compartment(s) in which the tumor has extended and in turn also obliterates the possibility of leaving any skip lesions causing recurrence.

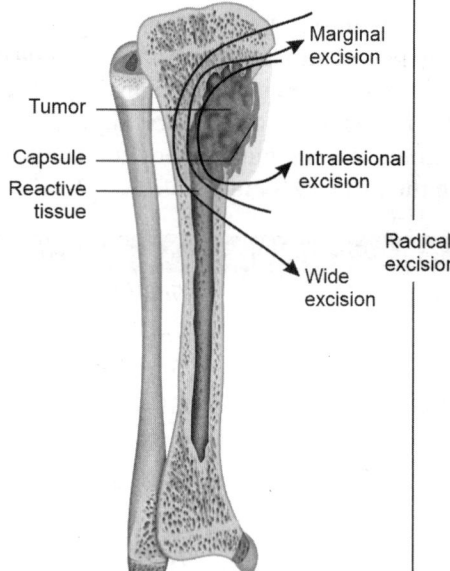

Fig. 5.2.1: Various surgical margins for tumor excision.

C. Limb Salvage Surgery for Osteosarcoma

The most important prerequisite for planning a limb sparing procedures is that LSS should be done only when the preoperative staging indicates that it would be possible to achieve wide surgical margins. To this effect contrary to what is commonly preached a pathologic fracture noted at diagnosis or during preoperative chemotherapy does not preclude LSS provided for sure that if wide surgical margins can be achieved. Mostly with advanced chemotherapy wide margins are adequate but r_0 resection should always be aimed at.

Reconstruction after surgery can be accomplished with many options including:
- Resection and arthrodesis ± bone lengthening
- Metallic endoprosthesis (and allograft-prosthetic composite)
- Allograft (and osteoarticular allograft) ± bone lengthening
- Vascularized autologous bone graft ± bone lengthening
- Rotationplasty—cosmetic deformity may not be acceptable to family
- Wide excision and autoclaved bone graft reconstruction

The choice of optimal surgical reconstruction is based on various identifiable factors, including the site and size of the primary tumor, the involvement or sparing (or possible reconstruction) of neurovascular supply of the distal extremity, the patient's age, and hence potential for additional growth after surgery. One must also try to address the needs and desires of the patient and family as may be involving specific function like participation in sports or future profession, etc. It is now a known fact however that delay or prohibition in resumption of systemic chemotherapy after LSS may endanger the chance for cure (increased recurrence), which is quite common when complicated reconstructions are planned for this tumor. This entails making a balanced plan that does not jeopardize chances of tumor-free life over function. Systematic review of retrospective analyses has shown that delay in resuming chemotherapy following definitive surgery is deleterious and is associated with increased tumor recurrence and death. Though considered mutilating and often the last option "to resort to, amputation" remains the optimal choice for saving life of patient and curing him of the primary tumor in some. This is strongly considered if histopathological examination of surgical specimen shows inadequate margins—plan an immediate amputation. The case is further strengthened if the histologic necrosis following preoperative chemotherapy was poor. The most sensitive indicator till now is response to preoperative (neoadjuvant) chemotherapy. Survival is directly related to chemotherapy response, those with a good response (>90% tumor necrosis) have 80–90% long-term survival while nonresponders (<90% tumor necrosis) survival is usually less than 15%.

8. Describe the prerequisites for limb salvage surgery in a malignant tumor.

Ans: A limb salvage surgery (LSS) is performed if:
- Adequate margin for resection of tumor can be obtained with low risk (<10%) of local recurrence.
- Functional outcome of the reconstructed limb is better than or comparable to that achieved by amputation and prosthetic fitting.
The above points can be described at will

9. What is Enneking classification of benign tumors?

Ans: The benign bone tumors of bone have been divided into three types by Enneking:
1. Latent
2. Active
3. Aggressive

10. Briefly describe methods to cover osseous defects after excision of primary malignant bone tumors of bone. What is extracorporeal irradiated tumor bone?

Ans: Sometimes the questions really bowl you out even if you know too much!!! Either the question means combined osseous and soft tissue reconstruction or it means reconstructing the osseous defect. In any case we describe both.

The management of bone and soft tissue defect after tumor resection involves principles of dead space management minus infection as is also practiced in management of chronic osteomyelitis. The following are the four common approaches in management:
1. Mobilize locally available tissue—most preferred if possible like in tibial shaft or lower tibial neoplasms. Fibula can be mobilized along with adjacent tissue.

2. *Microvascular reconstruction:* This is the most commonly deployed approach as local tissue is not always available. The most common combined bone and soft tissue reconstruction involves using osseofasciocutaneous or osseomyofasciocutaneous microvascular free flap.
3. Reconstruct the bone with implant/prosthesis or a bone-prosthesis composite and provide local or microvascular free tissue cover. The bone defect in this case may also be reconstructed with bone from bone bank, autoclaved or irradiated bone, and soft tissue reconstruction done over it.
4. Last is bone lengthening by Ilizarov method if sufficient soft tissue cover has been obtained. This method is not commonly followed as diaphyseal only lesions are not common to resect as intercalary resection and wide excision usually entails destruction of nearby joint. Ilizarov may be used to stabilize and obtain arthrodesis in a reconstruction instead.

Open bone grafting: This is an acceptable method of reconstructing small-to-moderate bone defects (up to 3 cm) in children. In upper limbs, defects in humerus can be adequately addressed with fibular (nonvascularized/vascularized) grafting. The results will be good if the growth plate is viable at the more severely affected end. In the forearm, small defects are usually bridged by open bone grafting. In lower limbs, a bone defect in femur in a small child may be treated with single or double fibular grafting. In tibia, open bone grafting, fibular grafting, and tibiofibular synostosis (single bone leg) are performed depending upon the length of the defect.

Microvascular graft osteosynthesis: Defects larger than 6 cm require vascularized grafts (less than that can be synthesized with autogenous cancellous bone graft). Advantages of vascularized bone grafts include:
- Good bone healing due to vascularity with simultaneous cortical bone support
- Can be used for larger defects >6 cm
- Can be used for previously failed cases tried with cancellous grafts
- They maintain their mass, architecture, and strength
- With endurance of load get hypertrophied (undergo remodeling).

Vascularized fibula graft is commonly used; however, vascularized rib, scapular, and ilium grafts have been described. The method requires skill and experience in microvascular surgery reconstruction else the success rate is low.

Huntington's procedure (ipsilateral fibula transfer and tibialization of fibula): Unlike transplanting a free fibula, the ipsilateral fibula can be transposed to the tibial defects (fibula-pro-tibia). The concept was first used by Kahn in 1884 for pseudoarthrosis of tibia. Huntington described the procedure for treating the tibial defect using the ipsilateral fibula transposition in 1903. The original procedure was described as having two steps (now often performed in one step). In the first stage the distal part of fibula is osteotomized and inserted into medullary canal of tibia or into a trough created on surface for fibula. The construct may be stabilized with cortical screws of K-wires. The second stage is done at 2–4 months where the proximal portion of the fibula is cut and approximated to tibial surface in a slot created for the same. This can also be stabilized with screws. The bone union occurs at around 6 months. Till then some protection is legible in the form of plaster cast or fixator.

Irradiated tumor bone reimplantation: The excised tumor tissue is swab-cultured immediately upon retrieval prior to processing. The soft tissues and periosteum are immediately stripped and cleaned. The bone is washed thoroughly with saline (betadine and peroxide solution are optional). Terminal sterilization is usually done by gamma irradiation. Gamma radiation is effective in killing bacteria, fungi, spores, and, to a lesser degree, viruses. Depending on the dose, however, gamma radiation can weaken the graft. Doses below 1.5 mrad do not adversely affect the tissue strength. A minimum dose of 2 mrad is required to kill bacteria and 4 mrad for killing viruses. After such high-dose irradiation the bone is discolored and fibrillar network of bone is destroyed. Solubility of collagen and proteoglycans increase reducing structural strength and inductive capacity is greatly reduced. Bone neoplasms are a special case as most of the tumors are radioresistant so high doses of irradiation are needed for killing the disease. High-energy X-rays are deployed and commonly 100 Gy irradiation is used for such sterilization (irradiation time is calculated depending on the output of source and bone volume). The irradiated bone is then reimplanted at the site for reconstruction of osseous defect.

The soft tissue coverage options depend on the following criteria (Heppert et al.):
- The type of osteosynthesis
- The site and size of the soft tissue defect

- The local vascular status
- Patient compliance.

The spectrum of treatment options for soft tissue coverage range from split skin grafts to free vascularized myocutaneous flaps depending on above factors.

11. Write a note on expandable megaprosthesis.

Ans: *Principle of expandable megaprosthesis:* A significant number of bone neoplasms are pediatric patients who have growing skeletons. Unfortunately, physis does not pose a significant barrier for most malignant neoplasms and surgical extirpation damages the growing ends of bone that need to be compensated for optimal functional outcome in future. For such patients especially with lower limb malignant tumors who are being considered for limb salvage, future limb-length inequality must be considered. For patients who are near skeletal maturity, the reconstructed limb can be lengthened 1 cm at the initial procedure. Also, epiphysiodesis of the contralateral limb can be done at the appropriate age to preserve limb-length equality (or to minimize inequality). For younger patients that have significant growth remaining, other options should be considered. Historically, amputation (followed by repeated larger prosthetic fitting) and rotationplasty were considered the only reasonable treatments for very young patients with bone sarcomas, advent, and use of expandable prostheses/megaprosthesis gained wide support and popularity. Presently at all centers this is the preferred modality of limb reconstruction following LSS.

Types of expandable prosthesis: Most endoprostheses are modular, allowing for incremental limb lengthening as an immature patient grows. A popular method is the use of Repiphysis® Expandable Prosthesis (Wright Medical Technology, Arlington, Tennessee). The surgical technique for implantation of this device is similar to that of other endoprostheses. The device is a spring-based technology where energy stored in a compressed spring is used for future expansion of the prosthesis as the child grows. When a leg-length discrepancy develops, the child is scheduled for an expansion. The procedure is done under fluoroscopy and light sedation. The locking mechanism on the prosthesis is identified using fluoroscopy, and an electromagnetic coil is placed over the patient's leg at that level. The electromagnetic coil is activated for 20 seconds generating a pulsed electromagnetic field which heats an element in the prosthesis through interference. The heated element melts a small segment of polyethylene and allowing controlled expansion of the imbibed spring lengthening the prosthesis. The leg lengths are re-evaluated under fluoroscopy, and the procedure is repeated one or two times as necessary. Normally lengths of 0.5–1.5 cm can be gained in each such session. Frequent lengthening sessions can be scheduled (say 3–4 weeks apart) if discrepancy is large or if one needs to "catch up" the shortening in operated leg. Patients usually can ambulate immediately without an assistive device.

The other technology used in expandable prosthesis is "screw" mechanism that is based on conversion of rotatory motion into linear motion. The prosthesis has inbuilt design of a threaded rod that slides inside of a counter threaded tube. Lengthening here is done in a short spinal anesthesia as the method is invasive. At the screw mechanism manual lengthening is done utilizing the threaded mechanism that is rotated in the given direction to gain prosthetic length. Usually, these expandable prostheses can gain up to 4–6 cm length in all.

The long-term complications of these prostheses include:
- *Polyethylene wear:* This is still the most limiting factor for articulating surfaces. Even if the prosthesis gains length the overall prosthesis survival is limited by the implanted device that has limited duration articulating surfaces and need to be replaced at appropriate interval.
- Fatigue fracture can occur at the rotating hinge
- Fatigue fracture at the base of the intramedullary stem where it attaches to the body of the prosthesis.

5.3 BIOPSY OF BONE TUMORS (Q12–14)

12. Explain types and principles of biopsy for musculoskeletal tumors.

Ans: *Types of bone biopsy:*
- Fine needle aspiration cytology (FNAC; not very useful for sarcomas)
- Core/trephine biopsy using a 14-gauge needle (usually recommended for most bone tumors)
- Incisional biopsy (for failed core biopsy, vascular bone tumors, and ABC)
- Excisional biopsy (usually done for small lesions <2–3 ms in the longest diameter).

Principles:
- Should be done at the conclusion of staging (to avoid radiological artifacts)
- Avoid sampling error, take multiple samples from the lesion (this is necessary for sarcomas but single specimens may suffice for carcinomas)
- The biopsy tract should be incorporated into the planned surgical incision
- Biopsy should be done from the representative tissue
- Biopsy tract should be the shortest way to tumor
- Should not violate more than one compartment
- Should not be done from intermuscular planes
- Should be remote from the main neurovascular bundle
- Try not to violate the cortex and take sample from the extracortical bone tissue (to prevent weakening the bone by creating a stress riser defect)
- Bone window should not have any sharp corners (avoiding stress risers)—prefer an oblong window
- Avoid transverse incisions (prefer longitudinal incisions)
- Do a sharp dissection, close with a subcuticular stitch
- Obtain meticulous hemostasis (to avoid hematoma formation); a drain if absolutely needed must be placed in the line of incision, or through the wound
- For an incisional biopsy take tumor tissue, reactive tissue, pseudocapsule, and capsule.
- Biopsy should be ideally done by the surgeon going to finally operate the patient.

13. **Explain biopsy in musculoskeletal tumors as well as advantages and limitations.**

Ans: Advantages of Biopsy in Musculoskeletal Tumors:
- **Definitive Diagnosis:**
  - Provides histopathological confirmation of tumor type (benign vs. malignant).
  - Helps to classify sarcomas (e.g., osteosarcoma, chondrosarcoma, and Ewing sarcoma) and soft-tissue tumors (e.g., liposarcoma and synovial sarcoma).
- **Guides Treatment Planning**
  - Determines the need for surgery, chemotherapy, or radiotherapy.
  - Helps in preoperative planning (e.g., limb-salvage vs. amputation in malignant cases).
- **Minimally Invasive Options Available**
  - *Core needle biopsy (CNB):* High accuracy (~90%) with minimal morbidity.
  - *Fine-needle aspiration (FNA):* Less invasive but lower diagnostic yield for some sarcomas.
- **Reduces Unnecessary Surgeries**
  - Avoids aggressive resection for benign or non-neoplastic lesions.
- **Allows Molecular and Genetic Testing**
  - Essential for tumors like Ewing sarcoma (EWSR1 translocation) or synovial sarcoma (SS18-SSX fusion).

Limitations and Risks of Biopsy:
- Sampling error and false negatives:
  - Heterogeneous tumors may yield nondiagnostic samples.
  - Small or necrotic areas may be missed.
- Risk of tumor seeding:
  - Improper technique can contaminate surrounding tissues, complicating future resection.
- Technical challenges:
  - Deep-seated or spinal tumors may require image guidance (USG/CT)
  - Vascular or neural injury risk in certain locations
- Pathologist expertise required:
  - Sarcoma diagnosis is complex; misinterpretation can lead to incorrect treatment.
- Potential complications:
  - Infection, hematoma, or fracture (especially in lytic bone lesions)

- Not always necessary:
  - Classic benign lesions (e.g., osteoid osteoma, and enchondroma) may not require biopsy.

14. Frozen section in orthopedics.

Ans: Frozen section is also called cryosection. This is a special type of biopsy that is requested at the time of surgery intraoperatively to better understand the completion of resection and tumor extirpation. If the margins remain positive, then resection will not be R0 type. So commonly multiple tissue samples are taken from the margin of resection to establish completeness of tumor resection. This technique is also being used in revision arthroplasty where it is imperative to remove all infected tissue that may otherwise compromise the success of procedure. The following are common indications of frozen section in orthopedics:

- Establish completeness of tumor resection during tumor excision and reconstruction—be it a primary surgery or done for recurrence of tumor.
- Establish the nature of abnormal mass/lesion identified during surgery. Sometimes suspicious tissue is identified in the surgical field—knowing the nature of tissue whether to keep or resect is guided by frozen section.
- Revision arthroplasty—intraoperative sterility of tissue and freeness from infection is better demonstrated by frozen section during revision arthroplasty for prosthetic joint infection. If the biopsy material contains >5–10 WBC per HPF, then it usually indicates infection. Result can be improved by taking multiple sections from operative field spanning all areas.

5.4 MAGNETIC RESONANCE IMAGING IN MANAGEMENT OF SPINAL TUMORS (Q15)

15. Explain the application of MRI in diagnosis and management of spinal tumors.

Ans: An MRI is an excellent modality for screening the spine for occult metastases, myeloma, or lymphoma. Both primary and metastatic diseases are seen well on T1-weighted sequences. Normal vertebral body marrow is well-delineated on T1-weighted images. Its signal progressively increases with age because of higher percentage of fatty marrow. In anemia, there is higher percentage of hematopoietic marrow, thus diffusely diminishing this T1-weighted signal. Vertebral tumor foci appear as discrete areas of diminished T1 signal. Tumor viability and response to chemotherapy can be judged by MRI to some extent. Viable tumor is generally bright on T2-weighted images. Signal intensity reduces on T2-weighted images after effective treatment. Uniformly dark signal on T2-weighted images predicts good to complete response but is rare and often the treated tissue appears bright. Neoplasms that diffusely involve vertebral marrow, such as multiple myeloma, are difficult to differentiate from hematopoietic marrow.

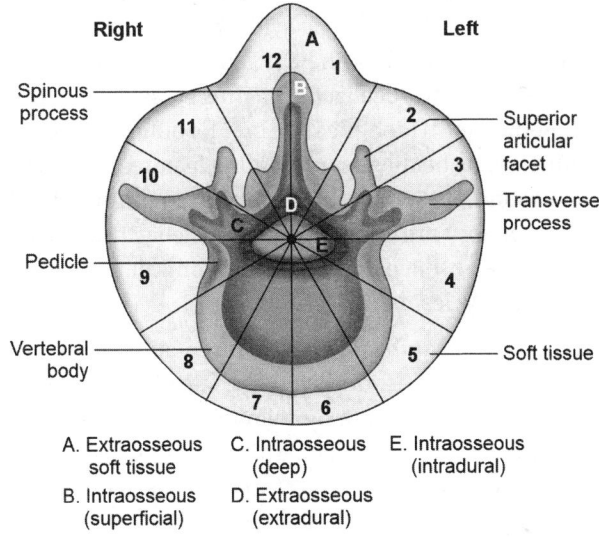

Fig. 5.4.1: Weinstein–Boriani–Biagini staging system.

Magnetic resonance imaging scan is highly sensitive to detect small skeletal metastases not detected on bone scans as it reveals abnormal bone marrow. Typical diagnostic feature of a metastatic lesion on MRI is focal low-signal intensity on a T1-weighted image, a mix-to-high intensity on a fat-suppressed T1-weighted image, and high intensity on a T2-weighted image due to marrow edema (high water content). MRI defines the anatomical extent of vertebral involvement quite precisely that can be used to stage the bony and extraosseous extent of tumor using the Weinstein–Boriani–Biagini staging system (**Fig. 5.4.1**) that was initially devised for primary vertebral tumors (an improvement over the McLain and Weinstein and Enneking system) but now also applied for spinal metastasis. This system divides the axial plane of the vertebral body into 5 concentric and 12 radiating segments (**Fig. 5.4.1**) and defines the axial tumor involvement of spine comprehensively.

5.5 CHONDROMYXOID FIBROMA AND OSTEOID OSTEOMA (Q16–17)

16. Explain clinical, radiological features, and management of:
  A. Chondromyxoid fibroma of distal femur.
  B. Osteoid osteoma (diagnosis and management) of femoral neck.

Ans:

A. *Chondromyxoid Fibroma of Distal Femur*

Clinical features: It occurs in males more commonly than females and is seen in 2nd to 3rd decades. Although seen in almost every bone, the common site of occurrence is around knee. A fourth of tumors occur in flat bones especially ilium. Pain usually mild and present for long time is the most common symptom. Flat bone lesions are most often discovered incidentally.

Radiological features: The lesions are geographical, lytic, and grow along the longitudinal axis of bone originating in metaphysis near physis. In a long bone, the location is typically metaphyseal, eccentric, sharply marginated oval lytic zone. In small bones, the lesion appears like a "flame-shaped" lytic lesion. Lesions may extend to epiphysis or diaphysis. Matrix mineralization is not seen (should be suspected for chondrosarcoma).

Management: Marginal excision with curettage and bone grafting [or polymethylmethacrylate (PMMA) packing] is the standard management of the tumor as the prognosis is excellent. Even recurrences which occur in approximately 15% of cases usually within first 2 years are treated similarly. In some lesions at periarticular sites, the lesion has to be managed with excision and joint reconstruction.

B. *Osteoid Osteoma*

Clinical features: Males in first three decades are affected more often than females, equalizing later in life. *Pain* is intermittent initially that becomes intensified later to disturb sleep. The localized pain is typically nocturnal and is relieved promptly by acetylsalicylic acid, characteristic of osteoid osteoma. Pain is due to high concentration (100–1,000 times normal) of prostaglandin E2 (PGE2) in the nidus that excites the abundant nerve endings in the nidus. There is often an area of exquisite, localized *tenderness* associated with the lesion, and there may be redness and localized swelling.

Radiological identification may be difficult in atypical forms like those in periarticular bones where joint contractures, stiffness may be the first presenting features.

Around 5–15% are intra-articular and infrequently respond to salicylates for pain relief. They may cause reactive inflammatory arthritis, secondary osteoarthritis, and ectopic ossification. They are difficult to diagnose radiologically and in the absence of typical symptoms, it may get delayed for months. Bone scan followed by MRI or CT would help diagnose the lesion.

Radiological features: Classical presentation on a plain radiograph is a small lucent round to ovoid lesion in a radiodense area of bone corresponding to the site of clinical pain. The central lucent lesion is commonly 0.5–1 cm in diameter but never more than 1.5 cm by definition.

Larger lesions usually harbinger osteoblastoma so should always raise suspicion. Uncommon lesions with central ossification may have "target" appearance. Radiological localization could be difficult in periarticular regions and in axial skeleton (so rely on modalities other than a plain radiograph). 99Tc-MDP bone scans consistently reveal hot spot at the osteoid osteoma and can be used to narrow down the site of involvement (especially in above-mentioned radiologically difficult locations). Noncontrast computed tomography (NCCT) is a very good investigation to localize the lesion in all planes especially for surgical or radioablation purpose.

On an NCCT, the typical features are small nidus that may have variably extending high-density area within. Reactive peripheral sclerosis surrounds the nidus as usual. Spinal lesions are common in neural arch and may be localized to apophyseal joint or even articular process. On MRI, the lesion appears isoechoic to muscle on T1-weighted images. The T2-weighted image has increased intensity but is still lower than the short tau-inverted images (STIR) sequence where it is hyperintense. Bone marrow edema is seen in around 60% of patients. Intra-articular osteoid osteoma may additionally have synovitis and effusion that is detected on MRI. MRI is better for diagnosis of cancellous bone osteoid osteoma but is inferior to cortical bone osteoid osteoma compared to NCCT. Hypervascularity of the nidus may be misinterpreted for aggressive lesions.

Management: Osteoid osteomas have been known to undergo spontaneous resolution and symptoms may subside over 3–4 years. Intralesional excision had been the standard approach however various recent modalities to minimize associated surgical trauma have been used. These include radiofrequency ablation (heating to 80°C) under CT or ultrasound guidance, laser-guided interstitial thermal therapy, laser photocoagulation, ethanol injection, and cryotherapy. During surgical excision, identification of the lesion is most important. Several different approaches have been tried. Overpenetrated films give fine detail.

Tetracycline labeling the lesion (giving preoperative tetracycline) and localization intraoperatively by ultraviolet light can be done but has low sensitivity. Intraoperative bone scan and using a portable gamma camera has been reported but is too cumbersome. Intraoperative CT scan (modern C-arm has the facility to do intraoperative CT also) identification is the best way to identify osteoid osteoma. This or at some centers ultrasonography is used for radiofrequency ablation. Microwave ablation or scanned marking are other strategies. It is anyway imperative to send the tissue for frozen section confirmation after excision. Additionally, cauterization of the surrounding bone using standard diathermy to ablate any remaining tissue can be done.

17. Differentiate between osteoid osteoma and osteoblastoma.

Ans: Table 5.5.1 Compares osteoma and osteoblastoma.

TABLE 5.5.1: Differentiation between osteoid osteoma and osteoblastoma.

Characteristics	Osteoid osteoma	Osteoblastoma
Size of nidus	<1.5 cm	>2 cm
Pain	More	Less
Effect of aspirin	Effective	Ineffective
Predilection for microscopically	Appendicular skeleton Orderly zonal pattern of central ossification	Axial skeleton Higher degree of trabecular haphazardness

5.6 FIBROUS LESIONS OF BONE (Q18–22)

18. Enumerate fibrous lesions of bone.

Ans:
- Nonossifying fibroma
- Cortical desmoid
- Benign fibrous histiocytoma
- Fibrous dysplasia (FD)
- Osteofibrous dysplasia (OFD)
- Desmoplastic fibroma.

19. Describe and compare:
  A. Fibrous dysplasia.
  B. Clinical features of fibrous dysplasia.
  C. Campanacci disease (Osteofibrous dysplasia).

Ans:

A. Fibrous Dysplasia

Fibrous dysplasia is a nonheritable, benign, fibro-osseous lesion that is commonly medullary monostotic (80%), or sometimes polyostotic (20%). Monostotic FD may be present at any age though it is most common in those aged below 30 years while polyostotic FD is seen much early and most commonly presents before puberty. There is equal sex distribution. It is considered that a developmental failure occurs during remodeling of woven so that mature lamellar bone fails to form. The bone also fails to remodel in response to mechanical stress (i.e., does not follow Wolff's law). Due to loss of maturation, an unorganized mass of immature trabeculae is left enmeshed in dysplastic fibrous tissue.

There is no complete failure or absence of remodeling but the turnover is so slow that completion of the remodeling process does not occur. The bone fails to follow Wolff's law and hence trabeculae do not align along the stress line, this is combined with insufficient mineralization causing significant loss in mechanical strength. This causes stress concentration and hence development of pain, progressive deformity, and even pathologic fractures. Any bone of the skeleton may be involved but generally four forms are considered:

1. Monostotic form affecting single bone (70–80% of cases). The disease is usually asymptomatic until 2nd to 3rd decades, but can be seen even during adulthood. The disease becomes inactive after puberty, and monostotic form has not been found to progress to polyostotic form. Ribs, craniofacial bones, and femur are commonly affected.
2. Polyostotic form affecting multiple bones (20–30% of cases). Usually, one side is predominantly involved rather than a uniform distribution. Lower extremity bones are the most common to be involved (femur, tibia, and pelvis).
3. Craniofacial affecting only the skull and facial bones.
4. Cherubism—distinct from FD in that it is inherited (autosomal dominant), occurs early in life (3–4 years of age), has predominant cosmetic changes in face (symmetric jaw fullness and upward turning of eyes due to bilateral expansile multiloculated cystic masses in mandible and maxilla) and histologically resemble giant cell granuloma. They often regress with age.

Associations of Fibrous Dysplasia
- About 2–3% of polyostotic FD with café-au-lait skin lesions, precocious puberty in girls, with or without fibromyxomatous soft tissue tumors: McCune–Albright syndrome (Albright syndrome).
- *Mazabraud syndrome:* The development of soft tissue or intramuscular myxoma (typically multiple) near most severely affected bone.

Etiopathogenesis
The abnormal replacement of bone with fibro-osseous tissue has been linked to mutation in the gene that encodes the α-subunit of a stimulatory G-protein (Gsα) located on chromosome 20 (*GNAS1* gene). This mutation is present in the lesional tissue only. Even the skin lesions in some cases have been found to have somatic mutations in the signal-transducing guanine nucleotide binding proteins.

In monostotic disease, the genomic mutation probably arises due to unknown factors later in life and producing single tumor. Depending on the cell type where it originates activated Gs produce differential effects like in the skin it causes hyperpigmentation while in the endocrine tissues, there is increased hormonal secretion. Altered local hormonal milieu in bone leads to local bone resorption, and the formation of dysplastic fibro-osseous tissue.

FD possibly represents a proliferation of somatically mutated spindle cells occurring either in a mosaic pattern (polyostotic), or at a localized site in bone (monostotic).

B. Clinical Presentation
It is an incidental finding in majority monostotic cases as the disease is more often than not asymptomatic. Otherwise pain, deformity, and pathological fracture are the most common presenting features. *Bone pain* has been reported in up to 81% of adults and 49% of children present in dysplastic areas with high stress. A reduction in pain and disease activity with age is seen in many lesions, with a possible reactivation at the time of pregnancy in female patients. Bones plastically *deform* under the mechanical pressure from body weight and the type of deformity depends on place and extent of lesion. *Shepherd's crook deformity* (resembling the kyphotic spine deformity of shepherd) is a lateral bow of proximal femur due to passage medially of body weight and developing characteristic deformity in polyostotic disease. Scoliosis develops similarly in spinal lesions. It results in limb shortening, limping and, occasionally, chronic fatigue fracture (seen as a Parrot's beak on medial cortex) accompanied by disabling pain.

Other deformities include tibial bow (even saber tibia), protrusio acetabuli, and Harrison's groove (a horizontal depression along the peripheral border diagram in lower thorax, corresponding to its costal insertion). Deformity in monostotic forms halts after skeletal maturity but in polyostotic forms usually continues to progress even after stopping of bone growth.

Swelling is palpable in subcutaneous bones. Jaw bones are most common site of involvement, appendicular skeleton is preferentially affected in females while males have predominant skull and ribs lesions.

Radiology
The lesions are intramedullary, geographic with well-defined, sclerotic margins, and a "ground-glass" matrix. "Ground-glass" matrix is an area with no or minimally discernable trabecular region having density similar to cancellous bone

(lighter compared to cortical region). With continued growth, the sharp cortical border is also lost giving a uniform look to area of lesion. The lesions are often expansile and may contain lucent areas of secondary ABC. Ribs are the most common site of monostotic FD and FD is the most common cause of benign expansile rib lesion. Endosteal scalloping is seen in large lesions and periosteal reaction is absent. Shepherd's crook deformity develops in proximal femur when the weight of the body acts through the mechanically weakened bone and causes severe varus in the proximal femur. Variegated appearance of skeletal lesions causes some lesions to appear more sclerotic or demonstrate calcified cartilage. Other lesions often show marked bony expansion especially lesions involving the ribs.

Bone Scintigraphy and Tomography
These are intensely hot on bone scans and may be used to locate the extent and distribution of disease. CT is useful in demonstrating the cortical involvement and continuity.

Magnetic Resonance Imaging
The lesion has intermediate-intensity on T1-weighted images and is a bit enhanced heterogeneously on T2-weighted images (but less than fluid or malignant tissue).

Secondary cysts have high-signal intensity. Due to high variability of lesions on MRI, it is not a useful investigation for differentiation of the disease from other lesions.

Histopathology
On gross examination, FD lesion appears firm with variable amount of "grittiness". Cyst formation, if present, is occasional and often secondary. Some lesions demonstrate cartilage areas grossly. Lesion is easily separable from the encircling shell of bone mostly. On microscopic examination discrete delicate trabeculae of immature woven bone are dispersed in a background of moderately cellular fibrous tissue. These trabeculae organize into variegated shapes of (Cs, Os) arranged haphazardly and are referred to as forming "Chinese-letters" or "alphabet soup" pattern. Osteoblasts are found interspersed in woven bone but do not rim the trabeculae (differentiating from OFD, fracture callus, or myositis ossificans). Occasionally, small foci of lamellar bone may also be seen in a few cases of FD. The background of fibrous stroma is variegated in appearance and is variably cellular, myxomatous, or show prominent collagenization. The fibroblasts in the lesion usually have plump ovoid nuclei. Nonspecific osteoclast-type giant cells may be also found. Cartilage in the form of long islands or rounded nodules with peripheral endochondral ossification is sometimes present (differentiating it from chondrosarcoma). Collections of foam cells are common (should not be confused for metastatic clear cell carcinoma).

Differential Diagnoses
- Radiological differential diagnosis includes Paget's disease (different demographics, histologically mosaic pattern on histology), neurofibromatosis type 1 (rare osseous lesions, often axial, ribbon ribs), OFD (exclusively tibial with anterior bow, cortical lesions), adamantinoma (mostly tibial), nonossifying fibroma, SBC (more radiolucent, expansile, thinner lamellar bone surrounding), and enchondromatosis.
- Pathological differentials include OFD (cortical location, well-organized zonation, and osteoblast rimming), reactive woven bone, well-differentiated intraosseous osteosarcoma (cytologic atypia and permeative growth pattern), and desmoplastic fibroma (extensively heavily collagenized).

Management
For incidental lesions observation is practiced after confirming that the lesion is FD only especially in monostotic forms as there is minimal risk of pathological fracture or deformity. For polyostotic disease, endocrinology evaluation should be done for endocrine abnormalities and appropriate management. Medical management includes mainly use of injectable [pamidronate (60 mg/day given for 3 days repeated every 6 months) and zoledronic acid] or equivalent oral bisphosphonate. The osteopenic lesions are thought to be mainly due to bone absorption by excess osteoclastic activity that can be effectively inhibited by bisphosphonates. Levels of alkaline phosphatase (ALP), fasting urinary hydroxyproline, and urinary type I collagen C-telopeptide are lower in treated patients and lesions heal in 1–3 years. Clinically, this reduces pain and improves bone strength. Surgical management is directed toward the treatment or prevention of its complications such as deformities and pathological fracture along with surgical extirpation of the disease. Simple curettage and bone grafting has high failure with local recurrence and reappearance of the lesion in polyostotic disease. Usually, wide procedures are hence adopted as the new bone formed is still dysplastic. For

proximal femoral deformity, corrective osteotomy (valgus) and fixation with extramedullary or intramedullary implants is usually done. Cancellous grafts are quickly replaced by dysplastic bones so contrary to the views cortical bone grafts and allografts have a special place in these patients. Reports of secondary neoplasia superimposed on FD are emerging. Malignant transformation into osteosarcoma, fibrosarcoma, malignant fibrous histiocytoma (MFH), and chondrosarcoma is seen in 0.4–4% cases. Radiation exposure for treatment or patients with Mazabraud's syndrome is at higher risk for malignant transformation.

C. Osteofibrous Dysplasia

Osteofibrous dysplasia is a rare, non-neoplastic fibro-osseous proliferation affecting the cortex of the tibial (commonly) or fibular diaphysis in children and infants.

In 1981, Campanacci and Laus studied 35 cases recognizing it as a benign disease and coined the term osteofibrous dysplasia of the tibia and fibula. "Dysplasia" is preferred over the use of historical "ossifying fibroma" because it is now considered to be of congenital origin and due to its resemblance to FD, histopathologically the term expands to osteofibrous dysplasia. The disease is apparently exclusive to tibia and fibula. Few researchers use term intracortical FD to emphasize its cortical location instead of using Campanacci's disease. Only rarely is OFD is also referred to as Campanacci syndrome possibly nonpragmatically. Occasional cases involving radius, humerus, and ulna have been reported. The disease is diagnosed in children <10 years of age, with a peak incidence reported among those between 1 year and 5 years. Several reports also exist noting there occurrence in newborn (hence thought to be congenital). Adults (oldest on record being 39 years of age) with de novo OFD have also been reported. Sex predilection is unclear, some studies do favor male predilection. The etiology of OFD, as well as the cell of origin, is unknown. Familial occurrence is not popular and only one description of such familial OFD is present in literature.

Etiopathogenesis

The most pertinent hypothesis of occurrence points to origin from a fibrovascular abnormality. Possibly OFD to adamantinoma reflect a spectrum of abnormalities, the two forming extreme ends. A relationship between OFD and adamantinoma has been proposed by Johnson on the basis of common origin of the two—namely, the fibrovascular defect. As proposed by this theory, OFD results from an abnormality in the Haversian canals, whereas adamantinoma is a product of defect of intramedullary vasculature. According to Komiya and Inoue, a deficiency in blood flow within the periosteum results in OFD. Relationship between adamantinoma and OFD is supported by the cytogenetic analysis and finding that both have some extent of chromosomal trisomy. Trisomy of chromosome 7, 8, 12, and 22 has been described in OFD while adamantinoma also has trisomy of chromosome 7 and 12. Strength to this association is provided by report by Sherman et al. coexistent adamantinoma and OFD in the same patient.

Clinical Presentation

The most common presentation is a painless, localized, firm swelling of the tibia. The tibia frequently is bowed anteriorly or anterolaterally. Pathological fracture may also be present but is uncommon. The symptoms are present for average of 14 months before diagnosis. Pain is present in around one-third of the patients. Some cases are noticed incidentally on radiographs taken for some other reason.

Radiology

The lesion is a cortically based, diaphyseal eccentric geographic lucency with well-defined sclerotic margins. There could be multiple lucencies in the cortex separated by areas of sclerosis (multilocular). The anterior cortical surface is usually involved. There could be anterior bowing of tibia. The cortex is often thickened and the lesion appears expansile. Periosteal reaction is rare and if present it is thick and solid type.

Histopathology

Grossly, the tissue is fibrous gritty contained by the periosteum. Microscopically, the characteristic feature is storiform (cartwheel pattern) fibrous background containing spicules of woven bony trabeculae that are lined by a layer of osteoblasts (osteoblast rimming). Rimming is absent in FD. OFD has additionally zonal architecture (zonification described by Campanacci and Laus) where the immature woven bone is more centrally located while the number and maturity of trabeculae increase toward periphery of lesion so that the center is more fibrous while periphery is more osseous. Focal cytokeratin positivity may be seen raising the possibility that OFD could represent a variant of extragnathic adamantinoma with poorly developed epithelial islands.

Differential Diagnosis

Differential diagnosis includes adamantinoma [soft tissue extension and intramedullary presence), FD (intramedullary, no osteoblastic rimming **(Table 5.6.1)**], and nonossifying fibroma. Other radiological differentials include chondromyxoid fibroma (CMF), ABC, unicameral bone cyst (UBC), eosinophilic granuloma (EOG), osteomyelitis, rarely chondrosarcoma, osteosarcoma, and hemangioendothelioma.

TABLE 5.6.1: Difference between fibrous and osteofibrous dysplasia.

Fibrous dysplasia	Osteofibrous dysplasia
Most commonly presents before puberty (polyostotic form) to up to 30 years (monostotic form)	Presents within 10 years
Can be found anywhere in skeleton—ribs most common	Exclusive to tibia and fibula very rare other sites reported
Intramedullary lesion	Intracortical lesion
Many bones can be involved simultaneously	Limited to one bone
Usually incidental in monostotic forms, else pain and deformity are the common presentations	Presents as a swelling of tibia with anterior or anterolateral bowing
May be associated with endocrine abnormalities	Not so
Geographical destruction with very fine or lost sclerotic cortical border with growth. Overall a ground glass appearance	Sharp well-defined cortical border around the lesion. Multilocular lesion may also be seen
Alphabet soup appearance on microscopy	Characteristic osteoblastic rimming and zonification seen

Treatment

For OFD, the current recommendation had been to avoid surgical intervention due to high recurrence rates and benign disposition of the lesion. Also, the lesion stops growing after skeletal maturity. So apart from biopsy, there is possibly no need for extirpation of lesion. Once the maturity is reached excision with bone grafting may be done. Some advice bracing for prevention of deformity. Surgical management may be done for extensive or deforming lesions or for those having pathological fracture. This view has been recently challenged by Lee et al. and they recommend initial aggressive extraperiosteal resection in all cases. This is typically based on the fact that there is quite a high chance of sampling error in biopsy and finding of high percentage of adamantinoma or adamantinoma-like OFD in resected specimens. Possibly a thorough representative biopsy and vigilant histopathological examination should save patient from such aggressive treatment methods. The prognosis of "true" OFD is excellent and no progression to adamantinoma is seen.

20. Write a note on fibrous dysplasia.

Ans: Kindly see Answer to Question above.

21. Discuss role and principles of various pharmacological agents in fibrous dysplasia.

Ans: Bisphosphonates as pharmacological agent has been written in Answer to Question above.

22. Describe nonossifying fibroma under clinical features, radiology, and treatment.

Ans: It is possibly the most common tumor of children originating from proliferation of fibrous tissue and histiocytes that present as intracortical, multilocular, and well-circumscribed lesion.

Clinical features: The most common presentation is an incidental finding in more than half of the cases in first three decades. There is slight male preference. The lesions are asymptomatic and mostly occur in the metaphyseal region of distal femur and distal tibia. When symptomatic, may present with palpable swelling near the affected area. Lesions less than 2 cm in greatest diameter are called fibrous cortical defect. Although any bone may be involved but femur and tibia involvement account for 85% of the cases (if fibula is also included then >90% cases will be covered), occurrence in upper limb is unusual. Pathologic fracture may be the initial presentation. A small percentage (<5%) cases are associated with neurofibromatosis or Jaffe-Campanacci syndrome with characteristic Café-au-lait spots. Multifocal lesions are still unusual. The lesions frequently heal after skeletal maturity progressing from area most distally in the lesion to region toward growth plate. The lesion may contain ABC that usually causes bony destruction.

Differential diagnosis: CMF, FD, desmoplastic fibroma, GCT of bone, ABC, MFH, and osteosarcoma.

Radiology: Nonossifying fibroma appears as a well-defined cortical, lytic, lobulated lesion located eccentrically in the metaphysis with surrounding sclerosis. If ABC is present, then it may appear expansile and sharply marginated. The long axis of the lesion is oriented along the long axis of bone. There is no periosteal reaction in the absence of a pathological fracture. Multiple lesions may be uncommonly seen. With ossification of the lesion bone fills in the defect and is denser than the innate bone.

Noncontrast computed tomography and MRI determine true extent of the lesion and expansile nature in case of ABC. Internal trabeculations are also easily seen. MRI usually presents with low-signal on T1 and variable heterogenecity on T2. MRI may better demonstrate associated ABC.

Treatment: As mentioned above most heal spontaneously by skeletal maturation. The lesions are asymptomatic and hence treatment is needed only if they threaten bony integrity and strength or if ABC eroding into bone is identified that would usually cause pain. Surgical resection is indicated if the lesion covers half of the bone in perpendicular extent (>50% of the bone diameter). The standard management is curettage and bone grafting that is curative. Most pathological fractures otherwise can be treated nonoperatively.

5.7 CHONDROBLASTOMA (Q23–24)

23. **Write a note on chondroblastoma of bone, its clinical features, diagnosis, and management in detail.**
Ans: (ICD-O 9230/0, Calcifying Giant Cell Tumor, Epiphyseal Chondromatous Giant Cell Tumor, Codman Tumor).

Chondroblastoma of bone is a benign cartilage-producing neoplasm accounts for <1% of the bone tumors. Codman confused this to chondromatous variant of GCT that was later corrected by Jaffe and Lichtenstein to chondroblastoma as a distinct entity. The tumor usually is seen in skeletally immature patients (10–25 years of age) and classically is located in the epiphysis or apophysis of bones. Metaphyseal or diaphyseal occurrence is unusual. Growth plate is not a barrier for tumor growth and the tumor is often seen crossing across to adjacent metaphysis, but joint penetration is rare if at all. Patients with flat bone (skull, etc.) chondroblastoma present late (3rd to 5th decade). The femur (distal and proximal), tibia, and humerus are the preferred sites but ilium, acetabulum, temporal bones in skull, and tarsal bones are also involved. Lower limb accounts for 70% cases and the proximal femur lesions characteristically involve the greater trochanter rather than the epiphysis. There is confusion as to the origin of tumor and though the most common view of chondrogenic origin is accepted, few researchers have proposed different pathogenesis. Absence of true cartilage matrix and presence of type 1 collagen portend it to be originally a bone-forming lesion (Aigner et al.). Some researchers have suggested the tumor to be akin to pigmented villonodular synovitis (PVNS) or GCT of tendon sheath where the tumor originates from intramedullary/endosteal cells similar to tendon sheath cells with preferential differentiation into chondroid tissue.

Clinical Presentation and Radiology
The lesions are solitary and mostly only one bone is involved (multifocal involvement is extremely unusual). Localized pain of long duration is the common presentation while soft tissue swelling and joint effusion can be occasionally seen. Patients with temporal bone lesions might develop tinnitus, vertigo, or hearing loss. The average duration of symptoms (delay in diagnosis) in patients with chondroblastoma is around 20 months. Radiologically the lesions are small (usually 3–5 cm), eccentrically located in the epiphysis, and mostly lytic (70% lesions, calcification is seen in less than one-third of patients) in a geographic pattern that occupy less than half of the epiphyseal width. The lesions are sharply demarcated with a thin sclerotic rim that differentiates them from GCT (sclerotic rim absent). The bone is usually not expanded, and there is no periosteal reaction. Secondary ABCs are common. Uncommon large lesions may deform especially in weight-bearing bones due to collapse of the wall. Rare chondroblastomas may metastasize to lungs however the excision of the metastasis suffices. These are called aggressive chondroblastomas. The metastasis, however, is nonprogressive.

Histopathology
Gross examination of tissue reveals blue-gray chondroid areas of chondroid tissue with yellow gritty areas of calcification or immature bone. Secondary ABCs may be seen. The chondroblasts are seen with numerous variations. Typically, the oval or polygonal cell with a round nucleus that contains prominent longitudinal groove is seen. Chondroblasts are commonly packed in pseudolobulated sheets arranged in a pavement-like pattern. S-100 protein is frequently demonstrable in the chondroblast. Some cells with abundant pink cytoplasm represent epithelioid variant. Syncytial variety lacks most of the typical features.

Interspersed are spindle, giant cells and macrophages that may be hemosiderin positive. Fine network of calcification present around the chondroblasts focally, especially in the necrotic areas results in characteristic "chicken wire" pattern of calcium deposition.

Differential Diagnosis
- *Radiologically:*
  - GCT
  - Chondrosarcoma (clear cell type and low grade)
  - Osteomyelitis (Brodie's abscess)
  - EOG
  - Intra-osseous ganglion (IOG)
- *Histopathologically:*
  - Osteosarcoma
  - Clear cell chondrosarcoma.

Management
Marginal excision with bone grafting or polymethylmethacrylate (PMMA) cement packing is the usual surgical management. Recurrence is seen in 14–18% cases and is seen within 2 years. Huvos et al. found increased recurrence in lesions associated with ABC though it is not substantiated. For reasons of incomplete curettage to avoid injury to growth plate, the recurrence is more common in pediatric epiphyseal lesions. The curettage can be extended with high-speed burr or cryoablation. Tissue contamination should be particularly avoided as this is the most common mode of recurrence. However, incomplete excision is the most common cause of recurrence (up to 50% within first 2 years) in flat bones. For aggressive chondroblastomas, wide excision with excision of metastasis usually suffices. Recently radiofrequency ablation (Rybak et al.) with a probe has been reported to provide prolonged pain relief in smaller lesions.

24. Write a note on Codman's tumor.
Ans: Kindly see Answer to Question 23.

5.8 DIAPHYSEAL ACLASIS (Q25)

25. Describe the pathology, clinical features, radiological features, and treatment of diaphyseal aclasis.
Ans: (Hereditary osteochondromatosis, hereditary deforming osteochondromatosis, hereditary chondrodysplasia, diaphyseal aclasis, metaphyseal aclasis, hereditary multiple exostoses, ICD-O 9210/1).

Multiple exostosis is the most common and least disfiguring of the skeletal dysplasias.

Clinical Features
The condition is usually discovered in childhood. Clinically most of the lesions are detected or noticed incidentally by parents and are asymptomatic, presenting just for worrisome swelling and found while bathing the child. If symptomatic, the most common presentation is that of a hard mass of longstanding duration symptoms (often related to the size and location of the lesion). Multiple osteochondromas usually present as limb growth disturbances. The more severely affected bones are abnormally short; this is seldom very marked but on measurement the lower body segment is shorter than the upper and span is less than height. In the forearm and leg, the thinner of the two bones (the ulna or fibula) is usually the more defective, resulting in typical deformities: Ulnar deviation of the wrist, bowing of the radius, subluxation of the radial head, valgus knees, and valgus ankles. As the child grows, these lumps enlarge and some may become hugely visible, especially around the knee. Bony lumps may cause pressure on nerves or vessels. Secondary complications (these are also often painful) are the common reason for surgical intervention and include:
- Mechanical obstruction
- Fracture of the stalk of the lesion
- Nerve impingement
- Pseudoaneurysm of an overlying vessel
- Bursa forming over the osteochondroma and bursitis
- Infarction of the osteochondroma

- Reactive myositis
- Increasing pain and/or rapidly growing mass (possible malignant transformation)

Malignant transformation of osteochondromas (also see secondary chondrosarcoma) has been reported in less than 1% in patients with solitary and approximately 1–3% in patients with multiple osteochondromas. The features that suggest this include:

- Mass becoming suddenly painful and tender or sudden increase in pain without above changes
- Increase in cartilage cap thickness more than 2 cm (seen on MRI or CT, also see histopathology below, and secondary chondrosarcoma for detailed description)
- Excessive cartilage type flocculent calcification seen on radiograph or CT scan
- Lucencies in the bony component or fuzzy border between cartilage and bone on radiograph
- Multiple recurrences in a well-excised lesion

There is often a generalized osseous remodeling defect distributed throughout the body and hence causing limb growth disturbances. Some uncommon syndromes are also associated with development of multiple osteochondromas and include Langer–Giedion (associated with facial dysmorphism and mental retardation) and Potocki-Shaffer (Defect-11) syndrome.

Pathology

The underlying fault in multiple exostosis is unrestrained transverse growth of the cartilaginous physis (growth plate). The condition affects only the endochondral bones. Grossly the specimens have a well-defined bony narrow or broad stalk (unless sessile) covered by a cartilage cap at the broader end. The cartilage cap is usually thicker in younger patients (adolescents) while a cap larger than 2 cm in an adult should raise suspicion of malignancy. Thickness as an absolute criterion is not very well accepted by experts and is more arbitrary (see also secondary chondrosarcoma). Conventionally, cartilage cap measuring <1 cm is designated for osteochondroma without any validating data. In fact, the mean thickness for cartilage cap has been reported to be 9 mm with a range of few mm to 2.5 cm. On the contrary chondrosarcomas have been shown to be present even in thinner caps 5–10 mm, so cap thickness is not a good criteria and what some call a "qualitative assessment" of the cartilage cap could better help in differentiation. Microscopically the chondrocytes show a zonification and superficial ones are more clustered and seen in lacunae. The lower ones near the base line-up like in growth plate. Some amount of large disorganized masses of cartilage in the stalk and amorphous calcification with focal necrosis of cartilage is common and should not be mistaken for chondrosarcoma. Chondrosarcomatous cartilage has prominent myxoid change and accentuated cellular and lobular appearance. Permeation of bone and entrapment is pathognomonic of chondrosarcoma.

Radiology

X-ray: Solitary osteochondromas may be pedunculated or sessile lesions often found in metaphyseal region despite their origin from physeal plate (shift due to continued growth). The characteristic feature is a projection of the cortex in continuity with the underlying bone. The continuity of marrow space into the lesion is evident on CT scan or MRI images. These modalities are also good imaging modalities to estimate the thickness of the cartilage cap that used to have treatment implications previously.

Management

Exostoses may need removal because of reasons mentioned above. Excision including the covering periosteum (extraperiosteal resection—the plane of dissection passes outside "extra" the periosteum, or to better remember—not only the tumor but its periosteum is also removed as "extra" precaution) is done for a symptomatic or cosmetically disabling lesion. Deformities of the legs or forearms may be severe enough to warrant treatment by corrective osteotomy or concomitant correction and lengthening by the Ilizarov technique. Physeal stapling or plating may be used to direct longitudinal growth. Exostoses should stop growing when the parent bone does; any subsequent enlargement suggests malignant change and calls for advanced imaging and wide local resection. The secondary malignancy requires wide excision for cure. Recurrence is common for:

- Incomplete excision (often the cartilage cap is left behind or pathological periosteum inadequately excised) is the most common cause of recurrence.

- The mature bony stalk should be excised completely with periosteum and flange of parent bone at the base, some palisaded cells (at base of stalk) in periosteum might reflect metaplasia and possible recurrence of tumor if not ablated or excised.
- Multiple recurrences in a well-excised lesion indicate malignancy.

5.9 OSTEOSARCOMA AND RELATED QUESTIONS (Q26–30)

26. Discuss osteogenic sarcoma: pathology, clinical features, and investigations.

Ans: *Pathology:* Section through bone reveals wide extension within the marrow cavity with variegated appearance. In the same lesion bluish areas of lobular cartilaginous growth and gritty bone with foci of hemorrhage and necrosis, and telangiectatic component may be seen. Rarely, skip areas (skip metastasis) can be found.

Clinical features: Osteosarcoma typically affects the metaphysis of long bones, most common being in frequency of involvement distal femur, proximal tibia, and proximal humerus. Coincidently these are also the most active physes during growth spurt. Pain without swelling is the most common presentation that is variably present for few weeks to months. The pain is intermittent to begin with but quickly becomes unremitting, deep, boring, and severe. Pain with a swollen tender mass is the next most common often seen in delayed presentation or referred cases. Decreased range of motion (ROM) and functional limitation are features of delayed neglected cases. Local warmth, telangiectasia, dilated veins, and a bruit on auscultation may be observed particularly in aggressive tumors. There is often a delay of 6–9 months from disease to diagnosis. Sudden increase in pain indicates hemorrhage in tumor, secondary changes like dedifferentiation and rapid growth, pathological fracture, or invasion into nearby neurological structures. Serum alkaline phosphatase (ALP) and lactate dehydrogenase (LDH) are not typically useful for diagnosis but a rise in ALP after tumor excision suggests recurrence.

Investigations: Based on the radiological presentation, osteosarcomas can be broadly classified into three categories: (1) sclerotic osteosarcomas (30%), (2) osteolytic osteosarcomas (25%) and (3) mixed pattern (45%). The classical radiologic appearance is an intramedullary combined lytic and sclerotic lesion with a commonly demonstrable cortical breach and is associated with bone matrix formation. There is commonly a pattern of permeative invasion of the surrounding bone and soft tissue with calcification. The borders are poorly defined but are not as aggressive as that of rapidly growing Ewing's sarcoma. Lifting of periosteum by rapidly growing mass produces the characteristic reactive bone formation—Codman's angle (also called Codman's triangle). MRI is the modality of choice for defining the intramedullary extent and surrounding infiltration by the tumor. The investigation guides the level of excision of the tumor and the muscle groups that can be spared to retain postoperative function. For staging purpose PET scan is commonly obtained.

27. Differentiate parosteal and periosteal osteosarcoma in terms of pathology, clinical features, treatment, and prognosis.

Ans: Table 5.9.1 shows difference between parosteal and periosteal osteosarcoma.

TABLE 5.9.1: Difference between parosteal and periosteal osteosarcoma.

Parosteal osteosarcoma	Periosteal osteosarcoma
More common surface osteosarcoma	Relatively rare form
Swelling without pain	Swelling quickly accompanied by pain
Metaphyseal femur	Diaphyseal location common
Wraps around the bone	Protrudes into soft tissue
Periosteal reaction uncommon	Periosteal reaction is often seen
Osteoid formation prominent	Chondroid features common
Zonation seen	Not evident

Parosteal osteosarcoma: The tumor arises from the cortical bone on bone surface as a protuberant multinodular mass in older age group (slight female predilection) and is the most common of the surface osteosarcoma. The tumor characteristically is seen on the posterior aspect of femur; other sites being tibia and proximal humerus. They are slow to grow and often present as a mass usually *not* associated with pain. Stiffness in the nearby joint might be the initial presentation. The tumor appears to encircle the bone circumferentially (partially or completely) and may even have a cartilaginous cap-like structure for very slow growing reasons. Periosteal reaction is rare if at all. Some aggressive ones infiltrate the surrounding tissues. Metastasis is late to occur as is intramedullary extension. The tumor shows centrifugal differentiation (immature periphery compared to base). Radiologically the tumor appears as a large, dense irregular exophytic mass attached to parent bone by a wide base. Lucencies within the dense calcification are rare and indicate dedifferentiation (to fibrosarcoma, MFH or osteosarcoma). Deep-seated lucencies indicate aggressiveness. CT is required to determine the intramedullary involvement and "wrapping around" tendency of the bone tumor. The lesion should be differentiated from osteochondroma, myositis ossificans, florid reactive periostitis, periosteal osteochondromatous proliferation (Nora's lesion) radiologically and conventional osteosarcoma and high-grade surface osteosarcoma histopathologically. The parosteal osteosarcoma does not have a contiguous medullary canal as is seen with osteochondroma and also the columnar arrangement of cartilage seen in osteochondroma is missing in parosteal osteosarcoma. Radiologically, the osteochondromas appear lucent in the center. Myositis ossificans shows a centripetal differentiation (periphery more mature, "zonation"). Periostitis is quite painful clinically and has relevant history.

The classical histopathological appearance (of parosteal osteosarcoma) is that of irregular osteoid seams surrounded by spindle cells and scattered innocuous fibroblasts, i.e., an overall well-differentiated tumor. Most tumors are grade 1 at diagnosis. Atypia and high-grade lesions correlate with intramedullary spread and metastasis. Parosteal variety differs from conventional variety in that there is one or supernumerary ring chromosome. Unless high grade, the treatment suffices with well-performed wide excision else neoadjuvant chemotherapy should be given. The prognosis is distinctly favorable with 75–85% survival at 5 years. Recurrences due to inadequate excision are common and are of concern as they are of higher grade that require combined chemotherapy and aggressive surgery for management.

Periosteal osteosarcoma (juxtacortical chondrosarcoma): They are also surface osteosarcomas (originating from cortex), but involve diaphysis of long bones and involve patients of age group similar to conventional osteosarcoma. They are typically described as intermediate-grade chondroblastic osteosarcoma arising on surface of bone. The tibial shaft is the commonly affected region. Clinically, they also initially present as a swelling usually painless to begin with but later develop pain. Rather than wrapping around the bone, they project into the soft tissue as well-circumscribed mass. The cortex is not destroyed but may be scooped and periosteal reaction in the form of Codman's triangle is often seen. Radiographically, the lesions are lucent without any intramedullary extension, and mineralization is more or less limited to the tumor base. The calcification occurs in radiating spiculated pattern. Gross examination of a specimen reveals cartilaginous grayish-blue lobulated mass that contains chondrosarcomatous areas microscopically (resembling intermediate-grade chondrosarcomas), but as per definition of osteosarcoma, there are at least some foci of osteoid formation (often thin and lacy) usually located in the center. High-grade surface osteosarcomas are differentiated on the basis of presence of high-grade anaplastic osteoblasts. Peripheral chondrosarcomas are metaphyseal and lack radiating spicules. The periosteal osteosarcoma should be managed like conventional osteosarcoma (wide local resection) with neo- and adjuvant chemotherapy.

28. Mention histopathological features of osteosarcoma.

Ans: Microscopically, they are high-grade anaplastic spindle cell tumors with mixed osteoblastic, chondroblastic and fibroblastic differentiation and presence of epithelioid, plasmacytoid, round and clear cells (pleomorphic) but by definition have definite osteoid production. Very rarely osteoid may be absent from primary tumor (telangiectatic osteosarcoma), but their metastasis has abundant osteoid production justifying the term osteosarcoma. Both malignant and benign osteoblast-like giant cells can be found in the stroma, abundance of latter is referred to as giant cell rich osteosarcoma and should be differentiated from GCT. In osteoblastic osteosarcoma, there is predominant production of malignant osteoid.

Predominance of malignant cartilage production will be identified as chondroblastic osteosarcoma. Fibroblastic osteosarcoma is characterized by large areas of proliferating fibroblasts arranged in intersecting fascicles representing fibrosarcomas, but foci of osteoid tissue will characterize it as osteosarcoma. Telangiectatic osteosarcoma contains multiple blood-filled cystic and sinusoidal spaces of variable size separated by thin septa. Phenomenon of "normalization" can be seen in osteosarcoma; this refers to osteoblasts becoming smaller and less pleomorphic (regression to normal) as they get incorporated into osteoid. Osteoblastic rimming is however characteristically absent helping differentiation of neoplastic (absent) from reactive osteoid or osteoblastoma (present). A thin, highly mineralized pattern (the filigreed pattern) is highly suggestive of neoplastic osteoid. There is a tendency of the osteosarcoma to grow in around vessels (angiocentric) giving an overall "basketweave" pattern to tumor.

29. Explain current concepts in management of osteosarcoma.

Ans: The most apt description is that without appropriate treatment the tumor is uniformly fatal, and till 1970s the 5-year survival for osteosarcoma was less than 20%. Conventional tumor has an aggressive local growth pattern and rapid hematogenous spread. Lung is the most common site of metastasis followed by bone although latter occurs only terminally. By the time primary tumor is diagnosed, micrometastasis to lungs is present so osteosarcoma is considered *a systemic disease* at diagnosis now. This is the utmost reason to start contemporary multidisciplinary therapy (chemotherapy-, radiotherapy, if required, surgery) focusing on both local and systemic manifestations of osteosarcoma. The drastic improvement in survival rates to 50% appeared after introduction of adjuvant chemotherapy. The initially used drugs like vincristine, bleomycin, or dactinomycin were quickly replaced by cisplatin, ifosfamide added to doxorubicin and methotrexate that further improved the survival to over 70% in nonmetastatic osteosarcoma. Patients on chemotherapy are put on protective weight bearing to prevent pathological fractures that could preclude limb-preserving surgery. "With advancements in chemotherapy the trend shifted to control the micrometastasis with the use of preoperative chemotherapy." This intensive preoperative chemotherapy regime so called neoadjuvant chemotherapy combined with assessment of the histological response allowed for better assessment of the surgical margins and early treatment of microscopic disease that would otherwise limit the surgical efficacy. This significant advancement in the current scenario of optimal management of the disease allowed limb-salvage procedures in more than 80–90% of the cases drastically reducing the need for amputation and producing tumor-free survival of 50–75% even for high-grade osteosarcoma. Analyzing the available data it is found, however, that survival rates improved only between 1973 and 1983 and between 1984 and 1993, but not significantly between 1993 and 2004. This has led some to believe that statistical improvements in "5-year survival" may simply delay the time to recurrence and metastasis that would eventually happen (after the measured 5- or 10-year) in most and also possibly the improvement in results could be mounted by increased intensity of chemotherapy that might still have higher propensity for later side-effects. Overall survival for patients with metastatic disease at presentation ranges from 10% to 40% only, recurrent disease still occurs in 30–40% of patients and more than 70% of them die of tumor. Even in the survivors of osteosarcoma there is a significantly increased risk of chronic medical conditions that arise as a result of osteosarcoma-related treatment. The most important prerequisite for planning limb-sparing procedures is that limb-sparing surgery (LSS) should be done only when the preoperative staging indicates that it would be possible to achieve wide surgical margins. To this effect contrary to what is commonly preached a pathologic fracture noted at diagnosis or during preoperative chemotherapy does *not* preclude LSS provided for sure that if wide surgical margins can be achieved. Although radical margins have been the preferred modality to achieve local control, the advances in chemotherapy have enabled *wide excision* to be the desired modality of surgical treatment and limb salvage.

Reconstruction after surgery can be accomplished with many options including:
- Resection and arthrodesis ± bone lengthening
- Metallic endoprosthesis (and allograft-prosthetic composite)
- Allograft (and osteoarticular allograft) ± bone lengthening
- Vascularized autologous bone graft ± bone lengthening
- Rotationplasty—cosmetic deformity may not be acceptable to family
- Wide excision and autoclaved bone graft reconstruction.

The choice of optimal surgical reconstruction is based on various identifiable factors, including the site and size of the primary tumor, the involvement or sparing (or possible reconstruction) of neurovascular supply of the distal extremity, the patient's age and hence potential for additional growth after surgery. One must also try to address the needs and desires of the patient and family as may be involving specific functions like participation in sports or future profession, etc. It is now a known fact however that delay or prohibition in resumption of systemic chemotherapy after LSS may endanger the chance for cure (increased recurrence), which is quite common when complicated reconstructions are planned for this tumor. This entails making a balanced plan that does not jeopardize chances of tumor-free life over function. Systematic review of retrospective analyses has shown that delay in resuming chemotherapy following definitive surgery is deleterious and is associated with increased tumor recurrence and death. Though considered mutilating and often the last option "to resort to, amputation" remains the optimal choice for saving life of patient and curing him of the primary tumor in some. This is strongly considered if histopathological examination of surgical specimen shows inadequate margins—plan an immediate amputation.

The case is further strengthened if the histologic necrosis following preoperative chemotherapy was poor. The most sensitive indicator till now is response to preoperative (neoadjuvant) chemotherapy. Survival is directly related to chemotherapy response, those with a good response (>90% tumor necrosis) have 80–90% long-term survival while nonresponders (<90% tumor necrosis) survival is usually less than 15%. One exception to improved survival of responders in osteosarcoma is possibly telangiectatic form where despite extreme sensitivity of the tumor to chemotherapy the survival may not be improved. Current chemotherapy protocols include combinations of the following agents: high-dose methotrexate, doxorubicin, cyclophosphamide, cisplatin, ifosfamide, etoposide, and carboplatin. As for tubercular chemotherapy regimens containing three active chemotherapy agents against osteosarcoma have been found superior to regimens containing two active agents, and also regimens that include high-dose methotrexate are superior. Pulmonary metastasis and secondary complications are the most common cause of death. Local recurrence in particular is associated with a high risk for death from osteosarcoma.

The factors that are associated with increased incidence of local recurrence are:
- Pelvic primary site of tumor
- Doing biopsy at an institution different from the institution performing definitive surgery
- LSS
- Soft-tissue infiltration of the tumor beyond periosteum
- Poor histological response (necrosis) to initial chemotherapy
- Failure/delay in completing planned chemotherapy.

It is a known fact that patients who undergo an amputation have lower local recurrence rates than patients undergoing LSS (although not by any means this suggests amputation for all patients). The functional outcome has been similar between amputation and LSS group of patients; this is however a strong point in favoring amputation at sites where LSS would be difficult or too complex to jeopardize chemotherapy. Radiation therapy is recommended in most patients with osteosarcoma of the head and neck that have been left with positive or uncertain resection margins.

30. **Describe the chemotherapy and advances for osteosarcoma.**

Ans: Current chemotherapy protocols for osteosarcoma include combinations of the following agents: High-dose methotrexate, doxorubicin, cyclophosphamide, cisplatin, ifosfamide, etoposide, and carboplatin. As for tubercular chemotherapy regimens containing three active chemotherapy agents against osteosarcoma have been found superior to regimens containing two active agents, and also regimens that include high-dose methotrexate are superior. Most commonly the chemotherapy is administered after local control of the tumor (as adjuvant) to kill the remaining micrometastasis. The neoadjuvant chemotherapy has become quite popular these days to downstage the tumor primarily making it better resectable. For patients with unresectable tumors, palliative chemotherapy may be given. Neoadjuvant chemotherapy has resulted in good local tumor control and higher rates of limb salvage. The chemotherapy should be administered through intravenous (IV) route (conventional) or intra-arterial (usually Adriamycin/cyclophosphamide) and can be combined with radiation therapy. University of California and Los Angeles regime involves use of intravenous (continuous infusion for 48 hours) or intra-arterial Adriamycin and cisplatin (two cycles), along with ifosfamide (two cycles) and three doses of radiotherapy (2800 cGy). In other centers, usually ifosfamide and Adriamycin in 1st cycle followed by two cycles of cisplatin and Adriamycin are given in neoadjuvant regime (aimed to downstage tumor and enhance chances of LSS) followed by surgery and adjuvant therapy of remaining 4, 5, and 6 cycles given after 21 days comprising of ifosfamide and Adriamycin.

Advances in management of osteosarcoma:
- *Radiotherapy:*
  - *Intensity-modulated radiation therapy:* The radiation beams are modulated to give maximum dose to the tumor area and sparing the surrounding tissues. The sensitive tissues can also be differentially spared.

- *Proton beam therapy:* Protons do tissue damage after they pass certain distance in soft tissues so that the normal tissue can be spared by adjusting the beam strength. The protons then deliver energy quickly to the tissue.
- *Carbon ions:* These are heavier protons causing more damage to cancer cells but the treatment is available at select centers (mostly Japan).
- Chemotherapy:
  - *Mifamurtide [biological compound muramyl tripeptide phosphatidylethanolamine encapsulated in liposomes (L-MTP-PE)]:* The drug is used along with chemotherapy and surgery to improve event-free survival (EFS) in patients with nonmetastatic disease. The drug stimulates innate immunity against osteosarcoma. It is suitable for patients aged 2–30 years following surgical resection of nonmetastatic disease.
  - *Targeted therapy:* Saracatinib affecting bone metabolism, bevacizumab and sorafenib affecting angiogenesis in tumors and drugs such as temsirolimus and everolimus against mTOR protein are being studied. COG-ADVL 1115 is a phase I study of trebananib, an angiopoietin-neutralizing peptibody, in children with relapsed or refractory solid tumors; also COG-ADVL 1014 studying wild type reovirus (reolysin) is underway for relapsed or refractory solid tumors.
  - Zoledronic acid has been found to act synergistically to paclitaxel in chemotherapeutic regimens against osteosarcomas.

5.10 GIANT CELL LESIONS (Q31–35)

31. Explain giant cell variants.

Ans: This is again a bouncer question!! Either it means the types of microscopic giant cells or it means GCT variants!

Several bone tumors have giant cells as a histological component and are called giant cell lesions. They are not GCT per se:
- NOFs (nonossifying fibroma, metaphyseal fibrous defect)
- Chondroblastoma
- Chondromyxoid fibroma
- Unicameral and ABCs
- Hyperparathyroidism
- Paget's disease
- Reparative giant cell granulomas/solid ABC

Histopathologically, various giant cells are found in different conditions. The following are some of the commonly recognized giant cells:
- *Physiological giant cells:*
  - Osteoclasts
  - Syncytiotrophoblast
  - Megakaryocytes
- *Macrophage derived:*
  - *Langhans giant cells:* These cells have horse shoe-shaped nuclei arrangement. The nuclei are usually 15 or more but depending on the virulence of organism they may be less also. The giant cells are characteristic of granulomatous inflammation as seen in:
    - Tubercular granuloma
    - Leprosy (TT Type mainly)
    - Late syphilis
    - Deep fungal infection
    - Sarcoidosis
    - Leishmaniasis
    - Crohn's disease
  - *Foreign body giant cells (FBGCs):* The nuclei are randomly scattered throughout the cytoplasm and are formed by the fusion of macrophage in an attempt to ward off the foreign material.

- *Touton giant cells: Xanthelasmatic giant cells:* They are formed by fusion of epithelioid cells and contain a ring of nuclei surrounded by foamy cytoplasm, seen in xanthomas, fat necrosis, xanthogranulomatous inflammation, and dermatofibroma.
- *Epidermal cell derived:* Tzanck giant cells—multinucleated epidermal giant cell formed in response to viral infection (herpes, varicella, etc.) with molding of the ground glass appearing with marginated chromatin nuclei as they are crowded together.
- *Melanocyte derived:*
  - Starburst giant cells
  - Balloon cells in melanocytes
  - Giant nevus cells of melanocytes
- *Other giant cells:*
  - Floret-like multinucleated giant cells—seen in gynecomastia, neurofibromatosis-1, etc.
  - Giant cells of astrocytoma
  - Reed–Sternberg cells seen in Hodgkins lymphoma
  - Warthin–Finkeldey giant cell of measles

32. Describe giant cell.

Ans: Please see the Answer to Question above.

33. Define GCT of bone. Describe clinical features, diagnosis, and management principles of GCT for upper end of tibia.

Ans: *Definition:* It is a locally aggressive benign neoplasm characterized by large numbers of osteoclast-like giant cells, distributed uniformly in sheets of *neoplastic* ovoid mononuclear cells (plump epithelioid or spindle cells).

Clinical features: Patients usually present with painful swelling. Juxta-articular tumors may additionally have restriction of joint motion and/or joint effusion. Most patients with GCTs have progressive pain that often is related to activity initially and only later becomes evident at rest. The pain is rarely severe, unless a pathological fracture has occurred. Pathological fractures are seen in around 10% of patients.

The tumor is not uncommon representing around 4–5% of all primary bone neoplasms, and more than 20% of benign primary bone tumors. It occurs slightly more often in females than in males. Young adults are commonly affected and peak incidence is seen around 20–45 years of age. The most common location for this tumor is the distal femur, followed closely by the proximal tibia and is often solitary lesions. In the distal radius (the third most common location), these tumors frequently are more aggressive. The primary areas of involvement are ends of long bones commonly the distal femoral condyles, proximal tibial plateau, proximal humerus, and styloid process of distal radius. In axial skeleton (vertebrae and sacrum) anterior column is predominantly involved. The tumor commonly originates from the epiphyseal scar near metaphyseo-epiphyseal junction. Multifocal GCTs (synchronous or metachronous) are known to occur (1–2% of all cases) and are more aggressive than conventional form.

Diagnosis: Radiologically, the characteristic appearance of GCTs is an eccentric geographical lytic lesion without matrix formation typically involving epiphysis and extending to metaphysis. The tumors show a well-defined sclerotic transition between the lesion and host bone. Bone response to the pathology in the form of periosteal elevation or reactive bone formation is rare unless a pathological fracture is present. The cortex is expanded and thinned with frequent breach and soft tissue extension. Soft tissue extensions have thin "egg-shell" of bone remaining. Benign and less aggressive forms have multiple thin trabeculae running as septae across the lytic lesion giving a "soap-bubble" appearance (seen in around 20% cases). The margins of the lesion also vary and hence the tumor has been classified by Campanacci into three radiological subtypes (there is no histopathological correlation though of these radiological subtypes):

- *Type 1 (Quiescent lesions):* Well-defined margin with surrounding sclerosis and little, if any, cortical involvement.
- *Type 2 (Active tumors):* Well-defined margins, but lack surrounding sclerosis. Thin and expanded cortex but no breach.
- *Type 3 (Aggressive tumors):* Ill-defined margins often with cortical breakthrough and soft tissue extension.
  Computed tomography scan provides a good evaluation of cortical continuity.

Magnetic resonance imaging is the investigation of choice for surgical planning especially in axial lesions and aggressive forms or longstanding tumors where soft tissue extension needs accurate assessment.

Giant cell tumor typically shows low-to-intermediate signal intensity on T1-weighted images and intermediate-to-high intensity on T2 images. Hemosiderin is associated with attenuation of signals on both T1 and T2 images. Patients usually present with painful swelling. Juxta-articular tumors may additionally have restriction of joint motion and/or joint effusion. Pathological fractures are seen in around 10% of patients.

Management principles: GCT has propensity to locally recur after treatment (currently 10–20%) but has a low metastatic potential. Tumors that recur multiple times are also prone to malignant transformation. This makes imperative that GCT is managed with utmost care to prevent such complication.

Simple curettage, with or without bone grafting, has a significantly high rate of local recurrence of up to 60%. These intralesional and marginal procedures without adjuvants are associated with higher recurrences (the recurrence is actually "persistence" of original disease) due to inability to completely remove the microscopic disease, and recurrence is not correlated with grade or site of lesion.

- Modern treatment of GCT with extended curettage (making a wide window, using head lamps or dental mirror, angled curettes and high-speed burrs and pulsatile lavage) and cryosurgery (using liquid nitrogen) to the tumor cavity has achieved a recurrence rate of <3%. Routine use of adjuvants is recommended.
- Cryotherapy with liquid nitrogen popularized by Marcove has various side effects and has been effectively abandoned due to frostbite of soft tissues and bone necrosis.
- Bone cement has a tumor kill effect by exothermic reaction and possible chemical reaction (solvent aerosol is cytotoxic) that produces necrosis of tissue for 1–2 mm from contact area. Some people have used methotrexate and Adriamycin in the bone cement to augment cytotoxic effect. Bone cement has the advantage of filling the defect and having tumoricidal effect. Advantages of cementing include:
  - Cytotoxic (exothermic and monomer aerosol)
  - Radiographic detection of recurrence is easier—as a clear lucent line around the cement
  - Good structural support and early weight bearing
- There has been a concern for poor functional outcome in lesions involving large articular surfaces; the larger the articular surface involved the poorer the function. Wide local excision for such larger tumors can be done followed by reconstruction using megaprosthesis (provide mobility but prone to loosening and late failure), arthrodesis (stability but immobility). Arthrodesis reconstruction of limb can be done using standard procedures (internal/external fixation), Ilizarov method, osteoarticular allografts, and microvascular bone grafts.

34. What is the management for recurrence of GCT?

Ans: *Recurrences of GCT* occur within 2 years and is less in Campanacci grade 1 and 2 (7%) compared to grade 3 (29%). Total serum acid phosphatase (TCAP) can be used as a tumor marker for monitoring response to the treatment of GCT. TCAP correlates with initial tumor size and normalizes after resection; reappearing with recurrence of tumor. Late recurrence (>5 years) should be suspected for sarcomatous transformation. The recurrences are treated in similar fashion as for primary tumor. Radiation therapy (megavoltage 35–70 Gy) has been used for additional clearance of surgical margins in cases that are difficult to adequately manage surgically (lesions of spine and sacrum) or for aggressive recurrent tumors. Multiple recurrences and use of radiation have been linked to development of malignancy in GCT (secondary malignant transformation apart from primary cases).

35. A. Describe the pathogenesis and classification of "Giant cell tumor of bone".
   B. Explain the concept of extended curettage.
   C. Discuss role and schedule of denosumab in the treatment of appendicular bone GCT.

Ans: Answers to parts (A) and (B) already covered in above questions.

C. Role of Denosumab in Appendicular GCT

1. Neoadjuvant therapy (presurgical):
   - Reduces tumor size, facilitating less morbid surgery (e.g., curettage instead of resection)
   - May help to preserve joint function in periarticular tumors.
2. Adjuvant therapy (postsurgical):
   - Reduces recurrence risk after incomplete resection.

- Definitive therapy for unresectable or metastatic GCT:
  - Used when surgery is not feasible (e.g., sacral/spinal GCT) or in metastatic disease.

Dosing Schedule of Denosumab for GCT
- Standard regimen:
  - 120 mg subcutaneously (SC) on days 1, 8, 15, and 29, followed by maintenance doses every 4 weeks.
- Modified regimens:
  - Some protocols use 120 mg SC weekly for 3 weeks, then monthly.
- Duration of treatment:
  - Neoadjuvant: Typically 3–6 months before surgery.
  - Adjuvant/Definitive: Continued until maximal response (often 6–12+ months).
  - Long-term therapy may be needed for unresectable/metastatic cases.

5.11 PRIMITIVE NEUROECTODERMAL TUMORS AND EWING'S SARCOMA (Q36–39)

36. Explain primitive neuroectodermal tumors.

Ans: Primitive neuroectodermal tumors (PNETs) are a group of malignant tumors characterized by small round cells of neuroectodermal origin. Batsakis et al., in 1996, divided the PNET tumors into three groups based on the tissue of origin:
1. *Central nervous system (CNS) PNETs:* Neoplasms derived from the CNS
2. *Neuroblastoma:* These are neoplasms derived from the autonomic nervous system
3. *Peripheral PNETs (pPNETs):* These neoplasms originate from tissues outside the central and autonomic nervous system and are of interest to orthopedic surgeon as cytogenetically they belong to Ewing's sarcoma (EWS) family of tumors with translocation of *EWS* gene (22q12) and *FLI-1* (11q24) seen in 85% of cases.

The pPNETs usually manifest in the thoracopulmonary region (Askin tumor), pelvis, abdomen, and extremities while less common sites include head and neck. The pPNETs usually present in the second decade of life, with a slight male preponderance. The common symptoms based on the origin of neoplasia include pain and swelling of the surrounding structures due to mass effect. Other site-specific symptoms include individual cranial neuropathies, exophthalmos, epistaxis, nasal obstruction, anosmia, neck masses, and headache. A large number of tumors have metastasized by presentation. The most common sites of metastases include the lung, bone, and bone marrow.

Differential diagnosis: Malignant lymphoma, poorly differentiated salivary gland tumors, rhabdomyosarcoma, neuroblastoma, and undifferentiated nasopharyngeal carcinoma.

Pathology: PNETs need differentiation from round cell tumors and that usually needs immunohistochemical profiling or in rare cases electron microscopy or cytogenetic studies. On light microscopy pPNETs have a monotonous collection of small, round, darkly stained cells that is quite unremarkable and even rhabdomyosarcoma, neuroblastoma, and non-Hodgkin lymphoma exhibit the same albeit Homer-Wright rosettes are seen in latter. Immunohistochemistry can be used to detect antibodies to FLI-1 in the gene fusion product (typically MIC2 antigen) of EWS. Identification of MIC2 consistently identifies both Ewing sarcoma and pPNETs and is absent in CNS PNET and neuroblastomas. In addition, in pPNET also coexpress CD99 (the glycoprotein MIC2) and vimentin and nonspecific markers include S-100, neuron-specific enolase, CD75, and synaptophysin.

Investigation: NCCT of head and neck and MRI are usually done for head and neck neoplasia; HRCT of chest is needed in neoplasia of the chest. Abdominal tumors are diagnosed best by NCCT abdomen. A full metastatic work-up [including bone scan or positron emission tomography (PET) scan] is needed as most of these tumors have metastasized by presentation.

Prognosis: Tumors of head and neck region have better prognosis than tumors of thorax and scapula while abdominal tumors have worst prognosis.

Treatment: Surgical excision of tumor with R0 resection is recommended to extirpate the local disease. This may be precluded in aggressive tumors that have spread diffusely or vital structures are involved. Chemotherapy and radiation are most important adjuncts in management. Both adjuvant and neoadjuvant chemotherapy are used with a regimen based on vincristine, doxorubicin, and cyclophosphamide with ifosfamide and etoposide similar to Ewing's tumor. Metastatic disease needs similar chemotherapy combined with radiotherapy to surgical site and sites of gross disease. The significant disadvantage to use of radiotherapy is the development of secondary sarcomas related to radiotherapy the risk of which can be mitigated by use of fractionated therapy.

37. Enumerate various round cell tumors of bone.
Ans: Vide Answer to Question above please.

38. Explain clinical features, pathology, radiological features, and management of (upper end humerus) EWS.
Ans: Ewing's sarcoma

Clinical features: On an average it has been seen that there is a delay in diagnosis of approximately 6 months from the onset of symptoms in 50% patients. Pain and a local tender swelling in the involved area are the most common clinical symptoms. The pain precedes swelling by several months. Overlying skin may be red, inflamed, and edematous. Fever (remittent and moderate grade), anemia, leukocytosis, and increase in sedimentation rate are often seen. This may confuse the surgeon to osteomyelitis and has been responsible for few surgeries mistakenly performed to decompress the bone (for acute osteomyelitis). To utter surprise even pus (liquefied tumor) may be found at the time of surgery further reconciling the surgeon for bone infection.

Systemic signs often reflect malignant disease that has metastasized. Pathological fracture is an uncommon complication but may be seen in neglected cases or those with delayed presentation. Metastatic disease to bone if extensive may lead to petechiae or purpura due to thrombocytopenia. Pulmonary metastasis may be clinically identified with asymmetric breath sounds, pleural rub, etc.

Etiopathogenesis: The *MIC2* gene product, *CD99*, is a surface membrane protein that is expressed in most cases of EWS. The detection of a consistent translocation involving the *EWSR1* locus [a member of the TET family (TLS/EWS/TAF15) of RNA-binding proteins] on chromosome 22 band q12 and any one of a number of partner chromosomes [number 11 band q24 (*FLI1*), number 21 band q22 (*ERG*), number 7 (*ETV1*) or number 17 (*E1AF*)] is the key feature in the diagnosis of EWS. The characteristic consistent translocations that result thus include recurrent t(11;22) (q24;q12) chromosomal translocation, t(21;22), t(7;22) and t(17;22). Virtually all of these appear to express some form of *EWS/ETS* gene fusion. *EWS/FLI1* has potent oncogenic activity and the fusion product function as aberrant transcription factors binding to *ETS* target genes. One target is downregulation of expression of TGF-β type II receptor which is a potent tumor suppressor. TGF-β signaling induces apoptosis in many cell types. Apart from the above-mentioned aberrations that are quite consistent, other abnormalities are also found that involve the *EWSR1* gene at 22q12. There is a growing consensus that trisomy 20 and *CDKN2A* mutations may indicate a more aggressive subset of EWS tumors. As molecular diagnosis of EWS is quite consistent and reproducible efforts are on to commercially produce a molecular test based on reverse transcriptase polymerase chain reaction (RT-PCR) and restriction analysis of PCR products that can be performed on a small tissue sample and offer the opportunity to markedly simplify the detection and definition of EWS.

Gross and Histopathology
Grossly the tumor is firm, glistening, or more liquefied like pus. Hemorrhage and cystic changes are usual. Microscopically, the classic form comprises of cellular sheets and nests of uniform, small, typical round to polygonal cells with scanty cytoplasm. Areas of necrosis show perivascular cuffing. Rosettes pattern is seen in few patients and have no diagnostic value as they are not at all characteristic. Paying too much attention on them may cause a misdiagnosis of metastatic neuroblastoma. When stained by periodic acid-Schiff cytoplasmic glycogen is demonstrated in many (but not all) cases. The glycogen is more prominent if the tumor is fixed in 80% alcohol. MIC2 (*CD99*) shows membranous positivity in the large majority of EWS and PNETs in contrast to cytoplasmic positivity in rhabdomyosarcomas and cells from acute lymphoblastic leukemia. Few histopathological variants of the above classic pattern have been noted including a large cell type variant and a filigree pattern.

- Large cell variant demonstrated larger cells, and may also have prominent nucleoli.
- In the filigree pattern, however, the architecture is bicellular (made of two types of cells) that are separated by stroma.

Radiological features: An ill-defined osteolytic lesion involving the diaphysis or metaphysis (or both) of a long tubular bone is the most common feature. Epiphyseal involvement is extremely rare. Poorly marginated permeative or moth-eaten bone destruction (76%) often associated with "onion skin" like multilayered laminated periosteal reaction (57%) is characteristic. Occasionally Codman's triangle or sunburst appearance may be seen. The cortex overlying the tumor is irregularly thinned or thickened (40%) and even cystic spaces may be seen in some. A large, ill-defined soft tissue mass is a frequent association in Ewing's tumor. CT scan and MRI are useful investigations and ideally both should be done for staging. Whole body MRI may be done in select cases to guide treatment plan. On T1 images, the tumor appears low-to-intermediate signal, and on T2-weighted images, there is heterogeneously high signal often with hair-on-end low-signal striations. Gadolinium contrast shows heterogeneous but prominent signal enhancement.

Management: EWS is considered a systemic disease at presentation to control local disease and kill metastatic disease simultaneously. With current regimens for therapy for localized EWS, the prognosis is good and patients achieve EFS and an overall survival rate of nearly 70% at 5 years. Current *chemotherapy* regime includes VAdriaC [vincristine, Adriamycin (doxorubicin), and cyclophosphamide] for 2 days alternating with IE (ifosfamide and etoposide) for 5 days given every 2 weeks (interval compression) or 3 weeks (traditional method). High initial dose of Adriamycin (dose intense regime) has better outcome. Addition of topotecan to above chemotherapy is being studied. Local control has been deemed to be better with surgery than radiation due to associated growth retardation in young children with radiotherapy. Also surgically resected specimen can be subjected to assess the tumor necrosis that can be then utilized to prognosticate or change chemotherapy (high-dose chemotherapy with stem cell rescue). Positive surgical margins have a poor prognosis.

The specific reconstruction technique deployed is determined by the location of tumor, patient's age, and the requirement of additional modalities for comprehensive management (i.e., chemotherapy and/or radiation). Allografts and autogenous vascularized bone grafts in conjunction with endoprosthesis or alone may be used. Autogenous grafts are associated with donor-site morbidity. Allografts are a biological solution without donor-site morbidity and will last for lifetime if incorporated. The major drawback is incorporation and union of allografts. Metallic endoprosthetic provides immediately stable reconstruction for mobilization.

Radiation therapy, though has been effective especially for unresectable tumors, but there remains always a risk of secondary neoplasms developing in future. Despite these drawbacks that are not certain in all patients who have residual microscopic disease or in whom margins were inadequate, or those who demonstrate viable tumor on histopathological examination of resected tumor specimen should receive adjuvant radiation therapy.

For *metastatic disease* to lungs standard radiotherapy should be given. For metastatic sites of disease in bone and soft-tissues fractionated radiation therapy doses totaling 45–56 Gy should be given. Pulmonary metastases are managed with whole-lung irradiation (12–15 Gy) even if chemotherapy has given complete resolution of overt pulmonary metastasis. Currently for patients with metastatic disease, use of high-dose chemotherapy with stem cell rescue for metastatic disease is being studied. Recurrence of tumor usually occurs within 2 years (80%) compared to those with primary EWS (mean age 22.5 years) and are likely to have neoplastic lesions in axial skeleton or extraskeletal site. Some predictors for outcome are as follows:

- *Tumor metastases* (detected in about 25% of patients): It is the *most powerful* predictor of outcome individually. Even considering the distribution of metastasis, if it is solely pulmonary, it fares better than in patients with metastasis outside the lungs.
- *Cytogenetics:* The *EWS-FLI1* translocation breakpoint is not associated with adverse outcome as had been considered previously.
- *Molecular markers:*
  - Detectable fusion transcripts by RT-PCR in morphologically normal marrow is associated with higher recurrence.
  - Poor prognosis has been associated with overexpression of the p53 protein, expression of Ki67, and loss of long-arm chromosome (16q deletion)
  - Increased microsomal glutathione S-transferase expression is associated with resistance to doxorubicin and hence inferior response to chemotherapy.

Treatment Response to Preoperative Therapy
A good response to preoperative chemotherapy is evident in the form of minimal (<5%) or no residual viable tumor left after presurgical chemotherapy that obviously is correlated to significantly improved EFS when compared to patients

having residual larger volume of viable tumor left. Better histologic response to preoperative chemotherapy is seen in females and younger patients. PET scans can help evaluate the response to chemotherapy being a metabolic indicator; decreased PET uptake seen in patients who underwent preinduction and postinduction chemotherapy and were evaluated by PET at both times, correlates well with good histologic response and better outcome.

Histology: Tumors that demonstrate histological variants like filigree pattern have an unfavorable prognosis. However, the degree of neural differentiation has no prognosticating value in EWS.

39. How will you treat a case of Ewing's tumor arising from lower end of femur in a 15-year-old boy?

Ans: Kindly see Answer to Question 38 above and formulate a similar answer for distal femur instead of humerus.

5.12 CYSTIC LESIONS OF BONE (Q40–44)

40. Describe the differential diagnosis of cystic lesions in upper end of humerus in a 10-year-old child. Describe the management of SBC in the same child.

Ans:

Differential diagnosis:

- Unicameral bone cyst (UBC)
- ABC
- Intraosseous ganglion cyst
- Hydatid disease.

Management of SBC

Diagnosis: The cysts are visualized as oval or ovoid lytic lesions with thinned cortices in metaphyseal or metadiaphyseal region of the long tubular bones with their long axis aligned parallel to the long axis of bone. The margins are clear and distinct, cortical breach may occur in fast growing cysts or with trauma. Fallen fragments of bone may be seen within the cyst.

Treatment: Many unicameral cysts heal either spontaneously or following trauma. Pathologic fractures through cyst often heal with healing of cyst unintervened. Impending fracture may be treated with immobilization and aspiration of the cyst along with hydrocortisone injections. For some uncommon cases, curettage with or without bone grafting or cementing may be done (especially if failed to heal by injection or for larger cysts). Excision is reserved for recurrent cysts (10% of cases).

41. Explain the following:
   A. Gross histopathological and radiological features of ABC.
   B. Differential diagnosis of ABC in a flat bone.
   C. Outline management of ABC of scapula in an adult.

Ans:

A. *Histopathological features:* Microscopically, there are anastomosing cavernous areas filled with blood that represent the gross honey-combed structure. These spaces are, however, walled by thin fibrous tissue containing fibroblasts, myofibroblasts, osteoid and chondroid tissue, and osteoclast-like giant cells in varying proportions (instead of smooth muscle wall or endothelial cells of blood vessels of true cavernous vascular spaces). In one-third cases, characteristic reticulated lacy chondroid-like material (described as calcified matrix with a chondroid aura) is seen that histologically represents reparative tissue (Campanacci et al.). This has led to the acceptance of ABC as a secondary reparative lesion in primary pathologies.

Radiological features: The radiological features vary with the developmental four stages of ABC also called evolution of ABC. In the incipient phase (usually identified incidentally), there is a small nonexpansile intramedullary (often eccentric) lytic lesion that may have permeative margins. There is distinctive elevation of periosteum. During growth phase, there is rapid growth and lysis of bone that may present as cortical blowout in "accelerated" phenomenon of ABC. The Codman's triangles may be prominent at the ends. In the stable phase, there is expanded bone with a "shell" around the lesion along with trabeculations coursing within it (coarse soap-bubble appearance). The healing cyst (self-resolution or following treatment) shows progressive ossification, resulting in a coarsely trabeculated bony mass often with mineralized matrix. Fluid/blood levels (requires minimum 10 minutes of patient in still position) with multiple internal septae on MRI are a characteristic finding. There is increased T1-signal in dependent fluid (due to methemoglobin) while septations are more prominent on T2-weighted images. The cyst may invaginate into normal bone and to epiphysis through growth plate or extend into soft tissue. Capanna et al. described five "morphologic types" (separate from grades mentioned in treatment) based on the radiographic findings:

- *Type I:* Central metaphyseal lesion well-contained within bone with intact bone cortices.
- *Type II:* Lesion gives an inflated appearance to bone with cortical thinning.
- *Type III:* Eccentric metaphyseal location with unaffected cortex.
- *Type IV:* Subperiosteal extension but cortex intact rarely seen in the diaphysis.
- *Type V:* Metadiaphyseal location blowout appearance, cortical breach present and cyst may invaginate into nearby bone.

B. *Differential diagnosis:* Telangiectatic osteosarcoma, ossifying hematoma, and hemophilic pseudotumor.

C. After histopathological diagnosis, the treatment options are multiple and best one for a patient needs to be individualized. Active and aggressive ABCs are treated by one of the following treatments depending on surgeon's preference.

- Percutaneous methods for inducing sclerosis in the cyst and secondary mineralization (healing)—for localized lesions that do not contain any secondary malignancy this appears to be appropriate treatment provided patient accepts that it will not cause obliteration of the deformity. Also, the method is good for small-to-moderate tumor size—volume <20 cm³ (for spherical tumors radius <3–4 cm). Multiple injections are often needed especially for larger lesions.
- Curettage and bone grafting had been the gold standard of treatment that especially for larger lesions involving scapula. The curettage can be supplemented with the use of high-speed burr, or extended curettage has been proposed using various adjuvants [peroxide, phenol, cryotherapy, zinc chloride, hypochlorite, polymethyl methacrylate (PMMA) bone cement] to reduce recurrence rate. Selective arterial embolization is recommended for reducing the blood loss in large cysts. Lesions of acromion may be excised and reconstructed using mesh.
- If the lesion is very large expansile and aggressive with demonstrated or doubtful areas of possible other malignancies, then it is better to perform marginal en bloc excision and do prosthetic reconstruction.

42. **What are the clinical and radiological features and management of ABC of distal femur?**

Ans: Clinical features: Although, the cyst can be seen in any age (especially secondary ABC), the primary ABC is typically seen to affect the individuals in first two decades. The metaphyseal regions in long bones such as femur are commonly affected by the *de novo* lesion; however, secondary ABC has site predilection according to the primary lesion. The lesion is usually solitary; however, multiple site involvement in same patients has also been reported and can be seen in 5% of patients. Patients commonly have pain and swelling at the site. Unusually patients may present with a pathological fracture at the site of ABC.

Radiological features: The radiological features vary with the developmental four stages of ABC also called evolution of ABC. In the incipient phase (usually identified incidentally), there is a small nonexpansile intramedullary (often eccentric) lytic lesion that may have permeative margins. There is distinctive elevation of periosteum. During growth phase, there is rapid growth and lysis of bone that may present as cortical blowout in "accelerated" phenomenon of ABC.

The Codman's triangles may be prominent at the ends. In the stable phase, there is expanded bone with a "shell" around the lesion along with trabeculations coursing within it (coarse soap-bubble appearance. The healing cyst (self-resolution or following treatment) shows progressive ossification, resulting in a coarsely trabeculated bony mass often with mineralized matrix. Fluid/blood levels (requires minimum 10 minutes of patient in still position) with multiple internal septae on MRI are a characteristic finding. There is increased T1-signal-independent fluid (due to methemoglobin) while septations are more prominent on T2-weighted images. The cyst may invaginate into normal bone and to epiphysis through growth plate or extend into soft tissue.

Management: After histopathological diagnosis, the treatment options are multiple and best one for a patient needs to be individualized. Some guide can be taken from Capanna classification of ABC radiologically into three "grades." The inactive cysts have complete periosteal shell and sclerotic bone margins. In contrast, active cysts have incomplete shell and aggressive lesions have indefinite margins. Inactive lesions may be observed as spontaneous regression has been observed. Active and aggressive ABCs are treated by one of the following treatments depending on surgeon's preference:

Percutaneous methods for inducing sclerosis in the cyst and secondary mineralization (healing) have become recently popular for treatment of extremity and pelvic regions. They have advantage particularly in the juxtaphyseal location and difficult surgical sites. Alcoholic solution of zein has been investigated by various authors and has good efficacy, but the side effects of percutaneous fistulation, local abscess formation, and sometimes embolization have raised concerns. Polidocanol is an effective, cheap, and reasonably safe alternative that has shown good success in some large studies focused on ABC treatment. Sclerotherapy possibly acts by mechanism same as its role in varicose veins treatment wherein the walls of the cyst containing the active spindle cells are inactivated and the lytic effects subside. Healing of bone then takes precedence, healing the cyst in due course of 6–18 months depending on the size of initial lesion.

Use of demineralized bone particle instilled into the lesion as a paste of allogenic bone powder and autogenous bone marrow has been reported to induce healing. No curettage or extensive surgery is done, particulated bone allograft is easy to handle and introduce into an irregular cavity. It is expected that the bone grafting material promoting ossification at a pace faster that the native rate of ABC expansion. It also utilizes the repair potential of conventional ABC, in-effect reversing the lesion.

The percutaneous methods are not to be used in patients with rapid expansion of the cyst causing local and distal neurological or vascular symptoms as the time to healing is quite long. It should also be not used in impending fractures and patients allergic to drug.

Curettage and bone grafting has been the gold standard of treatment that is still used to compare efficacy of other methods. The curettage can be supplemented with the use of high-speed burr, or extended curettage has been proposed using various adjuvants [peroxide, phenol, cryotherapy, zinc chloride, hypochlorite, and polymethyl methacrylate (PMMA) bone cement] to reduce recurrence rate. The rates of recurrence are quite unacceptable (7–50%) in various series with the use of conventional curettage alone with or without bone grafting, so extended curettage is recommended. Selective arterial embolization has been used for reducing the blood loss in large cysts that are at difficult surgical location but should not be used to rely upon for inducing healing. Growth plate can get damaged while treating the juxtaphyseal lesions.

43. Explain unicameral bone cyst.

Ans: Simple bone cyst also called unicameral, juvenile, or essential bone cyst. The cyst is primarily a metaphyseal intramedullary lesion that enlarges slowly and is commonly seen in first two decades of life. With growth of the child, the cyst may "artifactually" come to lie in diaphysis of bone. The lesion is usually unilocular cavity generally filled with clear or straw-colored fluid though septations may develop in irregular growing cysts or in cancellous bone or with healing of cortical breaches. The lining is composed of thin fibrovascular tissue membrane.

Etiopathogenesis
Simple cysts are considered either a developmental abnormality (hamartoma) or recently the hemodynamic pressure measurements suggest some form of venous obstruction though the chain of events leading to cyst formation are not clear. The normal bone intraosseous pressure is usually around 5–15 mm Hg while intracystic pressure ranges from 15 mm Hg to 40 mm Hg. The normal bone pressure curves are smooth without any notches while transduced pressure traces from UBC depict systolic, diastolic, and dicrotic notches.

Clinical features
The proximal humerus and femur are the most common sites (80%) affected followed by proximal tibia, ilium, and calcaneus. Quite a few are recognized incidentally on radiographs done for other purpose otherwise pain at the site is the most common presentation. Pathologic fractures occur often in young teenagers due to trivial injury while playing, stiffness as a presenting feature is uncommon.

Radiology
The cysts are visualized as oval or ovoid lytic lesions with thinned cortices in metaphyseal or metadiaphyseal region of the long tubular bones with their long axis aligned parallel to the long axis of bone. The margins are clear and distinct, cortical breach may occur in fast growing cysts or with trauma. Fallen fragments of bone may be seen within the cyst.

Gross and Histopathology

Grossly the cyst is a dilated region of bone containing straw-colored fluid. The walls are generally smooth. The lining of cyst consists of irregular fragments of membranous fibrovascular tissue. Hemosiderin (due to injury), granulation tissue, uncommon giant cells, or scattered chronic inflammatory cells may be additionally present.

Management and Prognosis

Many unicameral cysts heal either spontaneously or following trauma. Pathologic fractures through cyst often heal with healing of cyst unintervened. Impending fracture may be treated with immobilization and aspiration of the cyst along with hydrocortisone injections. For some uncommon cases curettage, with or without bone grafting or cementing may be done (especially if failed to heal by injection or for larger cysts). Excision is reserved for recurrent cysts (10% of cases).

44. Explain osteitis fibrosa cystica.

Ans: It is the bony manifestation of primary hyperparathyroidism which occurs in 10–20% of patients (Brown tumor). Histologically, there are increased giant multinucleated osteoclasts in scalloped areas on the surface of the bone (Howship's lacunae) and the normal cellular and marrow elements are replaced by fibrous tissue. Radiological changes usually include areas of subperiosteal cortical resorption which is evident radiologically replacement of the usual sharp cortical outline of the bone in the digits by an irregular outline. There is also resorption of the phalangeal tufts. Other findings include loss of lamina dura dentes, mineralization of soft tissues, development of bone cysts, and an overall reduction in bone density.

Other Signs and Symptoms

Classical patients with stones (renal), abdominal groans, psychiatric moans, bones are rare to find and most patients are now asymptomatic at detection. The classical manifestations are mentioned below:
- *Renal manifestations:* Deposition of calcium in renal parenchyma (nephrocalcinosis) or recurrent nephrolithiasis, diabetes insipidus, and renal failure.
- *Abdominal groans:* Constipation, vomiting, peptic ulcer disease [may be associated with Zollinger-Ellison syndrome (MEN)], and acute pancreatitis.
- *Psychiatric moans:* Result from memory loss, fatigue, depression, and delirium.

Diagnosis
- Elevated immunoreactive parathyroid hormone (PTH) level in asymptomatic hypercalcemia
- Hypercalcemia, hypophosphatemia, increased urinary phosphate, increased alkaline phosphate, and increased excretion of hydroxyproline in the urine.

Treatment: Usually, the asymptomatic patients are managed conservatively with adequate hydration and reduced calcium intake. The patients should be followed annually for serum calcium levels, bone mineral density (BMD) test, and serum creatinine. There is a growing concern for cardiovascular deterioration, neuropsychiatric dysfunction, the adverse effects of osteoporosis, and reduced bone quality favoring early surgery. Prophylactic parathyroidectomy is, however, debated and there is no clear consensus. Currently, surgery is indicated in patients with sustained serum calcium more than 1 mg/dL above normal, creatinine clearance <60 mL/min, age <50 years, and bone density t-score less than −2.5 (or a z-score of <2.0 if age is <20 years) at any of the three sites. Surgical removal of the functional parathyroid lesion results in a rapid decrease in circulating PTH levels, due to rapid bone formation by uninhibited osteoblasts ("hungry bone"). It may acutely result in severe hypocalcemic tetany since the half-life of PTH in plasma is approximately 20 minutes. Postoperatively, if hypercalcemia persists for a week or more or recurs after showing initial improvement one should suspect a second adenoma or metastases from carcinoma.

5.13 SCHWANNOMA (Q45)

45. What is a schwannoma, elaborate on the clinical features and diagnosis?

Ans: Schwannoma is a commonly benign nerve sheath tumor arising from Schwann cells of the peripheral nerves. They are also known as neurilemmoma. They can arise from both cranial as well as spinal nerves. The most common location of occurrence of the tumor is in the inner ear where they present as vestibular schwannoma also known as acoustic neuromas. They are commonly seen in orthopedic practice with neurofibromatosis type 1 (Von Recklinghausen's disease). In NF-1 the gene-encoding neurofibromin is responsible in most of the cases. Neurofibromin is expressed at higher levels in the neural crest during development. Cells from the neural crest migrate to become pigmented cells of the skin, parts of the brain, spinal cord, peripheral nerves, and adrenals, thus explaining the common sites of abnormalities in the disorder. Most commonly arise in 8th cranial nerve and 2nd most common is 5th cranial nerve. At both sites the tumor is intradural.

When these tumors are malignant, they are called malignant schwannomas or malignant peripheral nerve sheath tumors or neurofibrosarcomas. These arise commonly in sciatic nerve, brachial plexus, and sacral plexus. There are few variants of schwannoma as follows:
- Ancient schwannoma
- Cellular schwannoma
- Melanotic schwannoma
- Plexiform schwannoma.

Clinical features: These occur in adults except in von Recklinghausen's disease where they are diagnosed in first decade itself. When they occur in patients with neurofibromatosis type 2 (NF2), schwannomas usually present by the 3rd decade. They occur as a solitary nodule on any sheathed sensory, motor or autonomic nerve (commonly in vagus nerve). Multiple schwannomas are uncommon and occur in von Recklinghausen's disease. The following are the common locations of origin of schwannoma:
- Intracranial schwannomas:
  - Cranial nerves
  - Intracerebral (very rare)
- Spinal schwannoma
- Trunk:
  - Intercostal nerves
  - Posterior mediastinum
  - Retroperitoneum
  - Gastrointestinal schwannoma
- *Limbs:*
  - Ulnar and peroneal nerves.

Common symptoms include hearing loss (vestibular schwannoma), back pain that increases in supine position, paresthesias in lower limb, numbness, weakness of the lower limb, and sciatica.

Diagnosis: The diagnosis is made by investigating according to the presentation. MRI of head and neck will be needed for evaluation of hearing loss in a child. MRI of lumbar and lumbosacral spine is needed in lower back pain with associated symptoms. The schwannoma appears iso- or hypointense on T1-weighted images while it shows intense enhancement on contrast T1 images. On T2-weighted images it is heterogeneously hyperintense and larger schwannomas show cystic degeneration. Large tumors also have areas of hemosiderin due to intramural hemorrhages (5% cases). "Split-fat sign" is seen in non-fat-suppressed images where a thin rim of fat embraces along the long axis of lesion. Target sign comprising of peripheral high signal with low central signal and "fascicular sign" comprising of multiple small ring-like structures are seen in peripheral large schwannomas.

Treatment: The vestibular schwannoma is primarily a domain of ENT surgeon and neurosurgeon. Spinal schwannomas are usually managed by surgery for weakness, numbness or pain. Microsurgery is preferred with intraoperative electrophysiological monitoring. The nerve is opened, and the tumor is carefully excised. Large tumors are managed in addition by radiotherapy (stereotactic spine radiosurgery) that utilizes highly focused radiation beams to target spinal tumor. This is beneficial in the sense that the surrounding tissue is spared of ill-effects of radiation with nearly instant recovery.

5.14 MULTIPLE MYELOMA (Q46)

46. Describe clinical features, diagnosis, and treatment of multiple myeloma.

Ans: Multiple Myeloma

Clinical Features

Myeloid marrow-containing bones in adults are the most frequently involved: vertebrae, ribs, skull, pelvis, femur, clavicle, and scapula. The skeletal lesions are typically well-demarcated osteolytic (osteosclerotic form is also recognized), extensive and cause *bone pain (70% patients), pathological fractures, hypercalcemia,* and anemia. *Thoracolumbar pain or a compression fracture* is usually the first symptom. Neurologic *symptoms* due to compression of roots or cord often occur and may result from extraosseous extension of the tumor or from a pathological fracture. The osteosclerotic variant of multiple myeloma commonly presents with *peripheral neuropathy* but this is rare with classic PCM. Loss of bone marrow causes anemia that is exaggerated by amyloid deposition in kidneys causing *renal damage* (and failure) depleting erythropoietin. An M-component (electrophoresis) in γ-globulin region is present in 99% of the patients (serum or urine). Immunoelectrophoresis (qualitative analysis) determines the monoclonal nature. The monoclonal proteins are mainly IgG (50% of the cases) or IgA class (25–20%) and, rarely, of the IgM, IgD or IgE classes. Antibody concentration of 5 g/L (corresponding to 109 cells producing the antibody) is required for accurate determination and quantification by electrophoresis. A monoclonal light chain (Bence Jones protein) is found in the serum in 75% of the patients that results in *renal failure* from light chain proteinuria. *Recurrent bacterial infections* are common due to lack of effective globulin component and ineffective utilization of cells to produce redundant globulins only.

Diagnosis

Diagnostic criteria for symptomatic multiple myeloma and associated disorders.

Symptomatic Multiple Myeloma

- Clonal plasma cells >10% on bone marrow biopsy or (in any quantity) in a biopsy from other tissues (plasmacytoma)
- A monoclonal protein (paraprotein, M-protein) in either serum or urine (except in cases of true non-secretory myeloma)
- Evidence of end-organ damage felt related to the plasma cell disorder (*related organ or tissue impairment*, ROTI, commonly referred by the acronym "CRAB"):
    - Hypercalcemia (corrected calcium >2.75 mmol/L)
    - Renal insufficiency attributable to myeloma
    - Anemia (hemoglobin <10 g/dL)
    - Bone lesions (lytic lesions or osteoporosis with compression fractures)

Asymptomatic (smoldering) multiple myeloma:
- M-protein (serum) >30 g/L and/or
- Clonal plasma cells >10% on bone marrow biopsy, and
- No myeloma-related organ or tissue impairment

Monoclonal gammopathy of undetermined significance (MGUS):
- M-protein <30 g/L and
- Clonal plasma cells <10% on bone marrow biopsy and
- NO myeloma-related organ or tissue impairment (ROTI)

Solitary plasmacytoma of bone:
- No M-protein in serum and/or urine
- Single area of bone destruction due to clonal plasma cells
- Bone marrow not consistent with multiple myeloma
- Normal skeletal survey (and MRI of spine and pelvis if done)
- No related organ or tissue impairment (no end-organ damage other than solitary bone lesion)

Radiology

Lesions erode the cortex and periosteal new bone formation is not seen. Expansile lesion is usually seen in bones with a small diameter, such as the ribs. Skull radiographs demonstrate the earliest and more severe changes as also evident later in vertebrae, ribs, and pelvis. Generalized osteoporosis may be present in few at presentation. Solitary plasmacytoma lesions are also typically lytic and may also expand the bone. Presence of sclerotic lesions points typically to the very rare POEMS syndrome that stands for an uncommon cluster of clinical findings—polyneuropathy, organomegaly, endocrinopathy, monoclonal gammopathy, skin changes. Bone scan is usually negative.

Histopathological

Histopathologically, the round cells of PCM show variable features of cellular maturity that is closely linked to prognosis. Well-differentiated tumors demonstrate sheets of closely packed cells (resembling normal plasma cells) with little intercellular matrix. These cells have abundant, dense eosinophilic cytoplasm with eccentric nucleus that has characteristic peripherally clustered chromatin in a "cartwheel pattern". Intracytoplasmic aggregation of immunoglobulins gives a morular appearance termed "Mott cells". "Russell bodies" is the term used for similar extracellular globules of polymerized immunoglobulins.

Immunophenotype

Myeloma cells express distinct plasma cell-associated antigen (PCA, CD38). Malignant lesions express monotypic kappa or lambda immunoglobulin. PCM characteristically expresses monotypic cytoplasmic immunoglobulin and lacks surface immunoglobulin. PCM usually lack the pan-B cell antigens (characteristically the CD19 and CD20), while CD38 and the immunoglobulin-associated antigen CD79a are expressed mostly.

Management

Hematological investigations usually reveal anemia on complete hemogram. Erythrocyte sedimentation rate is prominently elevated and is often around or more than 100 mm in 1st hour. Other parameters like the serum calcium (bone absorption), blood urea nitrogen (catabolism), serum creatinine, and uric acid levels (purine and pyrimidine metabolism) are also often elevated. The most common method to diagnose PCM is by serum protein electrophoresis and measurement of serum immunoglobulins and free light chains. These reveal the characteristic M-spikes which is a sensitive marker though its absence does not rule out myeloma. Bence Jones protein can be detected in urine but 24-hour urine should be collected. *ALP (marker of bone formation) is usually normal* even with extensive bone involvement because of the absence of osteoblastic activity. Plasma cell dyscrasias can be comfortably divided into premalignant and malignant conditions. Monoclonal gammopathy of undetermined significance (MGUS) represents a premalignant condition that may (or may not) progress to MM as opposed to asymptomatic MM and active MM that are frankly malignant counterparts. Of these malignant components, asymptomatic MM is distinguished from active myeloma by absence of end-organ compromise identified by the acronym "CRAB". MGUS is approximately 80–100 times more common than MM and is found in 3–5% of general population aged 70 years or older. The MGUS has been found to progress to MM at a rate of around 1% per year. Although similar cytogenetic abnormalities (translocations and deletions) have been observed in patients with MGUS and MM; however no obvious clinical or conclusions could be drawn based on these chromosome abnormalities. MGUS patients can be stratified to high- or low-risk based on their immunoglobulin isotype; the level of their paraprotein secretion, and the ratio of serum-free light chains. A patient with monoclonal immunoglobulin concentration 1.5 g/dL other than IgG and an abnormally high serum-free light chain ratio would be classified as high risk with 58% risk of progression of MGUS to MM than in one if none of these factors are present. Low-risk MGUS patients can be followed yearly while high-risk MGUS patients should be followed every 3–6 months. Serum β2-microglobulin has specific role in staging and should be quantitated in all diagnosed cases. The International *Staging System* for myeloma published by the International Myeloma Working Group in 2005 is based on β2-microglobulin concentration:

- *Stage I:* β2-microglobulin (β2M) <3.5 mg/L, albumin ≥3.5 g/dL
- *Stage II:* β2M <3.5 mg/L, and albumin <3.5 g/dL; or β2M 3.5–5.5 mg/L irrespective of the serum albumin
- *Stage III:* β2M ≥5.5 mg/L

Multiple myeloma is generally an incurable disease (median survival 3 years; 10% survival at 10 years). β2-microglobulin are the single most strong predictor of prognosis with higher levels associated with shorter survival. Other factors that predict poor or shorter survival include a higher stage at diagnosis, renal involvement causing insufficiency, hypoploidy, chromosome 13q and 17p deletion, translocations t(4;14) and t(14;16), replacement of marrow by neoplastic cells, histopathologically demonstrable cellular immaturity and atypia on bone marrow examination and high Ki-67 proliferation antigen levels. 10% patients have smoldering disease and require treatment only when symptomatic. Chemotherapy and autologous stem cell transplantation is the mainstay of treatment. Dexamethasone, bortezomib (proteasome inhibitor that targets 26S proteasome), thalidomide and its immunomodulatory derivative lenalidomide are currently employed in varying combinations in patients planned for future stem cell transplantation. Melphalan, prednisolone, and lenalidomide are used in patients not planned for transplantation. Radiation therapy (4,500–5,000 cGy) is effective for solitary plasmacytoma. Autologous hematopoietic stem cell transplantation provides the best chance of EFS in most patients. High-dose chemotherapy followed by transplantation can be beneficial even in refractory patients. Sequential planned tandem hematopoietic stem cell transplantation with high-dose therapy is an innovative approach that has been quite successful and nearly doubled the sustained remission rates. Newer agents targeting therapy in myeloma patients have been developed. Peferisone is a synthetic alkyl phospholipid that interacts and induces cytotoxicity in MM triggered by c-Jun NH2-terminal kinase by inhibiting the Akt/protein kinase B activity (important for MM cell survival and anti-apoptosis). Geldanamycin and tanespimycin are HSP-90 (heat shock protein) inhibitors that show promising results with bortezomib. NPI-0052 is another proteasome inhibitor like bortezomib but with earlier onset of action and different kinetics. Tocilizumab is an interleukin-6 inhibitor that has been shown effective in murine MM model; other therapies targeting surface receptors includes the anti-CD40, anti-CD56, anti-CD138, anti-CS-1, anti-CD70, TGF-β inhibitor, etc. Supportive care is required in patients with respect to the osteolytic lesions, hypercalcemia and associated pain. Bisphosphonates, especially the injectable, form have been found effective in this regard. For anemia, erythropoietin has been found effective. Similarly, prophylaxis, evaluation and treatment are required for patients at risk of developing deep vein thrombosis and infections.

5.15 PYKNODYSOSTOSIS (Q47)

47. Discuss pyknodysostosis.

Ans: Pyknodysostosis ["pucnos" (dense), "dys" (defective) and "ostosis" (bone condition)] is a rare autosomal recessive disorder of bones and is called osteopetrosis acro-osteolytica or Toulouse-Lautrec syndrome. The name Toulouse-Lautrec syndrome is derived from the French impressionist, Henri Marie Raymond de Toulouse-Lautrec-Monfa who was a victim of this unusual disorder.

Clinical features include:
- Shortness of stature (prominently acromelia)
- Short broad hands with stubby fingers
- Onychohypoplasia (hypoplasia of nails)
- Nasal beaking and relative proptosis on observing face from side
- Delayed closure of fontanels causing frontal and occipital bossing
- Underdevelopment of the mandible (with relative prognathism) and abnormal dentition (persistence of primary teeth).

The presence of blue sclerae and propensity to fracture may cause confusion with osteogenesis imperfecta. The condition is caused by a lysosomal disorder due to genetic deficiency in cathepsin K (essential for normal osteoclast function) which has been mapped to chromosome 1q21 and is inherited as an autosomal recessive trait.

Radiologically: The bones are dense (osteosclerosis) with narrowed medullary canal in a generalized fashion; the skull is enlarged, with wide suture lines, calvarial thickening and open fontanels, but the facial bones and mandible are hypoplastic, thus accounting for the typical "triangular" facies. Mandible has prominent obtuse angle. There may be partial agenesis of terminal phalanges of fingers appearing as acro-osteolysis. There is delayed bone age radiologically. Spine demonstrates increased lumbar lordosis, vertebral body sclerosis, and vertebral segmentation abnormalities in upper cervical and lower lumbar region. The most important radiological differential is osteopetrosis.

Management: Despite appearances, it causes little trouble (apart from the odd pathological fracture) and needs no treatment.

5.16 SYNOVIAL CHONDROMATOSIS (Q48–49)

48. Discuss synovial chondromatosis—diagnosis and management.

Ans: Synovial chondromatosis.

Diagnosis: Plain radiographs are usually normal unless there is calcification in the loose bodies. Uncalcified loose bodies appear as foci with opacity similar to that of water especially in lateral projections of the knee. Finding calcified loose bodies usually entails late disease where degeneration has already set in. Classically air contrast arthrogram used to be done to reveal the cartilaginous loose bodies but is obsolete now. MRI has taken precedence now that reveal cartilaginous nodules with intermediate signal intensity on T1-weighted MRI and high signal intensity on T2-weighted images. Arthrocentesis is commonly done to reduce joint fluid pressure and one must obtain cell count, crystal examination, Gram staining, and cultures for thorough evaluation. Although increased levels of interleukin (IL)-6, vascular endothelial growth factor (VEGF)-A, and chondrocalcin have been reported but their role in establishing diagnosis is limited, if at all.

Management: Radiographs may show several rounded calcifications within the joint cavity. Surgical management is indicated in patients having recurrent painful effusions, mechanical symptoms, or both as a consequence of synovial chondromatosis. Treatment is synovectomy; however, the tumor may recur and patient should be warned that osteoarthritis is present at any stage of diagnosis, so knee would ultimately get worn off. The only controversies in management are whether to go for complete or incomplete synovectomy and what approach to use—arthroscopic versus open. In view of the current evidence with the easy availability of arthroscopy it is preferred modality for all joints amenable to this management (commonly knee, hip, shoulder, elbow, and possibly ankle). For all other joints and location of disease not approachable with arthroscope, open approach would be legible. Also, arthroscopic approach is somewhat debatable in ankle joint where open approach might be preferred. Surgeons well trained in surgical dislocation of the hip may prefer open to arthroscopic approach, especially if there is need for secondary procedure like labral repair or so for addressing femoroacetabular impingement which is commonly associated. Complete synovectomy is associated with unacceptable joint stiffness later in course of rehabilitation so should be restricted for failed recalcitrant cases. Menisci are usually damaged and removed in the same sitting. With the development of osteoarthritis joint replacement with synovectomy is the management of choice with good results.

49. Describe pathology and clinical features of synovial chondromatosis.

Ans: Pathology: At sites of synovial reflection in the stratum synovial, there is transformation into hyaline cartilage. A number of white, glistening chondroid nodules are seen protruding into the joint. These may be loose in the joint space, but some are pedunculated with tethering to the synovium deriving nutrition from same. The nodules may fuse to form multinodular masses. Segments of cartilage or the spheroidal masses themselves break loose and continue to grow as loose bodies deriving nutrition from fluid. When calcification and ossification of loose bodies occur, the disorder is referred to as *synovial osteochondromatosis*. Microscopically, the cartilage has a distinct multinodularity and presence of smaller cellular areas that are thought to represent the proliferative foci.

The absence of this multifocality should question the diagnosis. Eventually, the constant friction and damage to native cartilage leads to development of osteoarthritic changes. Initially, the chondrogenic process was thought to be metaplasia of primitive mesenchymal cells lying beneath the synovial membrane. More recently, clonal cytogenetic findings with recurring but nonidentical changes in chromosome 6 have been reported, suggesting that this is, in fact, a neoplastic cartilage tumor. Loss of Rab23, an essential negative regulator of the sonic hedgehog signaling pathway, has been demonstrated in synovial chondromatosis. In addition, loss of *collagen X* and *collagen IX* genes has been implicated in the pathogenesis. The multifocal nature of chondrocyte growth is explained by the observation that only a subpopulation of cells proliferate and that these cells demonstrate an autocrine growth factor loop consisting of fibroblast growth factor (FGF)-9 and FGF receptor 3.

Clinical features: Symptoms are dull pain, swelling, and stiffness of the joint. Knee is the most common joint affected. Locking and intermittent grating sensation present initially may transform into degenerative arthritis over time and disease progression. Other large joints such as hip, elbow, and shoulder and very occasionally small joints can be affected. The joint is tender to palpation with nodules palpable as free small marbles along with crepitus. There is usually already an early set-up of degenerative arthritis suggested by joint line tenderness and terminal restriction of 10–15° of movements.

5.17 ONCOGENIC OSTEOMALACIA (Q50)

50. Oncogenic osteomalacia.

Ans: [Tumor-induced osteomalacia (TIO), oncogenic hypophosphatemic osteomalacia]. This is a paraneoplastic syndrome characterized by bone pain, fractures, and muscle weakness. There is increased renal phosphate excretion, hypophosphatemia, and low levels of circulating 1,25-dihydroxy vitamin D. The condition is primarily caused by increased levels of phosphate and vitamin D-regulating hormone, fibroblast growth factor-23 (FGF-23). In majority of the patients, a fibronectin-1 (FN-1) and fibroblast growth factor receptor-1 (FGFR-1) fusion gene has been identified that may be responsible for high FGF-3 levels.

The patients present with bone pain, fractures, gait abnormalities, and muscle weakness. Because of nonspecific symptoms misdiagnosis into various rheumatologic, orthopedic or neuropsychiatric cases is common. Often in investigations no significant abnormality is revealed as also most panels do not include phosphate levels so patient is long treated symptomatically without benefit. The condition can be seen with benign, malignant or metastatic neoplasms. In any case histopathologically a primitive mesenchymal cell has been identified that has the ability to secrete the hormone.

Management

The treatment is primarily based on two lines—one is the normalization of hematological parameters like correction of serum inorganic phosphate, correction of serum vitamin D levels [and, in turn, the serum parathyroid hormone (PTH) levels]. The other is identification of the neoplastic lesion. As soon as clinical suspicion is made, diagnosis is made by hematological investigations and demonstration of renal tubular wasting of phosphate and exclusion of familial forms must be done [Fanconi syndrome, Fanconi-Bickle syndrome, X-linked hypophosphatemic (XLH) rickets and autosomal dominant/recessive hypophosphatemic rickets (ADHR/ARHR) by *PHEX, FGF-23, DMP-1* gene identification]. While FGF-23 is elevated in XLH, ADHR and ARHR, it is found normal or low in Fanconi syndrome, Dent's disease and XLHR. Tumor localization is done by functional imaging (PET scan or ^{111}Indium octreotide scintigraphy + SPECT) followed by anatomical imaging with MRI/CT scan. ^{68}Ga-DOTANOC PET/CT may be more sensitive to identify TIO. Radiographs usually demonstrate generalized osteopenia and "reactivation" of growth plate as transverse lucent lines in the region of physeal scar. Venous sampling (for FGF-23) from the draining site may be added for more assurance if needed. The identified lesion should be excised on standard procedure for type of neoplasm.

If no neoplasm is identified, then corrective treatment is continued in the form of phosphate [15–60 mg/kg/day (~1–3 g/day for adults); divided into 4–5 times/day to improve tolerance] and vitamin D supplementation to achieve target serum phosphate and vitamin D/PTH levels. The monitoring is done every 3 months in the form of serum calcium, phosphorus, PTH, urinary calcium (UCa), and creatinine (UCr). Relocalization of tumor is attempted after 1 year.

5.18 MUSCULOSKELETAL MANIFESTATIONS OF NEUROFIBROMATOSIS (Q51–60)

51. Describe musculoskeletal manifestations of neurofibromatosis.

Ans: *The following are the common musculoskeletal and associated manifestations of neurofibromatosis:*

- Abnormal skeletal development (seen in 15–20% patients). These comprise bony dysplasia, bony erosion (scalloping), demineralizing osteoporosis, nonossifying fibroma, and scoliosis. Patients might exhibit mild anisomelia to massive gigantism and overgrowth is commonly seen that may range from single digit to entire limb.
- Fractures and bony deformities are present in 5–10% patients (especially boys).
- Pseudarthrosis is common even after fracture treatment.
- Radiographs of pelvis demonstrate coxa valga of various degrees and may also show protrusio acetabuli.
- Patients with neurofibromatosis type 1 (NF1) may develop cystic lesions in long bones and congenital tibial dysplasia. Congenital tibial dysplasia includes a spectrum from anterolateral tibial bowing to pseudarthrosis. Congenital pseudarthrosis (distal tibia and/or fibula) is difficult to treat in such cases.
- Osteoporosis has been reported in around 50% cases. This metabolic bone disease is similar to hypophosphatemic rickets/osteomalacia.

- Short, sharp, single thoracic, angular scoliosis is seen in 15–20% cases though other forms of scoliosis are also seen making overall percentage of the scoliosis even higher. The typical curve is associated with distortion of the ribs and vertebrae. The onset is early in childhood, and it is relentlessly progressive. The risk of malignancy is increased in a patient with NF1 and includes a 10% lifetime risk of a malignant peripheral nerve sheath tumor, which typically arises within a plexiform neurofibroma. Pheochromocytoma, astrocytoma, and brainstem glioma also occur. Hypertension may develop due to renal artery stenosis or pheochromocytoma.

Management
Management of orthopedic manifestations is as follows:
- *Long bone pseudarthrosis (see also congenital pseudarthrosis of tibia):* To prevent fracture, prophylactic application of a total contact ankle-foot orthosis is indicated before a child reaches walking age.
- After the child begins walking, a knee-ankle-foot orthosis is needed. The definitive treatment consists of pseudarthrosis excision, bone grafting, intramedullary fixation, or ilizarov reconstruction. Vascularized bone grafting, typically from the contralateral fibula, has been attempted in a limited fashion.
- Scoliosis occurs in approximately 20% of patients with NF1. The curves are classified as dystrophic or nondystrophic. Nondystrophic curves have radiographic features similar to those of idiopathic scoliosis and are treated similarly. Nondystrophic curves can evolve into dystrophic curves (70% chance) which are:
  – Short (fewer than six segments)
  – Sharp
  – Enlarged neural foramina
- These dystrophic curves typically occur in patients who are:
  – Younger than 6 years
  – Have an apical vertebra with associated scalloped end plates
  – Radiological rib penciling
  – High Cobb angle
  – Curve located in middle to lower thoracic region

The curves are dangerous as they progress rapidly, are resistant to bracing, and may have an associated sagittal plane deformity. Surgical treatment is done using growing rod instrumentation in younger children or combined anterior and posterior fusion in older children. The risk of pseudarthrosis after spine surgery is higher in NF than idiopathic scoliosis. It is preferable to do circumferential fusion to prevent this. Preoperative CT and MRI are helpful to identify defective pedicles and dural ectasias. One should be also vigilant of the developing anterolateral meningoceles due to outpouching of the dura that can erode the pedicle and may lead to weakening (they may also cause dislocations in cervical spine).

52. What are the techniques of biopsy in aggressive (potentially malignant) bone tumors?
Ans: Kindly see Answer to Question 12 above.

53. Discuss briefly the management of GCT of distal end of femur.
Ans: Kindly see Answer to Question 33 above.

54. Discuss differential diagnosis and approach to confirm diagnosis in a lytic metaphyseal long bone lesion in an 8-year-old child.
Ans: The differential diagnosis of lytic metaphyseal lesion in an 8-year-old child in order of possibility is as follows:
- Aneurysmal bone cyst
- Simple bone cyst
- Chondromyxoid fibroma
- Nonossifying fibroma
- Giant cell tumor
- Desmoplastic fibroma
- Osteosarcoma
- Osteoblastoma
- Osteomyelitis

- Cortical desmoid
- Intraosseous lipoma
- Enchondroma
- Chondrosarcoma
- Metastases

Further radiology of cystic lesions, GCT, osteosarcoma, osteomyelitis can be written from answers described in specific questions. Ultimately biopsy confirms diagnosis and some characteristic histopathological features can be described.

(Kindly read details of few important ones from Essential Orthopedics: Principles and Practice, chapter on Orthopedic Oncology)

55. What is alloprosthetic composite?

Ans: It is a combination of allograft and endoprosthesis. This is a versatile type of reconstruction. It can be used in a variety of patients including children and patients who have received chemotherapy.

Allograft is selected and implanted to replace the segment of bone resected. The articular surfaces of the graft are excised and replaced using conventional techniques of total joint arthroplasty. These composites restore both anatomy and function.

Advantages:
- Allograft provides source of bone stock and anchorage for soft tissues such as tendon insertions
- Prosthesis provides a reliable and stable mobile joint and provides some support for allograft
- Not susceptible to osteoarthritis
- Lower fracture rates and period of immobilization than allograft alone
- Useful in situations where remaining proximal host bone is inadequate to accept prosthesis stem.

56. What is custom megaprosthesis?

Ans: Megaprostheses are defined as special segmental bone and joint prostheses which bridge large defects of joints and bones. Nowadays, megaprostheses are available for all major anatomical regions of the body, i.e., scapula, shoulder joint, proximal humerus, elbow, portions of the pelvis, hip joint and proximal femur, knee joint including proximal tibia and distal femur. Also, total replacements of femur as well as humerus including the adjacent joints are feasible.

Megaprostheses are available as custom made and modular types. Custom-made types are individually manufactured for each patient and therefore give an accurate fit. However, they have to be ordered, made, and delivered and delays can occur. Modular types are always available and allow variable resections due to their multicomponent designs.

As implantation of megaprostheses is a demanding and risky procedure, the following considerations should be taken into account:
- If in malignant bone tumors, a wide or radical resection cannot be achieved then megaprostheses should not be used.
- For a successful implantation, sufficient blood vessels, nerves, and muscles must be retained and additional reconstructive procedures, e.g., microvascular flaps and tendon/muscle transfers must be workable.
- Is the patient suitable for a long-lasting operation and rehabilitation? Does he really need this prosthesis for a better quality of life? Consider age, risk factors such as vascular disease, diabetes, prolonged chemotherapy, and pregoing infection.
- Is the performing surgeon sure that megaprostheses are better than arthrodesis, allograft, rotationplasty, and amputation with regard to final function, complications, hospital stay, and costs?
- Are the skills and facilities present to perform the surgery?

Features:
- Cemented stem fixation-early ambulation and weight bearing
- Circumferential porous coating—permits ingrowth of bone
- Multiple diameter stems—proper largest-sized stem used. Minimal fracture risk
- Rotating hinge-enable joint movement in the absence of ligaments
- Metal loops to permit soft-tissue reattachment and fibrous ingrowth into the prosthesis

Despite all precautions, the overall complication rate is there including early flap complications such as wound healing problems, superficial and deep infections, dislocations, nerve palsy and thrombosis. Late complications such as loosening, stem breakage, and other prosthetic complications.

57. What are the principles of gamma camera? Mention the radioactive substances used in gamma camera. What are the indications and uses of gamma camera?

Ans: Gamma camera detects gamma rays and reconstruct their line of flight. It works on principle of Compton effect and photoelectric effect.

- *Compton effect:* The scattering of a photon by a charged particle, usually an electron at rest is called Compton scattering. It results in a decrease in energy (increase in wavelength) of the photon (which may be an X-ray or gamma ray photon) called the Compton effect.
- *Photoelectric effect:* Emissions of electrons when electromagnetic rays (light) hit a material. This is attributed to transfer of energy from light to electron.

A gamma camera consists of one or more flat crystal planes (detectors) optically coupled to an array of photomultiplier tubes in an assembly mounted on a gantry. Gantry is connected to computer that controls operation of camera and acquires images. It stores data about number of gamma photons that are absorbed by the crystal in camera.

The crystal scintillates in response to incident gamma radiation. When a gamma photon leaves the patient (who has been injected with a radioactive drug), it knocks an electron loose from an elemental atom (usually iodine) in the crystal and a faint flash of light is produced when that excited electron again loses energy to attain minimal state. The initial phenomena of excited electron are similar to photoelectric effect and Compton effect. The flash of light is detected by photomultiplier tubes present behind the crystal and computer then sums the counts. Data reconstruction shows a 2D image reflecting the distribution and concentration of tracer elements in organ or tissue under study.

Radioactive substances used in gamma camera:
Technetium 99 in single photon imaging and F-18 in positron imaging.

Indications and uses of gamma camera:
Gamma camera has been used for thyroid, brain, and kidney scanning. In orthopedics, gamma camera is used in PET scan studies and bone scan.

58. What is Turret exostosis? Outline its management briefly.

Ans: Turret exostosis is an unusual case of reactive periostitis developing into a benign osteocartilaginous lesion so also called acquired osteochondroma. The lesion arises after relatively mild trauma from reactive periosteum as a smooth dome-shaped parosteal bone proliferation. The common site for the lesion is phalanges but unusually talus has also been reported.

Histopathology: Microscopically a central area of mature trabecular bone maturing via enchondral ossification with a thin hypocellular peripheral rim of cartilage is seen. The absence of a periosteal layer, abundant "blue bone," bizarre metaplastic cartilage, or marked cytologic atypia confirms benign nature of disease.

Radiology: The growth is well-circumscribed osseous mass occurring in close relationship to underlying cortex without any connection to the medullary canal.

Management: The mass produces unsightly swelling that is commonly painful due to friction and impingement to nearby structures. Erosion of the overlying structures and skin may cause ulceration and in neglected cases infection. The lesion swelling may cause bony block-limiting motion at nearby joint-like hallux rigidus in foot. Simple excision of the bony lesion results in disappearance of symptoms. Recurrence is uncommon but it is considered to cauterize the periosteum around the base similar to excision of osteochondroma.

59. Write salient features of Ollier's disease. Write differentiating features from Maffucci syndrome.

Ans:
Salient features: The enchondromatosis here has a tendency toward unilaterality. Even in bilateral cases one side of body is predominantly involved. Ollier's disease is a developmental disorder where there is a failure of normal ossification.

The large tumors form extensively in the metaphyseal region of multiple bones with varying deformity. Some studies implicate parathormone receptor and PTH-related peptide gene to Ollier's disease.

Differentiating features between Ollier's disease and Maffucci syndrome are presented in **Table 5.18.1**.

TABLE 5.18.1: Differences between Ollier's disease and Maffucci syndrome.

	Ollier's disease	Maffucci syndrome
Characteristic features	Multiple enchondromas	Multiple osteochondromas, secondary chondrosarcoma, secondary osteosarcoma
Skin lesions	Absent	Cavernous hemangiomas on skin are progressive and do not necessarily occur over bony lesions
Bone lesions	Develop after 5 years of age and are prominent by adolescence. Stop with skeletal maturity	Lesions develop early 1–3 years and are more diffuse. In 40% cases, lesions may be unilateral and affect growth of individuals
Risk of malignancy	20–30%	40–50%, may be more

60. Describe secondary chondrosarcoma and its likely causes. Discuss in brief its radiological, histopathological features, and management principles.

Ans: This chondrosarcoma arises in benign precursors [solitary osteochondroma (<2%)/osteochondromatosis (5–30%)], Ollier's and Maffucci syndrome (25–30%).

Risk factors and identifying features for development of secondary chondrosarcoma:

Hereditary conditions: Ollier's disease, Maffucci syndrome, hereditary multiple exostosis (*EXT1, EXT2,* and *EXT3* mutations)

Radiological features:
- Size of osteochondroma > 5 cm
- Cartilage cap > 2 cm in adults (in adolescents the cap is already quite thick averaging 3 cm in most studies)
- Blurring of osseous border at osteocartilaginous junction suggests invasiveness and is more important than cap thickness.
- Inhomogeneous mineralization of cartilage cap

Histopathological features: Secondary chondrosarcoma is composed entirely of cartilaginous tissue, and it is usually a low-grade malignancy. Furthermore, though very rare but dedifferentiated chondrosarcoma can arise in secondary chondrosarcomas.

Management principles: Management of secondary chondrosarcoma involves a combination of surgical and supportive therapies. Here are some key principles in managing secondary chondrosarcoma:

1. Diagnosis and staging:
- *Imaging studies:* Utilize X-rays, MRI, and CT scans to assess the tumor's size, location, and extent of involvement.
- *Biopsy:* Obtain a tissue sample for histological examination to confirm the diagnosis and differentiate from other types of sarcomas.
- *Staging:* American Joint Committee on Cancer (AJCC) classification system to determine the stage of the tumor based on size, location, and presence of metastasis.

2. Surgical management:
- Wide resection: The primary treatment for chondrosarcoma is surgical excision. A wide resection with clear margins is necessary to reduce the risk of local recurrence.
- Limb-sparing surgery: When possible, strive for limb-salvage procedures rather than amputation.
- Assessment of bone integrity: Evaluate the need for reconstruction using bone grafts or prosthetics after resection.

5.19 SOFT-TISSUE SARCOMA (Q61)

61. A. Classify appendicular soft-tissue sarcoma.

B. Describe principles of resection of appendicular soft-tissue sarcoma.

C. Describe concept of "external beam radiation therapy" and/or "brachytherapy" in its treatment.

Ans:

A. Classification of Appendicular Soft-tissue Sarcoma

Appendicular soft-tissue sarcomas (STS) are rare malignant tumors arising from mesenchymal tissues (e.g., muscle, fat, nerves, and blood vessels) in the extremities (upper and lower limbs).

1. Classification by Histological Type (WHO, 2020)

Soft-tissue sarcomas are classified based on tissue of origin and histological features. Common appendicular STS include:

- Adipocytic tumors:
  - Liposarcoma (e.g., well-differentiated, myxoid, and pleomorphic).
- Fibroblastic/Myofibroblastic tumors:
  - Fibrosarcoma, myxofibrosarcoma, and low-grade fibromyxoid sarcoma.
- Smooth muscle tumors:
  - Leiomyosarcoma
- Skeletal muscle tumors:
  - Rhabdomyosarcoma (embryonal, alveolar, and pleomorphic)
- Vascular tumors:
  - Angiosarcoma and epithelioid hemangioendothelioma
- Peripheral nerve sheath tumors:
  - Malignant peripheral nerve sheath tumor (MPNST)
- Undifferentiated/Unclassified sarcomas:
  - Undifferentiated pleomorphic sarcoma (UPS, formerly malignant fibrous histiocytoma).
- Synovial and Tendon sheath tumors:
  - Synovial sarcoma (monophasic or biphasic)
- Others:
  - Clear cell sarcoma, alveolar soft part sarcoma, and epithelioid sarcoma.

2. Classification by Staging (AJCC 8th Edition, 2017)

Staging integrates tumor size, grade, lymph node involvement, and metastasis:

- *T (Tumor)*:
  - T1: ≤5 cm
  - T2: >5 cm and ≤10 cm
  - T3: >10 cm and ≤15 cm
  - T4: >15 cm
- *N (Node)*:
  - N0: No regional lymph node metastasis
  - N1: Regional lymph node metastasis (rare in STS)
- *M (Metastasis)*:
  - M0: No distant metastasis
  - M1: Distant metastasis (e.g., lungs, common in appendicular STS)
- *Grade (G):* G1, G2, or G3 (per FNCLCC)
- *Stages:*
  - Stage IA: T1, N0, M0, G1.
  - Stage IB: T2–T4, N0, M0, G1.

- Stage II: T1, N0, M0, G2–3.
- Stage IIIA: T2, N0, M0, G2–3.
- Stage IIIB: T3–T4, N0, M0, G2–3.
- Stage IV: Any T, N1 or M1, any G.

B. Key Principles of Resection of Appendicular Soft-tissue Sarcoma

1. *Wide local excision with negative margins:*
- *Goal:* Complete removal of the tumor with a margin of normal tissue (typically 1–2 cm) to achieve R0 resection (no microscopic residual disease).
- *Rationale:* Negative margins reduce local recurrence risk [5–10% with R0 vs. 20–30% with R1 (microscopic residual)].
- *Technique:* En bloc resection includes the tumor, its pseudocapsule, and surrounding normal tissue, avoiding tumor violation to prevent seeding.

2. *Limb-sparing surgery:*
- *Goal:* Preserve functional limb anatomy while achieving oncologic clearance.
- *Rationale:* Limb-sparing resection is feasible in 90–95% of appendicular STS cases, avoiding amputation unless critical structures (e.g., major nerves, and vessels) are involved.
- *Approach:* Careful planning to preserve muscles, nerves, and vessels unless encased by tumor; use of flaps or grafts for soft tissue coverage.

3. *Preoperative planning with imaging:*
- *Goal:* Define tumor extent and relationship to critical structures (neurovascular bundles and bone).
- *Rationale:* MRI delineates tumor size, depth (superficial vs. subfascial), and involvement of adjacent structures for precise surgical planning.
- *Adjuncts:* CT chest for metastasis staging; core needle biopsy for histological diagnosis and grading.

4. *Multidisciplinary approach:*
- *Goal:* Optimize oncologic and functional outcomes through collaboration.
- *Rationale:* Involves surgical oncologists, radiation oncologists, medical oncologists, and pathologists to tailor treatment (e.g., neoadjuvant radiation for high-grade tumors).
- *Decision-making:* Assess tumor grade (FNCLCC G1–G3), size (>5 cm higher risk), and depth for adjuvant therapies.

5. *Adjuvant therapies to enhance resection:*
- *Neoadjuvant radiation:* Shrinks large (>5 cm) or high-grade tumors, facilitating resection and reducing recurrence (used in 50–60% of cases).
- Intraoperative radiation: For close margins near critical structures.
- *Chemotherapy:* Considered for high-grade, large, or metastatic STS (e.g., synovial sarcoma, rhabdomyosarcoma).
- *Rationale:* Improves local control and resectability, especially in deep tumors.

6. *Management of critical structures:*
- *Goal:* Balance oncologic clearance with function preservation.
- *Approach:* Sacrifice minor muscles if involved; preserve major nerves/vessels unless encased (may require vascular reconstruction). Bone resection is rare unless it is directly invaded.
- *Rationale:* Functional limbs improve quality of life; amputation reserved for unresectable cases (<5%).

7. *Reconstruction and rehabilitation:*
- *Goal:* Restore soft-tissue coverage and function postresection.
- *Techniques:* Primary closure, skin grafts, or flaps (e.g., fasciocutaneous and muscle flaps) for defects; tendon transfers or nerve grafts, if needed.
- *Rehabilitation:* Early physiotherapy to restore range of motion and strength, tailored to resection extent.

C. Concept of External Beam Radiation Therapy and Brachytherapy in Appendicular Soft Tissue Sarcoma Treatment: External Beam Radiation Therapy (EBRT) and brachytherapy are adjuvant treatments used in appendicular soft-tissue sarcoma (STS) to improve local control, reduce recurrence, and facilitate limb-sparing surgery.

External Beam Radiation Therapy

Concept: External beam radiation therapy (EBRT) delivers high-energy radiation (X-rays or protons) from an external source (e.g., linear accelerator) to the tumor bed or surgical site to destroy residual cancer cells. In appendicular STS, it targets microscopic disease postresection or shrinks tumors preresection to enable limb preservation.

Principles:
- *Mechanism:* Ionizing radiation damages DNA in cancer cells, preventing replication and causing cell death.
- *Delivery:* Focused beams are shaped to the tumor/surgical bed, sparing surrounding healthy tissues (e.g., skin, bone, and nerves).
- *Timing:*
  - *Neoadjuvant:* Presurgery to shrink large (>5 cm) or high-grade tumors, improving resectability.
  - *Adjuvant:* Postsurgery to eliminate microscopic residual disease, especially with close (<1 cm) or positive margins.
- *Indications*:
  - High-grade STS (FNCLCC G2–G3)
  - Large tumors (>5 cm) or deep (subfascial) tumors
  - Close or positive margins after resection (R1/R2)
  - Tumors near critical structures (e.g., neurovascular bundles) to avoid amputation
- *Dosage*:
  - *Neoadjuvant:* 50 Gy in 25 fractions (5 weeks).
  - *Adjuvant:* 60–66 Gy in 30–33 fractions, with a boost (10–16 Gy) for positive margins.
- *Salient features*:
  - Reduces local recurrence by 15–20% (from ~30% to ~10–15% with surgery alone).
  - *Techniques:* Intensity-modulated radiation therapy (IMRT) or proton therapy for precise targeting, minimizing damage to adjacent structures.
  - *Side effects:* Skin erythema, fibrosis, edema, joint stiffness, or wound complications (more common with neoadjuvant EBRT).
  - *Advantage:* Noninvasive, widely applicable; improves limb-sparing outcomes.
  - *Limitation:* Delayed wound healing (neoadjuvant) or long-term fibrosis affecting function.

Brachytherapy

Concept: Brachytherapy involves placing radioactive sources (e.g., iridium-192) directly into or near the tumor bed, delivering high-dose radiation locally with minimal exposure to surrounding tissues. In appendicular STS, it is typically used postresection to target the surgical bed.

Principles:
- *Mechanism:* Radioactive implants emit continuous, localized radiation, causing DNA damage in residual cancer cells.
- *Delivery:* Catheters or seeds are placed intraoperatively or percutaneously in the tumor bed, removed after treatment (temporary) or left permanently (rare).
- *Timing:* Primarily adjuvant, immediately postresection, targeting the surgical bed.
- *Indications:*
  - High-grade STS with close or positive margins
  - Recurrent STS after prior surgery or EBRT
  - Tumors where EBRT is contraindicated (e.g., prior radiation exposure)
  - Smaller, superficial tumors with accessible surgical beds
- *Dosage*:
  - 20–30 Gy over 4–6 days (low-dose-rate brachytherapy) or 10–15 Gy in 1–2 fractions (high-dose-rate)
  - Often combined with EBRT (e.g., 45 Gy EBRT + 15–20 Gy brachytherapy boost).
- *Salient features*:
  - Reduces local recurrence by ~10–15%, similar to EBRT, but with less exposure to healthy tissues.

- *Techniques:* Temporary catheters placed intraoperatively, removed after 4–6 days; high-dose-rate (HDR) brachytherapy allows outpatient treatment.
- *Side effects:* Wound complications (10–15%), infection, or nerve irritation; lower rates of fibrosis compared to EBRT.
- *Advantage:* High local dose, spares distant tissues, shorter treatment duration.
- *Limitation:* Invasive, requires surgical expertise, less effective for large or deep tumors.

Role in Appendicular STS Treatment
- *EBRT:* Preferred for large, deep, or high-grade STS, either pre- or postresection. Neoadjuvant EBRT facilitates limb-sparing surgery by shrinking tumors; adjuvant EBRT reduces recurrence with close margins.
- *Brachytherapy:* Used as an adjuvant boost for high-risk surgical beds or in recurrent cases. Less common than EBRT but effective for superficial tumors or when EBRT is limited.
- *Combination:* Brachytherapy may supplement EBRT for positive margins or high-grade tumors, delivering a boost to the tumor bed.
- *Outcomes:* Both reduce local recurrence to ~10–15% at 5 years; limb preservation achieved in 90–95% of cases.
- *Choice*: EBRT for broader applicability; brachytherapy for targeted, high-risk beds or recurrent disease.

CHAPTER 6

Miscellaneous Topics and Recent Advances

6.1 NANOTECHNOLOGY (Q1)

1. What is nanotechnology? Describe the role in orthopedics. Also, explain the recent advances in detection of periprosthetic joint infections.

Ans: Nanotechnology is a science dealing with objects functional on extremely small scale of the size from 1 nanometer to 100 nanometers. In 1959, Richard Feynman first introduced the concept of nanotechnology. The technology is based on two thoughts—one is to miniaturize the functional objects/machines so that they occupy less space and the other is basically an inspiration from living organisms where the molecular interactions taking place at miniature scale are able to produce directed functions (e.g. enzymatic actions). These objects for sheer size are referred to as nanomolecules. Despite the rationality in thought and the widespread interest development encompasses lot of hurdles and technology progress is not a straight path. As with quantum physics that does not follow the laws of particle physics, nanomolecules have unique chemical and physical properties that do not follow the laws of macromolecules/larger objects. Understanding the same is the primary reason for delay and limitation because control of these parameters has produced a new scientific field, experts of which are still evolving. The molecular interactions in human body occur at 4–400 atomic units measured in nanometers. Nanotechnology heralds to reproduce/produce/manipulate such processes on a scale of <100 nm by integration of nanoscopic materials into macro/microscopic systems. In general, two approaches are used for nanoscience evolution, one uses the bottom-up approach where the simpler smaller elements are arranged in the designated patterns (e.g. in 3D printing) to produce complex molecules and expected to have predefined function while the other approach is called the top-down approach where miniaturization comes to work and smaller and smaller objects are developed that can work similar to their larger predecessors. Nanophase describes conventional matter at very small sizes (<100 nm) but preserved atomic structure. At such small sizes the physical properties behave in terms of quantum (in simple terms both wave + particle properties) physics instead of particle physics. The prominent characteristic exploited by biological systems for nanoparticles is its markedly enhanced surface area as we know that with reduction in size the surface area increases. Such large surface area provides for faster and much higher magnitude of reactions/processes to occur. So for orthopedic implants modified by nanotechnology the interaction with bone cells and mesenchymal cells would enhance by multiple times. This is expected to produce better cell adsorption, differentiation, growth and ultimately osseointegration and other desired properties.

Despite the limitations there are potential applications of nanotechnology that may be pertinent to the medical field for the resemblance to molecular mechanisms that occur at same scale. In orthopedics the development of nanomedicine has currently focused on devices and implants for surface characteristics, molecular structure, bonding with bone, etc. while the typical clinical application is still limited to tissue-engineering, diagnostic aspects of musculoskeletal infection and oncology. Therapeutic applications are still far away in orthopedic field. The current application of nanomedicine pertaining to orthopedics in nanoscale surface modification and tissue engineering is vastly expanding opening new horizons. If specific nanotopographical features are developed on implants that resemble biological surfaces, viz. type X collagen initiating endochondral ossification; complications like loosening and implant subsidence may be ameliorated. The major focus of nanotechnology in orthopedics is to reduce the complications associated with operative procedures namely—aseptic loosening and periprosthetic osteolysis, infection, scar tissue formation and management of bone defects; a spillover effect of technology is seen in cartilage regeneration, drug delivery system, etc.

The specific surface modifications presently studied include: Nanophase ceramics (like nanophase hydroxyapatite), aluminum oxide and titanium dioxide, carbon, selenium, titanium, and nanocrystalline diamond. These are further supplemented by the use of fibronectin and vitronectin in a controlled manner that facilitates osteoblast activation, adhesion, and recruitment to a biomaterial. The currently used polished implants are smooth in nanoterms while the osseous inorganic phase has sizes of 50 nm × 25 nm × 4 nm; interaction of these produces fibrous interface. Nanoscience surface modification aims to roughen the implant surfaces so that bone-implant interface interacts in a productive way to get better integration. Surface modification by conjugation of substances such as bone morphogenetic protein-2 (BMP-2) to chitosan membranes also produced a significantly increased proliferation of osteoblasts, alkaline phosphatase activity, and calcium deposition. Nanocomposites have been created utilizing the above described nanoinorganic phase coupled to nanophase collagen improving osseointegration.

Bone defects: Nanocrystalline hydroxyapatite paste has been found to be efficient filler for bone defects. It has been used for filling distal radius defects and cavity after elevation of tibial plateau. The defects can be bioengineered by 3D printing using the nanohydroxyapatite "ink" and implanted into defects.

Cartilage regeneration and osteochondral defects: The underlying basis is synthesis of 3D mirror scaffolds that precisely control intercellular, cell-matrix and cell-growth factor interactions to provide milieu suitable to hyaline cartilage growth/formation. Additionally, the matrix should adhere to the underlying surface with a pore size larger than diameter of the osteoblasts (10 μm) so that cell penetration and neovascularization can happen. Nanocomposite biological implants can be used as scaffolds to treat the cartilage and osteochondral defects. For the latter a trilayer composite scaffold has been synthesized that comprises a cartilage layer formed from 100% type I collagen and a bone layer composed of nanocrystalline hydroxyapatite (70%) + type I collagen (30%); these are separated by an intermediate transition layer of collagen rich (60%) nanocrystalline hydroxyapatite (40%).

Orthopedic oncology: Nanometric selenium potentiates chemotherapeutic agents and when applied to titanium implants it inhibits the malignant osteoblasts. Similarly, nanocrystalline hydroxyapatite induces the apoptosis of osteosarcoma cells. Biodegradable nanocapsules containing small interfering ribonucleic acid (siRNA) targeting the oncogene inhibited tumor growth in mouse model of Ewing's sarcoma.

Orthopedic infection: Nanophase silver is a powerful bacteriostatic and bactericidal agent that can be specific use in open fractures. Nanophase silver deployed on surface of implants into titanium nanotubes is a strong bactericidal agent and also prevents bacterial adhesion for up to 30 days. This finds special use in revision arthroplasty and implant related infections.

Peripheral nerve injury: Nanophase silver impregnated type I collagen significantly reduces the time to nerve regeneration by increasing the quantity of adsorbed neurotropic proteins that produce thicker myelin sheath and improves nerve conduction.

Drug delivery: Gold has been shown to be an efficient transcutaneous drug delivery system for iontophoresis. Diclofenac administered with 30 nm gold nanopartcicles produced marked anti-inflammatory properties than plain form in transcutaneous system. Nanophase poly-L-lactic acid (PLLA) is also a nanoscopic drug delivery system as has been shown to heal large calvarial bony defects when used as delivery system for BMP-2. Such drug delivery systems (polypeptide nanofilms) when used with total joint prosthesis have shown marked reduction in bacterial load and improved osteoblastic response.

Diagnosis of periprosthetic joint infection (PJI): Apart from the conventional serological markers, current research is ongoing to study the synovial biomarkers like IL-6, IL-8, C-reactive protein (CRP), alpha-2 macroglobulins to rapidly diagnose PJI from samples.
- Alpha-defensin is an emerging and promising marker to this effect. It is an antimicrobial peptide released by neutrophils in the presence of bacteria and has a sensitivity and specificity of 100% and 96% respectively if detected positive. Only deterrent is its high cost. The test is also not influenced by antibiotic treatment.
- Leukocyte esterase is an enzyme secreted by neutrophils at the site of infection and inflammation and is simple and cheap to perform. It is available for diagnosing urinary tract infection as a reagent strip test where neutrophils from the sample get lysed and release the esterase causing color change of the dye.
- Nucleic acid amplification tests like polymerase chain reaction (PCR) amplification (for specific microorganisms like staphylococci, streptococci, anaerobes or a broad battery covering many organisms) and sequencing analysis of 16S

rRNA (for negative culture of PCR panel), and reverse transcription PCR are newer tools in the armamentarium of detection of infection.
- Matrix-assisted laser desorption ionization time-of-flight mass spectrometry (MALDI-TOF-MS) can rapidly detect staphylococci in patients of PJI with great accuracy.
- Microcalorimetry is another emerging tool that measures the heat intensity produced by proliferating organisms in relation to their metabolism in real time. This can provide a real time microbiological assay of biofilms.

(For further details, kindly refer to Chapter 11 of the book Essential Orthopedics: Principles and Practice, 2nd edition.)

6.2 STEM CELL AND ITS ROLE IN ORTHOPEDICS (Q2–3)

2. What are stem cells? How are stem cells procured for therapeutic use? What are the indications of stem cell therapy in orthopedics? What is the role of stem cell therapy in avascular necrosis (AVN) of head femur?

Ans: Stem cells are unique undifferentiated cells of a multicellular organism, which are capable of giving rise to indefinitely (theoretically at least) more cells of the same type (self-renewal), and from which certain other kinds of cell arise by differentiation in specific physiological or research controlled conditions. Stem cells are uniquely different from other cell types, as they possess three distinctive characteristics:

1. *Nonspecialization:* These cells have no tissue-specific structure or function that they would perform in human body. This repair characteristic is one of the most important distinctions that differentiate living from nonliving.
2. *Self-renewal and theoretical unlimited proliferation:* Stem cells are capable of dividing and renewing themselves for long periods without losing their basic identity and without differentiating.
3. *Ability to differentiate:* Stem cells can produce specialized cells under specific circumstances (chemokine or physical influence through contact from neighboring cells or microenvironment).

There are two broad types of stem cells:
1. Embryonic stem cells
2. *Somatic stem cells or tissue specific stem cells:*
   - iPS cells (induced pluripotent stem cells)
   - SCNT (somatic cell nuclear transfer).

Procuring stem cells:
- Mesenchymal stem cells can be derived from a number of sources but optimization is lacking and we are in process of identifying the best source for them. The commonly used/studied sources of stem cells for orthopedic research use are:
  - *Bone marrow-derived mesenchymal stem cells (BM-MSCs):* MSCs from the bone marrow (BM-MSCs) has been the most popular source of stem cells, although the yield is small and the procedure is painful. For a long time, BM-MSCs have been used as plain aspirate from iliac crest or greater trochanter for treating nonunions/delayed unions. The cells behave as multipotent cells capable of differentiating into trabecular bone, articular cartilage, ligament, and tendon.
  - *Bone marrow concentrate:* This is just a centrifuge of bone marrow aspirate from iliac crest containing a higher percentage of BM-MSCs.
- *Adipose-derived mesenchymal stem cells (AD-MSCs):* AD-MSCs can be easily harvested in good numbers through lipoaspiration and they can resist serum–deprivation-induced apoptosis well.
- *Cortical bone fraction stem cells (CBF-MSCs):* Cortical bone is the more potent than bone marrow as a stromal source for MSCs. Although bone marrow can produce a subset of clonogenic, multilineage cells; they are outnumbered and outperformed by an equivalent harvest of CBF-MSCs.
- Lineage-depleted CBF-MSCs have shown greater than 150-times enrichment of colony forming unit–fibroblasts (CFU-F) per cell incidence compared to bone marrow-derived MSCs.
- *Synovial tissue-derived mesenchymal stem cells (ST-MSCs):* The stem cells are scarce, as their availability is limited and has been used for potential regeneration of cartilage.

- *Peripheral blood-derived mesenchymal stem cells (PB-MSCs):* The stem cells are obtained by automated cell separator from peripheral blood. The stem cells have also been used for cartilage regeneration.
- Amnion, tendon, and skin have been also studied as source of stem cells but the usage is limited to specific research.

Orthopedic indications:
- *Cartilage synthesis and regeneration:* Newer techniques of using MSCs in natural matrices hence demand exacting engineering to provide optimal milieu (mechanical stability) for ideal differentiation of the implanted cells into hyaline cartilage. This mechanical stability (protecting from axial and shear stress) imparts important cell-matrix interactions (enough porosity to allow nutrient diffusion while maintaining adequate adhesion), so that functional tissue growth can happen. MSC-based constructs use (as described by various authors) poly (vinyl alcohol)/polycaprolactone (PVA/PCL) nanofibers or alginate or collagen gel/powder covered with periosteum or hyaluronic acid membrane, while free injection of MSCs has also been done. Various studies performed utilizing different combinations claim variable success in obtaining hyaline cartilage. Some of the methods include combining BM-MSCs with transwell permeable membrane (Murdoch et al.), BM-MSCs with connective tissue growth factor (Zhu et al.), BM-MSCs with TGF-β (Guo et al.), etc.
- *Nonunions and delayed unions:* MSCs have been used by Libergall et al. [MSC + PRP (platelet rich plasma) + DBM (demineralized bone matrix)] and Giannotti et al. (iliac crest MSC with induction to osteogenic differentiation in culture). The studies showed good bone formation in the treated patients but as a technical challenge critics put forward the challenge to prove that the regenerated bone comes from implanted cells. Hernigou et al. demonstrated correlation between callus volume and number of progenitor cells used thus quality of bone marrow aspirate would also have bearing when using alone.
- *Treating bone defects:* Masquelet technique is favored by and large for management of bone defects as is Ilizarov apparatus, the former relying mostly on MSCs in the second stage. It has been postulated that supplementation of bone graft with MSCs may help in enhancing the healing potential of the cancellous bone.
- *Tendon and ligament repair:* Ideal carrier is unknown and inhomogeneous results restrict its clinical translation. For ligament repair, anterior cruciate ligament (ACL) has been the primary contender, as it is commonly injured and has significant morbidity, if not reconstructed. Studies have been done in animals where partially transected ACL showed good recovery and healing in the knees injected with MSCs as compared to controls. Repair of Achilles tendon has been attempted with the use of BM-MSCs showing some nonstandardized support to its use.
- *Osteonecrosis (or AVN):* Decompression of a structurally maintained femoral head has been commonly practiced and advised, but the results are often variable with decompression alone and it is difficult to arrest collapse. Often the "forage" is combined with fibular grafting or cancellous grafting depending on the experience of surgeon. Hernigou et al. produced the largest case series of autologous bone marrow concentrate in 2002 and 2009 suggesting that results are very good in early stages and the progenitor cells home well in the transplanted bone. The relation is also proportional to the number of progenitor cells with higher the number of cells higher is the chance of cellular homing. The clinical improvement is in terms of reduced pain and slower progression of the disease.

Other less commonly studied indications for use of stem cells are:
- Spinal fusion
- Treating bone cysts and bone defects
- Osteogenesis imperfecta
- Osteoarthritis
- Nerve injury and spinal cord injury.

(For further reading and details, kindly refer to Regenerative Medicine and Stem Cell Research in Orthopedics in the book Essential Orthopedics: Principles and Practice, 2nd edition.)

3. Write the advantages and disadvantages of mesenchymal stem cells in trauma and orthopedics.

Ans:

Advantages:
- They not only differentiate into tissue-specific cell lines (cartilage, bone, fat, fibroblast, etc.) replacing the lost cells but also modulates inflammatory process.

- They have low immunoreactivity and high immunosuppressive properties.
- They have proven to be anti-inflammatory such as inhibiting maturation of helper T, cytotoxic T, dendritic and B-cells, and having immunosuppressive properties by secretion of transforming growth factor β-1 (TGF-β1), nitric oxide (NO), prostaglandin-E2, human leukocyte antigen G (HLA-G), hepatocyte growth factor (HGF), and interleukin 10 (IL-10).

Disadvantages: These stem cells are found in nearly all tissues but are very few in number and located in remote deep-seated places of the tissue often difficult to access, isolate, and grow in laboratory.

6.3 RECENT ADVANCES (Q4–25)

A. Cup and Stem Designs of Cemented and Uncemented Hips

4. What are the recent advances in cup and stem designs of cemented and uncemented hips?

Ans: As such the designing of acetabular cup (shell) and femoral stem has more-or-less stabilized in total hip prosthesis. Only two areas of active research are rapidly progressing—one is with respect to the bearing surfaces (this is also stabilizing) and the other one is regarding surface treatment of the prosthesis for improving bone integration and averting loosening (gaining attention of nanotechnology also).

Cementless Total Hip Prosthesis

Acetabular cups and press-fit design: Press-fit cups are 1–4 mm larger than reamed bone to impress bone implant bonding by adjusting hoop stresses. We are using third generation cup design where the liner is flush with the shell rim and does not protrude out. The congruity of the liner and acetabular cup has improved to allow placing ceramic, metal and highly cross-linked polyethylene (PE) liners all in single design. The first generation liners used to protrude from the acetabular cups and got easily damaged by impingement causing loss of locking mechanism and liner subluxation. The congruity was also not well maintained with empty area between the cup and liner causing liner failure in case thin poly was used. Ceramic liners were incompatible in this scenario. Second generation liners were also extruded but were much thicker to endure impingement, this however did not make them fail proof. The current contention in acetabular shell design involves improving the surface by specialized treatment to form trabecular tantalum bone or nanotreated surface that induces just enough roughness to stimulate osteogenesis and osteointegration (kindly see the above answer on nanotechnology).

The new introduction has been "dual mobility" head where femoral head articulates within a retentive PE. The PE is free to move in metal-back shell in a nonretentive way (in a bipolar prosthesis there is no movement between the poly liner and the shell and instead the shell is smooth that moves within acetabulum). Both the surfaces are mobile but outer bearing moves only in extremes of movements (nonphysiological ranges). The outer cup is surface modified for osteointegration and acetabular fixation. The main advantage is dual mobility design is reduced dislocation rate as it is the ever-concerning complication of a total hip replacement (THR). One should not be obsessed with dual mobility cups as they are not a substitute for classic hip design and are specifically indicated. The indications of dual mobility cup are typically:
- Situations in which primary hip is more likely to dislocate (elderly, patients with poor muscle mass and build, dementia)
- Revision hip arthroplasty
- Total hip replacement in developmental dysplasia of the hip (DDH), rheumatoid patients, and deformed hips
- Hyperlaxity, neuromuscular disease.

Intraprosthetic dissociation is a unique complication of this design which has to be reduced by open methods. The other disadvantage is inability to visualize acetabular floor during cup impaction as this is a monolithic cup.

Acetabular component is most susceptible to osteolysis, one of the factors for which is stress shielding due to rigid acetabular shells. Few modifications in materials and design have been produced to reduce the stress-shielding as follows:
- *Cambridge cup®* (Howmedica, Staines, UK): This is a horseshoe-shaped all polymer acetabular construct of ultra-high molecular weight polyethylene (UHMWPE) liner and carbon fiber reinforced polybutylene terephthalate shell with hydroxyapatite (HA) coating to fix to acetabulum.
- MITCH PCR cup (Stryker SA, Montreux Switzerland), a second-generation horseshoe-shaped cup made of polyetheretherketone (PEEK)/carbon fiber composite articulating with alumina femoral head.

Cementless femoral stem designs: The stems available are either unibody or bi-body (SROM type). The unibody designs vary with respect to the porous coating (proximal, distal, complete, tantalum, HA coated, etc.). The bi-body designs offer advantage as to improved adjustment of anteversion and offset, also it traps the particulate debris that develops at the interface without allowing it to percolate down once integration occurs. Slim anteroposterior designs have been developed but real advantage is unclear. Recently custom designs have been introduced. The custom stem can be prepared intraoperative (time consuming and limits the porous coating that can be provided) or preoperative customization using the radiological templating. Advantages over off-the-shelf stems have yet to come. The first generation cementless femoral stems of the hip arthroplasties include anatomic medullary locking (AML) (DePuy/Johnson & Johnson, Warsaw, IN, USA), the porous-coated anatomic (PCA) femoral stem (Howmedica, Rutherford, JN, USA), and the anatomic femoral stem (Zimmer, Warsaw, IN, USA) suffered from pain in the femur, the stress shielding phenomenon in the distal femur, osteolysis, dissociation, and difficulties in removal during revision. Second generation femoral stems were designed to fit firmly into the femoral proximal area by the concept of the tapered shape design, and maintain the hoop stress continuously to avoid stem subsidence. The tapered design did not match the shape of the femoral endosteum, and thus weight and stress transduction gets focused on special areas leading to formation of distal femoral shelf. Plasma sprayed stem surfaces tend to have less thigh pain than bead sintered stem designs. The most preferred stem design currently incorporates the following features:

- Proximally coated single wedge stems with wide proximal portions
- Collarless stem
- Shortened distal part by approximately 4–5 cm, compared to conventional stems
- The lateral shoulder of the proximal stem is inclined to make a slope to encourage bone preservation
- The neck is designed to minimize collision between liners and acetabular cups
- Reduce elasticity of distal stem by making long grooves on both the anterior and posterior sides of distal parts of stems, parallel to the vertical axis
- The lateral part of stem tips is partially removed to reduce contacts with lateral cortical bone to reduce thigh pain.

Cemented cups and stems: It is the improvements in cementing technique that has produced improvements in cemented hip arthroplasty rather than much changes in stem or cup designs. Only introduction of highly cross-linked poly is a major change in cup. In stem design the introduction of cement-in-cement revision stems has helped in cemented revisions otherwise the contemporary designs have not met major changes.

B. Anterior Cruciate Ligament Reconstruction

5. Discuss recent advances in arthroscopic anterior cruciate ligament (ACL) reconstruction with reference to creation of femoral tunnel and femoral fixation methods.

Ans: The placement of femoral tunnel and fixation methods have been a concern. Over a period of time the current recommendations are:

- Though double bundle technique has been envisaged to provide better rotational control, the clinical differences are yet to be proven. Single bundle technique by using anteromedial portal to create femoral tunnel more anatomically possibly yields similar results.
- Femoral tunnel placement should be at 10:30 position for right knee or 1:30 for left knee.
- The femoral tunnel should embrace the posterior cortex that can be achieved by 7 mm offset drill guide.
- It is better to widen the femoral notch so that it looks like a smooth inverted U "roman arch" rather than a pointed "gothic arch".

The femoral fixation devices have advanced to the following types:

- Compressive fixation (these produce compressive forces to the longitudinal axis of the graft pushing them against the bony tunnel). The commercial devices for such fixation are various interference screws that may be metallic (steel or titanium), bioabsorbable screws (polyglycolic acid, poly-L-lactic acid, poly-D, L-lactic acid, polyglycolic acid with trimethylene carbonate, poly-L-lactic acid with HA and poly-L-lactic acid with tricalcium phosphate). Bioabsorbable screws (available since 1995) instead are more compatible with ligament fixation and get absorbed in the body over a period of time. The PEEK cages have been introduced that provide strong fixation of soft tissue grafts with circumferential aperture compression.

- Expansive fixation (these devices produce a bulging effect of the graft again compressing it against the bony tunnel). The cross pin (Rigifix®) system has been a popular technique among expansion mechanisms that utilizes two bioabsorbable (poly-L-lactide) cross pins inserted across the graft through two parallel drill holes from the lateral femoral condyle perpendicular to the femoral socket made by a guide. The system has good stability and a high failure load, easier revision surgery and overall lower complication rate. The problem, however, is higher cost and guide misfire after prolonged usage. Expansion bolt is another expansive fixation device.
- Suspension of the graft (suspending the graft into the femoral tunnel). The suspension mechanism may be located within the graft bone interface (as in transfix) or may be located more or less far away from the knee joint. Depending on the type of bone the fixation system latches into, three divisions can be made:
  1. *Cortical:* This system is most common in practices and utilizes buttons (endobutton®, tightrope®, etc.), Swing Bridge, or Ligament Plate as fixation device
  2. *Cortical-cancellous:* These suspension devices consist of cross pin and bone mulch screw
  3. *Cancellous:* Cancellous fixation is very near to or just abutting the graft as is used with Linx-HT, PEEK cage fixation device or tape locking screw (TLS) screw system.

(For further details, kindly refer to chapter on 'Sports medicine: Knee' of the book Essential Orthopedics: Principles and Practice, 2nd edition.)

6. **Discuss the role of fixation devices in cruciate ligament reconstruction.**
Ans: Femoral fixation devices have been already described above.

Tibial side: Two broad categories of fixation methods are utilized for fixation of graft on tibial side:
1. *Intratunnel fixation:* These are the primary methods of fixation deployed in most reconstructions and mainly comprise interference screw (metallic or bioabsorbable) providing fixation by compression. Evolgate® system utilizes titanium-based components for fixation of graft on tibial side by reinforcing the tunnel wall with a coil while metallic screw provides interference fit and a washer gives stable cortical fixation. Xenogenic spongiosa cylinders have also been used as bone plugs to provide interference fit. Intrafix system (compressive fixation) provides relatively more secure fixation, while cross pins and CentraLoc® has also been used for expansive fixation. Tape locking system (TLS)® system or polyetheretherketone (PEEK) cage fixation suspends the graft within the tunnel.
2. *Extratunnel fixation:* Most surgeons use this as a supplementary fixation method to intratunnel fixation. Common methods are using a cancellous/cortical screw as a post, staples, or ligament washers.

C. Diagnosis of *Mycobacterium (M) Tuberculosis*

7. **A. Discuss recent advances in detection of *M. tuberculosis*.**
   B. Enumerate various newer methods with their sensitivity and specificity.
   C. GeneXpert/CB-NAAT and its specific advantages.

Ans: A. To rapidly diagnose tubercular infection, direct diagnostic measures are rapidly advancing that can demonstrate the bacterium in the specimen with high certainty. The gold standard is microscopic demonstration of the organism or formation of "central caseating necrotic granulomas" on histopathological examination (though other uncommon causes forming such granulomas also exist) as evidence of tubercular infection. As an extended application demonstration using nucleic acid amplification tests (NAAT) in the obtained sample from representative lesion should also be acceptable under proper clinical setup. Molecular diagnosis using NAAT is gaining popularity for rapid diagnosis (few hours to less than 1 day), high sensitivity, and specificity. The specimens sent to the laboratory are directly subjected to amplification of specific *M. tuberculosis* DNA sequences using one of the many available techniques such as polymerase chain reaction (PCR), real-time PCR or strand displacement amplification. These are highly sensitive and specific to confirm in acid-fast bacilli (AFB) positive cases and even in AFB negative extra-pulmonary tuberculosis (EPTB) cases DNA-PCR is, however, unable to differentiate between viable and nonviable bacillus and cost is also a prohibiting factor. The mRNA-based reverse transcriptase-PCR (RT-PCR) can differentiate viable from nonviable *M. tuberculosis* and is a rapid diagnostic method for EPTB too. RT-PCR has also been used to monitor drug resistance. Bacterial mRNA has a mean half-life of 3–5 minutes only, thus demonstrating positive mRNA signal would indicate viable organisms.

B. Newer targets have been studied for differentiation of latent from virulent and active organisms. Alpha crystallin (α-crystallin, *acr*) protein encoded by *acr* gene (also known as *hspX, Rv2031*) is such a marker; this protein is synthesized by mycobacterium under stress (reduced oxygen, immune response or treatment by antibiotics) and is associated with increased bacterial wall thickness. Synthesis of *acr* exponentially increases when bacterium undergoes transition from log phase to stationary mandating that the protein is essential for survival of stationary phase bacteria. Demonstration of *acr* is hence a new tool to identify latent infection, this can be done both in the tissue samples and even in patient serum. In contrast, the early secreted antigenic target-6 (ESAT-6) and culture filtrate 10 protein (CFP-10) act as virulence factors in *M. tuberculosis*, and contribute to pathogenicity. ESAT-6 and CFP-10 are particularly expressed by *M. tuberculosis* but not by Bacillus Calmette–Guérin (BCG) strains so *in vitro* T cell responses to ESAT-6 and CFP-10 appear to be highly sensitive and specific for the detection of infection with *M. tuberculosis* even in those immunized by BCG. Th1 proinflammatory cytokines are expressed at high levels when challenged with CFP-10 and ESAT-6 presentation in patients with active TB. Another method to diagnose active TB due to virulent bacteria expressing CFP-10 and ESAT-6 is to identify the CFP-10/ESAT-6 fusion protein using enzyme-linked immunospot (ELISPOT) assay for diagnosis of active TB either in tissue samples or patient sera.

C. The GeneXpert test (I personally recommend this test for diagnosis of active infection): Under the EXPAND-TB (expanding access to new diagnostics for TB) project a collaboration between WHO, foundation for innovative new diagnostics (FIND), and STOP-TB partnership's global drug facility (GDF) and global laboratory initiative (GLI) the Xpert MTB/ rifampin (RIF) assay was introduced to 6 EXPAND-TB countries (Azerbaijan, Ethiopia, India, Myanmar, Swaziland and Uzbekistan) in 2012 covering 21 countries in 2013. Xpert MTB/RIF is a fully automated diagnostic molecular test (applied on the tissue or sputum sample) using the NAAT. It simultaneously detects TB and rifampicin (R) drug resistance (*rpoB* gene) in less than 2 hours offering treatment opportunity same day. WHO strongly recommends the test to be used as the initial diagnostic test in individuals suspected of multidrug-resistant (MDR)-TB or HIV/TB. Conditionally, it is recommended as a follow on test to microscopy in settings where MDR-TB or HIV is of lesser concern especially in smear negative cases (like OATB). Line probe assay (DNA strip test) for first-line drugs (approved by WHO 2008) is recommended (encouraged) for diagnosis of MDR-TB (resistance to isoniazid (H) and/or (R)) and is a good supplement to diagnosis in MDR-TB regions but requires rigorous setup. Still WHO recommends conventional culture methods and drug susceptibility testing (DST) to determine extended drug resistant (XDR) cases in endemic regions. The beacon assay and line probe assay are extended form of the GeneXpert test that can be used for detection of drug-susceptibility/resistance.

[For further details, kindly refer to Chapter 11 Joint Disorders Including Inflammatory and Noninflammatory Arthritis and Infective Arthritides (Including Mycobacterial infection and Prosthetic Joint Infection) of Essential Orthopedics, Principles and Practice, 2nd edition.]

D. Management of Polytrauma Patient

8. **Describe recent advances in management of polytrauma patient highlighting the role of various investigative treatment modalities.**

Ans: Metabolic imbalances and oxidative stress influence the outcome of critically ill polytrauma patients. Most often just a damage to an organ does not indicate the true decompensation or hemodynamic compensation. The peripheral measures like blood pressure, pulse rate, and central measures like cardiac output and central venous pressure (CVP) are more or less approximations. Such cases are increasingly evaluated by evaluation of the microenvironment and molecular diagnosis. Some of the studied markers are mentioned in **Table 6.3.1**.

TABLE 6.3.1: Serum inflammatory markers.	
Acute-phase reactants	LBP, CRP, procalcitonin
Mediator activity	TNF, IL-1, IL-6, IL-10, IL-18
Cellular activity	TNF-RI, TNF-RII, IL-1R-I, IL-1R-II, IL-6-R, mIL-6-R, ICAM 1, E-selectin, CD11b, elastase, HLA-DR class-II

Lipopolysaccharide-binding protein (LBP) is of hepatic origin and has ability to bind bacterial lipopolysaccharide (LPS). LBP level rises during II or III day of trauma or sepsis, systemic inflammatory response syndrome (SIRS), and multiple organ dysfunction syndrome (MODS). LBP is significantly high in-patient with MODS with infection and can be used to differentiate SIRS from nonseptic MODS. C-reactive protein (CRP) has no role in polytrauma. Procalcitonin may indicate sepsis following SIRS. Development of SIRS followed by compensatory anti-inflammatory response (CARS) leads to activation of various inflammatory pathways. After CARS the patient may evolve into resolution or MODS depending on balance of pathways. Specifically, the activation of nuclear factor transcription-κB (NF-κB) modulates the activation of specific adhesion molecules, such as vascular cell adhesion molecules-1, intercellular adhesion molecules-1, and E selectin. Moreover, the activity of NF-κB is responsible for the modulation of some proinflammatory cytokines such as tumor necrosis factor-alpha (TNF-α) and interleukin-1-beta (IL-1β). IL-1 (difficult to detect due to short half-life of 6 minutes) appears to be a marker of traumatic insult, with significantly elevated levels occurring within 1–4 hours after trauma, and correlates with the severity of illness. IL-6 helps in identifying patients who are less likely to survive. Increased concentrations of IL-6 associated with a poor outcome in patients with acute respiratory distress syndrome (ARDS). IL-6 is not predictive of septic complications, but rather correlates with the magnitude of the injury. IL-6 seems to be the most reliable marker systemic inflammation while LBP appears to be an accurate and early marker of infection. The use of these two markers together may offer the ability to detect the onset of SIRS and allows early intervention to prevent MODS. In polytrauma patients, the recognition of high levels of inflammatory markers favors the damage control orthopedics (DCO) application, in order to prevent the effects of the "second hit" inflammatory reaction. IL-6 is considered the most specific prognostic indicator (discussed later) and early high levels of IL-6 have been associated with the development of organ failure (measuring IL-6 has become a routine in dedicated trauma centers).

Micro-RNA: As we know that primary and secondary injuries both contribute to reduced survival of polytrauma patients, it becomes imperative at directing the molecular analysis to identify this aspect. Numerous studies have been conducted regarding the identification of expression of micro-RNAs in the different traumas. Significant among studied are 17–92 micro-RNA, micro-RNA-181, micro-RNA-146a, micro-RNA-155, micro-RNA-511, micro-RNA-132, micro-RNA-122, micro-RNA-21, micro-RNA-125b, micro-RNA-187, and micro-RNA-223 that modulate activity of antigen-presenting cells or T cells correlating with increased TNF-α and IL-1 levels. Additionally, expression of micro-RNA-181b is found to be greatly reduced in critically ill polytrauma patients.

(For further details, kindly refer to Chapter 120 "Polytrauma, Mass Casualties and Disaster" of Essential Orthopedics: Principles and Practice, 2nd edition.)

E. Reducing Recurrence of Giant Cell Tumor

9. **Describe recent advances in reduction of recurrence of giant cell tumor (GCT) with emphasis on the medical treatment.**

Ans: Simple curettage, with or without bone grafting, has a significantly high rate of local recurrence of up to 60%. The intralesional and marginal procedures without adjuvants are associated with higher recurrences (the recurrence is actually "persistence" of original disease) due to inability to completely remove the microscopic disease, and recurrence is not correlated with grade or site of lesion. Modern treatment of GCT with extended curettage (making a wide window, using headlamps or dental mirror, angled curettes and high-speed burrs and pulsatile lavage) and cryosurgery (using liquid nitrogen) to the tumor cavity has achieved a recurrence rate of less than 3%. Routine use of adjuvants is recommended. Cryotherapy with liquid nitrogen popularized by Marcove has various side effects and has been effectively abandoned due to frostbite of soft tissues and bone necrosis. Photoablation with an argon laser is another therapy that can lead to successful tumor necrosis.

Bone cement has a tumor kill effect by exothermic reaction and possible chemical reaction (solvent aerosol is cytotoxic) that produces necrosis of tissue for 1–2 mm from contact area. Some people have used methotrexate and adriamycin in the bone cement to augment cytotoxic effect. Bone cement has the advantage of filling the defect and having tumoricidal effect.

Bisphosphonates especially the newer forms (zoledronic acid and pamidronate) have been proposed to reduce the osteopenia due to osteoclastic effect of giant cells and can be used as adjuvant to extended curettage. Also, they have been shown to have *in vitro* tumoricidal action. With the recognition of osteoclast differentiation factor receptor activator of nuclear factor kappa B (NF-κβ) ligand (RANKL) on tumor cells, targeted therapy against the receptor has been shown to be promising. Denosumab is the first agent licensed to be used for this purpose by Food and Drug Administration (FDA) in 2013. Denosumab is indicated in the US for treatment of adults and skeletally mature adolescents with giant-cell tumor of bone (GCTB) that is unresectable or where surgical resection is likely to result in severe morbidity.

The increased expression of several angiogenic growth factors observed in GCT led to the use of interferon alpha (IFN-α) as an anti-angiogenic agent. Pegylated (PEG)-IFN has also been shown to have anti-GCT activity.

(For further details, kindly refer to Chapter 5 "Bone Tumors, Common Soft Tissue Tumors and Heterotopic Ossification" of Essential Orthopedics: Principles and Practice, 2nd edition.)

F. Advances in Biomaterials

10. **Discuss recent advances in biomaterials in joint replacement to increase their longevity?**
Ans: Kindly see Answers to Questions 1, 3, and 13 for detail.

G. Management of Infected Persistent Wounds

11. **Discuss recent advances in the management of infected persistent wounds.**
Ans: The following are some of the recent additions in management of chronic persistent wound infections.

Use of sliver and nanoactivated silver topically: Newer forms of delivery aim to increase the efficacy while minimizing side effects. It has a favorable broad-spectrum coverage [Yeast, Fungi, Methicillin-resistant *Staphylococcus aureus* (MRSA), vancomycin-resistant enterococci (VRE)] even against antibiotic resistant organisms. Nanoactivated silver ions interact readily with negatively charged particles such as proteins, DNA, RNA, and chloride ions inhibiting the respiratory chain at the cytochrome level, interfering with electron transport, denaturing nucleic acids, inhibiting DNA replication, and altering cell membrane permeability. The pathogens are immediately killed upon contact due to this multi-pronged attack. Wound healing is also improved due to inhibition of zinc ions [hence matrix metalloproteinases (MMP)], and it has inhibitory effect on release of proinflammatory cytokines and TNF-α reducing inflammation in wound. Nanocrystalline silver dressings have two layers of high-density PE net sandwiching a layer of rayon/polyester gauze. The outer layer is coated with a nanocrystalline (<20 nm), noncharged form of silver (Ag^+), and the inner layer helps maintain a moist environment for wound healing.

Negative pressure wound therapy (NPWT): Vacuum-assisted closure (VAC) is recommended to be used as a comprehensive treatment plan in indicated acute or chronic wounds especially those that fail (or show delay) to heal normally and are challenging. It incorporates the use of negative pressure to optimize conditions for wound healing and has been found to reduce the need for frequent dressing changes, improve patient comfort, and reduce associated costs. Controlled negative pressure (50–125 mm Hg) is applied by an adjustable vacuum pump which reduces interstitial fluid accumulation and edema formation helping minimize bacterial colonization of the wound and increase proliferation of the granulation tissue by arteriolar dilation in negative pressure. The noted benefits of VAC therapy are:
- Removal of exudate from the wound and reduction in interstitial edema.
- Increased local microvascular flow and improved vascularity (arteriolar dilation).
- Increased controlled production of granulation tissue formation by reduction in the exposure to proteolytic enzymes. Vacuum also puts shear force producing cellular hyperplasia.
- Reduction in the need of antibiotics.

Improvements in dressing materials: Various advanced dressing materials have been introduced to improve wound healing—
- *Hydrocolloids:* These are impermeable to water, bacteria and other contaminants but permeable to water vapor.
- *Alginates:* They act as fillers for undermined and tunneled wounds and promote angiogenesis.
- *Foams:* These are nonadherent, easy to apply and remove, and are meant for highly exuding wounds.
- *Collagen:* It is chemotactic for fibroblasts and macrophages and also provide a temporary scaffold to allow in growth of tissue.
- *Hydrogels:* They are best suited for dry wounds or those with minimal exudates but need additional dressing.
- *Hydrofibers:* They maintain a moist environment and allow autolytic debridement so highly suitable for pressure ulcers.

Skin substitutes: They are available for wound coverage and are of various composite materials depending on type of wound. Bioengineered cellular therapies like Apligraf® (bilayered construct consisting of a bovine collagen matrix seeded with living human neonatal fibroblasts and a neonatal keratinocyte neoepidermis) and Dermagraft® [human fibroblast-derived dermal substitute (HFDS) comprising a cryopreserved, absorbable, three-dimensional polyglactin mesh substrate seeded with living neonatal dermal fibroblasts] are available for specific purpose. Human dermal allografts have become increasingly popular in recent years for augmenting tissue regeneration in chronic lower extremity wounds.

Growth factors and biologic wound products: Biological therapies refer to tissue-based treatments (acellular and cellular), autologous platelet-rich plasma (PRP), as well as recombinant human growth factor therapies. These aim to accelerate healing by augmenting or modulating inflammatory mediators viz. prostaglandin E1, cytokines like chemokines, lymphokines, monokines, interleukins, colony-stimulating factors, and interferons. Becaplermin (Regranex) is a combination of recombinant human platelet-derived growth factor (rhPDGF) and recombinant human epidermal growth factor (rhEGF). Topical insulin has been found trophic for wounds and is being increasingly used in combinations.

Wound debridement systems and pressure irrigation: Ultrasonic and powerful jet-based wound debridement systems are available for removing dead and infected material from wound providing clean surface for further intervention. Power-jets of compressed oxygen combined with minimal amount of saline solution produce fast and virtually painless debridement compared to other mechanical debridement methods.

Extracorporeal shock wave therapy (ESWT): Promote a cascade of cytokine and growth factor upregulation leading to enhanced neovascularization, anti-inflammatory response, and tissue regeneration expediting wound repair.

Hyperbaric oxygen and ozone therapy: While ozone is delivered by "bagging" technique locally, hyperbaric oxygen therapy (HBOT) is given in 100% high pressure oxygen tanks for patients to breathe. Ozone therapy is beneficial for diabetic infected wounds. HBOT is beneficial for a wide variety of chronic wounds by increasing tissue oxygen tension, angiogenesis, fibroblast proliferation, collagen deposition, and enhanced bacterial killing.

Stem cell therapy: Mesenchymal stem cells (MSCs) (bone marrow or placental) can directly differentiate into mesenchymal tissues, such as bone, tendon, and cartilage but need paracrine trophic function for cutaneous repair. MSCs produce growth factors, such as TGF-β3, to limit excessive scarring as well as modulate the balance between MMP and tissue inhibitors of metalloproteinases while regulating collagen deposition.

(For further details, kindly refer to chapter on wound healing and principles of wound care of the book Essential Orthopedics: Principles and Practice, 2nd edition.)

H. Management of Prolapsed Intervertebral Disks

12. **Discuss recent advances in management of prolapsed intervertebral disks.**

Ans: Prolapsed intervertebral disks (PIVD) causing intractable pain can be managed by a number of interventions apart from conventional microscopic or endoscopic diskectomy, fusion and disk replacement as follows:
- *Lumbar epidural steroid injections (transforaminal or caudal):* It is usually indicated after thorough evaluation for acute radicular pain due to irritation or inflammation, symptomatic herniated disk with failed conservative therapy, acute exacerbation of diskogenic pain or pain of spinal stenosis, neoplastic infiltration of roots, epidural fibrosis, chronic LBP with acute radicular symptoms. The drug is deposited in posterior epidural space in a blind procedure similar to giving epidural anesthesia/analgesia.
- *Selective nerve root block:* It is preferred for management of radiculopathy in patients with equivocal neurological finding or discrepancy between clinical and radiological examination. It can also be done in patients with unexplainable or recurrent pain.
- *Epidural adenolysis or percutaneous decompressive neuroplasty:* Epiduroscopy (a fiber-optic scope to visualize epidural space) helps in establishing the diagnosis of adhesions and also site of these adhesions. These adhesions can be managed by adhesiolysis during epiduroscopy under vision.
- *Trigger point (TP) injection:* The iliopsoas and quadratus lumborum are two muscles commonly involved in the origin of low back pain in the lumbar region. Neutralization of TP is the treatment of choice. TP injection with local anesthetic, depo steroid, ozone gas or even dry needling gives pain relief.
- *Botox paraspinal muscle injection:* This relieves the intractable muscle spasm associated with unrelieved low back pain and breaks the cycle of pain → spasm → deformity → neural compression → pain.

- *Facet joint or pericapsular injection and medial branch block:* Relief from intra-articular local anesthetic injection or medial branch block with 0.5–1.5 mL local anesthetic confirms diagnosis of facet joint as source of pain. Radiofrequency (RF) ablation procedure of medial branch gives good and sustained pain relief. Therapeutic facet joint injection with steroid/RF ablation of medial branch of dorsal rami gives long-term relief.
- *Spine prolotherapy and manipulation:* It is done with normal saline, hypertonic saline with/without hyaluronidase.
- *Gray ramus block:* Gray ramus block (GRB) is effective to relieve low back pain caused by diskogenic pain. This procedure is used when surgery is not an option to relieve pain from disk.
- Percutaneous disk decompression:
    - *Laser diskectomy:* Holmium:yttrium-aluminum-garnet (Ho:YAG) laser is most commonly used. Nucleus pulposus is vaporized, intradiskal pressure decreases, allowing the disk to return to its normal state. Best candidates for laser diskectomy include those with back and leg pain with a confirmed disk herniation.
    - Radiofrequency coblation (plasma diskectomy)
    - *Mechanical disk decompression:* This procedure is usually performed under fluoroscopic guidance using a disposable, self-contained, battery operated handpiece connected to a helical probe (dekompressor®). Percutaneous diskectomy has a reported success rate of 60–87%.
    - *Percutaneous endoscopic diskectomy:* Percutaneous nucleotomy by means of arthroscopy instruments for disk removal for the treatment of posterior or posterolateral lumbar disk herniation under local anesthesia was demonstrated by Hijikata et al. in 1975. This technique is based on arthroscopic visualization of the herniation via the posterolateral approach for diskectomy of contained herniations. Ideal patient for this procedure is one who has paramedian, foraminal, or extraforaminal contained herniation.
- *Annuloplasty:*
    - *Intradiskal electrothermy(IDET):* Intradiskal electrothermy is based on modification of collagen making it thicker and causing it to contract decreasing its ability to revascularize. This in turn also prohibits the reinnervation and inflammation which may be causing root irritation.
    - *Radiofrequency posterior annuloplasty:* This is a minimally invasive method of delivering radiofrequency thermal energy to the disk to treat diskogenic lower back pain. Ideal candidates for this procedure are patients with intervertebral disc disease (IDD) grade 3/4/5 as per CT classification with chronic low back pain.
    - *Biacuplasty:* Intradiskal biacuplasty utilizes a bipolar system that includes two cooled radiofrequency electrodes placed on the posterolateral sides of the intervertebral annulus fibrosus to produce shrinkage.
- *Augmentation of nucleus pulposus and nucleus replacement:* Nucleus replacement arthroplasty aims to replace the intervertebral disk (IVD) nucleus while preserving the annulus and vertebral endplates. This would prevent disk height loss and the associated biomechanical and biochemical changes.
- *Gene therapy and stem cell-based therapies:* These are aimed to improve the intradiskal environment and production of healthy matrix. The gene-vector complex is directly injected into the target tissue producing the requisite growth factor. Various other approaches (cell based) are also under study but have limited success rates.

(*For further details, kindly refer to Chapters 86, 87, 88 and 89 of the book Essential Orthopedics: Principles and Practice, 2nd edition.*)

13. **A. Disc replacement surgery.**
    B. Navigation in spine surgery.

Ans:

A. In this procedure, the biological injured or degenerated disc material is removed, and an artificial disc is implanted in the spine. Total disc replacement (TDR) technology is not totally new, and first attempts were made in the 1950s using the Fenstrom steel-ball endoprosthesis. The technology has been used for many years in Europe but is still mostly in trial stages in the United States of America, more than 100 designs were developed but only few are in use. More widespread application of TDR followed after the mid-80s developments of a TDR designed at the Charite Hospital in Berlin, Germany. The principle of replacing almost the entire IVD is based on the success of hip and knee replacements. Proponents of TDR view, it as a technology to treat back pain while attempting to decrease adjacent segment disease. The initial excitement with TDR got tampered by the realization that specific cause of LBP is still not known, so complete relief in all patients is far-fetched expectation and the fact that mechanical failure of devices were quickly reported.

Aims of Total Disc Replacement
- Restore the physiological kinematics of the IVD
- Relieve pain
- Improve stability and resist wear
- Protecting the adjacent discs and facet joints from undue degeneration.

Indications: The classic indication for TDR includes failure of aggressive conservative treatment with disabling LBP attributed to the lower lumbar spine affecting no more than two discs. Other indications are like those of fusion.

Prerequisite:
- Demonstrable disc degeneration as the cause of pain
- Intact facet joints posteriorly and no other pain generators demonstrated

Contraindications:
- Lumbar spinal stenosis
- Facet disease
- Old fractures
- Previous laminectomy
- Instability as seen in spondylolisthesis
- Osteoporosis
- Pars fracture
- Infection

Relative contraindication—patients with a steep lumbosacral angle at the intended TDR level. It is difficult to implant disc in such situation.

Total Disc Repair Designs

The materials that have been used for TDR are similar to those that have been employed in other major joint arthroplasties (e.g. polyethylene, chrome cobalt, titanium). And to this effect, the replacement designs are also available in varying conformities:
- Unconstrained
- Semi-constrained
- Constrained

The surgical approach is like the one used to obtain an anterior lumbar interbody fusion and carries similar rates of vascular complications.

Outcome of implantation: The reports have been encouraging and, in most cases, have not been found to be inferior to fusion surgery. The long-term complications and benefits of TDR are yet to be realized, especially in terms of preventing adjacent level disc degeneration.

Complications:
- Osteolysis
- Implant fracture or wear
- Vertebral body fracture
- Failure of ingrowth
- Instability with dislocation

The revision surgery is technically difficult as there is prominent anterior fibrosis after the procedure increasing the chances of vascular injury and other complications.

B. Navigation in spine surgery

Safety and efficiency during spine surgery is of paramount importance due to the sensitive nature of the neurovascular structures involved. The complexity of the three-dimensional anatomy of the spine innovative and modern techniques that improve 3D orientation and guidance during surgery have gained popularity. Intraoperative computer-aided navigation (CAN) during spine surgery has been classically used for pedicle screw placement that gets smoothly incorporated into minimally invasive spinal surgery procedures to reduce intraoperative radiation exposure and enhance surgical accuracy. To combat the relative inaccuracy of traditional methods of pedicle screw placement and involved high stakes (neurovascular injury), CAN was introduced as a means to improve accuracy. Now the computer-based navigation systems guide surgeons while placing instrumentation and also for noninstrumented cases. CAN uses novel computer-based technologies, including stereotaxy, navigated surgery and robotics.

Basic Components of Navigation System
- *Image acquisition and processing unit:* High-resolution images are obtained either preoperatively or intraoperatively. Due to the anatomical changes between image acquisition (usually supine position) and actual operative procedure (prone position), re-registration of landmarks intraoperatively is essential. Intraoperative images are acquired using fluoroscopy, CT scan or MRI.
- *Referencing system:* The intraoperative landmarks are referenced to the image/navigation database using referencing system. This consists of:
  - *Dynamic reference frame/array (DRA):* DRA is attached to fixed landmark (spinous process/iliac crest) which should remain undisturbed throughout surgery. Preoperative image is taken along with the fixed DRA to synchronize between the virtual navigated images and anatomical landmarks.
  - *Light emitting diodes (LED):* Emit (positive array-like DRA) or reflect light (passive array—instruments), which is tracked by an electro-optical camera and are known as active arrays to provide a real-time tracking of the exact location of these devices over the surgical field.
  - *Tracking system:* Optical (more accurate), mechanical, acoustic or electromagnetic systems calculate the location and provide real-time 3D positional data of the handheld surgical instruments in relation to the surgical field.

Registration process: This synchronizes virtual images to real anatomy. *Three types:*
1. Paired point registration
2. Surface matching
3. Automatic registration

Generations of CAN system:
a. First generation—image acquisition using thin-slice CT scan, manual point-matching referencing (long and tedious).
b. Second generation—intraoperative reconstruction images of the spinal anatomy using 2D and 3D (isocentricity based concept) fluoroscopy. Improved versions used cone-based CT that have better image quality, larger vertebral span and automatic registration.
c. Third generation—intraoperative CT scan with subsequent automatic registration, screening whole spine, total navigated spine surgery and complete support to minimally invasive techniques are some of its salient features.

Clinical applications:
- Cervical spine pedicle screw and lateral mass screw placement, Hangman fracture osteosynthesis and occipitocervical surgeries in congenital defects.
- Minimally invasive surgery—the accuracy and safety of pedicle screw placement is highly improved over free-hand technique.
- Correction of spinal deformity (osteotomy) and fixation (pedicle screw placement in dysmorphic pedicles).
- Spinal tumor surgery—better localization of tumor and clearer- defined margin for resection + safety of displaced sensitive neurovascular structures.
- Complex lumbosacral trauma osteosynthesis—placement of S1, S2, alar and iliac screws.

Advantages of navigation-assisted spine surgery:
- Accuracy and improved safety
- Reduced surgeon fatigue
- Reduced operative time (depends on familiarity with system however)
- Minimal radiation exposure

Disadvantages (areas of improvement):
- Wobbling and motion-related artefacts
- Altered accuracy due to distance from reference array.

I. Diagnosis and Management of Rheumatoid Arthritis

14. Elaborate recent advances in diagnosis and management of rheumatoid arthritis.

Ans: Specific diagnostic tests do not exist for definitive diagnosis of rheumatoid arthritis (RA). The diagnosis is mainly clinical but to speed up the diagnosis few tests act as supportive measures as follows:

- *Anti-cyclic citrullinated peptide (CCP) antibody:* The second generation anti-CCP assay is recommended as a routine work-up of patients clinically diagnosed as (RA).
- *Anti-mutated citrullinated vimentin (MCV) antibody:* These are associated with more severe RA. The assay may prove to be of high specificity for the diagnosis of RA and is likely to be useful in clinical practice due to its simplicity.
- Ultrasonography and MRI scan are being increasingly used to determine synovitis and joint erosion to implement specific therapy.

European League Against Rheumatism (EULAR) new criteria (2010) for clinical diagnosis **(Table 6.3.2):**

TABLE 6.3.2: European League Against Rheumatism criteria (2010) for clinical diagnosis.

Joint involvement (0–5)	
1 medium-large joint	0
2–10 medium-large joints	1
1–3 small joints (with or without involvement of large joints)	2
4–10 small joints (with or without involvement of large joints)	3
>10 joints (at least one small joint)	5
Serology (0–3)	
Negative rheumatoid factor and negative anti-citrullinated protein antibodies	0
Low positive rheumatoid factor or low positive anti-citrullinated protein antibodies	2
High positive rheumatoid factor or high positive anti-citrullinated protein antibodies	3
Acute phase reactants	
Normal C reactive protein and normal erythrocyte sedimentation rate	0
Abnormal C reactive protein or abnormal erythrocyte sedimentation rate	1
Duration of symptoms	
<6 weeks	0
≥6 weeks	1

These criteria are intended for patients with at least 1 joint with definite clinical synovitis (swelling, not just tenderness), and in whom the synovitis is not explained by another disease such as psoriasis, systemic lupus erythematosus, or gout. Patients are considered to have RA if they have a score of at least 6.

Management aspect: Biologic agents refer to complex protein molecules produced by using molecular biology methods in prokaryotic or eukaryotic cell cultures. It is now well validated that biologic therapies have changed the way RA is managed. These directed therapies act either on the cytokines or their receptors.

Anti-TNF agents: These improve symptoms while reducing radiographic progression of joint erosions and are the most commonly deployed biological agents for management of RA. A number of them (etanercept, adalimumab, infliximab, golimumab, and certolizumab pegol) are available and others being actively developed for improvement in specific activity. There is a demonstrable benefit of early treatment with TNF inhibitors and methotrexate, suggesting that early intervention may have lasting benefits to patients with regards to disease progression.

Interleukin-1 (IL-1) antagonist (Anakinra) has demonstrated improvement in symptoms but is not commonly used due to its comparatively low efficacy as against anti-TNF agents.

Inhibitors of T-cell costimulation: Abatacept blocks T-cell activation through inhibition of CD28-B7 mediated costimulation of the T-cell and has been effective in patients not responding to anti-TNF agents.

IL-6 receptors antagonist (Tocilizumab): This agent is approved for management of moderate to severe RA showing inadequate response to anti-TNF agents.

Anti-B-cell agent (Rituximab): This is also approved for patients failing on anti-TNF agents. These are not associated with risk of tuberculosis reactivation and are not contraindicated in previous history of cancer.

Kinase inhibitors: These are under development novel agents that are different from conventional biological agents in that they target intracellular molecules that are involved in signal transduction instead of cytokines or receptors. In particular, janus kinases (JAKs), spleen tyrosine kinase (SyK), and p38 mitogen-activated protein kinases (MAPKs) as targets are under study.

Apart from above lots of molecules are under developments that target various integrated and intermediary pathways like IL-15, IL-17, IL-32, lymphotoxins, and B-lymphocyte stimulator (BLyS).

[A detailed description on the use of biological agents and diagnostics is provided in the chapter on Joint Disorders Including Inflammatory and Noninflammatory Arthritis and Infective Arthritides (Including Mycobacterial Infection and Prosthetic Joint Infection) of the book Essential Orthopedics: Principles and Practice, 2nd edition.]

J. Total Hip Arthroplasty

15. **Discuss recent advances in total hip arthroplasty.**

Ans: Total hip replacement has established itself as a successful orthopedic intervention for management of specific hip disorders beyond doubt. Attempts have been and are being made to improve the outcomes still further. The recent advances have been made specifically in bearing surfaces, improving longevity, stem and cup designing (limited), cementing techniques and resolving controversies for hip exposure technique. Methods to ameliorate infection are applicable to all joint arthroplasties and osteosynthesis in general.

Bearing surfaces: Currently this has moved in a circle with various advances not proving significantly advantageous in general over standard metal-on-poly (MOP) articulation. Some alternative bearing surfaces do have indications in specific situations.

Ceramic (alumina or zirconia) on poly: When envisaged this was considered a superior counterpart of MOP bearing, but this has not been consistently proven. Oxidized zirconium (Oxinium®, Smith and Nephew) has been specifically produced for this articulation but wear properties are not very impressive (compared to available materials). The oxinium improves the wear characteristics of zirconium while simultaneously utilizing the hardness and its fracture resistance. This has also allowed the use of large heads as the volumetric wear would be less ultimately while increasing stability. Alumina seems to have outpaced zirconia in the race against wear as it has reduced wear rates than the latter. The inconsistent reports of sometimes increased and at other times reduced wear would be explained by presence of third-body wear. This also explains the imperative need of hardened poly as a safety measure to be used against harder femoral head bearings (hence preferring highly cross-linked poly). The newer highly cross-linked PE show annual linear wear at 45% of conventional UHMPE in prosthesis implanted for 5 years. This indicates that osteolysis may not possibly occur at all.

Ceramic-on-ceramic (COC) bearings: While alumina remains the most widely used ceramic and is preferred for COC bearings, zirconia is utilized as a replacement for alumina femoral heads for COP bearings (UHMWPE acetabular liner). This is reasoned on the fact that zirconia is stronger than alumina and therefore it can resist higher degrees of stress. The advantages conferred by zirconia include superior mechanical strength posing a reduction in bearing fracture risk. The advantages on COC bearings are minimal wear and virtually no osteolysis due to inert nature of alumina wear particles, alumina ceramics are highly oxidized so they cannot be further oxidized and are biologically inert and resistance to surface damage.

Ceramic-on-metal (COM) bearings: The wear for alumina COM articulations is very favorable, but the articulation should be ceramic femoral heads 28 mm in diameter articulating against acetabular cups manufactured from medical-grade, high carbon-wrought cobalt-chromium alloy. In addition, this bearing also appears to produce less stripe wear with edge loading than metal-on-metal (MOM) or COC implants. The potential advantage of this novel COM bearing is thus lower wear and the production of significantly reduced metal particles quantitatively.

Metal-on-metal (MoM) bearing: MOM bearing has been withdrawn world over since around 2010 for concerns of ill-effects of metal ions and untoward biological response including cancer risk.

Silicon nitride bearing surfaces: Si_3N_4 shows good fracture toughness, high-flexural strength, and resistance to hydrothermal degradation (like alumina). Si_3N_4 is currently used in aerospace bearings and in high-temperature places like in diesel engines. When studied for THA, the Si_3N_4 cups have been shown to highly reduce the wear rates when used against Co-Cr or Si_3N_4 femoral heads. The Si_3N_4-Si_3N_4 bearings have very low friction coefficient of 0.001 even when compared COC alumina bearing of 0.08.

Carbon-fiber polymeric composites and PEEK bearings are under study and would need substantial time for clinical development and acceptability.

Recent advances in cup and stem designs of cemented and uncemented hips—see Question 3 above for details. *Improvements in surface finish and design to improve implant longevity* is discussed in Answer to Question 1 above.

Recent advances in cementing technique and bone cements: Apart from the standard hand mixing and pressurization of bone cement advancements have been made to provide a composite cement mantle devoid of deficiencies and having uniformity. The third-generation cementing technique involves:

- Use of vacuum-centrifugation for cement preparation to reduce porosity
- Pulsatile lavage irrigation of femoral canal and packing with adrenaline soaked swabs
- Insertion of the cement in a retrograde fashion and cement pressurization using proximal pressurizers
- Adrenaline-soaked sponges for femoral canal
- Prosthesis is inserted using distal and proximal centralizers to ensure optimal position and even cement mantle.

Cartridge mixing and delivery is a further improvement using a universal power mixer that quickly mixes and then injects nearly all types of bone cement. It has the advantage of reduced mixing times and consistency of the mixture. Also, the operating room personnel are spared of toxic fumes.

Composite cements are being produced for improving bone cement interface characteristics. Polymer fibers are added to poly (methyl methacrylate) (PMMA) for improving fracture toughness and fatigue strength. The following are currently studied additives:

- Carbon fibers as multiwalled carbon nanotubes
- Glass fibers
- Kevlar (used in F1 racing car's petrol tanks)
- Oriented PMMA
- Rubber impregnated PMMA
- Ultra-high-molecular-weight polyethylene
- Polyethylene terephthalate
- Aramid
- Graphite
- Nano-sized titanium fibers
- Embedded continuous stainless steel coils
- Zirconia fibers with and without acrylic coating.

For improving cement integration into bone mixing the 40% w/w calcium phosphate (Brushite) into two-solution pseudoplastic system (non-Newtonian material where the viscosity decreases as the shear rate increases) to yield highly viscous, injectable, bioactive cement with high compressive strength and has shown encouraging results *in vitro*. Osteoconduction can also be improved by addition of bioactive ceramics.

Heat generation in bone cement can be reduced by adding 1-dodecyl mercaptan, ammonium nitrate, zeolytes or N-acetyl cysteine as appropriate.

Recent advances in diagnosing periprosthetic joint infections are discussed in Answer to Question 1.

Advances in preventing and managing the DVT after arthroplasty is discussed in Chapter 1 elaborately.

Advances in surgical exposure of hip: Direct anterior approach and minimally invasive surgery (MIS) are new contenders for surgical exposure of hip joint. The anterior approach has been proposed to avoid damage to abductor function (lateral approach) and also reduce dislocation rates after THA (posterior approach). The MIS anterior approach has been found to have longer operative time, higher blood loss, four intraoperative conversions to posterolateral, more complications and the same length of stay in hospital with no functional difference. Currently no systematically performed study demonstrates superiority of any approach and possibly the approach in which the surgeon is most comfortable and trained should be used.

(Details on various advances discussed can be read from Chapters 58, 60 and 61 of the book Essential Orthopedics: Principles and Practice, 2nd edition.)

K. Articular Tissue Engineering

16. Discuss advances in articular cartilage tissue engineering.

Ans: Articular cartilage tissue engineering requires the integration of stem-cell therapy, 3D printing and surgical modifications to come together. Principle is culturing chondrocytes in an implantable biological matrix with ideal properties—biocompatible, biodegradable and bioactive while preserving the phenotypic characteristics, thus favoring the cellular proliferation and synthesis of the extracellular matrix (ECM), which is permeable, easy to use and inexpensive. The matrix is bioengineered using 3D printing technology. Innovative approach is to use a combination of structures that use "force dissipation pattern" utilizing stem cells or chondroblasts that can be influenced by the mechanical stimuli. "Smart scaffold designs" are created by combining different biomaterials that influence deposition of extracellular matrix by influencing cellular alignment. These constructs have to be, however, grown in a controlled environment in a bioreactor into functional tissue that then matures in the body. The process has been taken a step further by trying to incorporate the functions of tissue into synthesized construct itself. Construct such as cell-laden heterogeneous hydrogel can be produced with 3D printing to be potentially used as osteochondral grafts. Decellularized extracellular matrix (dECM) has been bioprinted that can provide microenvironment to chondrons for induction of cartilage tissue growth by providing crucial signals for cell engraftment, survival, and future functions. To mimic the zonal (three zones of native hyaline cartilage) construct of cartilage combination of polymers have been used like polyethylene glycol (PEG), hyaluronic acid, chondroitin sulfate, and metalloprotease-sensitive peptides that encapsulate single lineage of MSCs.

Mesenchymal stem cells are the work-horse for providing the source cells that could regenerate into cartilage but it is easier said than done. Newer techniques of using MSCs in natural matrices demand exacting engineering to provide optimal milieu (mechanical stability) for ideal differentiation of the implanted cells into hyaline cartilage. This mechanical stability (protecting from axial and shear stress) imparts important cell-matrix interactions (enough porosity to allow nutrient diffusion while maintaining adequate adhesion), so that functional tissue growth can happen. MSC-based constructs use (as described by various authors) poly (vinyl alcohol)/polycaprolactone (PVA/PCL) nanofibers or alginate or collagen gel/powder covered with periosteum or hyaluronic acid membrane, while free injection of MSCs has also been done.

(For further details, kindly refer to Chapters 10, 130 and 131 of the book Essential Orthopedics: Principles and Practice, 2nd edition.)

L. Management of Periarticular Fractures

17. Discuss the advances in management of periarticular fractures.

Ans: The periarticular fractures are managed on primary principle of accurate joint line restoration and alignment. If intra-articular extension is seen, then anatomic reduction and absolute stability needs to be added. The most important concern is the articular surface depression and compaction into the subchondral cancellous bone in associated intra-articular extension and common finding of comminution at the metadiaphyseal interface. So the goals of osteosynthesis are:
- Joint line alignment in anatomical position (with respect to the mechanical/anatomical axis)
- Joint surface (articular surface) restoration
- Adequate stability to allow early joint mobility to prevent stiffness.

To achieve all three goals usually the joint surface is to be lifted that leaves a void in the supporting cancellous area. Also, the implant construct need to provide good stability over a prolonged period to support rehabilitation. The following are the advances in current practice supporting this end:

Filling of cancellous bone defect: Apart from the conventional autogenous and allogenic bone graft synthetic materials have been introduced to act as bone fillers. Most of the current available synthetic bone graft substitutes can be grouped into HA products, soluble calcium-based blocks and granules, or injectable cements. Injectable calcium phosphate cement may leak through intra-articular defects and harden in the articular surface causing arthrosis of joint so injectable resorbable calcium sulfate cement is favorable. The biodegradable calcium sulfate cement has been designed to harden with the defect and provide intraoperative stabilization. It can be drilled through and receive self-tapping screws after hardening without hindering material strength or integrity properties.

Use of 3D-printed blocks as bone defect spacers: 3D printed biocompatible porous 3D matrix scaffolds allow conducive environment for cell attachment, migration, incorporation of growth factors, and encouraging vascular ingrowth. These scaffolds apart from above properties should be sufficiently mechanically stable providing requisite strength at the site of usage. For cellular growth, it has been found that in a hydrogel model (alginate scaffold) addition of peptide like arginine-glycine-aspartic acid increases bone formation. PEG hydrogel as also demonstrated promising results in terms of its properties for supporting cellular growth. 3D printing controls the precise form, architecture, and disposition of scaffold producing clinically optimal combinations.

Arthroscopic assisted-reduction and fixation: The arthroscopically-assisted reduction and internal fixation (ARIF) techniques has advantages of accurate diagnosis of the fracture and associated soft tissue involvement, the potential for concomitant treatments (removal of loose fragments/ligament reconstruction), anatomical reduction and minimal invasiveness. This is especially useful in minimally invasive plate osteosynthesis (MIPO) technique where accurate reduction can be effected by intra-articular manipulation of the displaced fragments to align them anatomically. The "PART" and "dry technique" are further advancements where complex fractures can also be addressed.

Use of hybrid fixators: In high energy trauma where skin condition is unfavorable hybrid fixation with wire frame combined to regular fixator may serve the purpose. The reduction can be improved by arthroscopic techniques.

Use of locked plate constructs: Anatomical locked plates with fixed angle screws have drastically improved the stability of periarticular osteosynthesis. The plates have further gone advancements like variable locked screw plate constructs where the screw can be locked in different positions as needed by surgeon and design improvements for matching the anatomy.

Use of allograft-plate construct: This is rarely used in cases with bone loss but repairable tissues where osteoarticular allograft is first fixed to the locked plate and the composite can be used for osteosynthesis.

Custom printed implants: This is a new frontier opened by the 3D-printed technique where patient specific implants can be printed using data from CT scans preoperatively, facilitating application and osteosynthesis.

18. **Recent advances in various imaging modalities in orthopedics?**

Ans: This would need a complied answer [the reader is encouraged to read the positron emission tomography *(PET) scan, magnetic resonance imaging (MRI), and ultrasonography* from chapters—123, 125, and 126, respectively of the book *Essential Orthopedics—Principles and Practice*]. There have been subtle changes only in advances of imaging such as zero-ECHO MRI. Some additional details are written below:

- *Magnification radiography:* Magnification radiography is occasionally used to enhance bony details not well appreciated on the standard radiographic projections. This technique may help is detecting early arthritic changes and some metabolic disorders. Very rarely it may be useful in demonstrating subtle fracture lines otherwise not seen on routine projections.
- *Digital radiography:* Digital (computed) radiography (DR) is the name given to the process of digital image acquisition using an X-ray detector comprising a photostimulable phosphor imaging plate and an image reader-writer that processes the latent image information for subsequent brightness scaling and laser printing on film.
- *Tomography:* Tomography is a body-section radiography that permits more accurate visualization of lesions too small to be noted on conventional radiographs or demonstrates anatomic detail obscured by overlying structures. Newly developed tomographic units can localize the image more precisely and have aided greatly in the ability to detect lesions as small as approximately 1 mm.
    - *Computed tomography (CT):* The newest advances in sophisticated software-enabled 3D reconstruction, which is helpful in analyzing regions with complex anatomy, such as the face, pelvis, vertebral column, foot, ankle, and wrist. New computer systems now permit the creation of plastic models (3D printing) of the area of interest based

on 3D images. These models facilitate operative planning and allow rehearsal surgery of complex reconstructive procedures. High-resolution flat-panel volume CT (fpVCT) uses digital flat-panel detectors and provides volumetric coverage as well as ultra-high spatial resolution in two-dimensional (2D) and 3D projections. It reduces metal and beam hardening artifacts and fpVCT also allows dynamic imaging of time-varying processes. 3D CT-angiography is effectively used to determine the presence or absence of injury to the vessels near the fractured bones.

19. Discuss various considerations, pros and cons and future perspective of day care surgery in orthopedics.

Ans: The Royal College of Surgeons' definition for day care surgery is when the surgical day case patient is admitted for investigation or operation on a planned nonresident basis and who nonetheless requires facilities for recovery. It is a part of ambulatory surgery but is different from outpatient surgery in that some degree of postoperative specialized nursing care/observation is needed during postoperative recovery. The definition also includes 'extended' (23 hours 59 minutes admission) stay surgeries based on individual patient needs. Commonly performed orthopedic surgeries include Dupuytren's release, carpal tunnel release, ganglion excision, arthroscopy, bunion surgery, implant removal, etc.

Considerations:
- Patient selection
    - For GA, patients must preferably be American Society of Anesthesiologists (ASA) classes I or II. ASA class III and IV are only taken up in a well-established experienced Day Care Surgical Centre.
    - Psychologically stable patients are preferred who understand the pros and cons and are not just monetarily inclined.
    - Obese, elderly and frail are generally better managed on an inpatient basis.
    - Operations should be so chosen that have minimal blood loss and produce mild to moderate (bearable) postoperative pain.
    - Operations should preferably be of <1 hour duration.
- *Contraindications:*
    - Unstable cardiovascular patients—Angina, recent MI, on blood thinners, uncontrolled hypertension, and cardiac failure
    - Pulmonary complications—acute respiratory infection, COAD/ILD like emphysema, chronic bronchitis, and asthma.
    - BMI > 35
    - IDDM
    - Psychologically unstable on medications, anxious patient
    - Patient living far from the center who may not return fast enough should any complication arise.

Advantages (Pros)
- To patient:
    - Less likely to be cancelled due to prebooking and minimal impact of emergency surgeries due to dedicated facility.
    - Shorter waiting lists
    - Minimal disruption of patient's personal life and easier domestic arrangements
    - Earlier mobilization
    - Earlier return to normalcy and work (job)
    - Reduced risk of cross-infection
    - Less psychological disturbances in children
- To hospital:
    - Economic savings
        - Less staff and facilities needed.
        - Minimal/no need of night staff
        - Lass capital intensive than a regular hospital bed
        - Reduces the number of in-patient beds need of hospital
    - Happy staff due to less shift work

Disadvantages (cons):
- There is additional need for a responsible/understanding person at home to oversee the patient for first 24–48 hours.
- The day case surgery needs experienced senior staff due to high turnover where junior staff may keep fumbling on trivial logistical arrangements.
- Extra work for the medical officer in the postoperative period
- Cost-effectiveness of the unit is reduced if less complex cases (that may be managed in outpatient surgical care) are dealt with on a day-care basis.

Future perspective: Considering the advantage to the patients and reduction in economic burden, the list of day care surgeries is increasing. This is also in-line with the much pushed affordable health care in developing countries where hospitals struggle to cope-up with the expenditures they have to make compared to the limited returns from government schemes. Now the scope of day-care surgeries is being extended in orthopedics to all surgeries that can be done under regional anesthesia like fixation of peripheral uncomplicated fractures, arthroscopies, simple deformity corrections, etc.

20. **Discuss the current concepts in treatment of osteomyelitis.**

Ans: The recent advances in osteomyelitis deal with pathogenic mechanisms and novel therapeutic strategies. The latter especially deal with novel local delivery materials with appropriate mechanical properties, lower exothermicity, and controlled release of antibiotics, and absorbable scaffolding for bone regeneration is progressing rapidly. Emerging strategies for prevention, early diagnosis of low-grade infections, and innovative treatments of osteomyelitis such as biofilm disruptors and immunotherapy are also described.

Pathogenic mechanisms of bone infection (novel descriptions): The description describes the development of chronic osteomyelitis from acute osteomyelitis involving three distinct mechanisms:
1. Staphylococcal abscess communities in the local soft tissue and bone marrow
2. Glycocalyx formation on implant hardware and necrotic tissue
3. Colonization of the osteocyte-lacunocanalicular network (OLCN) of cortical bone

In contrast, *Staphylococcus aureus* intracellular persistence in bone cells has not been substantiated *in vivo*, which challenges this mode of chronic osteomyelitis.

Management of osteomyelitis (recent trends):
Diagnostics:
- Direct measurement of bacterial burdens from infected specimens is increasingly possible due to advances in protocols for bone homogenization.
- Micro-computed tomography (microCT) is a high-resolution, 3D imaging modality frequently used in the field of bone biology because of its ability to calculate bone density and volume. MicroCT is used to quantify pathogen-induced changes in bone remodeling during osteomyelitis, including both bone destruction and aberrant new bone formation.
- Blood-serum-based *S. aureus*-specific antibodies as diagnostic marker:
    - Antibody responses against iron-sensing determinant proteins (IsdA, IsdB, IsdH) could be predictors of infection outcomes in patients with *S. aureus* prosthetic joint infection (PJI), and that higher serum anti-IsdA and anti-IsdB IgG levels in patients are associated with increased mortality.
    - IgG levels in serum against a cell division protein called autolysin (Atl) was protective against *S. aureus* infections in patients undergoing orthopedic surgeries.
    - Pathogen-specific B-cells stimulated in germinal centers of lymph nodes proliferate, secrete their antibodies and enter the circulation. These plasmablasts, often called antibody-secreting cells (ASCs), emerge early in an infection and are circulating in the blood as long as the infecting pathogen remains active.
    - Media enriched for newly synthesized antibodies (MENSA) represent a measurable and accessible way to detect acute immune responses to ongoing infections. MENSA levels are direct indicators of ongoing infections as they develop and as the infections wane under the attack of the host's immune responses. MENSA evaluation could be used as a prognostic tool to guide clinical decisions in orthopedic infections.

Some of the current treatment methods are:
- *Immunotherapies* may be effective adjuvants with antibiotics for combating hard-to-treat osteomyelitis. Passive immunization involving monoclonal antibodies (mAbs) is an evolving method to treat *S. aureus* osteomyelitis. A benefit of passive immunization with mAbs is their high antigen-neutralizing specificity. Some examples include mAbs that target fibrinogen-binding cell surface protein (ClfA), cell wall components [lipoteichoic acid (LTA), poly-N-acetylated glucosamine (PNAG)] and secreted toxin, such as α-hemolysin. The second generation of immunotherapy target multiple antigens with essential functions for *S. aureus* immunoevasion, colonization, intracellular growth, and persistence within the host cells. Examples of these include mAbs that target the B-cell antigen staphylococcal protein A, the immunodominant surface protein IsaA, 170 and the immune-stimulatory staphylococcal superantigen SEB.
- *Antibiotic-coated implants and nanotechnology surface-modified implants to kill pathogens and disrupt the biofilms:* Intramedullary nail-coated nanoparticles with antibiotic and its growth factor.
- *Formulation and development of composite biodegradable scaffolds as antibiotic delivery system and also a regenerative device for bone:* The major focus is developing a combined 3D system that induces bone regeneration + a drug delivery system (3D-DDs). The 3D-DDs can be taken as injectable or moldable, which composed of a biocompatible, biodegradable polymer, with a combination of decellularized bone matrix [bovine bone substitute (BBs)] and with the antibiotic drug (aminoglycoside/vancomycin microparticles). The moldable 3D scaffold is formulated in such a way that it can be separated by cutting into desirable length, hydrated, and can be remodeled by a surgeon according to their specification, for fitting and curing the bone defect. The injectable composite scaffold is obtained with the method of lyophilization and also results in high porosity, and the obtained spongy structure of lyophilized scaffolds allows fast hydration of scaffold in blood or any physiological fluids of the body, without any change in the physical structure. Certain advantages of 3D-DDS are: it is ready to be used at any time, administration can be done through cannula or can be administered into the defected part through surgical procedures, easy to insert into irregular body spaces or cavities caused due to the disease or caused due to fracture and perfectly fit in the defected site of the bone, keeping the physical integrity stable throughout.
- *Bioactive hydrogels for bone regeneration:* Bioactive hydrogels are polymer scaffolds with several advantages for repairing bone defects. Hydrogels are the formation of 3D hydrophilic polymer chains, which are having high mechanical strength and provides nutrient environments suitable for the growth of endogenous cells.
- *Formulation and development of vancomycin-incorporated chitosan/gelatin coatings coupled with the TiO_2–SrHAP surface-modified Cp-titanium for the osteomyelitis treatment:* This method improves the implant material providing a biointeractive surface that will restrict or obstruct the growth site bacterial agents and increase the biological activity.

There are two layers: In the first layer, there is a combination of TiO_2 metal oxide and SrHAP ceramic oxide (increases electrochemical resistance). The second layer is a formation of the drug, i.e. vancomycin, which is encapsulated with chitosan/gelatin coating.
- *Single-stage treatment of diabetic calcaneal osteomyelitis with an absorbable gentamicin-loaded calcium sulfate/hydroxyapatite biocomposite: The Silo Technique*—in recent studies, it has been seen that using of calcium sulfate (CAS), combining with hydroxyapatite (HA) in a synthetic and injectable mixture has become "the new era bone substitute" that can be fortified with antibiotics.
- *Biodegradable polyurethane (PUR) scaffolds* have shown promise for dual delivery of both an antibiotic and bone regenerating small molecule during experimental osteomyelitis. PUR scaffolds have also been shown to promote biofilm dispersal and resolution of infection when loaded with D-amino acids.
- *Newer home-based antibiotic medications (currently unavailable in India):* Telavancin has shown good antimicrobial activity against methicillin-resistant *S. aureus* (MRSA) and its biofilm as compared to vancomycin. It also inhibits formation of biofilms at concentrations below each isolate's respective maximum inhibitory concentration (MIC). Telavancin is a semisynthetic derivative of vancomycin, exhibits concentration-dependent bactericidal activity via a dual mechanism of action involving inhibition of bacterial cell wall synthesis as well as disruption of cell membranes. It has broad anti-staphylococcal activity, including activity against isolates with methicillin resistance, and intermediate vancomycin susceptibility. Dose for therapy is 10 mg/kg/day for 30 days. Dose adjustments are needed as per renal function. Adverse effects are nausea, anemia of chronic disease, vomiting, metallic taste, diarrhea, infusion reaction,

pruritus, red man syndrome, aspartate transaminase (AST) or alanine (transaminase) ALT greater than 3 times upper limit of normal, serum creatinine increase of 2 times baseline or estimated glomerular filtration rate (eGFR) decrease of 50%. Oritavancin is a long-acting semisynthetic second-generation lipoglycopeptide approved by the Food and Drug Administration (FDA) in treatment. Pharmacokinetic/pharmacodynamic data shows single 1200 mg dose as intravenous (IV) infusion per week for 2–3 weeks is safe, well tolerated and optimizes concentration-dependent killing against several gram-positive organisms. It demonstrated potent *in vitro* activity against *Staphylococcus, Streptococcus,* and *Enterococcus* species.

21. **What is the effect of COVID-19 pandemic on orthopedic surgery? Describe the various precautions which you will take in avoiding complications during surgery in such cases?**

Ans: Presently, I would say that there is no effect of COVID-19 pandemic on orthopedic surgeries barring possibly elective surgeries in COVID-19 positive patients. There was an initial panic phase during the pandemic onset and progression, where it became extremely difficult to formulate guidelines, and hence all surgeries especially generating aerosols were prohibited. Only the emergencies and nondeferrable conditions were allowed by various agencies and organizations in their interim recommendations. Pathologies considered nondeferrable electives were septic arthritis, malignant tumor, risk of impeding pathological fractures, neurological symptoms, traumatic tendon injury, dislocations and aseptic loosening of total joint replacement, and loose bodies/joint locking. It was generally considered that orthopedic surgeries should be very rare for COVID-19 patients. As a result many fractures went on to develop mal- or nonunion and joint stiffness. Now the effect of COVID-19 disease is limited to seropositive symptomatic patients undergoing surgery. If elective surgery, then it is postponed till patient becomes sero-negative while for emergency surgeries assessment is based on disease severity and taking universal precautions while operation procedure. The following precautions are legible:

- Both patients and providers should be educated and follow hand hygiene.
- Wearing a mask and social distancing should be the norm.
- Waiting rooms should be avoided.
- High contact surfaces cleaned regularly.
- Visitors should have restricted access, and be updated by phone.
- Patients should be housed in single rooms.

22. **Musculoskeletal symptoms associated with SARS-CoV-19 virus infection and their management.**

Ans: The following are the commonly reported symptoms in patients with SARS-CoV-19:

- Myalgia
- Fatigue
- Arthralgia
- Rarely arthritis

Management: The management is on standard procedures for symptom control and prevention of aggravation using NSAIDs, short-term low-dose steroids, if former fail and supplementation with vitamin D. Ice packs for arthralgias and arthritis helps. Arthritis per se from the disease has not been promptly reported and mostly represents aggravation of symptoms of underlying joint disease.

23. **Discuss current advancements in the treatment of chronic lateral ankle instability.**

Ans: *Conservative management:* Due to prolonged peroneal reaction times in these patients structured rehabilitation program for improving proprioception and coordination of peronei improves patients with dynamic instability component (nearly half of the patients).

Operative management: This is done in patients with mechanical instability and failed conservative management.

- *Anatomical:* Brostrom repair augmented by Gould (inferior retinaculum pull-up) modification—Gold standard still.
    - Suture-tape extracapsular augmentation of the Brostrom repair {Internal Brace® or LARS (ligament advanced reconstruction system)}

- Autograft/allograft ligamentous reconstructions—in cases of revision surgery or long-standing instability where no ligaments are available for repair using anchor sutures.
- Using artificial ligament (Leeds-Keio ligament) for reconstruction
- Nonanatomical procedures—fallen out of favor
- *Minimally invasive—low-quality evidence:*
  - Arthroscopic repairs and reconstructions:
    1. Arthroscopically assisted—repair/reconstruction
    2. All-inside repair
    3. Inside-out repair
  - Percutaneous reconstructions only

24. **Discuss recent advances in management of osteochondritis dissecans in knee joint.**

Ans: Apart from the conventional techniques like microfracture, loose fragment fixation, mosaicplasty, OATS, allograft implantation various new techniques have emerged that are being increasingly used for reconstruction of the defect of osteochondritis dissecans.

Autologous chondrocyte implantation: Autologous chondrocyte implantation (ACI) is a first-generation cell-based therapy that involves transplantation of autogenous chondrocytes/chondrospheres into articular cartilage defects. The specific advantage is that it promises to provide complete hyaline repair tissues for articular cartilage repair.

The main drawbacks of ACI are:
- Need for large open arthrotomy
- The two-stage procedure (one for cell harvesting and the other for implantation)
- The prolonged period of time required to expand sufficient numbers of chondrocytes *in vitro*
- High cost of cell culture system

Collagen-covered autologous chondrocyte implantation: The collagen membrane has a compact layer to prevent diffusion of the cells out of the pouch and an inner porous layer to encourage cell invasion and attachment. This adaptation avoids the second incision needed in the classic ACI technique.

Matrix-assisted chondrocyte implantation: This is an advancement over the use of membranes. It is logical to use a scaffold for cells to colonize and develop into tissue rather than just using the membranes. The technique uses adaptation from tissue engineering. MACI is a second-generation approach for articular cartilage reconstruction where chondrocytes are combined to a three-dimensional scaffold (matrix) replicating the defect.

Third-generation chondrocyte grafting: This is still under evaluation and basically involves chondrocyte and matrix culture system. Principle is culturing chondrocytes in an implantable biological matrix with ideal properties—biocompatible, biodegradable, and bioactive while preserving the phenotypic characteristics, thus favoring the cellular proliferation and synthesis of the ECM, which is permeable, easy to use, and inexpensive.

Gene therapy: Gene transfer delivers a therapeutic protein to a target cell or tissue that after incorporation starts acting as a local source of the particular growth factor. This provides a constant and regular source for the desired growth factor. Most commonly a plasmid DNA containing a specific reporter gene that can stimulate a desired gene expression (to synthesize a growth factor) is used for incorporation through a virus vector.

(Each technique has specific details that can be read from Chapter 8 of the Essential Orthopedics: Principles and Practice, 3rd edition. Also, students should mention role of scaffolds in third generation chondrocyte grafting and gene therapy)

25. **A. What is industry 5.0 technology?**

B. Discuss role of 5.0 technology capabilities in trauma and orthopedics.

Ans: (A) *Industry 5.0: The Human-Centric Industrial Revolution:*

Core concept: Industry 5.0 advances beyond Industry 4.0's automation focus by integrating human expertise, sustainability, and collaborative technologies to create resilient, value-driven ecosystems.

Key Pillars:
- Human-machine collaboration
  - *Cobots:* Enhance productivity by handling repetitive tasks while humans focus on creativity and problem-solving.
  - *Artificial intelligence (AI)/machine learning* (ML): Supports decision-making with predictive analytics and real-time process optimization.
  - *Augmented reality (AR)/virtual reality (VR):* Enables immersive training and remote assistance, improving safety and efficiency.
- Sustainability
  - Circular economy principles, energy-efficient processes, and waste reduction are central to production.
- Workforce empowerment
  - Prioritizes upskilling, well-being, and ethical labor practices to harness human ingenuity alongside automation.

Challenges:
- Workforce adaptation, ethical AI use, and cybersecurity risks in interconnected systems.

Impact: Drives competitive advantage through innovation, employee engagement, and eco-conscious operations, ensuring long-term industrial resilience.

(B) The Role of Industry 5.0 Technology Industry 5.0 in Trauma and Orthopedics:
- Robotic-assisted surgery
  - *Precision:* AI-guided robotic systems enhance accuracy in complex procedures (e.g. joint replacements, fracture fixation).
  - *Haptic feedback:* Provides tactile sensitivity during minimally invasive surgeries, reducing complications.
- AR/VR for surgical planning and training
  - *Preoperative visualization:* 3D reconstructions from CT/MRI enable virtual rehearsals of surgeries.
  - *Intraoperative navigation:* AR overlays anatomical markers in real time for safer execution.
  - *Education:* Immersive simulations train surgeons without risk to patients.
- AI and predictive analytics
  - *Personalized care:* Machine learning analyzes patient data (imaging, genetics) to optimize surgical plans.
  - *Risk prediction:* Identifies high-risk patients for complications (e.g. infections, delayed healing).
  - *Postoperative monitoring:* AI tracks recovery trends and flags deviations (e.g. implant failure).
- Smart rehabilitation
  - *Wearables:* Sensors monitor mobility, gait, and muscle activity, tailoring rehab protocols.
  - *AI-driven adjustments:* Adapts exercises in real time based on recovery progress.
- Ethical and security challenges
  - *Data privacy*: Secure handling of sensitive health records [General Data Protection Regulation (GDPR)/Health Insurance Portability and Accountability Act (HIPAA) compliance].
  - *Human oversight*: Ensures AI supports—not replaces—clinical judgment.
  - *Impact*: Faster recovery, fewer complications, and patient-centric care through human-machine collaboration.

Index

Page numbers followed by b refer to box, f refer to figure, fc refer to flowchart, and t refer to table.

A

Abaloparatide 118
Abatacept 316
Abduction lurch gait 627
Abductor
   insufficiency 168
   pollicis longus 521, 533
Aberrant epiphysis 268
Abrasion chondroplasty 695
Abscess 229, 236
   cold 753, 757
   spread of 756f
   types of 756
Absorbable gentamicin-loaded calcium
    sulfate 888
Absorbable sutures 328t
Acetabular cup 650t
   designing of 871
Acetabular defects 662t
   management of 661
   types of 661
Acetabular dysplasia 567
Acetabular fossa 618
Acetabular fractures 424
   classification of 448
   combination of 451t
   management of 448, 449
   radiological assessment of 448
Acetabular index 569
Acetabular injuries 450
Acetabular osteotomy 567
   types of 569
Acetabular quadrant system 618f
Acetabular reconstruction, principles
    of 661
Acetabuloplasty 621, 660
Acetabulum 566, 570, 618
   fractures, modified Stoppa approach
    for 208
Achilles tendinopathy 266, 309, 751
Achilles tendon
   chronic painful mid portion
    tendinopathy of 724
   disorders of 722
   lengthening 306
   rupture 723, 751
Achilles tenotomy 598
   roles of 598
Acid-fast bacilli 186, 873
Acidic fibroblast growth factors 83
Acidosis 40, 58
Acquired immunodeficiency syndrome
    168
Acrobot systems 230
Acromegaly 81, 115
Acromioclavicular joint injuries 345,
    347
Acromion
   morphology of 475
   process, morphology of 475
Actinomadura pelletieri 190
Actinomycetoma trimethoprim 190
Acute compartment syndrome,
    pathophysiology of 289
Acute distal radius fractures 506
Acute hematogenous osteomyelitis 162
   clinical features of 157
Acute knee dislocation, management
    of 405
Acute odontoid fractures
   clinical features of 439
   management of 439
Acute respiratory distress syndrome 36
Acute spinal cord injury
   pathophysiology of 428
   pharmacological treatment of 428
Acute tubular necrosis 294
Adalimumab 316
Adaptability 74
Adaptive carpal instability 515
Adductor tenotomy 566
Adenolysis, epidural 877
Adhesions 520
Adipocytic tumors 863
Adipose derived mesenchymal stem
    cells 869
Adjunctive therapies 717
Adjustable length foot abduction
    brace 286
Adolescent coxa vara 565
Adriamycin 842
Adson's test 29
Advanced cardiac life support 44, 46
Aglietti system 721
Airway 51
Alcohol
   abuse 639
   consumption 65
Alendronate 118, 126, 127
Algodystrophy 13
Alkaptonuria 110, 146
   clinical features of 145
   etiopathogenesis of 145
   management of 145
Alkphos 130
Allen–Ferguson classification 437, 437f
Allis method 383, 615
Allograft 253, 696, 841
   bone 103
     antigenicity of 104
     characteristics of 104
     types of 103
   endoprosthetic reconstruction 824
   freeze-dried 103
   fresh-frozen 103
   harvest 109
   healing 103
   indications of use of 108
   plate construct, use of 885
   processing of 105
   role of 108
   structural 103
   tissue 681, 683
Alloprosthetic composite 860
Allopurinol 60
Alonso-lames triceps sparing
    approach 357
Alpha-defensin 868
Alsberg angle 600
Altered scapulohumeral rhythm 468
Alternative fusion techniques 796

Alumina 882
  ceramics 654
Aluminum oxide 654
American Spinal Injury Association
    score 777
Amikacin 187, 188, 190, 766
Aminoglycosides 459
Amoxicillin 188, 190
Amphotericin 647
Amputation 181, 191, 194, 560, 717
  complications of 191
  indications of 191, 193
  level of 193
  osteomyoplasty 193
  principles of 191
Anal tone 436
Analgesia
  epidural 299
  patient-controlled 299
  preventive 299
Analgesics 640
  topical 702
Anatomical condylar locking plate 397
Anchor funicular suture technique 526
Andersson lesion 147
Andren-Von-Rosen line 568
Aneurysmal bone cyst 859
  gross histopathological features of 849
Aneurysms, aortic 13
Angiogenesis 706
Angiography 498
Angiotensin-converting enzyme 14
Angle of Wiberg 569
Angular deformity, surgical correction
    of 269
Angulation osteotomy 632, 639
Anion gap 10
Ankle
  arthrodesis 726
  foot orthosis 286
  fractures 406, 410
  instability, chronic lateral 889
  joint 726
    biomechanics of 725
  osteochondritis dissecans of 717
  plantar flexion weakness 200
  valgus 614
Ankylosing spondylitis 65, 146, 148, 239,
    802, 806
Ankylosing spondylosis 146
Ankylosis 271, 271t
Annular ligament 355
Annuloplasty 878
  radiofrequency posterior 878
Anterior column fixation 449
Anterior cruciate ligament 235, 405, 686
  injuries 681
  reconstruction 872
  rehabilitation 688

Anterior dislocations 386
Anterior fractures, modified Stoppa
    for 454
Anterior hip
  dislocation 615b
  impingement 648
Anterior inferior iliac spine 570
Anterior interosseous nerve
  compression of 549
  syndrome 548-550
Anterior odontoid screw 440
Anterior superior iliac spine 221
Anterior wedge compression
    fracture 437
Anteversion, combined angle
    of 647, 653
Antiapoptotic pathways, activation
    of 430
Anti-B-cell agent 882
Antibiotic 647
  bone cement 645
  coated implants 888
  impregnated cements 256
  medications, newer home-based 888
  prophylaxis 175
  therapy 181, 717, 743
Antibody responses against iron-sensing
    determinant proteins 887
Anticoagulant 6fc
  medications 30
Anti-cyclic citrullinated peptide
    antibody 881
Antifibrinolytic hemostatic drug 75
Antigen 155
Antigenicity 103, 104
Antiglide plate 260
Anti-inflammatory cytokines,
    attenuation of 427, 430
Anti-inflammatory drugs 703
Anti-mutated citrullinated vimentin
    antibody 881
Antiplatelet drugs 4, 62
Antiprotrusio rings 661
Antisepsis 175
Antituberculous therapy 766
Anti-tumor necrosis factor agents 881
AO classification 375, 396f
Apical vertebra 794
Apixaban 9
Apley's distraction test 679
Aponeurosis 535
Apoptosis, inhibition of 427
Appendiceal lesions 758
Appendicitis 322
Appendicular soft-tissue sarcoma 863
  classification of 863
  role of 866
Approximation test 672
Aramid 883

Arch
  bone of 727
  intact, posterior 440
  suspension 728
Arcus juvenilis 150
Areflexic bladder 775
Arterial spasm 290
Arterial thoracic outlet syndrome,
    treatment of 30
Arterial vascular injuries, role of 76
Artery 194
Arthritis
  advanced 669
  early 669
  inflammatory 64
  reactive 170
  true tubercular 759
Arthrocentesis 320
Arthrochalasis 154
Arthrodesis 63, 271, 481, 670, 732, 740, 841
  general principles of 272
  role of 789, 749
  triple 748
Arthrography 207
Arthrogryposis 227
Arthropathies, inflammatory 312
Arthroplasty 318, 652, 664, 722
  excisional 670
  resection 717
  revision 652
Arthroscopic anterior cruciate ligament
    688, 872
Arthroscopic assisted-reduction and
    fixation 885
Arthroscopic lavage 704
Arthroscopic medial imbrication 582
Arthroscopic repair 473, 474, 476
Arthroscopic staging system 719
Arthroscopic surgery 266
Arthroscopy 335, 341, 677, 886
  assistive 677
Arthrotomy 621
  traumatic 674
Articular branches 529
Articular cartilage 84, 84f
  defect reconstruction 206
  morphology of 84
  tissue engineering 884
Articular disorders 236
Articular fractures, nonoperative
    treatment of partial 361
Articular lesions, classification of 85t
Articular surface fracture 350
Articular tissue engineering 884
Articularis genu 329
Artificial intelligence 891
Aseptic technique 176
Aspartate transaminase 889
Aspirate hip joint 207

Asporin gene 706
Assistive devices 306, 812
Astrocytoma, giant cell of 844
Atavistic epiphysis 268
Atlantoaxial instability 155
Augment acetabulum 660
Augmentation techniques 474
Autoantibody 155
Autograft 109, 696
   tissue 681, 683
Autoimmune diseases 238
Autologous blood 309
   product, use of 704
Autologous chondrocyte implantation 273, 696, 890
   matrix-induced 696
Autologous donation, preoperative 55
Autonomous bladder, management of 769
Autonomous robotic systems 230
Avascular necrosis 514, 616, 638, 639
   indications of 638
Avascular nonunion 23, 24
Axial skeleton injury 424
Axonotmesis 525, 540, 541
Azithromycin 187

B

Babinski sign 821
Bacillus Calmette-Guerin strains 874
Baclofen 302, 304
Bacterial seeding leads 162
Bacteriophages 717
Ballistics 778
Balloon cells 844
Balloon kyphoplasty 121, 435
   contraindications of 121
Balloon-assisted vertebroplasty 121
Bankart lesion 481, 482, 485, 493, 494
Barlow's test 568
Basic cardiac life support 44
Basic fibroblast growth factors 83
Bath ankylosing spondylitis disease activity index 147
Battered baby syndrome 32
Bazedoxifene 118
Bearing surfaces 882
Behçet syndrome 2
Beighton scoring system 488, 488t
Belly press 472
Below-knee
   amputation 592
   prosthesis 203
Bernard-Soulier syndrome 62
Bernese periacetabular osteotomy 571
Bevacizumab 843
Biacuplasty 878
Bicortical pins 262

Bicycle test 778
Bigelow maneuver, reverse 616
Bigelow method 383, 384
Bikini incision 209
Bilateral facet dislocation 439
Biliary system 18
Bioabsorbable biomaterials 247
Bioabsorbable implants 258
   use of 259
Bioabsorbable screws 872
Bioactive hydrogels 888
Bioceramics 248
Biochemical theory 21
Biocomposite materials 247
Biodegradable antibiotic delivery systems 159
Biodegradable polyurethane scaffolds 888
Biodegradable systems 161
Bioengineered grafts 696
Biofilm
   disruptors 887
   formation 157fc
   management of 156
   regulation 156
   role of 156
Biologic wound products 877
Biological compound muramyl tripeptide phosphatidylethanolamine encapsulated 843
Biomaterials 246, 247, 876
   fibrin-based 248
Biomedical waste
   disposal 78
   management 77
   categorization of 77t
   types of 78t
Bionic hand 202
Biophysical methods 99
Biopolymer hydrogel implants 697
Biopsy 642, 643, 670, 827, 828
   limitations of 828
   risks of 828
   techniques of 859
Bipedicular approach 120
Bisphosphonates 111, 118, 123, 126, 128, 129, 150, 225, 640, 821, 822, 833, 856, 875
   induced subtrochanteric fractures 127
   injectable 821
Bladder
   augmentation 775
   automatic 772
   dysfunction 343
      types of 775t
   injuries 444, 445
      management of 444
   paralysis 772

Bleeding
   disorders 62, 64
   excessive 75
Block apoptotic trigger 430
Blood
   clotting, increased risk of 76
   component therapy 55
   conservation strategies 55
   fractions 55
      uses of 55
   supply 379
   tests 751
   transfusion 56
   values 136
Blount's disease 604
Blount's lesion 610
Blunt trauma 342
Body cast syndrome 245
Bone 88, 126, 133, 193, 458, 825
   anatomical parts 87
   bank 106
      protocol 106
      quality control of 108
   biopsy 814
      types of 827
   block
      procedures 740
      supply of 88, 89f
   bridge 194
   broad constituents of 86fc
   callus formation, repair with 96
   cartilage, anatomy of 78
   cells 887
   cellular elements of 87
   cement 247, 255, 645
      properties of 256
   chondroblastoma of 836
   closure of 194
   cutting cone healing of 96f
   cystic lesions of 849
   cysts 870
      simple 859
      unicameral 849, 851
   defects 318, 868, 870
      spacers 885
   disorders, congenital 151
   effects of reaming of 282
   electrical charges of 92
   fibrous lesions of 831
   fixation 197
   formation 90
      biochemical markers of 124
      types of 88
   giant cell tumor of 844, 845
   grafting 163, 309, 653
      autologous 722
      nonvascularized 514
      open 159, 826

posterolateral 22
substitutes 99, 101, 102
types of 101, 253t
vascularized 514
healing
  direct 95
  secondary 96
infection, pathogenic mechanisms of 887
inflammatory diseases of 146
lengthening 151
  technique of 278
loss 461, 812
marrow 253, 877
  aspirate 102, 267
  derived mesenchymal stem cells 869
  evaluation 239
  fat, embolization of 282
mass measurement 110, 111
metabolic
  disease of 125, 239
  disorders of 110
metabolism 843
metastasis, management of 815fc, 821
microstructure of 87f
mineral density 114, 116
minimal disturbance of 258, 260
morphogenetic protein 100
  role of 100
pain 832
patellar tendon 686
regeneration 888
remodeling unit 98, 129
  traverses across compressed fracture 96f
repair
  features of 640
  types of 97t
round cell tumors of 847
scan 240, 242, 642, 643, 821
  limitations of 241
  three-phase 241t
  types of 240
scintigraphy 241, 479, 833
  conventional 240
shape of 728
solitary plasmacytoma of 854
specific alkaline phosphatase 124
structure of 86
surgeries 306
transfer 824
tumors 241, 859
  biopsy of 827
  differential diagnosis of 236
  primary malignant 825
  staging of 822
Bony anatomy 354f, 618
Bony component 80, 82
Bony defect 486

Bony injury 326
Borderline polytrauma 48
Botox paraspinal muscle injection 877
Botulinum toxin 302
Boutonnière deformity 555
  mild 556
  moderate 556
  pathoanatomy of 555
  pathological anatomy 313
Bovine bone substitute 888
Bow knee 628
Bow leg 628
Bowel dysfunction 343
Boyd amputation 195, 591
Boyd and Griffin classification 391f
Boyes brachioradialis transfer 530, 531
Brachial artery injury, management of 361
Brachial plexus 550
  anatomy of 551
  formation 551f
  injury
    birth-related 552t
    classification of 208
    types of 552
  palsy, birth-related 553
  primary involvement of 552
  upper trunk of 208
Brachytherapy 239, 863, 865, 866
Bracing 795
  spine 805
Brackett procedure 566
Brain injury 200
Breast cancer 820
Breathing 51
Bridle procedure 737, 740
Briefcase grip 518
Bristow-Latarjet operation 486
Broström procedure 726
Broström repair 726, 889
Brown–Séquard syndrome 426
Bryan–Morrey approach 207, 357
Buckle fractures 344
Bunion surgery 886
Bursae, pathoanatomy of 523
Bursitis 227, 228, 299
Burst fracture 433
  L1, clinical presentation of 436
  stable 434
  unstable 434
Butyl methacrylate 256

C

Caffey's disease 161
Cahill and Berg classification 693
Calcaneal fracture 418, 420, 751
  complications of 418
  treatment of 419
Calcaneal osteomyelitis 419

Calcaneocuboid joints 593
Calcaneofibular ligament 595
Calcaneoplasty 736
Calcaneovalgus deformity 729, 733
Calcaneum 595
  fractures 420t
Calcaneus, osteotomy of 597
Calcimimetic cinacalcet 822
Calcitonin 111, 129
Calcium 111
  deficiency 141
  influx, prevention of 430
  metabolism 110, 134
    physiology of 131
  phosphate 253
    homeostasis 131
  supplementation 124
Calf
  muscle 200
  pain 3
  tenderness 3
Callotasis 270, 271
Callus formation 96
Calvarium 109
Cambridge cup 871
Campanacci disease 831
Campbell triceps splitting approach 357
Canadian C-spine rule 431, 432, 433fc
Cancellous allografts 103, 253, 636
Cancellous bone defect, filling of 885
Cancellous chips, multiple 101
Cancer, colorectal 818, 820
Cannulated cancellous screws, multiple 388
Capitellum, fracture of 361
Capreomycin 187, 188, 766
Capsular ligament 367
Carbon
  fibers 883
  ions 843
Cardinal principles 259
Cardiovascular system 18, 19
Caries spine, neurological deficit in 757
Carpal bones, disorders of 511
Carpal instability 515
Carpal tunnel
  anatomy 542f
  syndrome 525, 536, 539
    clinical features of 536
    development of 536
    diagnosis of 536
    etiopathogenesis of 536
    management of 536
Cartilage
  defect, management of 692
  grafting 695, 697
    technique 696t, 697t
    types of 696
  injury 85

model formation 90
regeneration 868
structure 83*f*
synthesis 870
types of 82
Cartilaginous growth plate 79
Cast
   layers for 338*t*
   syndrome 245
Catterall classification 574
Cauda equina syndrome 427, 790, 792
Cavernous hemangiomas, large 13
Cavus deformity, classification of 650
Cefotaxime 190
Ceftazidime 647
Cefuroxime 647
Cell salvage, intraoperative 55
Cellulitis 174, 229
   clinical features of 173
   management of 173
   organism of 173
   pathogenesis of 173
Cement creep behavior 256
Cemented hips 871
Cemented technique 265, 318, 646
Cementless acetabular
   components 651
   cups, first-generation 660
   implantation, principles of 660
Cementless femoral
   components 650
   stem designs 871
Cementless modular acetabular cups,
   third-generation 660
Cementless total hip prosthesis 871
Central canal stenosis 782
Central cord syndrome 426
Central lesions 758
Central nervous system 18, 541, 846
Central tears 506
Cephalomedullary nail 390, 393, 394
Ceramic-on-alumina 654
Ceramic-on-ceramic bearings 882
Ceramic-on-metal
   articulation 656
   bearings 882
Ceramic-on-polyethylene bearings 656
Ceramics 247
   mechanical properties of 654
Cerebral palsy 200, 300, 303, 488, 535,
   600, 611, 627
   anatomical classification of 304*t*
   gross motor function classification
      system of 304*t*
   pharmacological treatment in 302
   physiological classification of 303*t*
   treatment of 303
Cerebral signs 21

Cerebrospinal fluid 320
Certolizumab pegol 316
Cervical lesions 756
Cervical osteotomy 802, 803
Cervical rib 31
Cervical spine 437, 755, 808
   injury 437
      Allen–Ferguson classification
         of 437*f*
   instability 432*t*
   lower 431, 432
   tuberculosis 757
   whiplash injury of 430
Cervicodiaphyseal angle 600
Chandler–Penenberg classification 662
Charcot's foot 743
Charcot's joints 739
   clinical features of 747
   etiology of 747
   pathology of 747
   principles of management of 747
Charcot's neuroarthropathy 745
Charnley's low friction arthroplasty 645
   principles of 665
Cheilectomy 621
Chemical synovectomy 63
Chemotherapy 842, 843, 864
Chest 49
Child abuse 32
Chlorhexidine body wash 172
Chondral injuries 665
Chondroblastoma 836, 843
Chondroblasts 90, 836
Chondrocalcinosis 61, 132
Chondrocyte
   culture 275
   grafting, third-generation 890
   hypertrophy, zone of 80
   implantation, matrix-assisted 890
   proliferation, zone of 79
Chondrodiastasis 268, 269
Chondrolysis 160
Chondromalacia patellae 322
Chondromyxoid fibroma 830, 843, 859
Chondroplasty 677
   principles of 695
Chondrosarcoma 860
   juxtacortical 840
   pathognomonic of 838
   secondary 862
Chromium 654
Chronaxie 544
Chronic anterior cruciate ligament
   deficiency, management of 406
Chronic compartment syndrome 294
Chronic osteomyelitis 156, 159, 163*t*
   anatomical classification of 163
   management of 157, 158

pathology of 164
radiological classification of 163
Cineradiograms 810
Ciprofloxacin 187
Circular economy principles 891
Circulations 51
Circumferential deficiency 663
Clarithromycin 187
Claudication 778
Clavicle hypoplasia 468
Clavulanic acid 190
Claw hand deformity
   causes of 530
   pathogenesis of 532
Cleidocranial dysostosis 467
Clindamycin 647
Clodronate 126
Clofazimine 188, 766
Clopidogrel 4
Clostridial collagenase injection 560
Clostridial myonecrosis 174
Clostridium perfringens 185
Club foot 227
   orthosis in 286
Coagulation pathway, abnormal
   activation of 1, 2
Coagulopathy
   dilutional 41
   rapid identification of 41
Cobalt-chromium alloy 656
Cobb method 794
Codman's triangles 850
Codman's tumor 837
Cold abscess 753, 757
   clinical features of 755
   etiopathogenesis of 755
   management of 753
   operative treatment of 753
   peripheral 753
Cold curing cements 256
Coleman lateral block test 729
Collagen
   fibers, loss of 787
   microspheres 249
Collagen-covered autologous
   chondrocyte implantation 890
Collarless stem 872
Collateral ligament, lateral 354, 355*t*
Colles' fracture, simple 371
Colony-stimulating factor 83
Column acetabular fractures, surgical
   management of posterior 454
Comminuted Colles' fracture 371
Common peroneal nerve 737
   branches of 737*f*
Compact bone formation 90
Compartment syndrome 288, 290, 327, 360
   etiology of 288*t*
   management of 290

Complete cord injuries 425
Complete radial nerve palsy 527, 546, 547
Complex femoroacetabular impingement deformities 206
Complex regional pain syndrome 13, 417
  stages of 15
Composite biodegradable scaffolds
  development of 888
  formulation of 888
Compound palmar ganglion 189
Compression
  fractures 433
  molding 254
  test 672
Compressive fixation 872
Computed tomography angiography 233
Condylar buttress plate 397
Condylocephalic nails 394
Congenital scoliosis 797, 799
  classification of 793
  management of 797
Congenital talipes equinovarus 594, 598
  severity classification of 598
Conjoined nerve roots 790
Contemporary orthopedic practice 667
Control complex regional pain syndrome 17fc
Conus medullaris syndrome 427
Conus terminalis 776
Convex hemiepiphysiodesis 798
Cord
  branches of 552
  compression, red flags for 820
  injuries
    incomplete 425
    types of 425
  lateral 552
Core decompression 639, 722
Core needle biopsy 828
Coronoid fixation 358
Cortical allografts 104, 253
Cortical bone fraction stem cells 869
Cortical desmoid 831, 860
Corticospinal tracts 426
Corticosteroid 177, 315, 538, 560, 703, 752
Corticotomy 260, 261
  use of 258
Corynebacterium 180
Counter-regulatory anti-inflammatory response syndrome 39
COVID-19 pandemic, effect of 889
Coxa
  breva 669
  profunda 631
  valga 600
  vara 322, 564, 565, 634

congenital 565
infantile 564
Craig test 601
Cranial fractures 285
C-reactive protein 54
Crescent sign 644
Crescentic osteotomy 632
Critical neurovascular structures 355
Crohn's disease 843
Cross-arm adduction test 348
Cross-leg flap, principles of 215
Crouch gait 223, 300, 611, 612
  clinical features of 612
  management of 612
Cruciate ligament
  reconstruction 873
    failure of primary anterior 685
  role of posterior 714
Crush injury, severe 198
Crush syndrome 291-293
Crutch walking gait 224
Crystal arthritis 672
Cubitus valgus 493
Cuboid bone 595
Cuff tear arthroplasty, pathophysiology of 478
Curvularia lunata 190
Cushing's syndrome 82, 110
Custom fabricated shoes 287
Custom megaprosthesis 860
Custom printed implants 885
Custom-made prosthesis 824
Cut flexor tendons, treatment of 319
Cycloserine 188, 766
Cyst
  around joints 227
  hemophilic 63
Cystic fibrosis 110
Cystic lesions 849, 860
  differential diagnosis of 849
Cytogenetics 848
Cytokines
  inflammatory 318
  upregulation of 139
Cytomegalovirus 317
Cytotoxic chemotherapy 98

D

Dabigatran etexilate 6
Damage control
  orthopedics 34, 48
  surgery 38
Danis–Weber system of classification 409, 409f
Dantrolene sodium 302, 305
Dapsone 190
Daptomycin 165

Davis law 595
de Quervain's tenovaginitis
  clinical features of 521
  diagnosis of 521
  treatment of 521
Death, terrible triad of 57
Decompression, laminectomy for 764
Decubitus ulcer 219
  development of 220fc
  management of 221
Deep fungal infection 843
Deep gluteal syndrome 666
Deep space infections
  etiology of 523
  treatment of 523
Deep tissue dissection 206, 622
Deep vein thrombosis 2
  chemical prophylaxis of 4
  clinical features of 3
  management of 3
  pathogenesis of 1, 1f
Defective endochondral ossification 565
Defluoridation 139
Deformity 99, 821
  components 674
  correction 264, 269
  higher grade of 631
  magnitude of 603
Dega osteotomy 570
Degenerative joint disease 635
Delbet and Colonna classification 387f
Dementia 297
Demineralized bone matrix 103, 108, 253
Denis Browne bar 569
Denosumab 118, 129, 822
Dent disease 142
Dental abnormalities 468
Deoxyribonucleic acid 186
Dermatosparaxis 154
Dermis, superficial 219
Dermofasciectomy 560
Desensitization 16
Desmoplastic fibroma 831, 859
Developmental dysplasia of hip 81, 228, 563, 567, 569, 573, 624, 871
  management principles of 566
Devil's claw extract 703
DEXA measurement 244
DEXA T-score 114
Diabetes mellitus 178
Diabetic calcaneal osteomyelitis, treatment of 888
Diabetic foot 743, 744
  infections 238, 242
  lesions of 743
Diacerein 703
Dial test 691
Dialysis, indications of 293

Diaphyseal aclasis 837
  clinical features of 837
  pathology of 837
  radiological features of 837
  treatment of 837
Diaphyseal gap nonunion, management of 21
Diarthrodial joint 347
Diastematomyelia 731
Diastrophic dwarfism 268
Diazepam 305
Diffuse idiopathic skeletal hyperostosis 806
Digital radiography 885
Dillwyn Evans procedure 599
Diplegia 611, 612
Direct thrombin inhibitor 6
Disability, reduction of 122
Disaster 875
Disc
  degeneration, nutritional pathways of 788
  replacement surgery 878
Discectomy 787
Discitis 236, 320
  postoperative 790, 792
Discoid meniscus 675, 676
  clinical features of 675
  management of 675
Disease modifying antirheumatic drugs 315, 703
  conventional 178
Dislocated irreducible knee 579
Disseminated idiopathic skeletal hyperostosis 226
Disseminated intravascular coagulation 9, 12, 292
  pathogenesis of 12*fc*
Dissociative carpal instability 515
Distal femoral fractures 423
  classification of 395
  management of 395
Distal femur
  chondromyxoid fibroma of 830
  fracture of 398
  Gustilo Anderson fracture of 457
  osteosarcoma of 822
Distal fractures 515
Distal humerus 354
  condylar fractures of 253
  fractures 356, 423
  functional anatomy of 354
  supracondylar fractures of 353
  surgical anatomy of 354
Distal interphalangeal joint 532
Distal radial fractures, anatomy of 506
Distal radioulnar joint 341, 503
  anatomy of 503, 504*f*

disruption, management of 506
injuries replacement 510
Distal radioulnar ligament, disposal of 504*f*
Distal radius fracture 372, 507
Distal scaphoid 375
Distal third tibia 214
Distal tibial fractures 423
Distraction
  histiogenesis 258, 259
  osteogenesis 258
    clinical application of 264
  test 672
Distractive flexion 438
Dobb's method 593
Dog bite, categorization of 380*t*
Donor
  selection 107
  tissue 696
Dorsal blocking splint 380
Dorsal intercalated segment instability 370
  pathoanatomy of 507
Dorsal radiocarpal ligament 374
Dorsal radioulnar ligament 504
Dorsal root rhizotomy, principles of 302
Dorsal spine 755, 757
Dorsal translocation 370
Dorsalis pedis flap 217
Dorsiflexion 201
  eversion test 742
Double crush syndrome 791
Double-line sign 642
Dowel grafts 101
Down's syndrome 154, 488
  musculoskeletal manifestations of 154, 155
Doxycycline 315, 703
Drawer test 481
  anterior 679, 684
  posterior 680
  posterolateral 691
Drop arm test 472
Drugs 188, 503
  class 118
  therapy 110
Drug-susceptibility testing 187
Drummond's criterion 804
Dry technique 885
Dual mobility hips, principle of 649
Dual onlay cortical bone graft 101
Dual plate fixation 369
Dual-energy X-ray absorptiometry
  peripheral 111
  scan 116, 243
Duchenne muscular dystrophy 273, 580
  clinical features of 580
  investigations of 580
  pathology of 580

Dupuytren's contracture 557
Dupuytren's fracture dislocation 412
Dural tears 792
Durkan's direct median nerve 537
Dwyer's osteotomy 597, 599
Dynamic compression 252
  screw 457
Dynamic condylar screw 397
Dynamic hip screw 388, 391
Dysplasia 566
Dyspnea 57
Dysreflexia, autonomic 342

E

Early tendon transfer 530
  principles of 530
Edema 3, 16
E-fast 234
Eggshell osteotomy 803
Ehlers–Danlos syndrome 110, 146, 152, 488
Eikenella corrodens 525
Elastic modulus 246
Elbow
  arthroplasty, complications of 495
  constraints of 355
  dislocation 366
  disorders, miscellaneous 492
  intercondylar fracture of 358
  joint
    bony anatomy of 354*f*
    ligaments of 367
    transfixation of 369
  post-traumatic ankylosis of 492
  radiographs of 497
  sideswipe injuries of 368
  trash
    injuries of 367
    lesions 367
Electrical stimulation 99, 774
Electrolyte abnormalities 292
Electromyography 550
Ellis–Van Creveld syndrome 607
Ely's test 582
Emactuzumab 325
Embolization, role of 239
Embryonic stem cells 869
Enchondral ossification 97
Enchondroma 860
Enchondromatosis 861
Endemic fluorosis 139
Endochondral ossification 90
Endochondral repair 96
Endocrine diseases 115
Endoprosthetic reconstruction 824
Endoscopic spinal surgery technique 789
Endplate fibrillation potentials 543, 546

Endplate osteophytes 781
Energy consumption 202
Enneking classification 825
Enneking system 822, 822t
Enoxaparin 5
Enthesopathy 227
Entrapment syndrome 550
Enzymatic activity 787
Enzyme-linked immunosorbent assay 182
Epicondylitis, lateral 266
Epidermal cell derived 844
Epidermal growth factor 266
Epidermal nevus 142
Epimetaphyseal system 94
Epiperineurorrhaphy 526
Epiphyseal injury 88, 344
Epiphyseolysis 140
Epiphysiodesis 268, 270, 278, 606
  lateral 160
Epiphysis 88
  types of 268
Epoxy resins, use of 249
Epstein classification 615b
Epstein–Barr virus 317
Equines contracture, types of 612
Equinocavovarus deformity 613
Equinoplanovalgus deformity 612, 614
Equinus
  deformity 613, 738
  foot 740
Erb's palsy 552
Ertl osteomyoplastic procedure 194
Erysipelas
  clinical features of 173
  management of 173
  organism of 173
  pathogenesis of 173
Erythrocyte sedimentation rate 54
Erythromycin 647
Essex-Lopresti classification 418
Estrogens 2, 111, 703
  receptor modulators, selective 111, 129
Etanercept 316
Ethambutol 188, 754, 755, 760, 766
Ethionamide 188, 766
Etidronate 126, 225
Etodolac 59
Etoricoxib 59
Eumycetoma 190
Evans classification 391, 391f
Evans lateral column lengthening 731
Everolimus 843
Evidence-based medicine 71, 72
  pyramid 73f
Ewing's sarcoma 828, 846
Ewing's tumor 849

Exercises
  strengthening 588
  types of 295
Exertional compartment syndrome 295
Exostoses 838
Extensive radical fasciectomy 560
Extensor carpi
  radialis brevis 533
  ulnaris 504
Extensor digitorum longus 214
Extensor pollicis
  brevis 533
  longus 197
Extensor tendon relocation 556
External beam radiation therapy 863, 865
External fixation devices 278
External fixator 282
  assembly of 280
  complications of 262
External rotation
  injury 407f, 408f
  lag test 472
  recurvatum test 680, 691
  stress test 472
External tibial torsion 582
Extra-articular deformity 605f
  pure 605f
Extra-articular distal radius fracture, management of 370
Extracapsular arterial ring 210, 619
Extracorporeal irradiated tumor bone 825
Extracorporeal shockwave
  therapy 99, 877
  treatment 744
Extractable nuclear antigen test 154, 155
Extraperiosteal resection 838
Extratunnel fixation 873
Exudate, removal of 876

F

F wave 544
Facet dislocation, unilateral 425
Facet joint 878
  separation of 768
Factor Xa direct inhibitors 5
Failure to thrive 321
Fairbank fragment 565
Fallacies 627
Fanconi syndrome 858
Fanconi–Bickle syndrome 858
Farnesyl diphosphate 821
Fascia 458
  slip of 364
Fasciectomy 560
  open 560
  regional 560

Fasciocutaneous flap 214, 216, 218
Fat
  embolism
    pathophysiology of 21
    syndrome 19, 21, 48
  globules, demonstration of 20
  pad syndrome, clinical signs of 588
Fatigue behavior 256
Feagin modification 679
Febuxostat 60
Felon 522, 522f
Femoral anteversion 229, 582, 599, 601
Femoral artery, medial circumflex 206
Femoral bone stock deficiency 662
Femoral circumflex, lateral 210
Femoral condyles, osteochondritis dissecans of 692
Femoral defect 663, 663t
Femoral deficiency, congenital 563
Femoral derotation osteotomy 306
Femoral epiphysis, slipped upper 268, 565
Femoral fixation devices 872
Femoral head 566
  avascular necrosis of 640
  blood supply of 211
  center 645
  fractures 206, 253, 384, 386
    classification of 385
  osteonecrosis of 640, 642, 642t
  preservation of 657
  small 646
  vascular anatomy of 210f
Femoral intramedullary nails, types of 394
Femoral nails, retrograde 397
Femoral neck 830
  anteversion 600
  fracture 638
    fixation of 388t
    type of neglected 637
  nonunion 636
  osteotomy 633
  shaft angle 645
  stress fractures of 389
  system 388, 389
    concept of 389
Femoral pelvic abnormalities 563
Femoral reconstruction, principles for 661
Femoral shaft after total hip arthroplasty, periprosthetic fractures of 462
Femoral shortening 563, 564
Femoral stem 871
  offset for 665
Femoral version, radiological measurement of 616

Femoroacetabular impingement 629, 665
  management of 631
  surgery for 631
Femorotibial alignment 602
Femur 619
  fracture
    fixation 404
    head 384
    neglected neck of 423, 637, 638
    proximal third of 390
    shaft of 673
  head 869
  individual axis of 599
  malunited fracture of 628
  nonunion fracture neck of 634, 636fc
  proximal end of 563
Fever
  causes of postoperative 185
  high grade 320
Fibers, discontinuity of 227
Fibrin gel 254
  role of 254
Fibrinogen 20
  binding cell surface protein 888
  levels 41
Fibrinolytics, overdose of 75
Fibromyalgia-like syndrome 170
Fibronectin 787
Fibrous bands 471
Fibrous dysplasia 126, 239, 591, 831, 835, 835t
  associations of 832
  clinical features of 831
Fibrous sheath 80
Fibrous tissue formation 96
Fibula 109
  exposure of 272
  supramalleolar fracture of 409
  tibialization of 722, 723, 826
Fibular collateral ligament 690
Fibular head graft 101
Fibular osteotomy, proximal 707
Fibulectomy, partial 22
Ficat and Arlet classification 642t
Filum terminale syndrome 808
Fine-needle aspiration 828
Fingers 500
  extensor expansion of 313f
  fibrous flexor sheaths of 519
Fingertip
  injuries, treatment of 381, 382
  unstable painful 522
Firecracker hand injury, first aid management of 380
Fish and Dunn osteotomy 579
Fisher classification 375
Fitzgerald's acetabular labral tests 630

Fix pilon fractures 414
Fixation devices, role of 873
Fixed angle devices 389
Fixed lumbar lordosis 653
Flaccid paralysis 342
Flail chest 27
  treatment of 26
Flap reconstruction 214
Flat feet 155
Flexed scaphoid 513
Flexible flatfoot 731
Flexible guide wire 688
  concept of 688
Flexible pes planus 731
Flexible reamer 688
Flexion
  abduction external rotation test 672
  contractures 15
  deformity 674
  dislocations 434
  rotation injuries 436
Flexor carpi radialis 533
  transfer 547
Flexor carpi ulnaris 533
  transfer 530, 547
Flexor digitorum profundus 533
Flexor pollicis longus 524
Flexor tendon injury 319, 561
Flexural stability 336
Floating knee 403, 404
  injury, assessment of 404
Floor reaction orthosis 200, 223
Floret-like multinucleated giant cells 844
Fluid
  accumulation 76
  normal 312
  replacement 48, 51
  resuscitation 48
Fluorescence in situ hybridization 182
Fluorodeoxyglucose-positron emission tomography scan 182, 814
  principle of 238
Fluoroquinolones 98, 181, 188, 766
Fluoroscopy 395
Fluorosis 110, 115, 138
Focal dome osteotomy, principles of 608
Fondaparinux 5, 8
Foot
  amputations 194
  arches of 727
  atypical 598
  drop 738, 740
  principles of stabilization of 729
  single-axis 203
  skin temperature 747
  stabilization, principles of 727
  trauma, unsalvageable 199

Foraminal stenosis 782
Forced plantar flexion 593
Forces transmitted across hip joint 626
Forearm, radiographs of 497
Forefoot
  amputations 194
  deformities 417
Fortin's finger test 672
Fracture 390, 393, 616
  around
    elbow 352
    hip 816
  atypical insufficiency 127
  complex 151, 422
  dislocation 379, 434f
  displaced 515
  extra-articular 418
  femoral 663
  fix unstable 451
  fixation 336
  geriatric 123
  healing 98, 106, 239
    augmentation of 99
    primary 99
    secondary 99
    types of 95, 98
  humerus 495
  implant 879
  intertrochanteric 393
  intra-articular 251, 341, 418
  intracapsular 340
  intraoperative 462
  line, secondary 418
  management 514
  mechanism 435
  neck
    femur 386, 634, 635
    management of 364
  nondisplaced 395, 414
  nonossifying fibroma 577
  pattern 451
  pelvis 446
  postoperative 462
  proximal 515
  recurrent 151
  repair 95, 98, 100
  risk assessment 815
  scaphoid, nonunion of 513
  simple 448
  stabilization 21
  surgery 257
  surgical reduction of 261
  susceptibility 655
  three-column 401
  toughness 256
  types of 448
  ulna 495
  undisplaced 375, 376

unreconstructable 422
unstable 393
Fragility fractures, management of 123
Frax and Frax plus score 116
Free vascularized bone transplant 272
French osteotomy, modified 361
Frozen shoulder 470
Fulcrum test 481
Functional cast bracing, principles of 244
Fusion 507

G

Gait 221
   antalgic 222, 323fc, 669
   ataxic 305
   circumduction 222
   crouch 223, 300, 611, 612
   cycle 223
      phases of 221, 223
   disorders 303
   dyskinetic 305
   hand-to-knee 224f
   painless 323fcf
   training, robotic-assisted 306
Galeazzi sign 568
Gallium scans 158
Gallium-67 imaging 237
Gamma camera, principles of 861
GANGA trauma score 195, 458, 458t
Ganglia 227
Ganglion excision 886
Ganz antishock pelvic fixator 453
Ganz approach to hip, surgical anatomy of 206
Ganz C-clamp 451
Gap balancing technique 709, 710
Gap healing 95
Gapping test 672
Gas gangrene 173, 174, 185
Gaucher's disease 110, 268, 639
Gel phenomenon 147
Gene
   delivery systems 274fc
   therapy 273, 878, 890
Genetic testing 828
GeneXpert
   Mycobacterium tuberculosis 760
   test 186, 874
Gentamicin 190, 647
Genu valgum 155, 582, 606
Genu varum 322
   causes of 604
Geometric method 635
Geranylgeranyl diphosphate 821
Geriatric acetabular fractures 454
Giant cell 844
   lesions 843

tumor 845, 859
   recurrence of 875
   variants 843
Gigantism 115
Gigli saw 572
Gilula's lines, appearance of 516f
Girdlestone classification 757, 759
Girdlestone procedure 717
Glanzmann thrombasthenia 62
Glass fibers 883
Glenohumeral joint 487
Glenoid
   labrum 494
   posterior rim of 483
Global growth disorder 573
Glomerular rickets 131
Glucocorticoids 37, 114
   excess 115
   use 123
Glucosamine sulfate 703
Glutaraldehyde preservation 106
Gluteus
   maximus
      flap, role of 221
      muscle transposition 221
   medius weakness 222, 223
Glycerol preservation 106
Glycocalyx formation 887
Glycogen storage disorders 110
Glycosamine polysulfuric acid 703
Glycosaminoglycan peptide complex 703
Golimumab 316
Gout 61, 61t, 115
   diagnosis of 58
   management of 59
   pathogenesis of 59
Goutallier grading system 475
Gower sign 580
Gracilis muscle
   free flap 216
   transfer 498
Graft
   bone, excision of 107
   failure 219
   fixation 685
   freeze-dried 108
   fresh-frozen 108
   impingement 685
   sterilization of 107
   suspension of 873
   tensioning 685
   type 253, 683, 687, 688
Granuloma, tubercular 843
Gravity, center of 625
Gray ramus block 878
Gray-blue sclerae 150
Greater trochanteric pain syndrome 666
Green procedure 466

Groans, abdominal 133, 852
Groin flap 217
Ground reaction force 200f
Ground-glass matrix 832
Growing rods 794
Growth 151
   factors 92, 877
      transforming 83
   modulation 81
   plate 81f
      concerns 152
      histology of 79
   retardation 137
Guided growth
   method 604
   modulation, principles of 79
Gunshot injuries 326
Gunshot wounds 459
   pathophysiology of 460
Gustilo and Anderson classification 455
Gustilo and Anderson fracture 457

H

Haglund's deformity 751
Half-moon sign 641
Hallux valgus 751
   deformity 748
Halo-pelvic device 285
Halstead's maneuver 29
Hamstring lengthening 306
Hand
   bursae of 524
   disorders of 517
   flexor tendon zones of 561, 561f
   functions of 517
   hygiene 170
   plate 284
   potential spaces of 523
   suppurative flexor tenosynovitis of 183
Hanging cast 338
   technique 338
Hangman's fracture 424
Haptic robotic systems 230
Hard callus 97
Hardinge approach 623
Harpagoside 703
Harrison's groove 135
Haversian canals 162
Hawkins classification 420, 421f
Hawkins sign 420
Head-preserving procedures 636
Head-sacrificing procedures 637
Healed disease, paraplegia of 757
Healing
   rickets 134
   shoe 287
   stimulation 267

Health Insurance Portability and
　　Accountability Act compliance 891
Heel
　compression 201
　pain, treatment of posterior 751
　width 419
Hemarthrosis, management of 405
Hematocrit 20
Hematoma 229
　epidural 236
　formation 96
Hemiarthroplasty 484
Hemicylindrical grafts 101
Hemipelvis
　stable 452*f*
　unstable 452*f*
Hemiphysiodesis 604
Hemiplegia 611
　double 612
Hemivertebra
　excision 798
　incarcerated 797
Hemochromatosis 110
Hemodilution, acute normovolemic 55
Hemoglobinopathies 639
Hemoglobinuria 57
Hemolytic immediate transfusion
　　reactions 57
Hemophilia 62
　pseudotumor 64
Hemophilic arthropathy knee,
　　management of 62
Hemorrhagic shock 48, 49, 51
　classes of 54*t*
　different types of 54
Hemosiderin granules 324
Hemostatic resuscitation 48
Hemothorax 26
Herberts classification 375
Herberts screw 253
Herring's lateral pillar 574
Heterotopic ossification 384, 492
Hierarchical scratch collapse test 537
High efficiency particulate air filters 177
High fibular station 614
High fusion rates 109
High hip center 662
High kinetic energy 460
High muzzle velocity 460
High radial nerve palsy 527, 529,
　　546, 548
High temperature thermoplastic
　　splints 288
High tibia osteotomy 701
　indications of 705
　osteotomy 610, 699, 701*t*, 706-708, 722
　role of 701
　technique of 709

High ulnar nerve palsy 532, 533, 533*t*
High viscosity cements 255
Highly cross-linked polyethylene 255
Highly porous tantalum cones 711
Hilgenreiner's line 568
Hilgenreiner's physeal angle 565
Hill–Sachs defect, reverse 483
Hill–Sachs lesion 481-483
Hill–Sachs remplissage technique 487
Hindfoot
　amputations 194
　nail 727
　　indications of 727
Hinge
　abduction 576, 577
　technique 215
Hip 635
　anterolateral exposure of 623
　anteroposterior radiograph of 449
　arthrography 624
　arthroplasty 649, 665
　arthroscopy 665, 667
　　complications of 667
　　conventional 665
　　current status of 667
　　indications of 665
　　portals of 665
　　positioning of 665
　　techniques of 665
　biomechanics 625, 626*f*, 628
　cemented 871
　congenital dysplasia of 627
　developmental dysplasia of 81, 228,
　　563, 567, 569, 573, 624, 871
　dislocation 155, 656, 738
　　reduced risk of 658
　disorders 614
　dynamic compression screw 393
　fractures, complications of 383, 388
　hiking 222
　instability 648
　joint 617
　　arthrodesis of 579
　　clinical examination of 640
　　major structural abnormalities of
　　　206
　　surgical anatomy of 617
　　transient osteoporosis of 671
　　tuberculosis of 321
　movements of 619, 629
　of Voss, hanging 660
　pain 222
　posterior dislocation of 383
　preserving methods 640
　resurface arthroplasty, advantages
　　of 657
　　disadvantages of 657
　rotation, external 222

　sacrificing 640
　safe surgical dislocation of 210, 621
　septic arthritis of 166
　transient osteoporosis of 479, 671
　trochanteric fractures of 390
　tuberculosis of 667, 670
　uncemented 871
Histamine test 550, 554
Histiocytoma, benign fibrous 831
Hodgkins's lymphoma 844
Hodgson's classification 757
Hoffa's disease 588
Hoffa's fat pad 330
Hoffa's fracture 398
　bicondylar 399
Hoffa's syndrome 588
Holden's classification 500
Holdsworth classified thoracolumbar
　　fractures 433, 437
Holmium:yttrium-aluminum-garnet
　　laser 878
Holstein–Lewis injury 546
Holstein–Lewis lesion 351, 352
Homan's sign 3
Homocystinuria 2, 110, 114
Hook grip 518
Hormonal disorders 81
Hormone 573
　replacement therapy 124
Horn Blower's sign 472
Horner's syndrome 426, 550
Hospital waste disposal management 77
Howship's lacunae 133
Hueston table top test 559
Hueter-Volkmann law 81, 81*f*
Human chondrocyte culture, procedure
　　of 276
Human immunodeficiency virus 168,
　　169, 760
Humeral head, blood supply of 308
Humeral shaft, open fracture of 351
Humerus
　fracture
　　proximal 349, 423
　　shaft of 351
　supracondylar fracture of 359, 361
Hungry bone syndrome 133, 134
Hunka classification 167*f*
Hunter circulus articuli vasculosus 211
Huntington's procedure 723, 826
Hyaluronans, intra-articular 705
Hybrid external fixator 262, 263
Hybrid fixators, use of 885
Hybrid scanning techniques 241
Hydatid disease 849
Hydrocolloids 876
Hydrofibers 876
Hydrogels 876

Hydroxyapatite biocomposite 888
Hydroxychloroquine 315
Hyperadrenalism 115
Hyperbaric oxygen 877
   therapy 186, 717
   treatment 744
Hypercalcemia 126, 131, 812
Hypercalciuria
   chronic 132
   pre-existing 125
Hyperkalemia 293
Hyperlaxity 871
Hypermobile segment, prophylactic fusion of 811
Hypermobility 582, 650
   syndrome 488
Hyperparathyroidism 115, 843
Hyperprolactinemia 119
Hyperreflexia 821
Hyperthyroidism 115
Hypervascular nonunion 23, 24
Hypoadrenalism 115
Hypocalcemia 131, 293
Hypogonadism 115, 119
Hypoparathyroidism 115
Hypoperfusion 40, 50
   quantification of 51
Hypophosphatasia 110, 143, 144, 145t
Hypophosphatemic rickets 131, 137, 604, 858
   management of 137
   pathology of 137
   salient clinical features of 137
Hypopituitarism 115
Hypoplastic thumb 502
Hypotensive resuscitation 47, 48
Hypothermia, consequences of 57
Hypothyroidism 115
Hypotonia 155
Hypoventilation 25
Hypovolemia 292
Hypoxia 40
Hysteresis 257

I

Iatrogenic stenosis 783
Ibandronate 126
Idiopathic arthritis, juvenile 155
Idiopathic kyphoscoliosis, clinical features of 800
Idiopathic osteoporosis, juvenile 113
Idiopathic scoliosis 794
   infantile 793
   management of 795
Idiopathic thrombocytopenic purpura 62
Ifosfamide 842
Ilfeld orthosis 569

Iliac crest 109, 589
   anterosuperior 568
Ilioischial line 454
Iliotibial band 328
   anatomy of 329
Ilizarov apparatus 597
Ilizarov external fixator 264
Ilizarov hip
   principle of 280
   reconstruction 280
Ilizarov method 277, 589
Ilizarov spatial frame 23
Ilizarov technique 279
   primary applications of 264
Image-guided percutaneous cryoablation 814
Imatinib 325
Imipenem 188
Immobilization 114
Immune cells 312
Immunotherapies 888
Impaired temperature control 342
Impingement syndrome 469
Implant removal, reoperation for 390
Impression defects 484
Inadequate glenoid bone support 480
Indian Space Research Organization 74
Induced membrane technique 275
Inducible nitric oxide synthase inhibitors 704
Industry 5.0 technology 890
Indwelling catheterization 773
Infantile tibia vara
   classification of 609t
   clinical features of 610
   radiological features of 610
Infections 179, 219, 237, 390, 672
   assessment 170
   control of 19
   locoregional 156
   mode of 179
   postoperative 300
   prevention 196
Inferior end vertebra 794
Inferior tibiofibular diastasis, chronic 411
Inflammation, trauma-induced 41
Inflammatory diseases 146, 238
Infliximab 316
Infrapatellar fat pad 330
Infrapatellar tendon bursa 330
Ingrowth, failure of 879
Inhibitory concentration, minimum 161
Injury
   abdominal 233, 453
   around elbow 493
   chronic 347
   concurrent 692

   head 21, 38
   mechanism of 292, 362, 413, 439, 444
   secondary mechanisms of 429
   severity score 42b
   type 382
Inkjet printing 331
Inlay bone grafting 101
Innominate bone, osteotomy of 571
Inspired oxygen, fraction of 18
Instability
   chronic 417, 432
   complete 442
Instrumentation, patient-specific 664
Insulin-like growth factors 83
Intercalary deficiencies 563
Intercondylar fracture, management of 357
Intercostal chest tube drainage 28
Interferential therapy 296
Interleukin 706, 881
   inhibitor 856
   receptor 704
Interlocking nail 282
   applications of 281
   principles of 281
Internal fixation 300, 356
International Association for Study of Pain Diagnostic Criteria 16
International Cartilage Repair Society 85, 86
Interneural neurorrhaphy 526
Interosseous nerve, surgical anatomy of posterior 528
Interteardrop line 645
Intervertebral disk disease 235
In-toeing gait 614
   causes of 616
Intra-articular fractures, complex 379
Intracavity lavage 172
Intracorporeal bone grafting 435
Intradiskal electrothermy 878
Intramedullary growth rod
   advantages of 151
   disadvantages of 151
   indications of 151
   principle of 151
Intramedullary nailing 22, 394, 397
Intramedullary system 94
Intramembranous ossification 97
   steps of 90
Intraosseous ganglion cyst 849
Intraosseous lipoma 860
Intraosseous therapy 313
Intraprosthetic dissociation 871
Intrasubstance tears, partial articular-sided 472
Intrathecal therapy 305
Intratunnel fixation 873

Intravascular stimulus hypothesis 17
Intrinsic plus deformity, causes of 535
Intubation, indications of 42
Invasive surgical management 173
Ipsilateral fibula transfer 723, 826
Ischemia 196, 293
Ischemic foot 745
Ischioacetabular segment 454
Ischiofemoral impingement 666
Isokinetic exercises 296
Isokinetic training 296
Isolated phosphorus malabsorption 137
Isometric 295
Isoniazid 754, 760, 766
   susceptibility testing for 188
Isotonic contraction 296

J

Jaffe-Campanacci syndrome 835
Jaipur foot 201, 202, 202*t*
Janus kinases 882
Jerk test 481, 685
Jersey finger 379
   classification of 379*t*
Jobe's test 472, 481
Joint 79, 136, 458
   arthritis 748
   capsule, anatomy of 95
   compromising methods 659
   deformed 668
   depression fracture 418
   dislocation 347
   disorders 227
   effusions 229
   fusion 561
   hypermobility syndrome 488
   inflammatory diseases of 146
   involvement 881
   line alignment 884
   line convergence angle 600
   orientation angle 270
   reaction forces across patellofemoral joint 581
   replacement, timing after 179
   stiffness 160
   swelling 99
   tuberculosis 760
      treatment 760
Jones transfer 529, 547
Joshi's device 597
Judet classification 353, 448*f*
Jumbo cup 662
Jump flap 215
Jumper's knee 322
Jupiter sub-classification 354

K

Kanamycin 187, 188, 190, 766
Kanavel's sign 524
Kapandji procedure 504
Kaplan approach 209
Kasabach-Merritt syndrome 13
Kawasaki disease 320
Kegel exercises 772
Kicking sports 630
Kidney
   disease
      acute 293
      chronic 294
Kienböck's disease 511, 512
   classification of 512*t*
Kinase inhibitors 704, 882
Kirschner wires 197
Klein's line, failure of 577
Kleinman's shear test 516
Klippel-Feil syndrome 464, 810, 811
   classic features of 810
Klumpke's palsy 29, 553
Knee 674, 711
   angular deformity of 601
   ankle-foot orthosis 286
   arthritis 62, 674
      viscosupplementation for 702
   arthroplasty 403, 677, 714
      types of 677
   congenital dislocation of 579
   deformity of 674
   degenerative arthritis of 702
   dislocation, acute management of traumatic 405
   extensor mechanism of 329, 586
   flexion test 722
   gait 223
   hyperextended 579
   joint 695, 890
      arthroscopy of 677
      inflammatory arthritis of 698
      monoarticular arthritis of 701, 702*fc*
      traumatic arthrotomy of 674
      unicompartmental osteoarthritis of 698
   ligament assessment 404
   ligamentous injuries of 678
   malalignment 605*f*
   meniscal injuries of 683
   osteoarthritis 266, 309, 701
      management of 705
   posterolateral corner of 689, 690*f*
   replacement systems, robot-assisted unicompartmental 230
   spontaneous osteonecrosis of 717
   stiffness 281, 402
      management of postoperative 689
   triple deformity of 674
Kniest syndrome 268
Knuckle bender splint 283
Kocher approach 209
Kocher interval 357
Kocher posterolateral approach, conventional 478
Koshino and Aglietti staging systems 721, 721*t*
Küntscher Y-nail 394
Kuwada's classification 723
K-wire
   joystick 365
   placement 379
Kyphoplasty 121, 122, 266, 435
Kyphoscoliosis 153
Kyphosis 113, 135
Kyphotic deformity 436, 767

L

Labral tears 625, 665
Lachman test 679, 684
Lactate dehydrogenase 839
Lag screw 253
   principle 252*f*
Lamellar bone 87
   deposition 97
Laminar airflow, principle of 176
Langhans giant cells 843
   formation of 753*f*
Laser diskectomy 878
Latarjet procedure
   advantages of 487
   disadvantages of 487
   indications of 487
Lateral condyle fracture elbow, complications of 356
Lateral mass fixation technique 801
Latissimus dorsi 498
Lauge-Hansen classification 410, 412
Ledderhose disease 558
Leflunomide 316
Leg
   different compartments of 295
   length discrepancy 276, 601
   pain 3
Legg-Calve-Perthes disease 242, 321
Leiomyosarcoma 863
Leishmaniasis 843
Leprosy, reference to 287
Leptosphaeria senegalensis 190
Lesions
   anterolateral 718
   classic benign 829

complete 758
fracture of stalk of 837
multiple atypical 814
posterior 758
posteromedial 718
pre-ganglionic 550
treatment of 694
vascular 236
Less invasive stabilization system 251, 397
Letournel classification 448f
Leukemia 639
Leukocyte 311
count 311t
esterase 868
Levofloxacin 188
Lewinnek safe zone concept 648
Lewis and Rorabeck classification 461f
Lichtblau procedure 599
Ligament
healing 274
injuries 237, 677
lateral 367
reconstruction of 692
tears 235
Ligamentotaxis 340, 341
role of 335
role of 340
Ligamentous injury 378
Ligamentum flavum hypertrophy 808
Ligamentum teres, artery of 211, 619
Light emitting diodes 880
Limb 136
length discrepancy 160, 276, 390, 608
management of 277
length equalization, devices of 277
principles of 277
lengthening 264, 268, 278, 279
positioning 526, 615
reconstruction, modalities for 824
salvage surgery 458, 822, 825
in malignant tumor, prerequisites for 825
principles of 823
shortening 278
Limp, management of painful 320
Lindeque's criteria 20
Linezolid 166, 181
Lipid peroxidation, inhibition of 427, 430
Lipopolysaccharide-binding protein 874
Liposarcoma 863
Liposomes 843
Liquid culture 76
role of 76
Lisfranc fracture dislocation, complications of 417
Lisfranc injuries
chronic 416, 417
classification of 415

clinical features of 415
management of 415
pathoanatomy of 416
treatment of chronic 417
Lisfranc ligament bundle 416
Listhesis, fixation of 266
Little finger, adduction of 532
Liver 18
disease 7
Load-shift test 481
Lobenhoffer approach, steps of 211
Locked knee, management of 678
Locked plate constructs, use of 885
Locking compression plate 251, 252
Locking screws, proximal 395
Long bone 49
blood supply of 94, 94f
deformity 113, 151
fractures, nailing of 265
fragility fractures of 123
metaphyses 134
nonunion of 266
shafts of major 816
Longitudinal arch, lateral 727
Loose bodies 665, 678
etiology of 678
Looser's zones 138
Low backache 820
acute 789
chronic 789
Low radial nerve palsy 527, 546, 548
Low temperature thermoplastic splints 288
Low ulnar nerve palsy 533, 533t
transfers for 532
Low viscosity cements 255
Lower end radius, surgical anatomy of 506
Lower extremity 600f
alignment, normal parameters of 600
fractures, high-risk 339
malalignment 715
Lower limb 563, 599, 611, 626
length discrepancy 160
mechanical axis of 599, 599f
Lower motor neuron paralysis, ipsilateral 426
Low-molecular-weight heparin 5, 9
use of 5, 8
Lumbar
canal stenosis 782
clinical features of 780
diagnosis of 780
etiology of 780
investigations of 780
lateral 784
types of 782
discectomy 791

disk surgery, complications of 790
epidural steroid injections 877
lesions 756
lordosis 650, 786
accentuation of 135
osteotomy 802, 803
root anomalies, types of 790
spine 436, 755, 806
tuberculosis 757
spondylolisthesis 786
tubercular affection of 330
Lumbosacral lipomata 731
Lunate, decompression of 512
Lung cancer 820
Lunotriquetral ballottement test 515, 516
Lymph nodes, regional 823
Lymphatic, development of 219
Lymphoma 818
Lytic metaphyseal lesion 859
differential diagnosis of 859

M

Machine
learning 891
screw 253
Mackinnon's mixed injury 541
Macrophage inflammatory protein-1 beta 85
Madelung deformity 509
clinical features of 509
diagnosis of 509
pathology of 509
treatment of 509
Madelung disease, pathoanatomy of 510
Madigan's quadricepsplasty 582
Madura foot 190
clinical features 190
diagnosis 190
pathology 190
treatment 190
Maduramycosis 190
Madurella
grisea 190
mycetomati 190
Maffucci syndrome 861, 862, 862t
Malabsorption syndrome 7, 114, 115
Malalignment test 608
Malgaigne fracture 414
Malignancy 13, 114
hypercalcemia of 126
Malignant cartilage, predominance of 840
Malignant lesion, high grade of 817
Malleolus, posterior 411
Mallet fingers 377
Malnutrition 7, 178

Malunion 361, 366, 419, 443
Mangled extremity severity score 195, 195b
Marfan syndrome 110, 146, 154, 488
Marrow edema syndrome, management of 479
Mason classification 362f
Masquelet technique 275, 318, 870
Mass 229
   casualties 875
Matrix metalloproteinases 85
Matsen's unified concept 290
Mayo classification 375
Mazabraud syndrome 832
McCune-Albright syndrome 126, 142
McKay's procedure, modified 597
McLain and Weinstein and Enneking system 819
McMurray's osteotomy 632
Measles 844
Mechanical axis deviation 600
Mechanical chondroplasty 695
Mechanical disk decompression 878
Mechanical stimuli, response to 92
Mechanical tibiofemoral angle 603
Mechanotransduction underplays, process of 259
Medial branch block 878
Medial collateral ligament 711
   injury 711
Medial compartment osteoarthritis
   clinical features of 694
   pathogenesis of 694
Medial cord, branches of 552
Median nerve injury 540
Medical ethics, role of 69
Medoff plate 282, 393
Medullary grafts 101
Megakaryocytes 843
Megaprosthesis 827, 860
   principle of expandable 827
Melanocytes 844
   giant nevus cells of 844
Melanoma 820
Meningitis 320
Meniscal injuries 675, 683
Meniscal repair 677, 682
   different methods of 676
   in knee joint, role of 681
   indications of 676
   methods of 676
Meniscal tears 341
Meniscal transplantation 682
Meniscectomy 677
Meniscus, ramp lesion of 676
Menopause 730
Mesenchymal stem cells 90, 877
   advantages of 870

disadvantages of 870
   peripheral blood-derived 870
Messenger ribonucleic acid 186
Metabolic acidosis 10, 293
Metabolic diseases 115, 119
Metabolic disorders 110, 511
Metabolic syndrome 65
Metabolism 92
Metacarpophalangeal flexion 532
Metacarpophalangeal joint, knuckle stands for 283
Metaizeau technique 365
Metal
   implants 151
   ions 655
Metallic endoprosthesis 825, 841
Metallic implants 188
Metalloprotease-sensitive peptides 884
Metal-on-metal bearings 655
   disadvantages of 655
Metal-on-polyethylene bearings 656
Metaphyseal arteries 88
Metaphyseal chondrodysplasia 565
Metaphyseal femoral neck 211
Metaphyseal sleeve, concept of 710
Metaphyseal system 210
Metaphysis 80, 88
Metastatic bone tumor, laboratory diagnosis of 812, 813fc
Metastatic disease 818fc, 848
Metatarsals 595
Metatarsophalangeal joint 748
Metatarsus adductus 583
   complex 584
Methicillin-resistant *Staphylococcus aureus* infection 165
Methotrexate 315
Methyl methacrylate 883
Methyl prednisolone
   role of 427
   injectable 777
   succinate, role of 425
Microcurrent therapy 465
Microfractures 677
Microvascular fibular graft 589
Microvascular graft osteosynthesis 826
Microvascular repair 196
Midcarpal instability 517
Midfoot amputations 194
Midpalmar space infection 523
Mifamurtide 843
Milkman's syndrome 138
Milwaukee brace, principles of application of 286, 800
Milwaukee shoulder syndrome 61, 490
Mineral 111
   metabolism, regulation of 133

Minimally invasive
   fracture repair 265
   joint replacement surgery 266
   percutaneous plate osteosynthesis 258, 265, 398
   plate osteosynthesis 258
      advantages of 258
      disadvantages of 258
   spine surgery 266
   techniques 266
   techniques, increasing role of 265
Minocycline 766
Mirel's scoring system 816, 816t
Mitogen-activated protein 704
Mixed syndrome 427
Möberg key pinch procedure 518
Mobile nonunion 24
Modified staging system 667t
Modular fixators 263
Molecular markers 848
Molecular techniques 716
Molecular tests 186
Monoarthritis 64
Monoarticular arthritis 701, 702fc
Monoclonal antibody 325, 888
Monoclonal gammopathy 854
Mononuclear infiltrate 753f
Monoplegia 611
Monorail fixator 279
Monteggia fracture dislocation 354, 363, 364, 367
   management of 363
   types of 363
Morel-Lavallée lesion 424
Morrey procedure 369
Mosaicism 155
Motion, range of 364, 492, 575
Motor
   deficits 550, 615
   functions 426, 758
   march 548
   nerve fiber compression, evidence of 539
   paralysis 342
   paralytic bladder 771
Motorized intramedullary bone lengthening
   advantages of 279
   disadvantages of 279
   indications of 279
   principle of 279
Movement 667, 668
   related pain 817
Moxifloxacin 187, 188
Mucopolysaccharidoses 268
Multidrug-resistant tuberculosis 186, 187, 760, 761
Multifragmentary fractures 258

Multiligament knee injury 405, 683
Multilineage cells 869
Multimodal analgesia 299
Multiple myeloma 820, 854, 855
   clinical features of 854
   diagnosis of 854
   symptomatic 854
   treatment of 854
Multiple organ dysfunction syndrome 18, 18t
Multiple rib fractures 27
   management of 26
Multisystem organ failure 18
Muscle 326, 472
   around shoulder, functional classification of 489
   assessment of 228
   brachialis 226
   compartments act 245
   compression 293
   disorders 239
   dysfunction 716
   flaps 214
   group 53
   hypertrophy 471
   relaxants 431
   slide 498
Muscular anomalies 501
Muscular branches 528
Muscular diseases 274
Musculocutaneous flaps 216
Musculoskeletal disorders 242
   antenatal diagnosis of 227
Musculoskeletal effects 303
Musculoskeletal implications 304
Musculoskeletal manifestations 169, 303, 304
Musculoskeletal syndromes 169
   management of 169
Musculoskeletal tumors 827, 828
Mycetoma 190
Mycobacteria 76
   growth indicator tube 76
Mycobacterium tuberculosis 186, 765, 873
   diagnosis of 873
Mycoplasma 317
Myerson's classification 723
Myerson's modification 415
Myocardial infarction 76
Myocutaneous flaps 214
   rotational 215
Myoelectric prosthesis 205
   disadvantages of 205
   principle of 205
Myofibroblastic tumors 863
Myoglobin release 292
Myonecrosis 291

Myositis 239
   ossificans 225, 361
   reactive 838
Myotome indicating injury 53t

N

Nail bed
   anatomy of 381, 381f, 381t
   injuries
      complete spectrum of 381
      management of 382t
Nail impingement 390
Nail-plate construct 372
Nalebuff deformity 556
Nanoactivated silver topically 876
Nanocrystalline hydroxyapatite paste 868
Nanophase hydroxyapatite 868
Nanophase silver 868
Nanotechnology 867
   heralds 867
Napoleon test 472
Narakas group 552
Nasal beaking 856
Nasal decolonization 172
Navigation, role of 711
Navigation-assisted spine surgery, advantages of 880
Neck 566
   femur fracture
      complications of 388
      nonunion of 637
      stress of 389
   resorption ratio 636
   shaft angle 600
   shorter 629
Necrotizing fasciitis 174, 183
   clinical features of 172,173
   management of 172,173
   organism of 172,173
   pathogenesis of 172,173
Needle
   stick injuries, management of 170, 171fc
   test of O'brien 722
   thoracostomy 28
Neer's classification 349f
Neer-Hawkins test 472
Negative pressure wound
   therapy 212, 876
   use of 213
   treatment 744
Neoadjuvant radiation 864
Neonatal hip, clinical assessment of 572f
Neoplasia 812
Neotestudina rosatii 190
Nerve 193

   conduction studies 739
   conduction velocity 311, 544
   degeneration, process of 312
   entrapment 495
   funicular for small 526
   grafting 526
   harvesting 527
   impingement 837
   lesions, classification of 500
   paresthesias 495
Nerve injuries 369, 525, 525t, 543, 545, 616, 741, 870
   classification of 540t
   management of 360, 370
   mid-arm median 541
   Sunderland classification of 525
Nerve repair 197
   methods of 525
Nerve root
   block, selective 877
   injury 792
Neural foraminal stenosis 782
Neurapraxia 360, 525, 540
Neuroblastoma 322, 846
Neurofibromatosis 142, 591, 835, 858
   musculoskeletal manifestations of 858
   orthopedic manifestations of 323
Neuroforaminal canal, narrowed 781
Neurogenic bladder 770
Neurogenic shock 52, 53
Neurologic disease 651
Neurological claudication 778, 778t
Neurological deficits 436, 820
Neurological injuries 406
Neurology intact 763
Neuroma
   and painful stump, prevention of 194
   formation 199
Neuromuscular blockade 37
Neuromuscular disease 748, 871
Neuromuscular disorders 614
Neuromuscular factors 618
Neuropathic arthritis 745
Neuropathic foot 745
Neuropathic joint 745
   diagnosis of 746
Neuropathy, peripheral 204
Neuropraxia 496
Neurotmesis 525, 540, 541
Neurotropism 542
Neurovascular injury 384
Neurovascular structures 501
Neutrophil 311
   cell 311t
New Beighton criteria 489b
Newton's third law of motion 200
Nilotinib 325

Nitric oxide production, inhibition of 427
Nocturnal acroparesthesia 536
Nonarthroplasty surgical methods 639
Nonbiodegradable bone cements 161
Noncontrast computed tomography 836
Nondissociative carpal instability 515
Nonhemolytic reactions 57
Nonimmune-mediated reactions 57
Nonossifying fibroma 859
Nonsegmental hemivertebrae 797
Nonsteroidal anti-inflammatory drugs 6, 59, 98, 148, 168, 225, 346, 431, 469, 521, 706
Nonsurgical intervention 502
Nonunion 21, 264, 443, 870
   noninfected 24
   of fracture scaphoid, pathology of 513
   types of 23
Nonweight-bearing gait, three-point 224
Noyes flexion-rotation drawer test 680, 685
Nuclear factor
   inhibitors 704
   kappa-B ligand inhibitors, receptor activator of 111
Nuclear medicine 242
Nuclear scan studies, role of 241
Nucleic acid amplification test 186, 868, 873
Nucleus
   pulposus, augmentation of 878
   replacement 878
Nutritional rickets 604
   clinical features of 140
   diagnosis of 140
   management of 140

O

O'brien's active compression test 346, 348
O'Donoghue, injury of unhappy triad of 680
O'Driscoll, approach of 357
Oats 696
Ober's test 607, 680
Obligatory patellar dislocation 585
Oblique talus, category of 593
Obstructive shock 53
Occipital condyle fracture 285
Occupational therapy 559
Ochronotic arthritis 115
Ochronotic arthropathy 110, 146
Odontoid fractures 439
   acute 439
   classification of 439
   mechanism of injury of 439

Ofloxacin 187, 188
Ogden classification 345
Olecranon
   osteotomy 357
   pin traction 369
Oligoarthritis 64
Ollier's disease 861, 862, 862t
Ombredanne's line 568
Oncogenic hypophosphatemic osteomalacia 858
Oncogenic osteomalacia 858
One-column fracture 400
Onychohypoplasia 856
Open direct reduction and fixation, technique of 401
Open fracture 455, 456
   management 404
Open injury 455
Open reduction internal fixation 378, 454, 455
Operation
   theater 175
      etiquettes 175
   types of 486
Oral analgesics 703
Organ system 18
Organism, type of 184
Oritavancin 889
Orthobiologics 309
Orthofix technique 279
Orthopedic 38, 100, 226, 246, 254, 331
   disorders 126
   frozen section in 829
   implants, removal of 307
   infection 156, 868
   oncology 77, 868
   surgery 55, 815
      robotics of 226, 232
   sutures 328
   trauma 267, 335
      general aspects of 335
Orthosis 431
Orthostatic hypotension 125
Orthotic support 481
Orthotics devices 306
Ortolani and Barlow's sign 568
Ortolani test, modification of 568
Osgood–Schlatter disease 322, 587
Osseous
   pathological conditions 236
   pseudotumors 63
   structure 228, 618
Osteitis fibrosa cystica 852
Osteoanabolic therapy 125
Osteoarthritis 84, 98, 99, 99t, 274, 694, 695, 703, 706, 707, 870
   early 665
   management 706fc

   of knee, pathogenesis of primary 706
   post-traumatic 384, 616
   slow acting drugs for 703
Osteoarthrosis, high tibial osteotomy for 708
Osteoarticular incongruity 492
Osteoarticular tuberculosis 186-188, 766
   management of 76
Osteoblastic activity 821
Osteoblastoma 831, 831t, 859
Osteoblasts, transition from 91
Osteocalcin 124
Osteocartilaginous 678
Osteochondral allograft 104, 108, 722
   transplantation 696
Osteochondral defects 868
Osteochondral injuries 236
Osteochondral lesions, arthroscopic management of 693
Osteochondritis dissecans 693t
   arthroscopic grading of 693
   etiology of 693, 694
   magnetic resonance imaging grading of 693
   management of 890
   radiological staging of 693
   surgical staging of 693
Osteochondrodysplasia 227
Osteochondromas, Multiple 837
Osteochondromatosis 665
Osteoclasts 843
Osteocutaneous free flaps 218
Osteocyte 91
   lacunocanalicular network 887
Osteofasciocutaneous free flaps 218
Osteofibrous
   dysplasia 831, 834, 835, 835t
   imperfecta 110, 114, 126, 146, 149, 151, 600, 604, 870
Osteogenesis, electrically induced 93
Osteogenic potential 109
Osteogenic power 96
Osteogenic sarcoma 839
Osteoid osteoma 830, 831, 831t
Osteoinduction 252, 253
   property 109, 253t
Osteolysis 652, 879
   biology of 652
   mechanism of 652
   radiology of 652
Osteolytic lesions 653
Osteomalacia 115, 136, 137, 268
   classical lesion of 136
Osteomalacic bones, uncalcified cortex of 138
Osteomyelitis 28, 236, 238, 320, 321, 604, 859
   acute 156

chronic 156, 159, 163t
  recurrent multifocal 166
  hematogenous 157
  management of 887
  treatment of 887
Osteonecrosis 160, 384, 634, 671, 671t, 870
Osteopenia 114, 114t
Osteopenic lesions 833
Osteoplasty, femoral 621
Osteoporosis 110, 114, 114t, 116-118, 120, 126
  causes of 110
  development of 112
  diagnosis of 112
  management of 124
  pharmacotherapy for 118t
  regional migratory 479
  transient 479, 671, 671t, 804
    migratory 671
Osteoporotic fractures 128
Osteoporotic spine fractures, management of 120
Osteoporotic vertebral fracture, management protocol of 122
Osteosarcoma 839, 840, 859
  advances for 842
  limb salvage surgery for 825
  management of 841, 842
Osteosynthesis 590
  techniques of 388
  type of 826
Osteotomy 510, 570, 571, 632, 699, 704, 731
  around hip 632
    joint 632
  deformity correction 608
  double 584
  intertrochanteric 579
  location of proximal 632
  nondisplaced 261
  pemberton 570
  pericapsular dial 571
  resection 526
  rotational 639
  stabilization 281
  techniques 802
Oxidized zirconium 656
Oxygen
  debt 51
  partial arterial pressure of 20
  partial pressure of 18
Ozone therapy 877

P

P38 mitogen-activated protein kinases 882
Packed red blood cells 55

Paget's disease 126, 239, 843
Pain 290, 426, 520, 751
  control 16
  gate control theory of 11
  management 295, 481
    modalities of 299
  relief 122, 315
  severe 383
Painful arc
  syndrome 468
  test 469f
Painful area 297
Painful elbow 493
  diagnosis of 493
  etiology of 493
Painful prominent hardware 402
Paley classification 590
Palliative factors 778
Pallor 290
Palm component 283
Palmar
  arch 532
  deep fascia, anatomy of 518
  maintenance of 532
  triquetrum-hamate ligaments 517
Pamidronate 126, 833, 875
  therapy 150
Pan talar arthrodesis
  disadvantages of 750
  indications of 750
Pancoast tumor 28
Pangenome, development of 156
Pappas
  classes 563t
  classification 563
Paprosky classification 662t
Para-aminosalicylic acid 188
Paradiskal lesions, typical 756
Paradoxical reaction 760
Paraffin wax 298
Paralabral cysts 471
Paralysis 290
Paraplegia 612, 757, 763, 767, 767t, 775t
  degree of 767
  early-onset 767
  Girdlestone classification of onset of 757, 759
  late-onset 767, 767t
Paraplegic patient, sexual rehabilitation of 776
Parathormone
  analog 129
  therapy 125
Parathyroid
  disorders 81
  gland 133f
    anatomy of 133
    role of 134

hormone
  influence of 91
  role of 132
Paravertebral lesion, typical 311
Paresis 342
Paresthesia 290
Paronychia 522
Parosteal osteosarcoma 839, 839, 839t
Parvovirus 317
Patella 586
  alta 583
  congenital 585t
    dislocation of 583, 585
  dislocation of 586
  fractures 462
  habitual dislocation of 585, 585t
  hypermobility of 582
  maltracking of 715
  recurrent dislocation of 582, 583, 583fc, 586
Patellar height 707
Patellar tendinopathy 266, 309
Patellar tendon 330
Patellofemoral articulation 329
Patellofemoral joint
  biomechanics of 581
  kinematics of 581
Patellofemoral ligaments 330
Pathoanatomy 416, 444, 753
Pathological fracture, risk of 816t
Patient's own tissue 696
Patient-centered care 74
Patient-related factors 687
Patrick's sign 672
Pauwels osteotomy 389, 632
Pavlik harness 569, 580
Paxinos test 348
Peak bone mass 120
Pectus carinatum 113
Pediatric basic life support 45
Pediatric bone 88, 88t
  blood supply of 89f
Pediatric fractures, general aspects of 344
Pediatric hip fractures 387
Pediatric lateral condyle humerus fracture 353
Pediatric medial epicondyle fracture 353
Pediatric radial neck fracture classification 353
Pediatric supracondylar humerus fractures
  complications of 360
  management of 360
Pedicle grafts, vascularized 101
Pedicle subtraction osteotomy 803
Peg grafts 101
Pelken spur 134

Pelviacetabular disease 816
Pelviacetabular fractures, complex 422
Pelvic
   C-clamp, design of 451
   floor exercises 772
   incidence 649, 786
   region 570t
   section 800
   tilt 649, 786
   torsion test 672
   trauma 47, 453
Pelvic fracture 233, 234, 440, 444, 453fc
   classification of 440t
   management of 444fc
   open 453
   urethral injuries in 444
Pelvic injury 447fc
   tile classification of 441f
Pelvic osteotomy 576
   indications of 570
   principles of 570
   types of 567
Pelvic ring
   disruptions 443
   injury 453
   stable 441
Pelvic support osteotomy 633
   type of 634
Pelvis 49, 424, 627
   fractures 424
   open book injury of 446
Pentosan sulfate 703
Peptide nucleic acid 182
Percutaneous bone marrow injection 22
Percutaneous decompressive neuroplasty 877
Percutaneous endoscopic diskectomy 878
Percutaneous fixation 454
Percutaneous physiodesis 271
Percutaneous reduction 266
Percutaneous screw fixation 452
Periacetabular osteotomy 631, 632
Perianal sensation 436
Periarticular fractures, management of 884
Pericapsular injection 878
Perilunate dislocation 374
   fracture 373
Perilunate injury, classification of 374
Perineurorrhaphy 526
Periosteal osteosarcoma 839, 839t, 840
Periosteal system 94
Peripheral nerve
   cross-section of 539, 539f
   injuries 547, 771, 868
   regeneration following axonotmesis, pathophysiology of 541
   repair 317

sheath tumor, malignant 863
   system 541
Periprosthetic fractures 251, 461
   around knee 461
   around total knee replacement 714
Periprosthetic joint infection 883
   diagnosis of 868
   management protocol of 179
Periprosthetic osteolysis 867
Periprosthetic tibial fractures 461
Peritalar dislocation 421
Peritrochanteric fractures 282, 393
Perkin's line 568
Peroneal autograft 686
Peroneal nerve 741
   disorder 737
   injury 738
   palsy 741
Peroneal tendon
   disease 735
   disorders
      causes of 735
      diagnosis of 735
      treatment of 735
   irritation 419
Perren's guidelines 250
Perren's hypothesis 250
Persistent limp 321
Personal protective equipment 175, 333
Perthes disease 126, 322, 573, 621, 625, 670
   management of 575, 576, 576fc
Pes cavus 728
Pes planus 155, 582, 729
Petit's triangle 330, 756f
Pexidartinib 325
Peyronie's disease 558
Phalangeal component 283
Phalen's test, reverse 537
Phalen's wrist hyperflexion test 537
Phemister bone grafting 106
Phosphatonin, role of 137
Phrenic nerve damage 552
Physeal bar
   excision 268
   management of post-traumatic unilateral 268
Physeal closure, premature 388
Physeal distraction osteogenesis 590
Physeal fractures 88, 91f
Physeal injury 81
   classification of 81, 81t
   management of 82
   traumatic 604
Physical activity 120
Physical examination 596
Physical therapy 470, 480
Physician-patient relationship 69

Physiodesis 278, 510
   conventional 271
   temporary 270
Physiotherapy 295
Physis 81f
   components of 79f
   disorders of 268
   epiphysis complex 88, 91f
   structure of 81
Pigmented villonodular synovitis 207, 323, 324
Pilon fractures 414
Pin
   fixators 262
   orientation 451f
   site infection 262
   tract infection 281
Pincer impingement 629-631
Pincer lesion 631
Pinch grip 518
Pinless external fixator 262
Pipkin
   classification 385f
   fractures 206, 621
Pirani scoring 596, 596t
Pivot shift test 516
Plantar fasciitis 266, 309
Plantar flexion, causes of 734
Plantaris 724
   tendon
      anatomy of 724
      role of 724
Plasma
   fresh-frozen 55
   imbibition 219
Plaster cast
   general principles of 336
   techniques of 336
Plaster of Paris
   cast, advantages of 338
   cast, disadvantages of 338
   technique of applying 337
   use of 244
Plate and screw
   fixation 396
   stabilization 372
Plate osteosynthesis 173
   evolution of 249
Platelet 55
   abnormality 62
   count 20
   dysfunction 41
Platelet-derived
   endothelial growth factor 266
   growth factor 92, 259
Platelet-enriched plasma 266
Platelet-rich
   concentrate 266

plasma 266, 267, 309
   autologous 877
   therapy 752
   types of 267
Plexus injuries, pure lower 553
Pneumatic extrusion printing 331
Pneumatic tourniquet 326
Poloxamer 188 704
Polyarthritis 64
Polycythemia rubra vera 2
Polydactyly 591
Polyesters 249
Polyethylene 254, 653
  cup 646
  glycol 249
  high density 254
  terephthalate 883
  wear 827
Polyglycolic acid 248, 872
Polymerase chain reaction amplification 868
Polymethyl methacrylate 249
  antibiotic bead chains 159
  bone cement 183
Polymorphonuclear neutrophil 166
Polymyalgia rheumatica 239
Polymyositis 229
Polytrauma 33, 39, 42, 47, 48, 435, 875
  effects of 48
  management of 33, 36, 39, 56, 874
  patient 51
    management of 36
    pathophysiology of 34
    prehospital care of 35
  treatment of 47
  types of 41
  victims, hospital management of 40
Ponseti
  manipulation, steps of 594
  method 598
Pop slab 337
Positive end-expiratory pressure 18
Positron emission tomography scan 25, 186
  role of 237
Post-chikungunya arthritis 170
Post-COVID musculoskeletal syndrome 170
Posterior heel pain
  causes of 751
  clinical features of 751
  investigations of 751
Posterolateral corner injury
  management of 691
  symptoms of 692
Postganglionic brachial plexus injury 554
Postganglionic lesions 550
Postmenopausal osteoporosis, medical management of 113

Post-polio paralysis 200
Post-talofibular ligament 595
Post-tourniquet syndrome 327
Post-traumatic thumb reimplantation surgery
  principles of 196
  steps of 196
Postural kyphosis 806
Pott's paraplegia 311, 764
  diagnosis of 759
  management of 759
Pott's spine 756, 760
  pathophysiology of 755
Practice evidence-based medicine 73, 74
Precision grips 518
Predestructive stage 768
Preemptive analgesia 299
Prehospital and early management 292
Pressure
  epiphysis 268
  irrigation 877
Pretibial muscle weakness 222
Primary fracture
  healing 99
  line 418
Primitive neuroectodermal tumors 846
Printing technique, selection of 331
Procuring stem cells 869
Profundus tendon avulsion 379
  management of 378
Prognosticate osteoporosis 115
Proinflammatory cytokine 876
  expression 430
  presence of 318
Prolapsed intervertebral disk 787, 877
  management of 877
Proliferative synovium 324
Pronation abduction injury 408, 408f
Prophylactic fasciotomy 609
Prophylaxis, postexposure 380
Propionibacterium acnes 180
Prostate cancer 820
Prosthesis
  conventional 477
  types of expandable 827
Prosthetic feet, different designs of 203
Prosthetic joint infection 179, 181, 182, 238
  classification of 179t
  management of 182fc
Prosthetic replacement 512
Prosthetic titanium rib, vertical expandable 794
Proteasome 856
Protective in-toeing 614
Protein
  C deficiency 3
  S deficiency 3

Proteoglycan
  loss of 787
  low molecular weight 275
Prothionamide 188
Proton beam therapy 843
Protrusio acetabuli 645, 658, 660
Provocative tests 537
Proximal femoral
  capital physis 565
  focal deficiency 564
  fractures 392, 423
  nail 392
  osteotomy 632, 637, 638
  sagittal plane deformities of 630
  shortening 566
Proximal interphalangeal
  joint manipulation 556
  region 520
Proximal radius
  fresh fractures of 365
  malunited fractures of 366
Proximal tibia
  four columns of 401, 402f
  fracture 290, 423
    fixation 401
  osteotomy 708
  types of 708
Pseudarthrosis, congenital 588t
Pseudoachondroplasia 268
Pseudoaneurysm 837
Pseudoarthrosis 120
Pseudofractures 138
Pseudoglioma syndrome 114
Pseudogout 60, 61, 61t
Pseudorheumatoid disease 61
Pseudotrendelenburg test 223
Pseudotumor 63
  complications of 63
  rupture of 63
Psoas abscess 322, 330, 331, 756f
Psoriatic arthritis 238
  management of 64
Psychiatric moans 133, 852
Pulmonary artery disease 76
Pulmonary complications 886
Pulmonary dysfunction 19
Pulmonary embolism 790, 792
Pulsatile parathyroid hormone therapy, indications of 114
Pulse, radiofrequency 235
Pulselessness 290
Push-pull test 481
Putti-Platt operation 486
Pyknodysostosis 856
Pylon prosthesis 192
Pyogenic spondylitis 790, 792
Pyomyositis 174, 320
  clinical features of 173

management of 173
organism of 173
pathogenesis of 173
Pyrazinamide 188, 754, 760, 766
Pyroelectricity 93

Q

QFracture scores 115
Quad procedure, modified 553
Quadratus lumborum muscle 223
Quadriceps
    apparatus 329
    contracture, components of 586
    tendon tears 235
    weakness 221
Quadrilateral space, boundaries of 471
Quadrilateral syndrome, treatment of 471
Quadriplegia 611
Quasi-experimental research 73
Quénu and Küss classification 415f

R

Radial bone 109
Radial club hand 501
    classification of 501t
Radial collateral ligament 355, 367
Radial head
    and neck 209
        malunion 366
    excision of 493
    fractures 253, 478
        mechanism of injury of 362
    implants, types of 477
    malunions of 366
    prosthesis 477, 478
    replacement 477
Radial neck, malunions of 366
Radial nerve 356
    course of 527
    palsy 351, 530, 546
        diagnosis of 547
        management of 352, 352fc, 528, 528fc
Radial shaft, malunions of proximal 366
Radiation
    hazards 332
    therapy 848
Radiocapitellar contact 478
Radiofrequency
    ablation 814
    coblation 878
Radiography, conventional 479
Radionucleotide 63
Radiotherapy, primary 819
Radioulnar length adjustment 510

Radioulnar synostosis 366
Radius
    deformity, correction of 510
    fracture distal end of 371
Raloxifene 118
Ramp lesions, optional for 686
Randomized control
    study designs 67fc
    trial 66, 73
Range of motion, reduced 615
Reamed nail 283, 283t
Reconstructive ladder 456, 456f
    revised 456, 456fc
Rectus abdominis free flap 216
Rectus femoris 498
Recurrent dislocation 384, 616
    shoulder 485
Red active marrow 267
Red man syndrome 889
Reduction techniques 261
Reed–Sternberg cells 844
Referencing system 880
Reflex
    neurogenic bladder 771
    sympathetic dystrophy 13, 260, 479, 746
    voiding 774
Refrigerator temperature 198
Registration process 880
Rehabilitation 480, 687, 752, 772, 864
    postoperative 683, 692
    postsurgery 534
Reiter syndrome 155
Relapsed clubfoot 597
Remplissage procedure 487
Renal cell carcinoma 820
Renal failure 132, 132t
Renal losses 142
Renal manifestations 133, 852
Renal osteodystrophy 110, 604
    clinical features of 140
    diagnosis of 140
    etiology of 140
    treatment of 140
Renal rickets 131
Renal system 18
Renal tubular acidosis 132, 132t
Repair flexor pollicis longus 197
Reperfusion injury 291
Reperfusion syndrome 327
Research literacy 74
Resin cast, technique of 336, 338
Respiratory dysfunction 342
Respiratory physiology 48
Respiratory system 18
Retinacular arteries 210
Retinacular system 210
Retinal vein clotting 76

Retract flexor pollicis longus tendon 373
Retracted tendon level 379
Retrocalcaneal bursitis 751
Retroclavicular spurling's test 29
Retroperitoneum 49
Retropharyngeal abscess 756
Retropulsion, posterior 768
Revascularization procedures 512, 636
Reverse shoulder
    arthroplasty, contraindications of 478
    replacement, principles of 476
Rhabdomyolysis 293, 327
Rheobase 544
Rheumatoid arthritis 98, 99, 99t, 148, 178, 238, 274, 313, 317, 535
    diagnosis of 881
    etiopathogenesis of 317
    juvenile 495
    management of 881
    treatment of 313
Rheumatoid hand 554
    deformities of 555
Rheumatoid synovitis 207
Rheumatologic diseases 154, 155
Rhomboid muscles 554
Ria system 261
Rib 109, 589, 808
    vertebral angle 793, 793f
Rickets 88, 91f, 114, 115, 129
    causes, types of standard 133
    classification of 142
    clinical features of 135
    etiological classification of 129b, 142b
    hypophosphatemic 131, 137, 604, 858
    radiological features of 134
    types of 130t
Rifabutin 188
Rifampicin 166, 188, 754, 760, 766
    topical 717
Rigid cavus foot 339
Rigid metatarsus adductus 584
Rigid pes planus 732
    deformity
        signs of 592
        symptoms of 592
Ring fixators 279
Risser-Ferguson method 794
Rituximab 316, 882
Rivaroxaban 9
Robotic arm interactive orthopedic system 230
Robotic surgery
    advantages of 230
    limitations of 231
Rocking horse effect, management of 480
Rod bending 152
Rod migration 152

Roos test 29
Root anomalies 787
Rostral sparing 573
Rotational stability 336
Rotationplasty 624, 825, 841
   principles of 624
Rotator cuff 471
   anatomy of 472f
   impingement syndrome 468
   pathology 468
   repair 266, 309
     open 473
   tendinosis 474
Rotator cuff tear 228, 471, 479
   chronic full thickness 474
   clinical tests for 472t
   conservative management of 476
   full thickness 475
   pathogenesis of 475
   surgical treatment options for 476
Rotator interval 475
Rotatory instability, posterolateral 368
Rubber composition 202
Rubella virus 317
Rüedi and Allgöwer classification 413
Run-in wear period 655
Russe classification 375
Russell-Taylor classification 391
Ryder test 601

S

Sach foot 201, 202, 202t
   use of 201
Sacral cord injury 771
Sacral fractures 452
Sacral nutation 789, 790
Sacral rhizotomy, posterior 774
Sacral slope 649, 786
Sacroiliac joint injection, technique of 672
Sacroiliitis 65, 672
   etiology of 672
   management of 672
Sacrum, fracture of 452
Saddle point 645
S-adenosylmethionine 703
Sagittal vertical axis 650
Sailor's gait 568
Salter's osteotomy 570, 571
Salter-Harris
   classification 81t, 344, 345
     rang modified 345
   epiphyseal injury, management of 344
   fractures 352
   injury 345, 377
Salvage procedure 579, 637, 750
Sandifer syndrome 464
Saracatinib 843

Sarcoidosis 239, 843
Sarcoma 816
Sarcopenia 116, 118
   pharmacotherapy for 118t
Sarmiento's modification 199
SARS-CoV-19 virus infection 889
Scaphoid bone, blood supply of 374, 375f
Scaphoid fracture 374
   displaced 374
   fixation 253
   undisplaced 374
Scaphoid nonunion 514fc
Scaphoid osteotomy 507
Scapholunate incompetence 516
Scapho-Trapezio-trapezoidal joint 61
Scapula
   protractors of 489
   retractors of 489
   rotators of 489
Scapular depressors 489
Scapular dyskinesia 468
Scapular elevators 489
Scapular osteotomy, vertical 467
Scar tissue formation 867
Scedosporium apiospermum 190
Schanz
   osteotomy 634, 634f
   screws 263
Schatzker classification 399, 400, 400f
Scheuermann's disease 803
   differential diagnosis of 806
   pathology of 806
Scheuermann's kyphosis 805
Schmorl's nodes 804
Schober's test, modified 147
Schonfeld's criteria 20, 20t
Schroth method 795
Schwann cells 541, 542
Schwannoma 852
Sciatic nerve 741
   pathoanatomy of 741
Scintigraphy 241
   scanning 641
SCIWORA 343
   pathophysiology of 343
Sclerotic fracture 513
Scoliosis 113, 135, 155, 792, 793
   classification of 792t
   congenital 797, 799
   functional 793
   idiopathic 794
   structural 793
Scoliotic surgery 792
Scratch collapse test 537
Screw density 251
Screw-rod mechanism 284

Scurvy 88, 91f, 115
   clinical features of 135
   etiopathology of 135
   management of 135
   radiological features of 134
Seatbelt type injury 434
Second hit phenomena 39, 39f
Second-generation cups 660
Sectoral sign 640
Seinsheimer 395
Senile osteoporosis, management of 118
Sensory 15
   branches 529
   deficits 615
   examination 53
   loss 820
   nerve fiber compression, evidence of 539
   neurogenic bladder 771
Separates patellofemoral 399
Septic
   complications, classification of 716
   hip 167
   shock 54, 54t
   tenosynovitis 523
Septic arthritis 229, 312, 320, 321, 321t
   development of 160
   late sequelae of 167, 167f
Septicemia
   gram-negative 17
   markers for 17
Sequestrum, different types of 164
Serum
   inflammatory markers 874t
   markers 716
   protein electrophoresis 821
Sever's disease 751
Sexual and bladder rehabilitation 773
Sexual dimorphism 308
Sexual dysfunction 343
Shear forces, minimizing 665
Shear test, posterior 672
Shearing movements 219
Shell allografts 108
Shepherd's crook deformity 832
Sherman plates 249
Shilla procedure 794
Shock 17, 51, 292
   hypovolemic 51, 54, 54t
   management of 51
   reversal of 343
   traumatic 52
Shoe modification 287, 731
Short broad hands 856
Short tau inversion recovery 344
Short-stiff nonunions 24
Shortwave diathermy 298

Shoulder 474
  adhesive capsulitis of 471
  anterior dislocation of 481
  arthrodesis 489
    techniques for 490
  arthroplasty, conventional 476
  capsule, excessive laxity of 485
  dislocation, traumatic 483
  osteoarthritis 266
  posterior dislocation of 483
  recurrent anterior dislocation of 484
  stability of 482
  trauma series of affected 482
Shoulder girdle 816
  afflictions, congenital 464
  to hand 345
Shoulder instability 481, 487
  management of 488
Shoulder joint
  multidirectional instability of 487
  old unreduced dislocation of 484
  posterior dislocation of 482
  stabilizers of 482
Shoulder–hand syndrome 13
Shuck test 515, 516
Shy-Drager syndrome 771
Sickle cell disease 146
Sideswipe injury 368
  classification of 369fc
Side-to-side grip 518
Signet ring, appearance of 516f
Silfverskiold test 741
  reverse 723
Silicate-based grafts 102
Silicon nitride bearing surfaces 883
Simulated metatarsal movement 202
Singh's index 635
Single joint effusions 315
Single onlay cortical grafts 101
Sinus tarsi 420
  approach 420
Skeletal dysplasia 151, 604
Skeletal fluorosis
  radiological stages of 139
  spine surgery in 140
Skeletal growth 344
Skeletal immature patient 510
Skeletal limb deficiencies, congenital 563
Skeletal manifestations 115
Skeletal mature patients 510
Skeletal maturity 733
Skeletal metastasis 812
  management of 814
Skeletal muscle tumors 863
Skeletal structures 458
Skeletal variations 511
Skew foot 584
  complex 584

Skin 458
  closure 197
  flap 192
  graft 218
    complications of 219
    delayed 218
    primary 218
    split-thickness 218
  infection 165
  loss, management of 370
  substitutes 876
Slap lesions 479, 480, 758
Sliding hip screw 388
Slipped capital femoral epiphysis 321, 383, 577
  clinical features of 577
  pathophysiology of 577
Sliver, use of 876
Slocum anterior rotary drawer test 679
Smith's fractures 372
Smith–Petersen osteotomy 802
Smoking 65, 639
Smooth muscle tumors 863
Soft callus 97
Soft-tissue 197, 239
  contracture 492, 595
  coverage 826
  dissection 621
  imbalance 480
  infections of 229
  injuries 616
  procedure 732
  quadriceps 686
  sarcomas 863
  support system 504, 505
  surgery 306, 597
Solid ankle 202
  cushioned heel 203
Solid keel 202
Solitary osteochondromas 838
Soluble cell adhesion molecule 182
Somatic stem cells 869
Somi brace 284
Song classification 353
Sonication 181
  protocol 181fc
Sorafenib 843
Sorenson's criteria 804
Soybean unsaponifiables 703
Spasmodic torticollis 467
Spastic
  bladder 775
  diplegia 306
  quadriplegic gait 305
Spasticity 301, 343, 821
  comparison of 301t
  treatment of 303
Speed's V-Y muscleplasty 366

Sphygmomanometer test 722
Spina
  bifida 200, 731
  ventosa 189
Spinal canal 121
  stenosis 778, 779
    anatomical classification of 779t
Spinal cord 310, 311f
  cross-section of 428, 429f
  injury 53, 200, 236, 342, 425, 772, 777, 777f, 870
    acute 428
  lesions 769, 771
  level 11
  syndromes 778
  tumors 236
  zone of 310
Spinal curve progression 797
Spinal dysraphism 731
Spinal fusion 796, 870
Spinal infections 237, 238, 242
Spinal injury 436
  Denis three column concept of 436, 436f
  traumatic 777
Spinal instability 821
Spinal lesions 229
Spinal metastasis 817, 820
Spinal osteotomy
  complications of 802
  indications of 802
Spinal shock 335, 342
Spinal stability, concept of 431
Spinal tuberculosis 188, 765
  management 760
Spinal tumor 763
  management of 829
  syndrome 759
Spine 424, 753, 768
  ballistic injuries of 778
  complex fractures of 422
  immobilization of 344
  injuries 437
    classification of 437
  metastatic disease of 818fc
  oncology study group 817
  prolotherapy 878
  stable 763
  surgery, navigation in 878
  tubercular affection of 753
Spinopelvic kinematics, role of altered 648
Spinopelvic relationship 649
  concept of 649
Spinopelvic sagittal balance 786
  radiological features of 786
Spinopelvic stiffness 650
Spinopelvic tilt 649

Spinothalamic tracts 426
Spleen tyrosine kinase 882
Splint, layers for 337, 338t
Spondyloarthropathy 239, 672
Spondylodiscitis 238
Spondylolisthesis 784
Spongiosa
   primary 82
   secondary 82
Sports-specific feet 205
Sprengel deformity, surgical correction of 811
Sprengel shoulder 466
   deformity 464
Sprinting sports 630
Stainless steel 656
Standard skeletal survey 32
Staphylococcal
   abscess communities 887
   colonization 177, 178
Staphylococcus aureus 162, 177, 522
   intracellular persistence 887
Starburst giant cells 844
Stasis, role of 1
Static cerebral palsy, management of 302
Static compression 252
Statins 129, 315
Statistical proficiency 74
Stature, shortness of 856
Steel, blanch sign of 577
Steenbeek brace 296
Steinberg classification 643t
Steinmann pin 452f
Stem cell 869
   indications of use of 870
   therapy 306, 877, 878
Stem cementing, generations of 646t
Stener lesion 378, 378f
Stenosis
   degenerative 783
   traumatic 783
Stereolithography 331
Sterilization 175
Sternocleidomastoid muscle, classical surgical division of 466
Steroids 119
Stickler syndrome 488
Stiff elbow, causes of 492
Stiff knee, causes of painful 713
Stiffness, management of 370
Stiles–Bunnell FF4T phasic transfer, modified 531
Stimson method 383, 384, 616
Stoppa
   approach, modified 208
   modification 208
Stoss therapy 130

Stove-in chest 25
Straight leg raising test, interpretation of 789
Strain 249, 299
Strength-duration curve 544f, 545f
Streptococcus pyogenes 184
Streptomyces somaliensis 190
Streptomycin 188, 190, 754, 766
Stress 249
   fracture 322, 339, 751
   relaxation 256
   shielding 250
Stretch test 432
Stroke 535
Strontium 129
   oxides 654
Structural deformity, primary 748
Stubby fingers 856
Stulberg classification 573, 573t
Subacromial impingement syndrome 468
Subacromial space, anatomy of 475, 475f
Subaxial spine, tuberculosis of 768
Subcutaneous fasciotomy 560
Sublaminar wiring techniques 440
Sublimis transfer 531
Subluxated knee 579
Subluxating ulnar nerve 549
Subsynovial intra-articular arterial ring of Chung 211
Subtalar arthritis 419
Subtalar dislocation, open reduction of 422
Subtrochanteric osteotomy 633
Subtrochanteric valgus osteotomy 566
Sudeck's atrophy 13
Sudeck's osteodystrophy 13
Sudomotor 15, 16
Sulcus test 475
Sulfamethoxazole 190
Sulfasalazine 316
Sunderland classification 525t
Sunderland grades 525, 540
Superficial dissection 206
Supination adduction injury 407f
Supination external rotation injury 406
   management of 409
Supine position arthroscopy 666
Suppurative flexor tenosynovitis, management of 183, 524
Supracondylar fracture 352, 353
   femur 461
   management of 359, 359fc
Suprapatellar fat pad 588
Sural communicating nerve 737
Sural nerve injury 419
Surgery
   effects of 94
   indications of 478, 762, 764

Surgical site infection 173
   prevention of 177
   prophylaxis to prevent 178
Surgical sterility 176
Surgical technique, principles of 281
Suture hook repair 677
Suzuki frame 379
   functioning of 378
Swan neck deformity 313, 314, 555
   pathoanatomy of 555
Swashbuckler approach 399
Swelling, management of 588
Swing-through gait 224
Syme amputation 198, 199, 591
   demerits of 199
   principle of 199
Syncytiotrophoblast 843
Syndesmophytes 808
Syndesmotic injuries 411
Synovectomy 557
Synovial chondromatosis 207, 857
   clinical features of 857
   management of 323
   pathology of 857
Synovial disease 665
Synovial fluid
   analysis 311, 312t, 716
   culture 716
Synovial joint pathologies 311t
Synovial pathology 235
Synovial tissue-derived mesenchymal stem cells 869
Synoviorthesis 63
Synovitis 669
   transient 321, 321t
Synthetic grafts 696
Synthetic resin cast 338
Syphilis, late 843
Systemic inflammatory response syndrome 39
Systemic lupus erythematosus 2
Systemic vascular resistance 54

T

T1 pelvic angle 650
Talectomy 748
   demerits of 750
   indications of 750
   merits of 750
Talipes equinovarus, congenital 594, 598
Talocalcaneonavicular joint 596
Talocalcaneus capsule 595
Talonavicular joints 593
Talus
   blood supply of 724
   fracture of neck of 420
Tantalum augments 183

Tardy ulnar nerve palsy 548
Tarsal tunnel syndrome 741
Tarsometatarsal joint complex 416
Tartrate-resistant acid phosphatase 124
Taylor spatial frame 23, 263, 264, 279
T-cell costimulation, inhibition of 881
Tear
    full thickness 475
    massive unreparable 474
Teardrop
    line, vertical 645
    lysis 662
Technetium methylene diphosphonate 242
Technetium-99 bone
    scan 814
    scintigraphy 578
Technetium-99 scan, indications of 240
Technetium-99m phosphate imaging, standard technique of 240
Teicoplanin 181
Telavancin 166, 888
Telemedicine 74
    advantages of 74
    delivery, methods of 75
Temperature sensation 426
Templating, role of 645
Temsirolimus 843
Tendinitis 227, 235
Tendinopathy 236
    chronic 310
Tendinoscopy 266
Tendinosis 227
Tendo-Achilles 595, 722
    contracture 593
    signs of neglected 722
    symptoms of neglected 722
Tendon 520
    disorders 227
    focal thinning of 227
    grafting 319
        two-stage 562
    injury 236
    regeneration 310
    repair 197
    tears 227
        partial 227
    transfer 525, 529, 531, 532, 598, 737, 740
        principles of 529
Tennis
    elbow, recalcitrant 493
    leg 723
Tenosynovitis 227, 299
Tensile strength 256
Tension band
    principle 257, 257f
    wiring 257

Tension pneumothorax 27
Tensor fascia lata 209
    flap 217
Teriparatide 111, 118, 125, 128
Terizidone 188
Terrible triad
    elbow 358
    injuries, principles of managing 357
Terry-Thomas sign 516, 516f
Testosterone 118
Tethered cord syndrome 229
Thalidomide 225
Therapeutic knee arthroscopy 677
Therapeutic studies 72
Thermal ablation, radiofrequency 695
Thermal processing 255
Thermoplastic splints 288
Thiacetazone 188
Thigh thrust test 672
Thioacetazone 187, 766
Third tibia, proximal 214
Thompson-Simmonds-Doherty test 722
Thoracic disease, cold abscess of 757
Thoracic kyphosis 650, 786
Thoracic outlet syndrome 28
    etiopathogenesis of 30
    pathoanatomy of 31
Thoracic spine 808
Thoracolumbar injury
    classification 435t
    Denis classification of 434f
Thoracolumbar spine 437
    fractures, management of 437
    injuries 433
        classification of 440
Thrombin generation 9
Thromboembolism 384, 443
Thrombolytic medications 30
Thrombophlebitis 790, 792
Thromboprophylaxis 7
Thumb 500
    adduction 531, 532
    deformity 557
    ligamentous injury of 378
    reconstruction 503
    reimplantation surgery, steps of 196
    Stener lesion of 378
Thumb-index finger 532
Thyroid 81
    cancer 820
    shields 334
Thyrotoxicosis 119
Tibia 109, 588t, 628
    bowing of 591
    congenital
        anterolateral bowing of 591
        bowing of 591
        pseudoarthrosis of 276, 588-591

    deficiency of 591
    fracture fixation 404
    individual axis of 599
    mechanical axis of 599, 602
    middle third 214
    nonunion of 22
    open fracture of 458, 459
    over femoral condyles, external rotation of 674
    posterolateral subluxation of 674
    vara 604, 608
        classification of 608
Tibial angle
    medial proximal 600
    posterior proximal 600
Tibial condylar fractures, potential complications of 402
Tibial fractures 461
    open 459, 459t
Tibial hemimelia 591, 592
    classification of 592
    clinical features of 592
    management of 592
Tibial nerves 741
Tibial nonunion 402
Tibial pilon fracture, classification of 413
Tibial plafond fractures 401
Tibial plateau fracture 399, 400
    classification for 400
    reduction, technique for 341
Tibial pseudoarthrosis 589
Tibial shaft axis 599, 602
Tibial side 873
Tibial slope 707
Tibial tendon dysfunction, posterior 729
Tibial version, radiological measurement of 616
Tibialis
    anterior 214
        affect gait, paralysis of 223
        transfer 598
    posterior dysfunction 736
    posterior tendon
        anatomical disposition of 733f
        anatomy of 733
Tibiofemoral angle 603
Tibiotalar arthrodesis 412
Tibiotalar capsule 595
Tibiotalarcalcaneal nail
    contraindications of 726
    indications of 726
Tigecycline 166
Tile's type B injury, principles of treating 447
Tillaux fracture 414, 415f
Tillaux-Chaput avulsion fracture 414
Tinel's sign 537
Tip pinch 532

Tissue
   cultures, intraoperative 716
   functional 458
   loss 382
   oxygenation, maintenance of 19
   plasminogen activator, release of 12
   specific stem cells 869
   type of 526
Titanium 246
   alloy 656
   fibers, nano-sized 883
Tizanidine 302, 304
Tobramycin 647
Tocilizumab 316, 856
Tokuhashi prognostic score, revised 819t
Tom Smith arthritis 185
Tomograms 810
Tomography 833, 885
Tongue-type fracture 418
Toppling sign 768
Torsion wedge nonunion 24
Torticollis 464
   benign paroxysmal 464
   classification of 464
   congenital 467
Torus fractures 344, 352
Tossy–Rockwood
   AC joint dislocation classification 345
   classification 346f
Total angular deformity 605f
Total ankle arthroplasty, current status of 725
Total contact casts, advantages of 745
Total disc replacement 878
Total elbow arthroplasty 369
   contraindications of 494
   indications of 494
Total hip arthroplasty 254, 601, 621, 637, 645, 882
   acute 454, 455
   complications of 663
   recent advances in 882
Total hip replacement 645, 646t, 871
Total joint arthroplasty 63, 181, 659, 709, 722
Total knee
   arthroplasty 711
   replacement 7, 182fc, 653, 709, 714
      design 714
      septic complications of 716
Total plexus palsy 553
Total shoulder arthroplasty 477, 480
Tourniquet 192
   paralysis 327
Touton giant cells 844
Toxic release 293
Trabecular metal 657
Trabeculations 850

Traction epiphysis 268
Tranexamic acid 41, 55, 75
   mechanism of action of 75
   principle of 56
Transarticular screw fixation 440
Transcapitellar pin fixation 365
Transcutaneous electrical nerve stimulation, salient features of 335
Transcutaneous nerve stimulation 11, 297
Transepiphyseal separations 387
Transepiphyseal vessels 167
Transfusion mismatch 56
Translational injuries 434
Transpositional osteotomy 632
Trans-scaphoid perilunate fracture dislocation 373
Trans-scaphoperilunate dislocation 373
Transtendinous in situ repair 473
Transthoracic transpleural approach 764
Transurethral sphincterotomy 774
Transverse arch 727
Trauma 2, 763
   associated coagulopathy 40
   high energy 35
   neglected 727
   penetrating 342
Traumatic anterior hip dislocation
   classification of 615
   clinical features of 615
   potential complications of 615
Trebananib 843
Trendelenburg
   gait 222, 223, 565, 625, 627
   sign 627
   test 223, 223f
Trethowan's sign 577
Triangle tilt 554
Triangular fibrocartilage complex 504
Tribology 265
Triceps fascia, central slip of 364
Trigger finger 519, 520f
Trigger point injection 877
Trigger thumb 521
   infantile 521
   surgical management of 519
Trimalleolar fracture, mechanism of 412
Triple attack technique 636
Triradiate cartilage, surgical closure of 660
Trochanteric deficiency 663
Trochanteric displacement osteotomy 633
Trochanteric flip osteotomy 617
Trochanteric fracture, unstable 393
Trough sign 483
Trummerfeld zone 134
Tscherne classification 459t
T-score classification 112

Tubercle 753
   microscopic appearance of 753f
Tubercular infection 156
Tuberculoma 754
Tuberculosis
   apophyseal 758
   drug-resistant 188
   extrapulmonary 186
   treatment of
      drug-resistant 188t
      drug-susceptible 188t
Tuberculosis hip
   clinical features of 669
   diagnosis of 669
   management of 669
   stage of 667
Tuberculosis spine 762, 764
   anterolateral decompression of 764
   diagnosis of 758
Tuberculous
   paraplegia, classification of 758t
   tetraplegia, classification of 758t
Tumor 28, 238, 242, 604
   benign 825
   excision 824f
   fibroblastic 863
   imaging 236
   induced osteomalacia 858
   induced rickets 142
   intra-articular 823
   markers 821
   metastases 848
   necrosis factor 39, 83, 704, 706
      alpha 875
   primary 823
   seeding, risk of 828
   type 817
   vascular 863
Turner syndrome 114, 509
Turret exostosis 861
Two-column fractures 401
Tzanck giant cells 844

U

Ulcers, diabetic 743b
Ulna shortening 510
Ulnar claw hand 531
Ulnar collateral ligament 354, 354t, 355, 378
Ulnar impingement syndrome 508
Ulnar nerve 355, 533
   anatomy of 533
   decompression 534
   palsy 532
      management of 533
   transposition 534
Ulnar paradox 534, 535
Ulnar styloid nonunion 508

Ulnar translocation 370
Ulnar wrist pain, causes of 507
Ulnohumeral joint, widening of 368
Ultrahigh molecular weight polyethylene 247, 883
Ultrasonography
  principles of 232
  role of 226
Undreamed nail 283
Unhappy triad of O'donoghue 405
Unicompartmental arthritis 698
Unicompartmental knee arthroplasty 699, 701t
  advantages of 700
  disadvantages of 700
Unicompartmental osteoarthritis, management of 699
Unifacetal fracture dislocation 425
Unilateral coxa vara
  clinical features of 565
  differential diagnosis of 565
  management principles of 565
  radiological features of 565
Uninhibited neurogenic bladder 771
Unreamed nail 283, 283t
Upper limb 205, 464, 816
  injuries 345
  trauma 383
Upper motor neuron paralysis, ipsilateral 426
Urethra 444
Urethral injury 447fc
  anterior 444, 445
  management of 444
  posterior 444, 445
Uric acid, renal excretion of 59
Uricosuric agents 59, 60
Urinary bladder
  anatomy 769
  nerve supply of 769, 770f
Urinary calcium 858
Urinary diversion 775
Urinary incontinence varies, treatment of 771
Urolithiasis 125

V

Vacant glenoid sign 483
Vaccine
  intradermal administration of 380
  intramuscular administration of 380
Vacuum-assisted closure 212, 876
  therapy 456
    indications of 213
Valgus
  deformity 711, 713
  intertrochanteric osteotomy 660

osteotomy
  indications of 634
  steps of 635
  stress 355
  test 678
Valvular heart disease 76
van Gordner approach 357
Vancomycin 165, 647
  incorporated chitosan
    development of 888
    formulation of 888
Vancouver classification 462t
Vancouver type fractures 463
Varus derotation osteotomy 575
Varus stress 355
  test 678
Vascular claudication 778, 778t
Vascular complications 228, 616
Vascular endothelial growth factor 182
  effect of 96
Vascular injuries 406
Vasogenic shock 52
Vasomotor 15, 16
Vasopressors, role of 49, 51
Veins 194
Venous blood stasis 1
Venous hypertension theory 289
Venous thoracic outlet syndrome, treatment of 30
Venous thromboembolism
  recurrence 4
Vertebra, superior end 794
Vertebral anomalies 464
Vertebral artery embolism 344
Vertebral body 120
  anterior inferior portion of 758
  fracture 879
Vertebral canal, tracking posteriorly into 755, 756
Vertebral fracture injury management, treatment of 437
Vertebral kyphoplasty 817
Vertebral metastasis 820
Vertebral osteoporotic fractures, management of 122
Vertebral stapling 794
Vertebral tethering 794
Vertebroplasty 122, 266, 435, 817
  complications of 121
  indications of 120
Vertical excursion control 202
Vertical talus, congenital 594
Vessel injuries 369
Vessel wall, abnormalities of 1
Vestibular schwannoma 853
Vickers ligament release 510
Villi stroma 324
Viral infection, prevention of 170

Virchow's triad 1f
  role of 1
Virtual reality 891
Vitamin D 111, 129, 133
  deficiency 136
  dependent rickets 141-143, 143t
    clinical features of 143
    laboratory findings of 143
    pathology of 143
    radiographic findings of 143
  dietary lack of 137
  disorders 142
  high-dose 131
  resistant rickets 142, 143, 143t, 144
  supplementation 124
Vitamin E 704
Vitamin K antagonists 4
Volar Barton's fracture, management of 372
Volar intercalated segmental instability, management of 370
Volar locking plate, principles of 251
Volar sensations 532
Volkmann's canals 162
Volkmann's ischemic contracture 361, 496
  clinical features of 496
  etiopathogenesis of 496
  management of 496
  prevention of 496
Volkmann's sign 497
Volkmann's splint 284
Volkmann's turnbuckle splint 284
von Rosen splint 569

W

Wagner's classification 743b
Wagner's device 278, 597
Waist fractures 515
Waiter's tip posture 208
Wake-up test 796
Walking uphill 778
Wallerian degeneration 311, 312
Warthin-Finkeldey giant cell 844
Waste
  category 78
  content 77, 78
Watson's test 516
Weakness 820
Weaver-Dunn procedure 348
Wedge compression fractures 434
Weight-bearing exercise 117
  promotion of 124
Weight-bearing three-point gait, partial 224
Weinstein-Boriani-Biagini staging system 817, 819, 829f

Wet leather sign 521
Wheaton's type braces 286
Whiteside's technique 290
Whitman's operation 168
Wider pelvis 629
Wilson's disease 114
Wimberger's line 135
Wimberger's ring sign 134
Winquist 282
Wire fixators 262
Wnt pathway 125
Woodward procedure 466
Workforce empowerment 891
Wound
    ballistics 325
        pathoanatomy of 325
    complications 419, 664
    condition, poor 219
    debridement 457
    debridement
        principles of 213
        systems 877
    healing, dressings for 172
    infected persistent 876
    infection 790, 792
        and breakdown 402
    infiltration, local 299
    irrigation 172
    management 211
    problems 495
    therapy, technique of applying negative pressure 213
    toileting 213
    vacuum-assisted closure closure of 458
Woven bone 87
Wright's hyperabduction test 29
Wrightington approach 209
Wrist 500
    arthroplasty 557
    biomechanics, abnormal 511
    fusion 503, 557
    joint 557
    radial deviation of 555
    radiological indices of 370

X

Xanthelasmatic giant cells 844
Xenograft 253
X-linked hypophosphatemia 144, 144t

Y

Young–Burgess classification 440, 441t, 442f

Z

Zanca view 346
Zancolli 314, 499
    capsulodesis 535
        indications of 535
        surgical method of 535
    functional classification 500t
    Lasso 531
Zero-column fracture 400
Zickel subtrochanteric nail 394
Zirconia 654, 882
    ceramics 654
    fibers 883
Zoledronate 118, 126, 821
Zoledronic acid 128, 590, 821, 843, 875